Bring Your
Nutrition Course
Into

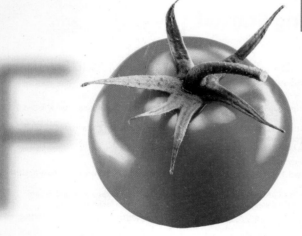

FOCUS

New and Expanded
Learning **Tools**

The Fourth Edition of **Nutrition: An Applied Approach** provides students with practical, accessible tools and resources to help them personalize the content and make deeper connections in their understanding.

NEW! Behavior Change...Getting Started

This engaging new feature, posted near the end of all main chapters, provides students with a useful tool to help them achieve better nutritional awareness and put their knowledge to immediate use in their own lives.

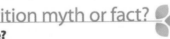

✳behavior change. . .getting started!

Now that you've read this chapter, try making these changes:

For yourself:
- Read the Nutrition Facts panel of your favorite snacks and change your usual selections to ones that are lower in sodium, total fat, or saturated fat.
- Log on to the MyPlate website (see Web Resources) and design a healthy food plan that will help you maintain your present weight or lose weight.
- Follow the Mediterranean Diet for one full day and see how you like it!

For your community:
- Offer to teach your family and friends how to read food labels to help them make healthier choices.
- Approach the manager of your campus dining hall or favorite restaurant and inquire about his or her willingness to provide nutrition information for all menu items.

nutrition myth or fact?

Is Pellagra an Infectious Disease?

In the first few years of the 20th century, Dr. Joseph Goldberger successfully controlled outbreaks of several fatal infectious diseases, from yellow fever in Louisiana to typhus in Mexico. So it wasn't surprising that, in 1914, the U.S. Surgeon General chose him to tackle another disease, thought to be infectious, that was raging throughout the South. Called *pellagra,* the disease was characterized by a skin rash, diarrhea, and mental impairment. At the time, it afflicted more than 50,000 people each year, and in about 10% of cases it resulted in death.[1]

Goldberger began studying the disease by carefully observing its occurrence in groups of people. He asked, if it is infectious, then why would it strike children in orphanages and prison inmates yet leave their nurses and guards unaffected? Why did it overwhelmingly affect impoverished millworkers and sharecroppers while leaving their affluent (and well-fed) neighbors healthy? Could a dietary deficiency cause pellagra?

To confirm his hunch, he conducted a series of trials in which he fed afflicted orphans and prisoners—who had been consuming a limited, corn-based diet—a variety of nutritious foods, including meats. They recovered. Moreover, orphans and inmates who did not have pellagra and ate the new diet did not develop the disease. Finally, Goldberger recruited eleven healthy prison inmates, who, in return for a pardon of their sentence, agreed to consume a limited, corn-based diet. After

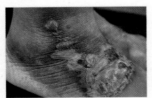

Pellagra is characterized by a scaly skin rash.

5 months, six of the eleven developed pellagra.

Still, many skeptics were unable to give up the idea that pellagra was an infectious disease. To prove that pellagra was not spread by germs, Goldberger and his colleagues deliberately injected themselves with and ingested patients' scabs, nasal secretions, and other body fluids. He and his team remained healthy.

Although Goldberger could not identify the precise component in the new diet that cured pellagra, he eventually found an inexpensive and widely available substance, brewer's yeast, that when added to the diet prevented or reversed the disease. Shortly after Goldberger's death in 1937, scientists identified the component that is deficient in the diet of pellagra patients: niacin, one of the B-vitamins, which is plentiful in brewer's yeast.[1]

CRITICAL THINKING QUESTIONS

1. What issues arise from the research done by Dr. Goldberger and his colleagues?
2. Do you think that this research would be considered ethical and acceptable by today's standards? Why or why not?
3. Identify a disease linked to nutrition that you feel deserves substantial attention from researchers. What makes you choose this disease?

NEW! Critical Thinking Questions

These stimulating new content tools have been added to every main chapter *Nutrition Debate* as well as to the *Nutrition: Myth or Fact* feature, to help students incorporate the information and encourage them to make connections and think independently.

CRITICAL THINKING QUESTIONS

1. Many ranchers feed antibiotics to livestock to quickly increase the animals' weight. Explain a possible mechanism for this weight gain.
2. At the beginning of this debate, we referred to the "miracle of antibiotics." Are antibiotics a miracle cure? Why or why not?

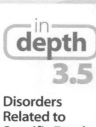

in depth 3.5

Disorders Related to Specific Foods

Trying to decide between two brands of energy bars, you compare their lists of ingredients. You notice that one of the bars, although it contains no nuts, says, "Produced in a facility that processes peanuts." The other warns, "Contains wheat, milk, and soy." Why all the warnings? The reason is that, to some people, consuming these normally healthful foods can be dangerous, even life-threatening.

Disorders related to specific foods can be clustered into three main groupings: food intolerances, food allergies, and a genetic disorder called celiac disease. We discuss these disorders **In Depth** here.

learning objectives

After studying this In Depth, you should be able to:

1. Identify the most common physiologic problem underlying food intolerances, including lactose intolerance, p. 103.

2. Describe how an immune hypersensitivity to food proteins such as those in peanuts, eggs, or milk can produce the symptoms commonly associated with an allergic reaction, pp. 103–105.

3. Identify the site of the tissue damage that occurs in celiac disease and the food protein that provokes the response, pp. 105–106.

math review

11. Hannah goes to a sandwich shop near the university at least once a week to buy what she considers a healthy lunch, which includes a chicken breast sandwich, garden salad (with Ranch dressing), and a diet cola. Recently, the shop started posting the Calorie and fat content of its menu items. Hannah discovers the following about the Calorie and fat content of the items in her "healthy lunch":

• Chicken sandwich—317 Calories, 4 g fat
• Garden salad—49 Calories, 1 g fat
• Ranch dressing (1 packet)—280 Calories, 28 g fat
• Diet cola—0 Calories, 0 g fat

Based on this information, what is the total Calorie and fat content of Hannah's lunch? What is the percentage of Calories from fat for this lunch? Which food item is contributing the highest amount of fat to Hannah's lunch, and what can she do to make a healthier change to this lunch?

Answers to Review Questions and Math Review are located at the back of this text and in the MasteringNutrition Study Area.

NEW! and Expanded Learning Tools!

The Fourth Edition now includes end-of chapter **Math Review** questions in all applicable chapters, and **Learning Objectives** included at the start of all In Depth chapters.

These expanded pedagogic tools enable instructors to track student learning and create better assessments, in addition to assisting students in understanding key topics.

Focus Figures

Clarify Tough Topics

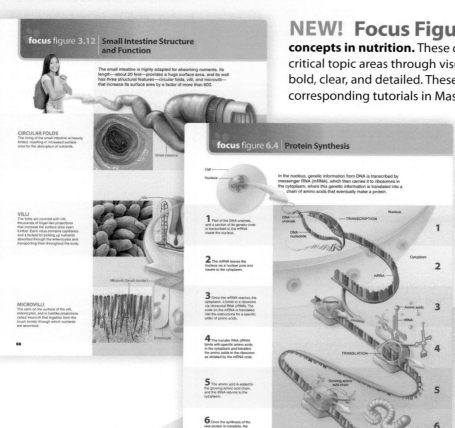

NEW! **Focus Figures** teach students key concepts in nutrition.

These colorful, full-page figures highlight critical topic areas through visually engaging displays that are bold, clear, and detailed. These dynamic new figures also have corresponding tutorials in MasteringNutrition™

■ Focus Figures include **introductory text** that explains how the figure is central to concepts the students will cover throughout the text.

■ Students **get clear directions via text and stepped-out art** that guide the eye through complex processes, breaking them down into manageable pieces that are easy to teach and understand.

■ Focus Figures provide **dynamic illustrations—often paired with photographs**—that make key and difficult topics come alive.

■ Intuitive layouts facilitate comparison and comprehension of related processes.

■ Large layout enables micro-to-macro levels of explanation for complex topics.

Put a Focus on
Student **Assessment**

MasteringNutrition™ | **Mastering** is the most effective and widely-used online homework, tutorial, and assessment system for the applied sciences. It delivers self-paced tutorials that focus on your course objectives, provide individualized coaching, and responds to each student's progress.

FOR STUDENTS Proven, assignable, and automatically graded nutrition activities reinforce course learning objectives.

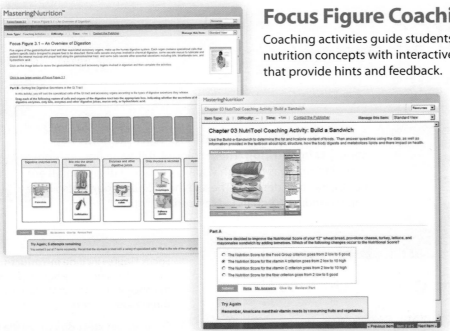

Focus Figure Coaching Activities

Coaching activities guide students through key nutrition concepts with interactive mini-lessons that provide hints and feedback.

NutriTools Build-A-Meal Activities

These unique activities allow students to combine and experiment with different food options and learn firsthand how to build healthier meals.

Nutrition Animations

Animations built specifically for nutrition help students master tough topics with assessment and feedback.

Other automatically graded nutrition activities include:

- MyDietAnalysis Case Study Coaching Activities
- Calculation Corner Activities
- Reading Quizzes
- *ABC News* Videos
- Chapter Tutor Session MP3s
- *Get Ready for Nutrition*

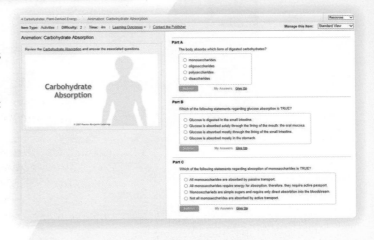

DO YOUR STUDENTS WANT TO PRACTICE ON THEIR OWN?

MasteringNutrition also provides students with the tools to study effectively and practice on their own time at their own pace.

eText

The Pearson eText gives students access to the text whenever and wherever they can access the Internet. The eText can be viewed on PCs, Macs, and tablets, including iPad and Android.

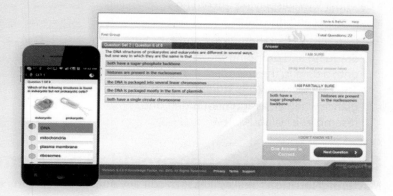

NEW! Dynamic Study Modules

enable students to study effectively on their own in an adaptive format. Students receive an initial set of questions with a unique answer format asking them to indicate their confidence level. Once completed, reviews include explanations using materials taken directly from the text. These modules can be accessed on smartphones, tablets, and computers.

Study Area

Students can access the Study Area for use on their own or in a study group.

The Study Area also includes: Cumulative Test, RSS Feeds, Audio Case Studies, *ABC News* Videos, Animations and book specific activities.

MyDietAnalysis

MyDietAnalysis is now available as a single sign on to **MasteringNutrition**.

For online users, a new mobile website version of **MyDietAnalysis** is available. Students can track their diet and activity intake accurately, anytime and anywhere, from their mobile device.

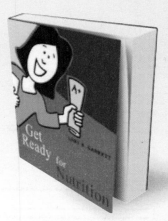

Get Ready for Nutrition

helps students get up to speed for their course by covering study skills, basic math, chemistry, and biology basics.

Easy to Get Started, Use, and
Make **Your Own**

MasteringNutrition™

FOR INSTRUCTORS Mastering Nutrition
helps instructors maximize class time with easy-to-assign, customizable, and automatically graded assessements that motivate students to learn outside of the class and arrive prepared for lecture.

Calendar Feature for Instructors and Students

The Course Home default page now features a Calendar View displaying upcoming assignments and due dates.

- Instructors can schedule assignments by dragging and dropping the assignment onto a date in the calendar.
- The calendar view lets students see at-a-glance when an assignment is due, and resembles a syllabus.

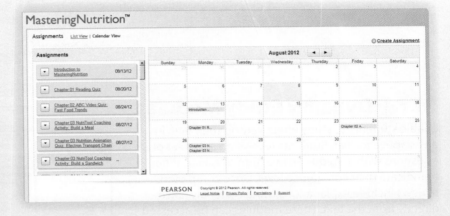

Customize publisher-provided problems or quickly add your own

MasteringNutrition™ makes it easy to edit any questions or answers, import your own questions, and quickly add images or links to further enhance the student experience.

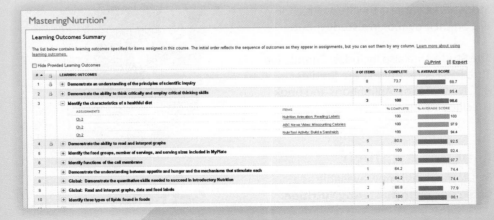

Learning Outcomes

Tagged to book content and tied to Bloom's Taxonomy, Learning Outcomes are designed to let Mastering do the work in tracking student performance against your learning outcomes. Mastering offers a data supported measure to quantify students' learning gains and to share those results quickly and easily:

- Add your own or use the publisher-provided learning outcomes.
- View class performance against the specified learning outcomes.
- Export results to a spreadsheet.

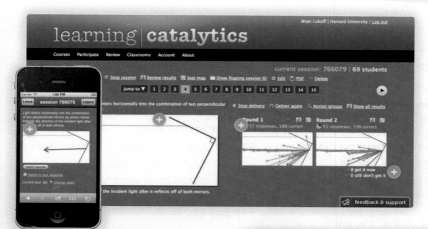

NEW! Learning Catalytics™

Learning Catalytics allows students to use their smartphones, tablets, or laptops to respond to questions in class. With Learning Catalytics you can:

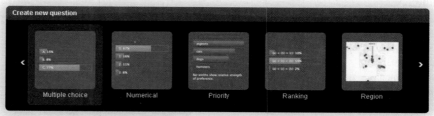

Use a wide variety of question types to engage students: multiple choice, word clouds, sketch a graph, annotate art, highlight a passage, compute a numeric answer, and more.

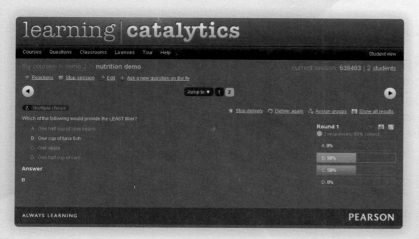

Use multiple question types to get into the minds of students to understand what they do or don't know and adjust lectures accordingly.

- Access rich analytics to understand student performance.
- Add your own questions to make Learning Catalytics fit your course exactly.
- Assess and improve students' critical-thinking skills, and so much more.

Learning Catalytics is included with the purchase of **MasteringNutrition** with **MyDietAnalysis**.

Everything You Need to Teach
In One Place!

Teaching Toolkit DVD for *Nutrition: An Applied Approach*

The **Teaching Toolkit DVD** replaces the former printed Teaching Toolbox by providing everything you need to prep for your course and deliver a dynamic lecture in one convenient place. Included on 3 disks are these valuable resources:

Disk 1
Robust Media Assets for Each Chapter

- 36 *ABC News* Lecture Launcher videos
- Nutrition Animations
- Nutritools
- PowerPoint® Lecture Outlines
- Media Link PowerPoint slides for easy importing of videos, animations, and Nutritools
- PowerPoint clicker questions and Jeopardy-style quiz show questions
- Files for all illustrations and tables and selected photos from the text
- Transparency Masters

Disk 2
Comprehensive Test Bank

- Test Bank in Word and RTF formats
- Computerized Test Bank, which includes all the questions from the test bank in a format that allows you to easily and intuitively build exams and quizzes

Disk 3
Additional Innovative Supplements for instructors and students

For Instructors:

- Instructor's Resource Support Manual
- Introduction to MasteringNutrition
- Introductory video for Learning Catalytics

For Students:

- *Eat Right! Healthy Eating in College and Beyond*
- *Food Composition Table*

TEACHING TOOLKIT

Nutrition
An Applied Approach

FOURTH EDITION

Janice Thompson • Melinda Manore

User's Quick Guide for *Nutrition: An Applied Approach*, Fourth Edition

This easy-to-use printed supplement accompanies the Teaching Toolkit and offers easy instructions for both experienced and new faculty members to get started with the rich Toolkit content, how to access assignments within MasteringNutrition, and how to "flip" the classroom with Learning Catalytics.

Nutrition
An Applied Approach
FOURTH EDITION

Janice Thompson, Ph.D., FACSM
University of Birmingham

Melinda Manore, Ph.D., RD, CSSD, FACSM
Oregon State University

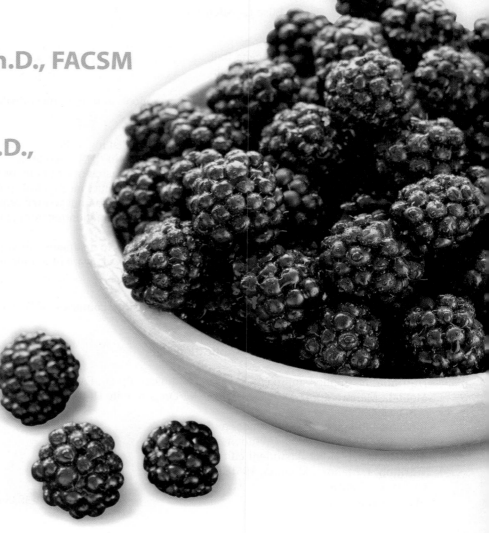

PEARSON

Boston   Columbus   Indianapolis   New York   San Francisco   Upper Saddle River
Amsterdam   Cape Town   Dubai   London   Madrid   Milan   Munich   Paris   Montreal   Toronto
Delhi   Mexico City   São Paulo   Sydney   Hong Kong   Seoul   Singapore   Taipei   Tokyo

Executive Editor: Sandra Lindelof
Director of Development: Barbara Yien
Program Manager: Susan Malloy
Project Editor: Susan Scharf
Developmental Editor: Laura Bonazzoli
Art Development Editors: Kari Hopperstead, Kelly Murphy
Editorial Assistants: Briana Verdugo, Tu-Anh Dang-Tran
Senior Managing Editors: Deborah Cogan, Mike Early
Assistant Managing Editor: Nancy Tabor
Production Project Manager: Michael Penne
Media Content Producer: Lauren Hill
Production Management and Composition: S4Carlisle Publishing Services
Photo Manager: Maya Melenchuck
Photo Research: PreMediaGlobal
Design Manager: Marilyn Perry
Art Director: Derek Bacchus
Interior and Cover Designer: Elise Lansden
Illustrators: Precision Graphics
Manufacturing Buyer: Stacey Weinberger
Executive Marketing Manager: Neena Bali
Cover Photo Credit: Picsfive/Shutterstock

Library of Congress Cataloging-in-Publication Data
Thompson, Janice
    Nutrition: an applied approach / Janice Thompson, Ph.D., FACSM, University of Birmingham;
Melinda Manore, Ph.D., RD, CSSD, FACSM, Oregon State University. — Fourth edition.
        pages cm.
    Includes bibliographical references and index.
    ISBN-13: 978-0-321-91039-4 (student edition)
    ISBN-10: 0-321-91039-7 (student edition)
1. Nutrition. I. Manore, Melinda, 1951-II. Title.
    QP141.T467 2015
    612.3—dc23   2013035636

5   16

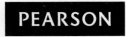

ISBN 10: 0-321-91039-7; ISBN 13: 978-0-321-91039-4
(Student edition)
ISBN 10: 0-321-94903-X; ISBN 13: 978-0-321-94903-5
(Instructor Review copy)

"To our Moms—your consistent love and support are the keys to our happiness and success. You have been incredible role models."

"To our Dads—you raised us to be independent, intelligent, and resourceful. We miss you and wish you were here to be proud of, and to brag about, our accomplishments."

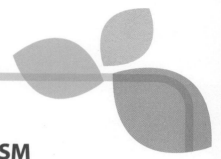

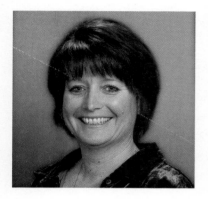

Janice Thompson, Ph.D., FACSM

University of Birmingham

Janice Thompson earned her Ph.D. at Arizona State University in exercise science with an emphasis in exercise physiology and nutrition. She is currently a professor in the School of Sports and Exercise Sciences at The University of Birmingham, U.K. Her work in the United Kingdom focuses on developing nutrition and physical activity interventions to reduce the risk for cardiovascular disease and type 2 diabetes in high-risk populations. Janice has retained her U.S. affiliation as a nutrition and exercise research consultant with the Office of Native American Diabetes Programs at the University of New Mexico Health Sciences Center.

Janice is a fellow of the American College of Sports Medicine (ACSM) and a member of the American Society for Nutrition (ASN), the British Association of Sport and Exercise Science (BASES), and The Nutrition Society. Janice won an undergraduate teaching award while a faculty member at the University of North Carolina, Charlotte.

Janice publishes two other nutrition books with Pearson: the higher-level majors text, *The Science of Nutrition* (just published in its 3rd edition), and the consumer-level book, *Nutrition for Life,* 3rd edition. In addition, Janice co-authored *Sport Nutrition for Health and Performance,* with Melinda Manore (published by Human Kinetics).

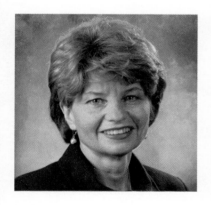

Melinda Manore, Ph.D., RD, CSSD, FACSM

Oregon State University

Melinda Manore earned a doctorate in human nutrition with a minor in exercise physiology at Oregon State University, and a master's degree in health education from the University of Oregon. She is currently a professor in the Department of Nutrition and Exercise Sciences at Oregon State University, where she teaches and conducts research in the area of nutrition and exercise. She served as Chair and Professor in the nutrition department until late 2004, when it combined with the exercise sciences department and she stepped down from her Chair position. Before coming to Oregon State, she taught at Arizona State University for 17 years. Melinda's areas of specialization include nutritional requirements and issues for active women, nutrition assessment, and the role that nutrition and exercise play in health, energy balance, obesity, and disordered eating.

A registered dietitian, Melinda is an active member of the American Dietetic Association (ADA). She is Past Chair of the ADA Research Committee and the Research DPG (Dietetic Practice Group). Melinda is a member of the American Society of Nutritional Sciences (ASNS), the American Society for Clinical Nutrition (ASCN), the North American Association for the Study of Obesity (NAASO), the National Academy of Sciences Committee on Military Nutrition Research, and a Fellow of the American College of Sports Medicine (ACSM).

Melinda writes a nutrition column for and is an associate editor for ACSM's *Health and Fitness Journal,* and she has won numerous awards for excellence in research and teaching. While at Arizona State University, she was nominated for the Distinguished Mentor of Women Award (1996), and the College of Liberal Arts & Sciences Alumni Association Outstanding Teaching Award (1998, 2000). In 2001, she received the SCAN Excellence in Practice Award.

Melinda co-authored *The Science of Nutrition,* 3rd edition with Janice Thompson and Linda Vaughan; *Nutrition for Life,* 3rd edition with Janice Thompson; and co-authored the Human Kinetics title *Sport Nutrition for Health and Performance* with Janice.

Welcome to *Nutrition: An Applied Approach,* Fourth Edition!

Why We Wrote This Book

Nutrition gets a lot of press. Go online or pick up a magazine and you'll read the latest debate over which weight-loss diet is best; turn on the TV or stream a video and you'll hear a celebrity describe how she lost 50 pounds without exercising; scan the headlines or read some blogs and you'll come upon the politics surrounding the creation of new, enhanced "designer" foods. How can you evaluate these sources of nutrition information and find out whether the advice they provide is reliable? How do you navigate through seemingly endless recommendations and arrive at a way of eating that's right for *you*—one that supports your physical activity, allows you to maintain a healthful weight, and helps you avoid chronic diseases?

Nutrition: An Applied Approach began with our conviction that students and instructors would both benefit from an accurate and clear textbook that links nutrients to their functional benefits. As authors and instructors, we know that students have a natural interest in their bodies, their health, their weight, and their success in sports and other activities. By demonstrating how nutrition relates to these interests, this text empowers students to reach their personal health and fitness goals. Throughout the text, material is presented in a lively narrative that continually links the facts to students' circumstances, lifestyles, and goals. Information on current events and research keeps the inquisitive spark alive, illustrating that nutrition is truly a "living" science, and a source of considerable debate. The content of *Nutrition: An Applied Approach* is appropriate for non-nutrition majors, but also includes information that will challenge students who have a more advanced understanding of chemistry and math. We present the "science side" in a contemporary narrative style that's easy to read and understand, with engaging features that reduce students' apprehensions and encourage them to apply the material to their lives. Also, because this book is not a derivative of a majors text, the writing and the figures are cohesive and always level-appropriate.

As teachers, we are familiar with the myriad challenges of presenting nutrition information in the classroom, and we have included the most comprehensive ancillary package available to assist instructors in successfully meeting these challenges. We hope to contribute to the excitement of teaching and learning about nutrition: a subject that affects all of us, a subject so important and relevant that correct and timely information can make the difference between health and disease.

New to the Fourth Edition

In this edition we are pleased to introduce all-new, colorful **Focus Figures**. Appearing in bold displays covering fifteen critical topics, these full-page visual displays help instructors to more easily teach, and students to better understand, some of the toughest topics in nutrition, with clear, easy-to-follow graphics and text. These dramatic visual spreads also appear as tutorials within MasteringNutrition™, with hints and wrong answer feedback that can be assigned and graded.

This Fourth Edition of *Nutrition: An Applied Approach* also now features the **MasteringNutrition**™ online homework, tutorial, and assessment system which delivers self-paced tutorials and activities that provide individualized coaching, a focus on course objectives, and tools enabling instructors to respond individually to each student's progress. The proven Mastering system provides instructors with customizable, easy-to-assign, automatically graded assessments that motivate students to learn outside of class and arrive prepared for lecture. Key MasteringNutrition™ features include:

- **Personalized learning** to help students quickly master key concepts using self-paced tutorials that include wrong-answer feedback and hints
- **Focus Figure Coaching Activities** that guide students through key nutrition concepts with interactive mini-lessons that supply hints and feedback.
- **NutriTools Build-A-Meal Coaching Activities** that enable students to apply nutrition concepts through interactive mini-lessons that supply hints and feedback.
- **Math Activities** that provide hands-on practice for important calculations along with helpful wrong-answer feedback.
- *ABC News* **Videos** that bring nutrition to life with up-to-date topics in the nutrition field, and include multiple choice questions with wrong-answer feedback.
- **Nutrition Animations** that elucidate big-picture concepts and provide a helpful visual overview of complex topics in nutrition.
- An online **Study Area** that is broken out into learning areas and which includes videos, animations, MP3s, and other resources.
- Additional graded activities include chapter-based **Reading Quizzes, MP3s, Math Review, and MyDietAnalysis Case Study Activities**.

Other exciting new features include a new **Behavior Change** feature box, appearing near the end of every main chapter, that provides a personalized and useful tool for improving students' nutritional awareness and their ability to incorporate positive nutritional changes into their lives. We have also updated and expanded the chapter-opening **Learning Objectives** throughout the text, in addition to adding them to each In Depth feature. **Critical Thinking Questions** have been added to every main chapter Nutrition Debate box, and new topic areas have been added. **Hot Topics** is an engaging new feature appearing throughout the text that provides snapshots of important and trending topics in nutrition.

We have also reorganized and enhanced numerous chapter topics and treatments, including expanding coverage of Functional Foods; reorganizing and expanding content in Chapter 10 on Nutrients Involved in Energy Metabolism and Blood Health; revising, updating, and reorganizing the content in Chapter 13 and In Depth 13.5, covering Food Safety and Technology and issues related to Food Ethics; and added a new In Depth (Chapter 2.5) on Eating Wisely that focuses on recent developments in the areas of mindful eating and the practical aspects of eating well. Note that the Find the Quack feature from previous editions can now be found in the MasteringNutrition Study Area.

The Visual Walkthrough located at the front of this text provides an overview of these and other important features in the Fourth Edition. For specific changes to each chapter, please see below.

Chapter 1 and In Depth 1.5:

- Added new Learning Objectives matched to main (A-level) sections of the chapter.
- Changed the title of chapter to more accurately reflect revised content.
- Added new Focus Figure 1.9 on Dietary Reference Intakes (replaces previous Figures 1.9–1.11).
- Added new section on *Healthy People 2020*.
- Added new Nutrition Debate, "Are There Such Things as Good Foods and Bad Foods?"
- Added Nutrition Online links.
- Revised text to include more references to the Internet.
- Revised section title and added new information within section, "How Can You Interpret the Results of Research Studies?"
- Revised and tightened the Quick Tips on detecting media hype.
- Updated Figures 1.3 and 1.4 with more recent statistics on causes of death and obesity rates, respectively.

- Simplified the You Do The Math box context.
- Added the new Behavior Change feature.
- Added an end of chapter Math Review question.
- Added new In Depth, "New Frontiers in Nutrition and Health."
- Added new Learning Objectives to the In Depth.

Chapter 2 and In Depth 2.5:

- Added new Learning Objectives matched to main (A-level) sections of the chapter.
- Added additional information on cultural influences on food choices.
- Updated discussion related to proposed changes to food labels and the Nutrition Facts panel.
- Updated information on the Dietary Guidelines for Americans, the USDA Food Patterns, and MyPlate.
- Deleted the Nutrition Label Activity related to Health Claims on Food Labels.
- Dropped the figures of Latin American, Asian, and Mediterranean food pyramids.
- Added new Figures 2.5 (MyPlate), 2.6 (MyPlate can be easily used to design a Mediterranean-style diet), and 2.11 (MiPlato).
- Developed a new Hot Topic, "Does Calorie-Labeling Influence Food Choice?"
- Wrote a new Nutrition Debate, "Will MyPlate Promote America's Health?"
- Added in a brief section discussing healthy eating plans (DASH diet and the exchange system).
- Added Nutrition Online links.
- Added a second You Do The Math box on determining the healthiest food choices when eating out.
- Added the new Behavior Change feature.
- Developed an entirely new In Depth on Eating Wisely.
- Added an end of chapter Math Review question.
- Added new Learning Objectives to the In Depth.

Chapter 3 and In Depth 3.5:

- Added new Learning Objectives matched to main (A-level) sections of the chapter.
- Moved content on appetite and eating cues from the section "Why Do We Want to Eat What We Want to Eat?" to In Depth 2.5.
- Expanded the discussion of hormones involved in hunger and satiation.
- Added two new Focus Figures (Figures 3.4 and 3.12) to provide a more comprehensive overview of digestion and of the absorption of nutrients at the enterocytes.
- Moved the figure of the role of enzymes in the human body from Chapter 6 to this chapter.
- Discussed and added a math box (You Do The Math) on the pH scale, with a figure.
- In the disorders section, added discussions of vomiting and of GI cancers. We also added a new figure of a colonoscopy.
- Added a new Hot Topic on digestion simulators, removing the old one on prescription appetite suppressants.
- Also in the disorders section, we completely updated the discussion of GERD.
- Replaced a previous Nutrition: Myth or Fact? feature on ulcers with a more comprehensive Nutrition Debate on ulcers, "*H. pylori:* Could the Same Germ Make Us Sick and Keep Us Well?", which discusses research into the helpful role of *H. pylori* in childhood as well as its role in ulcers and stomach cancer.
- Deleted the previous Nutrition Debate on colon cleansing.
- Added the new Behavior Change feature.
- Added an end of chapter Math Review question.
- Added new Learning Objectives to the In Depth.

Chapter 4 and In Depth 4.5:

- Added new Learning Objectives matched to main (A-level) sections of the chapter.
- Introduced the terms *glycogenesis* and *glycogenolysis*.

- Added two new Focus Figures—one on carbohydrate digestion (Figure 4.8) and one on regulation of blood glucose (Figure 4.10).
- Added new Focus Figure 2 on Diabetes in In Depth.
- Added a new section on "What Makes a Whole Grain Whole," which includes new Figure 4.13.
- Added a new Quick Tips feature on reducing added sugar intake, "Slashing Your Sugar Intake."
- Enhanced the section on diabetes by adding *prediabetes* as a key term, adding the blood glucose range values for diagnoses of normal, prediabetes, and diabetes, and expanding information on the management of diabetes.
- Expanded the information on high-fructose corn syrup by adding it as a boldfaced term and discussing it in more detail in the section on sugar and obesity.
- Updated and revised the Nutrition Debate to encompass the role of all added sugars in the obesity epidemic.
- Added the new Behavior Change feature.
- Added an end of chapter Math Review question.
- Added new Learning Objectives to the In Depth.

Chapter 5 and In Depth 5.5:

- Added new Learning Objectives matched to main (A-level) sections of the chapter.
- Added three new Focus Figures: Figure 5.10 on lipid digestion, Figure 1 on atherosclerosis in In Depth 5.5 and Figure 3 on lipoprotein transport and distribution in In Depth 5.5.
- Added the new Behavior Change feature.
- Added an end of chapter Math Review question.
- Added new Learning Objectives to the In Depth.

Chapter 6 and In Depth 6.5:

- Added new Learning Objectives matched to main (A-level) sections of the chapter.
- Moved the figure on proteins acting as enzymes to Chapter 3 (it is now Figure 3.6) where the concept is first introduced.
- Expanded the section on how genes regulate amino acid binding and protein synthesis.
- Added two new Focus Figures—one on protein synthesis (Figure 6.4) and one on protein digestion (Figure 6.11).
- Expanded the information on the functions of proteins, including their role in the transport and storage of nutrients, as neurotransmitters, and in blood clotting.
- Updated and expanded the section examining whether eating too much protein is harmful.
- Deleted the figure of the Vegetarian Food Pyramid, and added a new section on using MyPlate to design a vegetarian diet.
- Updated the section on kwashiorkor, highlighting recent research implicating the role of dysfunctional GI bacteria in this disorder.
- Added a new section addressing disorders related to genetic abnormalities, including PKU, sickle cell anemia, and cystic fibrosis.
- Updated and revised the Nutrition Debate to focus on climate change and the current controversies surrounding meat consumption and livestock production.
- Added the new Behavior Change feature.
- Added an end of chapter Math Review question.
- Updated the In Depth on vitamins and minerals.
- Added a Quick Tips feature on "Retaining the Vitamins in Foods."
- Added new Learning Objectives to the In Depth.

Chapter 7 and In Depth 7.5:

- Added new Learning Objectives matched to main (A-level) sections of the chapter.
- Added the new Behavior Change feature.
- Added a new Focus Figure (Figure 7.4) on fluid and electrolyte balance in the cell membrane.

- Added an end of chapter Math Review question.
- Added new Learning Objectives to the In Depth.

Chapter 8 and In Depth 8.5:

- Added new Learning Objectives matched to main (A-level) sections of the chapter.
- Enhanced the matching of examples of foods high in specific nutrients in the written text with examples provided in the figures (specifically Figures 8.6, 8.7, 8.10, 8.12, and 8.16).
- Added a new figure on selenium and glutathione peroxidase (now Figure 8.9).
- Expanded information related to antioxidant supplementation and risk for various cancers and cardiovascular disease.
- Added additional information on the conversion of units of beta-carotene and vitamin A in both food and supplement forms.
- Updated, revised, and reorganized the content on vitamin A.
- Added a new Focus Figure on vitamin A's role in vision (Figure 8.14).
- Added the new Behavior Change feature.
- Added an end of chapter Math Review question.
- Updated the In Depth on cancer, and enhanced information on the role of diet in cancer prevention.
- Added new Learning Objectives to the In Depth.

Chapter 9 and In Depth 9.5:

- Added new Learning Objectives matched to main (A-level) sections of the chapter.
- Revised and updated content on parathyroid hormone and its role in increasing blood calcium.
- Revised Figure 9.5 to illustrate the mechanism and action of parathyroid hormone in increasing blood calcium.
- Updated the new RDA information for calcium and vitamin D.
- Updated the Hot Topic feature on the role of calcium in weight loss.
- Revised the latitude line (from 40° to 37°) at which sun exposure is/is not adequate for vitamin D conversion during the winter in Figure 9.9.
- Updated content on the link between soft drink intake and bone mineral density.
- Provided recent recommendations on vitamin D supplementation to prevent vitamin D insufficiency and deficiency in children and adults.
- Added the new Behavior Change feature.
- Added an end of chapter Math Review question.
- Updated and revised current recommendations and associated risks for the use of calcium and vitamin D supplements to prevent and treat osteoporosis.
- Updated the latest research into the risks and benefits of medications used to treat osteoporosis, including bisphosphonates and hormone replacement therapy.
- Added new Learning Objectives to the In Depth.

Chapter 10 and In Depth 10.5:

- Added new Learning Objectives matched to main (A-level) sections of the chapter.
- Added the new Behavior Change feature.
- Added an end of chapter Math Review question.
- Added new Learning Objectives to the In Depth.

Chapter 11 and In Depth 11.5:

- Added new Learning Objectives matched to main (A-level) sections of the chapter.
- Updated research on possible protective effects of having a body mass index in the overweight category, and included a new Hot Topic on this issue.
- Expanded information on energy balance and introduced the concept of dynamic (versus static) energy balance and its role in body weight regulation.
- Added a new Focus Figure (Figure 11.5) illustrating energy balance.

- Added a section describing Non-Activity Thermogenesis (NEAT).
- Added information on the FTO gene and obesity.
- Expanded the information describing metabolic and physiologic factors that influence weight loss and gain.
- Added a section on cultural and economic factors that influence food choice and body weight.
- Expanded the information on how to design a healthy weight loss plan.
- Added a section on underweight and how to healthfully gain weight.
- Added a section on obesity and its related health risks.
- Added a new figure on abdominal obesity (Figure 11.10).
- Updated information on current medications used to treat obesity, and on the sleeve gastrectomy surgical procedure.
- Revised and updated the Nutrition Debate on High Carbohydrate, Moderate-Fat Diets.
- Added the new Behavior Change feature.
- Added two new end of chapter Math Review questions.
- Added new Learning Objectives to the In Depth.

Chapter 12 and In Depth 12.5:

- Added new Learning Objectives matched to main (A-level) sections of the chapter.
- Added new Figure 12.1 highlighting benefits of physical activity.
- Added a new section describing how to assess your current level of fitness.
- New What About You? feature on "Taking the President's Challenge Adult Fitness Test."
- Expanded information on the factors that influence a person's motivations to be physically active.
- Updated and expanded content on the FITT principle (frequency, intensity, time, and type) for appropriately overloading the body to achieve fitness gains.
- Added new Figure 12.4—heart rate training chart to estimate heart rate training range for goal setting.
- Added new Focus Figure (Figure 12.7) on What Fuels Our Activities?
- Expanded information on the intensity of exercise needed to decrease body fat.
- Added a new Hot Topic feature, "Should Athletes 'Train Low' with Carbohydrate?"
- Revised and updated the Nutrition Debate, "How Much Physical Activity Is Enough?"
- Added the new Behavior Change feature.
- Added an end of chapter Math Review question.
- Added a new In Depth chapter on Ergogenic Aids, which includes a new table providing an overview of commonly used ergogenic aids, their claimed mechanism of action, whether or not they are effective, and side effects.
- Added new Learning Objectives to the In Depth.

Chapter 13 and In Depth 13.5:

- All Learning Objectives are matched to main (A level) sections of the chapter.
- Replaced the chapter-opening discussion with a discussion of norovirus specifically, because of the many recent outbreaks.
- Updated information on the Food Safety Modernization Act.
- Expanded and separated with subheadings the discussions of the microorganisms involved in foodborne illness.
- Expanded and separated with subheadings the discussions of toxins involved in foodborne illness.
- Added Figure 13.7 on the "danger zone" of temperature within which microorganisms readily multiply in food.
- Removed previous Table 13.3 (A Guide to Thawing Poultry) and Figure 13.8 ("Thermy").
- Condensed the information on food preservation.
- Expanded the discussion of genetically modified foods.
- Expanded the discussion of organic foods.

- Added the new Behavior Change feature.
- Added an end of chapter Math Review question.
- Replaced the prior In Depth on Global Nutrition with a new In Depth called Food Ethics: Sustainability, Equity, and the New Food Movement, which covers the impact of corporate farming on the environment and on food diversity; various initiatives such as CSAs and school gardens; food insecurity; fair trade; and what consumers can do to help.
- Added new Learning Objectives to the In Depth.

Chapter 14 and In Depth 14.5:

- Added new Learning Objectives matched to main (A-level) sections of the chapter.
- Added the new Behavior Change feature.
- Added an end of chapter Math Review question.
- Added new Learning Objectives to the In Depth.

Chapter 15 and In Depth 15.5:

- Added new Learning Objectives matched to main (A-level) sections of the chapter.
- Added the new Behavior Change feature.
- Added an end of chapter Math Review question.
- Added new Learning Objectives to the In Depth.

Appendices and Back Matter:

- Moved the USDA Food Guide Evolution to Appendix A.
- Data for Appendix C—"Foods Containing Caffeine"—has been revised and updated.
- References for all chapters and In Depth features are now located and centralized at the back of the text.
- Answers to Review Questions and Math Review have been revised and updated to reflect the new edition's changes.
- Glossary terms have been revised and expanded as needed.

nutri-case | You Play the Expert!

Our Nutri-Case scenarios enable students to evaluate the nutrition-related beliefs and behaviors of five people representing a range of backgrounds and nutritional challenges. Take a moment to get acquainted with our Nutri-Case characters here.

HANNAH

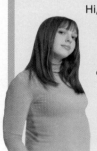

Hi, I'm Hannah. I'm 18 years old and in my first year at Valley Community College. I'm 5'6" and right now I weigh 171 lbs. I haven't made up my mind yet about my major. All I know for sure is that I don't want to work in a hospital like my mom! I got good grades in high school, but I'm a little freaked out by college so far. There's so much homework, plus one of my courses has a lab, plus I have to work part-time because my mom doesn't have the money to put me through school. . . . Sometimes I feel like I just can't handle it all. And when I get stressed out, I eat. I've already gained 10 pounds and I haven't even finished my first semester!

THEO

Hi, I'm Theo. Let's see, I'm 21, and my parents moved to the Midwest from Nigeria 11 years ago. I'm 6'8" tall and weigh-in at 200 lbs. The first time I ever played basketball, in middle school, I was hooked. I won lots of awards in high school and then got a full scholarship to the state university, where I'm a junior studying political science. I decided to take a nutrition course because, last year, I had a hard time making it through the playing season, plus keeping up with my classes and homework. I want to have more energy, so I thought maybe I'm not eating right. Anyway, I want to figure out this food thing before basketball season starts again.

LIZ

I'm Liz, I'm 20, and I'm a dance major at the School for Performing Arts. I'm 5'4" and currently weigh about 103 lbs. Last year, two other dancers from my class and I won a state championship and got to dance in the New Year's Eve celebration at the governor's mansion. This spring, I'm going to audition for the City Ballet, so I have to be in top condition. I wish I had time to take a nutrition course, but I'm too busy with dance classes, rehearsals, and teaching a dance class for kids. But it's okay, because I get lots of tips from other dancers and from the Internet. Like last week, I found a website especially for dancers that explained how to get rid of bloating before an audition. I'm going to try it for my audition with the City Ballet!

JUDY

I'm Judy, Hannah's mother. I'm 38 years old and a nurse's aide at Valley Hospital. I'm 5'5" and weigh 200 lbs. Back when Hannah was a baby, I dreamed of going to college so I could be a registered nurse. But then my ex and I split up, and Hannah and me, we've been in survival mode ever since. I'm proud to have raised my daughter without any handouts, and I do good work, but the pay never goes far enough and it's exhausting. I guess that's partly because I'm out of shape, and my blood sugar's high. Most nights, I'm so tired at the end of my shift that I just pick up some fast food for supper. I know I should be making home-cooked meals, but like I said, I'm in survival mode.

GUSTAVO

Hello. My name is Gustavo. I'm 69 years young at the moment, but when I was 13 years old I came to the United States from Mexico with my parents and three sisters to pick crops in California. Now I manage a large vineyard. They ask me when I'm going to retire, but I can still work as hard as a man half my age. Health problems? None. Well, maybe my doctor tells me my blood pressure is high, but that's normal for my age! I guess what keeps me going is thinking about how my father died 6 months after he retired. He had colon cancer, but he never knew it until it was too late. Anyway, I watch the nightly news and read the papers, so I keep up on what's good for me, "Eat less salt" and all that stuff. I'm doing great! I'm 5'5" tall and weigh 166 lbs.

Throughout this text, students will follow these five characters as they grapple with various nutrition-related challenges. As they do, the characters might remind students of themselves, or of people they may know. Our hope is that by applying the information learned in this course to their own circumstances, students will deepen their understanding of the importance of nutrition in achieving a healthful life.

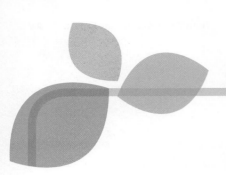

acknowledgments

It is always eye-opening to author a textbook and to realize that the work of so many people contributes to the final product. There are numerous people to thank, and we'd like to begin by extending our gratitude to our contributors. Our deep gratitude and appreciation goes to Dr. Linda Vaughan, of Arizona State University, who revised and updated the fluid and electrolyte balance chapter and the lifecycle chapters, as well as the In Depth features on alcohol, the fetal environment, and strategies to combat aging. Our enduring thanks as well goes to the many contributors and colleagues who made important and lasting contributions to earlier editions of this text. We also extend our sincere thanks to the able reviewers who provided much important feedback and guidance for this revision.

We would like to thank the fabulous staff at Pearson for their incredible support and dedication to this book. Our Acquisitions Editor, Sandra Lindelof, has provided unwavering support and guidance throughout the entire process of writing and publishing this book. We could never have written this text without the exceptional skills of our Developmental Editor, Laura Bonazzoli, whom we have been fortunate enough to have had on board for multiple editions. In addition to providing content guidance, Laura revised and updated the chapters on digestion and food safety and technology, as well as the In Depth features on disorders related to specific foods and food ethics. She also wrote the new In Depth feature on new frontiers in nutrition. Laura's energy, enthusiasm, and creativity significantly enhanced the quality of this textbook. Susan Scharf, our Project Editor, kept us on course and sane with her humor, organizational skills, and excellent editorial instincts, and made revising this book a pleasure rather than a chore. We are also deeply indebted to Art Development Editors Kari Hopperstead and Kelly Murphy for their work on the Focus Figures in this edition. Briana Verdugo and Tu-Anh Dang-Tran, Editorial Assistants, provided invaluable editorial and administrative support that we would have been lost without. Multiple talented players helped build this book in the production and design processes as well. Michael Penne and Nancy Tabor kept manuscripts and proofs moving, and ensured that the many production-related aspects flowed smoothly. Maya Melenchuck supervised the photo program, assisted by Kerri Wilson and Divya Narayanan who researched the important photo permissions. Elise Lansden created both the beautiful interior design and our glorious cover, under the expert guidance of Derek Bacchus. We would also like to thank the professionals at S4Carlisle Publishing Services, especially our Compositor Lynn Steines, for their important contributions to this text. Our thanks as well to Patricia Longoria for her excellent work on developing and updating the comprehensive Test Bank.

We also can't go without thanking the marketing and sales teams, especially Neena Bali, Executive Marketing Manager, and her talented marketing team, who ensured that we directed our writing efforts to meet the needs of students and instructors, and who worked so hard to get this book out to those who will benefit most from it.

We would also like to thank the many colleagues, friends, and family members who helped us along the way. Janice would like to thank her co-author Melinda Manore, who has provided unwavering support and guidance throughout her career and is a wonderful life-long friend and colleague. She would also like to thank her family and friends, who have been so incredibly supportive throughout her career. They are always there to offer a sympathetic ear and endless encouragement. She would also like to thank her students because they are the reason she loves her job so much.

Melinda would specifically like to thank her husband, Steve Carroll, for the patience and understanding he has shown through this process—once again. He has learned that there is always another chapter due! Melinda would also like to thank her family, friends, graduate students, and professional colleagues for their support and listening ear throughout this whole process. They all helped make life a little easier during this incredibly busy time. Finally, she would like to thank Janice, a great friend and colleague, who makes working on the book fun and rewarding.

reviewers

Lenore Boccia
The Restaurant School at Walnut Hill College

Carol Bradley
Stephen F. Austin State University

Diane Carson
California State University, Long Beach

Melissa Chabot
University at Buffalo, The State University of New York

Dorothy C. Chen-Maynard
California State University, San Bernardino

James F. Collins
University of Florida

Christine Coy
Saddleback Community College

Heather Graham-Williams
Truckee Meadows Community College

Shahla Khan
University of North Florida

Shannon Seal
University of Northern Colorado

Donna Zoss
Purdue University

Nancy Zwick
Northern Kentucky University

MasteringNutrition reviewers

Brain Barthel
Utah Valley College

Melissa Chabot
University at Buffalo, The State University of New York

Julia Erbacher
Salt Lake Community College

Carol Friesen
Ball State University

Urbi Ghosh
Oakton Community College

Judy Kaufman
Monroe Community College

Michelle Konstantarakis
Univeristy of Nevada–Las Vegas

Milli Owens
College of the Sequoias

Janet Sass
Northern Virginia Community College

Dana Sherman
Ozarks Technical Community College

Priya Venkatesan
Pasadena City College

brief contents

contents

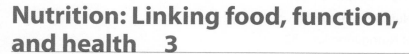

1

Nutrition: Linking food, function, and health 3

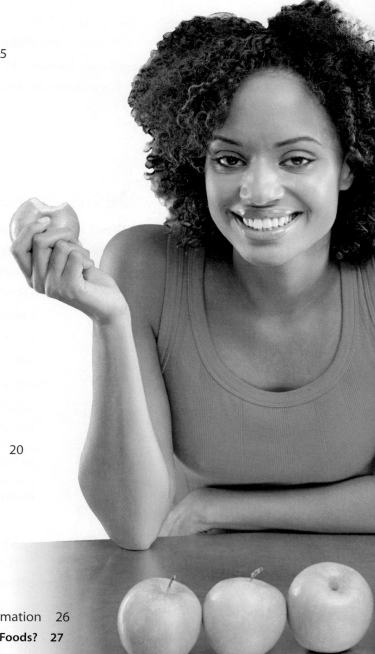

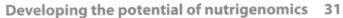

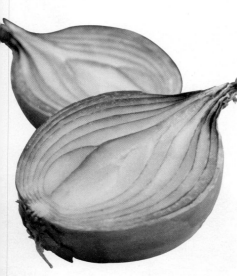

2

Designing a Healthful Diet   39

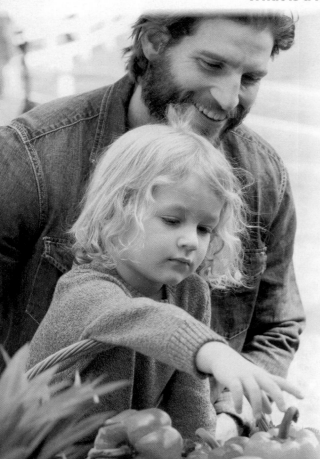

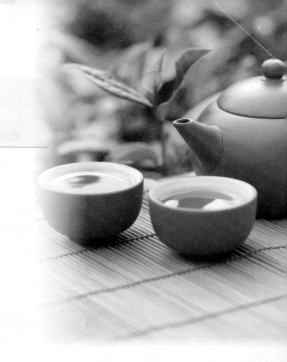

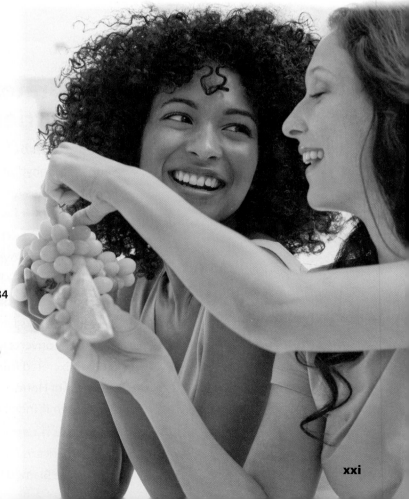

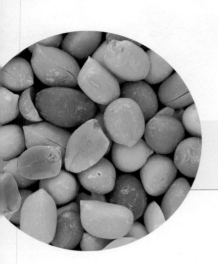

4

Carbohydrates: Plant-derived energy nutrients 109

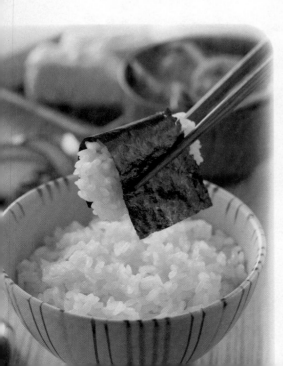

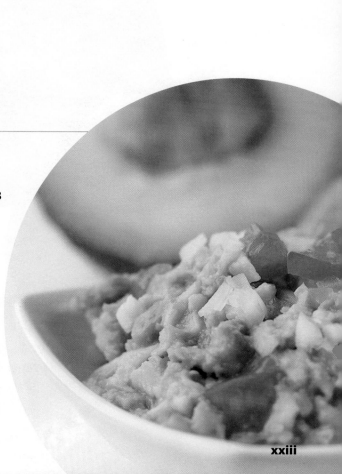

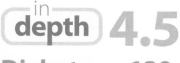

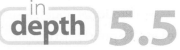

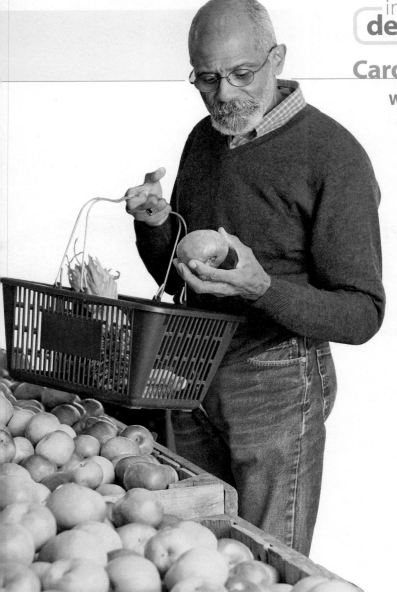

6

Proteins: Crucial components of all body tissues   191

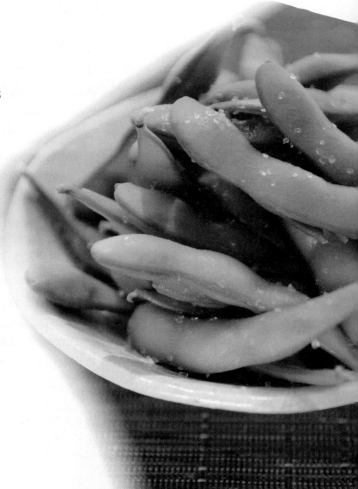

in
depth 6.5

Vitamins and Minerals: Micronutrients with Macro Powers 224

7

Nutrients Involved in Fluid and Electrolyte Balance   235

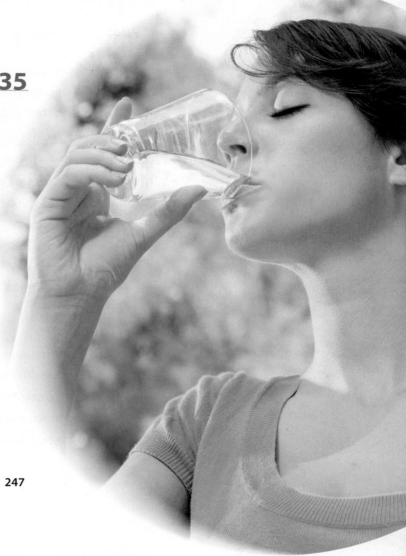

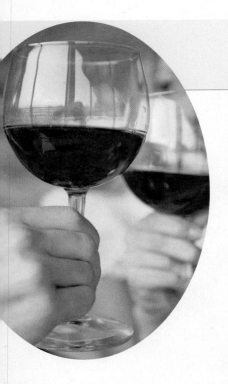

8

Nutrients Involved in Antioxidant Function and Vision 275

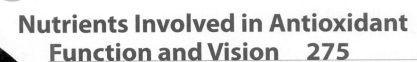

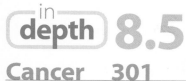

Cancer   301

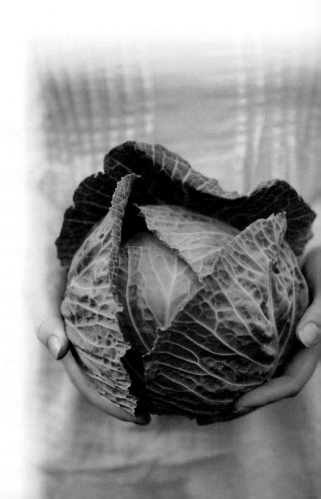

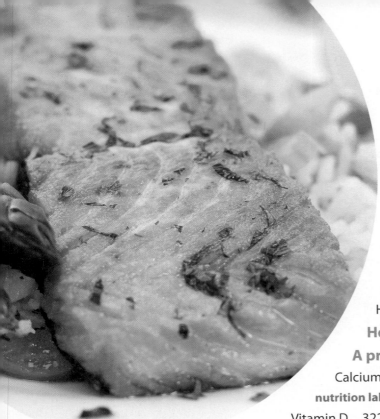

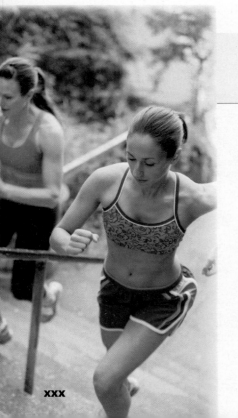

10

Nutrients Involved in Energy Metabolism and Blood Health   347

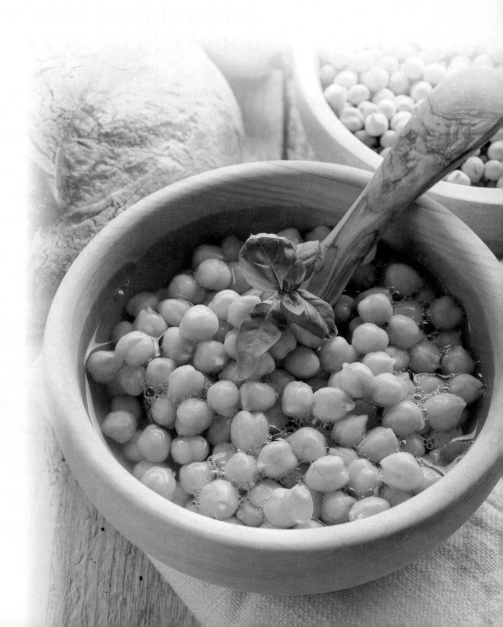

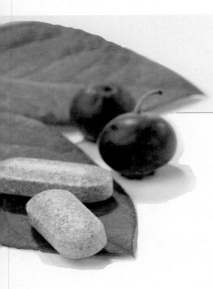

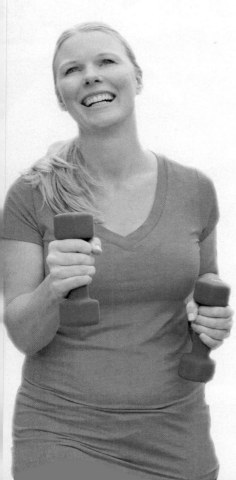

in
depth 11.5

Disordered Eating 429

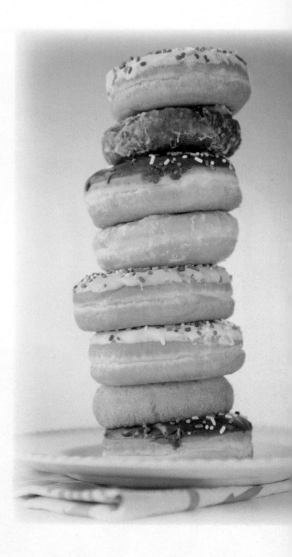

12

Nutrition and Physical Activity: Keys to good health   441

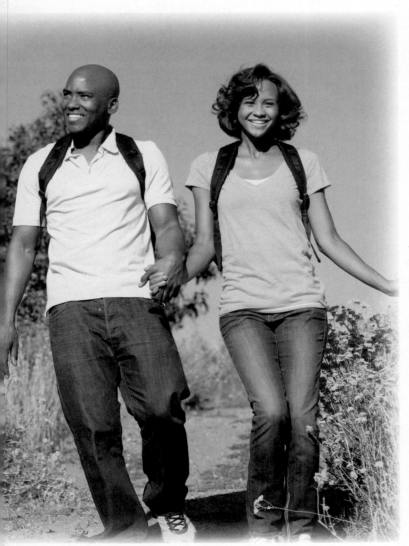

in depth 12.5
Do Active People Need Ergogenic Aids? 471

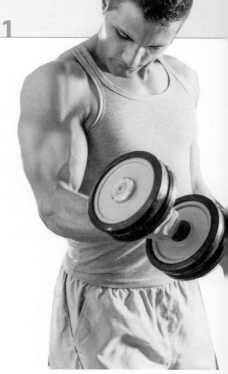

13
Food Safety and Technology: Impact on consumers 477

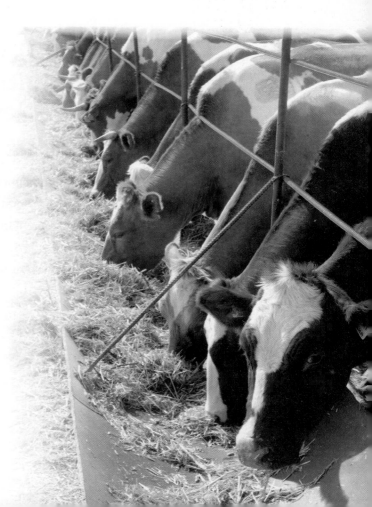

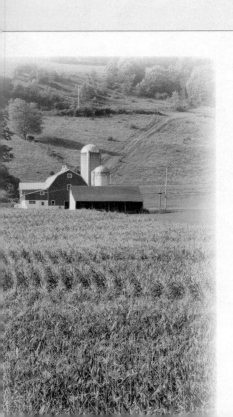

in depth 13.5

Food Ethics: Sustainability, Equity, and the New Food Movement   505

14

Nutrition Through the Life Cycle: Pregnancy and the first year of life   513

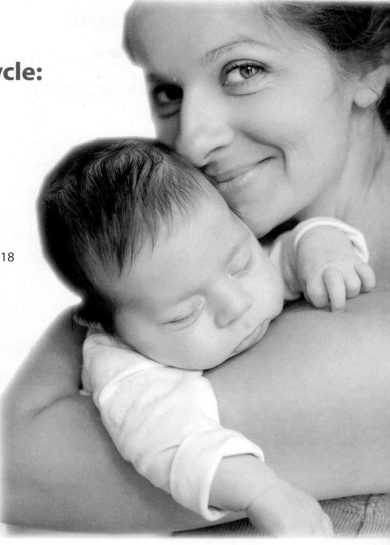

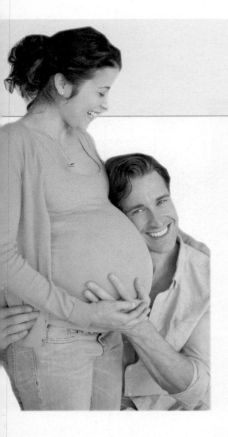

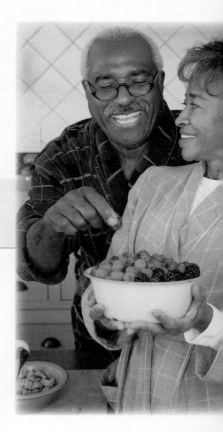

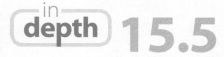

depth 15.5

Searching for the Fountain of Youth   587

Appendices

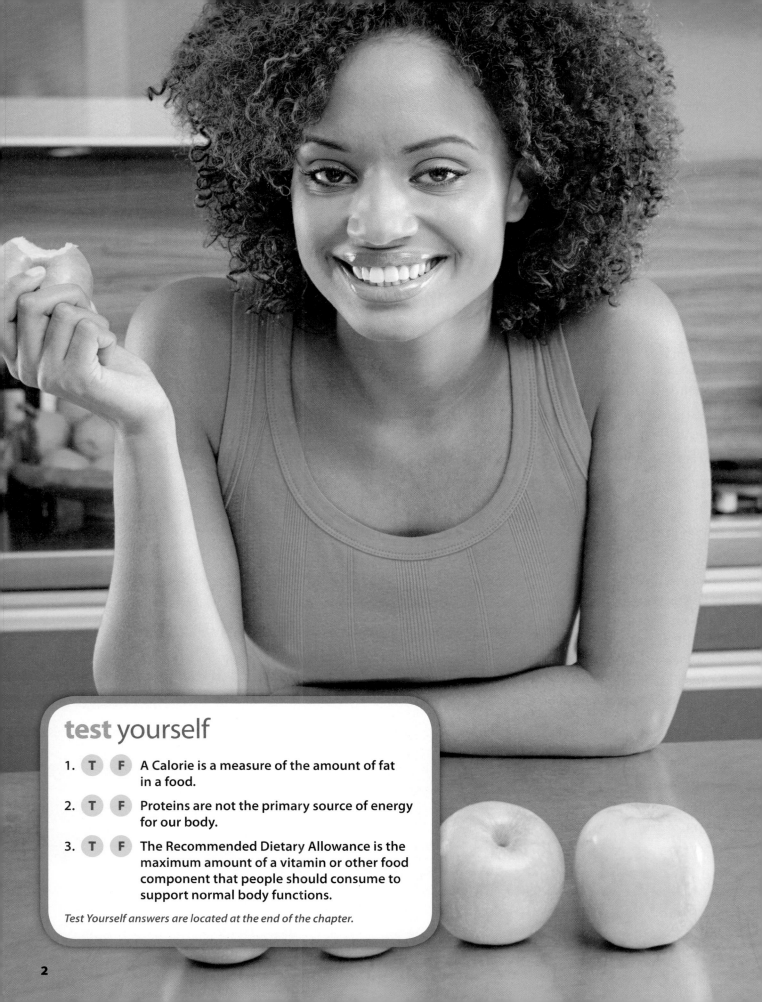

test yourself

1. **T F** A Calorie is a measure of the amount of fat in a food.

2. **T F** Proteins are not the primary source of energy for our body.

3. **T F** The Recommended Dietary Allowance is the maximum amount of a vitamin or other food component that people should consume to support normal body functions.

Test Yourself answers are located at the end of the chapter.

Nutrition
Linking food, function, and health

1

learning objectives

After studying this chapter you should be able to:

1 Define the term *nutrition* and describe its evolution as a science, p. 4.

2 Discuss why nutrition is important to health, pp. 4–8.

3 Identify the six classes of nutrients essential for health, pp. 8–13.

4 Identify the Dietary Reference Intakes for nutrients, pp. 14–17.

5 Describe the steps of the scientific method used in research studies, pp. 17–23.

6 List at least four sources of reliable and accurate nutrition information, pp. 24–26.

Miguel hadn't expected college life to make him feel so tired. After classes, he just wanted to go back to his dorm and sleep. Plus, he'd been having trouble concentrating and was worried that his first-semester grades would be far below those he'd achieved in high school. Scott, his roommate, had little sympathy. "It's all that junk food you eat!" he insisted. "Let's go down to the organic market for some real food." Miguel dragged himself to the market with Scott. A woman wearing a white lab coat approached him and introduced herself as the market's staff nutritionist. "You're looking a little pale," she said. "Anything wrong?" Miguel explained that he had been feeling tired lately. "I don't doubt it," the woman answered. "I can see from your skin tone that you're anemic. You need to start taking an iron supplement." She took a bottle of pills from a shelf and handed it to him. "This one is the easiest for you to absorb, and it's on special this week. Take it twice a day, and you should start feeling better in a day or two." Miguel bought the supplement and began taking it that night with the meal his roommate had prepared. He took it twice the next day as well, just as the nutritionist had recommended, but didn't feel any better. After 2 more days, he visited the university health clinic, where a nurse drew some blood for testing. When the results came in, the doctor told him that his thyroid gland wasn't making enough of the hormone he needed to keep his body functioning properly. She prescribed a medication and congratulated Miguel for catching the problem early. "If you had waited," she said, "it would only have gotten worse, and you could have become seriously ill." Miguel asked if he should continue taking his iron supplements. The doctor looked puzzled. "Where did you get the idea that you needed iron supplements?"

Continued next page

MasteringNutrition™

Build your knowledge—and nutrition— in the MasteringNutrition Study Area with a variety of online tools! Go to www.masteringhealthandnutrition.com (or www.pearsonmastering.com).

Continued—

Like Miguel, you've probably been offered nutrition-related advice from well-meaning friends and self-professed "experts." Perhaps you found the advice helpful, or maybe, as in Miguel's case, it turned out to be all wrong. Where can you go for reliable advice about nutrition? What exactly *is* nutrition, and why does what we eat have such an influence on our health? In this chapter, we'll begin to answer these questions, and you'll gain a deeper understanding as you work through the rest of this book. You'll also learn how to evaluate nutrition-related research studies, as well as how to distinguish science from scams. Our goal is that, by the time you finish this course, you'll be the expert on your own nutritional needs!

What is nutrition?

Although many people think that *food* and *nutrition* mean the same thing, they don't. **Food** refers to the plants and animals we consume. It provides the chemicals our body needs to maintain life and support growth and health. **Nutrition**, in contrast, is the science that studies food and how food nourishes our body and influences our health. It encompasses how we consume, digest, absorb, and store the chemicals in food, and how these chemicals affect our body. Nutrition also involves studying the factors that influence our eating patterns, making recommendations about the amount we should eat of each type of food, attempting to maintain food safety, and addressing issues related to the global food supply. You can think of nutrition, then, as the discipline that encompasses everything about food.

When compared with other scientific disciplines such as chemistry, biology, and physics, nutrition is a relative newcomer. Although food has played a defining role in the lives of humans since the evolution of our species, an appreciation of the importance of nutrition to our health has developed slowly only during the past 400 years. Early research in nutrition focused on making the link between dietary deficiencies and illness. For instance, the cause of scurvy, which is a vitamin C deficiency, was discovered in the mid-1700s. At that time, however, vitamin C had not been identified—what was known was that some ingredient found in citrus fruits could prevent scurvy. Another early discovery in nutrition is discussed in the accompanying **Nutrition Myth or Fact?** box about a disease called pellagra.

Nutrition research continued to focus on identifying and preventing deficiency diseases through the first half of the 20th century. Then, as the higher standard of living after World War II led to an improvement in the American diet, nutrition research began pursuing a new objective: supporting health and preventing and treating **chronic diseases**—that is, diseases that come on slowly and can persist for years, often despite treatment. Chronic diseases of particular interest to nutrition researchers include obesity, heart disease, type 2 diabetes, and various cancers. This new research has raised as many questions as it has answered, and we still have a great deal to learn about the relationship between nutrition and chronic disease.

In recent decades, advances in technology have contributed to the emergence of several exciting new areas of nutrition research. For example, reflecting our growing understanding of genetics, *nutrigenomics* seeks to uncover links between our genes, our environment, and our diet. The **In Depth** following this chapter describes this and other new frontiers in nutrition and health.

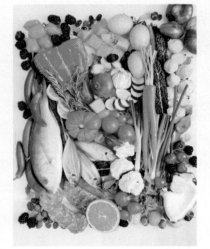

◆ Nutrition is the science that studies all aspects of food and its influence on our body and health.

food The plants and animals we consume.

nutrition The science that studies food and how food nourishes our body and influences our health.

chronic diseases Diseases that come on slowly and can persist for years, often despite treatment.

How does nutrition contribute to health?

Think about it: If you eat three meals a day, by this time next year, you'll have had more than a thousand chances to influence your body's makeup! As you'll learn in

nutrition myth or fact?

Is Pellagra an Infectious Disease?

In the first few years of the 20th century, Dr. Joseph Goldberger successfully controlled outbreaks of several fatal infectious diseases, from yellow fever in Louisiana to typhus in Mexico. So it wasn't surprising that, in 1914, the U.S. Surgeon General chose him to tackle another disease, thought to be infectious, that was raging throughout the South. Called *pellagra,* the disease was characterized by a skin rash, diarrhea, and mental impairment. At the time, it afflicted more than 50,000 people each year, and in about 10% of cases it resulted in death.[1]

Goldberger began studying the disease by carefully observing its occurrence in groups of people. He asked, if it is infectious, then why would it strike children in orphanages and prison inmates yet leave their nurses and guards unaffected? Why did it overwhelmingly affect impoverished millworkers and sharecroppers while leaving their affluent (and well-fed) neighbors healthy? Could a dietary deficiency cause pellagra?

To confirm his hunch, he conducted a series of trials in which he fed afflicted orphans and prisoners—who had been consuming a limited, corn-based diet—a variety of nutritious foods, including meats. They recovered. Moreover, orphans and inmates who did not have pellagra and ate the new diet did not develop the disease. Finally, Goldberger recruited eleven healthy prison inmates, who, in return for a pardon of their sentence, agreed to consume a limited, corn-based diet. After

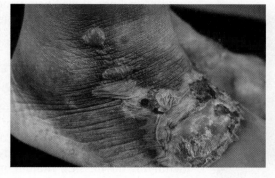

Pellagra is characterized by a scaly skin rash.

5 months, six of the eleven developed pellagra.

Still, many skeptics were unable to give up the idea that pellagra was an infectious disease. To prove that pellagra was not spread by germs, Goldberger and his colleagues deliberately injected themselves with and ingested patients' scabs, nasal secretions, and other body fluids. He and his team remained healthy.

Although Goldberger could not identify the precise component in the new diet that cured pellagra, he eventually found an inexpensive and widely available substance, brewer's yeast, that when added to the diet prevented or reversed the disease. Shortly after Goldberger's death in 1937, scientists identified the component that is deficient in the diet of pellagra patients: niacin, one of the B-vitamins, which is plentiful in brewer's yeast.[1]

CRITICAL THINKING QUESTIONS

1. What issues arise from the research done by Dr. Goldberger and his colleagues?
2. Do you think that this research would be considered ethical and acceptable by today's standards? Why or why not?
3. Identify a disease linked to nutrition that you feel deserves substantial attention from researchers. What makes you choose this disease?

---

this text, you really are what you eat: the substances you take into your body are broken down and reassembled into your brain cells, bones, muscles—all of your tissues and organs. The foods you eat also provide your body with the energy it needs to function properly. In addition, proper nutrition can improve your health, prevent certain diseases, achieve and maintain a desirable weight, and maintain your energy and vitality. Let's take a closer look at how nutrition supports health and wellness.

Nutrition Is One of Several Factors Supporting Wellness

Wellness can be defined in many ways. Traditionally considered simply the absence of disease, wellness has been redefined as we have learned more about our body and what it means to live a healthful lifestyle. Wellness is now considered to be *multidimensional*, including physical, emotional, social, occupational, and spiritual health (**FIGURE 1.1**, page 6). Wellness is not an endpoint in our lives, but an active process we work on every day.

In this book, we focus on two critical aspects of physical health: nutrition and physical activity. The two are so closely related that you can think of them as two sides of the same coin: our overall state of nutrition is influenced by how much energy we expend doing daily activities, and our level of physical activity has a major impact on how we use the food we eat. We can perform more strenuous activities for

wellness A multidimensional, lifelong process that includes physical, emotional, social, occupational, and spiritual health.

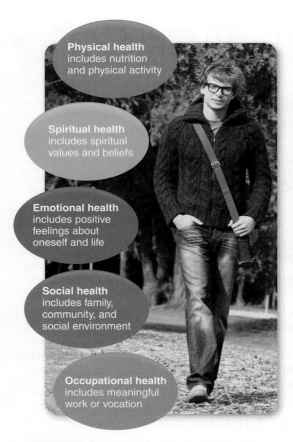

Physical health
includes nutrition
and physical activity

Spiritual health
includes spiritual
values and beliefs

Emotional health
includes positive
feelings about
oneself and life

Social health
includes family,
community, and
social environment

Occupational health
includes meaningful
work or vocation

FIGURE 1.1 Many factors contribute to our wellness. Primary among these are a nutritious diet and regular physical activity.

longer periods when we eat a nutritious diet, whereas an inadequate or excessive food intake can make us lethargic. A poor diet, inadequate or excessive physical activity, or a combination of these also can lead to serious health problems. Finally, several studies have suggested that healthful nutrition and regular physical activity can increase feelings of well-being and reduce feelings of anxiety and depression. In other words, wholesome food and physical activity just plain feel good!

A Healthful Diet Can Prevent Some Diseases and Reduce Your Risk for Others

Nutrition appears to play a role—from a direct cause to a mild influence—in the development of many diseases (FIGURE 1.2). As we noted earlier, poor nutrition is a direct cause of deficiency diseases, such as scurvy and pellagra. Early nutrition research focused on identifying the missing vitamin or other food substance behind such diseases and on developing guidelines for intake levels that are high enough to prevent them. Over the years, nutrition scientists successfully lobbied for the fortification of foods with the substances of greatest concern. These measures, along with a more abundant and reliable food supply, have almost completely wiped out the majority of nutritional deficiency diseases in developed countries. However, they are still major problems in many developing nations.

In addition to causing disease directly, poor nutrition can have a subtle influence on our health. For instance, it can contribute to the development of brittle bones (a disease called *osteoporosis*) as well as to the progression of some forms of cancer. These associations are considered mild; however, poor nutrition is also strongly associated with three chronic diseases—heart disease, stroke, and diabetes—which are among the top ten causes of death in the United States (FIGURE 1.3).

It probably won't surprise you to learn that the primary link between poor nutrition and mortality is obesity. Fundamentally, obesity is a consequence of eating more Calories than are expended. At the same time, obesity is a well-established risk factor for heart disease, stroke, type 2 diabetes, and some forms of cancer. Unfortunately, the prevalence of obesity has dramatically increased throughout the United States during the past 25 years (FIGURE 1.4). Throughout this text, we will discuss in detail how nutrition and physical activity affect the development of obesity.

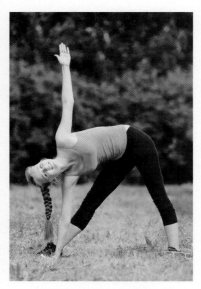

Our level of physical activity has a major impact on how we use the foods we eat.

Diseases in which nutrition plays some role	Osteoporosis Osteoarthritis Some forms of cancer
Diseases with a strong nutritional component	Type 2 diabetes Heart disease High blood pressure Obesity
Diseases caused by nutritional deficiencies or toxicities	Pellagra Scurvy Iron-deficiency anemia Other vitamin and mineral deficiencies and toxicities

FIGURE 1.2 The relationship between nutrition and human disease. Notice that, whereas nutritional factors are only marginally implicated in the diseases of the top row, they are strongly linked to the development of the diseases in the middle row and truly causative of those in the bottom row.

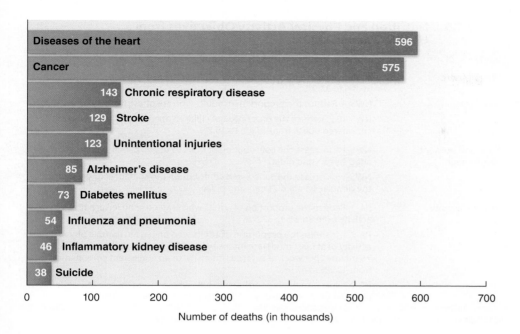

◀ **FIGURE 1.3** Of the ten leading causes of death in the United States in 2011, three—heart disease, stroke, and diabetes—are strongly associated with poor nutrition. In addition, nutrition plays a limited role in the development of some forms of cancer.
Data from: "Deaths: Preliminary Data for 2011" (U.S. Department of Health and Human Services).

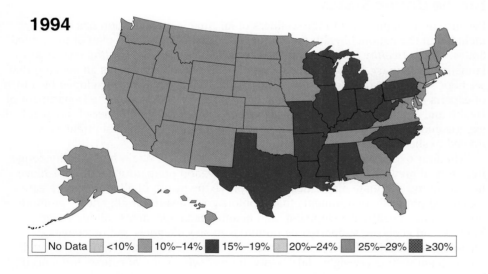

◀ **FIGURE 1.4** These diagrams illustrate the increase in obesity rates across the United States from 1994 to 2011 as documented in the Behavioral Risk Factor Surveillance System. Obesity is defined as a body mass index greater than or equal to 30, or approximately 30 lb overweight for a 5'4" woman.
Graphics and data from: "Prevalence of Self-Reported Obesity among U.S. Adults" and "Percent of Obese (BMI=30) in U.S. Adults: 1994" (Centers for Disease Control and Prevention).

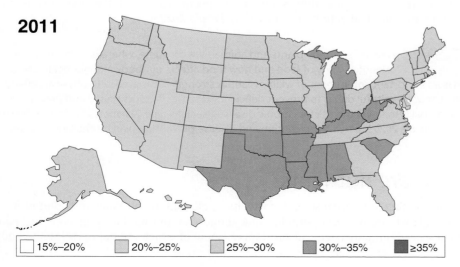

TABLE 1.1 Nutrition and Physical Activity Objectives from
Healthy People 2020

Topic	Objective Number and Description
Weight status	NWS-8. Increase the proportion of adults who are at a healthy weight from 30.8% to 33.9%.
	NWS-9. Reduce the proportion of adults who are obese from 34.0% to 30.6%.
	NWS-10.2. Reduce the proportion of children aged 6 to 11 years who are considered obese from 17.4% to 15.7%.
Food and nutrient composition	NWS-14. Increase the contribution of fruits to the diets of the population aged 2 years and older.
	NWS-15. Increase the variety and contribution of vegetables to the diets of the population aged 2 years and older.
Physical activity	PA-1. Reduce the proportion of adults who engage in no leisure-time physical activity from 36.2% to 32.6%.
	PA-2.1. Increase the proportion of adults who engage in aerobic physical activity of at least moderate intensity for at least 150 minutes per week, or 75 minutes per week of vigorous intensity, or an equivalent combination from 43.5% to 47.9%.
	PA-2.3. Increase the proportion of adults who perform muscle-strengthening activities on 2 or more days of the week from 21.9% to 24.1%.

Data adapted from: "Healthy People 2020" (U.S. Department of Health and Human Services).

Want to see how the prevalence of obesity has changed in the United States over the past 25 years? Go to www.cdc.gov and enter "obesity data trend maps" into the search bar.

Healthy People 2020 Identifies Nutrition-Related Goals for the United States

Because of its importance to the wellness of all Americans, nutrition has been included in the national health promotion and disease prevention plan of the United States. Called *Healthy People,* the plan is revised every decade. *Healthy People 2020*, launched in January 2010, identifies a set of goals and objectives (as an agenda) that we hope to reach as a nation by the year 2020.[2] This agenda was developed by a team of experts from a variety of federal agencies under the direction of the Department of Health and Human Services. Input was gathered from a large number of independent experts and national and state health organizations, and the general public was invited to share ideas.

The four overarching goals of *Healthy People* are to "1) attain high-quality, longer lives free of preventable disease, disability, injury, and premature death; 2) achieve health equity, eliminate disparities, and improve the health of all groups; 3) create social and physical environments that promote good health for all; and 4) promote quality of life, healthy development, and healthy behaviors across all life stages." These broad goals are supported by hundreds of specific goals and objectives, including many related to nutrition. Other objectives address physical activity and the problem with overweight and obesity, both of which are, of course, influenced by nutrition. **TABLE 1.1** identifies some of the specific goals and objectives related to nutrition and physical activity from *Healthy People 2020*.

recap *Food* refers to the plants and animals we consume, whereas *nutrition* is the scientifiic study of food and how food affects our body and our health. Nutrition is an important component of wellness and is strongly associated with physical activity. One goal of a healthful diet is to prevent deficiency diseases, such as scurvy and pellagra; a second goal is to lower the risk for chronic diseases, such as type 2 diabetes and heart disease. *Healthy People 2020* is a health promotion and disease prevention plan for the United States.

What are nutrients?

We enjoy eating food because of its taste, its smell, and the pleasure and comfort it gives us. However, we rarely stop to think about what our food actually contains. Foods are composed of many chemical substances, some of which are not useful to the body

SIX GROUPS OF ESSENTIAL NUTRIENTS

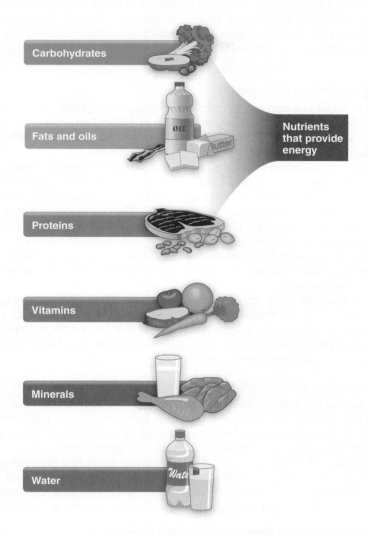

and others of which are critical to our growth and function. These latter chemicals are referred to as **nutrients**. The six groups of nutrients found in foods are (**FIGURE 1.5**):

- carbohydrates
- fats and oils (two types of lipids)
- proteins
- vitamins
- minerals
- water

The term *organic* is commonly used to describe foods that are grown with little or no use of synthetic chemicals. But when scientists describe individual nutrients as **organic**, they mean that these nutrients contain both carbon and hydrogen, fundamental units of matter that are common to all living organisms. Carbohydrates, lipids, proteins, and vitamins are organic. Minerals and water are **inorganic**. Organic and inorganic nutrients are equally important for sustaining life but differ in their structures, functions, and basic chemistry. You will learn more about these nutrients in subsequent chapters; a brief review is provided here.

Macronutrients Provide Energy

Carbohydrates, fats, and proteins are the only nutrients that provide energy. By this we mean that our body breaks down these nutrients and reassembles their

nutrients Chemicals found in foods that are critical to human growth and function.

organic A substance or nutrient that contains the elements carbon and hydrogen.

inorganic A substance or nutrient that does not contain carbon and hydrogen.

components into a fuel that supports physical activity and basic functioning. Although taking a multivitamin might be beneficial in other ways, it will not provide you with the energy for a 20-minute session on the stair-climber! These energy-yielding nutrients are also referred to as **macronutrients**. *Macro* means "large," and our body needs relatively large amounts of these nutrients to support normal function and health.

Energy Is Measured in Kilocalories

The energy in foods is measured in units called *kilocalories (kcal)*. A kilocalorie is the amount of heat required to raise the temperature of 1 kilogram (about 2.2 lb) of water by 1 degree Celsius. We can say that the energy found in 1 gram of carbohydrate is equal to 4 kcal.

You've certainly also seen the term *Calorie*. What's the difference? Well, technically, 1 kilocalorie is equal to 1,000 Calories. *Kilo-* is a prefix used in the metric system to indicate 1,000 (think of *kilometer*). For the sake of simplicity, nutrition labels use the term *Calories* to indicate kilocalories. Thus, if the wrapper on an ice cream bar states that it contains 150 Calories, it actually contains 150 kilocalories.

In this textbook, we use the term *energy* when referring to the general concept of energy intake or energy expenditure. We use the term *kilocalories (kcal)* when discussing units of energy. We use the term *Calories* only when presenting information about foods.

Both carbohydrates and proteins provide 4 kcal per gram, alcohol provides 7 kcal per gram, and fats provide 9 kcal per gram. Thus, for every gram of fat we consume, we obtain more than twice the energy derived from a gram of carbohydrate or protein. Refer to the **You Do the Math** box to learn how to calculate the energy contribution of carbohydrates, fats, and proteins in a given food.

Carbohydrates Are a Primary Fuel Source

Carbohydrates are the primary source of fuel for our body, particularly for our brain and during physical exercise (**FIGURE 1.6**). *Carbo-* refers to carbon, and *-hydrate* refers to water. You may remember that water is made up of hydrogen and oxygen. Thus, carbohydrates are composed of chains of carbon, hydrogen, and oxygen.

Carbohydrates are found in a wide variety of foods, including rice, wheat, and other grains, as well as vegetables and fruits. Carbohydrates are also found in *legumes* (foods that include lentils, beans, and peas), seeds, nuts, and milk and other dairy products. (Carbohydrates and their role in health are the subject of Chapter 4.)

Fats Provide Energy and Other Essential Nutrients

Fats are another important source of energy for our body (**FIGURE 1.7**). They are a type of *lipids*, a diverse group of organic substances that are insoluble in water. Like carbohydrates, fats are composed of carbon, hydrogen, and oxygen; however, they

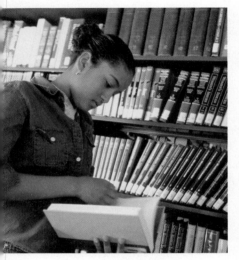

☛ Carbohydrates are the primary source of fuel for our body, particularly for our brain.

macronutrients Nutrients that our body needs in relatively large amounts to support normal function and health. Carbohydrates, fats, and proteins are macronutrients.

carbohydrates The primary fuel source for our body, particularly for our brain and for physical exercise.

fats An important energy source for our body at rest and during low-intensity exercise.

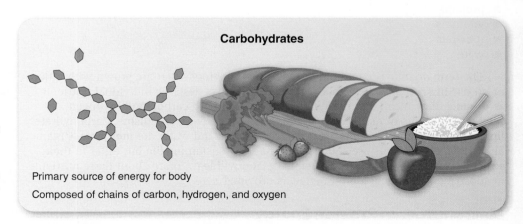

Carbohydrates

Primary source of energy for body
Composed of chains of carbon, hydrogen, and oxygen

☛ **FIGURE 1.6** Carbohydrates are a primary source of energy for our body and are found in a wide variety of foods.

you do the math

Calculating the Energy Contribution of Carbohydrates, Fats, and Proteins

The energy in food is used for everything from maintaining normal body functions—such as breathing, digesting food, and repairing damaged tissues and organs—to enabling you to perform physical activity and even to read this text. So how much energy is produced from the foods you eat?

To answer this question, you need to know the following information:

▪ Carbohydrates should make up the largest percentage of your nutrient intake, about 45–65%; they provide 4 kcal of energy per gram of carbohydrate consumed.

▪ Proteins also provide 4 kcal of energy per gram; they should be limited to 10–35% of your daily energy intake.

▪ Fats provide the most energy, 9 kcal per gram; they should make up 20–35% of your total energy intake.

In order to figure out whether you're taking in the appropriate percentages of carbohydrates, fats, and proteins, you will need to use a little math.

1. Let's say you have completed a personal diet analysis, and you consume 2,500 kcal per day. You consume 300 g of carbohydrates, 90 g of fat, and 123 g of protein.

2. To calculate your percentage of total energy that comes from carbohydrate, you must do two things:

a. Multiply your total grams of carbohydrate by the energy value for carbohydrate.

300 g of carbohydrate $\times$ 4 kcal/g
= 1,200 kcal of carbohydrate consumed

b. Take the kcal of carbohydrate consumed, divide this by the total kcal consumed, and multiply by 100. This will give you the percentage of the total energy you consume that comes from carbohydrate.

(1,200 kcal/2,500 kcal) $\times$ 100 = 48% of total energy comes from carbohydrate

3. To calculate your percentage of total energy that comes from fat, you follow the same steps but incorporate the energy value for fat:

a. 90 g of fat $\times$ 9 kcal/g = 810 kcal of fat

b. (810 kcal/2,500 kcal) $\times$ 100 = 32.4% of total energy comes from fat

Now try these steps to calculate the percentage of the total energy you consume that comes from protein.

Also, have you ever heard that alcohol provides "empty Calories"? Alcohol contributes 7 kcal per gram. You can calculate the percentage of kcal from alcohol in your daily diet, but remember that it is not considered an energy nutrient.

These calculations will be very useful throughout this course as you learn more about how to design a healthful diet and how to read labels to help you meet your nutritional goals. Later in this book you will learn how to estimate your unique energy needs.

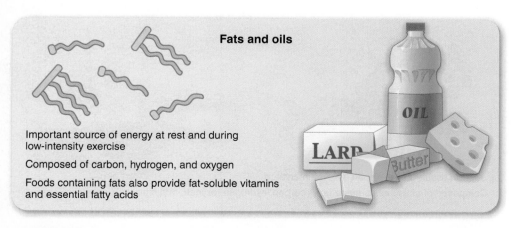

Fats and oils

Important source of energy at rest and during low-intensity exercise

Composed of carbon, hydrogen, and oxygen

Foods containing fats also provide fat-soluble vitamins and essential fatty acids

◆ **FIGURE 1.7** Fats are an important energy source during rest and low-intensity exercise. Foods containing fats also provide other important nutrients.

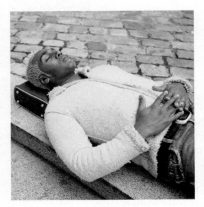

⬆ Fats are an important source of energy for our body, especially when we are at rest.

contain proportionally much less oxygen and water than carbohydrates do. This quality allows them to pack together tightly, which explains why they yield more energy per gram than either carbohydrates or proteins.

Fats are an important energy source for our body at rest and during low-intensity exercise. Our body is capable of storing large amounts of fat as adipose tissue. These fat stores can then be broken down for energy during periods when we are not eating—for example, while we are asleep. Foods that contain fats are also essential for the transportation into our body of certain vitamins that are soluble only in fat.

Dietary fats come in a variety of forms. Solid fats include such things as butter, lard, and margarine. Liquid fats, referred to as *oils,* include vegetable oils, such as canola and olive oils. Cholesterol is a form of lipid that our body can produce independently, and it can also be consumed in the diet. (Chapter 5 provides a thorough discussion of lipids.)

Proteins Support Tissue Growth, Repair, and Maintenance

Proteins also contain carbon, hydrogen, and oxygen, but they differ from carbohydrates and fats in that they contain the element *nitrogen* (**FIGURE 1.8**). Within proteins, these four elements assemble into small building blocks known as amino acids. We break down dietary proteins into amino acids and reassemble them to build our own body proteins—for instance, the proteins in our muscles and blood.

Although proteins can provide energy, they are not usually a primary energy source. Proteins play a major role in building new cells and tissues, maintaining the structure and strength of bone, repairing damaged structures, and assisting in regulating the breakdown of foods and fluid balance.

Proteins are found in many foods. Meats and dairy products are primary sources, as are seeds, nuts, and legumes. We also obtain small amounts from vegetables and whole grains. (Proteins are the subject of Chapter 6.)

Micronutrients Assist in the Regulation of Body Functions

Vitamins and minerals are referred to as **micronutrients**. That's because we need relatively small amounts of these nutrients to support normal health and body functions.

Vitamins are organic compounds that help regulate our body's functions. Contrary to popular belief, vitamins do not contain energy (kilocalories); however, they are essential to energy **metabolism**, the process by which the macronutrients are broken down into the smaller chemicals that our body can absorb and use. So vitamins assist with releasing and using the energy in carbohydrates, fats, and proteins. They are also critical in building and maintaining healthy bone, muscle, and blood; supporting our immune system so that we can fight infection and disease; and ensuring healthy vision.

proteins The only macronutrient that contains nitrogen; the basic building blocks of proteins are amino acids.

micronutrients Nutrients needed in relatively small amounts to support normal health and body functions. Vitamins and minerals are micronutrients.

vitamins Organic compounds that assist us in regulating our body's processes.

metabolism The process by which large chemicals, such as carbohydrates, fats, and proteins, are broken down via chemical reactions into smaller chemicals that can be used as fuel, stored, or assembled into new compounds the body needs.

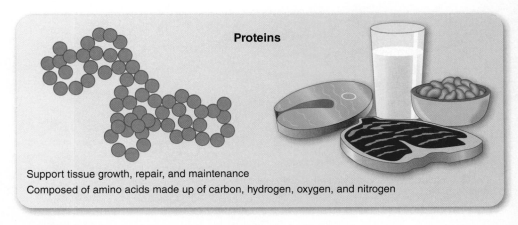

Proteins

Support tissue growth, repair, and maintenance
Composed of amino acids made up of carbon, hydrogen, oxygen, and nitrogen

⬆ **FIGURE 1.8** Proteins contain nitrogen in addition to carbon, hydrogen, and oxygen. Proteins support the growth, repair, and maintenance of body tissues.

TABLE 1.2   Overview of Vitamins

Type	Names	Distinguishing Features
Fat-soluble	A, D, E, and K	Soluble in fat Stored in the human body Toxicity can occur from consuming excess amounts, which accumulate in the body
Water-soluble	C, B-vitamins (thiamin, riboflavin, niacin, vitamin B$_6$, vitamin B$_{12}$, pantothenic acid, biotin, and folate)	Soluble in water Not stored to any extent in the human body Excess excreted in urine Toxicity generally only occurs as a result of vitamin supplementation

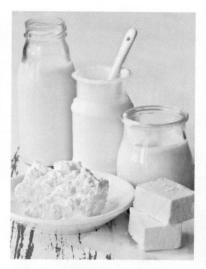

Fat-soluble vitamins are found in a variety of fat-containing foods, including dairy products.

Vitamins are classified as two types: **fat-soluble vitamins** and **water-soluble vitamins** (TABLE 1.2). This classification reflects how vitamins are absorbed, transported, and stored in our body. Both types of vitamins are essential for health and are found in a variety of foods. (Learn more about vitamins in the **In Depth** essay following Chapter 6. Chapters 7 through 10 discuss individual vitamins in detail.)

Minerals include sodium, potassium, calcium, magnesium, and iron. They are classified as inorganic because they do not contain carbon and hydrogen. In fact, they do not "contain" other substances at all. Minerals are single elements, so they already exist in the simplest possible chemical form. Thus, they cannot be broken down during digestion or when our body uses them to promote normal function; and unlike certain vitamins, they can't be destroyed by heat or light. All minerals maintain their structure no matter what environment they are in. This means that the calcium in our bones is the same as the calcium in the milk we drink, and the sodium in our cells is the same as the sodium in our table salt.

Minerals have many important functions in our body. They assist in fluid regulation and energy production, are essential to the health of our bones and blood, and help rid our body of the harmful by-products of metabolism.

Minerals are classified according to the amounts we need in our diet and according to how much of the mineral is found in our body. The two categories of minerals in our diet and body are the **major minerals** and the **trace minerals** (TABLE 1.3). (Learn more about minerals in the **In Depth** following Chapter 6. Chapters 7 through 10 discuss individual minerals in detail.)

Water Supports All Body Functions

Water is an inorganic nutrient (it contains oxygen and hydrogen, but not carbon) that is vital for our survival. We consume water from many sources; in its pure form; in juices, soups, and other liquids; and in solid foods, such as fruits and vegetables. Adequate water intake ensures the proper balance of fluid both inside and outside our cells, and assists in the regulation of nerve impulses and body temperature, muscle contractions, nutrient transport, and the excretion of waste products. (Chapter 7 focuses on water and its function in our body.)

fat-soluble vitamins Vitamins that are not soluble in water but are soluble in fat. These include vitamins A, D, E, and K.

water-soluble vitamins Vitamins that are soluble in water. These include vitamin C and the B-vitamins.

minerals Inorganic substances that are not broken down during digestion and absorption and are not destroyed by heat or light. Minerals assist in the regulation of many body processes and are classified as major minerals or trace minerals.

major minerals Minerals we need to consume in amounts of at least 100 mg per day and of which the total amount in our body is at least 5 g.

trace minerals Minerals we need to consume in amounts less than 100 mg per day and of which the total amount in our body is less than 5 g.

TABLE 1.3   Overview of Minerals

Type	Names	Distinguishing Features
Major minerals	Calcium, phosphorus, sodium, potassium, chloride, magnesium, sulfur	Needed in amounts greater than 100 mg/day in our diet Amount present in the human body is greater than 5 g (5,000 mg)
Trace minerals	Iron, zinc, copper, manganese, fluoride, chromium, molybdenum, selenium, iodine	Needed in amounts less than 100 mg/day in our diet Amount present in the human body is less than 5 g (5,000 mg)

recap The six essential nutrient groups are carbohydrates, fats, proteins, vitamins, minerals, and water. Carbohydrates, fats, and proteins are macronutrients and provide energy. Carbohydrates and fats are our main energy sources; proteins primarily support tissue growth, repair, and maintenance. Vitamins and minerals are micronutrients. Vitamins are organic compounds that assist in breaking down the macronutrients for energy and in many other functions. Minerals are inorganic units of matter essential to virtually all aspects of human health. Water is critical for regulating nerve impulses, body temperature, muscle contractions, nutrient transport, and the excretion of wastes.

How much of each nutrient do most people need?

Now that you know what the six classes of nutrients are, you're probably wondering how much of each you need each day. That depends on your gender, your age, your activity level, and many other factors. To get ready, you need to become familiar with the current standard intake recommendations that apply to most healthy people. (In Chapter 2, you'll learn how to plan a healthful diet that's just right for you.)

Use the Dietary Reference Intakes to Check Your Nutrient Intake

The United States and Canada share a set of standards defining the recommended intake values for various nutrients. These are called the **Dietary Reference Intakes (DRIs)** (FIGURE 1.9). The DRIs are dietary standards for healthy people only; they do not apply to people with diseases or to those who are suffering from nutrient deficiencies. For each nutrient (such as vitamin C or iron), the DRIs identify the amount needed to prevent deficiency diseases in healthy individuals as well as the amount that may reduce the risk for chronic diseases in healthy people. The DRIs also establish an upper level of safety for nutrient intake.

The DRIs for most nutrients consist of four values:

- Estimated Average Requirement (EAR)
- Recommended Dietary Allowance (RDA)
- Adequate Intake (AI)
- Tolerable Upper Intake Level (UL)

The standards for energy and the contribution of the macronutrients to total energy include the Estimated Energy Requirement (EER) and the Acceptable Macronutrient Distribution Range (AMDR). The definitions for each of these DRI values are presented in the following section.

The Estimated Average Requirement Guides the Recommended Dietary Allowance

The first step in determining our nutrient requirements is to calculate the EAR (see Figure 1.9). The **Estimated Average Requirement (EAR)** represents the average daily intake level estimated to meet the requirement of half the healthy individuals in a particular life stage and gender group.[3] As an example, the EAR for iron for women between the ages of 19 and 30 years represents the average daily intake of iron that meets the requirement of half the women in this age group. Scientists use the EAR to define the Recommended Dietary Allowance (RDA) for a given nutrient. Obviously, if the EAR meets the needs of only half the people in a group, then the recommended intake will be higher.

The Recommended Dietary Allowance Meets the Needs of Nearly All Healthy People

Recommended Dietary Allowance (RDA) was the term previously used to refer to *all* nutrient recommendations in the United States. The RDA is now considered one of many reference standards within the larger umbrella of the DRIs. The RDA represents

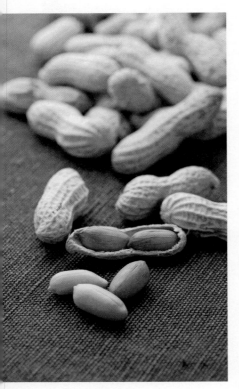

▲ Peanuts are a good source of the minerals magnesium and phosphorus, which play important roles in the formation and maintenance of our skeleton.

Dietary Reference Intakes (DRIs) A set of nutritional reference values for the United States and Canada that applies to healthy people.

Estimated Average Requirement (EAR) The average daily nutrient intake level estimated to meet the requirement of half the healthy individuals in a particular life stage or gender group.

Recommended Dietary Allowance (RDA) The average daily nutrient intake level that meets the nutrient requirements of 97–98% of healthy individuals in a particular life stage and gender group.

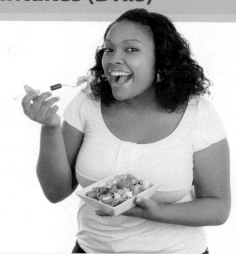

Dietary Reference Intakes (DRIs) are specific reference values for each nutrient issued by the United States National Academy of Sciences, Institute of Medicine. They identify the amounts of each nutrient that one needs to consume to maintain good health.

DRIs FOR MOST NUTRIENTS

EAR The Estimated Average Requirement (EAR) is the average daily intake level estimated to meet the needs of half the people in a certain group. Scientists use it to calculate the RDA.

RDA The Recommended Dietary Allowance (RDA) is the average daily intake level estimated to meet the needs of nearly all people in a certain group. Aim for this amount!

AI The Adequate Intake (AI) is the average daily intake level assumed to be adequate. It is used when an EAR cannot be determined. Aim for this amount if there is no RDA!

UL The Tolerable Upper Intake Level (UL) is the highest average daily intake level likely to pose no health risks. Do not exceed this amount on a daily basis!

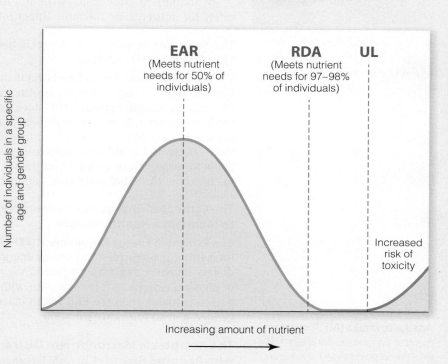

DRIs RELATED TO ENERGY

AMDR The Acceptable Macronutrient Distribution Range (AMDR) is the recommended range of carbohydrate, fat, and protein intake expressed as a percentage of total energy.

EER The Estimated Energy Requirement (EER) is the average daily energy intake predicted to meet the needs of healthy adults.

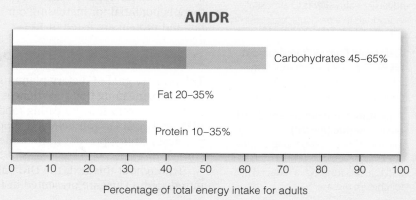

15

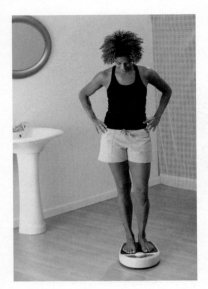

← Knowing your daily Estimated Energy Requirement (EER) is a helpful way to maintain an optimal body weight.

the average daily nutrient intake level that meets the requirements of 97–98% of healthy individuals in a particular life stage and gender group.[3] The graph in Figure 1.9 compares the RDA to the EAR. For example, the RDA for iron is 18 mg per day for women between the ages of 19 and 50 years. This amount of iron will meet the nutrient requirements of almost all women in this age group.

Again, scientists use the EAR to establish the RDA. In fact, if an EAR cannot be determined for a nutrient, then this nutrient cannot have an RDA. When this occurs, an Adequate Intake value is determined for the nutrient.

The Adequate Intake Is Based on Estimates of Nutrient Intakes

The **Adequate Intake (AI)** value is a recommended average daily nutrient intake level assumed to be adequate. It is based on observations or experiments involving healthy people, and it is used when an RDA cannot be determined.[3] Many nutrients have an AI value, including vitamin K, chromium, fluoride, and certain types of fats. More research needs to be done on human requirements for the nutrients assigned an AI value so that an EAR, and subsequently an RDA, can be established.

In addition to establishing RDA and AI values for nutrients, an upper level of safety for nutrients, or Tolerable Upper Intake Level, has also been defined.

The Tolerable Upper Intake Level Is the Highest Level That Poses No Health Risk

The **Tolerable Upper Intake Level (UL)** is the highest average daily nutrient intake level likely to pose no risk of adverse health effects to almost all individuals in a particular life stage and gender group.[3] This does not mean that we should consume this intake level or that we will receive more benefits from a nutrient by meeting or exceeding the UL. In fact, as our intake of a nutrient increases beyond the UL, the potential for toxic effects and health risks increases (see Figure 1.9). The UL value is a helpful guide to assist you in determining the highest average intake level that is deemed safe to consume. Note that there is not enough research to define the UL for all nutrients.

The Estimated Energy Requirement Is the Intake Predicted to Maintain a Healthy Weight

The **Estimated Energy Requirement (EER)** is defined as the average dietary energy intake that is predicted to maintain energy balance in a healthy individual. This dietary intake is defined by a person's level of age, gender, weight, height, and level of physical activity that is consistent with good health.[4] Thus, the EER for an active person is higher than the EER for an inactive person, even if all the other factors (age, gender, and so forth) are the same.

The Acceptable Macronutrient Distribution Range Is Associated with Reduced Risk for Chronic Diseases

The **Acceptable Macronutrient Distribution Range (AMDR)** is a range of intakes for a particular energy source that is associated with a reduced risk for chronic disease but provides adequate intakes of essential nutrients.[4] The AMDR is expressed as a percentage of total energy or as a percentage of total kilocalories. The AMDR also has a lower and an upper boundary; if we consume nutrients below or above this range, there is potential for increasing our risk for poor health. The AMDRs for carbohydrate, fat, and protein are listed in **TABLE 1.4**.

Diets Based on the DRIs Promote Wellness

The primary goal of dietary planning is to develop an eating plan that is nutritionally adequate, meaning that the chances of consuming too little or too much of any nutrient are very low. By eating foods that give you nutrient intakes that meet the RDA or AI values, you help your body maintain a healthful weight, support your daily physical activity, prevent nutrient deficiencies and toxicities, and reduce your risk for chronic disease.

Throughout this text, the DRI values are reviewed with each nutrient as it is introduced. (They are presented in full in Appendix A at the back of this text.) Find

Adequate Intake (AI) A recommended average daily nutrient intake level based on observed or experimentally determined estimates of nutrient intake by a group of healthy people.

Tolerable Upper Intake Level (UL) The highest average daily nutrient intake level likely to pose no risk of adverse health effects to almost all individuals in a particular life stage and gender group.

Estimated Energy Requirement (EER) The average dietary energy intake that is predicted to maintain energy balance in a healthy adult.

Acceptable Macronutrient Distribution Range (AMDR) The range of macronutrient intakes that provides adequate levels of essential nutrients and is associated with a reduced risk for chronic disease.

TABLE 1.4 **Acceptable Macronutrient Distribution Ranges (AMDRs) for Healthful Diets**

Nutrient	AMDR*
Carbohydrate	45–65%
Fat	20–35%
Protein	10–35%

*AMDR values are expressed as percentages of total energy or as percentage of total Calories.
Data from: *Dietary Reference Intakes for Energy Carbohydrates, Fiber, Fat, Fatty Acids, Cholesterol, Protein, and Amino Acids (Macronutrients).* National Academies Press. Reprinted by permission.

your life stage group and gender in the left-hand column; then simply look across to see each nutrient's value for you.) Using the DRI values in conjunction with diet-planning tools, such as the Dietary Guidelines for Americans or the USDA Food Guide, will ensure that you have a healthful and adequate diet. (Chapter 2 provides details on how you can use these tools to develop a healthful diet.)

recap The Dietary Reference Intakes (DRIs) are nutrient standards established for healthy people in a particular life stage and gender group. Whereas the Estimated Average Requirement (EAR) meets the requirements of half the healthy individuals in a group, the Recommended Dietary Allowance (RDA) meets the requirements of 97–98% of healthy individuals in a group. The Adequate Intake (AI) is an intake level assumed to be adequate. It is used when there is not enough information to set an RDA. The Tolerable Upper Intake Level (UL) is the highest daily nutrient intake level that likely poses no health risk. The Estimated Energy Requirement (EER) is the average daily energy intake that is predicted to maintain energy balance in a healthy adult. The Acceptable Macronutrient Distribution Range (AMDR) is a range of macronutrient intakes expressed as a percentage of total energy.

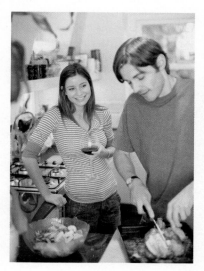

Eating foods that provide the recommended nutrients helps promote optimal wellness.

How can you interpret the results of research studies?

"Eat more carbohydrates! Fats cause obesity!"
"Eat more protein and fat! Carbohydrates cause obesity!"

Do you ever feel overwhelmed by the abundant and often conflicting advice in media reports related to nutrition? If so, you are not alone. How can you navigate this sea of changing information? What constitutes valid, reliable evidence, and how can you determine whether research findings apply to you?

To become a more informed critic of product claims and nutrition news, you need to understand the research process and how to interpret the results of different types of studies. Let's now learn more about research.

Research Involves Applying the Scientific Method

When confronted with a claim about any aspect of our world, from "The Earth is flat" to "Carbohydrates cause obesity," scientists must first consider whether the claim can be tested. In other words, can evidence be presented to substantiate the claim and, if so, what data would qualify as evidence? Scientists worldwide use a standardized method of looking at evidence called the *scientific method*. This method ensures that certain standards and processes are used in evaluating claims. The scientific method usually includes the following steps, which are described in more detail next and summarized in (**FIGURE 1.10**, page 18):

1. The researcher first makes an *observation* and a description of a phenomenon.
2. The researcher proposes a *hypothesis*, or an educated guess, to explain why the phenomenon occurs.

◗ FIGURE 1.10 The scientific method, which forms the framework for scientific research. The researcher makes an observation regarding a phenomenon. This leads the researcher to ask a question. A hypothesis is generated to explain the observations. The researcher conducts an experiment to test the hypothesis. Observations are made during the experiment, and data are generated and documented. The data may either support or refute the hypothesis. If the data support the hypothesis, more experiments are conducted to test and confirm support for the hypothesis. A hypothesis that is supported after repeated testing may be called a theory. If the data do not support the hypothesis, the hypothesis is either rejected or modified and then retested.

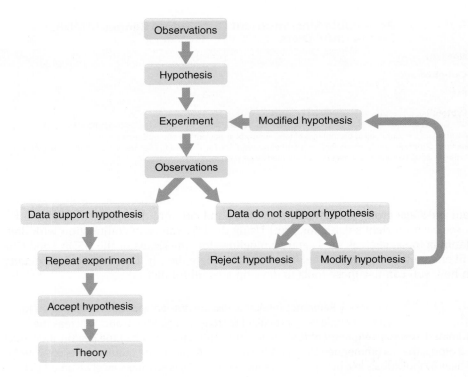

3. The researcher then develops an *experimental design* that will test the hypothesis.
4. The researcher *collects and analyzes data* that will either support or reject the hypothesis.
5. If the data do not support the original hypothesis, then an *alternative hypothesis* is proposed and tested.
6. If the data support the original hypothesis, then a *conclusion* is drawn.
7. The experiment must be *repeatable* so that other researchers can obtain similar results.
8. Finally, a *theory* is proposed offering a conclusion drawn from repeated experiments that have supported the hypothesis time and time again.

Observation of a Phenomenon Initiates the Research Process

The first step in the scientific method is to observe and describe a phenomenon. As an example, let's say you are working in a healthcare office that caters to mostly older clients. You have observed that many of these clients have high blood pressure, but some have normal blood pressure. After talking with a large number of clients, you notice a pattern developing in that those who report being more physically active are also those with lower blood pressure readings. This observation leads you to question a possible relationship that might exist between physical activity and blood pressure. Your next step is to develop a **hypothesis**, a possible explanation for your observation.

A Hypothesis Is a Possible Explanation for an Observation

A hypothesis is also sometimes referred to as a *research question*. In this example, your hypothesis might be "Adults over age 65 with high blood pressure who begin and maintain a program of 45 minutes of aerobic exercise daily will experience a decrease in blood pressure." A hypothesis must be stated so that it can be either supported or rejected. In other words, it must be testable.

An Experiment Is Designed to Test the Hypothesis

An *experiment* is a scientific study that is conducted to test a hypothesis. A well-designed experiment should have several key elements:

- The *sample size*—the number of people being studied—should be adequate to ensure that the results obtained are not due to chance alone. Would you be more likely to believe a study that tested 5 people or 500?

hypothesis An educated guess as to why a phenomenon occurs.

- Having a *control group* is essential for comparing treated to untreated individuals. A control group consists of people who are as much like the treated group as possible, except with respect to the *variable* being tested. For instance, in your study, 45 minutes of daily aerobic exercise would be the variable; the experimental group would consist of people over age 65 with high blood pressure who exercise, and the control group would consist of similar people who do not exercise. Using a control group helps a researcher judge whether a particular treatment has worked or not.

- A good experimental design also attempts to control for other variables that may coincidentally influence the results. For example, what if someone in your study is on a diet, smokes, or takes blood pressure–lowering medication? Because any of these factors can affect the results, researchers try to design experiments that have as many constants as possible. In doing so, they increase the chance that their results will be *valid*. To use an old saying, you can think of validity as "comparing apples to apples."

Data Are Collected and Analyzed to Determine Whether They Support or Reject the Hypothesis

As part of the design of the experiment, the researcher must determine the type of data to collect and how to collect them. For example, in your study the data being collected are blood pressure readings. These values could be collected by people or a machine, but because the data will be closely scrutinized by other scientists, they should be as accurate as technology allows. In this case, an automatic blood pressure gauge would provide more reliable and consistent data than blood pressure measurements taken by research assistants.

Once the data have been collected, they must be analyzed and subsequently interpreted. Often, the data will begin to make sense only after they have been organized and put into different forms, such as tables or graphs, to reveal patterns that at first were not obvious. In your study, you can create a graph comparing blood pressure readings from both your experimental group and your control group to see if there was a significant difference between the blood pressure readings of those who exercised and those who did not.

Most Hypotheses Need to Be Refined

Remember that a hypothesis is basically a guess as to what causes a particular phenomenon. Rarely do scientists get it right the first time. The original hypothesis is often refined after the initial results are obtained, usually because the answer to the question is not clear and leads to more questions. When this happens, an alternative hypothesis is proposed, a new experiment is designed, and the new hypothesis is tested.

An Experiment Must Be Repeatable

One research study does not prove or disprove a hypothesis. Ideally, multiple experiments are conducted over many years to thoroughly test a hypothesis. Indeed, repeatability is a cornerstone of scientific investigation. Supporters and skeptics alike must be able to replicate an experiment and arrive at similar conclusions, or the hypothesis becomes invalid. Have you ever wondered why the measurements used in scientific textbooks are always in the metric system? The answer is repeatability. Scientists use the metric system because it is a universal system and thus allows repeatability in any research facility worldwide.

Unfortunately, media reports on the findings of a research study that has just been published rarely include a thorough review of the other studies conducted on that topic. Thus, you should never accept one report in a newspaper, magazine, or online source as absolute fact on any topic.

A Theory May Be Developed Following Extensive Research

If the results of multiple experiments consistently support a hypothesis, then scientists may advance a **theory**. A theory represents a scientific consensus (agreement) as to why a particular phenomenon occurs. Although theories are based on data drawn from repeated experiments, they can still be challenged and changed as the

theory A conclusion, or scientific consensus, drawn from repeated experiments.

knowledge within a scientific discipline evolves. For example, at the beginning of this chapter, we said that the prevailing theory held that pellagra was an infectious disease. Experiments were conducted over several decades before their consistent results finally confirmed that the disease is due to niacin deficiency. We continue to apply the scientific method to test hypotheses and challenge theories today.

recap The steps in the scientific method are 1) observing a phenomenon, 2) creating a hypothesis, 3) designing and conducting an experiment, and 4) collecting and analyzing data that support or refute the hypothesis. If the data are rejected, then an alternative hypothesis is proposed and tested. If the data support the original hypothesis, then a conclusion is drawn. A hypothesis that is supported after repeated experiments may be called a theory.

Various Types of Research Studies Tell Us Different Stories

Understanding the role of nutrition in health requires constant experimentation. Depending on how the research study is designed, we can gather information that tells us different stories. Let's take a look at the various types of research.

Animal Versus Human Studies

In many cases, studies involving animals provide preliminary information that assists scientists in designing human studies. Animal studies also are used to conduct research that cannot be done with humans. For instance, researchers can cause a nutrient deficiency in an animal and study its adverse health effects over the animal's life span, but this type of experiment with humans is not acceptable. Drawbacks of animal studies include ethical concerns and the fact that the results may not apply directly to humans.

Over the past century, animal studies have advanced our understanding of many aspects of nutrition, from micronutrients to obesity. Still, some hypotheses can only be investigated using human subjects. The three primary types of studies conducted with humans are observational studies, case control studies, and clinical trials.

Observational Studies

observational studies Studies that indicate relationships between nutrition habits, disease trends, and other health phenomena of large populations of humans.

case control studies Complex observational studies with additional design features that allow us to gain a better understanding of factors that may influence disease.

Observational studies are used in assessing nutritional habits, disease trends, and other health phenomena of large populations and determining the factors that may influence these phenomena. However, these studies can only indicate *relationships* between factors; they do not prove or suggest that the data are linked by cause and effect. For example, smoking and low vegetable intake appear to be related in some studies, but this does not mean that smoking cigarettes causes people to eat fewer vegetables or that eating fewer vegetables causes people to smoke.

Case Control Studies

Case control studies are more complex observational studies with additional design features that allow scientists to gain a better understanding of things that may influence disease. They involve comparing a group of individuals with a particular condition (for instance, 1,000 elderly people with high blood pressure) to a similar group without this condition (for instance, 1,000 elderly people with normal blood pressure). This comparison allows the researcher to identify factors other than the defined condition that differ between the two groups. For example, researchers may find that 75% of the people in their normal blood pressure group are physically active but that only 20% of the people in their high blood pressure group are physically active. Again, this would not prove that physical activity prevents

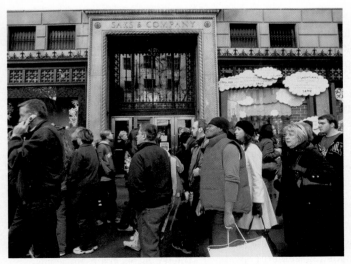

◆ Observational studies are used in assessing the habits, trends, and other phenomena in large populations of people.

high blood pressure. It would merely suggest a significant relationship between these two factors.

Clinical Trials

Clinical trials are tightly controlled experiments in which an intervention is given to determine its effect on a certain disease or health condition. Interventions include medications, nutritional supplements, controlled diets, and exercise programs. In clinical trials, people in the experimental group are given the intervention, but people in the control group are not. The responses of the two groups are compared. In the case of the blood pressure experiment, researchers could assign one group of elderly people with high blood pressure to an exercise program and assign a second group of elderly people with high blood pressure to a program where no exercise is done. Over the next few weeks, months, or even years, researchers could measure the blood pressure of the people in each group. If the blood pressure of those who exercised decreased and the blood pressure of those who did not exercise rose or remained the same, the influence of exercise on lowering blood pressure would be supported.

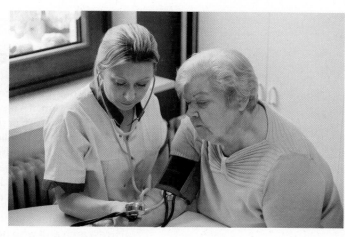

▲ In a clinical trial, an intervention is given to determine its effect on a health condition or disease.

Two important questions to consider when evaluating the quality of a clinical trial are whether the subjects were randomly chosen and whether the researchers and subjects were blinded:

- **Randomized trials.** Ideally, researchers should *randomly* assign research participants to intervention groups (who get the treatment) and control groups (who do not get the treatment). Randomizing participants is like flipping a coin or drawing names from a hat; it reduces the possibility of showing favoritism toward any participants and ensures that the groups are similar on the factors or characteristics being measured in the study. These types of studies are called *randomized clinical (controlled) trials*.

- **Single- and double-blind experiments.** If possible, it is also important to *blind* both researchers and participants to the treatment being given. A *single-blind experiment* is one in which the participants are unaware of or *blinded* to the treatment they are receiving, but the researchers know which group is getting the treatment and which group is not. A *double-blind experiment* is one in which neither researchers nor participants know which group is really getting the treatment. Double blinding helps prevent the researcher from seeing only the results he or she wants to see, even if these results do not actually occur. In the case of testing medications or nutrition supplements, the blinding process can be assisted by giving the control group a placebo. A **placebo** is an imitation treatment that has no effect on participants; for instance, a sugar pill may be given in place of a vitamin supplement. Studies like this are referred to as *placebo-controlled double-blind randomized clinical trials*.

There has been substantial interest in the "placebo effect." This refers to an improvement in health—for instance, pain reduction—in people given a placebo treatment. Although the placebo effect does not occur for all people or across the full range of human diseases, it is an intriguing phenomenon that suggests that personal beliefs, attitudes, expectations, and emotions can influence the body's responses.

Use Your Knowledge of Research to Help You Evaluate Nutrition Claims

Now that you've increased your understanding of scientific research, you're better equipped to discern the truth or fallacy of nutrition-related claims. Keep the nearby **Quick Tips** in mind when evaluating the findings of research studies and the claims made on commercial websites.

clinical trials Tightly controlled experiments in which an intervention is given to determine its effect on a certain disease or health condition.

placebo An imitation treatment having no active ingredient that is sometimes used in a clinical trial.

QuickTips

Detecting Media Hype

Consider the source of the information. If a report is written or reported by a person or group who may financially benefit from selling the products, you should be skeptical. Also, many people who write for popular magazines and newspapers are not trained in science and are capable of misinterpreting research results.

Find out who conducted the research and who paid for it. Was the study funded by a company or entity that stands to profit from certain results? Do the researchers have investments in such a company, or are they receiving money or perks from the research sponsor? If the answer to any of these questions is yes, there exists a conflict of interest between the researchers and the funding agency.

Evaluate the content. Is the report based on reputable research studies? Did the research follow the scientific method, and were the results reported in a reputable scientific journal? Ideally, the journal is peer-reviewed; that is, are the articles critiqued by other specialists working in the same scientific field? A reputable report should include the reference, or source of the information, and should identify researchers by name.

Watch for red flags. Is the report based on testimonials about personal experiences? Testimonials are fraught with bias. Are sweeping conclusions made from only one study? Remember that one study cannot prove any hypothesis. Are the claims made in the report too good to be true? If something sounds too good to be true, it probably is.

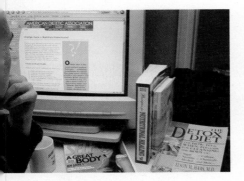

▲ To become a more educated consumer and informed critic of nutrition reports in the media, you need to understand the research process and how to interpret study results.

Beware of Conflict of Interest

You probably wouldn't think it strange to see an ad from your favorite brand of ice cream encouraging you to "Go ahead. Indulge." It's just an ad, right? But what if you were to read about a research study in which people who ate your favorite brand of ice cream improved the density of their bones? Could you trust the study results more than you would the ad?

To answer that question, you'd have to ask several more, such as who conducted the research and who paid for it. Specifically:

- Was the study funded by a company that stands to profit from certain results?
- Are the researchers receiving a stipend (payment), goods, personal travel funds, or other perks from the research sponsor, or do they have investments in companies or products related to their study?

If the answer to either of these questions was yes, a *conflict of interest* would exist between the researchers and the funding agency. This could seriously compromise the researchers' ability to conduct unbiased research. A *bias* is any factor—such as investment in the product being studied or gifts from the product manufacturer—that might influence the researcher to favor certain results.

Recent media investigations have reported widespread bias in studies funded by pharmaceutical companies testing the effectiveness of their drugs for medical treatment. These studies are more likely to report positive results than are studies that were independently financed.[5,6] Overall, reputable research journals have been found less likely to publish negative results (that is, study results suggesting that a therapy is not effective). This has serious implications: if ineffectiveness and side effects are not fully reported, healthcare providers may be prescribing medications that are ineffective or even harmful. The seriousness of this issue has inspired researchers around the world to demand reforms such as making all research results available to the public.

Determine a Website's Reliability

The Internet provides almost limitless access to a wide variety of health and nutrition information. But how can you determine if the advice given on a website is reliable? Here are some tips to assist you in separating Internet fact from fiction:

HOT TOPIC

Do You Respond to Spam?

If you have an e-mail account, you're probably familiar with spam ads that promise weight-loss miracles for "only $19.99!" Do you delete them unread? A study from Brooklyn College of the City University of New York found that, in the course of 1 year, 42% of students with weight problems had opened spam e-mails touting weight-loss products, and almost 19% had placed an order! Lead researchers were shocked by the findings and advised physicians to discuss with patients the potential risks of using weight-loss products marketed via spam e-mails.[7]

- Look at the credentials of the people sponsoring and providing information for the website. Is the individual, group, or company responsible for the website considered a qualified professional in the area of emphasis? Are the names and credentials of those contributing to the website available? Are experts reviewing the content of the website for accuracy and currency?
- Look at the date of the website. Is it fairly recent? Because nutrition and medical information are constantly changing, websites should be updated frequently, and the date of the most recent update should be clearly identified on the site.
- Look at the three letters following the "dot" in an Internet (www or "world wide web") address. Government addresses (ending in ".gov"), academic institutions (ending in ".edu"), and professional organizations (ending in ".org") are considered to be generally reliable sources of information. However, lecture notes, PowerPoint slides, and student assignments that can be found on university websites may not be reliable. Addresses ending in ".com" designate commercial and business sites; some may be reliable, but many are not. Check the qualifications of those contributing to the site to see if their primary motivation is to get you to buy a product or service.

As you may know, **quackery** is the promotion of an unproven remedy, usually by someone unlicensed and untrained, for financial gain. Throughout this text we provide information to assist you in recognizing quackery in its many guises. You'll learn about food labeling guidelines, explore both sides of nutrition debates, and find out whether various nutrition topics are myths or facts. Armed with the information in this book, plus plenty of opportunities to test your knowledge, you will become more confident and knowledgable when evaluating nutrition claims.

> To learn more about how to spot quackery, go to www.quackwatch.com, enter "spot quack" in the search box, and then click on "Critiquing Quack Ads."

recap Studies involving animals provide preliminary information that assists scientists in designing human studies. Human studies include observational studies, case control studies, and clinical trials. Each type of study can be used to gather a different kind of data. When evaluating research studies, consider whether a conflict of interest exists, and check the credentials, date, and address of websites. Quackery is the promotion of an unproven remedy, usually by someone unlicensed and untrained, for financial gain.

nutri-case | LIZ

"Am I ever sorry I caught the news last night right before going to bed! They reported on this study that just came out, saying that ballet dancers are at some super-high risk for fractures! I couldn't sleep, thinking about it, and then today in dance class every move I made was freaking me out about breaking my ankle. I can't go on being afraid like this!"

What information should Liz find out about the fracture study to evaluate its merits? Identify *at least two factors* she should evaluate. Let's say that her investigation of these factors leads her to conclude that the study is trustworthy: what else should she keep in mind about the research process that might help her take a more balanced perspective when thinking about this single study?

quackery The promotion of an unproven remedy, such as a supplement or other product or service, usually by someone unlicensed and untrained.

Whom can you trust to help you choose foods wisely?

Miguel, the young man from our opening story, was a victim of quackery. He probably would not have purchased that iron supplement if he had understood that the woman claiming to be a "nutritionist" was not qualified to diagnose or treat his condition. If you are wondering how to determine whether an "expert" is trustworthy, the following discussion should help.

Trustworthy Experts Are Educated and Credentialed

It is not possible to list here all of the types of health professionals who provide reliable and accurate nutrition information. The following is a list of the most common groups:

- **Registered dietitian (RD).** To become a registered dietitian requires, minimally, a bachelor's degree, completion of a supervised clinical experience, a passing grade on a national examination, and maintenance of registration with the Academy of Nutrition and Dietetics (formerly the American Dietetic Association). There is now an optional change to the RD designation—*RD/Nutritionist*. This designation indicates that anyone who has earned an RD is also a qualitified nutritionist, but not all nutritionists are qualified dietitians (see below). Individuals who complete the education, experience, exam, and registration are qualified to provide nutrition counseling in a variety of settings. For a reliable list of RDs in your community, contact the Academy of Nutrition and Dietetics (see Web Resources).

- **Licensed dietitian.** A licensed dietitian is a dietitian meeting the credentialing requirement of a given state in the United States to engage in the practice of dietetics.[8] Each state has its own laws regulating dietitians. These laws specify which types of licensure or registration a nutrition professional must obtain in order to provide nutrition services or advice. Individuals who practice nutrition and dietetics without the required license or registration can be prosecuted for breaking the law.

- **Nutritionist.** This term generally has no definition or laws regulating it. In some cases, it refers to a professional with academic credentials in nutrition who may also be an RD.[8] In other cases, the term may refer to anyone who thinks he or she is knowledgeable about nutrition. There is no guarantee that a person calling himself or herself a nutritionist is necessarily educated, trained, and experienced in the field of nutrition. It is important to research the credentials and experience of any individual calling himself or herself a nutritionist. In the chapter-opening scenario, how might Miguel have determined whether or not the "nutritionist" was qualified to give him advice?

- **Professional with an advanced degree (a master's degree [MA or MS] or doctoral degree [PhD]) in nutrition.** Many individuals hold an advanced degree in nutrition and have years of experience in a nutrition-related career. For instance, they may teach at colleges or universities or work in fitness or healthcare settings. Unless these individuals are licensed or registered dietitians, they are not certified to provide clinical dietary counseling or treatment for individuals with disease. However, they are reliable sources of information about nutrition and health.

- **Physician.** The term *physician* encompasses a variety of healthcare professionals. A medical doctor (MD) is educated, trained, and licensed to practice medicine in the United States. However, MDs typically have very limited experience and training in the area of nutrition. Medical students in the United States are not required to take any nutrition courses throughout their academic training, although some may take courses out of personal interest. On the other hand, a number of individuals who started their careers in nutrition go on to become medical doctors and thus have a solid background in nutrition. Nevertheless, if you require a dietary plan to treat an illness or a disease, most medical doctors will refer you to an RD. In contrast, an osteopathic physician, referred to as a doctor of osteopathy (DO), may have studied nutrition extensively, as may a naturopathic physician, a homeopathic physician, or a chiropractor. Thus, it is prudent to determine a physician's level of expertise rather than assuming that he or she has extensive knowledge of nutrition.

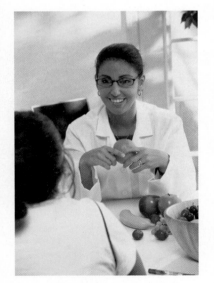

Your medical doctor may have limited experience and training in the area of nutrition but can refer you to a registered dietitian (RD) or licensed nutritionist to assist you in meeting your dietary needs.

Government Agencies Are Usually Trustworthy

Many government health agencies have come together to address the growing problem of nutrition-related disease in the United States. These agencies are funded with taxpayer dollars, and many provide financial support for research in the areas of nutrition and health. Thus, these agencies have the resources to organize and disseminate the most recent and reliable information related to nutrition and other areas of health and wellness. A few of the most recognized and respected of these government agencies are discussed here.

The Centers for Disease Control and Prevention Protects the Health and Safety of Americans

The **Centers for Disease Control and Prevention (CDC)** is considered the leading federal agency in the United States that protects human health and safety. Located in Atlanta, Georgia, the CDC works in the areas of health promotion, disease prevention and control, and environmental health. The CDC's mission is to promote health and quality of life by preventing and controlling disease, injury, and disability. Among its many activities, the CDC supports two large national surveys that provide important nutrition and health information.

The National Health and Nutrition Examination Survey (NHANES) is conducted by the National Center for Health Statistics and the CDC. The NHANES tracks the food and nutrient consumption of Americans. Nutrition and other health information is gathered from interviews and physical examinations. The database for the NHANES survey is extremely large, and an abundance of research papers have been generated from it. To learn more about the NHANES, see Web Resources at the end of this chapter.

The Behavioral Risk Factor Surveillance System (BRFSS) was established by the CDC to track lifestyle behaviors that increase our risk for chronic disease. The world's largest telephone survey, the BRFSS gathers data at the state level at regular intervals. Although the BRFSS includes questions related to injuries and infectious diseases, it places a particularly strong focus on the health behaviors that increase our risk for the nation's leading killers: heart disease, stroke, cancer, and diabetes. These health behaviors include:

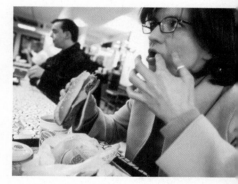

Lifestyle behaviors, such as eating an unhealthful diet, can increase your risk for chronic disease.

- Not consuming enough fruits and vegetables
- Being overweight
- Using tobacco and abusing alcohol
- Not getting medical care that is known to save lives, such as regular flu shots and screening exams

These behaviors are of particular interest because it is estimated that 50–60% of deaths in the United States can be attributed to smoking, alcohol misuse, lack of physical activity, and an unhealthful diet.[9]

The National Institutes of Health Is the Leading Medical Research Agency in the World

The **National Institutes of Health (NIH)** is the world's leading medical research center, and it is the focal point for medical research in the United States. The NIH is one of the agencies of the Public Health Service, which is part of the U.S. Department of Health and Human Services. The mission of the NIH is to uncover new knowledge that leads to better health for everyone. This mission is accomplished by supporting medical research throughout the world and by fostering the communication of this information. Many institutes within the NIH conduct research into nutrition-related health issues. Some of these institutes are:

- National Cancer Institute (NCI)
- National Heart, Lung, and Blood Institute (NHLBI)
- National Institute of Diabetes and Digestive and Kidney Diseases (NIDDK)
- National Center for Complementary and Alternative Medicine (NCCAM)

To find out more about the NIH, see Web Resources at the end of this chapter.

Centers for Disease Control and Prevention (CDC) The leading federal agency in the United States that protects the health and safety of people. Its mission is to promote health and quality of life by preventing and controlling disease, injury, and disability.

National Institutes of Health (NIH) The world's leading medical research center and the focal point for medical research in the United States.

Professional Organizations Provide Reliable Nutrition Information

A number of professional organizations represent nutrition professionals, scientists, and educators. These organizations publish cutting-edge nutrition research studies and educational information in journals that are accessible in most university and medical libraries. Some of these organizations are:

- **The Academy of Nutrition and Dietetics.** This is the largest organization of food and nutrition professionals in the world. Their mission is to promote nutrition, health, and well-being. (The Canadian equivalent is Dietitians of Canada.) The Academy of Nutrition and Dietetics publishes a professional journal called the *Journal of the Academy of Nutrition and Dietetics* (formerly the *Journal of the American Dietetic Association*).
- **The American Society for Nutrition (ASN).** The ASN is the premier research society dedicated to improving quality of life through the science of nutrition. The ASN fulfills its mission by fostering, enhancing, and disseminating nutrition-related research and professional education activities. The ASN publishes a professional journal called the *American Journal of Clinical Nutrition.*
- **The American College of Sports Medicine (ACSM).** The ACSM is the leading sports medicine and exercise science organization in the world. The mission of the ACSM is to advance and integrate scientific research to provide educational and practical applications of exercise science and sports medicine. Many members are nutrition professionals who combine their nutrition and exercise expertise to promote health and athletic performance. *Medicine and Science in Sports and Exercise* is the professional journal of the ACSM.
- **The North American Association for the Study of Obesity (NAASO).** NAASO is the leading scientific society dedicated to the study of obesity. It is committed to encouraging research on the causes and treatments of obesity and to keeping the medical community and public informed of new advances. The official NAASO journal is *Obesity Research*, which is intended to increase knowledge, stimulate research, and promote better treatment of people with obesity.

For more information on these organizations, see Web Resources at the end of this chapter.

recap The Centers for Disease Control and Prevention (CDC) is the leading federal agency in the United States that protects human health and safety. The CDC supports two large national surveys that provide important nutrition and health information: the National Health and Nutrition Examination Survey (NHANES) and the Behavioral Risk Factor Surveillance System (BRFSS). The National Institutes of Health is the leading medical research agency in the world. The Academy for Nutrition and Dietetics, the American Society for Nutritional Sciences, the American College of Sports Medicine, and the North American Association for the Study of Obesity are examples of professional organizations that provide reliable nutrition information.

✳behavior change ... getting started!

Now that you've read this chapter, try making these changes:

For yourself:

- Identify the components of wellness that you could focus on more often to promote your health and well-being.
- Conduct your own investigation into a nutritional product or food that is being promoted by celebrity testimonials, and identify the weaknesses of the claims being made.

For your community:

- Create a "how-to" list focusing on steps to determine which media reports and information sources are trustworthy, and share this list with your family and friends.
- Try writing a blog for your school's website highlighting how to determine if a nutrition-related website is reliable.

Are There Such Things as Good Foods and Bad Foods?

We are bombarded every day with messages regarding what we should and shouldn't eat. Terms such as *junk foods, super foods,* and *good* and *bad* foods dominate the news. At the same time, our food environments promote cheap and easy access to the "bad" foods we're warned to avoid—such as pizza, chips, doughnuts, french fries, and sugared soft drinks—while keeping "good" foods like fresh fruits and vegetables more expensive and less accessible.

Several questions are raised by the high-fat, high-sugar, low-cost, fast-food environment in which we live. First, can all foods fit into a healthful diet, or are there certain "bad" foods that we really should avoid entirely? Many dietitians and professional groups share the philosophy that all foods can fit into a healthful diet.[10] Although it is a fact that some foods are indeed more healthful than others, even "junk" foods can provide energy and some nutrients. As we'll discuss throughout this book, simple changes can often transform a "bad" food into a nutritious choice. For example, pizza made with a whole-grain crust, tomato sauce, fresh vegetables, and a moderate amount of low-fat cheese is a healthful lunch. And even high-sugar or high-fat versions of foods—such as sausage pizza—can fit into a healthful diet as long as they're just an occasional treat and portion control is exercised.

A second key question is, what type of food recommendations should nutrition professionals make? Should they advise people to avoid specific foods?

On one side of this question, nutrition professionals argue that consumers have a right to know which foods protect against disease and which increase their risk for disease. Some of them support U.S. Food and Drug Administration regulations requiring restaurants (including fast-food outlets) to publish the nutrient composition of their meals alongside the price in their menu. Some within this group also argue that unhealthful foods should be taxed in the same way that we tax alcohol and cigarettes, as a way to reduce purchases of these foods and promote better health.[11]

On the other side of the debate are the politics of food and food preferences. Every nutrition professional recognizes that, even among consumers who know it does not promote their health, low-cost fast food sells extremely

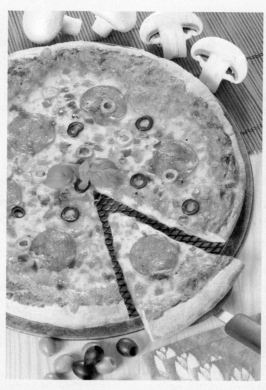

Can all foods fit into a healthful diet, or should some foods be avoided entirely?

well.[11] McDonald's alone enjoys annual global sales of over $34 billion, an average of $2.5 million per store.[12] Thus, many nutrition professionals attempt to work with clients' food preferences, and time and budget constraints, to develop an overall more healthful approach to eating. Thus, they look at a client's total diet and dietary patterns, including portion sizes, and not at individual foods. They also advise against assigning moral qualitities to foods, and believe their responsibility is to communicate positive nutrition messages that inspire people to make food choices that promote health.

Nutrition professionals on this side of the debate also point out that telling people to stop eating their favorite foods doesn't change their behavior. Instead, a significant percentage of people advised to make dramatic dietary changes get discouraged and give up. They also point to studies showing that, in restaurants that post Calorie and nutrient data for their meals, patrons' choices don't change.[13] Therefore, they believe it's more effective to encourage clients to make small steps toward changing their eating patterns, such as by choosing less healthful foods less often and in smaller portions.

Research conducted in controlled environments, in which nutrition messages are reinforced by increased availability of low-cost, appealing, and healthful foods, may indeed help people to improve their diet. But the real world is not a laboratory, and we have limited control over the food environments outside of our home. More research is needed to determine what strategies might really help people choose more healthful foods more often.

CRITICAL THINKING QUESTIONS

1. Do you frequently eat foods that you think of as "bad" or "junk" foods? On the other hand, are there foods that you avoid completely? Why or why not?
2. Should nutrition professionals warn people against "bad" foods? Why or why not?
3. Some cities in the United States have proposed imposing a tax on soda and other "junk" foods. What are the pros and cons of this proposition?

chapter **review**

test yourself | answers

1. **False.** A Calorie is a measure of the energy in a food. More precisely, a kilocalorie is the amount of heat required to raise the temperature of 1 kilogram of water by 1 degree Celsius.

2. **True.** Carbohydrates and fats are the primary energy sources for our body.

3. **False.** The Recommended Dietary Allowance is the *average daily intake* of a vitamin or other food component that meets the requirements of 97–98% of healthy individuals in a particular group.

MasteringNutrition™

Check out these additional resources in the MasteringNutrition Study Area at www.masteringhealthandnutrition.com (or www.pearsonmastering.com):

- Read It: Chapter Summary and RSS Feeds
- See It: ABC News videos and nutrition animations
- Hear It: MP3s
- Study It: Get Ready for Nutrition Math and Chemistry review
- Do It: NutriTools and "Find the Quack" feature
- Review It: Quizzes, flashcards, and glossary

review questions

1. Early nutrition research focused on
   a. improving crop yields.
   b. classifying plants as edible or inedible.
   c. identifying and preventing diseases caused by dietary deficiencies.
   d. uncovering links between genes, environment, and diet.

2. Which of the following statements is true?
   a. Pellagra is caused by a nutrient deficiency.
   b. Osteoporosis is caused by a nutrient deficiency.
   c. Scurvy is caused by a nutrient toxicity.
   d. Osteoporosis is caused by a nutrient toxicity.

3. Vitamins A and C, thiamin, calcium, and magnesium are considered
   a. water-soluble vitamins.
   b. fat-soluble vitamins.
   c. energy-yielding nutrients.
   d. micronutrients.

4. For good health, you should aim to consume
   a. the EAR for vitamin C.
   b. the RDA for vitamin C.
   c. the UL for vitamin C.
   d. within the AMDR for vitamin C.

5. Which of the following statements about hypotheses is true?
   a. Hypotheses can be proven by clinical trials.
   b. "Many inactive people have high blood pressure" is an example of a hypothesis.
   c. If the results of multiple experiments consistently support a hypothesis, it is confirmed as fact.
   d. "A high-protein diet increases the risk for porous bones" is an example of a hypothesis.

6. The world's leading medical research center is the
   a. Centers for Disease Control and Prevention.
   b. National Institutes of Health.
   c. American Medical Association.
   d. National Health and Nutrition Examination Survey.

7. **True or false?** Nutrition significantly affects a person's risk for heart disease.

8. **True or false?** Carbohydrates, fats, and proteins all contain carbon, hydrogen, and oxygen.

9. **True or false?** The Adequate Intake represents the average daily intake level known to meet the requirements of almost all healthy individuals in a group.

10. **True or false?** Nutrition-related reports in the *American Journal of Clinical Nutrition* are usually trustworthy.

math review

11. Kayla meets with a registered dietitian recommended by her doctor to design a weight-loss diet plan. She is shocked when a dietary analysis reveals that she consumes an average of 2,200 kcal and 60 grams of fat each day. What percentage of Kayla's diet comes from fat, and is this percentage within the AMDR for fat?

Answers to Review Questions and Math Review are located at the back of this text and in the MasteringNutrition Study Area.

web resources

www.eatright.org
The Academy of Nutrition and Dietetics (formerly the American Dietetic Association)

Obtain a list of registered dietitians in your community from the largest organization of food and nutrition professionals in the United States.

www.cdc.gov
Centers for Disease Control and Prevention

Visit this site for additional information about the leading federal agency in the United States that protects the health and safety of people.

www.cdc.gov/nchs
National Center for Health Statistics

Visit this site to learn more about the National Health and Nutrition Examination Survey (NHANES) and other national health surveys.

www.nih.gov
National Institutes of Health

Find out more about the National Institutes of Health, an agency under the U.S. Department of Health and Human Services.

www.ncbi.nlm.nih.gov
PubMed Central

Search for PubMed at the National Library of Medicine for summaries of research studies on health topics of your choice.

www.nutrition.org
American Society for Nutrition

Learn more about the American Society for Nutrition and its goal to improve quality of life through the science of nutrition.

www.acsm.org
American College of Sports Medicine

Obtain information about the leading sports medicine and exercise science organization in the world.

www.naaso.org
The North American Association for the Study of Obesity

Learn about this interdisciplinary society and its work to develop, extend, and disseminate knowledge in the field of obesity.

www.iom.edu
Institute of Medicine of the National Academies

Learn about the Institute of Medicine's history of examining the nation's nutritional well-being and providing sound information about food and nutrition. Enter "global topics food nutrition" into the search box for more details.

in depth 1.5

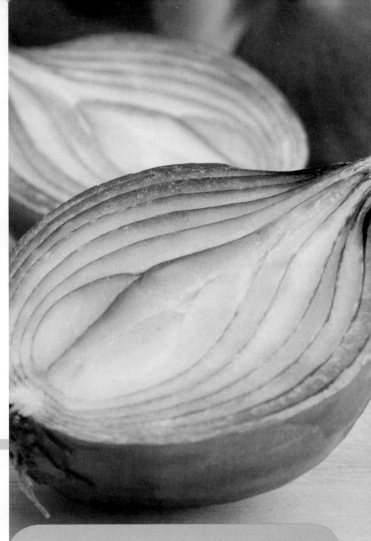

New Frontiers in Nutrition and Health

Imagine a patient visiting his physician for his annual exam. He is 20 pounds overweight and his blood pressure is elevated. The physician takes a blood sample for genetic testing, then sends the patient to a technician to extract a sample of the microbes living in his colon. At the close of the visit, she hands her patient a prescription: *2 servings of fresh fruits, 2 servings of fresh vegetables, a bowl of oatmeal, a cup of soy milk, and 2 cups of yogurt daily*. The patient accepts the prescription gratefully, assuring his physician as he says goodbye, "I'll stop at the market on my way home!"

Sound unreal? As researchers uncover more evidence of a link between our genes, microbes, functional foods, and health, it's possible that scenarios like this could become familiar. Here, we explore these new frontiers **In Depth**. Who knows? When you finish reading, you might find yourself writing up your own health-promoting grocery list!

learning objectives

After studying this In Depth, you should be able to:

1 Discuss the potential benefits and challenges of nutrigenomics, pp. 31–32.

2 Explain how research into the human microbiome is influencing our understanding of nutrition and health, pp. 32–33.

3 Identify some of the health benefits of three types of non-nutrient components of functional foods, pp. 33–37.

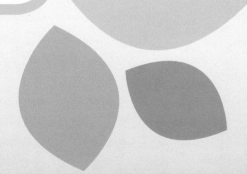

Developing the potential of nutrigenomics

Agouti mice are bred for scientific studies. These mice are normally yellow in color, obese, and prone to cancer and diabetes. When agouti mice breed, these traits are passed on to their offspring. Look at the picture of the agouti mice on this page; do you see a difference? The mouse on the right is obviously brown and of normal weight, but what you can't see is that it did not inherit its parents' susceptibility to disease. What caused this dramatic difference between parent and offspring? The answer is diet!

In 2003, researchers at Duke University reported that when they changed the mother's diet just before conception, they could "turn off" the agouti gene, and any offspring born to that mother would appear normal.[1] As you might know, a *gene* is a segment of DNA, the substance responsible for inheritance, or the passing on of traits from parents to offspring, in both animals and humans. An organism's *genome* is its complete set of DNA, which is found packed into the nucleus of its body cells. Genes are precise regions of DNA that encode instructions for making specific proteins. The agouti gene, for example, encodes the assembly of the pigment proteins that produce yellow fur. (Genes and proteins are covered in more detail in Chapter 6.)

The Duke University researchers fed a female agouti mouse a diet that was high in a compound thought to affect the agouti gene. Sure enough, this dietary compound attached to the gene and, in essence, turned it off. When the mother conceived, her offspring still carried the agouti gene on their DNA, but their cells no longer used the gene to make proteins. So the traits such as yellow fur and obesity that were linked to the agouti gene did not appear in the offspring. These studies were some of the first to directly link a change in diet to a genetic modification, and they led to the emerging science of *nutrigenomics*.

What Is Nutrigenomics?

Nutrigenomics is a scientific discipline studying the interactions between genes, the environment, and nutrition.[2] Scientists have known for some time that diet and environmental factors can contribute to disease, but what has not been understood before is *how*—namely, by altering how cells use genes. A key theory behind nutrigenomics is that foods and environmental factors can act like a "switch" in body cells, turning on some genes while turning off others. When a gene is activated, it will instruct the cell to assemble a protein that will show up as a physical characteristic or functional ability, such as a protein that facilitates the storage of fat. When a gene is switched off, the cell will not create that protein, and the organism's form or function will differ. Some of the factors thought most likely to affect gene activation include tobacco, alcohol, environmental toxins, radiation, exercise, and the foods most common to an individual's diet.

In addition, nutrigenomics scientists are discovering that what we expose our genes to can affect our future children. In the Duke University study, switching off the agouti gene caused beneficial changes in the offspring mice. But

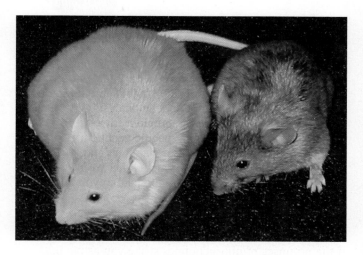

Prompted only by a change in her diet before she conceived, an inbred agouti mouse (left) gave birth to a young mouse (right) that differed not only in appearance but also in its susceptibility to disease.

sometimes flipping the switch can be harmful, as when a man's exposure to radiation causes changes in his sperm cells that increase the likelihood of birth defects in his children.

As you can see, nutrigenomics is an intriguing theory—but beyond the agouti study, what evidence supports it?

Evidence for Nutrigenomics

Several observations over many decades certainly suggest that the theory has merit. For example, it has long been noted that people following the same diet and exercise program will lose very different amounts of weight or will even gain weight. The varying results may reflect how the foods in the diet affect the study participants' genes. Scientists also point to evidence from population studies of the relationship between genes and risk for cardiovascular disease. Moderate alcohol intake reduces the risk for cardiovascular disease in people with a particular set of genes, but it doesn't benefit people who don't have these genes.[2] Similarly, when different ethnic groups are exposed to a high-fat Western diet, the percentage of cardiovascular disease increases in some populations significantly more than in others.[2]

Evidence of nutrigenomics influencing future generations includes the breakthrough study of agouti mice, as well as recent research suggesting that when mothers experience a food surplus during critical periods of fetal development, their offspring are more likely to develop type 2 diabetes.

Promises of Nutrigenomics

One promise of nutrigenomics is that it can help people improve their health by reducing their risk of developing diet-related diseases and possibly even by treating existing conditions through diet alone. For example, some research

---

nutrigenomics A scientific discipline studying the interactions between genes, the environment, and nutrition.

is now studying how chemical components of vegetables and certain spices may regulate important genes that suppress cancer.[3]

Another promise of nutrigenomics is personalized nutrition. In the future, your healthcare provider might send a sample of your tissue for genetic analysis. The results would guide the provider in creating a diet tailored to your specific genetic makeup. By identifying both foods to eat and foods to avoid, this personalized diet would help you to turn on genes that could be beneficial to you and turn off genes that could be harmful.

Challenges of Nutrigenomics

If the promises of nutrigenomics strike you as pie in the sky, you're not alone. Many researchers caution, for example, that dietary "prescriptions" to prevent or treat chronic diseases are unrealistic for several reasons. First, the **human genome** contains about 25,000 genes, and we don't yet know the function of many thousands of them.[4] Second, interpretation of measurements of thousands of genes, with millions of genetic variations, some of which have effects on hundreds or thousands of the chemicals involved in metabolism, will require new approaches in biology and statistics that are almost unimaginably complex.[4] Third, other factors such as age, gender, and lifestyle also affect how different foods interact with different genetic pathways. In short, in order to develop a fundamental knowledge base for this young discipline, the number of variables that will have to be considered is staggering.[4]

This means that nutrigenomics is—for now—more dream than reality. But that hasn't stopped companies from offering naïve consumers nutrigenomics products and services. A scientific review of online genomic profiling found little evidence that it is useful in measuring genetic risk for common diseases or in developing personalized recommendations for disease prevention.[5] One study of online sales of nutrigenomics services called such services premature.[6]

How Might Nutrigenomics Contribute to Healthcare?

For the reasons just noted, decades may pass before nutrigenomics is able to contribute to human health. Consumers might first encounter nutrigenomics in diagnostic testing. In this process, a tissue sample of DNA will be genetically analyzed to determine how foods interact with that individual's genes and how a change in diet might affect those interactions. It's also likely that consumers will begin to see more specialized foods promoted for specific conditions, and food packages of the future might even be coded for certain genetic profiles. Before these ideas can become a reality, however, scientists will have to untangle yet another web of interactions affecting our nutrition and health: the role of the human microbiome.

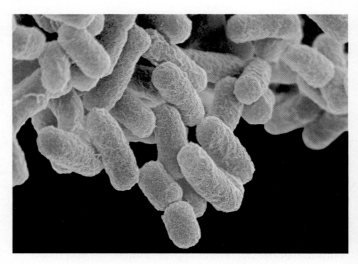

The human body is a microbial ecosystem containing about 100 trillion microscopic organisms, such as this gut bacteria.

Exploring the human microbiome

We like to think of ourselves as discrete, individual organisms, but it's not true. We're actually "super-organisms." The human body is a lush microbial ecosystem containing about 100 trillion *microorganisms* (microscopic organisms such as bacteria), whose collective genome, the **human microbiome**, contains 100-fold more genes than the entire human genome.[7] These microorganisms and their genes interact with our human cells and genes in a dizzying number of ways that affect our health. Although microorganisms live on our skin, in our urinary tract, and elsewhere in our body, here we'll focus on the *GI flora*; that is, the helpful bacteria in our gastrointestinal (GI) tract. Our GI tract includes the stomach, intestines, and other organs that enable us to digest food, absorb nutrients, and eliminate wastes.

Researchers have identified many ways in which the GI flora benefit human health. For example, genes carried by these bacteria enable humans to digest foods and absorb nutrients that otherwise would be unavailable to us.[8] It seems likely that genes in our GI flora complement the functions of human genes required for biological pathways involved in digestion—genes that may be missing or incompletely encoded in the human genome.[9] Moreover, GI flora directly[10,11]:

- Manufacture chemicals (called enzymes) that help us digest our food and absorb nutrients from food
- Supply key nutrients used to replace worn-out components of the GI tract

human genome The complete set of genes making up the DNA in the nucleus of a human cell.

human microbiome The complete set of genes belonging to the trillions of microorganisms that inhabit the human body.

- Produce certain essential vitamins
- Degrade potential carcinogens (cancer-causing agents) in foods

Furthermore, studies suggest that species among the GI flora may protect us against or predispose us to obesity, by either increasing or decreasing our "harvesting" of energy from the foods we eat, and our tendency to build up deposits of fat.[7] Many (but not all) studies suggest a link between depletion of the GI flora and the development of obesity as well as type 2 diabetes.[9,11,12] The GI flora also produce chemicals that oppose the inflammatory response, thereby protecting us against disorders characterized by inflammation, such as infectious diarrhea, certain GI cancers, esophagitis and gastritis (inflammation of the esophagus and stomach, respectively), inflammatory bowel disorders, eczema, and asthma and allergies.

Given this research, you're probably wondering how you can maintain a large and healthy population of microorganisms in your GI tract. That's where probiotics and prebiotics, two types of functional foods, come in.

Identifying the benefits of functional foods

Public health agencies define **functional foods** as components of the usual diet that may have biologically active ingredients with the potential to provide health benefits beyond basic nutrition.[13] Also called *nutraceuticals*, functional foods include **whole foods**, such as nuts, oats, and blueberries, as well as **processed foods**, including fortified, enriched, or enhanced foods. Examples of processed functional foods include orange juice with added calcium and vitamin D, or bread enriched with folate. Sometimes, the health-promoting substances are developed in a functional food by altering the way in which the food is produced. For example, eggs with higher levels of omega-3 fatty acids (fats that help protect against heart disease) result from feeding hens a special diet. And fruits and vegetables can be genetically engineered to contain higher levels of nutrients. As you can appreciate, the range of functional foods is vast. Here, we discuss three types that are often in the news.

Probiotics and Prebiotics: Growing Your Microbiome

The last time you ate a cup of creamy, fruity yogurt, did you think about the fact that you were also eating *bacteria*? Don't worry—these microorganisms are part of the human microbiome. Yogurt is one of a group of substances called **probiotics**: foods or food supplements containing microorganisms that beneficially affect consumers by improving the intestinal microbial balance.[13]

Interest in probiotics was sparked in the early 1900s with the work of Elie Metchnikoff, a Nobel Prize-winning scientist. Dr. Metchnikoff linked the long, healthy lives of Bulgarian peasants with their consumption of fermented

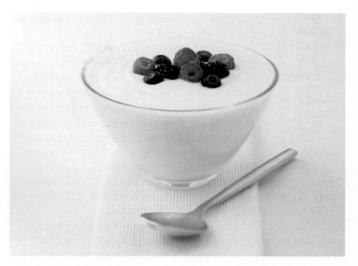

Beneficial bacteria, such as those found in yogurt or kefir, are a part of probiotic foods.

milk products, such as yogurt. Subsequent research identified the bacteria in fermented milk products as the factor that promoted health. These bacteria were characterized as *probiotic*, meaning "pro-life."

In the United States, probiotics include fortified milk, yogurt, and a creamy beverage called *kefir*, which is made from fermented milk. Probiotics are also sold in supplement form. The bacterial species most frequently used in these foods and supplements are *Lactobacillus* and *Bifidobacterium*.

When a person consumes probiotics, the bacteria adhere to the intestinal wall for a few days. There, they are thought to exert the beneficial actions identified with the GI flora. For example, results from several randomized controlled clinical trials show the benefits of probiotics in the treatment of a variety of GI diseases, and some lab studies have shown that probiotics can help reduce the inflammatory response.[9]

It is important to remember that, in order to be effective, a minimum number of bacteria must be present in probiotic foods or supplements. Commerical yogurts meeting the National Yogurt Association Standards contain 100 million live and active cultures per gram. So a 1-cup serving (8 oz, or 227 grams) of yogurt contains more than

functional foods Components of a typical diet which may have biologically active ingredients that provide health benefits beyond basic nutrition.

whole foods Foods that have been modified as little as possible, remaining in or near their natural state.

processed foods Foods that have been manipulated in some way to transform raw ingredients into products for consumption.

probiotics Foods or food supplements containing microorganisms that beneficially affect consumers by improving the intestinal microbial balance.

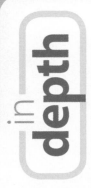

in depth

22 billion bacteria. This is considered more than the estimated effective dose.

Bacteria live only for a short time. This means that probiotic foods and supplements should be consumed on a daily basis to be most effective. They must also be properly stored and consumed within a relatively brief period to confer maximal benefit. In general, refrigerated foods containing probiotics have a shelf life of 3 to 6 weeks, whereas refrigerated supplements keep about 12 months. However, because the probiotic content of foods is much more stable than that of supplements, yogurt and other probiotic foods may be a better health bet.

Now that you know a little more about probiotics, you may be wondering how they're related to prebiotics. We've said that probiotics contain living and helpful bacteria that boost the population count in your GI tract. In contrast, **prebiotics** are nondigestible food ingredients (typically carbohydrates) that benefit the consumer by stimulating the growth and/or activity of these helpful bacteria.[13] By doing so, they improve digestion and metabolism, help regulate the inflammatory response, and in general complement the action of probiotics.

An example is inulin, a carbohydrate found in a few fruits, onions and certain green vegetables, and some grains. Like other prebiotics, inulin travels through the GI tract without being digested or absorbed until it reaches the colon, where it nourishes colonies of helpful resident bacteria. In other words, prebiotics don't feed you, but they do feed your microbiome.

In addition to whole prebiotic foods, many processed foods claim to be prebiotics. For example, inulin is added to certain brands of yogurt, milk, and cottage cheese, some fruit juices, cookies, and fiber bars and supplements. Watch out, though, that your desire to feed your flora doesn't cause you to overindulge. Cookies, sweet granola bars, and other products touted as prebiotics may have just as many Calories and just as much fat as regular versions of the same foods.

Phytochemicals: Another Advantage of Plants

As noted, whole-food prebiotics are plants. In addition, plant foods are loaded with nutrients, including carbohydrates, vitamins, minerals, and water. They're also a great source of dietary fiber. But another advantage of plants is their phytochemicals. *Phyto* means "plant," so **phytochemicals** are literally plant chemicals. While plants are growing, these naturally occurring compounds are believed to protect them from pests, the UV radiation they capture, and the oxygen they produce. What makes them important to nutrition scientists is that phytochemicals are believed to have health-promoting properties for humans who consume them.

To date, more than 10,000 different phytochemicals have been identified.[14] They're present in whole grains, fruits, vegetables, coffee, tea, wine, beer, herbs, and spices. Any one food can contain hundreds. **FIGURE 1** identifies a few of the most common phytochemical groups.

Like probiotics and prebiotics, phytochemicals are not classified as nutrients—that is, substances necessary for sustaining life. Yet eating an abundance of phytochemical-rich foods has been shown to reduce the risk for a number of diseases as well as age-related functional decline.[14] For example, phytochemicals are thought to:

- Reduce inflammation, which is linked to the development of cardiovascular disease, cancer, and Alzheimer's disease and is symptomatic of allergies and arthritis.[14,15]
- Impede the initiation and progression of cancer by enhancing the activity of chemicals that detoxify carcinogens, slowing tumor cell growth, inhibiting communication among cancer cells, and instructing cancer cells to self-destruct.[14,16]
- Combat infections by enhancing our immune function, reducing bacterial resistance to antibiotics, and acting as antibacterial and antiviral agents.[17]
- Protect against cardiovascular disease by modulating blood lipids and reducing platelet aggregation, blood clotting, and blockage of blood vessels.[18]
- Inhibit lipid synthesis and increase lipid metabolism, thereby potentially acting as an "antiobesity" agent.[19,20]

nutri-case | HANNAH

"On my way home from school today, I was really hungry, and when I passed a convenience store about halfway home, I just had to go in. I looked around for something healthy, like a banana or an apple, but they didn't have anything fresh. So I bought some pretzels. I know pretzels aren't exactly a health food, but at least they're low fat, right?"

Hannah and her mother live in an urban neighborhood that has eleven different fast-food outlets and four convenience stores but lacks a grocery store. There is no local farmer's market or community garden. In order to buy fresh produce, they have to travel to a more affluent neighborhood several miles away. Given the importance of phytochemicals to a healthful diet, can you think of at least two strategies Hannah and her mother could use to increase their access to affordable produce?

prebiotics Nondigestible food ingredients that beneficially affect the consumer by selectively stimulating the growth and/or activity of one or a limited number of bacteria in the colon.

phytochemicals Compounds found in plants believed to have health-promoting effects in humans.

34

Phytochemical	Health Claims	Food Source	
Carotenoids: alpha-carotene, beta-carotene, lutein, lycopene, zeaxanthin, etc.	Diets with foods rich in these phytochemicals may reduce the risk for cardiovascular disease, certain cancers (e.g., prostate), and age-related eye diseases (cataracts, macular degeneration).	Red, orange, and deep-green vegetables and fruits, such as carrots, cantaloupe, sweet potatoes, apricots, kale, spinach, pumpkin, and tomatoes	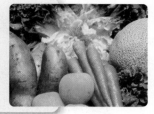
Flavonoids:[1] flavones, flavonols (e.g., quercetin), catechins (e.g., epigallocatechin gallate or EGCG), anthocyanidins, isoflavonoids, etc.	Diets with foods rich in these phytochemicals are associated with lower risk for cardiovascular disease and cancer, possibly because of reduced inflammation, blood clotting, and blood pressure and increased detoxification of carcinogens or reduction in replication of cancerous cells.	Berries, black and green tea, chocolate, purple grapes and juice, citrus fruits, olives, soybeans and soy products (soy milk, tofu, soy flour, textured vegetable protein), flaxseed, whole wheat	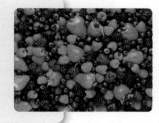
Phenolic acids:[1] ellagic acid, ferulic acid, caffeic acid, curcumin, etc.	Similar benefits as flavonoids.	Coffee beans, fruits (apples, pears, berries, grapes, oranges, prunes, strawberries), potatoes, mustard, oats, soy	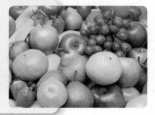
Phytoestrogens:[2] genistein, diadzein, lignans	Foods rich in these phytochemicals may provide benefits to bones and reduce the risk for cardiovascular disease and cancers of reproductive tissues (e.g., breast, prostate).	Soybeans and soy products (soy milk, tofu, soy flour, textured vegetable protein), flaxseed, whole grains	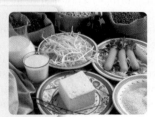
Organosulfur compounds: allylic sulfur compounds, indoles, isothiocyanates, etc.	Foods rich in these phytochemicals may protect against a wide variety of cancers.	Garlic, leeks, onions, chives, cruciferous vegetables (broccoli, cabbage, cauliflower), horseradish, mustard greens	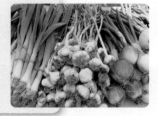

[1] Flavonoids, phenolic acids, and stilbenes are three groups of phytochemicals called phenolics. The phytochemical Resveratrol is a stilbene. Flavonoids and phenolic acids are the most abundant phenolics in our diet.
[2] Phytoestrogens include phytochemicals that have mild or anti-estrogenic action in our body. They are grouped together based on this similarity in biological function, but they also can be classified into other phytochemical groups, such as isoflavonoids.

FIGURE 1 Health claims and food sources of phytochemicals.

In addition, research over the past decade has shown that certain phytochemicals can increase the effectiveness of certain medications. When administered in concentrated doses, these phytochemicals work synergistically to enhance or prolong the effectiveness of the medications. Most such research is still in the stage of clinical trials, but this synergistic effect has been shown in the treatment of bacterial infections that have developed resistance to traditional antibiotics as well as with chemotherapy drugs in the treatment of cancer.[14,17,21]

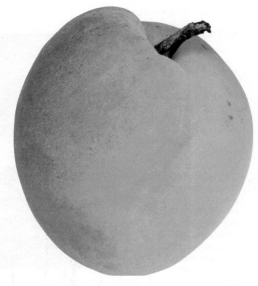

Apricots contain carotenoids, a type of phytochemical.

Although you might assume that the more phytochemicals you consume the better, that's somewhat simplistic. They appear to be beneficial in the low doses commonly provided by foods, but they may be ineffective or even harmful when consumed as supplements. This may be due to their mode of action: instead of *protecting* our cells, phytochemicals might benefit our health by *stressing* our cells, causing them to rev up their internal defense systems. Cells are very well equipped to deal with minor stresses, but not with excessive stress, which may explain why clinical trials with phytochemical supplements may not show the same benefits as high intakes of plant foods.[22]

So are phytochemical supplements harmful? Generally speaking, taking high doses of anything is risky. A basic principle of toxicology is that any compound can

HOT TOPIC

Will a PB&J Keep the Doctor Away?

Whole-grain bread, natural peanut butter, and grape jelly: how could a food that tastes so good be good for the body, too? We've known for decades about the fiber, micronutrients, and healthful fats a PB&J provides. But recently, research has revealed that the comforting PB&J is a good source of resveratrol, a phytochemical being studied in labs worldwide. Research has linked resveratrol to protective effects against cancer, heart disease, obesity, viral infections, and neurologic diseases like Alzheimer's.

A flavonoid, resveratrol is found in the skins of dark grapes, in dark grape juice, in most red wines, and in dark berries such as blueberries and cranberries. But fruits are not the only source: resveratrol also happens to be plentiful in peanuts, including peanut butter. Still, no one knows what an effective "dose" of resveratrol looks like, nor whether the amounts in a PB&J qualify. We also don't yet know whether high doses, such as those found in supplements, could be harmful.

If you decide to add resveratrol to your diet, we hope you'll bypass supplements in favor of the humble PB&J. Although the jury is still out on the benefits of its resveratrol content, it makes a highly nutritious meal or snack, doesn't need refrigeration, is inexpensive, and tastes great.

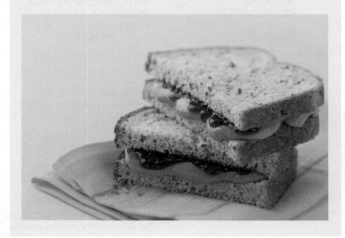

be toxic if the dose is high enough. Dietary supplements are no exception. For example, a classic study found that supplementing with 20 to 30 mg/day of beta-carotene for 4 to 6 years *increased* lung cancer risk by 16% to 28% in smokers.[23,24] Based on these and other results, experts recommend against beta-carotene supplementation.[25] In short, whereas there is ample evidence to support the health benefits of a plant-based diet, phytochemical supplements should be avoided.

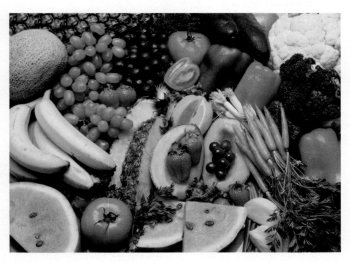

Avoid phytochemical supplements in favor of whole foods.

So what's the take-home message from all this new research into nutrition and health? Eat sensibly—for your genes, your microbiome, and your health. Consume a plant-based diet consisting of as many whole foods as possible. Prebiotic-rich whole foods include wheat and oats, tofu and soy milk, garlic, onions, leeks, and several dark green vegetables. Probiotics aren't plant foods, of course, but they, too, should be part of your daily diet. If you find yogurt too sour or watery, try the Greek kind, which is more creamy. Or pour yourself a glass of kefir, which tastes like a yogurt smoothie. Both are rich in probiotics. In short, a probiotic-rich plant-based diet may be just the prescription you need for better health.

MasteringNutrition™

Check out these additional resources in the MasteringNutrition Study Area:

- Read It: Chapter Summary and RSS Feeds
- See It: ABC News videos and nutrition animations
- Hear It: MP3s
- Study It: Get Ready for Nutrition Math and Chemistry review
- Do It: NutriTools and "Find the Quack" feature
- Review It: Quizzes, flashcards, and glossary

web resources

www.commonfund.nih.gov
The Human Microbiome Project

Click on "HMP" in the search box to find out more about the microbes that live within you—and help you live!

www.isapp.net
International Scientific Association for Probiotics and Prebiotics

Click on links from the home page to find consumer guides to probiotic and prebiotic foods.

www.aicr.org
American Institute for Cancer Research

Search for "phytochemicals" to learn about the AICR's stance and recommendations on the role of these substances in cancer prevention.

http://lpi.oregonstate.edu
Linus Pauling Institute

This extensive website covers phytochemicals as well as nutrients and other cutting-edge health and nutrition topics.

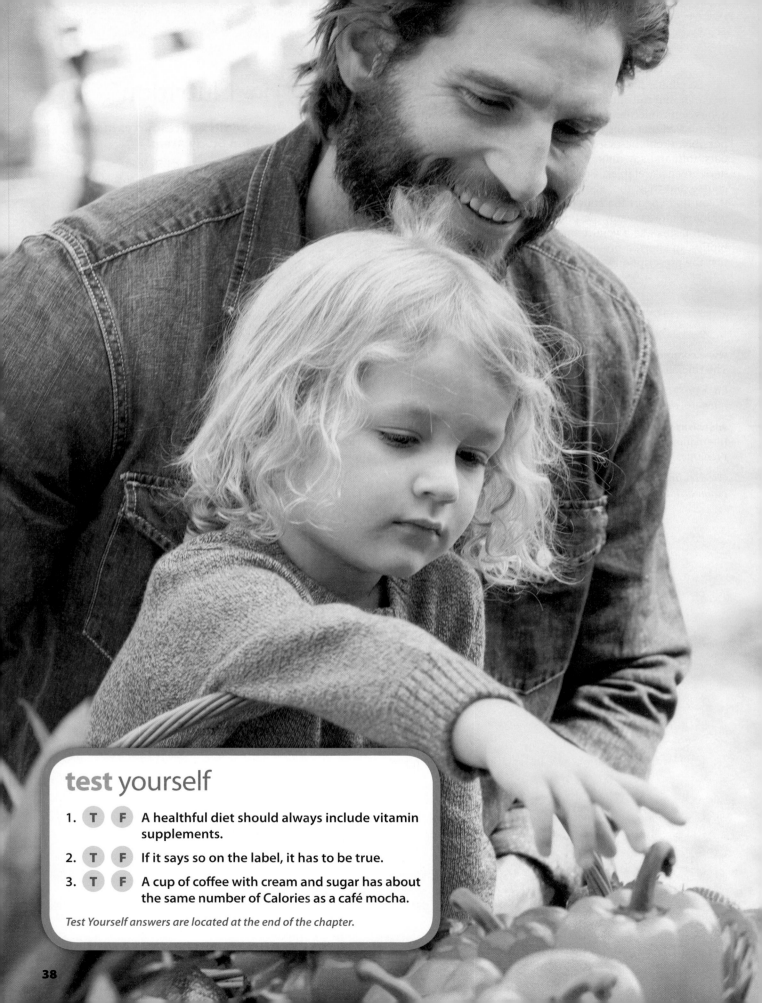

test yourself

1. **T** **F** A healthful diet should always include vitamin supplements.

2. **T** **F** If it says so on the label, it has to be true.

3. **T** **F** A cup of coffee with cream and sugar has about the same number of Calories as a café mocha.

Test Yourself answers are located at the end of the chapter.

Designing a Healthful Diet

2

learning objectives

After studying this chapter you should be able to:

1 Identify the characteristics of a healthful diet, pp. 40–41.

2 Name five components that must be included on food labels and use the Nutrition Facts panel to determine the nutritional adequacy of a given food, pp. 42–43.

3 Describe the Dietary Guidelines for Americans and discuss how these Guidelines can be used to design a healthful diet, pp. 47–50.

4 Identify the food groups and recommended equivalent amounts included in MyPlate, pp. 51–53.

5 Discuss similarities and differences between serving sizes identified in the USDA Food Patterns, serving sizes on food labels, and portions you serve yourself, pp. 52–56.

6 Explain how MyPlate accommodates ethnic and other dietary preferences, pp. 55, 57.

7 List at least four ways to practice moderation and apply healthful dietary guidelines when eating out, pp. 58–61.

Sigrid and her parents moved to the United States from Scandinavia when she was 6 years old. Although she was delicate in comparison to her American peers, Sigrid was healthy and energetic, excelling in school and riding her new bike in her suburban neighborhood. By the time Sigrid entered high school, her weight had caught up to that of her American classmates. Now a college freshman, she has joined the almost 17% of U.S. teens who are overweight.[1] Sigrid explains, "Back home, our diet is largely fish and vegetables, and people do much more walking and get daily exercise. Desserts are only for special occasions. When we moved to America, I wanted to eat like all the other kids: hamburgers, french fries, sodas, and sweets. I gained a lot of weight on that diet, and now my doctor says my cholesterol level, my blood pressure, and my blood sugar level are all too high. I wish I could start eating like my relatives again, but they don't serve our traditional foods at the dorm cafeteria."

What influence does diet have on health? What exactly qualifies as a "poor diet," and what makes a diet healthful? Is it more important to watch our total Calories or what kinds of foods we choose? What do national guidelines advise, and do they apply to "real people" like you?

Many factors contribute to the confusion surrounding healthful eating. First, although we have made substantial discoveries in the area of nutrition during the past century, nutritional research is still considered to be in its infancy. Thus, new findings on the benefits of foods and nutrients are discovered almost daily. These new findings contribute to regular changes in how a healthful diet is defined. Second (as stated in Chapter 1), the popular media typically report the results of only selected studies, usually the most

Continued next page

Continued—recent. This practice does not give a complete picture of all the research conducted in any given area. Indeed, the results of a single study are often misleading. Third, there is no one right way to eat that is healthful and acceptable for everyone. We are individuals with unique needs, food preferences, and cultural influences. Thus, there are literally millions of different ways to design a healthful diet to fit individual needs.

Given all this potential confusion, it's a good thing there are nutritional tools to guide people in designing a personalized healthful diet. In this chapter, we introduce these tools, including food labels, the Dietary Guidelines for Americans, the U.S. Department of Agriculture Food Patterns (and its accompanying graphic, MyPlate), and others. Before exploring the question of how to design a healthful diet, however, it is important to understand what a healthful diet *is*.

What is a healthful diet?

A **healthful diet** provides the proper combination of energy and nutrients. It has four characteristics: it is adequate, moderate, balanced, and varied. No matter if you are young or old, overweight or underweight, healthy or ill, if you keep these characteristics in mind, you will be able to select foods that provide you with the optimal combination of nutrients and energy each day.

A Healthful Diet Is Adequate

An **adequate diet** provides enough of the energy, nutrients, and fiber to maintain a person's health. A diet may be inadequate in only one area, or many areas. For example, many people in the United States do not eat enough vegetables and therefore are not consuming enough of the fiber and micronutrients vegetables provide. However, their intake of protein, fat, and carbohydrate may be adequate. In fact, some people who eat too few vegetables are overweight or obese, which means that they are eating a diet that, although inadequate in one area, exceeds their energy needs. On the other hand, a generalized state of undernutrition can occur if an individual's diet contains an inadequate level of several nutrients for a long period.

A diet that is adequate for one person may not be adequate for another. For example, the energy needs of a small woman who is lightly active are approximately 1,700 to 2,000 kilocalories (kcal) each day, whereas a highly active male athlete may require more than 4,000 kcal each day to support his body's demands. These two individuals differ greatly in their activity level and in their quantity of body fat and muscle mass, which means they require very different levels of fat, carbohydrate, protein, and other nutrients to support their daily needs.

A Healthful Diet Is Moderate

Moderation is one of the keys to a healthful diet. **Moderation** refers to eating any foods in moderate amounts—not too much and not too little. If we eat too much or too little of certain foods, we cannot reach our health goals. For example, some people drink as much as 60 fluid ounces (three 20-oz bottles) of soft drinks on some days. Drinking this much contributes an extra 765 kcal of energy to a person's diet. In order to allow for these extra kcal and avoid weight gain, most people would need to reduce their food intake significantly. This could mean eliminating many healthful food choices. In contrast, people who drink mostly water or other beverages that contain little or no energy can consume more nourishing foods that will support their wellness.

A Healthful Diet Is Balanced

A **balanced diet** contains the combinations of foods that provide the proper proportions of nutrients. As you will learn in this course, the body needs many

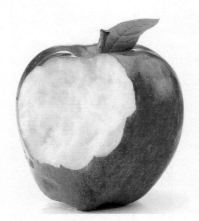
⬆ A healthful diet can help prevent disease.

healthful diet A diet that provides the proper combination of energy and nutrients and is adequate, moderate, balanced, and varied.

adequate diet A diet that provides enough of the energy, nutrients, and fiber needed to maintain a person's health.

moderation Eating any foods in moderate amounts—not too much and not too little.

balanced diet A diet that contains the combinations of foods that provide the proper proportions of nutrients.

types of foods in varying amounts to maintain health. For example, fruits and vegetables are excellent sources of fiber, vitamin C, potassium, and magnesium. Meats don't provide much of these, but they are excellent sources of protein, iron, zinc, and copper. By eating the proper balance of all healthful foods, including fruits, vegetables, and meats or meat substitutes, we can be confident that we're consuming the balanced nutrition we need to maintain health.

A Healthful Diet Is Varied

Variety refers to eating many different foods from the different food groups on a regular basis. With thousands of healthful foods to choose from, trying new foods is a fun and easy way to vary your diet. Eat a new vegetable each week or substitute one food for another, such as raw spinach on your turkey sandwich in place of iceberg lettuce. Selecting a variety of foods increases the likelihood that you will consume the multitude of nutrients your body needs. As an added benefit, eating a varied diet prevents boredom and helps you avoid getting into a "food rut." Later in this chapter, we'll provide suggestions for eating a varied diet.

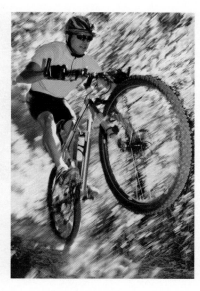

A diet that is adequate for one person may not be adequate for another. A woman who is lightly active may require fewer kilocalories of energy per day than a highly active male.

recap A healthful diet provides adequate nutrients and energy, and it includes sweets, fats, and salty foods in moderate amounts only. A healthful diet includes an appropriate balance of nutrients and a wide variety of foods.

What tools can help you design a healthful diet?

Many people feel it's not possible for them to eat a healthful diet. They may mistakenly believe that the foods they would need to eat are too expensive or not available to them, or that they're too busy to do the necessary planning, shopping, and cooking. But is it really that difficult to eat healthfully?

Although designing and maintaining a healthful diet is not as simple as eating whatever you want, most of us can do it with a little practice and a little help. Let's look at some tools to get you started.

Food Labels

To design and maintain a healthful diet, it's important to read and understand food labels. It may surprise you to learn that prior to the 1970s, there were no federal regulations for including nutrition information on food labels. The U.S. Food and Drug Administration (FDA) first established such regulations in 1973. Throughout the 1970s and 1980s, consumer interest in food quality grew substantially, leading the U.S. Congress to pass the Nutrition Labeling and Education Act in 1990. This act specifies which foods require a food label, provides detailed descriptions of the information that must be included on the label, and describes the companies and food products that are exempt from publishing complete nutrition information on food labels. For example, detailed food labels are not required for meat or poultry because these products are regulated by the U.S. Department of Agriculture, not the FDA. In addition, foods such as coffee and most spices are not required to follow the FDA labeling guidelines because they contain insignificant amounts of all nutrients that must be listed in nutrition labeling.

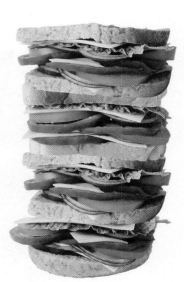

The serving size on a nutrition label may not be the same as the amount you eat.

variety Eating many different foods, from different food groups, regularly.

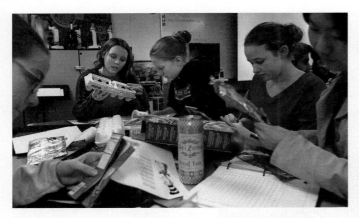

In this text you will learn how to read food labels, a skill that can help you meet your nutritional goals.

The FDA is reported to be considering changes to the current format and content of food labels.[2] Some of the potential changes being considered include more accurate serving size information, a greater emphasis on Calories, and less emphasis on nutrients such as fat, carbohydrate, and sodium. These changes have yet to be formally announced by the FDA. The information provided next reflects the components and information currently included on food labels.

Five Components Must Be Included on Food Labels

The FDA requires that the following five types of information be included on food labels (**FIGURE 2.1**):

1. **A statement of identity.** The common name of the product or an appropriate identification of the food product must be prominently displayed on the label. This information tells us very clearly what the product is.
2. **The net contents of the package.** The quantity of the food product in the entire package must be accurately described. Information may be listed as weight (such as "grams"), volume (such as "fluid ounces"), or numerical count (such as "4 each").
3. **Ingredient list.** The ingredients must be listed by their common names, in descending order by weight. This means that the first product listed is the predominant ingredient in that food. This information can be very useful in many situations, such as when you are looking for foods that are lower in fat or sugar or when you are attempting to identify foods that contain whole-grain flour instead of processed wheat flour.
4. **The name and address of the food manufacturer, packer, or distributor.** You can use this information to find out more details about a food product and to contact the company if there is something wrong with the product or you suspect that it has caused an illness.

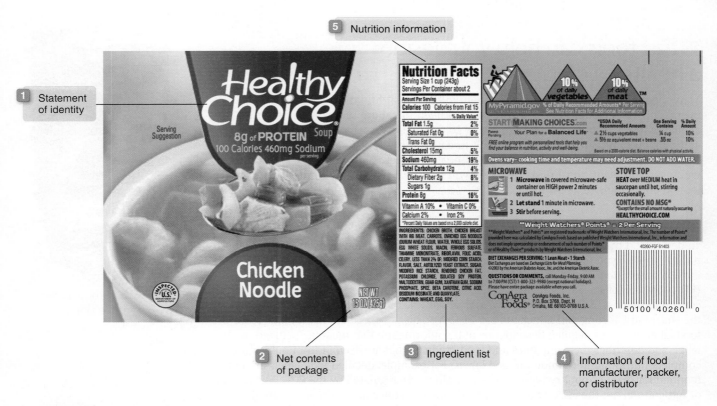

FIGURE 2.1 The five primary components that are required for food labels.
(© ConAgra Brands, Inc.)

5. **Nutrition information.** The Nutrition Facts panel contains the nutrition information required by the FDA. This panel is the primary tool to assist you in choosing more healthful foods. An explanation of the components of the Nutrition Facts panel follows.

How to Read and Use the Nutrition Facts Panel on Foods

FIGURE 2.2 shows an example of a **Nutrition Facts panel**. You can use the information on this panel to learn more about an individual food, and you can use the panel to compare one food to another. Let's start at the top of the panel and work our way down to better understand how to use this information.

1. **Serving size and servings per container.** This section describes the serving size in a common household measure (such as a cup) and a metric measure (such as grams), as well as how many servings are contained in the package. The FDA has defined serving sizes based on the amounts of each food people typically eat. However, keep in mind that the serving size listed on the package may not be the same as the amount *you* eat. You must factor in how much of the food you eat when determining the amount of nutrients that this food contributes to your diet.

2. **Calories and Calories from fat per serving.** This section describes the total number of Calories and the total number of Calories that come from fat in 1 serving of that food. By looking at this section of the label, you can determine whether a food is relatively high in fat. For example, 1 serving of the food on this label (as prepared) contains 320 total Calories, with 90 of those Calories coming from fat. This means that this food contains 28% of its total Calories as fat (90 fat Calories ÷ 320 total Calories).

Think you understand how to read the Nutrition Facts panel? Take an interactive quiz and find out at **www.sparkpeople.com**; enter "resources" and then "quizzes" in the search box to get started.

Nutrition Facts panel The label on a food package that contains the nutrition information required by the FDA.

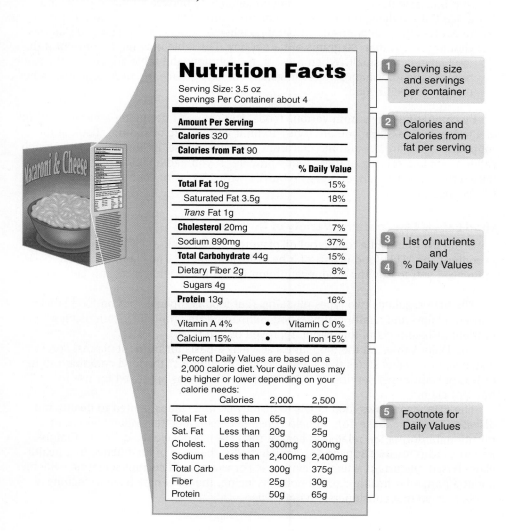

Nutrition Facts

Serving Size: 3.5 oz
Servings Per Container about 4

Amount Per Serving	
Calories 320	
Calories from Fat 90	

	% Daily Value
Total Fat 10g	15%
Saturated Fat 3.5g	18%
Trans Fat 1g	
Cholesterol 20mg	7%
Sodium 890mg	37%
Total Carbohydrate 44g	15%
Dietary Fiber 2g	8%
Sugars 4g	
Protein 13g	16%

Vitamin A 4%	•	Vitamin C 0%	
Calcium 15%	•	Iron 15%	

*Percent Daily Values are based on a 2,000 calorie diet. Your daily values may be higher or lower depending on your calorie needs:

	Calories	2,000	2,500
Total Fat	Less than	65g	80g
Sat. Fat	Less than	20g	25g
Cholest.	Less than	300mg	300mg
Sodium	Less than	2,400mg	2,400mg
Total Carb		300g	375g
Fiber		25g	30g
Protein		50g	65g

1 Serving size and servings per container

2 Calories and Calories from fat per serving

3 List of nutrients and
4 % Daily Values

5 Footnote for Daily Values

◀ **FIGURE 2.2** The Nutrition Facts panel contains a variety of information to help you make more healthful food choices.

Want to learn how to use the Nutrition Facts panel to make informed food choices? Go to www.fda.gov, enter "make calories count consumers" in the search box, and click on "Nutrition Facts Label Programs and Materials."

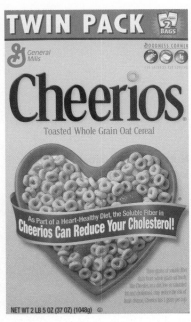

◆ This cereal box is an example of an approved health claim.

3. **List of nutrients.** This section states the nutrients this food contains. In this food, the nutrients listed toward the top, including total fat, saturated fat, *trans* fat, cholesterol, and sodium, are generally the nutrients you should strive to limit in a healthful diet. Some of the nutrients listed toward the bottom, including fiber, vitamins A and C, calcium, and iron, are those you should try to consume more of.

4. **Percent Daily Values (%DVs).** The **Percent Daily Values (%DVs)** section tells you how much a serving of food contributes to your overall intake of the nutrients listed on the label. For example, 10 grams of fat constitutes 15% of your total daily recommended fat intake. Because we are all individuals, with unique nutritional needs, it is impractical to include nutrition information that applies to each person consuming a food. That would require thousands of labels! Thus, when defining the %DV, the FDA based its calculations on a 2,000-Calorie diet. Even if you do not consume 2,000 Calories each day, you can still use the %DV to figure out whether a food is high or low in a given nutrient. For example, foods that contain less than 5% DV of a nutrient are considered low in that nutrient, whereas foods that contain more than 20% DV are considered high in that nutrient. If you are trying to consume more calcium in your diet, select foods that contain more than 20% DV for calcium. In contrast, if you are trying to consume lower-fat foods, select foods that contain less than 5% or 10% fat. By comparing the %DV of foods for any nutrient, you can quickly decide which food is higher or lower in that nutrient without having to know how many Calories you need.

5. **Footnote (lower part of the panel).** This section tells you that the %DV are based on a 2,000-Calorie diet and that your needs may be higher or lower based on your caloric needs. The remainder of the footnote includes a table with values that illustrate the differences in recommendations between 2,000-Calorie and 2,500-Calorie diets; for instance, someone eating 2,000 Calories should strive to eat less than 65 grams of fat per day, whereas a person eating 2,500 Calories should eat less than 80 grams of fat per day. The table may not be present if the food label is too small. When present, the footnote and table are always the same, because the information refers to general dietary advice for all Americans, rather than to a specific food.

By comparing labels from various foods, you can start designing a more healthful diet today. Let's assume you are trying to limit your intake of sodium. Look at the soup label in Figure 2.1 and the macaroni and cheese label in Figure 2.2. How much sodium would a serving of these foods provide? If you had a choice of either of these products for lunch, or a veggie burrito with 280 mg of sodium, which would you choose?

Food Labels Can Contain a Variety of Nutrient Claims

Have you ever noticed a food label displaying a claim such as "This food is low in sodium" or "This food is part of a heart-healthy diet"? The claim may have influenced you to buy the food, even if you weren't sure what it meant. Let's take a look.

The FDA regulates two types of claims that food companies put on food labels: nutrient claims and health claims. Food companies are prohibited from using a nutrient or health claim that is not approved by the FDA.

The Daily Values on the food labels serve as a basis for nutrient claims. For instance, if the label states that a food is "low in sodium," the food contains 140 mg or less of sodium per serving. **TABLE 2.1** defines the terms approved for use in nutrient claims.

The FDA also allows food labels to display certain claims related to health and disease (**TABLE 2.2**, page 46). To help consumers gain a better understanding of nutritional information related to health, the FDA has developed a Health Claims Report Card (**FIGURE 2.3**, page 46), which grades the level of confidence in a health claim based on current scientific evidence. For example, if current scientific evidence about a particular health claim is not convincing, the label may have to include a disclaimer, so that consumers are not misled.

Percent Daily Values (%DVs) Information on a Nutrition Facts panel that identifies how much a serving of food contributes to your overall intake of the nutrients listed on the label; based on an energy intake of 2,000 Calories per day.

TABLE 2.1 **U.S. Food and Drug Administration (FDA)–Approved Nutrient-Related Terms and Definitions**

Nutrient	Claim	Meaning
Energy	Calorie free	Less than 5 kcal per serving
	Low Calorie	40 kcal or less per serving
	Reduced Calorie	At least 25% fewer kcal than reference (or regular) food
Fat and Cholesterol	Fat free	Less than 0.5 g of fat per serving
	Low fat	3 g or less fat per serving
	Reduced fat	At least 25% less fat per serving than reference food
	Saturated fat free	Less than 0.5 g of saturated fat **AND** less than 0.5 g of *trans* fat per serving
	Low saturated fat	1 g or less saturated fat and less than 0.5 g *trans* fat per serving **AND** 15% or less of total kcal from saturated fat
	Reduced saturated fat	At least 25% less saturated fat **AND** reduced by more than 1 g saturated fat per serving as compared to reference food
	Cholesterol free	Less than 2 mg of cholesterol per serving **AND** 2 g or less saturated fat and *trans* fat combined per serving
	Low cholesterol	20 mg or less cholesterol **AND** 2 g or less saturated fat per serving
	Reduced cholesterol	At least 25% less cholesterol than reference food **AND** 2 g or less saturated fat per serving
Fiber and Sugar	High fiber	5 g or more fiber per serving*
	Good source of fiber	2.5 g to 4.9 g fiber per serving
	More or added fiber	At least 2.5 g more fiber per serving than reference food
	Sugar free	Less than 0.5 g sugars per serving
	Low sugar	Not defined; no basis for recommended intake
	Reduced/less sugar	At least 25% less sugars per serving than reference food
	No added sugars or without added sugars	No sugar or sugar-containing ingredient added during processing
Sodium	Sodium free	Less than 5 mg sodium per serving
	Very low sodium	35 mg or less sodium per serving
	Low sodium	140 mg or less sodium per serving
	Reduced sodium	At least 25% less sodium per serving than reference food
Relative Claims	Free, without, no, zero	No or a trivial amount of given nutrient
	Light (lite)	This term can have three different meanings: (1) a serving provides one-third fewer kcal than or half the fat of the reference food; (2) a serving of a low-fat, low-Calorie food provides half the sodium normally present; or (3) lighter in color and texture, with the label making this clear (for example, light molasses)
	Reduced, less, fewer	Contains at least 25% less of a nutrient or kcal than reference food
	More, added, extra, or plus	At least 10% of the Daily Value of nutrient as compared to reference food (may occur naturally or be added); may be used only for vitamins, minerals, protein, dietary fiber, and potassium
	Good source of, contains, or provides	10% to 19% of Daily Value per serving (may not be used for carbohydrate)
	High in, rich in, or excellent source of	20% or more of Daily Value per serving for protein, vitamins, minerals, dietary fiber, or potassium (may not be used for carbohydrate)

*High-fiber claims must also meet the definition of low fat; if not, then the level of total fat must appear next to the high-fiber claim.

Data adapted from: "Food Labeling Guide" (U.S. Food and Drug Administration).

In addition to nutrient and health claims, labels may also contain structure–function claims. These are claims that can be made without approval from the FDA. Although these claims can be generic statements about a food's impact on the body's structure and function, they cannot refer to a specific disease or symptom. Examples of structure–function claims include "Builds stronger bones," "Improves memory," "Slows signs of aging," and "Boosts your immune system." It is important to remember that these claims can be made with no proof, and thus there are no guarantees that any benefits identified in structure–function claims are true about that food. So, just because something is stated on the label doesn't guarantee it is always true!

TABLE 2.2 **U.S. Food and Drug Administration–Approved Health Claims on Labels**

Disease/Health Concern	Nutrient	Example of Approved Claim Statement
Osteoporosis	Calcium	Regular exercise and a healthy diet with enough calcium help teens and young white and Asian women maintain good bone health and may reduce their high risk for osteoporosis later in life.
Coronary heart disease	Saturated fat and cholesterol Fruits, vegetables, and grain products that contain fiber, particularly soluble fiber Soluble fiber from whole oats, psyllium seed husk, and beta glucan soluble fiber from oat bran, rolled oats (or oatmeal), and whole-oat flour Soy protein Plant sterol/stanol esters Whole-grain foods	Diets low in saturated fat and cholesterol and rich in fruits, vegetables, and grain products that contain some types of dietary fiber, particularly soluble fiber, may reduce the risk for heart disease, a disease associated with many factors.
Cancer	Dietary fats Fiber-containing grain products, fruits, and vegetables Fruits and vegetables Whole-grain foods	Low-fat diets rich in fiber-containing grain products, fruits, and vegetables may reduce the risk for some types of cancer, a disease associated with many factors.
Hypertension and stroke	Sodium Potassium	Diets containing foods that are a good source of potassium and that are low in sodium may reduce the risk of high blood pressure and stroke.*
Neural tube defects	Folate	Healthful diets with adequate folate may reduce a woman's risk of having a child with a brain or spinal cord defect.
Dental caries	Sugar alcohols	Frequent between-meal consumption of foods high in sugars and starches promotes tooth decay. The sugar alcohols in [name of food] do not promote tooth decay.

*Required wording for this claim. Wordings for other claims are recommended model statements but not required verbatim.

Data adapted from: "Food Labeling Guide" (U.S. Food and Drug Administration).

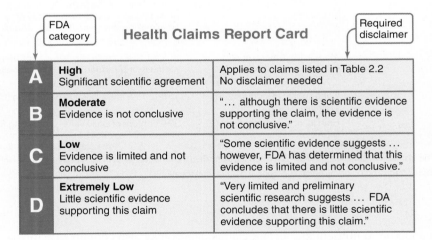

FIGURE 2.3 The U.S. Food and Drug Administration's Health Claims Report Card.

recap The ability to read and interpret food labels is important for planning and maintaining a healthful diet. Food labels must list the identity of the food, the net contents of the package, the contact information for the food manufacturer or distributor, the ingredients in the food, and a Nutrition Facts panel. The Nutrition Facts panel provides specific information about Calories, macronutrients, and selected vitamins and minerals. Food labels may also contain claims related to nutrients, health, and body structure and function.

nutri-case | GUSTAVO

"Until last night, I hadn't been inside a grocery store in about 10 years. But then my wife broke her hip and had to go to the hospital. On my way home from visiting her, I realized I needed to do some food shopping. Was I ever in for a shock! I don't know how my wife does it, with her English skills kind of shakey, choosing between all the different brands, and reading those long labels. I bought a frozen chicken pie for dinner, but it didn't taste right, so I got the package out of the trash and read all the labels, and that's when I saw there wasn't any chicken in it at all . . . it was made out of tofu! This afternoon, my daughter is picking me up, and we're going to do our grocery shopping together."

Given what you've learned about FDA food labels, what parts of a food package would you advise Gustavo to be sure to read before he makes a choice? What other advice might you give him to make his grocery shopping easier? Imagine that, like Gustavo's wife, you have only limited skills in mathematics and reading. In that case, what other strategies might you use when shopping for nutritious foods?

Dietary Guidelines for Americans

The **Dietary Guidelines for Americans** are a set of principles developed by the U.S. Department of Agriculture and the U.S. Department of Health and Human Services to promote health, reduce the risk for chronic diseases, and reduce the prevalence of overweight and obesity among Americans through improved nutrition and physical activity.[3] They are updated approximately every 5 years. The 2010 Dietary Guidelines for Americans include twenty-three recommendations for the general population, but you don't have to remember all twenty-three! Instead, they encourage you to focus on the following four main ideas.

Balance Calories to Maintain Weight

Consume adequate nutrients to promote your health while staying within your energy needs. This will help you maintain a healthful weight. You can achieve this by controlling your Calorie intake; if you are overweight or obese, you will need to consume fewer Calories from foods and beverages. At the same time, increase your level of physical activity and reduce the time you spend in sedentary behaviors, such as watching television and sitting at the computer.

An important strategy for balancing your Calories is to consistently choose **nutrient-dense foods** and beverages—that is, foods and beverages that supply the highest level of nutrients for the lowest number of Calories. **FIGURE 2.4** (page 48) compares 1 day of meals that are high in **nutrient density** to meals that are low in nutrient density. As you can see in this figure, skim milk is more nutrient dense than whole milk, and a peeled orange is more nutrient dense than an orange soft drink. This example can assist you in selecting the most nutrient-dense foods when planning your meals.

Limit Sodium, Fat, Sugars, and Alchohol

The Dietary Guidelines suggest that we reduce our consumption of the following foods and food components. Doing so will help us maintain a healthy weight and lower our risk for chronic diseases.

Sodium Excessive consumption of sodium, a major mineral found in salt, is linked to high blood pressure in some people. Eating a lot of sodium also can cause some people to lose calcium from their bones, which can increase their risk for bone loss and bone fractures. Although table salt contains sodium and the major mineral chloride, much of the sodium we consume comes from processed and prepared

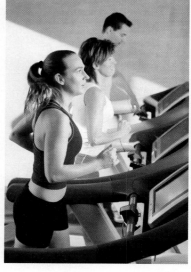

Being physically active for at least 30 minutes each day can reduce your risk for chronic diseases.

Dietary Guidelines for Americans A set of principles developed by the U.S. Department of Agriculture and the U.S. Department of Health and Human Services to assist Americans in designing a healthful diet and lifestyle.

nutrient-dense foods Foods that provide the most nutrients for the least amount of energy (Calories).

nutrient density The relative amount of nutrients per amount of energy (or number of Calories).

A Day of Meals: Low vs. High Nutrient Density

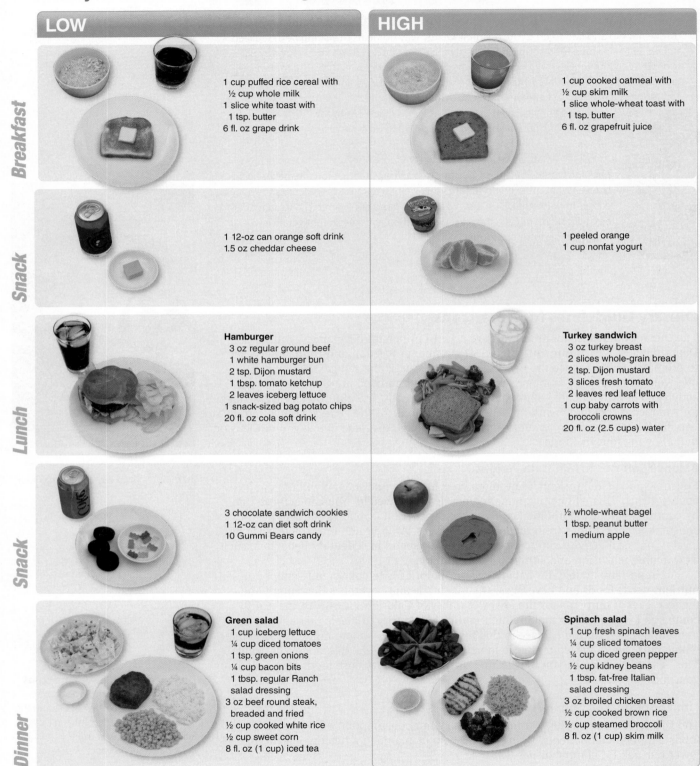

LOW

HIGH

Breakfast

1 cup puffed rice cereal with
½ cup whole milk
1 slice white toast with
  1 tsp. butter
6 fl. oz grape drink

1 cup cooked oatmeal with
½ cup skim milk
1 slice whole-wheat toast with
  1 tsp. butter
6 fl. oz grapefruit juice

Snack

1 12-oz can orange soft drink
1.5 oz cheddar cheese

1 peeled orange
1 cup nonfat yogurt

Lunch

Hamburger
3 oz regular ground beef
1 white hamburger bun
2 tsp. Dijon mustard
1 tbsp. tomato ketchup
2 leaves iceberg lettuce
1 snack-sized bag potato chips
20 fl. oz cola soft drink

Turkey sandwich
3 oz turkey breast
2 slices whole-grain bread
2 tsp. Dijon mustard
3 slices fresh tomato
2 leaves red leaf lettuce
1 cup baby carrots with
  broccoli crowns
20 fl. oz (2.5 cups) water

Snack

3 chocolate sandwich cookies
1 12-oz can diet soft drink
10 Gummi Bears candy

½ whole-wheat bagel
1 tbsp. peanut butter
1 medium apple

Dinner

Green salad
1 cup iceberg lettuce
¼ cup diced tomatoes
1 tsp. green onions
¼ cup bacon bits
1 tbsp. regular Ranch
  salad dressing
3 oz beef round steak,
  breaded and fried
½ cup cooked white rice
½ cup sweet corn
8 fl. oz (1 cup) iced tea

Spinach salad
1 cup fresh spinach leaves
¼ cup sliced tomatoes
¼ cup diced green pepper
½ cup kidney beans
1 tbsp. fat-free Italian
  salad dressing
3 oz broiled chicken breast
½ cup cooked brown rice
½ cup steamed broccoli
8 fl. oz (1 cup) skim milk

FIGURE 2.4 A comparison of 1 day's meals containing foods high in nutrient density to meals with foods low in nutrient density.

foods. Key recommendations include keeping your daily sodium intake below 2,300 milligrams (mg) per day. This is the amount in just 1 teaspoon of table salt! If you are African American; if you have high blood pressure, diabetes, or chronic kidney disease; or if you are over age 50, you should aim for a daily sodium intake below 1,500 mg. Some ways to decrease your sodium intake include the following:

- Eat fresh, plain frozen, or canned vegetables without added salt.
- Limit your intake of processed meats, such as cured ham, sausage, bacon, and most canned meats.
- When shopping for canned or packaged foods, look for those with labels that say "low sodium."
- Add little or no salt to foods at the table.
- Limit your intake of salty condiments, such as ketchup, mustard, pickles, soy sauce, and olives.

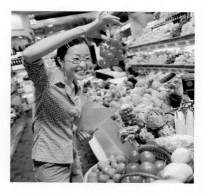

When grocery shopping, try to select a variety of fruits and vegetables.

Fat Fat is an essential nutrient and therefore an important part of a healthful diet; however, because fats are energy dense, eating a diet high in total fat can lead to overweight and obesity. In addition, eating a diet high in cholesterol and saturated fat (a type of fat abundant in meats and other animal-based foods) is linked to an increased risk for heart disease. For these reasons, less than 7–10% of your total daily Calories should come from saturated fat, and you should try to consume less than 300 mg per day of cholesterol. You can achieve this goal by replacing solid fats, such as butter and lard, with plant oils, as well as by eating meat less often and fish or vegetarian meals more often. Finally, replace full-fat milk, yogurt, and cheeses with low-fat or nonfat versions.

Sugars Limit foods and beverages that are high in added sugars, such as sweetened soft drinks and fruit drinks, cookies, and cakes. These foods contribute to overweight and obesity, and they promote tooth decay. Moreover, doughnuts, cookies, cakes, pies, and other pastries are typically made with unhealthful fats and are high in sodium.

Alcohol Alcohol provides energy but not nutrients. In the body, it depresses the nervous system and is toxic to liver and other body cells. Drinking alcoholic beverages in excess can lead to serious health and social problems; therefore, those who choose to drink are encouraged to do so sensibly and in moderation: no more than one drink per day for women and no more than two drinks per day for men, and only by adults of legal drinking age. Adults who should not drink alcohol are those who cannot restrict their intake, women of childbearing age who may become pregnant, pregnant and lactating women, individuals taking medications that can interact with alcohol, people with certain medical conditions, and people who are engaging in activities that require attention, skill, or coordination.

Consume More Healthful Foods and Nutrients

Another goal of the Dietary Guidelines is to encourage people to increase their consumption of healthful foods rich in nutrients while keeping their Calorie intake within their daily energy needs. Key recommendations for achieving this goal include the following:

- Increase your intake of fruits and vegetables. Each day, try to eat a variety of dark-green, red, and orange vegetables, along with beans and peas.
- Make sure that at least half of all grain foods—breads, cereals, pasta, and so on—that you eat each day are made from whole grains.
- Choose fat-free or low-fat milk and milk products, which include milk, yogurt, cheese, and fortified soy beverages.
- When making protein choices, choose protein foods that are lower in solid fat and Calories, such as lean cuts of beef or skinless poultry. Try to eat more fish and shellfish in place of traditional meat and poultry choices. Also choose eggs, beans and peas, soy products, and unsalted nuts and seeds.

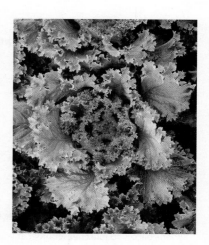

Nutrient-packed foods—such as kale, which is an excellent source of calcium—should be part of a well-rounded diet.

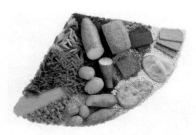

Eating a diet rich in whole-grain foods and fiber-rich fruits and vegetables can enhance your overall health.

- Choose foods that provide an adequate level of dietary fiber as well as nutrients of concern in the American diet, including potassium, calcium, and vitamin D. These nutrients help us maintain healthy blood pressure and reduce our risks for certain diseases. Healthful foods that are good sources of these nutrients include fruits, vegetables, beans and peas, whole grains, and low-fat milk and milk products.

Follow Healthy Eating Patterns

There is no one healthy eating pattern that everyone should follow. Instead, the recommendations made in the Dietary Guidelines are designed to accommodate diverse cultural, ethnic, traditional, and personal preferences and to fit within different individuals' food budgets. Still, the Guidelines offer several flexible templates you can follow to build your healthy eating pattern, including the U.S. Department of Agriculture (USDA) Food Patterns and the Mediterranean diet (both discussed shortly).

Building a healthy eating pattern also involves following food safety recommendations to reduce your risk for foodborne illnesses, such as those caused by microorganisms and their toxins. The four food-safety principles emphasized in the Dietary Guidelines are:

- *Clean* your hands, food contact surfaces, and vegetables and fruits.
- *Separate* raw, cooked, and ready-to-eat foods while shopping, storing, and preparing foods.
- *Cook* foods to a safe temperature.
- *Chill* (refrigerate) perishable foods promptly.

Another important tip is to avoid unpasteurized juices and milk products; raw or undercooked meats, seafood, poultry, and eggs; and raw sprouts.

TABLE 2.3 provides examples of how you can change your current diet and physical activity habits to meet some of the recommendations in the Dietary Guidelines.

recap The goals of the Dietary Guidelines for Americans are to promote health, reduce the risk for chronic diseases, and reduce the prevalence of overweight and obesity among Americans through improved nutrition and physical activity. This can be achieved by eating whole-grain foods, fruits, and vegetables daily; reducing intake of foods with unhealthful fats and cholesterol, salt, and added sugar; eating more foods rich in potassium, dietary fiber, calcium, and vitamin D; keeping foods safe to eat; and drinking alcohol in moderation, if at all.

TABLE 2.3   Ways to Incorporate the Dietary Guidelines for Americans into Your Daily Life

If You Normally Do This	Try Doing This Instead
Watch television when you get home at night	Do 30 minutes of stretching or lifting of hand weights in front of the television
Drive to the store down the block	Walk to and from the store
Go out to lunch with friends	Take a 15- or 30-minute walk with your friends at lunchtime 3 days each week
Eat white bread with your sandwich	Eat whole-wheat bread or some other bread made from whole grains
Eat white rice or fried rice with your meal	Eat brown rice or try wild rice
Choose cookies or a candy bar for a snack	Choose a fresh nectarine, peach, apple, orange, or banana for a snack
Order french fries with your hamburger	Order a green salad with low-fat salad dressing on the side
Spread butter or margarine on your white toast each morning	Spread fresh fruit compote on whole-grain toast
Order a bacon double cheeseburger at your favorite restaurant	Order a turkey burger or grilled chicken sandwich without the cheese and bacon, and add lettuce and tomato
Drink non-diet soft drinks to quench your thirst	Drink iced tea, ice water with a slice of lemon, seltzer water, or diet soft drinks
Eat salted potato chips and pickles with your favorite sandwich	Eat carrot slices and crowns of fresh broccoli and cauliflower dipped in low-fat or nonfat Ranch dressing

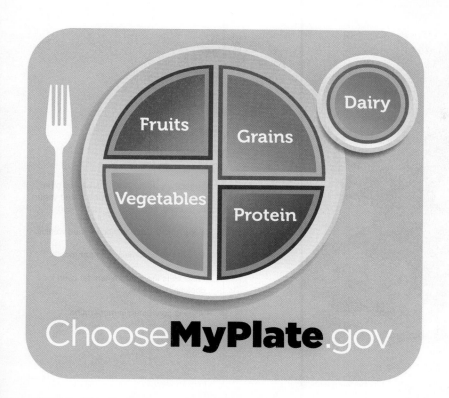

FIGURE 2.5 The USDA MyPlate graphic. MyPlate is an interactive food guidance system based on the 2010 Dietary Guidelines for Americans and the Dietary Reference Intakes from the National Academy of Sciences. Eating more fruits, vegetables, and whole grains and choosing foods low in fat, sugar, and sodium from the five food groups in MyPlate will help you balance your Calories and consume a healthier overall food pattern.
Data from: MyPlate graphic, U.S. Department of Agriculture.

The USDA Food Patterns

You can use the USDA Food Patterns to help you design a healthful diet. The visual representation of the USDA Food Patterns is called **MyPlate** (FIGURE 2.5). MyPlate, which was released in 2011, replaces the previous MyPyramid graphic (see Appendix A). It is an interactive, personalized guide that you can access on the Internet to evaluate your current diet and physical activity level and to plan appropriate changes. The MyPlate icon and its accompanying website help Americans to:

- eat in moderation to balance calories
- eat a variety of foods
- consume the right proportion of each recommended food group
- personalize their eating plan
- increase their physical activity
- set goals for gradually improving their food choices and lifestyle

MyPlate Incorporates Many of the Features of the Mediterrean Diet

MyPlate incorporates many of the features of the Mediterranean Diet. A Mediterranean-style diet has received significant attention for many years, largely because the rates of cardiovascular disease in many Mediterranean countries are substantially lower than rates in the United States. There is actually not a single Mediterranean diet because this region of the world includes Portugal, Spain, Italy, France, Greece, Turkey, and Israel. Each of these countries has different dietary patterns; however, there are many similarities. Aspects of the diet seen as more healthy than the typical U.S. diet include the following:

- Red meat is eaten only monthly, and eggs, poultry, fish, and sweets are eaten weekly, making the diet low in saturated fats and refined sugars.
- The primary fat used for cooking and flavor is olive oil, making the diet high in monosaturated fats.
- Foods eaten daily include grains, such as bread, pasta, couscous, and bulgur; fruits; beans and other legumes; nuts; vegetables; and cheese and yogurt. These choices make this diet high in vitamins and minerals, fiber, phytochemicals, probiotics, and prebiotics.
- Wine is included, in moderation.

MyPlate The visual representation of the USDA Food Patterns.

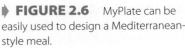

FIGURE 2.6 MyPlate can be easily used to design a Mediterranean-style meal.

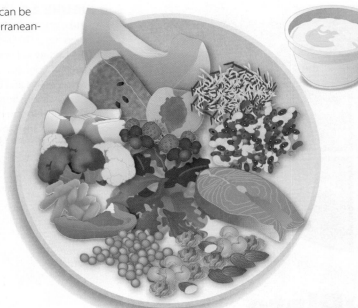

- Vegetables, fruits, nuts, beans and other legumes, whole grains, cheese and yogurt consumed daily.

- Eggs, poultry, and fish consumed weekly.

- Red meat consumed once per month.

- Olive oil is the predominant fat used for cooking and flavor.

- Wine is consumed in moderation.

As you'll discover, MyPlate does not make specific recommendations for protein food choices. In contrast, the Mediterrean diet recommends beans, other legumes, and nuts as daily sources of protein; fish, poultry, and eggs weekly; and red meat only about once each month. Also, for dairy choices, the Mediterrean diet recommends cheese and yogurt in moderation and suggests drinking water or wine (in moderation) rather than milk. There is currently not a MyPlate version available for the Mediterrean Diet, but as illustrated in **FIGURE 2.6**, it is easy to create a healthy Mediterranean-style meal using the principles of MyPlate.

Food Groups in the USDA Food Patterns

The five food groups emphasized in the USDA Food Patterns are grains, vegetables, fruits, dairy, and protein foods. They are represented in the plate graphic with segments of five different colors. **FIGURE 2.7** illustrates each of these food groups and provides detailed information on the nutrients they provide and recommended servings each day.

The Concept of Empty Calories

One concept emphasized in the USDA Food Patterns is that of **empty Calories**. These are Calories from solid fats and/or added sugars that provide few or no nutrients. The USDA recommends that you limit the empty Calories you eat to a small number that fits your Calorie and nutrient needs depending on your age, gender, and level of physical activity. Foods highest in empty Calories include cakes, cookies, pastries, doughnuts, soft drinks, fruit drinks, cheese, pizza, ice cream, sausages, hot dogs, bacon, and ribs.

High-sugar foods, such as candies, desserts, gelatin, soft drinks, and alcoholic beverages, are called *empty Calorie foods*. However, a few foods that contain empty Calories from solid fats and added sugars also provide important nutrients. Examples are sweetened applesauce, sweetened breakfast cereals, regular ground beef, and whole milk. To reduce your intake of empty Calories but ensure you get adequate nutrients, choose the unsweetened, lean, or nonfat versions of these foods.

Number and Size of Servings in the USDA Food Patterns

The USDA Food Patterns also help you decide *how much* of each food you should eat. The number of servings is based on your age, gender, and activity level. A term used

empty Calories Calories from solid fats and/or added sugars that provide few or no nutrients.

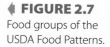

FIGURE 2.7
Food groups of the
USDA Food Patterns.

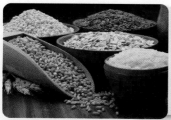

Grains

Make half your grains whole. At least half of the grains you eat each day should come from whole-grain sources.

Eat at least 3 oz of whole-grain bread, cereal, crackers, rice, or pasta every day.

Whole-grain foods provide fiber-rich carbohydrates, riboflavin, thiamin, niacin, iron, folate, zinc, protein, and magnesium.

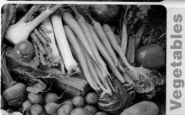

Vegetables

Vary your veggies. Eat a variety of vegetables and increase consumption of dark-green and orange vegetables, as well as dry beans and peas.

Eat at least 2½ cups of vegetables each day.

Vegetables provide fiber and phytochemicals, carbohydrates, vitamins A and C, folate, potassium, and magnesium.

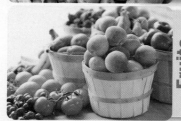

Fruits

Focus on fruits. Eat a greater variety of fruits (fresh, frozen, or dried) and go easy on the fruit juices.

Eat at least 1½ cups of fruit every day.

Fruits provide fiber, phytochemicals, vitamins A and C, folate, potassium, and magnesium.

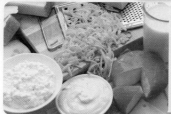

Dairy Foods

Get your calcium-rich foods. Choose low-fat or fat-free dairy products, such as milk, yogurt, and cheese. People who can't consume dairy foods can choose lactose-free dairy products or other sources, such as calcium-fortified juices and soy and rice beverages.

Get 3 cups of low-fat dairy foods, or the equivalent, every day.

Dairy foods provide calcium, phosphorus, riboflavin, protein, and vitamin B$_{12}$ and are often fortified with vitamins D and A.

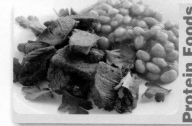

Protein Foods

Go lean with protein. Choose low-fat or lean meats and poultry. Switch to baking, broiling, or grilling more often, and vary your choices to include more fish, processed soy products, beans, nuts, and seeds. Legumes, including beans, peas, and lentils, are included in both the protein and the vegetable groups.

Eat about 5½ oz of lean protein foods each day.

These foods provide protein, phosphorus, vitamin B$_6$, vitamin B$_{12}$, magnesium, iron, zinc, niacin, riboflavin, and thiamin.

when defining serving sizes that may be new to you is **ounce-equivalent (oz-equivalent)**. It is defined as a serving size that is 1 ounce, or that is equivalent to an ounce, for the grains and meats and beans sections. For instance, both a slice of bread and 1/2 cup of cooked brown rice qualify as ounce-equivalents.

What is considered a serving size for the foods recommended in the USDA Food Patterns? **FIGURE 2.8** (page 54) identifies the number of cups or oz-equivalent servings recommended for a 2,000-Calorie diet and gives examples of amounts equal to 1 cup or 1 oz-equivalent for foods in each group. As you study this figure, notice the variety of examples for each group. For instance, an oz-equivalent serving from the grains group can mean one slice of bread or two small pancakes. Because of their low density, 2 cups of raw, leafy vegetables, such as spinach, actually constitute a 1-cup serving from the vegetables group. Although an oz-equivalent serving of meat is actually 1 oz, 1/2 oz of nuts also qualifies. One egg, 1 tablespoon of peanut butter, and 1/4 cup cooked legumes are also considered 1 oz-equivalents from the protein group.

ounce-equivalent (oz-equivalent)
A serving size that is 1 ounce, or equivalent to an ounce, for the grains and the protein foods sections of MyPlate.

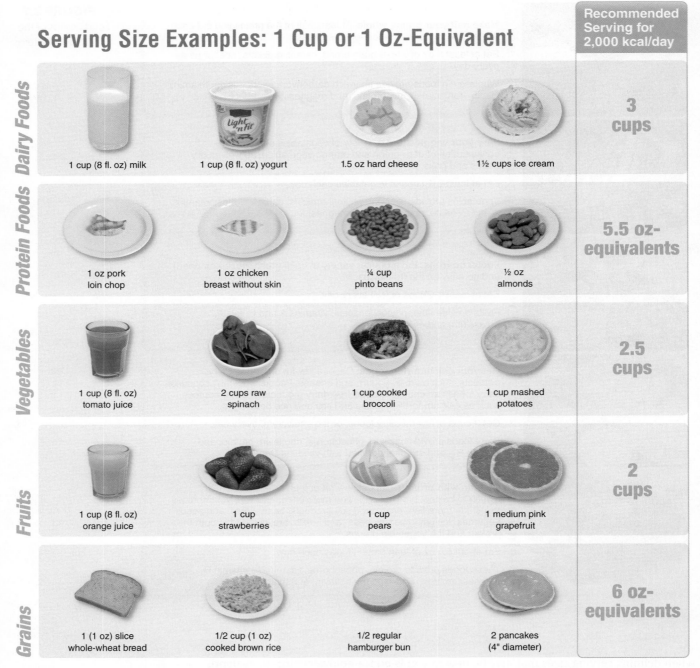

Serving Size Examples: 1 Cup or 1 Oz-Equivalent

				Recommended Serving for 2,000 kcal/day
Dairy Foods	1 cup (8 fl. oz) milk	1 cup (8 fl. oz) yogurt	1.5 oz hard cheese	1½ cups ice cream	**3 cups**
Protein Foods	1 oz pork loin chop	1 oz chicken breast without skin	¼ cup pinto beans	½ oz almonds	**5.5 oz-equivalents**
Vegetables	1 cup (8 fl. oz) tomato juice	2 cups raw spinach	1 cup cooked broccoli	1 cup mashed potatoes	**2.5 cups**
Fruits	1 cup (8 fl. oz) orange juice	1 cup strawberries	1 cup pears	1 medium pink grapefruit	**2 cups**
Grains	1 (1 oz) slice whole-wheat bread	1/2 cup (1 oz) cooked brown rice	1/2 regular hamburger bun	2 pancakes (4" diameter)	**6 oz-equivalents**

FIGURE 2.8 Examples of equivalent amounts for foods in each food group of MyPlate for a 2,000-kcal food intake pattern. Here are some examples of household items that can help you estimate amounts: 1.5 oz of hard cheese is equal to 4 stacked dice, 3 oz of meat is equal in size to a deck of cards, and half of a regular hamburger bun is the size of a yo-yo.

Although it may seem inconvenient to measure food servings, understanding the size of a serving is crucial to planning a nutritious diet. **FIGURE 2.9** shows you a practical way to estimate serving sizes.

No nationally standardized definition for a serving size exists for any food. Thus, a serving size as defined in the USDA Food Patterns may not be equal to a serving size identified on a food label. For instance, the serving size for crackers suggested in the USDA Food Patterns is three to four small crackers, whereas a serving size for crackers on a food label can range from five to eighteen crackers, depending on the size and weight of the cracker. Do you routinely check the serving size listed on a food label and measure out that exact amount of food? If not, try the nearby **Nutrition Label Activity** to find out how closely you're matching the serving size listed on the label.

The size of individual food items, such as muffins, frozen burgers, and bottled juices, as well as the portion size of foods served in restaurants, cafés, and movie theaters have grown substantially over the past 30 years (**FIGURE 2.10**, page 56). This "super-sizing" phenomenon, now widespread, indicates a major shift in accepted eating behaviors and is an important factor in the rise in obesity rates around the world. For over 10 years it has been recognized[4] that the size discrepancy between foods bought and consumed in the "real world" and USDA serving size standards is staggering— chocolate chip cookies have been reported as seven times larger than USDA standards, a serving of cooked pasta in a restaurant can be almost five times larger, and steaks are more than twice as large.[5] Thus, when using diet-planning tools, such as the USDA Food Patterns, learn the definition of a serving size for the tool you're using and *then* measure your food intake to determine whether you are meeting the guidelines. If you don't want to gain weight, it's important to become informed about portion size.

How much physical activity do you think you'd need to perform in order to burn off the extra Calories in a larger portion size? Try the nearby **You Do the Math** (page 56) and find out.

Despite efforts to improve upon the 2005 Dietary Guidelines for Americans (DGAs) and MyPyramid, the 2010 DGAs and MyPlate have met with some criticism. Refer to the **Nutrition Debate** (page 62) at the end of this chapter to learn more about this controversy.

Ethnic and Other Variations of MyPlate

As you know, the population of the United States is culturally and ethnically diverse, and this diversity influences our food choices. **FIGURE 2.11** (page 57) is a Spanish-language version of MyPlate. Like the English-language version, it recommends food groups, not specific food choices. As we illustrated with the Mediterranean Diet, MyPlate easily accomodates foods that we may consider part of an ethnic diet. You can also easily incorporate into MyPlate foods that match a vegetarian diet or other lifestyle preferences.

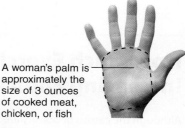

A woman's palm is approximately the size of 3 ounces of cooked meat, chicken, or fish

(a)

A woman's fist is about the size of 1 cup of pasta or vegetables (a man's fist is the size of about 2 cups)

(b)

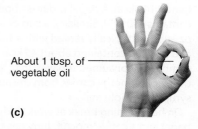

About 1 tbsp. of vegetable oil

(c)

FIGURE 2.9 Use your hands to help you estimate the amounts of common foods.

nutrition label activity

How Realistic Are the Serving Sizes Listed on Food Labels?

Many people read food labels to determine the energy (Caloric) value of foods, but it is less common to pay close attention to the actual serving size that corresponds to the listed Caloric value. To test how closely your "naturally selected" serving size matches the actual serving size of certain foods, try these label activities:

- Choose a breakfast cereal that you commonly eat. Pour the amount of cereal you would normally eat into a bowl. Before adding milk to your cereal, use a measuring cup to measure the amount of cereal you poured. Now read the label of the cereal to determine the serving size (for example, 1/2 cup or 1 cup) and the Caloric value listed on the label. How do your "naturally selected" serving size and the label-defined serving size compare?

- At your local grocery store, locate various boxes of snack crackers. Look at the number of crackers and total Calories per serving listed on the labels of crackers such as regular Triscuits, Reduced-fat Triscuits, Vegetable Thins, and Ritz crackers. How do the number of crackers and total Calories per serving differ for the serving size listed on each box? How do the serving sizes listed in the Nutrition Facts panel compare to how many crackers you would usually eat?

These activities are just two examples of ways to understand how nutrition labels can help you make balanced and healthful food choices. Because many people do not know what constitutes a serving size, they are inclined to consume too much of some foods (such as snack foods and meat) and too little of other foods (such as fruits and vegetables). This is a major influence behind some of the proposed changes to food labels currently being explored by the FDA.

you do the math

How Much Exercise Is Needed to Combat Increasing Food Portion Sizes?

Although the causes of obesity are complex and multifactorial, it is speculated that one reason obesity rates are rising globally is due to a combination of increased energy intake, reflecting expanding food portion sizes, and reduced overall daily physical activity. This math activity should help you better understand how portion sizes have increased over the past 20 years and how much physical activity you would need to do to expend the excess energy resulting from these larger portion sizes.

The two set of photos in Figure 2.10 give examples of foods whose portion sizes have increased substantially. A bagel 20 years ago had a diameter of approximately 3 inches and contained 140 kcal. A bagel today is about 6 inches in diameter and contains 350 kcal. Similarly, a cup of coffee 20 years ago was 8 fl. oz and was typically served with a small amount of whole milk and sugar. It contained about 45 kcal. A standard coffee mocha commonly consumed today is 16 fl. oz and contains 350 kcal; this excess energy comes from the addition of a sweet flavored syrup and whole milk.

On her morning break at work, Judy routinely consumes a bagel and a coffee mocha. Judy has type 2 diabetes, and her doctor has advised her to lose weight. How much physical activity would Judy need to do to "burn" this excess energy? Let's do some simple math to answer this question.

1. Calculate the excess energy Judy consumes from both of these foods:

   a. Bagel: 350 kcal in larger bagel – 140 kcal in smaller bagel = 210 kcal extra

   b. Coffee: 350 kcal in large coffee mocha – 45 kcal in small regular coffee = 305 kcal extra

   Total excess energy for these two larger portions = 515 kcal

2. Judy has started walking each day in an effort to lose weight. Judy currently weighs 200 lb. Based on her relatively low fitness level, Judy walks at a slow pace (approximately 2 miles per hour); it is estimated that walking at this pace expends 1.2 kcal per pound of body weight per hour. How long does Judy need to walk each day to expend 515 kcal?

   a. First, calculate how much energy Judy expends if she walks for a full hour by multiplying her body weight by the energy cost of walking per hour = 1.2 kcal/lb body weight × 200 lb = 240 kcal.

   b. Next, you need to calculate how much energy she expends each minute she walks by dividing the energy cost of walking per hour by 60 minutes = 240 kcal/hour ÷ 60 minutes/hour = 4 kcal/minute.

   c. To determine how many minutes she would need to walk to expend 515 kcal, divide the total amount of energy she needs to expend by the energy cost of walking per minute = 515 kcal ÷ 4 kcal/minute = 103.75 minutes.

Thus, Judy would need to walk for approximately 104 minutes, or about 1 hour and 45 minutes, to expend the excess energy she consumes by eating the larger bagel and coffee. If she wanted to burn off all of the energy in her morning snack, she would have to walk even longer, especially if she enjoyed her bagel with cream cheese!

Now use your own weight in these calculations to determine how much walking you would have to do if you consumed the same foods:

a. 1.2 kcal/lb × (your weight in pounds) = _____ kcal/hour

   (If you walk at a brisk pace, use 2.4 kcal/lb.)

b. _____ kcal/hour ÷ 60 minutes/hour = _____ kcal/minute

c. 515 extra kcal in bagel and coffee ÷ _____ kcal/minute = _____ minutes

20 Years Ago	Today

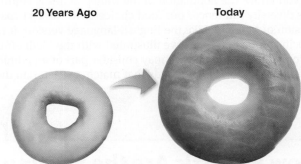

3-inch diameter, 140 Calories   6-inch diameter, 350 Calories

(a) Bagel

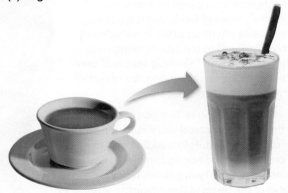

8 fluid ounces, 45 Calories   16 fluid ounces, 350 Calories

(b) Coffee

FIGURE 2.10 Examples of increases in food portion sizes over the past 20 years. **(a)** A bagel has increased in diameter from 3 inches to 6 inches; **(b)** a cup of coffee has increased from 8 fl. oz to 16 fl. oz and now commonly contains Calorie-dense flavored syrup as well as steamed whole milk.

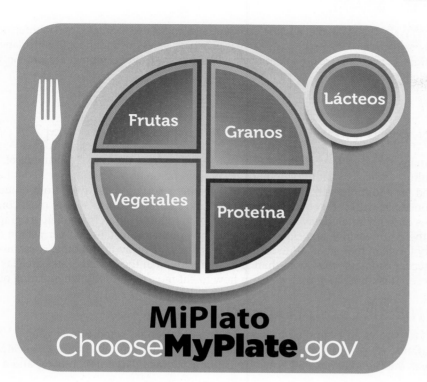

▲ **FIGURE 2.11** MiPlato is the Spanish language version of MyPlate. Data from: MiPlato graphic, U.S. Department of Agriculture.

recap The USDA Food Patterns can be used to plan a healthful, balanced diet that includes foods from the grains group, vegetables group, fruits group, dairy group, and protein foods group. The MyPlate graphic and website incorporates aspects of the Mediterranean Diet. The serving sizes in the USDA Food Patterns typically are smaller than the amounts we normally eat. The USDA Food Patterns and MyPlate can be easily adapted to accommodate a wide range of other ethnic preferences. This flexibility enables anyone to design a diet that meets the goals of adequacy, moderation, balance, variety, and nutrient density.

> Think you understand the relationship between portion sizes and the physical activity necessary to avoid weight gain? Find out by taking the National Heart, Lung, and Blood Institute's *Portion Distortion Quiz* at **www.hp2010.nhlbihin.net**; enter "portion distortion" into the search box to get underway.

Other Eating Plans

In addition to the USDA Food Patterns and MyPlate, there are other eating plans you can use to design a healthful diet. One example is the DASH diet, which stands for "Dietary Approaches to Stop Hypertension." The DASH diet plan is discussed in more detail in the **In Depth** on cardiovascular disease (starting on page 177).

The **exchange system** is another tool that can be used to plan a healthful diet. This system was originally designed for people with diabetes by the American Dietetic Association (now known as the Academy of Nutrition and Dietetics) and the American Diabetes Association. It has also been used successfully in weight-loss programs. Exchanges, or portions, are organized according to the amount of carbohydrate, protein, fat, and Calories in each food. There are six food groups, or exchange lists, and these lists contain foods that are similar in Calories, carbohydrate, fat, and protein content. The six exchange lists are starch/bread, meat and meat substitutes, vegetables, fruits, milk, and fat. In addition to these lists, there are other categories that can assist you in meal planning, including free foods (any food or drink less than 20 Calories per serving), combination foods (foods such as soups, casseroles, and pizza), and special-occasion foods (desserts such as cakes, cookies, and ice cream). Refer to Appendix D for more details about exchange lists for meal planning.

exchange system A diet planning tool in which exchanges, or portions, are organized according to the amount of carbohydrate, protein, fat, and Calories in each food.

The DASH diet and the exchange system are two examples of healthful food plans. The exchange system was originally designed for people with diabetes. Exchanges, or portions, are organized according to the amount of carbohydrate, protein, fat, and Calories in each food.

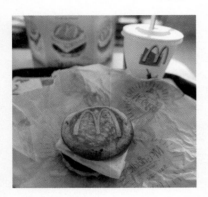

← Foods served at fast-food chains are often high in Calories, total fat, and sodium. The popular McDonald's sausage, egg, and cheese McGriddles breakfast sandwiches, for example, contain 550 kcal, 31 grams of fat, and 1,320 milligrams of sodium!

Can eating out be part of a healthful diet?

How many times each week do you eat out? A report from the U.S. Department of Agriculture indicates that buying foods away from home now accounts for about half of all food expenditures, and almost 75% of consumers surveyed eat away from home at least once per week.[6] Full-service restaurants and fast-food outlets are the most common sources of foods eaten away from home. Research indicates that, in a given geographic area, there is a positive association between the number of restaurants per person and obesity levels in that area.[7] With so many people eating away from home, combined with recent estimates that more than 35% of all adults in the United States are classified as obese,[1] it is imperative that we learn how to eat more healthfully when eating out.

The Hidden Costs of Eating Out

TABLE 2.4 shows an example of foods served at McDonald's and Burger King restaurants. As you can see, a regular McDonald's hamburger has only 250 kcal, whereas the Big Mac has 550 kcal. A meal of a Big Mac, large french fries, and a small

TABLE 2.4 **Nutritional Value of Selected Fast Foods**

Menu Item	kcal	Fat (g)	Fat (% kcal)	Sodium (mg)
McDonald's				
Hamburger	250	9	32	480
Cheeseburger	300	12	36	680
Quarter Pounder with Cheese	520	26	45	1,100
Big Mac	550	29	47	970
French fries, small	230	11	43	160
French fries, medium	380	19	45	270
French fries, large	500	25	45	350
Coke, large	310	0	0	0
McCafe Chocolate Shake (small)	560	16	26	240
McCafe Chocolate Shake (large)	880	24	25	370
Burger King				
Hamburger	260	9	31	500
Cheeseburger	300	14	42	710
Whopper	670	40	54	980
Double Whopper	900	57	57	1,050
Bacon Double Cheeseburger	520	31	54	1,180
French fries, small	340	15	40	480
French fries, medium	410	18	40	570
French fries, large	500	22	40	710

HOT TOPIC

Does Calorie-Labeling Influence Food Choice?

Many health and nutrition professionals have worked diligently to lobby for clear labeling of the nutritional content of foods on menus in restaurants to assist consumers in making healthier choices. A number of restaurant chains across the country have made voluntary changes to their menus as a result. Places such as King County, Washington, and New York City have taken the additional step of enforcing mandatory menu labeling in restaurants. But have these actions influenced Americans to make healthier food choices when eating out?

An overview of the research conducted in this area indicates that Calorie-labeling has not resulted in any consistent or substantive changes in food choices made by adults or children.[8] It also has not appeared to have any major impact on increasing the number of healthful menu options or reducing the Caloric-content of foods offered. Although some restaurants have reduced the Calories, fat, and sodium content of menu items, in most cases these foods still exceed the levels recommended for promoting health.

McCafé Chocolate Shake provides 1,610 kcal. This meal has enough energy to support an entire day's needs for a small, lightly active woman! A significant contributor to these Calories is the beverage: a large iced coffee, tea, orange juice, or soda is typically at least 270 Calories, and a large shake can cost you 650 or more. Similar meals at Burger King and other fast-food chains are also very high in Calories, not to mention total fat and sodium.

Fast-food restaurants are not alone in serving large portions. Most sit-down restaurants also serve large meals, which may include bread with butter, a salad with dressing, sides of vegetables and potatoes, and free refills of sugar-filled drinks. Combined with a high-fat appetizer like potato skins, fried onions, fried mozzarella sticks, or buffalo wings, it is easy to eat more than 2,000 kcal at one meal!

The Healthful Way to Eat Out

Does this mean that eating out cannot be a part of a healthful diet? Not necessarily. Most restaurants, even fast-food restaurants, offer lower-Calorie, lower-fat menu items that you can choose. For instance, eating a regular McDonald's hamburger, a small order of french fries, and a diet beverage or water provides 480 kcal and 20 g of fat (37.5% of kcal from fat). To provide some vegetables for the day, you could add a side salad with low-fat or nonfat salad dressing. Other fast-food restaurants also offer smaller portions, sandwiches made with whole-grain bread, grilled chicken or other lean meats, and side salads. Many sit-down restaurants offer "lite" menu items, such as grilled chicken and a variety of vegetables, which are usually a much better choice than eating from the regular menu.

Check out the **You Do the Math** box (page 60) for an example of how to make more healthful food choices when eating out. And for more suggestions on how to eat out in moderation, see the **Quick Tips** feature (page 61).

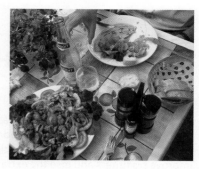

◀ Eating out can be a part of a healthful diet, if you are careful to choose wisely.

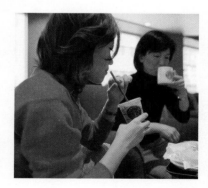

◀ When ordering your favorite coffee drink, avoid flavored syrups, cream, and whipping cream and request reduced-fat or skim milk instead.

recap Healthful ways to eat out include choosing smaller menu items, ordering meats that are grilled or broiled, avoiding fried foods, choosing items with steamed vegetables, avoiding energy-rich appetizers and desserts, and taking home for a later meal half of the food you are served.

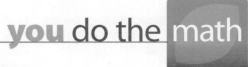

Determining the Healthiest Food Choices When Eating Out

Theo's friend and teammate, Jake, has put on extra weight over the basketball season. He had hoped to start more games this season, but their coach has made it clear that Jake needs to improve his fitness and lose the extra weight to be competitive as a starter.

Jake typically makes healthful food choices when he's on campus or at home, as he has a wide range of meals to choose from in the dining hall, and his family serves healthy foods when he visits them. But Jake really struggles to eat right when the team is on the road because they typically frequent fast-food outlets or sit-down restaurants that serve meals high in Calories, saturated fat, and salt. Jake knows that Theo is taking a nutrition class and asks him for help in selecting healthier menu items when they are ordering their meals on the road. Theo is happy to help. Fortunately, the fast-food restaurant where they stop for dinner has posted at the counter the nutrition values (Calories, total fat [g and %Daily Value], saturated fat [g and %Daily Value], and sodium [g]) for their menu items. They agree that Jake should order a chicken sandwich because Theo has learned that chicken has a much lower fat content than beef.

Jake's goal is to select food items that are lower in total Calories, % of Calories from fat, % of Calories from saturated fat, and sodium. As Theo examines these totals, he realizes that the %Daily Values for fat and saturated fat are based on a 2,000-Calorie-per-day intake—because Jake is a highly active male, this value is neither helpful nor appropriate. To determine the % of Calories from fat in the chicken sandwich, Theo does the following calculations:

a. Multiply the total fat (g) in the sandwich by 9 Calories (kcal)/g = 29 g × 9 Calories/g = 261 Calories from fat.

b. Divide the Calories from fat by the total Calories in the sandwich and multiply by 100 = (261 Calories ÷ 620 Calories) × 100 = 42% of total Calories from fat in the sandwich.

c. Multiply the saturated fat (g) in the sandwich by 9 Calories/g = 15 g × 9 Calories/g = 135 Calories from saturated fat.

d. Divide the Calories from saturated fat by total Calories in the sandwich = (135 Calories ÷ 620 Calories) = 21.8% of total Calories from saturated fat in the sandwich.

After thinking about these figures for % of Calories from fat and saturated fat, Jake decides to select a healthier sandwich that is lower in fat. He selects a grilled chicken club sandwich because it has only 460 Calories, 16 g of fat, and 6 g of saturated fat.

Now you do the math to calculate the % total Calories from fat and % total Calories from saturated fat in the grilled chicken club sandwich.

What other changes could Jake make to his menu selections to reduce his total intake of Calories, fat, saturated fat, and sodium?

The menu items that Jake selected are

Menu Item	Calories	Total Fat (g)	Total Fat (% Daily Value)	Saturated Fat (g)	Saturated Fat (% Daily Value)	Sodium (g)
Chicken club sandwich	620	29	45%	15	37%	1,200
Large french fries	500	25	38%	3.5	17%	350
Ketchup (4 packets)	60	0	0%	0	0%	440
Side salad	20	0	0%	0	0%	10
Salad dressing (1 packet)	170	15	23%	2.5	12%	530
Total	1,370	69	Not applicable	21	Not applicable	2,530

QuickTips

Eating Right When You're Eating Out

- Avoid all-you-can-eat buffet-style restaurants.

- Avoid appetizers that are breaded, fried, or filled with cheese or meat, or skip the appetizer altogether.

- Order a healthful appetizer instead of a larger meal as an entrée.

- Order your meal from the children's menu.

- Share an entrée with a friend.

- Order broth-based soups instead of cream-based soups.

- If you order meat, select a lean cut and ask that it be grilled or broiled rather than fried or breaded.

- Instead of a beef burger, order a chicken burger, fish burger, or veggie burger.

- Order a meatless dish filled with vegetables and whole grains. Avoid dishes with cream sauces and a lot of cheese.

- Order a salad with low-fat or nonfat dressing served on the side.

- Order steamed vegetables on the side instead of potatoes or rice. If you order potatoes, make sure to get a baked potato (with very little butter or sour cream on the side).

- Order beverages with few or no Calories, such as water, tea, or diet drinks. Avoid coffee drinks made with syrups as well as those made with cream, whipping cream, or whole milk.

- Don't feel you have to eat everything you're served. If you feel full, take the rest home for another meal.

- Skip dessert or share one dessert with a lot of friends, or order fresh fruit for dessert.

- Watch out for those "yogurt parfaits" offered at some fast-food restaurants. Many are loaded with sugar, fat, and Calories.

> For additional tips on how to make healthier choices when eating out, click on **www.today.msnbc.msn.com** and enter "ways to make eating out a healthy experience" into the search box for details.

✳**behavior change**… getting started!

Now that you've read this chapter, try making these changes:

For yourself:

- Read the Nutrition Facts panel of your favorite snacks and change your usual selections to ones that are lower in sodium, total fat, or saturated fat.
- Log on to the MyPlate website (see Web Resources) and design a healthy food plan that will help you maintain your present weight or lose weight.
- Follow the Mediterranean Diet for one full day and see how you like it!

For your community:

- Offer to teach your family and friends how to read food labels to help them make healthier choices.
- Approach the manager of your campus dining hall or favorite restaurant and inquire about his or her willingness to provide nutrition information for all menu items.

Will MyPlate Promote America's Health?

The Dietary Guidelines for Americans (DGAs) were updated in 2010, and the accompanying (MyPlate) graphic and website (www.chooseMyPlate.gov) were released in 2011 to replace the previous MyPyramid versions. But is MyPlate an improvement over MyPyramid, and will these revised tools halt the current obesity epidemic?

A recent editorial written by experts in public health nutrition highlights some of the progress that has been achieved in the revised DGAs and MyPlate:[9]

- More extensive use of high-quality evidence in developing the Guidelines
- Increased emphasis on eating more legumes and other vegetables, fruits, whole grains, and nuts
- Suggestions to replace red meat with fish and chicken
- Greater attention to replacing unhealthy fats with healthy fats

However, concerns about the limitations of these revised Guidelines and tools continue. These include the following:

- The new Guidelines still recommend that half of the grains we eat should be whole grains, and this continues to support eating half of our grains from refined, low-fiber sources. Some experts feel that the quality of the carbohydrates we consume needs more attention and specific guidance.[9]
- The new Guidelines recommend that Americans consume at least 3 servings of dairy foods per day. Some experts feel that this level of dairy consumption is unnecessary because some evidence suggests that dairy intake may not reduce the risk for bone fractures and could be associated with increased risk for ovarian and prostate cancers.[9,10]
- Although the revised Guidelines focus on reducing solid fats and added sugars, more targeted advice against the consumption of red meat, butter, cheese, and sugar may be needed to help people improve their dietary patterns.
- Although the DGAs address the benefits of regular physical activity, MyPlate does not illustrate this in any way. Some experts consider this a major oversight.

Given these limitations, it is unclear whether the revised DGAs and MyPlate can halt the current obesity epidemic or promote public health. Although the revisions are grounded in science, more research is needed on the impact of foods, rather than individual nutrients, on health outcomes. Such research should then inform the development of future recommendations. Experts have also called for moving the development of the Guidelines to the Centers for Disease Control and Prevention to avoid conflicts of interest that may arise within the USDA. They also recommend increased funding to allow for more frequent updates of nutrition information, including the DRIs, comprehensive reviews of current nutrition research, and recommendations about foods that should be avoided or reduced in the diet.[9]

Two alternative graphics to MyPlate have been developed: 1) The Harvard School of Public Health has developed a Healthy Eating Plate; and 2) The Physicians Committee for Responsible Medicine has proposed the Power Plate. (See Web Resources at the end of this chapter for the URLs.) Following the design of MyPlate, the Healthy Eating Plate highlights using healthy oils, consuming virtually all grains as whole grains, selecting healthy protein sources, and drinking water, tea, or coffee with little or no added sugar. It also emphasizes daily physical activity. The Power Plate emphasizes fruits, vegetables, whole grains, and legumes. Because the release of MyPlate and these alternatives has been so recent, no studies are yet available comparing their effectiveness in reducing risks for obesity and related chronic diseases.

As you can imagine, a great deal of time, effort, and money was invested in the new message, content, and design of MyPlate. In making this investment, nutrition experts at the USDA intend that MyPlate will help reduce the alarmingly high obesity and chronic disease rates in the United States. The primary assumption made by these experts is that people will actually use MyPlate to design their diets. In fact, however, the extent to which people will use MyPlate in their daily lives is debatable. Experts in the Department of Health and Human Services intended that the more user-friendly graphic and food group organization of MyPlate would help Americans eat a more healthful diet and maintain a healthier body weight. But until more evidence of their impact on the rates of obesity and chronic disease is assessed, the debate about their value will continue.

CRITICAL THINKING QUESTIONS

1. Do you think that the MyPlate graphic and website will help you design a more healthful diet?
2. Do you think that MyPlate can help reduce our nation's rates of obesity and chronic diseases? Why or why not?

chapter **review**

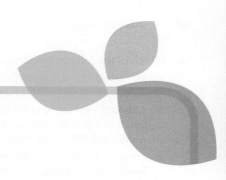

test yourself | answers

1. **False.** A healthful diet can be achieved by food alone; particular attention must be paid to adequacy, variety, moderation, and balance. However, some individuals may need to take vitamin supplements under certain circumstances.

2. **False.** The fact that something is stated on a food label doesn't guarantee it is true! Structure–function claims, such as "Supports healthy bones!" and "Promotes regularity!" are not regulated by the FDA and may or may not be backed with solid research evidence.

3. **False.** A cup of black coffee with a tablespoon of cream and a teaspoon of sugar has about 45 kcal. In contrast, a coffee mocha might contain from 350 to 500 kcal, depending on its size and precise contents.

MasteringNutrition™

Check out these additional resources in the MasteringNutrition Study Area at www.masteringhealthandnutrition.com:

- ▦ Read It: Chapter Summary and RSS Feeds
- ▦ See It: ABC News videos and nutrition animations
- ▦ Hear It: MP3s
- ▦ Study It: Get Ready for Nutrition Math and Chemistry review
- ▦ Do It: NutriTools and "Find the Quack" feature
- ▦ Review It: Quizzes, flashcards, and glossary

review questions

1. An adequate diet
   a. provides enough energy to meet minimum daily requirements.
   b. provides enough energy, nutrients, and fiber to maintain a person's health.
   c. provides a sufficient variety of nutrients to maintain a healthful weight and to optimize the body's metabolic processes.
   d. contains combinations of foods that provide healthful proportions of nutrients.

2. The Nutrition Facts panel identifies which of the following?
   a. all of the nutrients and Calories in the package of food
   b. the Recommended Dietary Allowance for each nutrient in the package of food
   c. a footnote identifying the Tolerable Upper Intake Level for each nutrient in the package of food
   d. the % Daily Values of select nutrients in a serving of the packaged food

3. The Dietary Guidelines for Americans recommend which of the following?
   a. choosing and preparing foods without salt
   b. consuming two alcoholic beverages per day
   c. replacing solid fats with vegetable oils
   d. following a vegetarian diet

4. Of the five food groups in MyPlate, which should make up half of your plate?
   a. grains
   b. vegetables
   c. fruits and dairy
   d. fruits and vegetables

5. An ounce-equivalent is
   a. a 1-ounce serving of bread, rice, or another grain, or a 1-ounce serving of a protein food.
   b. a serving that is 1 ounce or equivalent to an ounce for either grains or protein foods.
   c. a serving that is actually an ounce or is designated as a single serving on a food label for a grain or protein food.
   d. an ounce of a grain or protein food that you weigh and serve yourself.

6. Which of the following statements about MyPlate is true?

   a. MyPlate easily accommodates ethnic diets, vegetarian diets, and other healthful dietary variations.

   b. Although MyPlate can be adapted for ethnic, vegetarian, and other dietary variations, it recommends that Americans follow the Mediterranean Diet.

   c. Because MyPlate includes separate protein and dairy foods groups, it cannot fully accommodate individuals following a vegan diet.

   d. As long as individuals eat in moderation to balance Calories, MyPlate can accommodate their dietary preferences.

7. Which of the following statements about eating out is true?

   a. Almost 45% of consumers surveyed eat out at least once a week.

   b. Living in a neighborhood with a large number of fast-food restaurants causes obesity.

   c. At fast-food restaurants, a large beverage can provide a greater number of Calories than a hamburger.

   d. None of the above is true.

8. **True or false?** Structure–function claims on food labels must be approved by the FDA.

9. **True or false?** Empty Calories are the extra amount of energy a person can consume after meeting all essential needs through eating nutrient-dense foods.

10. **True or false?** The USDA classifies beans, peas, and lentils in both the vegetables group and the protein foods group.

math review

11. Hannah goes to a sandwich shop near the university at least once a week to buy what she considers a healthy lunch, which includes a chicken breast sandwich, garden salad (with Ranch dressing), and a diet cola. Recently, the shop started posting the Calorie and fat content of its menu items. Hannah discovers the following about the Calorie and fat content of the items in her "healthy lunch":

    • Chicken sandwich—317 Calories, 4 g fat

    • Garden salad—49 Calories, 1 g fat

    • Ranch dressing (1 packet)—280 Calories, 28 g fat

    • Diet cola—0 Calories, 0 g fat

    Based on this information, what is the total Calorie and fat content of Hannah's lunch? What is the percentage of Calories from fat for this lunch? Which food item is contributing the highest amount of fat to Hannah's lunch, and what can she do to make a healthier change to this lunch?

Answers to Review Questions and Math Review are located at the back of this text and in the MasteringNutrition Study Area.

web resources

www.fda.gov
U.S. Food and Drug Administration

Learn more about the government agency that regulates our food and first established regulations for nutrition information on food labels.

www.cnpp.usda.gov
2010 Dietary Guidelines for Americans

Use these guidelines to make changes in your food choices and physical activity habits to help reduce your risk for chronic disease. Scroll down to "dietaryguidelines" for details.

www.chooseMyPlate.gov
The USDA's MyPlate Home Page

Use the SuperTracker on this website to assess the overall quality of your diet and level of physical activity based on the USDA MyPlate.

www.diabetes.org
American Diabetes Association

Find out more about the nutritional needs of people living with diabetes as well as meal-planning exchange lists.

www.eatright.org
Academy of Nutrition and Dietetics

Visit the Public Information Center section of this website for additional resources to help you achieve a healthful lifestyle.

www.hsph.harvard.edu
Harvard School of Public Health

Scroll down to "nutritionsource" on this site to learn more about the Healthy Eating Plate, an alternative to the USDA MyPlate.

www.pcrm.org
Physicians Committee for Responsible Medicine

Visit this site to view the Power Plate, a vegetarian alternative to the USDA MyPlate. Scroll down to "health/diets/pplate/power-plate" for details.

in depth 2.5

Eating Wisely

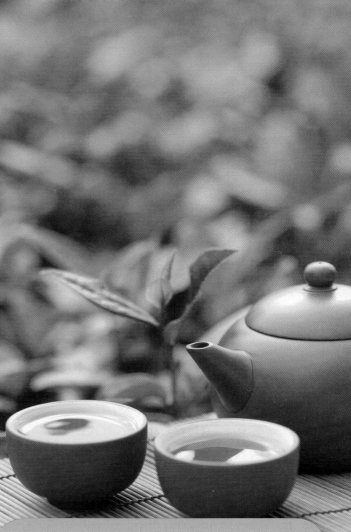

You've just finished dining at your favorite Thai restaurant. As you walk back to your car, you pass a bakery window displaying cakes and pies, each of which looks more enticing than the last, and through the open door wafts a complex aroma of coffee, cinnamon, and chocolate. You stop. You're not hungry, but you go inside and buy a slice of chocolate torte and an espresso anyway. Later that night, when the caffeine from the chocolate and espresso keeps you awake, you wonder why you succumbed.

Have you ever wondered what factors influence our food choices, and why we eat even when we aren't hungry? Here we take an **In Depth** look at what motivates our food choices, and provide an overview of tools you can use to help you eat more wisely.

learning objectives

After studying this In Depth, you should be able to:

1 Distinguish between hunger and appetite, p. 66.

2 Explain the role of sensory data; social, cultural, and emotional cues; and learning on appetite, pp. 66–67.

3 Identify two diet analysis programs and a government database that can be used to eat more wisely, pp. 68–69.

4 Define the concept of mindful eating and describe how it can be incorporated into a healthful eating plan, pp. 69–70.

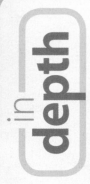

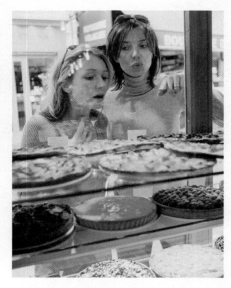

The sight, smell, and texture of foods stimulate our senses.

What's behind our food choices?

Two very different mechanisms induce us to seek food: hunger and appetite. Hunger is a basic biological urge to eat that occurs when our body senses that we need food. (The physiology of hunger is discussed fully in Chapter 3.) In contrast, **appetite** is a psychological desire to eat that is stimulated by the sight, smell, or thought of food. In the

opening scenario, it may have been hunger that influenced you to eat your Thai dinner . . . but it was appetite that stimulated your desire for dessert and espresso!

Whereas hunger is prompted by internal signals, appetite is triggered by aspects of our environment. The most significant factors influencing our appetite are sensory data; social, cultural, and emotional cues; and learning (**FIGURE 1**).

The Role of Sensory Data

Foods stimulate our five senses. Foods that are artfully prepared, arranged, or ornamented, with different shapes and colors, appeal to our sense of sight. The aromas of foods such as freshly brewed coffee and baked goods can also be powerful stimulants. **Olfaction**—our sense of smell—plays a key role in the stimulation of appetite and satiety.[1] Much of our ability to taste foods actually comes from our sense of smell. This is why foods are not as appealing when we have a stuffy nose. Certain tastes, such as sweetness, are almost universally appealing, while others, such as the astringent taste of some foods (for instance, spinach and kale), are quite individual. **Mouthfeel**, the tactile sensation of food in

---

appetite A psychological desire to consume specific foods.

olfaction Our sense of smell, which plays a key role in the stimulation of appetite and satiety.

mouthfeel The tactile sensation of food in the mouth; derived from the interaction of physical and chemical characteristics of the food.

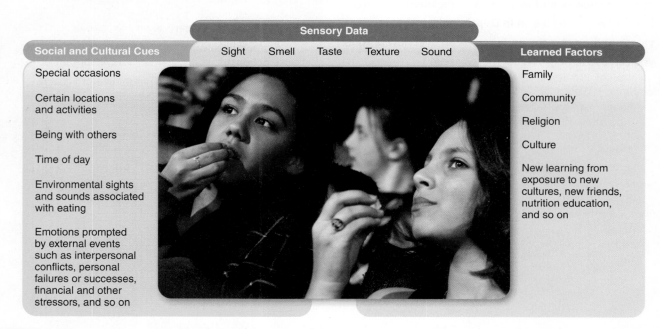

Social and Cultural Cues	Sensory Data					Learned Factors
	Sight	Smell	Taste	Texture	Sound	
Special occasions						Family
Certain locations and activities						Community
Being with others						Religion
Time of day						Culture
Environmental sights and sounds associated with eating						New learning from exposure to new cultures, new friends, nutrition education, and so on
Emotions prompted by external events such as interpersonal conflicts, personal failures or successes, financial and other stressors, and so on						

FIGURE 1 Appetite is a psychological drive to consume specific foods, such as wanting popcorn at the movies. It is aroused by social, cultural, and emotional cues and sensory data, and is influenced by learning.

the mouth, is also important in food choices because it stimulates nerve endings sensitive to touch in our mouth and on our tongue. Even our sense of hearing can be stimulated by foods, from the fizz of cola to the crunch of pretzels.

The Role of Social, Cultural, and Emotional Cues

In addition to sensory data, our brain's association with certain social events, such as birthday parties and holiday gatherings, can stimulate our appetite. At these times, our culture gives us permission to eat more than usual or to eat "forbidden" foods. Even when we feel full, these cues can motivate us to accept a second helping.

For some people, being in a certain location, such as at a baseball game or a movie theatre, can trigger appetite. Others may be influenced by activities such as watching television or at certain times of the day associated with mealtimes. Many people feel an increase or a decrease in appetite according to whom they are with; for example, they may want to eat more when at home with family members and less when out on a date.

The cultural group with which we identify strongly influences our food choices. A Japanese American, for example, might regularly cook with white rice, fish, and seaweed because these foods are readily available in, and part of the cuisine of, Japan. But even for recent immigrants, the dominant American food culture exerts a heavy influence in a variety of ways. These include the food advertisements we see every day, the types of restaurants in our community, and the availability of farm stands, farmer's markets, specialty markets, and supermarkets. The precise range of foods offered in these establishments dictates the variety of foods from which we can choose. The "culture" on a school campus can also encourage or discourage certain choices, inducing us to favor a popular brand of energy drink, for instance, or to snub the meals offered in the campus dining hall.

In some people, appetite masks an emotional response to an external event. For example, a person might experience a desire for food rather than a desire for emotional comfort after receiving a failing grade or arguing with a close friend. Many people crave food when they're frustrated, worried, or bored or when they're at a gathering where they feel anxious or awkward. Others subconsciously seek food as a "reward." For example, have you ever found yourself heading out for a burger and fries after turning in a term paper?

The Role of Learning

Pigs' feet, anyone? What about blood sausage, stewed octopus, eels, chicken feet, or tripe (the stomach lining of certain animals)? These are delicacies in various cultures around the world (as well as in some U.S. subcultures). Would you eat grasshoppers? If you'd grown up in certain parts of Africa or Central America, you might. That's because your preference

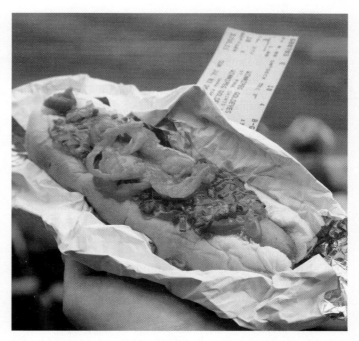

Certain locations or events, such as an outdoor baseball game at a stadium, can influence our appetite.

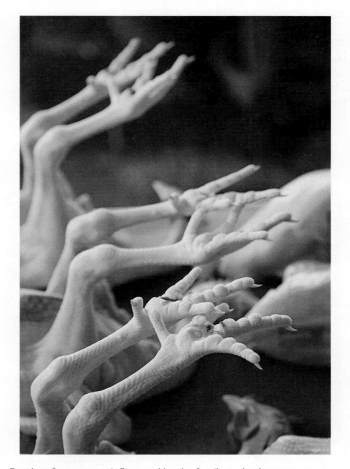

Food preferences are influenced by the family and culture you are raised in.

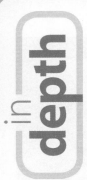

for particular foods is largely a learned response. The culture in which you are raised teaches you what plant and animal products are appropriate or desirable to eat. If your parents fed you cubes of plain tofu throughout your toddlerhood, then you are probably still eating tofu.

That said, early introduction to foods is not essential; we can learn to enjoy new foods at any point in our lives. For instance, you may never have tasted Ethiopian food before a restaurant opened in your neighborhood, but now it's your favorite cuisine. Many immigrants adopt a diet typical of their new home, especially when their traditional foods are not readily available (or they develop a blended diet of some of their traditional foods and foods found in their adopted country). This can also happen temporarily when traveling: the last time you were away from home, you probably looked forward to sampling dishes and foods that are not normally part of your diet.

Food preferences can also change when people learn what foods are most healthful. Chances are, as you learn more about the health benefits of specific types of carbohydrates, fats, and proteins, you'll start incorporating more of these foods in your diet.

We can also "learn" to dislike foods we once enjoyed. For example, a **conditioned taste aversion** to foods can occur as a result of illness, even if there is no relationship between the food and the illness. If we experience an episode of food poisoning after eating scrambled eggs, we might develop a strong distaste for all types of eggs.

Additionally, many adults who become vegetarians do so after learning about the treatment of animals in slaughterhouses: they might have eaten meat daily when young but no longer have any appetite for it.

Now that you understand the differences between appetite and hunger, as well as the influence of learning on food choices, you might be curious to investigate your own reasons for eating what and when you do. Use the **What About You?** box to find out if you eat in response to external or internal cues.

What tools can help us to eat more wisely?

You've learned how to design a healthful diet by reading food labels and following the Dietary Guidelines for Americans and the USDA Food Patterns. Here, we provide an overview of tools that can help you analyze your diet and determine the nutrient content of foods with or without labels. We also introduce you to the practice of mindful eating, which can help you to control your appetite and develop a more healthy relationship with food.

Take Advantage of Technology to Help You Analyze Your Diet

Many diet analysis programs are available to help you evaluate the quality of your diet. One example of a web-based tool available to the public is MyPlate Supertracker (see Web Resources at the end of this chapter). This tool allows you to analyze your current dietary intake and physical activity and to create personalized healthy eating and physical activity plans. It also provides access to information on the nutrient content of over 8,000 foods as well as tips to support you in making healthier choices. Using MyPlate Supertracker, you can track your current food intake and physical activity and compare it to targets you've set.

Students using this textbook also have access to MyDietAnalysis, a diet analysis software package developed by the nutrition database experts at ESHA Research. MyDietAnalysis is tailored for use in college nutrition courses, and it features a database of nearly 20,000 foods and multiple report options. This program is accurate, reliable, and easy-to-use in calculating the quality of your dietary intake.

In addition, anyone can access the U.S. Department of Agriculture's Nutrient Database for Standard Reference to find nutrient information on over 8,000 foods (see Web Resources at the end of this chapter). You can also

nutri-case | JUDY

"Ever since I was diagnosed with type 2 diabetes, I've felt like there's a 'food cop' always spying on me. Sometimes I feel like I have to look over my shoulder when I pull into the Dunkin' Donuts parking lot. My doctor says I'm supposed to eat fresh fruits and vegetables, fish, brown bread, brown rice . . . but I didn't tell him I don't like that stuff, and I don't have the money to buy it or the time to cook it even if I did. Besides, that kind of diet is for movie stars. All the real people I know eat the same way I do."

What do you think? Is the diet Judy's doctor described really just for movie stars and celebrities? Of the many factors influencing why and what we eat, identify at least two that might be affecting Judy's food choices. If you were to learn that Judy had not finished high school, would that fact have any bearing on your answer? If so, in what way?

conditioned taste aversion Avoidance of a food as a result of a negative experience, such as illness, even if the illness has no relationship with the food consumed.

Do You Eat in Response to External or Internal Cues?

Whether you're trying to lose weight, gain weight, or maintain your current weight, you might find it intriguing to keep a log of the reasons behind your decisions about what, when, where, and why you eat. Are you eating in response to internal sensations telling you that your body needs food, or in response to your emotions, your situation, or a prescribed diet? Keeping a "cues" log for 1 full week would give you the most accurate picture of your eating habits, but even logging 2 days of meals and snacks should increase your cue awareness.

Each day, every time you eat a meal, snack, or beverage other than water, make a quick note of the following:

- **When you eat:** Many people eat at certain times (for example, 6 PM) whether they are hungry or not.
- **What you eat, and how much:** Do you choose a cup of yogurt and a 6-oz glass of orange juice or a candy bar and a 20-oz cola?
- **Where you eat:** At home, watching television; on the subway; and so on.
- **With whom you eat:** Are you alone or with others? If with others, are they also eating? Have they offered you food?
- **Your emotions:** Some people overeat when they are happy, others when they are anxious, depressed, bored, or frustrated. Still others eat as a way of denying feelings they don't want to identify and deal with. For some, food becomes a substitute for emotional fulfilment.
- **Your sensations—what you see, hear, or smell:** Are you eating because you just saw a TV commercial for pizza, or smelled homemade cookies?

- **Any dietary restrictions:** Are you choosing a particular food because it is allowed on your current diet plan? Or are you hungry for a meal but drinking a diet soda to stay within a certain allowance of Calories? Are you restricting yourself because you feel guilty about having eaten too much at another time?
- **Your physiologic hunger:** Finally, rate your hunger on a scale from 1 to 5 as follows:
  - 1 = you feel uncomfortably full or even stuffed
  - 2 = you feel satisfied but not uncomfortably full
  - 3 = neutral; you feel no discernible satiation or hunger
  - 4 = you feel hungry and want to eat
  - 5 = you feel strong physiologic sensations of hunger and need to eat

After keeping a log for 2 or more days, you might become aware of patterns you'd like to change. For example, maybe you notice that you often eat when you are not actually hungry but are worried about homework or personal relationships. Or maybe you notice that you can't walk past the snack bar without going in. This self-awareness may prompt you to change those patterns. For instance, instead of stifling your worries with food, you could write down exactly what you are worried about, including steps you can take to address your concerns. And the next time you approach the snack bar, you could check with your gut: are you truly hungry? If so, then purchase a healthful snack, maybe a piece of fruit or a bag of peanuts. If you're not really hungry, then take a moment to acknowledge the strength of this visual cue—and then walk on by.

search on a specific nutrient (for instance, iron) to find out how much of that nutrient is present in a vast number of foods. The database even provides information on components of foods that are not classified as essential nutrients and are thus not typically included in diet analysis programs. These include, for example, caffeine, certain phytochemicals, and binders like oxalic acid that can inhibit nutrient absorption. The USDA's Nutrient Database is updated annually, and any errors are identified, corrected, and highlighted for users.

Apply the Principles of Mindful Eating

When you eat, how much do you think about what you are eating, especially how it smells, tastes, and feels? Do you typically rush through your meals or eat on the go? If you completed the **What About You?** feature (above), you've gained an increased awareness of what, why, and with

whom you eat. How can you use this increased awareness to eat more wisely, and possibly even benefit your health?

The concept of *mindfulness* refers to the nonjudgmental awareness of the present moment. The links between mindfulness and reduced stress were initially promoted by Dr. Jon Kabat-Zinn, a medical doctor who began teaching Mindfulness-Based Stress Reduction (MBSR) techniques in the late 1970s. Mindfulness is a learned skill that is associated with reduced stress, anxiety, and chronic pain, and improved immune function.[2,3]

Interest has been growing about the effects of applying mindfulness to our eating practices. **Mindful eating**

mindful eating The nonjudgmental awareness of the emotional and physical sensations one experiences while eating or in a food-related environment.

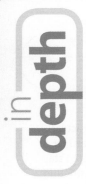

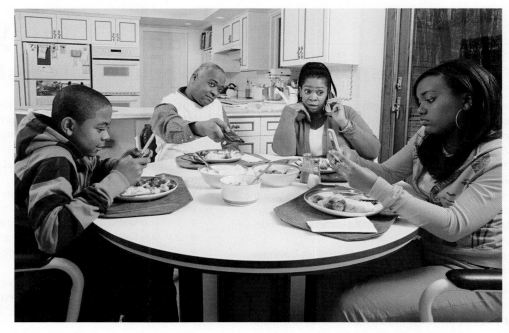

The concept of mindful eating means being present in the moment while consuming food, and concentrating on your emotional and physical sensations.

refers to a nonjudgmental awareness of the emotional and physical sensations one experiences while eating or in a food-related environment.[4] Because this is a relatively new area of research, there is limited information on the effectiveness of mindful eating on our health. However, several recently published pilot studies conducted with small numbers of participants have indicated that mindful eating may help to promote healthy eating practices when eating out; enhance weight loss and psychological well-being in people with obesity; and improve dietary intake and blood glucose control in adults with type 2 diabetes.[5–7]

Interested in exploring mindful eating practices? The **Quick Tips** box (shown here) can help get you started.

Incorporating mindful eating into your life doesn't have to be a chore. Try practicing mindful eating during one meal each week. With practice, you may be inspired to do it more often!

Quick Tips

Eating Mindfully

Focus only on eating: Turn off the television, put away your cell phone, tune out distractions, and focus on your food and the process of eating.

Savor each bite: Take your time, slow down, and chew slowly.

Recruit all of your senses: Focus your attention on the smell, taste, texture, and even the temperature of your food. Pay attention to any sensations of satisfaction or fullness.

Pause and rest between bites: Take a few breaths, sit back, and relax between each mouthful of food.

Try 10 minutes of silence: If eating with others, try to avoid conversations in order to enhance your ability to be more aware of your food and the experience of eating.

MasteringNutrition™

web resources

www.eatright.org
Academy of Nutrition and Dietetics

Explore a range of tips to help you eat more healthfully during holidays.

www.womenshealth.gov
womenshealth.gov

Visit this website to learn more about tools for eating wisely developed by the U.S. Departments of Health and Human Services and Agriculture. Click on "fitness nutrition" and then "how to eat for health" in the search box.

www.tcme.org
The Center for Mindful Eating

Learn more about the principles, practices, and potential benefits of mindful eating.

www.choosemyplate.gov
MyPlate Supertracker

Use this tool to develop a personalized food and physical activity plan, to analyze your current nutrient intake, and get tips to support healthy food choices. Search on "supertracker" once you get to the main website page.

www.ars.usda.gov
USDA National Nutrient Database for Standard Reference

To examine the nutrient content of over 8,000 foods, enter "nutrient database standard reference" into the home page search bar, then click on the top-most link on the page that appears.

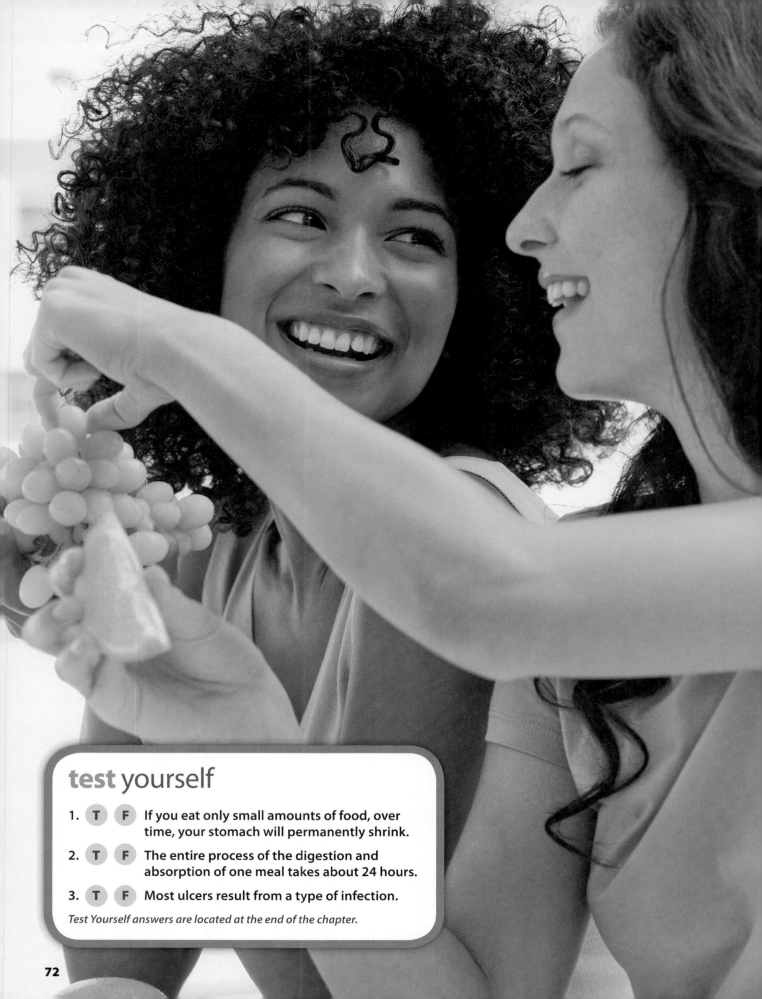

test yourself

1. **T** **F** If you eat only small amounts of food, over time, your stomach will permanently shrink.

2. **T** **F** The entire process of the digestion and absorption of one meal takes about 24 hours.

3. **T** **F** Most ulcers result from a type of infection.

Test Yourself answers are located at the end of the chapter.

The Human Body
Are we really what we eat?

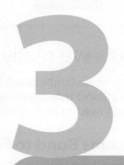

3

Two months ago, Andrea's lifelong dream of becoming a lawyer came one step closer to reality: she moved out of her parents' home in the Midwest to attend law school in Boston. Unfortunately, adjusting to a new city and new friends, and her intensive course work, has been more stressful than she'd imagined, and Andrea has been experiencing insomnia and exhaustion. What's more, her always "sensitive stomach" has been getting worse: after almost every meal, she gets cramps so bad she can't stand up, and twice she has missed classes because of sudden attacks of pain and diarrhea. She suspects that the problem is related to stress and wonders if she is going to experience it throughout her life. She is even thinking of dropping out of school if that would make her feel well again.

Almost everyone experiences brief episodes of abdominal pain, diarrhea, or other symptoms from time to time. Such episodes are usually caused by an infection. But do you know anyone who experiences these symptoms periodically for days, weeks, or even years? If so, has it made you wonder why? What are the steps in normal digestion and absorption of food, and at what points can the process break down?

We begin this chapter with a look at the contribution of the foods we eat to the cells of our body. We'll then discuss the physiology of hunger and the processes by which the body digests and absorbs food and eliminates waste. Finally, we'll look at some disorders that affect these processes.

MasteringNutrition™

Go online for chapter quizzes, pre-tests, Interactive Activities, and more!

Are we really what we eat?

You've no doubt heard the saying "You are what you eat." Is this scientifically true? To answer that question, and to better understand how we digest and process foods, we'll need to look at how our body is organized (**FIGURE 3.1**).

Atoms Bond to Form Molecules

Like all substances on earth, our body is made up of atoms. Atoms are tiny units of matter that cannot be broken down by natural means. Atoms almost constantly bind to each other in nature. When they do, they form groups called molecules. For example, a molecule of water is composed of two atoms of hydrogen and an atom of oxygen, which is abbreviated H_2O.

Not only the liquids we drink, but every bite of food we eat is composed of molecules. Rice, for instance, is composed of atoms of carbon, hydrogen, and oxygen grouped into large carbohydrate molecules. The actions of digestion break food down into molecules small enough to be absorbed easily through the wall of the intestine and transported in the bloodstream to every part of the body. We convert these molecules into the energy we need to live. We also use these molecules to help maintain supplies of the chemicals our body needs and to build, maintain, and repair our body structures. The smallest of these structures are the components of individual body cells.

Molecules Join to Form Cells

cell The smallest unit of matter that exhibits the properties of living things, such as growth, reproduction, and metabolism.

Cells are the smallest units of life. That is, cells can grow, reproduce, and perform certain basic functions, such as taking in nutrients, producing chemicals, and excreting wastes. The human body is composed of billions of cells, many of which

▶ **FIGURE 3.1** The organization of the human body. Atoms bind together to form molecules, and the body's cells are composed of molecules of the food we eat. Cells join to form tissues, one or more types of which form organs, such as the small intestine. Body systems, such as the gastrointestinal system, are made up of several organs, each of which performs a discrete function within that system.

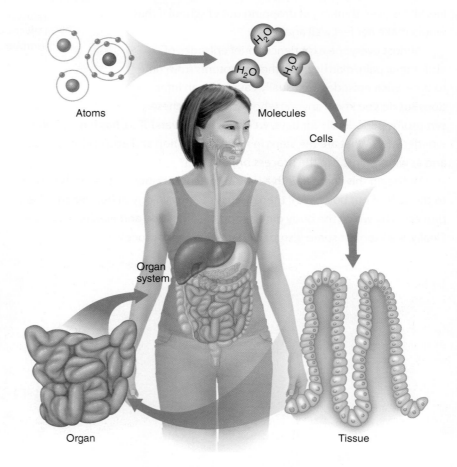

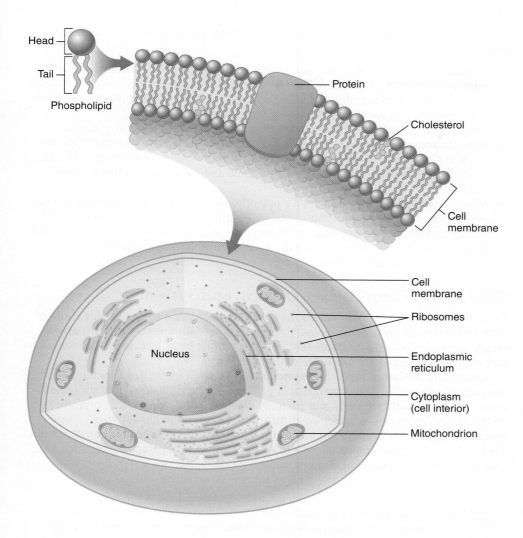

FIGURE 3.2 Representative enterocyte, showing the cell membrane, cytoplasm, and a variety of organelles. The cell membrane is a double layer of phospholipid molecules, aligned such that the lipid tails form a water-repellant interior, whereas the phosphate heads interact with the fluids inside and outside the cell. The fluid inside the cell is the cytoplasm. Within it are many different organelles.

have short life spans and must be replaced continually. For example, **enterocytes**, the cells lining the intestine, live only a few days (*entero-* is a prefix referring to the intestine, and *-cyte* means cell). To support this demand for new cells, we need a ready supply of nutrient molecules to serve as building blocks. All cells, whether of the intestine, bones, or brain, are made of the same basic nutrient molecules, which are derived from the foods we eat.

Cells Are Encased in a Functional Membrane

Cells are encased by a thin covering called a **cell membrane** (FIGURE 3.2). This membrane defines the cell's boundaries: it encloses the cell's contents and acts as a gatekeeper, either allowing or denying the entry and exit of molecules, such as nutrients and wastes.

Cell membranes are composed of two layers of molecules called phospholipids, which consist of a long lipid "tail" that repels water, bound to a round phosphate "head" that interacts with water. Located throughout the membrane are molecules of another lipid, cholesterol, which helps keep the membrane flexible. The membrane is also studded with various proteins, which assist in the gatekeeper function, allowing the transport of nutrients and other substances across the cell membrane.

Cells Contain Organelles, Which Support Life

The cell membrane encloses the semiliquid **cytoplasm** (see Figure 3.2), which includes a variety of **organelles**. These tiny structures accomplish some surprisingly sophisticated functions. A full description of all the organelles and their roles is

enterocytes The cells lining the wall of the intestine.

cell membrane The boundary of an animal cell that separates its internal cytoplasm and organelles from the external environment.

cytoplasm The interior of an animal cell, not including its nucleus.

organelle A tiny "organ" within a cell that performs a discrete function necessary to the cell.

beyond the scope of this book. In terms of nutrition, the most important are the following:

- **Nucleus.** The nucleus is where our genetic information, in the form of deoxyribonucleic acid (DNA), is located. The cell nucleus is darkly colored because DNA is a huge molecule that is tightly packed within it. A cell's DNA contains the instructions that the cell uses to make certain proteins.
- **Ribosomes.** Ribosomes use the instructions from DNA to assemble proteins.
- **Endoplasmic reticulum (ER).** Proteins assembled on the ribosomes enter this network of channels and are further processed and packaged for transport. The ER is also responsible for the breakdown of lipids and for storage of the mineral calcium.
- **Mitochondria.** Often called the cell's powerhouses, mitochondria produce the energy molecule adenosine triphosphate (ATP) from basic food components. ATP can be thought of as a stored form of energy that can be drawn upon as we need it. Cells that have high energy needs—such as muscle cells—contain more mitochondria than do cells with low energy needs.

Cells Join to Form Tissues, Organs, and Systems

Cells of a single type, such as enterocytes, join to form functional sheets or cords of cells called **tissues**. In general, several types of tissues join together to form **organs**, which are sophisticated structures that perform unique body functions. The stomach and the small intestine are examples of organs.

Organs are further grouped into **systems** that perform integrated functions. The stomach, for example, is an organ that is part of the gastrointestinal system (*gastro-* refers to the stomach). It holds and partially digests a meal, but it can't perform all the system functions—digestion, absorption, and elimination—by itself. These functions require the cooperation of several organs. In the next section, we'll see how the organs of the gastrointestinal system work together to accomplish digestion and absorption of food and elimination of waste.

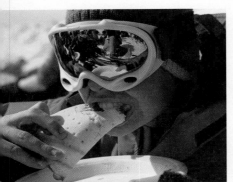

⬆ Hunger is a physiologic stimulus that prompts us to find food and eat.

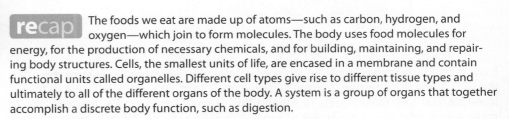

recap The foods we eat are made up of atoms—such as carbon, hydrogen, and oxygen—which join to form molecules. The body uses food molecules for energy, for the production of necessary chemicals, and for building, maintaining, and repairing body structures. Cells, the smallest units of life, are encased in a membrane and contain functional units called organelles. Different cell types give rise to different tissue types and ultimately to all of the different organs of the body. A system is a group of organs that together accomplish a discrete body function, such as digestion.

Why do we feel the urge to eat?

Two mechanisms prompt us to seek food: appetite and hunger. Whereas appetite is a desire to eat that is stimulated by the sight, smell, or thought of food, **hunger** is a physiologic drive to eat that occurs when our body senses that we need food.[1] If you've recently finished a nourishing meal, then hunger won't compel you toward dessert. Instead, the culprit is appetite, which we commonly experience in the absence of hunger. On the other hand, it is possible to have a physiologic need for food yet have no appetite. This state, called **anorexia**, can accompany a variety of illnesses, from infectious diseases to mood disorders. It can also occur as a side effect of certain medications, such as the chemotherapy used in treating cancer patients.

The Hypothalamus Regulates Hunger

Because hunger is a physiologic stimulus that drives us to find food and eat, we often feel it as a negative or unpleasant sensation. The primary organ producing that sensation is the brain. That's right—it's not our stomach but our brain that tells us

tissue A grouping of like cells that performs a function; for example, muscle tissue.

organ A body structure composed of two or more tissues and performing a specific function; for example, the esophagus.

system A group of organs that work together to perform a unique function; for example, the gastrointestinal system.

hunger A physiologic drive for food.

anorexia An absence of appetite.

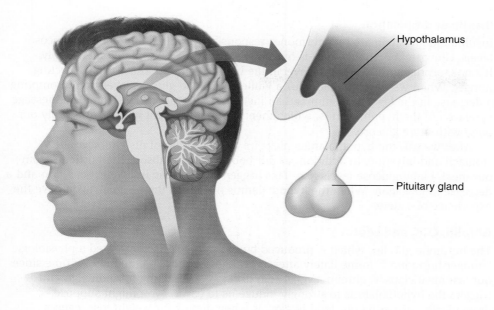

FIGURE 3.3 The hypothalamus triggers hunger by integrating signals from nerve cells throughout the body as well as from messages carried by hormones.

Hypothalamus

Pituitary gland

when we're hungry. The region of brain tissue responsible for prompting us to seek food is called the **hypothalamus** (**FIGURE 3.3**). It's located above the pituitary gland in the forebrain, a region that regulates many types of involuntary activity.

The hypothalamus contains a cluster of nerve cells known collectively as the *feeding center*. Stimulation of the feeding center triggers feelings of hunger that drive us to eat. In contrast, signals from a cluster of cells called the *satiety center* (**satiety** means fullness) inhibit the feeding center cells. This prompts us to stop eating.

The feeding and satiety centers work together to regulate food intake by integrating signals from three sources: nerve cells in the gastrointestinal system, chemicals called *hormones,* and the amount and type of food we eat. Let's review these three types of signals.

Nerve Cells in the Gastrointestinal System Signal the Hypothalamus

One important signal for both hunger and satiety comes from nerve cells lining the stomach and small intestine. These cells detect changes in pressure according to whether the organ is empty or distended with food. The cells then relay these data to the hypothalamus. For instance, if you have not eaten for many hours and your stomach and small intestine do not contain food, signals transmitted to the hypothalamus will suppress the satiety center, allowing the feeding center to dominate. This in turn will cause you to experience the sensation of hunger.

Nerve cells in the mouth, pharynx (throat), and esophagus (the tube leading to the stomach) also contribute to our feelings of hunger and satiety. Chewing and swallowing food, for example, stimulates these nerve cells, which then relay data to the satiety center in the hypothalamus. As a result, we begin to feel full.

Hormones Send Chemical Messages to the Hypothalamus

Hormones are molecules, usually proteins or lipids, that are secreted into the bloodstream by one of the many *glands* of the body. In the bloodstream, they act as chemical messengers, binding to and triggering a response in target cells far away from the gland in which they were produced. The relative levels of different hormones in the blood help regulate many body functions. Of the many hormones involved in food intake, the following are the most significant.

hypothalamus A region of the forebrain above the pituitary gland, where visceral sensations, such as hunger and thirst, are regulated.

satiety A physiologic sensation of fullness (from the Latin *satis* meaning enough, as in *satisfied*).

hormone A chemical messenger secreted into the bloodstream by one of the many glands of the body, which acts as a regulator of physiologic processes at a site remote from the gland that secreted it.

Insulin and Glucagon

Insulin and glucagon are two hormones responsible for maintaining blood glucose levels. Glucose (a carbohydrate) is our body's most readily available fuel supply. It's not surprising, then, that its level in the blood is an important signal affecting hunger. When we have not eaten for a while, our blood glucose levels fall, prompting a decrease in the level of insulin and an increase in glucagon. This chemical message is relayed to the hypothalamus, which then prompts us to eat in order to supply our body with more glucose.

After we eat, the hypothalamus picks up the sensation of distention in the stomach and intestine. In addition, as our body begins to absorb the nutrients from our meal, blood glucose levels rise. This triggers an increase in insulin secretion and a decrease in glucagon. When the hypothalamus integrates these signals, you have the experience of satiety.

Ghrelin, CCK, and Leptin

The hormone ghrelin, which is produced by the stomach, is considered a physiologic "hunger hormone."[2] Immediately after a meal, ghrelin levels plummet. As time since our last meal elapses, ghrelin levels begin to rise. A fast-acting hormone, ghrelin triggers the hypothalamus to strongly induce us to eat. As you might suppose, dramatically restricting our food intake, as when dieting for weight loss, causes ghrelin levels to surge.

Opposite in action to ghrelin is the hormone cholecystokinin (CCK), which is produced in the small intestine in response to food entry. CCK causes the transmission of signals to the hypothalamus that trigger satiety, reducing both how long we eat and how much.[2]

The hormones we've discussed so far act in short-term regulation of food intake. But our body produces other hormones that regulate food intake over time. One of the most important of these is leptin, a protein hormone produced by our adipose cells (fat cells). When we consume more Calories than we burn, the extra Calories are converted to fat and stored in adipose tissue. The more adipose tissue our body carries, the more leptin we produce. Leptin acts on the feeding and satiety centers of the hypothalamus to suppress hunger. Unfortunately, obese people appear to be leptin-resistant; therefore, attempts to administer leptin to help them reduce food intake and lose weight have not been successful.[2] (For more information about the role of hormones in weight management, see Chapter 11.)

The Amount and Type of Food Play a Role

Although the reason behind this observation is not understood, researchers have long recognized that foods containing protein have the highest satiety value.[3] This means that a ham and egg breakfast will cause us to feel satiated for a longer period than will pancakes with maple syrup, even if both meals have exactly the same number of Calories.

Another factor affecting hunger is how bulky the meal is—that is, how much fiber and water is within the food. Bulky meals tend to stretch the stomach and small intestine, which send signals back to the hypothalamus telling us that we are full, so we stop eating. Beverages tend to be less satisfying than semisolid foods, and semisolid foods have a lower satiety value than solid foods. For example, if you were to eat a bunch of grapes, you would feel a greater sense of fullness than if you drank a glass of grape juice providing the same number of Calories.

recap Hunger is a drive to eat triggered by the physiologic need for food. The feeding and satiety centers in the hypothalamus regulate food intake in response to cues about stomach and intestinal distention and the levels of certain hormones. High-protein foods make us feel satiated for longer periods, and bulky meals fill us up quickly, causing the distention that signals us to stop eating.

What happens to the food we eat?

When we eat, the food is digested, then the useful nutrients are absorbed, and, finally, the waste products are eliminated. But what does each of these processes really entail? In the simplest terms, **digestion** is the process by which foods are broken down into their component molecules, either mechanically or chemically. **Absorption** is the process of taking these products of digestion through the wall of the small intestine into the circulation. **Elimination** is the process by which the remaining waste is removed from the body.

Digestion, absorption, and elimination occur in the **gastrointestinal (GI) tract**, the organs of which work together to process foods. The GI tract is a long tube: if held out straight, an adult GI tract would be close to 30 feet long. Food within this tube is digested into molecules small enough to be absorbed by the cells lining the GI tract and thereby passed into the bloodstream.

The GI tract begins at the mouth and ends at the anus **(FIGURE 3.4)**. It is composed of several distinct organs, including the mouth, esophagus, stomach, small intestine, and large intestine. The flow of food between these organs is controlled by muscular **sphincters**, which are tight rings of muscle that open when a nerve signal indicates that food is ready to pass into the next section. Surrounding the GI tract are several accessory organs, including the salivary glands, liver, pancreas, and gallbladder, each of which has a specific role in digestion and absorption.

Now let's take a look at the role of each of these organs in processing the food we eat. Imagine that you ate a turkey sandwich for lunch today. It contained two slices of bread spread with mayonnaise, some turkey, two lettuce leaves, and a slice of tomato. Let's travel along with the sandwich and see what happens as it enters your GI tract and is digested and absorbed into your body.

Digestion Begins in the Mouth

Believe it or not, the first step in the digestive process is not your first bite of that sandwich. It is your first thought about what you want for lunch and your first whiff of turkey and freshly baked bread as you stand in line at the deli. In this **cephalic phase** of digestion, hunger and appetite work together to prepare the GI tract to digest food. The nervous system stimulates the release of digestive juices in preparation for food entering the GI tract, and sometimes we experience some involuntary movement commonly called "hunger pangs."

Now let's stop smelling that sandwich and take a bite and chew! Chewing moistens the food and breaks it down into pieces small enough to swallow **(FIGURE 3.5)**. Thus, chewing initiates the mechanical digestion of food. The tough coating surrounding the lettuce fibers and tomato seeds is also broken open, facilitating digestion. This is especially important when we're eating foods that are high in fiber, such as grains, fruits, and vegetables. Chewing also mixes everything in your sandwich together: the protein in the turkey; the carbohydrates in the bread, lettuce, and tomato; the fat in the mayonnaise; and the vitamins, minerals, and water in all of the foods.

The presence of food in your mouth also initiates chemical digestion. As your teeth cut and grind the different foods in your sandwich, more surface area is exposed to the digestive juices in your mouth. Foremost among these is **saliva**, which you secrete from your **salivary glands**. Saliva not only moistens your food but also begins the process of chemical breakdown. One component of saliva, called *amylase*, starts the process of carbohydrate digestion. Saliva also contains other components, such as antibodies that protect the body from foreign bacteria entering the mouth and keep the oral cavity free from infection.

Salivary amylase is the first of many **enzymes** that assist the body in digesting and absorbing food. Because we will encounter enzymes throughout our journey through the GI tract, let's discuss them briefly here. Enzymes are small chemicals, usually proteins, that act on other chemicals to speed up body processes **(FIGURE 3.6)**. Imagine them as facilitators: a chemical reaction that might take an hour to occur independently might happen in a few seconds with the help of one or more

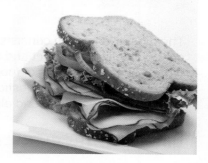

◆ Digestion of a sandwich starts before you even take a bite.

digestion The process by which foods are broken down into their component molecules, either mechanically or chemically.

absorption The physiologic process by which molecules of food are taken from the gastrointestinal tract into the circulation.

elimination The process by which undigested portions of food and waste products are removed from the body.

gastrointestinal (GI) tract A long, muscular tube consisting of several organs: the mouth, esophagus, stomach, small intestine, and large intestine.

sphincter A tight ring of muscle separating some of the organs of the GI tract and opening in response to nerve signals indicating that food is ready to pass into the next section.

cephalic phase The earliest phase of digestion, in which the brain thinks about and prepares the digestive organs for the consumption of food.

saliva A mixture of water, mucus, enzymes, and other chemicals that moistens the mouth and food, binds food particles together, and begins the digestion of carbohydrates.

salivary glands A group of glands found under and behind the tongue and beneath the jaw that release saliva continually as well as in response to the thought, sight, smell, or presence of food.

enzymes Small chemicals, usually proteins, that act on other chemicals to speed up body processes but are not apparently changed during those processes.

The digestive system consists of the organs of the gastrointestinal (GI) tract and associated accessory organs. The processing of food in the GI tract involves ingestion, mechanical digestion, chemical digestion, propulsion, absorption, and elimination.

ORGANS OF THE GI TRACT

MOUTH

Ingestion Food enters the GI tract via the mouth.

Mechanical digestion Mastication tears, shreds, and mixes food with saliva.

Chemical digestion Salivary amylase begins carbohydrate breakdown.

PHARYNX AND ESOPHAGUS

Propulsion Swallowing and peristalsis move food from mouth to stomach.

STOMACH

Mechanical digestion Mixes and churns food with gastric juice into a liquid called chyme.

Chemical digestion Pepsin begins digestion of proteins, and gastric lipase begins to break lipids apart.

Absorption A few fat-soluble substances are absorbed through the stomach wall.

SMALL INTESTINE

Mechanical Digestion and **Propulsion** Segmentation mixes chyme with digestive juices; peristaltic waves move it along tract.

Chemical digestion Digestive enzymes from pancreas and brush border digest most classes of nutrients.

Absorption Nutrients are absorbed into blood and lymph through enterocytes.

LARGE INTESTINE

Chemical digestion Some remaining food residues are digested by bacteria.

Absorption Reabsorbs salts, water, and vitamins.

Propulsion Compacts waste into feces and propels it toward the rectum.

RECTUM

Elimination Temporarily stores feces before voluntary release through the anus.

ACCESSORY ORGANS

SALIVARY GLANDS

Produce saliva, a mixture of water, mucus, enzymes, and other chemicals.

LIVER

Produces bile to emulsify fats.

GALLBLADDER

Stores bile before release into the small intestine through the bile duct.

PANCREAS

Produces digestive enzymes and bicarbonate, which are released into the small intestine via the pancreatic duct.

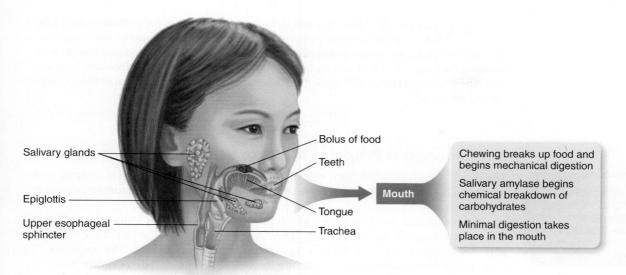

Salivary glands

Epiglottis

Upper esophageal sphincter

Bolus of food

Teeth

Tongue

Trachea

Mouth

Chewing breaks up food and begins mechanical digestion

Salivary amylase begins chemical breakdown of carbohydrates

Minimal digestion takes place in the mouth

◄ **FIGURE 3.5** Where your food is now: the mouth. Chewing moistens food and mechanically breaks it down into pieces small enough to swallow, while salivary amylase begins the chemical digestion of carbohydrates.

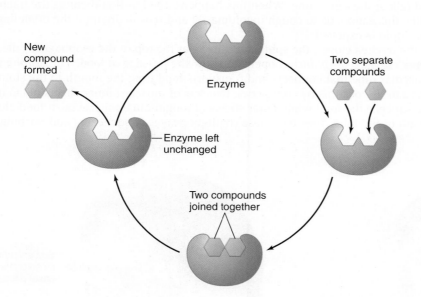

New compound formed

Enzyme

Two separate compounds

Enzyme left unchanged

Two compounds joined together

◄ **FIGURE 3.6** Enzymes speed up the body's chemical reactions, including many reactions essential to the digestion and absorption of food. Here, an enzyme joins two small compounds to create a larger compound. Notice that the enzyme itself is not changed in this process.

enzymes. Because they remain essentially unchanged by the chemical reactions they facilitate, enzymes can be reused repeatedly. The action of enzymes can result in the production of new substances or can assist in breaking substances apart. Our body makes hundreds of enzymes, and the process of digestion—as well as many other biochemical processes that go on in our body—could not happen without them. By the way, enzyme names typically end in –*ase* (as in *amylase*), so they are easy to recognize as we look at the digestive process.

In reality, very little digestion occurs in the mouth. This is because we do not hold food in the mouth for very long and because not all of the enzymes needed to break down food are present in saliva. Salivary amylase starts the digestion of carbohydrates in the mouth, and this digestion continues until food reaches the stomach. There, salivary amylase is destroyed by the acidic environment of the stomach.

recap Digestion, absorption, and elimination take place in the gastrointestinal (GI) tract. In the cephalic phase of digestion, hunger and appetite work together to prepare the GI tract for digestion and absorption. Chewing initiates mechanical digestion by breaking the food mass apart and mixing it together. The release of saliva moistens food and starts the process of chemical digestion of carbohydrates through the action of the enzyme salivary amylase.

The Esophagus Propels Food into the Stomach

The mass of food that has been chewed and moistened in the mouth is referred to as a **bolus**. This bolus is swallowed (**FIGURE 3.7**) and propelled to the stomach through the esophagus.

Most of us take swallowing for granted. However, it is a very complex process involving voluntary and involuntary motion. A tiny flap of tissue called the *epiglottis* acts as a trapdoor covering the entrance to the trachea (windpipe). The epiglottis is normally open, allowing us to breathe freely even while chewing (Figure 3.7a). As a food bolus moves to the very back of the mouth, the brain is sent a signal to temporarily raise the soft palate and close the openings to the nasal passages, preventing the aspiration of food or liquid into the sinuses (Figure 3.7b). The brain also signals the epiglottis to close during swallowing, so that food and liquid cannot enter the trachea.

Sometimes this protective mechanism goes awry—for instance, when we try to eat and talk at the same time. When this happens, food or liquid enters the trachea. Typically, this causes us to cough involuntarily and repeatedly until the offending food or liquid is expelled.

As the trachea closes, the sphincter muscle at the top of the esophagus, called the *upper esophageal sphincter*, opens to allow the passage of food. The **esophagus** is a muscular tube that connects and transports food from the mouth to the stomach (**FIGURE 3.8**). It does this by contracting two sets of muscles: inner sheets of circular muscle squeeze the food while outer sheets of longitudinal muscle push food along the length of the tube. Together, these rhythmic waves of squeezing and pushing are

To view a step-by-step animation of the complex process of swallowing, visit www.linkstudio.info. When the website link info is displayed on your search page, click on "Swallow," which takes you to the animated sequence.

bolus A mass of food that has been chewed and moistened in the mouth.

esophagus A muscular tube of the GI tract connecting the back of the mouth to the stomach.

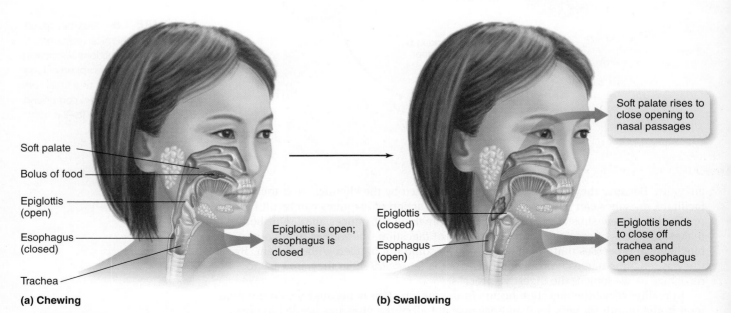

(a) Chewing

Soft palate
Bolus of food
Epiglottis (open)
Esophagus (closed)
Trachea

Epiglottis is open; esophagus is closed

(b) Swallowing

Soft palate rises to close opening to nasal passages

Epiglottis (closed)
Esophagus (open)

Epiglottis bends to close off trachea and open esophagus

FIGURE 3.7 Chewing and swallowing are complex processes. (a) During the process of chewing, the epiglottis is open and the esophagus is closed, so that we can continue to breathe as we chew. (b) During swallowing, the epiglottis closes, so that food does not enter the trachea and obstruct our breathing. Also, the soft palate rises to seal off our nasal passages to prevent the aspiration of food or liquid into the sinuses.

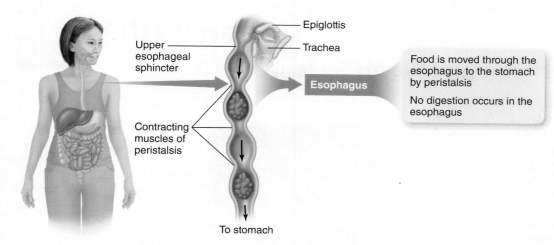

Upper esophageal sphincter

Epiglottis

Trachea

Esophagus

Food is moved through the esophagus to the stomach by peristalsis

No digestion occurs in the esophagus

Contracting muscles of peristalsis

To stomach

⬆ FIGURE 3.8 Where your food is now: the esophagus. Peristalsis, the rhythmic contraction and relaxation of both circular and longitudinal muscles in the esophagus, propels food toward the stomach. Peristalsis occurs throughout the GI tract.

called **peristalsis**. We will see later in this chapter that peristalsis occurs throughout the GI tract.

Gravity also helps transport food down the esophagus, which explains why it is wise to sit or stand upright while eating. Together, peristalsis and gravity can transport a bite of food from our mouth to the opening of the stomach in 5 to 8 seconds. At the end of the esophagus is a sphincter muscle, the *gastroesophageal sphincter*, which is normally tightly closed. When food reaches the end of the esophagus, this sphincter relaxes to allow the food to pass into the stomach. In some people, this sphincter is continually somewhat relaxed. Later in the chapter, we'll discuss this disorder and the unpleasant symptoms it causes.

The Stomach Mixes, Digests, and Stores Food

The **stomach** is a J-shaped organ. Its size varies with different individuals; in general, its volume is about 6 fluid ounces (or 3/4 cup) when it is empty. The stomach wall contains four layers, the innermost of which is crinkled into large folds called *rugae* that flatten progressively to accommodate food. This allows the stomach to expand to hold about 1 gallon of food and liquid.[4] As food is released into the small intestine, the rugae reform, and the stomach gradually returns to its baseline size.

Before any food reaches the stomach, the brain sends signals to the stomach to stimulate and prepare it to receive food. For example, the hormone *gastrin*, secreted by stomach-lining cells called *G cells*, stimulates gastric glands to secrete a digestive fluid referred to as **gastric juice**. Gastric glands are lined with two important types of cells—parietal cells and chief cells—that secrete the various components of gastric juice.

The parietal cells secrete:

- *Hydrochloric acid (HCl)*, which keeps the stomach interior very acidic. To be precise, the pH of HCl is 1.0, which means that it is ten times more acidic than pure lemon juice and a hundred times more acidic than vinegar! For a review of the calculations behind the pH scale, see the **You Do the Math** box (on page 84). The acidic environment of the stomach interior kills any bacteria and/or germs that may have entered the body with the sandwich. HCl is also extremely important for digestion because it starts to **denature** proteins, which means it breaks the bonds that maintain their structure. This is an essential preliminary step in protein digestion.
- *Intrinsic factor*, a protein critical to the absorption of vitamin B_{12} (discussed in more detail in Chapter 10). Vitamin B_{12} is present in the turkey.

peristalsis Waves of squeezing and pushing contractions that move food in one direction through the length of the GI tract.

stomach A J-shaped organ where food is partially digested, churned, and stored until it is released into the small intestine.

gastric juice Acidic liquid secreted within the stomach; it contains hydrochloric acid and other compounds.

denature The action of the unfolding of proteins in the stomach. Proteins must be denatured before they can be digested.

you do the math

Negative Logarithms and the pH Scale

Have you ever been warned that the black coffee, orange juice, or cola you enjoy is corroding your stomach? If so, relax. It's an urban myth. How can you know for sure? Take a look at the pH scale **(FIGURE 3.9)**. As you can see, the scale shows that hydrochloric acid (HCl) has a pH of 1.0 and gastric juice is 2.0, whereas soft drinks (including cola) are 3.0, orange juice is 4.0, and black coffee is 5.0. Not sure what all of these numbers mean?

An abbreviation for the *potential of hydrogen*, pH is a measure of the hydrogen ion concentration of a solution, or more precisely, the potential of a substance to release or to take up hydrogen ions in solution. Since an acid by definition is a compound that releases hydrogen ions, and a base (an alkali) is a compound that binds them, we can also say that pH is a measure of a compound's acidity or alkalinity. The precise measurements of pH range from 0 to 14, with 7.0 designated as pH neutral. Pure water is exactly neutral, and human blood is close to neutral, normally ranging from about 7.35 to 7.45.

The pH scale is a negative base-10 logarithmic scale. As you may recall from high school math classes, a base-10 logarithm ($\log_{10}$) tells you how many times you multiply by 10 to get the desired number. So for example, $\log_{10} (1000) = 3$ because to get 1000 you have to multiply 10 three times ($10 \times 10 \times 10$). The pH scale is a negative scale because an *increased* number on the scale identifies a corresponding *decrease* in concentration. These facts taken together mean that:

- for every increase of a single digit, the concentration of hydrogen ions decreases by tenfold.

- for every decrease of a single digit, the concentration of hydrogen ions increases by tenfold.

So, for example, milk has a pH of 6, which is one digit lower than 7. Milk is therefore ten times more acidic than pure water. Baking soda, at pH 9, is two digits higher than 7, and thus baking soda is 100 times less acidic than pure water: $2 = \log_{10}(100)$.

Now you do the math:

1. Is the pH of blood normally slightly acidic or slightly alkaline (basic)?

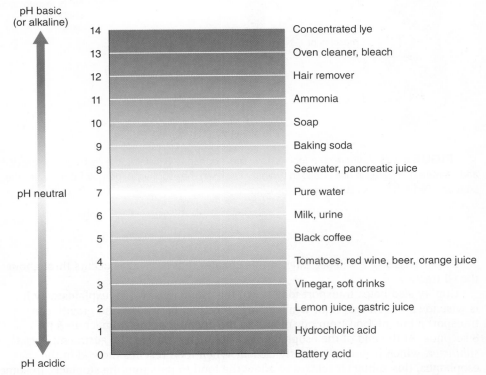

pH basic (or alkaline)

14 — Concentrated lye
13 — Oven cleaner, bleach
12 — Hair remover
11 — Ammonia
10 — Soap
9 — Baking soda
8 — Seawater, pancreatic juice

pH neutral — 7 — Pure water

6 — Milk, urine
5 — Black coffee
4 — Tomatoes, red wine, beer, orange juice
3 — Vinegar, soft drinks
2 — Lemon juice, gastric juice
1 — Hydrochloric acid
0 — Battery acid

pH acidic

▲ FIGURE 3.9 The pH scale identifies the levels of acidity or alkalinity of various substances. More specifically, pH is defined as the negative logarithm of the hydrogen–ion concentration of any solution. Each one-unit change in pH from high to low represents a tenfold increase in the concentration of hydrogen ions. This means that gastric juice, which has a pH of 2, is 100,000 times more acidic than pure water, which has a pH of 7.

2. Identify the relative acidity of black coffee as compared to pure water; as compared to HCl.

3. Identify the relative acidity of soft drinks as compared to pure water; as compared to HCl.

If you answered correctly, you can appreciate the fact that, because the tissues lining your stomach wall are adequately protected (by mucus and bicarbonate) from the acidity of HCl, they are not likely to be damaged by coffee, cola, or any other standard beverage. On the other hand, if you were to down an entire bottle of pure lemon juice (pH 2.0, the same as gastric juice), the release of all those additional hydrogen ions into the already acidic environment of your stomach would likely make you very sick. Your blood pH would drop, your breathing rate would increase, and you would almost certainly vomit. However, the juice would not corrode your stomach.

Answers to these questions can be found in the MasteringNutrition Study Area.

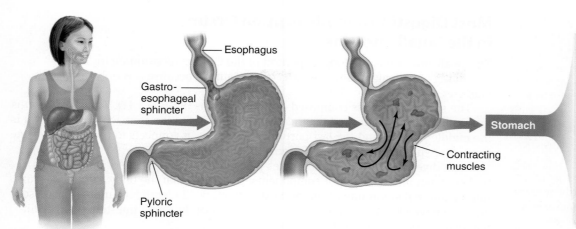

Mechanical digestion occurs when peristaltic waves mix contents of stomach

Gastric juice is secreted by stomach

Pepsin initiates protein digestion

Gastric lipase initiates lipid digestion

Small amounts of water, some minerals, drugs, and alcohol are absorbed

FIGURE 3.10 Where your food is now: the stomach. In the stomach, the protein and fat in your sandwich begin to be digested. Your meal is churned into chyme and stored until released into the small intestine.

The chief cells secrete:

- *Pepsinogen,* an inactive enzyme, which HCl converts into the active enzyme *pepsin.* Recall that salivary amylase begins to digest carbohydrates in the mouth. In contrast, proteins and lipids enter the stomach largely unchanged. Pepsin begins the digestion of protein and is considered one of the principal protein-digesting enzymes in the GI tract.
- *Gastric lipase,* an enzyme responsible for lipid digestion. Although gastric lipase begins to break apart the lipids in the turkey and mayonnaise in your sandwich, only minimal digestion of lipids occurs in the stomach.

Because gastric juice is already present in the stomach, chemical digestion of proteins and lipids begins as soon as food enters (**FIGURE 3.10**). The stomach also plays a role in mechanical digestion by mixing and churning the food with the gastric juice until it becomes a liquid called **chyme**. This mechanical digestion facilitates chemical digestion because enzymes can access the liquid chyme more easily than solid forms of food.

Despite the acidity of gastric juice, the stomach itself is not eroded because cells in gastric glands and in the stomach lining secrete a protective layer of mucus. Any disruption of this mucus barrier can cause gastritis (inflammation of the stomach lining) or an ulcer (a condition that is discussed later in this chapter). Other lining cells secrete bicarbonate, a base, which neutralizes acid near the surface of the stomach's lining.

Although most absorption occurs in the small intestine, some substances are absorbed through the stomach lining and into the blood. These include water, fluoride, some lipids, and some lipid-soluble drugs, including aspirin and alcohol.

Another of the stomach's jobs is to store chyme while the next part of the digestive tract, the small intestine, gets ready for the food. Remember that the capacity of the stomach is about 1 gallon. If this amount of chyme were to move into the small intestine all at once, it would overwhelm it. Chyme stays in the stomach for about 2 hours before it is released periodically in spurts into the duodenum, which is the first part of the small intestine. Regulating this release is the *pyloric sphincter* (see Figure 3.10).

For a fun animation explaining the concept of pH, visit www.johnkyrk.com. Then click on "pH" on the first-page menu and follow through the animation.

recap The esophagus is a muscular tube that transports food from the mouth to the stomach via waves of peristalsis. The stomach prepares itself for digestion by secreting a highy acidic gastric juice, components of which begin to digest proteins and lipids. It also secretes mucus to protect its lining. The stomach also churns food into a liquid called chyme. The stomach stores chyme and releases it periodically into the small intestine through the pyloric sphincter.

chyme A semifluid mass consisting of partially digested food, water, and gastric juices.

small intestine The longest portion of the GI tract, where most digestion and absorption take place.

gallbladder A sac-like accessory organ of digestion, which lies beneath the liver; it stores bile and secretes it into the small intestine.

bile Fluid produced by the liver and stored in the gallbladder; it emulsifies fats in the small intestine.

pancreas An accessory organ of digestion located behind the stomach; it secretes digestive enzymes as well as hormones that help regulate blood glucose.

Most Digestion and Absorption Occur in the Small Intestine

The **small intestine** is the longest portion of the GI tract, accounting for about two-thirds of its length. However, it is called "small" because it is only an inch in diameter.

The small intestine is composed of three sections **(FIGURE 3.11)**. The *duodenum* is the section that is connected via the pyloric sphincter to the stomach. The *jejunum* is the middle portion, and the last portion is the *ileum*. It connects to the large intestine at another sphincter, called the *ileocecal valve.*

Most digestion and absorption takes place in the small intestine. Here, food is broken down into its smallest components, molecules that the body can then absorb into its internal environment. In the next section, we'll identify a variety of accessory organs, enzymes, and unique anatomical features of the small intestine that permit maximal absorption of most nutrients.

The Gallbladder and Pancreas Aid in Digestion

We left your sandwich as chyme, being released periodically into the small intestine. As the chyme enters the duodenum, the hormone CCK, mentioned earlier for its role in promoting satiety, is released in response to the presence of protein and fat from the turkey and mayonnaise. The **gallbladder**, an accessory organ located beneath the liver (see Figures 3.4 and 3.11), stores a greenish fluid called **bile**, which the liver produces. The release of CCK signals the gallbladder to contract, sending bile through the *common bile duct* into the duodenum. Bile then *emulsifies* the fat; that is, it reduces the fat into smaller globules and disperses them, so that they are more accessible to digestive enzymes. If you've ever noticed how a drop of liquid detergent breaks up a film of fat floating at the top of a basin of greasy dishes, you understand the function of bile.

The **pancreas**, another accessory organ, manufactures, holds, and secretes different digestive enzymes. It is located behind the stomach (see Figures 3.4 and 3.11).

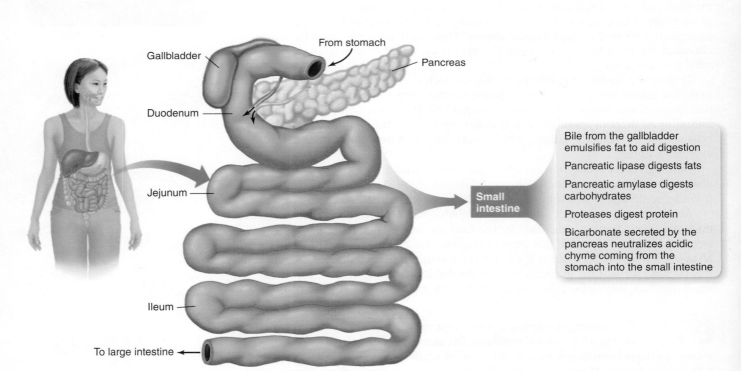

FIGURE 3.11 Where your food is now: the small intestine. Here, most of the digestion and absorption of the nutrients in your sandwich take place.

HOT TOPIC

Can Human Simulators Improve Research Ethics?

Advances in technology have led to the development of a variety of devices that can simulate the structure and functions of human organs. The Human Gastric Simulator (HGS), for example, consists of a latex chamber simulating the stomach. It is attached to a mechanized system of rollers, belts, and pulleys that mimic the peristaltic contractions of the stomach wall. By using devices such as these, researchers can simulate gastric secretions, and study how food particles are broken down and processed.

The HGS allows researchers to study human functions without using human beings. Currently, researchers can use tracers to study aspects of metabolism in living humans, but examining the digestive system overall is not possible.

As a result, many such studies use laboratory animals. But animal studies are technically challenging because the results can be affected by factors difficult to control, and differences in anatomy and physiology sometimes make findings from animal studies misleading or even irrelevant for humans. Animal studies are also expensive, and can be dangerous.

Certainly, many people find animal research ethically troubling, and most agree that study designs should avoid the use of animal subjects whenever possible.

For all these reasons, models of human organ functioning such as the HGS are welcome news.

Source: Nuffield Council on Bioethics. 2005, May. The ethics of research involving animals. Available at www.nuffieldbioethics.org/animal-research.

Enzymes secreted by the pancreas include *pancreatic amylase,* which continues the digestion of carbohydrates, and *pancreatic lipase,* which continues the digestion of fats. *Proteases* secreted in pancreatic juice digest proteins. The pancreas is also responsible for manufacturing hormones that are important in metabolism. Earlier we mentioned insulin and glucagon, two pancreatic hormones that help regulate the amount of glucose in the blood.

Another essential role of the pancreas is to secrete bicarbonate into the duodenum. Bicarbonate is a base; like all bases, it is capable of neutralizing acids. Recall that chyme leaving the stomach is very acidic. The pancreatic bicarbonate neutralizes the acidic chyme. This action helps the pancreatic enzymes work more effectively. It also ensures that the lining of the duodenum is not eroded.

Now the protein, carbohydrate, and fat in your sandwich have been processed into a liquid that contains molecules of nutrients small enough for absorption. This molecular "soup" continues to move along the small intestine via peristalsis, encountering the absorptive enterocytes of the intestinal lining all along the way.

A Specialized Lining Enables the Small Intestine to Absorb Food

The lining of the GI tract is especially well suited for absorption. If you were to look at the inside of the lining, which is also referred to as the mucosal membrane, you would notice that it is heavily folded (**FIGURE 3.12**). This feature increases the surface area of the small intestine and allows it to absorb more nutrients than if it were smooth. Within these larger folds, you would notice even smaller, finger-like projections called *villi,* whose constant movement helps them encounter and trap nutrient molecules. Inside each villus are *capillaries,* or tiny blood vessels, and a **lacteal**, which is a small lymph vessel. The capillaries absorb water-soluble nutrients directly into the bloodstream, whereas lacteals absorb fat-soluble nutrients into a watery fluid called *lymph.*

Covering the villi are enterocytes whose cell membrane is carpeted with hairlike projections called *microvilli.* Because this makes the cells look like tiny scrub brushes, the microvilli are sometimes referred to collectively as the **brush border**. The carpet of microvilli multiplies the surface area of the small intestine more than 500 times, tremendously increasing its absorptive capacity.

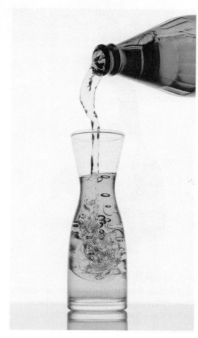

A small amount of vinegar emulsifies the oil in this container.

lacteal A small lymph vessel located inside the villi of the small intestine.

brush border The microvilli projecting from the membrane of enterocytes of the small intestine's villi. These microvilli tremendously increase the small intestine's absorptive capacity.

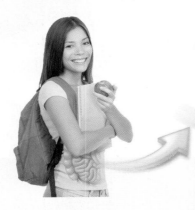

focus figure 3.12 | Small Intestine Structure and Function

The small intestine is highly adapted for absorbing nutrients. Its length—about 20 feet—provides a huge surface area, and its wall has three structural features—circular folds, villi, and microvilli—that increase its surface area by a factor of more than 600.

CIRCULAR FOLDS

The lining of the small intestine is heavily folded, resulting in increased surface area for the absorption of nutrients.

VILLI

The folds are covered with villi, thousands of finger-like projections that increase the surface area even further. Each villus contains capillaries and a lacteal for picking up nutrients absorbed through the enterocytes and transporting them throughout the body.

MICROVILLI

The cells on the surface of the villi, enterocytes, end in hairlike projections called microvilli that together form the brush border through which nutrients are absorbed.

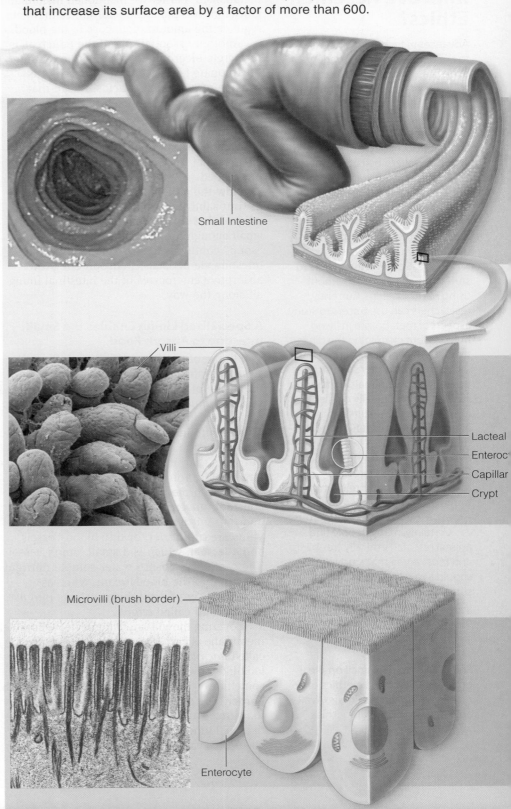

Small Intestine

Villi

Lacteal

Enteroc

Capillar

Crypt

Microvilli (brush border)

Enterocyte

Enterocytes Readily Absorb Vitamins, Minerals, and Water

The turkey sandwich you ate contained several vitamins and minerals in addition to protein, carbohydrate, and fat. The vitamins and minerals are not really "digested" in the same way that macronutrients are. Vitamins do not have to be broken down because they are already small enough to be readily absorbed. For example, the fat-soluble vitamins A, D, E, and K are absorbed into the enterocytes along with the fats in our foods. Water-soluble vitamins, such as the B-vitamins and vitamin C, typically use some type of transport process to cross the intestinal lining. Minerals don't need to be digested because they are already the smallest possible units of matter. Thus, they are absorbed all along the small intestine, and in some cases in the large intestine as well, by a wide variety of mechanisms.

Finally, a large component of food is water, and, of course, you also drink lots of water throughout the day. Water is readily absorbed along the entire length of the GI tract because it is a small molecule that can easily pass through the cell membrane. However, as we will see shortly, a significant percentage of water is absorbed in the large intestine.

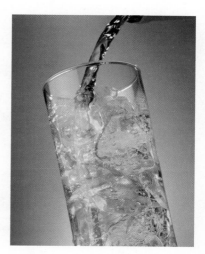

⬆ Water is readily absorbed along the entire length of the GI tract.

Blood and Lymph Transport Nutrients and Fluids

We noted earlier that, within the intestinal villi, capillaries and lacteals absorb water-soluble and fat-soluble nutrients, respectively, into blood and lymph. These two fluids then transport the nutrients throughout the body. Blood travels through the cardiovascular system, and lymph travels through the lymphatic system (FIGURE 3.13).

The oxygen we inhale into our lungs is absorbed by our red blood cells. This oxygen-rich blood then travels to the heart, where it is pumped out to the rest of the body. Blood travels to all of our tissues to deliver nutrients and other materials and pick up waste products. As blood travels through the GI tract, it picks up most of the nutrients, including water, that are absorbed through the brush border. This nutrient-rich blood is then transported to the liver. The role of the liver in packaging the arriving nutrients is described in the following section.

The lymphatic vessels pick up most fats, fat-soluble vitamins, and fluids that have escaped from the cardiovascular system and transport them in lymph. In its journey through the lymphatic vessels of the body, this lymph is filtered through *lymph nodes*, clusters of immune and other cells that trap particles and destroy harmful microbes. Eventually, lymph returns to the bloodstream in an area near the heart where the lymphatic and blood vessels join together.

Bear in mind that circulation also allows for the elimination of metabolic wastes. The waste products picked up by the blood as it circulates around the body are filtered and excreted by the kidneys in urine. In addition, much of the carbon dioxide remaining in the blood once it reaches the lungs is exhaled into the outside air, making room for oxygen to attach to the red blood cells and repeat this cycle of circulation.

The Liver Regulates Blood Nutrients

Once nutrients are absorbed from the small intestine, most enter the *portal vein*, which carries them to the **liver**. The liver is a triangular, wedge-shaped organ weighing about 3 pounds and resting almost entirely within the protection of the rib cage on the right side of the body (see Figure 3.4). It is not only the largest digestive organ but also one of the most important organs in the body, performing more than 500 discrete functions.

One function of the liver is to receive the products of digestion and then release into the bloodstream those nutrients needed throughout the body. The liver also processes and stores carbohydrates, fats, and amino acids and plays a major role in regulating their levels in the bloodstream. For instance, after we eat a meal, the liver picks up excess glucose from the blood and stores it as glycogen, releasing it into the bloodstream when we need energy later in the day. It also stores certain vitamins. But the liver is more than a nutrient warehouse: it also manufactures blood proteins

liver The largest accessory organ of digestion and one of the most important organs of the body. Its functions include the production of bile and the processing of nutrient-rich blood from the small intestine.

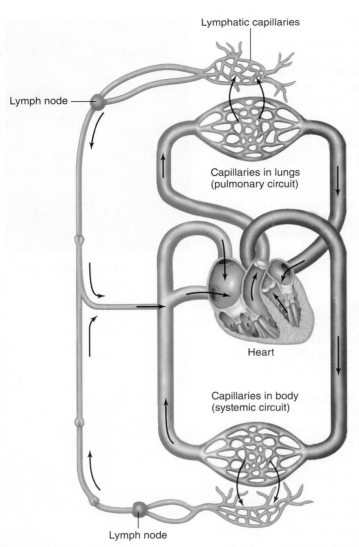

Lymphatic capillaries

Lymph node

Capillaries in lungs
(pulmonary circuit)

Heart

Capillaries in body
(systemic circuit)

Lymph node

◆ FIGURE 3.13 Blood travels through the cardiovascular system to transport water-soluble nutrients and pick up waste products. Lymph travels through the lymphatic system and transports most fats and fat-soluble vitamins.

large intestine The final organ of the GI tract, consisting of the cecum, colon, rectum, and anal canal and in which most water is absorbed and feces are formed.

and can even make glucose when necessary to keep our blood glucose levels constant.

Have you ever wondered why people who abuse alcohol are at risk for liver damage? It's because another of the liver's functions is to filter the blood, removing wastes and toxins such as alcohol, medications, and other drugs. When you drink, your liver works hard to break down the alcohol; but with heavy drinking over time, liver cells become damaged and scar tissue forms. The scar tissue blocks the free flow of blood through the liver, so that any further toxins accumulate in the blood, causing confusion, coma, and ultimately death.

Another important job of the liver is to synthesize many of the chemicals the body uses to carry out metabolic processes. For example, the liver synthesizes bile, which, as we just discussed, is then stored in the gallbladder until the body needs it to emulsify fats.

recap Most digestion and absorption occurs in the small intestine. Its three sections are the duodenum, the jejunum, and the ileum. The gallbladder stores bile, which emulsifies fats, and the pancreas synthesizes and secretes digestive enzymes that break down carbohydrates, fats, and proteins. The lining of the small intestine is heavily folded with the surface area expanded by villi and microvilli. Nutrients are absorbed across the mucosal membrane. The liver processes all the nutrients absorbed from the small intestine and stores and regulates energy nutrients.

The Large Intestine Stores Food Waste Until It Is Excreted

The **large intestine** (also called the *colon*) is a thick, tubelike structure that frames the small intestine on three-and-a-half sides **(FIGURE 3.14)**. It begins with a tissue sac called the *cecum*, which explains the name of the sphincter—the *ileocecal valve*—that connects it to the ileum of the small intestine. From the cecum, the large intestine continues up along the right side of the small intestine as the *ascending colon*. Beneath the liver, it flexes nearly 90° to continue as the *transverse colon* along the top of the small intestine. It then flexes downward, and continues as the *descending colon* along the left side of the small intestine. The *sigmoid colon* is the last segment of the colon; it extends from the bottom left corner to the *rectum*. The last segment of the large intestine is the *anal canal*, which is about an inch and a half long.

What has happened to your turkey sandwich? The undigested food components in the chyme finally reach the large intestine. By this time, the digestive mass entering the large intestine does not resemble the chyme that left the stomach several hours before. This is because most of the nutrients have been absorbed, leaving mainly nondigestible food material, such as fiber, bacteria, and water. As in the stomach, cells lining the large intestine secrete mucus, which helps protect it from the abrasive materials passing through it.

The GI tract hosts a population of trillions of bacterial cells, more than the number of cells making up the human body. Collectively called the *GI flora*, most of these live in the large intestine, where they perform several beneficial functions. First, they finish digesting some of the nutrients remaining in food residues. The by-products of

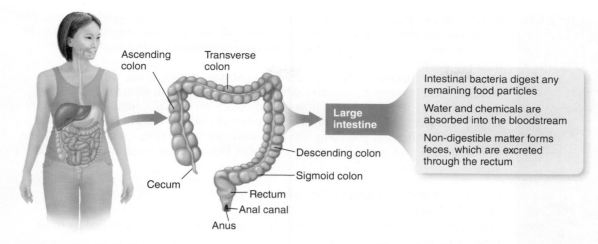

Ascending colon
Transverse colon
Intestinal bacteria digest any remaining food particles
Water and chemicals are absorbed into the bloodstream
Non-digestible matter forms feces, which are excreted through the rectum
Large intestine
Descending colon
Sigmoid colon
Cecum
Rectum
Anal canal
Anus

FIGURE 3.14 Where your food is now: the large intestine. Most water absorption occurs here, as does the formation of food wastes into semisolid feces. Peristalsis propels the feces to the body exterior.

this bacterial digestion are reabsorbed into the body, where they return to the liver and are either stored or used as needed. In addition, the GI flora synthesize certain vitamins, stimulate the immune system, inhibit the growth of harmful bacteria, and reduce the risk of diarrhea.[5] In fact, these bacteria are so helpful that many people consume them deliberately in so-called *probiotic* foods such as yogurt. On the other hand, they can be wiped out by the use of broad-spectrum antibiotics, as well as by harsh "colon-cleansing" treatments such as frequent enemas, colonics (in which the colon is "washed"), and certain dietary supplements. (For more information about the role of bacteria in human health, see **In Depth: New Frontiers in Nutrition and Health** following Chapter 1, pages 30–37.) No other digestion occurs in the large intestine. Instead, its main functions are to store the digestive mass for 12 to 24 hours and, during that time, to absorb water and other nutrients from it, leaving a semisolid mass called *feces*. Peristalsis occurs weakly to move the feces through the colon, except for one or more stronger waves of peristalsis each day, which force the feces more powerfully toward the rectum for elimination.

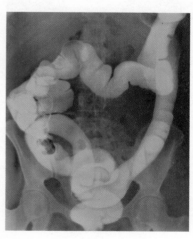

The large intestine is a thick, tubelike structure that stores the undigested mass exiting the small intestine and also absorbs any remaining nutrients, including water.

recap The large intestine is composed of seven sections: the cecum, ascending, transverse, descending, and sigmoid colon, rectum, and anal canal. Small amounts of undigested and indigestible food material, bacteria, and water enter the large intestine. Bacteria in the colon assist with the final digestion of any remaining food particles. The main functions of the large intestine are to store the digestive mass and to absorb any remaining nutrients, including water. A semisolid mass, called feces, is then eliminated from the body.

The Neuromuscular System Regulates the Activities of the GI Tract

Now that you can identify the organs involved in digestion, absorption, and elimination, and the job each performs, you might be wondering—who's the boss? In other words, what organ or system directs and coordinates all of these interrelated processes? The answer is the neuromuscular system. Its two components, the nervous and muscular systems, partner to regulate the activities of the GI tract.

The Muscles of the GI Tract Mix and Move Food

The purpose of the muscles of the GI tract is to mix food and move it in one direction—that is, from the mouth toward the anus. When food is present, nerves

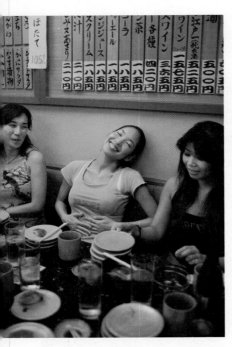

When we eat, both voluntary and involuntary muscles help us digest the food.

respond to the stretching of the tract walls and send signals to its muscles, stimulating peristalsis. As with an assembly line, the entire GI tract functions together so that materials are moved in one direction in a coordinated manner and wastes are removed as needed.

In order to process the large amount of food we consume daily, we use both voluntary and involuntary muscles. Muscles in the mouth are primarily voluntary; that is, they are under our conscious control. Once we swallow, involuntary muscles largely take over to propel food through the rest of the GI tract. This enables us to continue digesting and absorbing our food while we're working, exercising, and even sleeping. Let's now reveal the master controller behind these involuntary muscular actions.

Nerves Control the Contractions and Secretions of the GI Tract

The contractions and secretions of the gastrointestinal tract are controlled by three types of nerves:

- The **enteric nervous system (ENS)**, which is localized in the wall of the GI tract and is part of the *autonomic nervous system*, a group of nerves that regulates many unconscious, internal functions;
- Other branches of the autonomic nervous system outside the GI tract;
- The central nervous system (CNS), which includes the brain and spinal cord.

Some digestive functions are carried out entirely within the ENS. For instance, control of peristalsis is enteric, occurring without assistance from beyond the GI tract. In addition, enteric nerves regulate the secretions of the various digestive glands whose roles we have discussed in this chapter.

Enteric nerves also work in collaboration with other autonomic nerves and with the CNS. For example, we noted earlier in this chapter that in response to fasting, nerves in the stomach and intestinal walls (ENS nerves) trigger signals that travel along nerves beyond the GI tract all the way to the hypothalamus, which is part of the CNS. We then experience the sensation of hunger.

Finally, some functions, such as the secretion of saliva, are achieved without any enteric involvement. A variety of stimuli from the smell, sight, taste, and tactile sensations from food trigger special salivary cells in the CNS; these cells then stimulate increased activity of the salivary glands.

To click your way through the process of digestion, visit www.science .howstuffworks.com. Enter "digestive system" into the search bar, then click on the first video, "How the Digestive System Works" to get underway.

recap The coordination and regulation of digestion are directed by the neuromuscular system. Voluntary muscles assist us with chewing and swallowing. Once food is swallowed, the involuntary muscles along the entire length of the GI tract function together so that materials are processed in a coordinated manner. The enteric nerves of the GI tract work independently and in partnership with other nerves of the body to achieve the digestion, absorption, and elimination of food.

What disorders are related to digestion, absorption, and elimination?

Considering the complexity of digestion, absorption, and elimination, it's no wonder that sometimes things go wrong. Clinical disorders can disturb gastrointestinal functioning, as can merely consuming the wrong types or amounts of food for our unique needs. Whenever there is a problem with the GI tract, the absorption of nutrients can be affected and, over time, malnutrition can result. Let's look more closely at some GI tract disorders and what you might be able to do if they affect you.

enteric nervous system (ENS) The autonomic nerves in the walls of the GI tract.

Heartburn and Gastroesophageal Reflux Disease (GERD) Are Caused by Reflux of Gastric Juice

We noted earlier that, even as you're chewing your first bite of food, your stomach is starting to secrete gastric juice to prepare for digestion. When you swallow, the food is propelled along the esophagus, and the gastroesophageal sphincter relaxes to permit it to enter the stomach. As this occurs, it's normal for a small amount of gastric juice to flow "backwards" into the lower esophagus for a moment. This phenomenon is technically known as gastroesophageal reflux, or GER.

However, in some people, peristalsis in the esophagus is weak and the food exits too slowly, or the gastroesophageal sphincter is overly relaxed and stays partially open, allowing too much gastric juice to enter the esophagus. In either case, the result is that gastric juice isn't cleared from the lower esophagus quickly and completely.

Although the stomach is protected from the highly acidic gastric juice by a thick coat of mucus, the esophagus does not have this coating; thus, the gastric juice burns it (**FIGURE 3.15**). When this happens, the person experiences a painful sensation in the region of the chest behind the sternum (breastbone). This symptom is commonly called **heartburn**. Many people take over-the-counter antacids to raise the pH of the gastric juice, thereby relieving the heartburn. A non-drug approach is to repeatedly swallow: this action causes any acid pooled in the esophagus to be swept down into the stomach, eventually relieving the symptoms.

Occasional heartburn is common and not a cause for concern; however, heartburn is also the most common symptom of **gastroesophageal reflux disease (GERD)**, a chronic disease in which episodes of GER cause heartburn or other symptoms more than twice per week. These other symptoms of GERD include chest pain, trouble swallowing, burning in the mouth, the feeling that food is stuck in the throat, and hoarseness in the morning.[6]

The exact causes of GERD are unknown. However, a number of factors may contribute, including the following:[6]

- A hiatal hernia, which occurs when the upper part of the stomach lies above the diaphragm muscle. Normally, the horizontal diaphragm muscle separates the stomach from the chest cavity and helps keep gastric juice from seeping into the esophagus. Gastric juice can more easily enter the esophagus in people with a hiatal hernia.

heartburn A painful sensation that occurs over the sternum when gastric juice pools in the lower esophagus.

gastroesophageal reflux disease (GERD) A chronic disease in which episodes of gastroesophageal reflux cause heartburn or other symptoms more than twice per week.

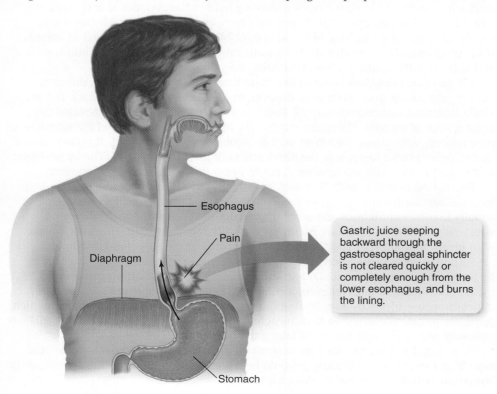

Gastric juice seeping backward through the gastroesophageal sphincter is not cleared quickly or completely enough from the lower esophagus, and burns the lining.

Esophagus

Pain

Diaphragm

Stomach

◀ FIGURE 3.15 The mechanism of heartburn and gastroesophageal reflux disease is the same: acidic gastric juices seep backward through the gastroesophageal sphincter into the lower portion of the esophagus and pool there, burning its lining. The pain is felt behind the sternum (breastbone), over the heart.

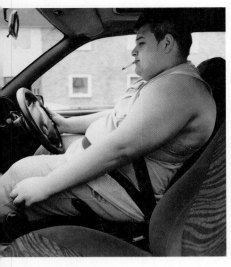

⬆ Although the exact causes of gastroesophageal reflux disease (GERD) are unknown, smoking and being overweight may be contributing factors.

- Cigarette smoking.
- Alcohol use.
- Overweight and obesity.
- Pregnancy.
- Foods such as citrus fruits, chocolate, caffeinated drinks, fried foods, garlic and onions, spicy foods, and tomato-based foods, such as chili, pizza, and spaghetti sauce.
- Large, high-fat meals. These meals stay in the stomach longer and increase stomach pressure, making it more likely that gastric juice will be pushed up into the esophagus.
- Lying down soon after a meal. In susceptible people, this is likely to bring on symptoms because it positions the body so it is easier for the gastric juice to back up into the esophagus.

One way to reduce the symptoms of GERD is to identify the types of foods or situations that trigger episodes, and then avoid them. Eating smaller meals also helps. After a meal, wait at least 3 hours before lying down. Some people relieve their nighttime symptoms by elevating the head of their bed 4 to 6 inches—for instance, by placing a wedge between the mattress and the box spring, or by raising their pillow. This keeps the chest area elevated and minimizes the amount of acid that can back up into the esophagus. People with GERD who smoke should stop, and, if they are overweight, they should lose weight. Taking an antacid before a meal can help prevent symptoms, and many other over-the-counter and prescription medications are now available to treat GERD.

It is important to treat GERD because it can lead to bleeding and ulcers in the esophagus. Scar tissue can develop in the esophagus, making swallowing very difficult. Some people can also develop a condition called Barrett's esophagus, which can lead to cancer. Asthma can also be aggravated or even caused by GERD.

An Ulcer Is an Area of Erosion in the GI Tract

A **peptic ulcer** is an area of the GI tract that has been eroded away by a combination of hydrochloric acid and the enzyme pepsin **(FIGURE 3.16)**. In almost all cases, it is located in the stomach area (*gastric ulcer*) or the part of the duodenum closest to the stomach (*duodenal ulcer*). It causes a burning pain in the abdominal area, typically 1 to 3 hours after eating a meal. In serious cases, eroded blood vessels bleed into the GI tract, causing vomiting of blood and/or blood in the stools as well as anemia. If the ulcer entirely perforates the tract wall, stomach contents can leak into the abdominal cavity, causing a life-threatening infection.

For decades, physicians believed that experiencing high levels of stress, drinking alcohol, and eating spicy foods were the primary factors responsible for ulcers. But in 1982, Australian gastroenterologists J. Robin Warren and Barry Marshall detected the same species of bacteria, *Helicobacter pylori* (*H. pylori*), in the majority of the stomachs of their patients with ulcers. Treatment with an antibiotic cured the ulcers. It is now known that *H. pylori* plays a key role in the development of most peptic ulcers. The hydrochloric acid in gastric juice kills most bacteria, but *H. pylori* thrives in acidic environments.

Preventing infection with *H. pylori,* as with any infectious microorganism, includes regular hand washing and safe food-handling practices. Ulcer treatment usually involves antibiotics and acid-suppressing medications. Special diets and stress-reduction techniques are no longer typically recommended. However, people with ulcers should avoid specific foods they identify as causing them discomfort.

Although most peptic ulcers are caused by *H. pylori* infection, some are caused by prolonged use of nonsteroidal anti-inflammatory drugs (NSAIDs); these drugs include the common pain relievers aspirin, ibuprofen, and naproxen sodium. They appear to cause ulcers by suppressing the secretion of mucus and bicarbonate, which normally protect the stomach from its acidic gastric juice. Ulcers caused by NSAID use generally heal once a person stops taking the medication.[7]

H. pylori is implicated not only in peptic ulcers, but also in stomach cancer and high blood sugar. So eradicating it would be a good idea, right? Find the answer in the **Nutrition Debate** at the end of this chapter.

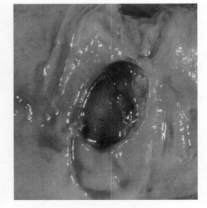

⬆ **FIGURE 3.16** A peptic ulcer.

peptic ulcer An area of the GI tract that has been eroded away by the acidic gastric juice of the stomach.

recap Gastroesophageal reflux is the seepage of gastric juices into the esophagus. It occurs commonly in most people and typically does not cause symptoms. Heartburn is the most common symptom of gastroesophageal reflux disease (GERD), a chronic condition that causes symptoms more than twice per week. Peptic ulcers are caused by erosion of the GI tract by hydrochloric acid and pepsin. The underlying cause in most cases is bacterial infection or use of nonsteroidal anti-inflammatory drugs.

Some Disorders Affect Intestinal Function

GERD and ulcers involve the upper GI tract. In this section, we'll discuss disorders affecting intestinal function.

Vomiting

Vomiting is the involuntary expulsion of the contents of the stomach and duodenum from the mouth. The reflex is triggered when substances or sensations stimulate a cluster of cells in the brain stem to signal a strong wave of "backwards" peristalsis that begins in the small intestine and surges upward. The sphincter muscles of the GI tract relax, allowing the chyme to pass.

One or two episodes of vomiting often accompany a gastrointestinal infection, typically with the norovirus, which is often spread via contaminated water or food. Vomiting triggered by infection is classified as one of the body's innate defenses because it removes harmful agents before they are absorbed. Certain medical procedures, medications, illicit drugs, motion sickness, and even severe pain can also trigger acute vomiting.

In contrast, *cyclic vomiting syndrome* (CVS) is a chronic condition characterized by recurring cycles of severe nausea and vomiting that can last for hours or days, alternating with symptom-free periods.[8] The vomiting may be severe enough to cause dehydration and the person may need to be hospitalized. The number of people affected is unknown, but the condition is thought to be somewhat common, and people of all ages can be affected.

Anxiety, excitement, allergies, infections, and a variety of other disturbances may trigger CVS. These triggers are similar to those involved in migraine headaches, and the same medications used for migraines are often prescribed for CVS, along with antinausea and antiemesis drugs.[8]

Diarrhea

Diarrhea is the frequent passage (more than three times in 1 day) of loose, watery stools. Other symptoms may include cramping, abdominal pain, bloating, nausea, fever, and blood in the stools. Diarrhea is usually caused by an infection of the gastrointestinal tract, a chronic disease, stress, or reactions to medications.[9] It can also occur as a reaction to a particular food or food ingredient. Disorders related to specific foods include food intolerances, allergies, and celiac disease. These are discussed in the **In Depth** section following this chapter.

Whatever the cause, diarrhea can be harmful if it persists for a long period because the person can lose large quantities of water and minerals and become severely dehydrated. **TABLE 3.1** reviews the signs and symptoms of dehydration, which is particularly dangerous in infants and young children. In fact, a child can die from dehydration in just a few days. Adults, particularly the elderly, can also become dangerously ill if severely dehydrated. A doctor should be seen immediately if diarrhea persists for more than 24 hours in children or more than 3 days in adults, or if diarrhea is bloody, fever is present, or there are signs of dehydration.

A condition referred to as *traveler's diarrhea* has become a common health concern due to the expansion in global travel. *Traveler's diarrhea* is experienced by people traveling to countries outside of their own and is usually caused by viral or

TABLE 3.1 Signs and Symptoms of Dehydration in Adults and Children

Symptoms in Adults	Symptoms in Children
Thirst	Dry mouth and tongue
Light-headedness	No tears when crying
Less frequent urination	No wet diapers for 3 hours or more
Dark-colored urine	High fever
Fatigue	Sunken abdomen, eyes, or cheeks
Dry skin	Irritable or listless
	Skin does not rebound when pinched and released

Data adapted from: *Diarrhea*, National Digestive Diseases Information Clearinghouse, NIH Publication No. 04-2749.

vomiting The involuntary expulsion of the contents of the stomach and duodenum from the mouth.

diarrhea A condition characterized by the frequent passage of loose, watery stools.

QuickTips

Avoiding Traveler's Diarrhea

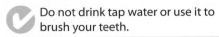

Do not drink tap water or use it to brush your teeth.

Do not drink unpasteurized milk or dairy products.

Do not use ice made from tap water. Freezing does not kill all microbes.

Avoid raw or rare meats and raw fruits and vegetables, including lettuce and fruit salads, unless they can be peeled and you peel them yourself.

Do not eat meat or shellfish that is not hot when served.

Do not eat food from street vendors.

Do drink bottled water. Make sure you are the one to break the seal, and wipe the top of the bottle clean before doing so. You can also safely choose canned carbonated soft drinks and hot drinks made with boiling water, such as coffee or tea.

Consult your doctor when planning your trip. Depending on where you are going and how long you will stay, your doctor may recommend that you take antibiotics before leaving to protect you from possible infection.

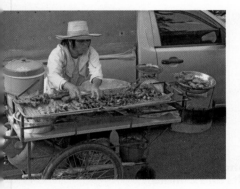

⬆ When traveling, it is wise to avoid food from street vendors.

bacterial infections, often a species of bacteria called *E. coli*. The large intestine and even some of the small intestine become irritated by the microbes and the body's defense against them. This irritation leads to increased secretion of fluid and increased motility of the large intestine, causing watery and frequent bowel movements.

People generally get traveler's diarrhea from consuming water or food that is contaminated with fecal matter. Very risky foods include any raw or undercooked fish, meats, and raw fruits and vegetables. Tap water, ice made from tap water, and unpasteurized milk and dairy products are also common sources of infection.

What can you do to prevent traveler's diarrhea? The accompanying **Quick Tips** from the National Institutes of Health should help.[9]

Constipation

At the opposite end of the spectrum from diarrhea is **constipation**, which is typically defined as a condition in which no stools are passed for 2 or more days; however, it is important to recognize that some people normally experience bowel movements only

constipation A condition characterized by the absence of bowel movements for a period of time that is significantly longer than normal for the individual. When a bowel movement does occur, stools are usually small, hard, and difficult to pass.

nutri-case | THEO

"My parents and I went to visit our family in Nigeria two years ago, during my winter break. We're planning to go again this year, but I'm not sure I'm looking forward to it. Don't get me wrong, I had a great time—after I got over being sick. We'd been there a couple of days when I came down with gut pain, nausea, and diarrhea so bad I had to stay within a few feet of a toilet. And it lasted for days! I'm thinking maybe I'll ask my doctor if I should start taking some antibiotics now so I can clean out my gut before we leave. I'd hate to go through all that again."

What do you think of Theo's idea about taking antibiotics to "clean out his gut" before he goes on his trip? Identify any potential benefits or drawbacks of such treatment. Is there a better approach Theo could take to reducing his risk for traveler's diarrhea? If so, what?

every second or third day. Thus, the definition of constipation varies from one person to another. In addition to being infrequent, the stools are usually hard, small, and somewhat difficult to pass.

Many people experience temporary constipation at some point, such as when they travel, when their regular schedule is disrupted, if they change their diet, or if they are on certain medications. Many healthcare providers suggest increasing fiber and fluid in the diet. Five to nine servings of fruits and vegetables each day and six or more servings of whole grains is recommended. If you eat breakfast cereal, make sure you buy a cereal containing at least 2 to 3 g of fiber per serving. (The dietary recommendation for fiber and the role it plays in maintaining healthy elimination are discussed in detail in Chapter 4.) Staying well hydrated is important when increasing your fiber intake. Regular exercise may also help reduce your risk for constipation.

Irritable Bowel Syndrome

Irritable bowel syndrome (IBS) is a group of symptoms caused by changes in the normal functions of the GI tract. It is one of the most common medical diagnoses, applied to an estimated 10% to 15% of the U.S. population, and it affects about twice as many women as men.[10] Symptoms include abdominal cramps, bloating, and either diarrhea or constipation: in some people with IBS, food moves too quickly through the GI tract, and in others, the movement is too slow.

IBS shows no sign of underlying disease that can be observed or measured. However, it appears that the GI tract is more sensitive to physiologic or emotional stress in people with IBS than in healthy people. Some researchers believe that the problem stems from conflicting messages between the central nervous system and the enteric nervous system. Infection may also trigger the syndrome. Many people with IBS report that certain foods and beverages cause episodes. Some of the foods linked to IBS include caffeinated tea, coffee, and colas; chocolate; alcohol; dairy products; and wheat. Certain medications may also increase the risk.

If you think you have IBS, it is important to have a complete physical examination to rule out any other health problems, including celiac disease. (See the **In Depth** essay following this chapter.) Treatment options include taking certain medications to treat diarrhea or constipation, managing stress, engaging in regular physical activity, eating smaller meals, avoiding foods that exacerbate symptoms, eating a higher-fiber diet, and consuming probiotics, whether in a dietary supplement or in whole foods such as yogurt.[10] Although IBS is uncomfortable, it does not appear to endanger long-term health. However, severe IBS can be disabling and can prevent people from leading normal lives; thus, an accurate diagnosis and effective treatment are critical.

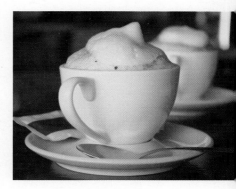

◀ Consuming caffeinated drinks is one of several factors that have been linked with irritable bowel syndrome.

Cancer Can Develop in Any Region of the GI Tract

Cancer can develop in any region of the GI tract; however, the regions most commonly affected are the oral cavity and pharynx, the pancreas, and the colon and rectum. (For information on the initiation and progression of cancer, see **In Depth: Cancer**, starting on page 301.)

Oral Cancer

Oral cancer affects the lips, tongue, mouth, or pharynx. About 40,000 Americans are diagnosed with oral cancer each year, and about 8,000 die.[11] Risk factors include smoking, the use of chewing tobacco, and heavy drinking. Excessive sun exposure increases the risk of cancer of the lips.

The classic symptom is a sore that doesn't heal. Treatment typically requires surgery, which may be disfiguring. Radiation and chemotherapy may be necessary. The best prevention measure is to avoid tobacco use and alcohol abuse. When out in the sun, coat your lips in a sun block.

Pancreatic Cancer

Pancreatic cancer is diagnosed in about 44,000 Americans each year, which is only slightly higher than the rate for oral cancer. However, the number of deaths due to pancreatic cancer is much higher, about 38,000.[11] This low survival rate reflects the

irritable bowel syndrome (IBS) A bowel disorder that interferes with normal functions of the colon.

fact that symptoms of pancreatic cancer rarely appear until the disease is too advanced to cure. Many patients feel entirely well but, on noticing that their skin looks yellowed (jaundiced), they visit their physician. Other common signs and symptoms include upper abdominal pain, ongoing dull lower-back pain, loss of appetite, and unexplained weight loss.

Some of the same risk factors involved in oral cancer—tobacco use and alcohol abuse—also increase the risk for pancreatic cancer. Unique risk factors include diabetes, lack of physical activity, and African American race. Because the cancer is usually advanced before it is detected, treatment is often focused on relieving symptoms rather than on a cure.

Colorectal Cancer

Colorectal cancer—cancer affecting the colon or rectum—is diagnosed in about 143,000 Americans annually, making it the third most common cancer in men as well as in women. It is also the third most deadly, killing about 50,000 Americans annually.[11]

Multiple factors have been identified as increasing the risk for colon cancer, including smoking and African American race. Research also implicates a high-fat diet, possibly because of correspondingly high levels of bile in chyme. Recall that the gallbladder releases bile into the chyme, where it begins to break apart fats; lining cells overexposed to bile have been shown to develop cancer.[12] In contrast, a diet high in whole grains, fruits, and vegetables appears to reduce the risk.

Symptoms of colorectal cancer include a persistent change in bowel habits, blood in the stool, unexplained weight loss, and abdominal pain or discomfort. Either of two screening tests are recommended for Americans beginning at age 50. An annual stool test looks for occult blood (hidden blood) in a stool sample. An internal imaging test called a *colonoscopy* is recommended every 5 to 10 years to look for polyps—small masses of malignant but noninvasive cells—as well as cancerous tumors. Polyps are typically removed during a colonoscopy. Larger tumors require surgery and possibly radiation and/or chemotherapy.

recap Cyclic vomiting syndrome is a pattern of recurring episodes of severe vomiting that can last hours or days. Diarrhea is the frequent passage of loose or watery stools. Constipation is failure to have a bowel movement within a time period that is normal for the individual. Irritable bowel syndrome causes abdominal cramps, bloating, and constipation or diarrhea. The causes are unknown. Cancer can develop in any region of the GI tract; however, the colon is more commonly affected than other sites.

*behavior change . . . getting started!

Now that you've read this chapter, try making these changes:

For yourself:

- Take better care of your GI tract! If you smoke or chew tobacco, stop! If you drink alcohol, keep your intake moderate—no more than one drink per day for women, and two for men. Keep up your fluids throughout the day, eat plenty of fruits, veggies, and whole grains, and stay active.

For your community:

- Start with your campus dining hall. Does it offer a wide variety of fresh fruits and vegetables, beans and other legumes, whole-grain breads and cereals, and probiotic foods such as yogurt? These foods are helpful in maintaining digestive health.
- Help combat quackery. If a friend is considering a colon-cleansing treatment or supplement, explain the importance of the GI flora. Suggest that your friend increase his or her intake of whole foods and probiotics and engage in more physical activity. These strategies are known to support digestive health and have no potentially harmful side effects.

H. pylori: Could the Same Germ Make Us Sick and Keep Us Well?

The bacterium *Helicobacter pylori* has resided in the human gastrointestinal tract for more than 50,000 years.[13] One hundred years ago, nearly every child on the planet had colonies of *H. pylori* inhabiting his or her stomach. Then came the "miracle of antibiotics," which not only toppled infectious disease from its place as the number-one cause of death in children, but also relieved childhood pain and suffering from *Strep* throat, ear infections, and a variety of other common bacterial diseases. These *broad-spectrum antibiotics*—medications effective against a wide variety of bacterial species—killed not only the targeted microbe, but also the *H. pylori* residing in children's stomachs. Today, the average American child receives a minimum of ten courses of antibiotics before age 18, and 95% of children no longer harbor *H. pylori*.[14]

Not long ago, the rapid decline of *H. pylori* was considered a triumph of modern medicine. After all, the bacterium increases our risk not only for ulcers, but also for stomach cancer and high blood glucose.[15] But over the past 20 years, researchers have become increasingly convinced that—at least throughout childhood—*H. pylori* can be a helpful, healthful member of our GI flora. Studies suggest that colonization of the GI tract with *H. pylori* might protect children against at least the following diseases:

- *Asthma and allergies.* Several epidemiological studies have found an inverse correlation between childhood *H. pylori* infection and childhood-onset asthma and allergies. That is, children whose GI tract is populated with *H. pylori* are less likely to suffer from these immune hypersensitivities. Recently, animal studies have provided experimental evidence that *H. pylori* colonization protects against the airway inflammation and other immune responses that are the hallmark of asthma. In one study, among mice exposed to dust mites and other allergens, all mice without *H. pylori* became ill, whereas mice with *H. pylori* did not.[16]
- *Gastroesophageal reflux disease and esophageal cancer.* Studies in the United States, Europe, and Asia have also found an inverse correlation between *H. pylori* colonization and both gastroesophageal reflux disease and esophageal cancer.[17] Although the precise mechanism for this relationship is not clear, some experimental studies suggest that the effect may occur because

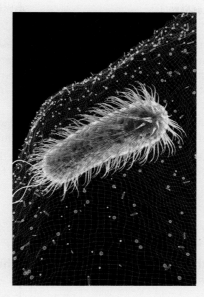

The *Helicobacter pylori* (*H. pylori*) bacterium plays a key role in the development of most peptic ulcers.

H. pylori reduces both the amount and acidity of gastric juice. Other researchers propose that, because obesity increases the risk for GERD, another contributing factor may be the role of *H. pylori* infection in protecting against obesity.[18]

- *Overweight and obesity.* Studies have shown that, in stomachs colonized by *H. pylori*, the production of the hormone ghrelin plummets after a meal. In contrast, in stomachs lacking *H. pylori*, ghrelin levels hold steady.[13] As we noted earlier, ghrelin is a "hunger hormone" that triggers the hypothalamus to strongly induce us to eat, so if levels don't fall after a meal, we're more likely to keep eating. Population studies have shown that children given antibiotics during early infancy (age 0 to 6 months) are 22% more likely to be overweight at age 3 than children not given antibiotics in early infancy.[19] Moreover, in animal studies, mice administered doses of antibiotics comparable to those given to American children to treat ear infections gained considerably more weight than control animals consuming the same diet.[14]

Despite these findings, no one denies that, in adults, *H. pylori* infection increases the risk of serious disease, from peptic ulcers to stomach cancer. But Martin J. Blaser, a leading researcher in *H. pylori*, cautions against eradication. Blaser acknowledges that, for some people, especially as they age, *H. pylori* poses a serious threat. But for most of us, its presence confers no risk and might be beneficial. Blaser is convinced that this is the case for children and proposes that, following a course of antibiotics, children be administered a therapeutic dose of *H. pylori*, allowing it to repopulate their GI tract. Then, in middle adulthood, patients could go to a clinic and have the bacteria destroyed.[14]

CRITICAL THINKING QUESTIONS

1. Many ranchers feed antibiotics to livestock to quickly increase the animals' weight. Explain a possible mechanism for this weight gain.
2. At the beginning of this debate, we referred to the "miracle of antibiotics." Are antibiotics a miracle cure? Why or why not?

chapter **review**

MasteringNutrition™

review questions

1. Which of the following represents the levels of organization in the human body from smallest to largest?
   a. cells, molecules, atoms, tissues, organs, systems
   b. atoms, molecules, cells, organs, tissues, systems
   c. atoms, molecules, cells, tissues, organs, systems
   d. molecules, atoms, cells, tissues, organs, systems

2. The cell membrane is composed of
   a. a somewhat rigid layer of cholesterol molecules.
   b. two flexible layers of phospholipid molecules.
   c. a flexible tissue containing multiple organelles.
   d. repeating atoms of various lipids.

3. The region of brain tissue that is responsible for prompting us to seek food is the
   a. pituitary gland.
   b. cephalic phase.
   c. hypothalamus.
   d. autonomic nervous system.

4. The jejunum is
   a. the first segment of the esophagus.
   b. the main portion of the stomach.
   c. the middle segment of the small intestine.
   d. the first segment of the large intestine.

5. Most digestion of carbohydrates, fats, and proteins takes place in the
   a. mouth.
   b. stomach.
   c. small intestine.
   d. large intestine.

6. The nerves of the GI tract are
   a. collectively known as the enteric nervous system.
   b. part of the central nervous system.
   c. incapable of acting independently of the brain.
   d. all of the above.

7. Heartburn is caused by pooling of
   a. gastric juice in the esophagus.
   b. gastric juice in the cardiac muscle.
   c. bile in the stomach.
   d. salivary amylase in the stomach.

8. **True or false?** Vitamins and minerals are digested in the small intestine.

9. **True or false?** Bile is produced by the gallbladder.

10. **True or false?** Diarrhea can be a normal, protective response to infection.

math review

11. Some people use baking soda as an antacid. The pH of baking soda is 9.0. The pH of gastric juice is 2.0. Baking soda is how many times more alkaline than gastric juice?

Answers to Review Questions and Math Review are located at the back of this text and in the MasteringNutrition Study Area.

web resources

www.digestive.niddk.nih.gov
National Institute of Diabetes and Digestive and Kidney Diseases (NIDDK)

Explore this site to learn more about disorders involving the gastrointestinal system.

www.cancer.gov
National Cancer Institute

Search this site to learn more about cancers affecting the gastrointestinal tract and its accessory organs.

www.ibsgroup.org
Irritable Bowel Syndrome Self-Help and Support Group

Visit this site for information on self-help measures and support for people diagnosed with IBS.

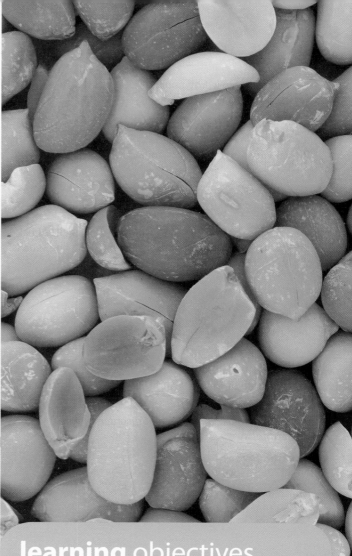

in depth 3.5

Disorders Related to Specific Foods

Trying to decide between two brands of energy bars, you compare their lists of ingredients. You notice that one of the bars, although it contains no nuts, says, "Produced in a facility that processes peanuts." The other warns, "Contains wheat, milk, and soy." Why all the warnings? The reason is that, for some people, consuming these normally healthful foods can be dangerous, even life-threatening.

Disorders related to specific foods can be clustered into three main groupings: food intolerances, food allergies, and a genetic disorder called celiac disease. We discuss these disorders **In Depth** here.

learning objectives

After studying this In Depth, you should be able to:

1 Identify the most common physiologic problem underlying food intolerances, including lactose intolerance, p. 103.

2 Describe how an immune hypersensitivity to food proteins such as those in peanuts, eggs, or milk can produce the symptoms commonly associated with an allergic reaction, pp. 103–105.

3 Identify the site of the tissue damage that occurs in celiac disease and the food protein that provokes the response, pp. 105–106.

Food intolerances

A **food intolerance** is a cluster of GI symptoms (often gas, pain, and diarrhea) that occur following the consumption of a particular food. Commonly, intolerance results when the body does not produce enough of the enzymes it needs to break down certain food components before they reach the colon. The immune system plays no role in intolerance, and, although episodes are unpleasant, they are usually transient, resolving after the offending food has been eliminated from the GI tract. People can have an intolerance to milk, wheat, soy, or other foods, but in all cases the symptoms can be prevented by avoiding the offending foods.

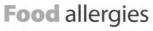

For those who are lactose intolerant, milk products, such as ice cream, are difficult to digest.

A common food intolerance is **lactose intolerance**, in which the enterocytes do not produce sufficient amounts of the enzyme lactase to digest foods containing the milk sugar *lactose*. Lactose intolerance should not be confused with a milk allergy. People who are allergic to milk experience an immune reaction to the proteins found in cow's milk. Symptoms of milk allergy include skin reactions, intestinal distress, and respiratory symptoms. In contrast, symptoms of lactose intolerance are limited to the GI tract and include intestinal gas, bloating, cramping, nausea, diarrhea, and discomfort. These symptoms resolve spontaneously within a few hours.

Although some infants are born with lactose intolerance, it is more common to see lactase enzyme activity decrease after 2 years of age. In fact, it is estimated that up to 70% of the world's adult population lose some ability to digest lactose as they age. In the United States, lactose intolerance is more common in Native American, Asian, Hispanic, and African American adults than in Caucasians.

Not everyone experiences lactose intolerance to the same extent. Many people who report being lactose intolerant are able to tolerate multiple small servings of dairy products without symptoms.[1] These people do not need to avoid all dairy products; they may simply need to eat smaller amounts and experiment to find foods that do not cause intestinal distress. Other people will experience symptoms after consuming minute amounts of lactose. These individuals should avoid not only all dairy products but also hidden sources of lactose in processed foods. If any of the following ingredients appears on a food label, the product contains lactose: milk, lactose, whey, curds, milk by-products, dry milk solids, nonfat dry milk powder. Lactose is also used in some prescription and over-the-counter medications.[1]

People with lactose intolerance need to find foods that can supply enough calcium for normal growth, development, and maintenance of bones. Many can tolerate specially formulated milk products that are low in lactose, whereas others take pills or use drops that contain the lactase enzyme when they eat dairy products. Calcium-fortified soy milk and orange juice are excellent substitutes for cow's milk. Many lactose-intolerant people can also digest aged cheese and yogurt with live and active cultures because the molds or bacteria used in these products break down the lactose during processing.

How can you tell if you are lactose intolerant? Many people discover that they have problems digesting dairy products by trial and error. But because intestinal gas, bloating, and diarrhea may indicate other health problems, you should consult a physician to determine the cause.

A common test for lactose intolerance in adults is a hydrogen breath test. First, the patient drinks a lactose-rich beverage. The breath is then analysed at regular intervals to measure the amount of hydrogen. Undigested lactose produces high levels of hydrogen, which suggests the diagnosis of lactose intolerance. In children, a stool sample is usually tested for levels of acids and other substances associated with undigested lactose.[1] For those diagnosed with lactose intolerance, a consultation with a registered dietitian may help in designing a diet that provides adequate nutrients.

Food allergies

A **food allergy** is a hypersensitivity reaction of the immune system to a particular component (usually a protein) in a food. This reaction causes the immune cells to release chemicals that cause either limited or systemic (whole-body) inflammation. About 5% of infants and young children and 2% of adults experience food allergies.[2] Although this makes them much less common than food intolerances, food allergies can be far more serious. Approximately 30,000 consumers require emergency department treatment and 150 Americans die each year because of allergic reactions to foods.[2]

---

food intolerance Gastrointestinal discomfort caused by certain foods that is not a result of an immune system reaction.

lactose intolerance A disorder in which the body does not produce enough lactase enzyme to break down the sugar lactose, which is found in milk and milk products.

food allergy An inflammatory reaction to food caused by an immune system hypersensitivity.

At the beginning of this **In Depth** chapter, we mentioned the warnings you see on food labels about wheat, soy, and other ingredients. These are technically referred to as *allergens* because they are capable of prompting an allergic reaction in susceptible people. What are the most common food allergens, and how can you recognize them? Check out the **Nutrition Label Activity** (below) to learn more.

You may have heard stories of people being allergic to foods as common as peanuts. This is the case for Liz. She was out to dinner with her parents, celebrating her birthday, when the dessert cart came around. The caramel custard looked heavenly and was probably a safe choice, but she asked the waiter just to be sure that it contained no peanuts. He checked with the chef, then returned and assured her that, no, the custard was peanut-free—but within minutes of consuming it, Liz's skin became flushed, and she struggled to breathe. As her parents were dialing 911, she lost consciousness. Fortunately, the paramedics arrived within minutes and were able to resuscitate her. It was subsequently determined that, unknown to the chef, the spoon that

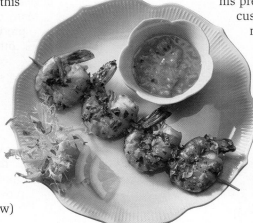

For some people, eating a meal of grilled shrimp with peanut sauce would cause a severe allergic reaction.

his prep cook had used to scoop the baked custard into serving bowls had been resting on a cutting board where he had chopped peanuts for a different dessert. Just this small exposure to peanuts was enough to cause a severe allergic reaction in Liz.

How can a food that most people consume regularly, such as peanuts, eggs, or milk, cause another person's immune system to react so violently? In Liz's case, a trace amount of peanut stimulated immune cells throughout her body to release their inflammatory chemicals. In some people, the inflammation is localized, so the damage is limited. For instance, some people's mouths and throats itch when they eat cantaloupe, whereas others develop a rash whenever they eat eggs. What made Liz's experience so terrifyingly different was that the inflammation was widespread, affecting essentially all of her body systems. Her blood vessels dilated, causing a sudden drop in her blood pressure. At the same time, her airways constricted, and the tissues in her throat swelled, making it difficult for her to breathe. Together, these and other responses sent her into a state called *anaphylactic shock*. Left untreated, anaphylactic shock is nearly always fatal, so many people with known food allergies carry with them a kit containing an injection of a powerful stimulant called

nutrition label activity

Recognizing Common Allergens in Foods

Beginning on January 1, 2006, the U.S. Food and Drug Administration (FDA) required food labels to clearly identify any ingredients containing protein derived from the eight major allergenic foods.[2] Manufacturers were required to identify "in plain English" the presence of ingredients that contain protein derived from milk, eggs, fish, crustacean shellfish (crab, lobster, shrimp, and so on), tree nuts (almonds, pecans, walnuts, and so on), peanuts, wheat, or soybeans.

Although more than 160 foods have been identified as causing food allergies in sensitive individuals, the FDA requires labeling for only these eight foods because together they account for over 90% of all documented food allergies in the United States and represent the foods most likely to result in severe or life-threatening reactions.[2]

These eight allergenic foods must be indicated in the list of ingredients; alternatively, adjacent to the ingredients list, the label must say "Contains" followed by the name of the

food. For example, the label of a product containing the milk-derived protein casein must use the term *milk* in addition to the term *casein,* so that those who have milk allergies can clearly understand the presence of an allergen they need to avoid.[2] Any food product found to contain an undeclared allergen is subject to recall by the FDA.

Look at the ingredients list from an energy bar, shown below. How many of the FDA's eight allergenic foods does this bar contain? If you were allergic to peanuts, would you eat this bar? Would you eat it if you were lactose intolerant? Explain your answers.

Ingredients: Soy protein isolate, rice flour, oats, milled flaxseed, brown rice syrup, evaporated cane juice, sunflower oil, soy lecithin, cocoa, nonfat milk solids, salt.

Contains soy and dairy. May contain traces of peanuts and other nuts.

---

epinephrine. This drug can reduce symptoms long enough to buy the victim time to get emergency medical care.

Physicians use a variety of tests to diagnose food allergies. Usually, the physician orders a skin test, commonly known as a "scratch test," in which a clinician swabs a small amount of fluid containing the suspected allergen onto the patient's skin, then lightly scratches or pricks the area so that the fluid seeps under the patient's skin. After 15–20 minutes, the clinician checks the area: redness and/or swelling indicates that the patient is allergic to the substance. However, people can have a positive response with allergy skin testing yet not have any problems with the specific substance in daily life.[3] Thus, some physicians will perform a blood test, in which a sample of the patient's blood is tested for the presence of unique proteins, called *antibodies,* that the immune system produces in a person with an allergy. In Liz's case, the blood test detected antibodies specific to peanut allergen.

Beware of e-mail spam, Internet websites, and ads in popular magazines attempting to link a vast assortment of health problems to food allergies. Typically, these ads offer allergy-testing services for exorbitant fees, then make even more money by selling "nutritional counseling" and sometimes supplements and other products they say will help you cope with your allergies. If you suspect you might have a food allergy, consult an MD.

Celiac disease

Celiac disease, also known as *celiac sprue*, is a disease that severely damages the lining of the small intestine and interferes with the absorption of nutrients. It is classified as an *autoimmune* disease; that is, the body's own immune system causes the destruction. Because there is a strong genetic predisposition to celiac disease, with the risk now linked to specific gene markers, it is also considered a genetic disorder. Specifically, celiac disease occurs in about 1 of 133 Americans, but in 1 of 22 Americans with a close relative diagnosed with the disorder.[4]

In celiac disease, the offending food component is *gliadin,* a fraction of a protein called *gluten* that is found in wheat, rye, barley, and triticale. When people with celiac disease eat one of these grains, their immune system triggers an inflammatory response that erodes the villi of the small intestine. If the person is unaware of the disorder and continues to eat gluten, repeated immune reactions cause the villi to become greatly decreased, and there is less absorptive surface area. As a result, the person becomes unable to absorb certain nutrients properly—a condition known as *malabsorption*. Over time, malabsorption can lead to malnutrition (poor nutrient status). Deficiencies of iron, folic acid, calcium, and vitamins A, D, E, and K are common in those suffering from celiac disease, as are inadequate intakes of protein and total energy.[4]

Symptoms of celiac disease often mimic those of other intestinal disturbances, such as irritable bowel syndrome, so the condition is often misdiagnosed. Some of the symptoms

nutri-case | LIZ

"I used to think of my peanut allergy as no big deal, but ever since I went to that restaurant last year, I've been pretty obsessed with it. For months after that one meal I had a reaction to, I didn't eat anything I hadn't prepared myself. I eat out again now, but always insist that the chef prepare my food personally, with clean utensils, and I avoid desserts; they're just too risky. Food shopping is harder, too, because I have to check every label. The worst, though, is eating at my friends' houses. I have to ask them if they have peanuts or peanut butter in their house. Some of them are sympathetic, but others look at me like I'm a hypochondriac! I wish I could think of something to say to make them understand this isn't something I have any control over!"

What could Liz say in response to friends who don't understand the cause and seriousness of her food allergy? Do you think it would help Liz to share her fears with her doctor and to discuss possible strategies? If so, why? In addition to shopping, dining out, and eating at friends' houses, what other situations might require Liz to be cautious about her food choices, and sources?

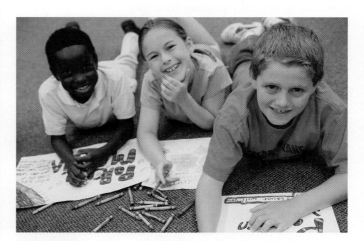

Schoolchildren may have celiac disease and not know it. Undiagnosed celiac disease can lead to physical and mental disorders as children grow.

---

celiac disease An autoimmune disorder characterized by an inability to absorb a component of gluten called *gliadin.* This causes an inflammatory immune response that damages the lining of the small intestine.

of celiac disease are fatty stools (due to poor fat absorption); frequent stools, either watery or hard, with an odd odor; cramping; anemia; pallor; weight loss; fatigue; and irritability. However, other puzzling symptoms do not appear to involve the GI tract. These include an intensely itchy rash called *dermatitis herpetiformis*, osteoporosis (poor bone density), infertility, seizures, anxiety, irritability, depression, and migraine headaches, among others.[4]

Diagnostic tests for celiac disease include a variety of blood tests that screen for the presence of antibodies to gluten, or for the genetic markers of the disease. Although the antibody test is considered generally reliable for diagnosing celiac disease, false negatives are not uncommon. Thus, the "gold standard" for diagnosis is a biopsy of the small intestine showing atrophy of the intestinal villi. Because one of the long-term complications of undiagnosed celiac disease is an increased risk for cancer of the small intestine, early diagnosis can be lifesaving. Unfortunately, celiac disease is widely underdiagnosed in the United States.[5] This is one reason that some researchers and healthcare professionals favor screening school-age children for celiac disease, as is common in several European countries.

Currently, there is no cure for celiac disease. Treatment is with a special diet that excludes all forms

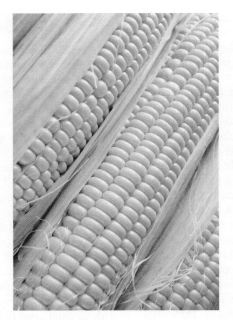

For people with celiac disease, corn is a gluten-free source of carbohydrates.

of wheat, rye, barley, and triticale. Oats are allowed, but they are often contaminated with wheat flour from processing, and even a microscopic amount of gluten can cause an immune response. The diet is made even more challenging by the fact that many binding agents and other unfamiliar ingredients in processed foods are derived from gluten. Thus, nutritional counseling is essential. Although many gluten-free foods are now available, they are typically more expensive and less palatable than traditional wheat-based foods. Someday, however, gluten-free foods may be unnecessary. Earlier we discussed the beneficial functions of certain types of bacteria in the GI tract. Now, researchers have discovered that beneficial mouth bacteria are able to degrade gluten.[6] Thus, researchers are looking into the potential of developing probiotic breads and other gluten-containing foods that would be safe for people with celiac disease to consume. Another line of research is exploring the use of certain combinations of enzymes that could break down gluten before it enters the small intestine.[4]

If you suspect you have celiac disease, consult your physician. Do not simply attempt to eliminate gluten from your diet because if you then decide to undergo antibody screening, being on a gluten-free diet will invalidate the results of the test. Moreover, a gluten-free diet is notoriously difficult to maintain without appropriate nutritional counseling and support.

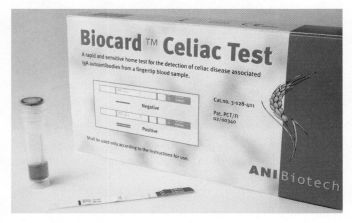

A simple blood test can identify celiac disease.

MasteringNutrition™

Check out these additional resources in the MasteringNutrition Study Area:

- Read It: Chapter Summary and RSS Feeds
- See It: ABC News videos and nutrition animations
- Hear It: MP3s
- Study It: Get Ready for Nutrition Math and Chemistry review
- Do It: NutriTools and "Find the Quack" feature
- Review It: Quizzes, flashcards, and glossary

web resources

www.medlineplus.gov
MEDLINE Plus Health Information

Search for "food allergies" to obtain additional resources as well as the latest news about food allergies.

www.ific.org
International Food Information Council Foundation

Scroll down to "Food Safety Information" and click on the link for "Food Allergies and Asthma" for additional information on food allergies.

www.foodallergy.org
The Food Allergy and Anaphylaxis Network

Visit this site to learn more about common food allergens.

www.americanceliac.org
American Celiac Disease Alliance

Learn more about the diagnosis and treatment of celiac disease, ongoing research, and living with celiac disease.

www.csaceliacs.org
Celiac Sprue Association—National Celiac Disease Support Group

Get information on the Celiac Sprue Association, a national educational organization that provides information and referral services for persons with celiac disease.

www.gfmall.com
Gluten-Free Mall

Find out where you can buy gluten-free products.

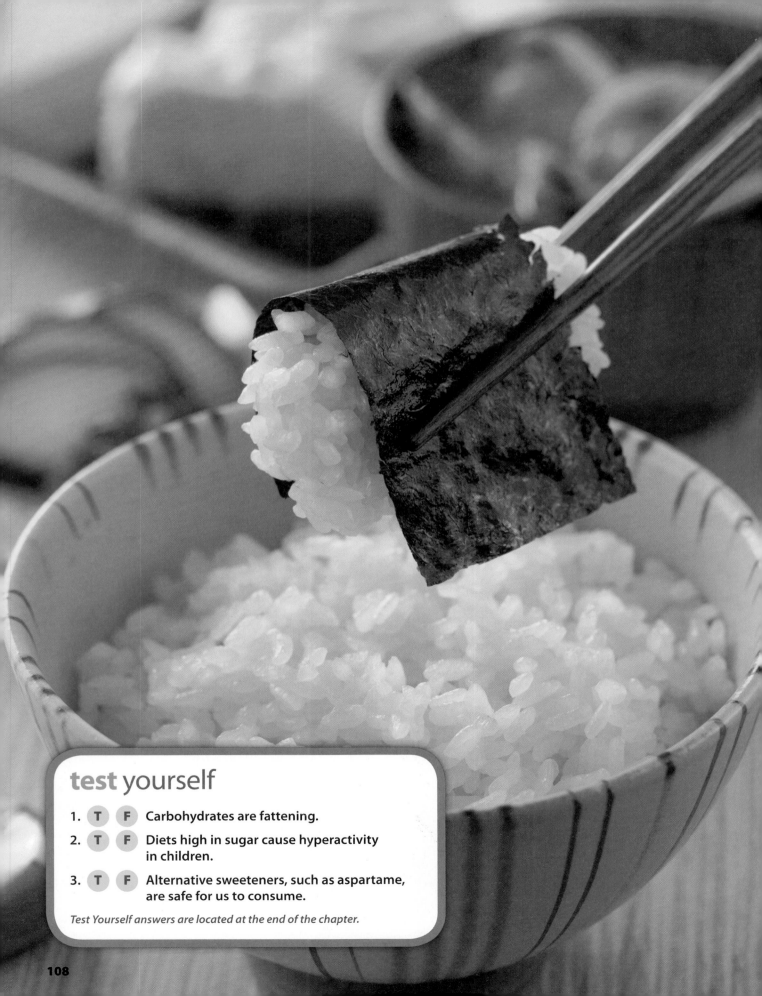

test yourself

1. **T** **F** Carbohydrates are fattening.

2. **T** **F** Diets high in sugar cause hyperactivity in children.

3. **T** **F** Alternative sweeteners, such as aspartame, are safe for us to consume.

Test Yourself answers are located at the end of the chapter.

Carbohydrates
Plant-derived energy nutrients

4

learning objectives

After studying this chapter you should be able to:

1 Distinguish between simple and complex carbohydrates, pp. 110–113.

2 List four functions of carbohydrates in our bodies, pp. 115–118.

3 Explain how carbohydrates are digested and absorbed by our bodies, pp. 118–121.

4 Define the glycemic index and glycemic load, pp. 123–124.

5 Define the Acceptable Macronutrient Distribution Range for carbohydrates, and the Adequate Intake for fiber, pp. 125 and 131.

6 Identify the most common dietary sources of added sugars and the potential health risks of a diet high in added sugars, pp. 125–128.

7 List five foods that are good sources of fiber-rich carbohydrates, pp. 128–129 and pp. 131–132.

8 Compare and contrast a variety of alternative sweeteners, pp. 132–135.

When Khalil lived at home, he snacked on whatever was around. That typically meant fresh fruit or his mom's homemade flatbread and either plain water or skim milk. His parents never drank soda, and the only time he ate sweets was on special occasions. Now Khalil is living on campus. When he gets hungry between classes, he visits the snack shack in the Student Union for one of their awesome chocolate-chunk cookies and washes it down with a large cola. Studying at night, he munches on cheese curls or corn chips and drinks more cola to help him stay awake. Not suprisingly, Khalil has noticed lately that his clothes feel tight. When he steps on the scale, he's shocked to discover that, since starting college 3 months ago, he's gained 7 pounds!

Several popular diets—including the Zone Diet, Sugar Busters, and Dr. Atkins' New Diet Revolution—claim that carbohydrates are bad for your health. They recommend reducing carbohydrate consumption and eating more protein and fat.[1–3] Is this good advice? Are carbohydrates a health menace, and is one type of carbohydrate "better" or "worse" than another?

In this chapter, we'll explore the differences between simple and complex carbohydrates and learn why some carbohydrates really are better than others. We'll also learn how the human body breaks down carbohydrates and uses them to maintain our health and to fuel activity and exercise. In the **In Depth** essay following this chapter, we'll discuss the relationship between carbohydrate intake and diabetes.

MasteringNutrition™

Go online for chapter quizzes, pre-tests, Interactive Activities, and more!

What are carbohydrates?

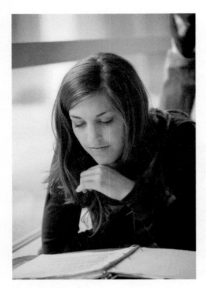

↞ Glucose is the preferred source of energy for the brain.

As noted earlier (in Chapter 1), carbohydrates are one of the three macronutrients. As such, they are an important energy source for the entire body and are the preferred energy source for nerve cells, including those of the brain. We will say more about their functions later in this chapter.

The term **carbohydrate** literally means "hydrated carbon." When something is said to be *hydrated*, it contains water, which is made of hydrogen and oxygen (H_2O). Thus, the chemical abbreviation for carbohydrate (CHO) indicates the atoms it contains: **c**arbon, **h**ydrogen, and **o**xygen.

We obtain carbohydrates predominantly from plant foods, such as fruits, vegetables, and grains. Plants make the most abundant form of carbohydrate, called **glucose**, through a process called **photosynthesis**. During photosynthesis, the green pigment of plants, called *chlorophyll*, absorbs sunlight, which provides the energy needed to fuel the manufacture of glucose. As shown in **FIGURE 4.1**, water absorbed from the earth by the roots of plants combines with the carbon dioxide present in the leaves to produce the carbohydrate glucose. Plants continually store glucose and use it to support their own growth. Then, when we eat plant foods, our bodies digest, absorb, and use the stored glucose.

Carbohydrates can be classified as *simple* or *complex*. These terms are used to describe carbohydrates based on the number of molecules of sugar present. Simple carbohydrates contain either one or two molecules, whereas complex carbohydrates contain hundreds to thousands of molecules.

carbohydrate One of the three macronutrients, a compound made up of carbon, hydrogen, and oxygen, that is derived from plants and provides energy.

glucose The most abundant sugar molecule, a monosaccharide generally found in combination with other sugars; it is the preferred source of energy for the brain and an important source of energy for all cells.

photosynthesis The process by which plants use sunlight to fuel a chemical reaction that combines carbon and water into glucose, which is then stored in their cells.

Energy from sun

Carbon dioxide from air

Glucose stored in plant

Water

↞ **FIGURE 4.1** Plants make carbohydrates through the process of photosynthesis. Water, carbon dioxide, and energy from the sun are combined to produce glucose.

Simple Carbohydrates Include Monosaccharides and Disaccharides

Simple carbohydrates are commonly referred to as *sugars*. Four of these sugars are called **monosaccharides** because they consist of a single sugar molecule (*mono* means "one," and *saccharide* means "sugar"). The other three sugars are **disaccharides**, which consist of two molecules of sugar joined together (*di* means "two").

Glucose, Fructose, Galactose, and Ribose Are Monosaccharides

Glucose, fructose, and *galactose* are the three most common monosaccharides in our diet. Each of these monosaccharides contains six carbon atoms, twelve hydrogen atoms, and six oxygen atoms **(FIGURE 4.2)**. Very slight differences in the arrangement of the atoms in these three monosaccharides cause major differences in their levels of sweetness.

Given what you've just learned about how plants manufacture and store carbohydrate in the form of glucose, it probably won't surprise you to discover that glucose is the most abundant sugar molecule in our diets and in our bodies. Glucose does not generally occur by itself in foods, but attaches to other sugars to form disaccharides and complex carbohydrates. In our bodies, glucose is the preferred source of energy for the brain, and it is a very important source of energy for all cells.

Fructose, the sweetest natural sugar, is found in fruits and vegetables. Fructose is also called *levulose*, or *fruit sugar*. In many processed foods, it comes in the form of **high-fructose corn syrup**. This syrup is manufactured from corn and is used to sweeten soft drinks, desserts, candies, and jellies.

Galactose does not occur alone in foods. It joins with glucose to create lactose, one of the three most common disaccharides.

Ribose is a five-carbon monosaccharide. Very little ribose is found in our diets; our bodies produce ribose from other carbohydrates we eat, and ribose is contained in the genetic material of our cells: deoxyribonucleic acid (DNA) and ribonucleic acid (RNA).

Lactose, Maltose, and Sucrose Are Disaccharides

The three most common disaccharides found in foods are *lactose, maltose,* and *sucrose* **(FIGURE 4.3)**. **Lactose** (also called *milk sugar*) consists of one glucose molecule and one galactose molecule. Interestingly, human breast milk has more lactose than cow's milk, making human breast milk taste sweeter.

Maltose (also called *malt sugar*) consists of two molecules of glucose. It does not generally occur by itself in foods but, rather, is bound together with other molecules. As our bodies break down these larger molecules, maltose results as a by-product. Maltose is also the sugar that is fermented during the production of beer and liquor

simple carbohydrate Commonly called *sugar;* can be either a monosaccharide (such as glucose) or a disaccharide.

monosaccharide The simplest of carbohydrates, consisting of one sugar molecule, the most common form of which is glucose.

disaccharide A carbohydrate compound consisting of two sugar molecules joined together.

fructose The sweetest natural sugar; a monosaccharide that occurs in fruits and vegetables; also called levulose, or fruit sugar.

high-fructose corn syrup A highly sweet syrup that is manufactured from corn and is used to sweeten soft drinks, desserts, candies, and jellies.

galactose A monosaccharide that joins with glucose to create lactose, one of the three most common disaccharides.

ribose A five-carbon monosaccharide that is located in the genetic material of cells.

lactose A disaccharide consisting of one glucose molecule and one galactose molecule. It is found in milk, including human breast milk; also called *milk sugar.*

maltose A disaccharide consisting of two molecules of glucose. It does not generally occur independently in foods but results as a by-product of digestion; also called *malt sugar.*

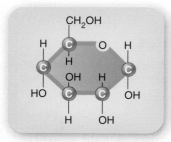

Glucose

Most abundant sugar molecule in our diet; good energy source

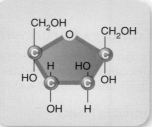

Fructose

Sweetest natural sugar; found in fruit, high-fructose corn syrup

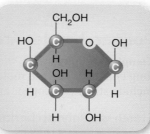

Galactose

Does not occur alone in foods; binds with glucose to form lactose

FIGURE 4.2 The three most common monosaccharides. Notice that all three monosaccharides contain identical atoms: 6 carbon, 12 hydrogen, and 6 oxygen. It is only the arrangement of these atoms that differs.

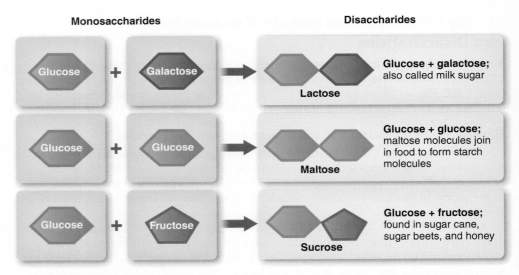

Monosaccharides   **Disaccharides**

Glucose + Galactose → **Lactose** Glucose + galactose; also called milk sugar

Glucose + Glucose → **Maltose** Glucose + glucose; maltose molecules join in food to form starch molecules

Glucose + Fructose → **Sucrose** Glucose + fructose; found in sugar cane, sugar beets, and honey

⬆ **FIGURE 4.3** Galactose, glucose, and fructose join together in different combinations to make the disaccharides lactose, maltose, and sucrose.

products. **Fermentation** is a process in which an agent, such as yeast, causes an organic substance to break down into simpler substances and results in the production of the energy molecule adenosine triphosphate (ATP). Maltose is formed during the breakdown of sugar in grains and other foods into alcohol. Contrary to popular belief, very little maltose remains in alcoholic beverages after the fermentation process is complete; thus, alcoholic beverages are not good sources of carbohydrate.

Sucrose is composed of one glucose molecule and one fructose molecule. Because sucrose contains fructose, it is sweeter than lactose or maltose. Sucrose provides much of the sweet taste found in honey, maple syrup, fruits, and vegetables. Table sugar, brown sugar, powdered sugar, and many other products are made by refining the sucrose found in sugarcane and sugar beets. Are honey and other naturally occurring forms of sucrose more healthful than manufactured forms? The **Nutrition Myth or Fact?** box investigates this question.

recap Carbohydrates contain carbon, hydrogen, and oxygen. Plants make one type of carbohydrate, glucose, through the process of photosynthesis. Simple carbohydrates include monosaccharides and disaccharides. Glucose, fructose, and galactose are monosaccharides; lactose, maltose, and sucrose are disaccharides.

Polysaccharides Are Complex Carbohydrates

Complex carbohydrates, the second major type of carbohydrate, generally consist of long chains of glucose molecules called **polysaccharides** (*poly* means "many"). They include starch, glycogen, and most fibers (**FIGURE 4.4**).

Starch Is a Polysaccharide Stored in Plants

Plants store glucose not as single molecules but as polysaccharides in the form of **starch**. The two forms of starch are *amylose* and *amylopectin*. Excellent food sources of starch include grains (wheat, rice, corn, oats, and barley), legumes (peas, beans, and lentils), and tubers (potatoes and yams). Our cells cannot use the complex starch molecules exactly as they occur in plants. Instead, our bodies must break them down into the monosaccharide glucose from which we can then fuel our energy needs.

Our bodies easily digest most starches; however, some starches in plants are not digestible and are called *resistant*. Technically, resistant starch is classified as a type

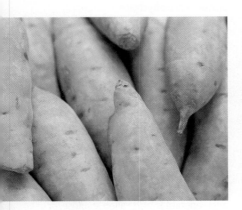

⬆ Tubers, such as these sweet potatoes, are excellent food sources of starch.

fermentation A process in which an agent causes an organic substance to break down into simpler substances and results in the production of ATP.

sucrose A disaccharide composed of one glucose molecule and one fructose molecule; sucrose is sweeter than lactose or maltose.

complex carbohydrate A nutrient compound consisting of long chains of glucose molecules, such as starch, glycogen, and fiber.

polysaccharide A complex carbohydrate consisting of long chains of glucose.

starch A polysaccharide stored in plants; the storage form of glucose in plants.

nutrition myth or fact?

Is Honey More Nutritious Than Table Sugar?

Liz's friend Tiffany is dedicated to eating healthful foods. She advises Liz to avoid sucrose and to eat foods that contain honey, molasses, or raw sugar. Like many people, Tiffany believes these sweeteners are more natural and nutritious than refined table sugar. How can Liz sort sugar fact from fiction?

Remember that sucrose consists of one glucose molecule and one fructose molecule joined together. From a chemical perspective, honey is almost identical to sucrose because honey also contains glucose and fructose molecules in almost equal amounts. However, enzymes in bees' "honey stomachs" separate some of the glucose and fructose molecules; as a result, honey looks and tastes slightly different from sucrose. As you know, bees store honey in combs, and they fan it with their wings to reduce its moisture content. This also alters the appearance and texture of honey.

Honey does not contain any more nutrients than sucrose, so it is not a more healthful choice than sucrose. In fact, per tablespoon, honey has more Calories (energy) than table sugar. This is because the crystals in table sugar take up more space on a spoon than the liquid form of honey, so a tablespoon contains less sugar. However, some people argue that honey is sweeter, so you use less.

It is important to note that honey commonly contains bacteria that can cause fatal food poisoning in infants. The more mature digestive system of older children and adults is immune to the effects of these bacteria, but babies younger than 12 months should never be given honey.

Are raw sugar and molasses more healthful than table sugar? Actually, the "raw sugar" available in the United States is not really raw. Truly raw sugar is made up of the first crystals obtained when sugar is processed. Sugar in this form contains dirt, parts of insects, and other by-products that make it illegal to sell in the United States. The raw sugar products in American stores have actually gone through more than half of the same steps in the refining process used to make table sugar. Raw sugar has a coarser texture than white sugar and is unbleached; in most markets, it is also significantly more expensive.

Molasses is the syrup that remains when sucrose is made from sugarcane. It is reddish brown in color with a distinctive taste that is less sweet than table sugar. It does contain some iron, but this iron does not occur naturally. It is a contaminant from the machines that process the sugarcane! Incidentally, blackstrap molasses is the residue of a third boiling of the syrup. It contains less sugar than light or dark molasses but more minerals.

TABLE 4.1 compares the nutrient content of white (or table) sugar, raw sugar, honey, and molasses. As you can see, none of them contains many nutrients that are important for health. This is why highly sweetened products are referred to as "empty Calories."

TABLE 4.1 Nutrient Comparison of Four Different Sugars

	Table Sugar	Raw Sugar	Honey	Molasses
Energy (kcal)	49	57	64	58
Carbohydrate (g)	12.6	14.27	17.3	14.95
Fat (g)	0	0	0	0
Protein (g)	0	0	0.06	0
Fiber (grams)	0	0	0	0
Vitamin C (mg)	0	0	0.1	0
Vitamin A (IU)	0	0	0	0
Thiamin (mg)	0	0	0	0.008
Riboflavin (mg)	0.002	0.003	0.008	0
Folate (µg)	0	0	0	0
Calcium (mg)	0	2	1	41
Iron (mg)	0.01	0.05	0.09	0.94
Sodium (mg)	0	0	1	7
Potassium (mg)	0	4	11	293

Note: Nutrient values are identified for 1 tablespoon of each product.

Data from: U.S. Department of Agriculture, Agricultural Research Service. 2012. USDA National Nutrient Database for Standard Reference, Release 25.

of fiber. When our intestinal bacteria ferment resistant starch, a fatty acid called *butyrate* is produced. Consuming resistant starch may be beneficial: some research suggests that butyrate consumption reduces the risk for cancer.[4] Legumes contain more resistant starch than do grains, fruits, or vegetables. This quality, plus their high protein and fiber content, makes legumes a healthful food.

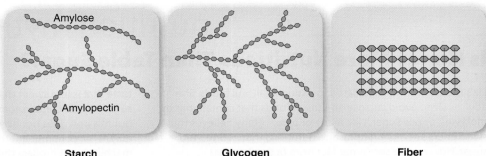

Starch
Storage form of glucose in plants; found in grains, legumes, and tubers

Glycogen
Storage form of glucose in animals; stored in liver and muscles

Fiber
Forms the support structures of leaves, stems, and plants

⬆ **FIGURE 4.4** Polysaccharides, also referred to as complex carbohydrates, include starch, glycogen, and fiber.

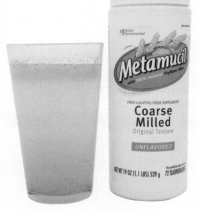

⬆ Dissolvable laxatives are examples of soluble fiber.

glycogen A polysaccharide; the storage form of glucose in animals.

dietary fiber The nondigestible carbohydrate parts of plants that form the support structures of leaves, stems, and seeds.

functional fiber The nondigestible forms of carbohydrates that are extracted from plants or manufactured in a laboratory and have known health benefits.

total fiber The sum of dietary fiber and functional fiber.

soluble fibers Fibers that dissolve in water.

viscous Having a gel-like consistency; viscous fibers form a gel when dissolved in water.

Glycogen Is a Polysaccharide Stored by Animals

Glycogen is the storage form of glucose for animals, including humans. After an animal is slaughtered, most of the glycogen is broken down by enzymes found in animal tissues. Thus, very little glycogen exists in meat. As plants contain no glycogen, it is not a dietary source of carbohydrate. We store glycogen in our muscles and liver; our bodies can metabolize this stored glycogen to glucose when we need energy. The storage and use of glycogen are discussed in more detail shortly.

Fiber Is a Polysaccharide That Gives Plants Their Structure

Like starch, fiber is composed of long polysaccharide chains; however, our bodies do not easily break down the bonds that connect fiber molecules. This means that most fibers pass through the digestive system without being digested and absorbed, so they contribute no energy to our diet. However, fiber offers many other health benefits, as we will see shortly.

There are currently a number of definitions of fiber. The Food and Nutrition Board of the Institute of Medicine propose three distinctions: *dietary fiber, functional fiber,* and *total fiber*.[5]

- **Dietary fiber** is the nondigestible parts of plants that form the support structures of leaves, stems, and seeds (see Figure 4.4). In a sense, you can think of dietary fiber as a plant's "skeleton."
- **Functional fiber** consists of the nondigestible forms of carbohydrates that are extracted from plants or manufactured in a laboratory and have known health benefits. Functional fiber is added to foods and is the form used in fiber supplements. Examples of functional fiber sources you might see on nutrition labels include cellulose, guar gum, pectin, and psyllium.
- **Total fiber** is the sum of dietary fiber and functional fiber.

Fiber can also be classified according to its chemical and physical properties as soluble or insoluble.

Soluble Fibers **Soluble fibers** dissolve in water. They are also **viscous**, forming a gel when wet, and fermentable; that is, they are easily digested by bacteria in the colon. Soluble fibers are typically found in citrus fruits, berries, oat products, and beans. Research suggests that the regular consumption of soluble fibers reduces the risks for cardiovascular disease and type 2 diabetes by lowering blood cholesterol and blood glucose levels. Soluble fibers include the following:

- *Pectins*, which contain chains of galacturonic acid and other monosaccharides. Pectins are found in the cell walls and intracellular tissues of many fruits and berries. They can be isolated and used to thicken foods, such as jams and yogurts.
- *Gums* contain galactose, glucuronic acid, and other monosaccharides. Gums are a diverse group of polysaccharides that are viscous. They are typically isolated from

seeds and are used as thickening, gelling, and stabilizing agents. Guar gum and gum arabic are common gums used as food additives.

■ *Mucilages* are similar to gums and contain galactose, mannose, and other mono-saccharides. Two examples are psyllium and carrageenan. Psyllium is the husk of psyllium seeds, which are also known as plantago or flea seeds. Carrageenan comes from seaweed. Mucilages are used as food stabilizers.

Insoluble Fibers   **Insoluble fibers** are those that do not typically dissolve in water. These fibers are usually nonviscous and typically cannot be fermented by bacteria in the colon. Insoluble fibers are generally found in whole grains, such as wheat, rye, and brown rice as well as in many vegetables. These fibers are not associated with reducing cholesterol levels but are known for promoting regular bowel movements, alleviating constipation, and reducing the risk for a bowel disorder called diverticulosis (discussed later in this chapter).

Examples of insoluble fibers include the following:

■ *Lignins* are noncarbohydrate forms of fiber. Lignins are found in the woody parts of plant cell walls and in carrots and the seeds of fruits and berries. Lignins are also found in brans (the outer husk of grains such as wheat, oats, and rye) and other whole grains.

■ *Cellulose* is the main structural component of plant cell walls. Cellulose is a chain of glucose units similar to amylose but, unlike amylose, cellulose contains bonds that are nondigestible by humans. Cellulose is found in whole grains, fruits, vegetables, and legumes. It can also be extracted from wood pulp or cotton, and it is added to foods as an agent for anticaking, thickening, and texturizing.

■ *Hemicelluloses* contain glucose, mannose, galacturonic acid, and other monosaccharides. Hemicelluloses are found in plant cell walls and they surround cellulose. They are the primary component of cereal fibers and are found in whole grains and vegetables. Although many hemicelluloses are insoluble, some are also classified as soluble.

Fiber-Rich Carbohydrates   Materials written for the general public usually don't refer to the carbohydrates found in foods as complex or simple; instead, resources such as the Dietary Guidelines for Americans 2010 emphasize eating *fiber-rich carbohydrates*, such as fruits, vegetables, and whole grains.[6] This term is important because fiber-rich carbohydrates are known to contribute to good health, but not all complex carbohydrate foods are fiber-rich. For example, potatoes that have been processed into frozen hash browns retain very little of their original fiber. On the other hand, some foods rich in simple carbohydrates (such as fruits) are also rich in fiber. So when you're reading labels, it pays to check the grams of dietary fiber per serving. And if the food you're considering is fresh produce and there's no label to read, that almost guarantees it's fiber-rich.

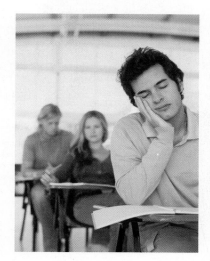

Our red blood cells, brain, and nerve cells primarily rely on glucose. This is why we get tired, irritable, and shaky when we have not eaten for a prolonged period.

recap   The three types of polysaccharides are starch, glycogen, and fiber. Starch is the storage form of glucose in plants, whereas glycogen is the storage form of glucose in animals. Fiber forms the support structures of plants. Soluble fibers dissolve in water, are viscous, and can be digested by bacteria in the colon, whereas insoluble fibers do not dissolve in water, are not viscous, and cannot be digested. Fiber-rich carbohydrates are known to contribute to good health.

Why do we need carbohydrates?

We have seen that carbohydrates are an important energy source for our bodies. Let's learn more about this and other functions of carbohydrates.

Carbohydrates Provide Energy

Carbohydrates, an excellent source of energy for all our cells, provide 4 kilocalories (kcal) of energy per gram. Some of our cells can also use fat and even protein for

insoluble fibers Fibers that do not dissolve in water.

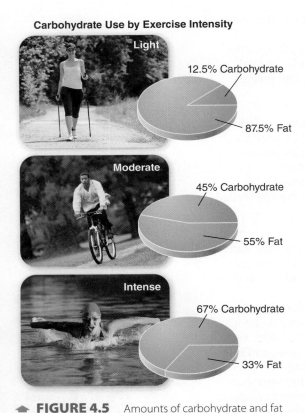

Carbohydrate Use by Exercise Intensity

Light
12.5% Carbohydrate
87.5% Fat

Moderate
45% Carbohydrate
55% Fat

Intense
67% Carbohydrate
33% Fat

FIGURE 4.5 Amounts of carbohydrate and fat used during light, moderate, and intense exercise. Data adapted from: "Regulation of endogenous fat and carbohydrate metabolism in relation to exercise intensity and duration" by Romijn et al., from *American Journal of Physiology*, September 1, 1993. Copyright © 1993 by The American Physiological Society. Reprinted with permission.

ketosis The process by which the breakdown of fat during fasting states results in the production of ketones.

ketones Substances produced during the breakdown of fat when carbohydrate intake is insufficient to meet energy needs. Ketones provide an alternative energy source for the brain when glucose levels are low.

ketoacidosis A condition in which excessive ketones are present in the blood, causing the blood to become very acidic, which alters basic body functions and damages tissues. Untreated ketoacidosis can be fatal. This condition is found in individuals with untreated diabetes mellitus.

gluconeogenesis The generation of glucose from the breakdown of proteins into amino acids.

energy if necessary. However, our red blood cells can use only glucose, and our brain and other nervous tissues rely primarily on glucose. This is why you get tired, irritable, and shaky when you haven't eaten any carbohydrate for a prolonged period.

Carbohydrates Fuel Daily Activity

Many popular diets—such as Dr. Atkins' New Revolution Diet and the Sugar Busters plan—are based on the idea that our bodies actually "prefer" to use fat and/or protein for energy. They claim that current carbohydrate recommendations are much higher than we really need.

In reality, we rely mostly on both carbohydrates and fat for energy. In fact, as shown in **FIGURE 4.5**, our bodies always use some combination of carbohydrates and fat to fuel daily activities. Fat is the predominant energy source used at rest and during low-intensity activities, such as sitting, standing, and walking. Even during rest, however, our brain cells and red blood cells rely on glucose.

Carbohydrates Fuel Exercise

When we exercise, whether running, briskly walking, bicycling, or performing any other activity that causes us to breathe harder and sweat, we begin to use more glucose than fat. Whereas fat breakdown is a slow process and requires oxygen, we can break down glucose very quickly either with or without oxygen. Even during very intense exercise, when less oxygen is available, we can still break down glucose very quickly for energy. That's why when you are exercising at maximal effort carbohydrates are providing almost 100% of the energy your body requires.

If you are physically active, it is important to eat enough carbohydrates to provide energy for your brain, red blood cells, and muscles. In general, if you do not eat enough carbohydrate to support regular exercise, your body will have to rely on fat and protein as alternative energy sources. One advantage of becoming highly trained for endurance-type events, such as marathons and triathlons, is that our muscles are able to store more glycogen, which provides us with additional glucose we can use during exercise. (See Chapter 12 for more information on how exercise affects our need, use, and storage of carbohydrates.)

Low Carbohydrate Intake Can Lead to Ketoacidosis

When we do not eat enough carbohydrate, our bodies seek an alternative source of fuel for our brain and begins to break down stored fat. This process, called **ketosis**, produces an alternative fuel called **ketones**.

Ketosis is an important mechanism for providing energy to the brain during situations of fasting, low carbohydrate intake, or vigorous exercise. However, ketones also suppress appetite and cause dehydration and acetone breath (the breath smells like nail polish remover). If inadequate carbohydrate intake continues for an extended period, the body will produce excessive amounts of ketones. Because many ketones are acids, high ketone levels cause the blood to become very acidic, leading to a condition called **ketoacidosis**. The high acidity of the blood interferes with basic body functions, causes the loss of lean body mass, and damages many body tissues. People with untreated diabetes are at high risk for ketoacidosis, which can lead to coma and even death (see the **In Depth** on diabetes following this chapter).

Carbohydrates Spare Protein

If the diet does not provide enough carbohydrate, the body will make its own glucose from protein. This involves breaking down the proteins in blood and tissues into amino acids, then converting them to glucose. This process is called **gluconeogenesis** ("generating new glucose").

When our bodies use proteins for energy, the amino acids from these proteins cannot be used to make new cells, repair tissue damage, support our immune system, or perform any other function. During periods of starvation or when eating a diet that is very low in carbohydrate, our bodies will take amino acids from the blood first, and then from other tissues, such as muscles and the heart, liver, and kidneys. Using amino acids in this manner over a prolonged period can cause serious, possibly irreversible, damage to these organs. (See Chapter 6 for more details on using protein for energy.)

Fiber Helps Us Stay Healthy

Although we cannot digest fiber, research indicates that it helps us stay healthy and may prevent many digestive and chronic diseases. The following are potential benefits of fiber consumption:

- May reduce the risk of colon cancer. Although there is some controversy surrounding this claim, many researchers believe that fiber binds cancer-causing substances and speeds their elimination from the colon. However, recent studies of colon cancer and fiber have shown that their relationship is not as strong as previously thought.
- Promotes bowel health by helping to prevent hemorrhoids, constipation, and other intestinal problems by keeping our stools moist and soft. Fiber gives gut muscles "something to push on" and makes it easier to eliminate stools.
- Reduces the risk for *diverticulosis,* a condition that is caused in part by trying to eliminate small, hard stools. A great deal of pressure must be generated in the large intestine to pass hard stools. This increased pressure weakens intestinal walls, causing them to bulge outward and form pockets (**FIGURE 4.6**). Feces and fibrous materials can get trapped in these pockets, which become infected and inflamed. This is a painful condition that must be treated with antibiotics or surgery.
- May reduce the risk of heart disease by delaying or blocking the absorption of dietary cholesterol into the bloodstream, a process depicted in **FIGURE 4.7**. In addition, when soluble fibers are digested, bacteria in the colon produce short-chain fatty acids that may reduce the production of low-density lipoprotein (LDL), a blood lipid that is associated with heart disease, to healthful levels.
- May enhance weight loss, as eating a high-fiber diet causes a person to feel more full. Fiber absorbs water, expands in our large intestine, and slows the movement of food through the upper part of the digestive tract. Also, people who eat a fiber-rich diet tend to eat fewer fatty and sugary foods.
- May lower the risk for type 2 diabetes. In slowing digestion and absorption, fiber also slows the release of glucose into the blood. It thereby improves the body's regulation of insulin production and blood glucose levels.

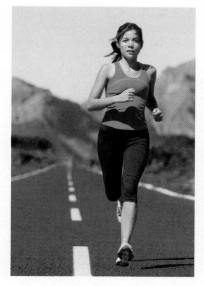

When we exercise or perform any activity that causes us to breathe harder and sweat, we begin to use more glucose than fat.

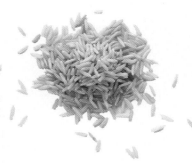

Brown rice is a good food source of dietary fiber.

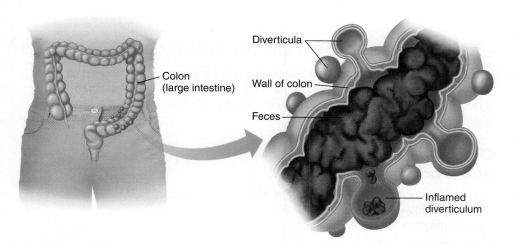

FIGURE 4.6 Diverticulosis occurs when bulging pockets form in the wall of the colon. These pockets become infected and inflamed, demanding proper treatment.

▶ **FIGURE 4.7** How fiber may help decrease blood cholesterol levels. **(a)** When eating a high-fiber diet, fiber binds to the bile that is produced from cholesterol, resulting in relatively more cholesterol being excreted in the feces. **(b)** When a lower-fiber diet is consumed, less fiber (and thus less cholesterol) is bound to bile and excreted in the feces.

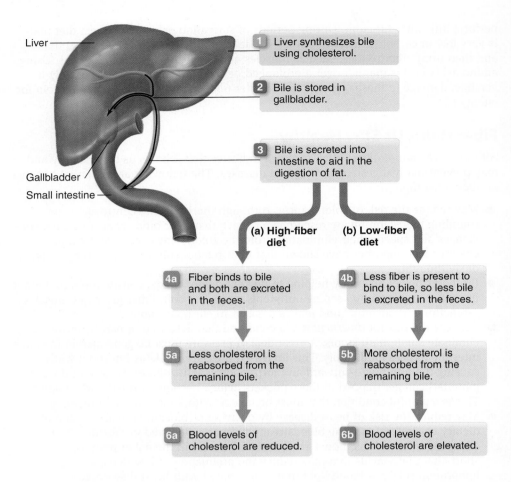

Liver

1 Liver synthesizes bile using cholesterol.

2 Bile is stored in gallbladder.

3 Bile is secreted into intestine to aid in the digestion of fat.

Gallbladder

Small intestine

(a) High-fiber diet

(b) Low-fiber diet

4a Fiber binds to bile and both are excreted in the feces.

4b Less fiber is present to bind to bile, so less bile is excreted in the feces.

5a Less cholesterol is reabsorbed from the remaining bile.

5b More cholesterol is reabsorbed from the remaining bile.

6a Blood levels of cholesterol are reduced.

6b Blood levels of cholesterol are elevated.

recap Carbohydrates are an important energy source at rest and during exercise, and they provide 4 kcal of energy per gram. Carbohydrates are necessary in the diet to spare body protein and prevent ketosis. Complex carbohydrates contain fiber and other nutrients that can reduce the risk for obesity, heart disease, and diabetes. Fiber helps prevent hemorrhoids, constipation, and diverticulosis; may reduce the risk for colon cancer and heart disease; and may assist with weight loss.

How do our bodies break down carbohydrates?

Glucose is the form of sugar that our bodies use for energy, and the primary goal of carbohydrate digestion is to break down polysaccharides and disaccharides into monosaccharides, which can then be converted to glucose. **FIGURE 4.8** provides a visual tour of carbohydrate digestion.

Digestion Breaks Down Most Carbohydrates into Monosaccharides

Carbohydrate digestion begins in the mouth as the starch in the foods you eat mixes with your saliva during chewing (see Figure 4.8). Saliva contains an enzyme called **salivary amylase**, which breaks starch into smaller particles and eventually into the disaccharide maltose. The next time you eat a piece of bread, notice that you can actually taste it becoming sweeter; this indicates the breakdown of starch into maltose. Disaccharides are not digested in the mouth.

salivary amylase An enzyme in saliva that breaks starch into smaller particles and eventually into the disaccharide maltose.

focus figure 4.8 | Carbohydrate Digestion Overview

The primary goal of carbohydrate digestion is to break down polysaccharides and disaccharides into monosaccharides that can then be converted to glucose.

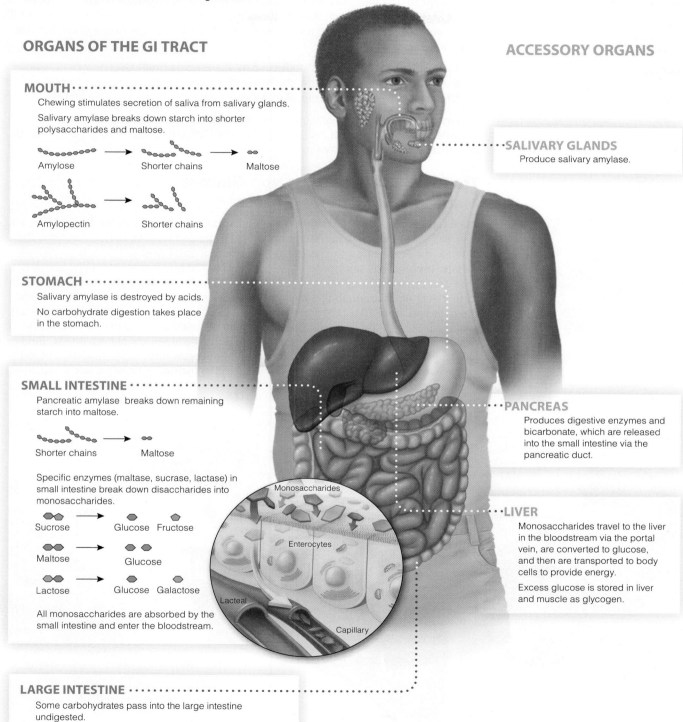

ORGANS OF THE GI TRACT

MOUTH
Chewing stimulates secretion of saliva from salivary glands.

Salivary amylase breaks down starch into shorter polysaccharides and maltose.

Amylose → Shorter chains → Maltose

Amylopectin → Shorter chains

STOMACH
Salivary amylase is destroyed by acids.

No carbohydrate digestion takes place in the stomach.

SMALL INTESTINE
Pancreatic amylase breaks down remaining starch into maltose.

Shorter chains → Maltose

Specific enzymes (maltase, sucrase, lactase) in small intestine break down disaccharides into monosaccharides.

Sucrose → Glucose Fructose

Maltose → Glucose

Lactose → Glucose Galactose

All monosaccharides are absorbed by the small intestine and enter the bloodstream.

LARGE INTESTINE
Some carbohydrates pass into the large intestine undigested.

Bacteria ferment some undigested carbohydrate.

Remaining fiber is excreted in feces.

ACCESSORY ORGANS

SALIVARY GLANDS
Produce salivary amylase.

PANCREAS
Produces digestive enzymes and bicarbonate, which are released into the small intestine via the pancreatic duct.

LIVER
Monosaccharides travel to the liver in the bloodstream via the portal vein, are converted to glucose, and then are transported to body cells to provide energy.

Excess glucose is stored in liver and muscle as glycogen.

Monosaccharides

Enterocytes

Lacteal

Capillary

119

pancreatic amylase An enzyme secreted by the pancreas into the small intestine that digests any remaining starch into maltose.

maltase A digestive enzyme that breaks maltose into glucose.

sucrase A digestive enzyme that breaks sucrose into glucose and fructose.

lactase A digestive enzyme that breaks lactose into glucose and galactose.

As the bolus of food leaves the mouth and enters the stomach, all digestion of carbohydrates ceases. This is because the acid in the stomach inactivates the salivary amylase enzyme.

The majority of carbohydrate digestion occurs in the small intestine. As the contents of the stomach enter the small intestine, an enzyme called **pancreatic amylase** is secreted by the pancreas into the small intestine. Pancreatic amylase continues to digest any remaining starch into maltose. Additional enzymes found in the microvilli of the mucosal cells that line the intestinal tract work to break down disaccharides into monosaccharides:

- Maltose is broken down into glucose by the enzyme **maltase**.
- Sucrose is broken down into glucose and fructose by the enzyme **sucrase**.
- Lactose is broken down into glucose and galactose by the enzyme **lactase**.

Once digestion of carbohydrates is complete, all monosaccharides are then absorbed into the mucosal cells lining the small intestine, where they pass through and enter into the bloodstream.

The Liver Converts Most Non-Glucose Monosaccharides into Glucose

Once the monosaccharides enter the bloodstream, they travel to the liver, where fructose and galactose are converted to glucose. If needed immediately for energy, the glucose is released into the bloodstream, where it can travel to the cells to provide energy. If glucose is not needed immediately for energy, it is stored as glycogen in our liver and muscles. Enzymes in liver and muscle cells combine glucose molecules to form glycogen in an anabolic, or building, process called *glycogenesis*. On average, the liver can store 70 g (280 kcal) and the muscles can store about 120 g (480 kcal) of glycogen. Stored glycogen can then be converted back into glucose in a catabolic, or destructive, process called *glycogenolysis* to supply the body's energy needs. Between meals, for example, our bodies draw on liver glycogen reserves to maintain blood glucose levels and support the needs of our cells, including those of our brain, spinal cord, and red blood cells **(FIGURE 4.9)**.

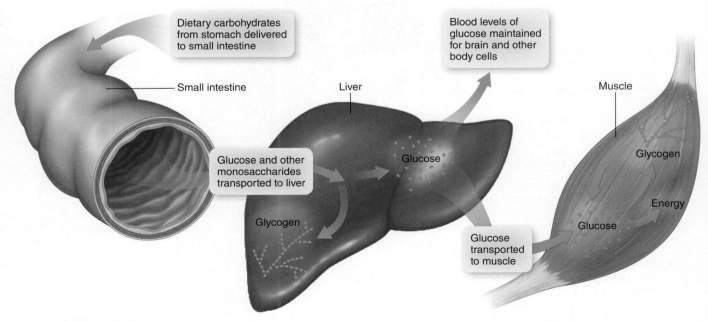

FIGURE 4.9 In the process of glycogenesis, glucose is stored as glycogen in both the liver and muscle. In the process of glycogenolysis, the glycogen stored in the liver is metabolized to maintain blood glucose between meals; muscle glycogen provides immediate energy to the muscle during exercise.

The glycogen stored in our muscles continually provides energy to our muscle cells, particularly during intense exercise. Endurance athletes can increase their storage of muscle glycogen from two to four times the normal amount through a process called *carbohydrate loading* (see Chapter 12). Any excess glucose is stored as glycogen in the liver and muscles and saved for such future energy needs as exercise. Once the storage capacity of the liver and muscles is reached, any excess glucose can be stored as fat in adipose tissue.

Fiber Is Excreted from the Large Intestine

As previously mentioned, humans do not possess enzymes in the small intestine that can break down fiber. Thus, fiber passes through the small intestine undigested and enters the large intestine, or colon. There, bacteria ferment some previously undigested carbohydrates, causing the production of gases and a few short-chain fatty acids. The cells of the large intestine use these short-chain fatty acids for energy. The fiber remaining in the colon adds bulk to our stools and is excreted in feces (see Figure 4.8). In this way, fiber assists in maintaining bowel regularity.

recap Carbohydrate digestion starts in the mouth and continues in the small intestine. Glucose and other monosaccharides are absorbed into the bloodstream and travel to the liver, where non-glucose sugars are converted to glucose. Glucose either is used by the cells for energy or is converted to glycogen and stored in the liver and muscle for later use.

A Variety of Hormones Regulate Blood Glucose Levels

Our bodies regulate blood glucose levels within a fairly narrow range to provide adequate glucose to the brain and other cells. A number of hormones, including insulin, glucagon, epinephrine, norepinephrine, cortisol, and growth hormone, assist the body with maintaining blood glucose.

When we eat a meal, our blood glucose level rises. But glucose in our blood cannot help our nerves, muscles, and other organs function unless it can cross into their cells. Glucose molecules are too large to cross cell membranes independently. To get in, glucose needs assistance from the hormone **insulin**, which is secreted by the pancreas (**FIGURE 4.10** top panel). Insulin is transported in the blood throughout the body, where it stimulates special molecules called glucose transporters, which are located in cells, to travel to the cell membrane and transport glucose into the cell. Insulin can therefore be thought of as a key that opens the gates of the cell membrane, enabling the transport of glucose into the cell interior, where it can be used for energy. Insulin also stimulates the liver and muscles to take up glucose and store it as glycogen.

When you have not eaten for some time, your blood glucose level declines. This decrease in blood glucose stimulates the pancreas to secrete another hormone, **glucagon** (Figure 4.10 bottom panel). Glucagon acts in an opposite way to insulin. It triggers glycogenolysis, in which the liver converts its stored glycogen into glucose, which is then secreted into the bloodstream and transported to the cells for energy. Glucagon also assists in the breakdown of body proteins to amino acids, so that the liver can stimulate gluconeogenesis, the production of new glucose from amino acids.

Epinephrine, norepinephrine, cortisol, and growth hormone are additional hormones that work to increase blood glucose. Epinephrine and norepinephrine are secreted by the adrenal glands and nerve endings when blood glucose levels are low. They trigger glycogen breakdown in the liver, resulting in a subsequent increase in the release of glucose into the bloodstream. They also increase gluconeogenesis. These two hormones are also responsible for our "fight-or-flight" reaction to danger; they are released when we need a burst of energy to respond quickly. Cortisol and growth hormone are secreted by the adrenal glands to act on liver, muscle, and adipose tissue. Cortisol increases gluconeogenesis and decreases the use of glucose by muscles and other body organs. Growth hormone decreases glucose uptake by our muscles,

insulin The hormone secreted by the beta cells of the pancreas in response to increased blood levels of glucose; it facilitates the uptake of glucose by body cells.

glucagon The hormone secreted by the alpha cells of the pancreas in response to decreased blood levels of glucose; it causes the breakdown of liver stores of glycogen into glucose.

focus figure 4.10 | Regulation of Blood Glucose

Our bodies regulate blood glucose levels within a fairly narrow range to provide adequate glucose to the brain and other cells. Insulin and glucagon are two hormones that play a key role in regulating blood glucose.

HIGH BLOOD GLUCOSE

1 **Insulin secretion:** When blood glucose levels increase after a meal, the pancreas secretes the hormone insulin from the beta cells into the bloodstream.

2 **Cellular uptake:** Insulin travels to the tissues. There, it stimulates glucose transporters within cells to travel to the cell membrane, where they facilitate glucose transport into the cell to be used for energy.

3 **Glucose storage:** Insulin also stimulates the storage of glucose in body tissues. Glucose is stored as glycogen in the liver and muscles (glycogenesis), and is stored as triglycerides in adipose tissue (lipogenesis).

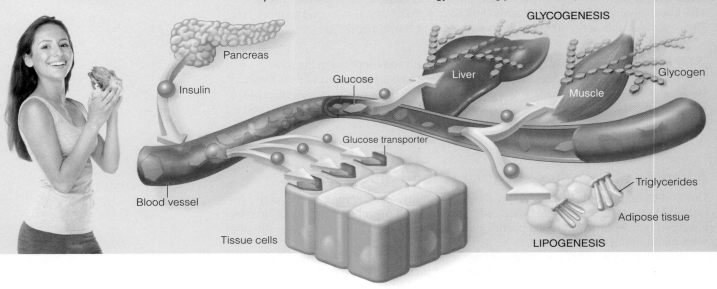

LOW BLOOD GLUCOSE

1 **Glucagon secretion:** When blood glucose levels are low, the pancreas secretes the hormone glucagon from the alpha cells into the bloodstream.

2 **Glycogenolysis:** Glucagon stimulates the liver to convert stored glycogen into glucose, which is released into the blood and transported to the cells for energy.

3 **Gluconeogenesis:** Glucagon also assists in the breakdown of proteins and the uptake of amino acids by the liver, which creates glucose from amino acids.

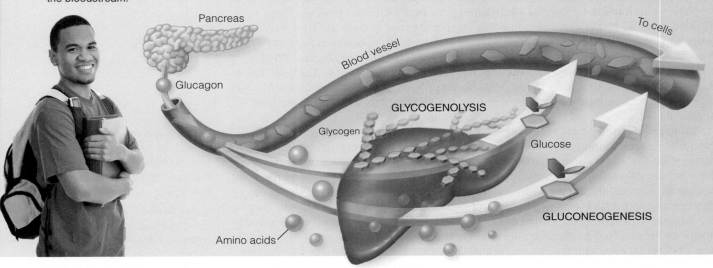

HOT TOPIC

Is it Hunger—or Hypoglycemia?

After going for several hours without eating, have you ever felt spaced out, shaky, irritable, and weak? And did the symptoms subside once you'd eaten? If so, maybe you wondered if your symptoms were due to hypoglycemia.

In **hypoglycemia**, blood glucose falls to lower-than-normal levels. This commonly occurs in people with diabetes who aren't getting proper treatment, but it can also happen in people who don't have diabetes if their pancreas secretes too much insulin after a high-carbohydrate meal. The characteristic symptoms usually appear about 1 to 4 hours after the meal and occur because the body clears glucose from the blood too quickly. People with this form of hypoglycemia must eat smaller meals more frequently to level out their blood insulin and glucose levels.

The trouble is, ordinary hunger can make you experience symptoms just like those of true hypoglycemia. So which is it— hunger or hypoglycemia? You can only find out for sure by getting a blood test, but unless you have diabetes it's probably not necessary. For most healthy people, eating regular meals and healthy snacks is the only "treatment" needed.

increases our mobilization and use of the fatty acids stored in our adipose tissue, and increases our liver's output of glucose.

Normally, the effects of these hormones balance each other to maintain blood glucose within a healthy range. An alteration in this balance can lead to health conditions such as diabetes (discussed **In Depth** following this chapter) or hypoglycemia.

The Glycemic Index Shows How Foods Affect Our Blood Glucose Level

The term **glycemic index** refers to the potential of foods to raise blood glucose levels. Foods with a high glycemic index cause a sudden surge in blood glucose. This in turn triggers a large increase in insulin, which may be followed by a dramatic drop in blood glucose. Foods with a low glycemic index cause low to moderate fluctuations in blood glucose. When foods are assigned a glycemic index value, they are often compared to the glycemic effect of pure glucose.

The glycemic index of a food is not always easy to predict. **FIGURE 4.11** ranks certain foods according to their glycemic index. Do any of these rankings surprise you? Most people assume that foods containing simple sugars have a higher glycemic index than starches, but this is not always the case. For instance, compare the glycemic index for apples and instant potatoes. Although instant potatoes are a starchy food, they have a glycemic index value of 85, whereas the value for an apple is only 38!

The type of carbohydrate, the way the food is prepared, and its fat and fiber content can all affect how quickly the body absorbs it. It is important to note that we eat most of our foods combined into a meal. In this case, the glycemic index of the total meal becomes more important than the ranking of each food.

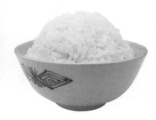
An apple has a much lower glycemic index value (38) than a serving of white rice (56).

For determining the effect of a food on a person's glucose response, some nutrition experts believe that the **glycemic load** is more useful than the glycemic index. A food's glycemic load is the number of grams of carbohydrate it contains multiplied by the glycemic index of that carbohydrate. For instance, carrots are recognized as a vegetable having a relatively high glycemic index of about 68; however, the glycemic load of carrots is only 3.[7] This is because there is very little total carbohydrate in a serving of carrots. The low glycemic load of carrots means that carrot consumption is unlikely to cause a significant rise in glucose and insulin levels.

Why do we care about the glycemic index and glycemic load? Foods and meals with a lower glycemic load are better choices for someone with diabetes because they will not trigger dramatic fluctuations in blood glucose. They may also reduce the risk for heart disease and colon cancer because they generally contain more fiber, and fiber

hypoglycemia A condition marked by blood glucose levels that are below normal fasting levels.

glycemic index The system that assigns ratings (or values) for the potential of foods to raise blood glucose and insulin levels.

glycemic load The amount of carbohydrate in a food multiplied by the glycemic index of the carbohydrate.

▶ FIGURE 4.11 Glycemic index values for various foods as compared to pure glucose. Data adapted from: "International Table of Glycemic Index and Glycemic Load Values," by Foster-Powell, K., S. H. A. Holt, and J. C. Brand-Miller from *American Journal of Clinical Nutrition*, 2002.

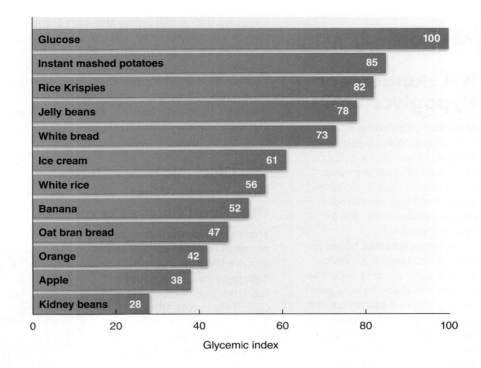

To find out the glycemic index and glycemic load of over 100 foods, visit **www.health.harvard.edu** , enter "newsweek" into the search bar, and then click on the link to "glycemic index and glycemic load for 100+ foods."

helps decrease fat levels in the blood. Recent studies have shown that people who eat lower glycemic index diets have higher levels of high-density lipoprotein, or HDL (a healthful blood lipid), and lower levels of low-density lipoprotein, or LDL (a blood lipid associated with increased risk for heart disease), and their blood glucose values are more likely to be normal.[8,9] Diets with a low glycemic index and load are also associated with a reduced risk for prostate cancer.[10]

Despite some encouraging research findings, the glycemic index and glycemic load remain controversial. Many nutrition researchers feel that the evidence supporting their health benefits is weak. In addition, many believe the concepts of the glycemic index/load are too complex for people to apply to their daily lives. Other researchers insist that helping people choose foods with a lower glycemic index/load is critical in the prevention and treatment of many chronic diseases. Until this controversy is resolved, people are encouraged to eat a variety of fiber-rich and less-processed carbohydrates, such as beans and lentils, fresh vegetables, and whole-wheat bread, because these forms of carbohydrates have a lower glycemic load and they contain a multitude of important nutrients.

recap Various hormones are involved in regulating blood glucose. Insulin lowers blood glucose levels by facilitating the entry of glucose into cells. Glucagon, epinephrine, norepinephrine, cortisol, and growth hormone raise blood glucose levels by a variety of mechanisms. The glycemic index is a value that indicates the potential of foods to raise blood glucose and insulin levels. The glycemic load is the amount of carbohydrate in a food multiplied by the glycemic index of the carbohydrate in that food. Foods with a high glycemic index/load cause surges in blood glucose and insulin, whereas foods with a low glycemic index/load cause more moderate fluctuations in blood glucose. Diets with a low glycemic index/load are associated with a reduced risk for chronic diseases.

How much carbohydrate should we eat?

Proponents of low-carbohydrate diets claim that eating carbohydrates makes you gain weight. However, anyone who consumes more Calories than he or she expends will gain weight, whether those Calories are in the form of simple or complex carbohydrates, protein, or fat. Moreover, fat is twice as "fattening" as carbohydrate: it contains 9 kcal per gram, whereas carbohydrate contains only 4 kcal per gram. In fact, eating carbohydrate sources that are high in fiber and micronutrients has been shown to reduce the overall risk for obesity, heart disease, and diabetes. Thus, all carbohydrates are not bad, and even foods with added sugars—in limited amounts—can be included in a healthful diet.

The Recommended Dietary Allowance (RDA) for carbohydrate is based on the amount of glucose the brain uses.[5] The current RDA for adults 19 years of age and older is 130 g of carbohydrate per day. It is important to emphasize that this RDA does not cover the amount of carbohydrate needed to support daily activities; it covers only the amount of carbohydrate needed to supply adequate glucose to the brain.

Carbohydrates have been assigned an Acceptable Macronutrient Distribution Range (AMDR) of 45% to 65% of total energy intake. This is the range of intake associated with a decreased risk for chronic diseases. **TABLE 4.2** compares the carbohydrate recommendations from the Institute of Medicine with the Dietary Guidelines for Americans related to carbohydrate-containing foods.[5,6] As you can see, the Institute of Medicine provides specific numeric recommendations, whereas the Dietary Guidelines for Americans are general suggestions about foods high in fiber and low in added sugars. Most health agencies agree that most of the carbohydrates you eat each day should be high in fiber, whole-grain, and unprocessed. As recommended in the USDA Food Guide, eating at least half your grains as whole grains and eating the suggested amounts of fruits and vegetables each day will ensure that you get enough fiber-rich carbohydrates in your diet. Although fruits are predominantly composed of simple sugars, they are good sources of vitamins, some minerals, and fiber.

◀ Eating the suggested daily amounts of vegetables and fruit, such as apricots, will ensure that you're getting enough fiber-rich carbohydrate in your diet.

Most Americans Eat Too Much Added Sugar

The average carbohydrate intake per person in the United States is approximately 50% of total energy intake. For some people, almost half of this amount consists of sugars. Where does all this sugar come from? Some sugar comes from healthful food sources, such as fruit and milk. Some comes from foods made with refined grains, such as soft white breads, saltine crackers, and pastries. Much of the rest comes from **added sugars**—that is, sugars and syrups that are added to foods during processing or preparation.[5] For example, many processed foods include high-fructose-corn syrup (HFCS).

The most common source of added sugars in the U.S. diet is sweetened soft drinks; we drink an average of 40 gallons per person each year. Consider that one 12-oz cola contains 38.5 g of sugar, or almost 10 teaspoons. If you drink the average amount, you are consuming more than 16,420 g of sugar (about 267 cups) each year! Other common sources of added sugars include cookies, cakes, pies, fruit drinks, fruit

added sugars Sugars and syrups that are added to food during processing or preparation.

TABLE 4.2 Dietary Recommendations for Carbohydrates

Institute of Medicine Recommendations*	Dietary Guidelines for Americans†
Recommended Dietary Allowance (RDA) for adults 19 years of age and older is 130 g of carbohydrate per day.	Limit the consumption of foods that contain refined grains, especially refined grain foods that contain solid fats, added sugars, and sodium.
	Reduce the intake of Calories from solid fats and added sugars.
The Acceptable Macronutrient Distribution Range (AMDR) for carbohydrate is 45–65% of total daily energy intake.	Increase vegetable and fruit intake. Eat a variety of vegetables, especially dark-green and red and orange vegetables and beans and peas.
Added sugar intake should be 25% or less of total energy intake each day.	Consume at least half of all grains as whole grains. Increase whole-grain intake by replacing refined grains with whole grains. Choose foods that provide more dietary fiber, as well as potassium, calcium, and vitamin D, which are nutrients of concern in American diets. These foods include vegetables, fruits, whole grains, and milk and milk products.

Data from: *Institute of Medicine, Food and Nutrition Board, 2005. *Dietary Reference Intakes for Energy, Carbohydrates, Fiber, Fat, Fatty Acids, Cholesterol, Protein, and Amino Acids (Macronutrients)*. Washington, DC: The National Academy of Sciences. Reprinted with permission.

Data from: †U.S. Department of Health and Human Services and U.S. Department of Agriculture. 2010. Dietary Guidelines for Americans.

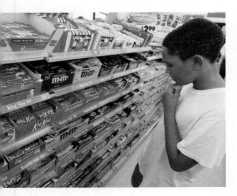

⬅ Candy and other foods with added sugars have lower levels of vitamins, minerals, and fiber than foods that naturally contain simple sugars.

punches, and candy. Even many nondessert items, such as peanut butter, yogurt, flavored rice mixes, and even salad dressing, contain added sugars.

If you want a quick way to figure out the amount of sugar in a processed food, check the Nutrition Facts panel on the box for the line that identifies "Sugars." You'll notice that the amount of sugar in a serving is identified in grams. Divide the total grams by 4 to get teaspoons. For instance, one national brand of yogurt contains 21 grams of sugar in a half-cup serving. That's more than 5 teaspoons of sugar! Doing this simple math before you buy may help you choose among different, more healthful versions of the same food.

Added sugars are not chemically different from naturally occurring sugars. However, foods and beverages with added sugars have lower levels of vitamins, minerals, and fiber than foods that naturally contain simple sugars. That's why most healthcare organizations recommend that we limit our consumption of added sugars. The Nutrition Facts panel includes a listing of total sugars, but a distinction is not generally made between added sugars and naturally occurring sugars. Thus, you need to check the ingredients list. Refer to **TABLE 4.3** for a list of terms indicating added sugars. To maintain a diet low in added sugars, limit foods in which a form of added sugar is listed as one of the first few ingredients on the label.

TABLE 4.3   Forms of Sugar Commonly Added to Foods

Name of Sugar	Definition
Brown sugar	A highly refined sweetener made up of approximately 99% sucrose and produced by adding to white table sugar either molasses or burnt table sugar for coloring and flavor.
Cane sugar	Sucrose that has been extracted from sugarcane, a tropical plant naturally rich in sugar.
Concentrated fruit juice sweetener	A form of sweetener made with concentrated fruit juice, commonly pear juice.
Confectioner's sugar	A highly refined, finely ground white sugar; also referred to as powdered sugar.
Corn sweeteners	A general term for any sweetener made with corn starch.
Corn syrup	A syrup produced by the partial hydrolysis of corn starch.
Dextrose	An alternative term for glucose.
Fructose	A monosaccharide that occurs in fruits and vegetables; also called levulose, or fruit sugar.
Galactose	A monosaccharide that joins with glucose to create lactose.
Granulated sugar	Another term for white sugar, or table sugar.
High-fructose corn syrup	A type of corn syrup in which part of the sucrose is converted to fructose, making it sweeter than sucrose or regular corn syrup; most high-fructose corn syrup contains 42% to 55% fructose.
Honey	A sweet, sticky liquid sweetener made by bees from the nectar of flowers; contains glucose and fructose.
Invert sugar	A sugar created by heating a sucrose syrup with a small amount of acid; inverting sucrose results in its breakdown into glucose and fructose, which reduces the size of the sugar crystals; because of its smooth texture, it is used in making candies and some syrups.
Levulose	Another term for fructose, or fruit sugar.
Mannitol	A type of sugar alcohol.
Maple sugar	A sugar made by boiling maple syrup.
Molasses	A thick, brown syrup that is separated from raw sugar during manufacturing; it is considered the least refined form of sucrose.
Natural sweeteners	A general term used for any naturally occurring sweeteners, such as fructose, honey, and raw sugar.
Raw sugar	The sugar that results from the processing of sugar beets or sugarcane; it is approximately 96% to 98% sucrose; true raw sugar contains impurities and is not stable in storage; the raw sugar available to consumers has been purified to yield an edible sugar.
Sorbitol	A type of sugar alcohol.
Turbinado sugar	The form of raw sugar that is purified and safe for human consumption; sold as "Sugar in the Raw" in the United States.
White sugar	Another name for sucrose, or table sugar.
Xylitol	A type of sugar alcohol.

Sugars Are Blamed for Many Health Problems

Why do sugars have such a bad reputation? First, they are known to contribute to tooth decay. Second, many people believe they cause hyperactivity in children. Third, eating a lot of sugar could increase the levels of unhealthful lipids in our blood, increasing our risk for heart disease. High intakes of sugar have also been blamed for causing diabetes and obesity. Let's learn the truth about these accusations.

Sugar Causes Tooth Decay

Sugars do play a role in dental problems, because the bacteria that cause tooth decay thrive on sugar. These bacteria produce acids, which eat away at tooth enamel and can eventually cause cavities and gum disease (**FIGURE 4.12**). Eating sticky foods that adhere to teeth—such as caramels, crackers, sugary cereals, and licorice—and sipping sweetened beverages over time are two behaviors that increase the risk for tooth decay. This means that people shouldn't suck on hard candies or caramels, slowly sip soda or juice, or put babies to bed with a bottle unless it contains water. As we have seen, even breast milk contains sugar, which can slowly drip onto the baby's gums. As a result, infants should not routinely be allowed to fall asleep at the breast.

To reduce your risk for tooth decay, brush your teeth after each meal, after drinking sugary drinks, and after snacking on sweets. Drinking fluoridated water and using a fluoride toothpaste will also help protect your teeth.

There Is No Link Between Sugar and Hyperactivity in Children

Although many people believe that eating sugar causes hyperactivity and other behavioral problems in children, there is little scientific evidence to support this claim. Some children actually become less active shortly after a high-sugar meal! However, it is important to emphasize that most studies of sugar and children's behavior have only looked at the effects of sugar a few hours after ingestion. We know very little about the long-term effects of sugar intake on the behavior of children. Behavioral and learning problems are complex issues, most likely caused by a multitude of factors. Because of this complexity, the Institute of Medicine has stated that, overall, there does not appear to be enough evidence to state that eating too much sugar causes hyperactivity or other behavioral problems in children.[5] Thus, there is no Tolerable Upper Intake Level for sugar.

High Sugar Intake Can Lead to Unhealthful Levels of Blood Lipids

Research evidence does suggest that consuming a diet high in added sugars is associated with unhealthful changes in blood lipids.[11] For example, higher intakes of added sugars are associated with higher blood levels of low-density lipoproteins (LDL) and lower levels of high-density lipoproteins (HDL). These are risk factors for heart disease. Two recent studies have shown that people who consume sugar-sweetened beverages have an increased risk of heart disease.[12,13] Although these recent findings illustrate a potential link between added sugar intake and heart disease, there is not enough evidence to prove that eating a diet high in sugar directly causes higher levels of heart disease. Still, based on current knowledge, it is prudent to eat a diet low in added sugars. Because added sugars are a component of many processed foods and beverages, careful label reading is advised.

High Sugar Intake Is Associated with Diabetes and Obesity

Recent studies suggest that eating a diet high in added sugars is associated with a higher risk for diabetes; this relationship is particularly strong between higher intakes of sugar-sweetened beverages and diabetes.[14-16] An observational study examined the relationship between diabetes and sugar intake across 175 countries and found that for every 150 kcal per person per day increase in availability of sugar (equivalent to about one can of soft drink per day), the prevalence of diabetes increased by 1.1%.[17] Although the exact mechansims explaining this relationship are not clear, experts have speculated that the dramatic increase in glucose and insulin levels that occur when we consume high amounts of rapidly absorbable carbohydrates (which includes any forms of sugar or high-fructose corn syrup) may stimulate appetite, increase food

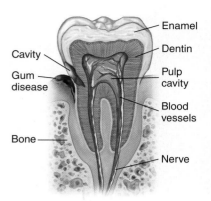

FIGURE 4.12 Eating sugars can cause an increase in cavities and gum disease. This is because bacteria in the mouth consume sugars present on the teeth and gums and produce acids, which eat away at these tissues.

QuickTips

Slashing Your Sugar Intake

When buying fruit, go for fresh, frozen, dried, or canned options packed in water or their own juice. Avoid fruits packed in light or heavy syrup.

Switch from drinking sweetened soft drinks, juice drinks, and energy drinks to diet drinks, or opt for water or unsweetened tea or coffee.

Limit the number of specialty coffees flavored with syrup that you drink— have these as an occasional treat.

Read food labels to increase your awareness of the sugar content of the foods you normally buy.

Reduce the amount of sugar you put into your coffee, tea, and cereal—try cutting the amount to half, then a quarter. Or consider using an alternative sweetener instead of sugar.

Choose snacks such as cookies, candies, and cakes less often, and replace more often with snacks with no added sugars, such as nuts, unsweetened yogurts, fresh and dried fruit, and vegetables.

---

intake, and promote weight gain, which increases our risk for diabetes. High-fructose corn syrup in particular has negative effects on how we metabolize and store body fat; this can lead to us being more resistant to the normal actions of insulin and increase our risk for diabetes.[18]

There is also evidence linking sugar intake with obesity. For example, a recent systematic review of randomized controlled trials and observational studies found that reducing intake of sugars in adults results in weight loss and increasing intake of sugars results in weight gain.[19] This increase in weight is due to the excess Calorie intake and not due to the sugars per se. This same review found that children who consume one or more servings of sugar-sweetened beverages per day had a 1.55 times higher risk of being overweight than those children consuming none or very little.

We know that if you consume more energy than you expend, you will gain weight. It makes intuitive sense that people who consume extra energy from high-sugar foods are at risk for obesity, just like people who consume extra energy from fat or protein. In addition to the increased potential for obesity, another major concern about high-sugar diets is that they tend to be low in nutrient density because the intake of high-sugar foods tends to replace that of more nutritious foods. The relationship between added sugars and obesity is highly controversial and is discussed in more detail in the **Nutrition Debate** (page 136).

If you're concerned about the amount of added sugars you consume, what can you do to cut down? See the **Quick Tips** feature for answers.

recap The RDA for carbohydrate is 130 g per day; this amount is only sufficient to supply adequate glucose to the brain. The AMDR for carbohydrate is 45% to 65% of total energy intake. Added sugars are sugars and syrups added to foods during processing or preparation. Sugar causes tooth decay but does not appear to cause hyperactivity in children. High intakes of sugars are associated with increases in unhealthful blood lipids and increased risks for heart disease, diabetes, and obesity.

Most Americans Eat Too Little Fiber-Rich Carbohydrates

Do you get enough fiber-rich carbohydrate each day? Most people in the United States eat only about two servings of fruits or vegetables each day, and most don't consistently choose whole-grain breads, pastas, and cereals. As explained earlier, fruits, vegetables, and whole-grain foods are rich in micronutrients and fiber. Whole-grains also have a lower glycemic index than refined carbohydrates; thus, they prompt a more gradual release of insulin and result in less severe fluctuations in both insulin and glucose.

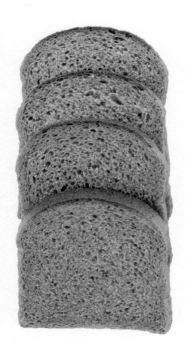

▲ Whole-grain foods provide more nutrients and fiber than foods made with enriched flour.

TABLE 4.4   Terms Used to Describe Grains and Cereals on Nutrition Labels

Term	Definition
Brown bread	Bread that may or may not be made using whole-grain flour. Many brown breads are made with white flour with brown (caramel) coloring added.
Enriched (or fortified) flour or grain	Enriching or fortifying grains involves adding nutrients back to refined foods. In order to use this term in the United States, a minimum amount of iron, folate, niacin, thiamin, and riboflavin must be added. Other nutrients can also be added.
Refined flour or grain	Refining involves removing the coarse parts of food products; refined wheat flour is flour in which all but the internal part of the kernel has been removed.
Stone ground	This term refers to a milling process in which limestone is used to grind any grain. Stone ground does not mean that bread is made with whole grain because refined flour can be stone ground.
Unbleached flour	Unbleached flour has been refined but not bleached; it is very similar to refined white flour in texture and nutritional value.
Wheat flour	This term refers to any flour made from wheat; it includes white flour, unbleached flour, and whole-wheat flour.
White flour	White flour has been bleached and refined. All-purpose flour, cake flour, and enriched baking flour are all types of white flour.
Whole-grain flour	This flour is made from grain that is not refined; whole grains are milled in their complete form with only the husk removed.
Whole-wheat flour	Whole-wheat flour is an unrefined, whole-grain flour made from whole-wheat kernels.

TABLE 4.4 defines the terms commonly used on nutrition labels for breads and cereals. Read the label for the bread you eat—does it list *whole-wheat* flour or just *wheat* flour? Although most labels for breads and cereals list wheat flour as the first ingredient, this term actually refers to enriched white flour, which is made when flour is processed. So check the ingredients label closely to make sure the first ingredient has the word "whole" in it. To gain a better understanding of the difference between a whole grain and processed grain products, it's important to learn about what makes a whole grain whole, and how whole grains are processed to reduce their fiber content.

What Makes a Whole Grain Whole?

Grains are grasses that produce edible kernels. A kernel of grain is the seed of the grass. If you were to plant a kernel of barley, a blade of grass would soon shoot up. Kernels of different grains all share a similar design. As shown in **FIGURE 4.13**, they consist of three parts:

- The outermost covering, called the *bran*, is very high in fiber and contains most of the grain's vitamins and minerals.
- The *endosperm* is the grain's midsection and contains most of the grain's carbohydrates and protein.
- The *germ* sits deep in the base of the kernel, surrounded by the endosperm, and is rich in healthful fats and some vitamins.

Whole grains are kernels that retain all three of these parts.

The kernels of some grains also have a *husk* (hull): a thin, dry coat that is inedible. Removing the husk is always the first step in milling (grinding) these grains for human consumption.

People worldwide have milled grains for centuries, usually using heavy stones. A little milling removes only a small amount of the bran, leaving a crunchy grain suitable for cooked cereals. For example, cracked wheat and hulled barley retain much of the kernel's bran. Whole-grain flours are produced when whole grains are ground and then recombined. Because these hearty flours retain a portion of the bran, endosperm, and germ, foods such as breads made with them are rich in fiber and a wide array of vitamins and minerals.

With the advent of modern technology, processes for milling grains became more sophisticated, with seeds being repeatedly ground and sifted into increasingly finer flours, retaining little or no bran and therefore little fiber and few vitamins and minerals. For instance, white wheat flour, which consists almost entirely of endosperm, is high in carbohydrate but retains only about 25% of the wheat's fiber, vitamins, and minerals. In the United States, manufacturers of breads and other baked goods made with white flour are required by law to enrich their products with vitamins and minerals to replace some of those lost in processing. **Enriched foods** are foods in which nutrients that were lost during processing have been added back, so the food meets

FIGURE 4.13   A whole grain includes the bran, endosperm, and germ.

enriched foods Foods in which nutrients that were lost during processing have been added back, so that the food meets a specified standard.

nutrition label activity

Recognizing Carbohydrates on the Label

FIGURE 4.14 shows labels for two breakfast cereals. The cereal on the left (a) is processed and sweetened, whereas the one on the right (b) is a whole-grain product with no added sugar. Which is the better breakfast choice? Fill in the label data below to find out!

■ Check the center of each label to locate the amount of total carbohydrate.

   1. For the sweetened cereal, the total carbohydrate is _____ g.

   2. For the whole-grain cereal, the total carbohydrate is _____ g for a smaller serving size.

■ Look at the information listed as subgroups under Total Carbohydrate. The label for the sweetened cereal lists all types of carbohydrates in the cereal: dietary fiber, sugars, and other carbohydrate (which refers to starches). Notice that this cereal contains 13 g of sugar—half of its total carbohydrates.

   3. How many grams of dietary fiber doees the sweetened cereal contain? _____

■ The label for the whole-grain cereal lists only 1 g of sugar, which is 4% of its total carbohydrates.

   4. How many grams of dietary fiber does the whole-grain cereal contain?

■ To calculate the percentage of Calories that comes from carbohydrate, do the following:

   a. Calculate the *Calories* in the cereal that come from carbohydrate. Multiply the total grams of carbohydrate per serving by the energy value of carbohydrate:

   26 g of carbohydrate $\times$ 4 kcal/g =
   104 kcal from carbohydrate

   b. Calculate the *percentage of Calories* in the cereal that come from carbohydrate. Divide the Calories from carbohydrate by the total Calories for each serving:

   (104 kcal $\div$ 120 kcal) $\times$ 100 =
   87% Calories from carbohydrate

Which cereal should you choose to increase your fiber intake? Check the ingredients for the sweetened cereal. Remember that they are listed in order from highest to lowest amount. The second and third ingredients listed are sugar and brown sugar, and the corn and oat flours are not whole grain. Now look at the ingredients for the other cereal—it contains whole-grain oats. Although the sweetened product is enriched with more B-vitamins, iron, and zinc, the whole-grain cereal packs 4 g of fiber per serving, not to mention 5 g of protein, and it contains no added sugars. Overall, it is a more healthful choice.

Nutrition Facts

Serving Size: 3/4 cup (30g)
Servings Per Package: About 14

Amount Per Serving	Cereal	Cereal With 1/2 Cup Skim Milk
Calories	120	160
Calories from Fat	15	15
	% Daily Value**	
Total Fat 1.5g*	2%	2%
Saturated Fat 0g	0%	0%
Trans Fat 0g		
Polyunsaturated Fat 0g		
Monounsaturated Fat 0.5g		
Cholesterol 0mg	0%	1%
Sodium 220mg	9%	12%
Potassium 40mg	1%	7%
Total Carbohydrate 26g	9%	11%
Dietary Fiber 1g	3%	3%
Sugars 13g		
Other Carbohydrate 12g		
Protein 1g		

INGREDIENTS: Corn Flour, Sugar, Brown Sugar, Partially Hydrogenated Vegetable Oil (Soybean and Cottonseed), Oat Flour, Salt, Sodium Citrate (a flavoring agent), Flavor added [Natural & Artificial Flavor, Strawberry Juice Concentrate, Malic Acid (a flavoring agent)], Niacinamide (Niacin), Zinc Oxide, Reduced Iron, Red 40, Yellow 5, Red 3, Yellow 6, Pyridoxine Hydrochloride (Vitamin B6), Riboflavin (Vitamin B2), Thiamin Mononitrate (Vitamin B1), Folic Acid (Folate) and Blue 1.

(a)

Nutrition Facts

Serving Size: 1/2 cup dry (40g)
Servings Per Container: 13

Amount Per Serving	
Calories	150
Calories from Fat	25
	% Daily Value*
Total Fat 3g	5%
Saturated Fat 0.5g	2%
Trans Fat 0g	
Polyunsaturated Fat 1g	
Monounsaturated Fat 1g	
Cholesterol 0mg	0%
Sodium 0mg	0%
Total Carbohydrate 27g	9%
Dietary Fiber 4g	15%
Soluble Fiber 2g	
Insoluble Fiber 2g	
Sugars 1g	
Protein 5g	

INGREDIENTS: 100% Natural Whole Grain Rolled Oats.

(b)

▲ **FIGURE 4.14** Labels for two breakfast cereals: **(a)** processed and sweetened cereal; **(b)** whole-grain cereal with no sugar added.

a specified standard. However, enrichment replaces only a handful of nutrients and leaves the product low in fiber. Notice that the terms *enriched* and *fortified* are not synonymous: **fortified foods** have nutrients added that did not originally exist in the food (or existed in insignificant amounts). For example, some breakfast cereals have been fortified with iron, a mineral that is not present in cereals naturally.

When choosing cereals, breads, and crackers and other baked goods, look for whole wheat, whole oats, or similar whole grains on the ingredient list. This ensures that the product contains the fiber and micronutrients that nature packed into the plant's seed. Try the nearby **Nutrition Label Activity** to learn how to recognize various carbohydrates on food labels.

We Need at Least 25 Grams of Fiber Daily

How much fiber do we need? The Adequate Intake for fiber is 25 g per day for women and 38 g per day for men, or 14 g of fiber for every 1,000 kcal per day that a person eats.[5] Most people in the United States eat only 12 to 18 g of fiber each day, getting only half of the fiber they need. Although fiber supplements are available, it is best to get fiber from food because foods contain additional nutrients, such as vitamins and minerals.

It's important to drink plenty of fluid as you increase your fiber intake because fiber binds with water to soften stools. Inadequate fluid intake with a high-fiber diet can actually result in hard, dry stools that are difficult to pass through the colon. At least eight 8-oz glasses of fluid each day are commonly recommended.

Can you eat too much fiber? Excessive fiber consumption can lead to problems such as intestinal gas, bloating, and constipation. Also, because fiber causes the body to eliminate more water in the feces, a very-high-fiber diet could result in dehydration. Fiber also binds many vitamins and minerals; thus, a diet with too much fiber can reduce our absorption of iron, zinc, calcium, and vitamin D. In children, some elderly, the chronically ill, and other at-risk populations, extreme fiber intake can even lead to malnutrition—they feel full before they have eaten enough to provide adequate energy and nutrients. So, although some societies are accustomed to a very-high-fiber diet, most people in the United States find it difficult to tolerate more than 50 g of fiber per day.

Food Sources of Fiber

Eating the amounts of whole grains, legumes and other vegetables, fruits, and nuts recommended in the USDA Food Guide will ensure that you eat enough fiber. **FIGURE 4.15** shows some common foods and their fiber content. You can use this information to design a diet that includes adequate fiber.

To help you eat right all day, see the menu choices high in fiber. Each of these choices is also packed with vitamins, minerals, and phytochemicals. For instance, a sweet potato is loaded with beta-carotene, a phytochemical the body converts to vitamin A.

See the **Quick Tips** feature (p. 133) for suggestions on selecting carbohydrate sources rich in fiber.

> To see a vast menu of high-fiber choices for each meal of the day, and find out how much fiber the foods you eat provide, visit the Fiber-o-Meter at www.webmd.com. Enter "fiber-o-meter" into the search bar to get to the page with a direct link.

fortified foods Foods in which nutrients are added that did not originally exist in the food, or which existed in insignificant amounts.

eating right all day

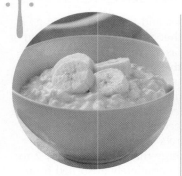

Breakfast
Oatmeal instead of sugary cereal!

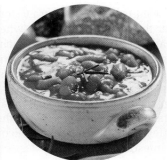

Lunch
Bean soup instead of pizza!

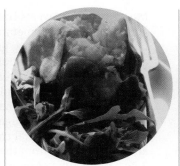

Dinner
Sweet potato instead of french fries!

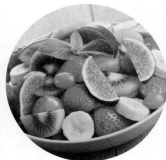

Snack
Fresh fruit instead of a candy bar!

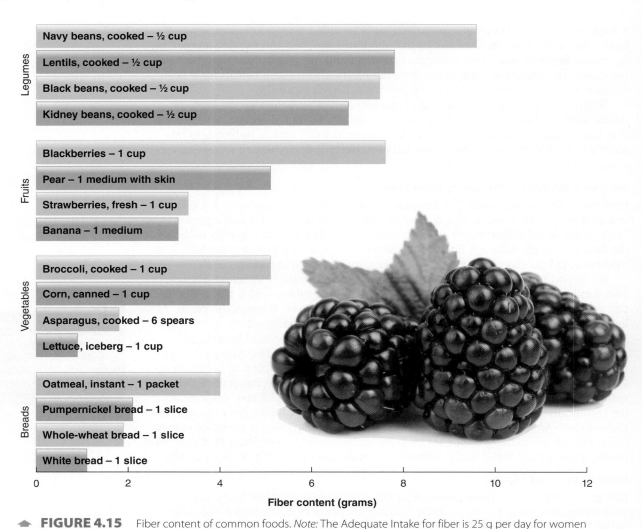

Legumes
- Navy beans, cooked – ½ cup
- Lentils, cooked – ½ cup
- Black beans, cooked – ½ cup
- Kidney beans, cooked – ½ cup

Fruits
- Blackberries – 1 cup
- Pear – 1 medium with skin
- Strawberries, fresh – 1 cup
- Banana – 1 medium

Vegetables
- Broccoli, cooked – 1 cup
- Corn, canned – 1 cup
- Asparagus, cooked – 6 spears
- Lettuce, iceberg – 1 cup

Breads
- Oatmeal, instant – 1 packet
- Pumpernickel bread – 1 slice
- Whole-wheat bread – 1 slice
- White bread – 1 slice

Fiber content (grams): 0 2 4 6 8 10 12

◆ **FIGURE 4.15** Fiber content of common foods. *Note:* The Adequate Intake for fiber is 25 g per day for women and 38 g per day for men.

Data from: U.S. Department of Agriculture, Agricultural Research Service. 2012. USDA National Nutrient Database for Standard Reference, Release 25. Nutrient Data Laboratory Home Page.

recap The Adequate Intake for fiber is 25 g per day for women and 38 g per day for men. Most Americans eat only half of the fiber they need each day. Foods high in fiber and nutrient density include whole grains and cereals, legumes and other vegetables, fruits, and nuts. The more processed the food, the fewer fiber-rich carbohydrates it contains.

What's the story on alternative sweeteners?

Most of us love sweets but want to avoid the extra Calories and tooth decay that go along with them. Remember that all carbohydrates, whether simple or complex, contain 4 kcal of energy per gram. Because sweeteners such as sucrose, fructose, honey, and brown sugar contribute energy, they are called **nutritive sweeteners**.

Other nutritive sweeteners include the *sugar alcohols* such as mannitol, sorbitol, isomalt, and xylitol. Popular in sugar-free gums, mints, and diabetic candies, sugar alcohols are less sweet than sucrose. Foods with sugar alcohols have health benefits that foods made with sugars do not have, such as a reduced glycemic response and decreased risk of dental caries. Also, because sugar alcohols are absorbed slowly and incompletely from the intestine, they provide less energy than sugar, usually 2 to 3 kcal of energy per gram. However, because they are not completely absorbed from the intestine, they can attract water into the large intestine and cause diarrhea.

A number of other products have been developed to sweeten foods without promoting tooth decay and weight gain. Because these products provide little or no energy, they are called **non-nutritive**, or *alternative*, **sweeteners.**

nutritive sweeteners Sweeteners, such as sucrose, fructose, honey, and brown sugar, that contribute Calories (energy).

non-nutritive sweeteners Manufactured sweeteners that provide little or no energy; also called *alternative sweeteners.*

QuickTips

Hunting for Fiber

✔ Select breads made with *whole* grains, such as wheat, oats, barley, and rye. Two slices of whole-grain bread provide 4–6 grams of fiber.

✔ Switch from a low-fiber breakfast cereal to one that has at least 4 grams of fiber per serving.

✔ For a mid-morning snack, stir 1–2 tablespoons of whole ground flaxseed meal (4 grams of fiber) into a cup of low-fat or nonfat yogurt. Or choose an apple or a pear, with the skin left on (approximately 5 grams of fiber).

✔ Instead of potato chips with your lunchtime sandwich, have a side of carrot sticks or celery sticks (approximately 2 grams of fiber per serving).

✔ Eat legumes every day, if possible (approximately 6 grams of fiber per serving). Have them as your main dish, as a side, or in soups, chili, and other dishes.

✔ Don't forget the vegetables! A cup of cooked leafy greens provides about 4 grams of fiber, and a salad is rich in fiber.

✔ Snack on a handful of almonds (about 4 grams of fiber) mixed with dried fruit.

✔ For dessert, try fresh, frozen, or dried fruit or a high-fiber granola with sweetened soy milk.

✔ When shopping, choose fresh fruits and vegetables whenever possible. Buy frozen vegetables and fruits when fresh produce is not available. Check frozen selections to make sure there is no sugar or salt added.

✔ Be careful when buying canned fruits, vegetables, and legumes because they may be high in added sugar or sodium. Select versions without added sugar or salt, or rinse before serving.

Limited Use of Alternative Sweeteners Is Not Harmful

Research has shown alternative sweeteners to be safe for adults, children, and individuals with diabetes. Women who are pregnant should discuss the use of alternative sweeteners with their healthcare provider. In general, it appears safe for pregnant women to consume alternative sweeteners in amounts within the Food and Drug Administration (FDA) guidelines.[20] These amounts, known as the **Acceptable Daily Intake (ADI)**, are estimates of the amount of a sweetener that someone can consume each day over a lifetime without adverse effects. The estimates are based on studies conducted on laboratory animals, and they include a 100-fold safety factor. It is important to emphasize that actual intake by humans is typically well below the ADI.

Saccharin

Discovered in the late 1800s, *saccharin* is about 300 times sweeter than sucrose. Concerns arose in the 1970s that saccharin could cause cancer; however, more than 20 years of subsequent research failed to link saccharin to cancer in humans. Based on this evidence, in May 2000 the National Toxicology Program of the U.S. government removed saccharin from its list of products that may cause cancer. No ADI has been set for saccharin, and it is used in foods and beverages and as a tabletop sweetener. It is sold as Sweet n' Low (also known as "the pink packet") in the United States.

Acesulfame-K

Acesulfame-K (acesulfame potassium) is marketed under the names Sunette and Sweet One. It is a Calorie-free sweetener that is 200 times sweeter than sugar. It is used to sweeten gums, candies, beverages, instant tea, coffee, gelatins, and puddings. The taste of acesulfame-K does not change when it is heated, so it can be used in cooking. The body does not metabolize acesulfame-K, so it is excreted unchanged by the kidneys. The ADI for acesulfame-K is 15 mg per kg body weight per day. For example, the ADI in an adult weighing 150 pounds (or 68 kg) would be 1,020 mg.

Acceptable Daily Intake (ADI) An FDA estimate of the amount of a nonnutritive sweetener that someone can consume each day over a lifetime without adverse effects.

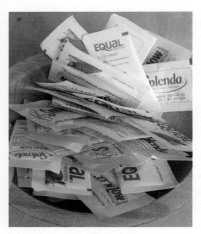

← Contrary to media reports claiming severe health consequences related to the consumption of alternative sweeteners, major health agencies have determined that these products are safe for us to consume.

Aspartame

Aspartame, also called Equal ("the blue packet") and NutraSweet, is one of the most popular alternative sweeteners currently in use. Aspartame is composed of two amino acids: phenylalanine and aspartic acid. When these amino acids are separate, one is bitter and the other has no flavor—but joined together, they make a substance that is 180 times sweeter than sucrose. Although aspartame contains 4 kcal of energy per gram, it is so sweet that only small amounts are used, thus it ends up contributing little or no energy. Heat destroys the bonds that bind the two amino acids in aspartame. Thus, it cannot be used in cooking because it loses its sweetness.

Although there are numerous claims that aspartame causes headaches and dizziness, and can increase a person's risk for cancer and nerve disorders, studies do not support these claims.[21] A significant amount of research has been done to test the safety of aspartame.

The ADI for aspartame is 50 mg per kg body weight per day. For an adult weighing 150 pounds (or 68 kg), the ADI would be 3,400 mg. **TABLE 4.5** shows how many servings of aspartame-sweetened foods would have to be consumed to exceed the ADI. Because the ADI is a very conservative estimate, it would be difficult for adults or children to exceed this amount of aspartame intake. However, drinks sweetened with aspartame, which are extremely popular among children and teenagers, are very low in nutritional value. They should not replace more healthful beverages such as milk, water, and 100% fruit juice.

There are some people who should not consume aspartame at all: those with the disease *phenylketonuria (PKU).* This is a genetic disorder that prevents the breakdown of the amino acid phenylalanine. Because the person with PKU cannot metabolize phenylalanine, it builds up to toxic levels in the tissues of the body and causes irreversible brain damage. In the United States, all newborn babies are tested for PKU; those who have it are placed on a phenylalanine-limited diet. Some foods that are common sources of protein and other nutrients for many growing children, such as meats and milk, contain phenylalanine. Thus, it is critical that children with PKU not waste what little phenylalanine they can consume on nutrient-poor products sweetened with aspartame.

Sucralose

Sucralose is marketed under the brand name Splenda and is known as "the yellow packet." It is made from sucrose, but chlorine atoms are substituted for the hydrogen and oxygen normally found in sucrose, and it passes through the digestive tract unchanged, without contributing any energy. It is 600 times sweeter than sucrose and is stable when heated, so it can be used in cooking. It has been approved for use in many foods, including chewing gum, salad dressings, beverages, gelatin and pudding products, canned fruits, frozen dairy desserts, and baked goods. Studies have shown sucralose to be safe. The ADI for sucralose is 5 mg per kg body weight per day. For example, the ADI of sucralose in an adult weighing 150 pounds (or 68 kg) would be 340 mg.

Neotame and Stevia

Neotame is an alternative sweetener that is 7,000 times sweeter than sugar. Manufacturers use it to sweeten a variety of products, such as beverages, dairy products, frozen desserts, and chewing gums.

Stevia was approved as an alternative sweetener by the FDA in 2008. It is produced from a purified extract of the stevia plant, native to South America. Stevia is 200 times sweeter than sugar. It is currently used commercially to sweeten beverages and is available in powder and liquid for tabletop use. Stevia is also called Rebiana, Reb-A, Truvia, and Purevia.

Using Artificial Sweeteners Does Not Necessarily Prevent Weight Gain

Remember that to prevent weight gain, you need to balance the total number of Calories you consume against

TABLE 4.5 Foods and Beverages That a Child and an Adult Would Have to Consume Daily to Exceed the ADI for Aspartame

Foods and Beverages	50-lb Child	150-lb Adult
12 fl. oz carbonated soft drink OR	7	20
8 fl. oz powdered soft drink OR	11	34
4 fl. oz gelatin dessert OR	14	42
Packets of tabletop sweetener	32	97

Data from: "Aspartame" from the Calorie Control Council website, 2013.

nutri-case | HANNAH

"Last night, my mom called and said she'd be late getting home from work, so I made dinner. I made vegetarian quesadillas with flour tortillas, canned green chilies, cheese, and sour cream, plus a few baby carrots on the side. Later on while I was studying, I got really hungry, so I had some sugar-free cookies. They're sweetened with sorbitol and taste just like regular cookies! I ate maybe three or four, but I didn't think it was a big deal because they're sugar-free. When I checked the package label this morning, I found out that each cookie has 90 Calories! I'm so mad at myself for blowing my diet!"

Without knowing the exact ingredients in Hannah's dinner and snack, would you agree that, prior to the cookies, she'd been making healthy choices? Why or why not? How might she have changed the ingredients in her quesadillas to increase their fiber content? And, if the cookies were sugar-free, how can you explain the fact that each cookie still contained 90 Calories?

the number you expend. If you're expending an average of 2,000 kcal a day and you consume about 2,000 kcal per day, then you'll neither gain nor lose weight. But if, in addition to your normal diet, you regularly indulge in "treats," you're bound to gain weight, whether they are sugar free or not. Consider the Calorie count of these artificially sweetened foods:

- One cup of nonfat chocolate frozen yogurt with artificial sweetener = 199 Calories
- One sugar-free chocolate cookie = 100 Calories
- One serving of no-sugar-added hot cocoa = 55 Calories

Does the number of Calories in these foods surprise you? *Remember, sugar-free doesn't mean Calorie-free.* Make it a habit to check the Nutrition Facts panel to find out how much energy is really in your food!

recap Alternative sweeteners can be used in place of sugar to sweeten foods. Most of these products do not promote tooth decay and contribute little or no energy. The alternative sweeteners approved for use in the United States are considered safe when consumed in amounts less than the Acceptable Daily Intake.

✳behavior change . . . getting started!

Now that you've read this chapter, try making these changes:

For yourself:

- Eat more high-fiber foods with each meal – including fruits, legumes and other vegetables, and whole-grain cereals and breads.
- Drink more water or other non-caloric beverages with every meal to reduce your energy intake and help you digest the higher amount of fiber you are eating.
- Brush your teeth more often throughout the day, particularly after eating sweet foods or sticky, starchy foods. This will reduce your risk for dental caries.

For your community:

- Write a blog for your school's website highlighting strategies to help people increase their fiber intake.
- Identify who on campus makes the decisions about the beverage and food content of vending machines, and inquire about his or her willingness to provide sugar-free and higher fiber options.

Are Added Sugars the Cause of the Obesity Epidemic?

Over the past 30 years, obesity rates have increased dramatically for adults and children. Obesity has become public health enemy number one because many chronic diseases, such as type 2 diabetes, heart disease, high blood pressure, and arthritis, go hand in hand with obesity.

Genetics cannot be held solely responsible for the rapid rise in obesity that has occurred. Our genetic makeup takes thousands of years to change; humans who lived 100 years ago had essentially the same genetic makeup as we do. We need to look at the effect of our lifestyle changes over the same period.

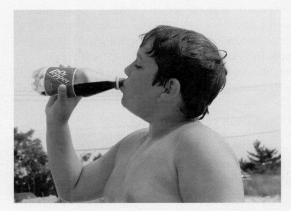

It is estimated that the rate of overweight in children has doubled since the mid-1970s.

One lifestyle factor that has come to the forefront of nutrition research is the contribution of added sugars to overweight and obesity. Consuming more energy than we expend causes weight gain. Consuming higher amounts of added sugars is a factor in weight gain for many people because they do not compensate for these increased Calories by increasing their energy expenditure through exercise or by reducing their energy intake from other foods.

The role of sugar-sweetened beverages in increasing our risk for obesity has received a great deal of attention in recent years. These beverages include soft drinks, fruit drinks, energy drinks, and vitamin water drinks. It is estimated that U.S. children's intake of sugar-sweetened beverages has increased threefold since the late 1970s, with approximately 10% of children's energy intake coming from these beverages.[19]

High-fructose corn syrup (HFCS), in particular, has garnered a great deal of attention because researchers have emphasized that HFCS is the sole caloric sweetener in sugared soft drinks and represents more than 40% of caloric sweeteners added to other foods and beverages in the United States.[22] These researchers have linked the increased use and consumption of HFCS with the rising rates of obesity since the 1970s, when HFCS first appeared. HFCS is made by converting the starch in corn to glucose and then converting some of the glucose to fructose, which is sweeter. Unfortunately, fructose is metabolized differently than glucose because it is absorbed farther down in the small intestine, and, unlike glucose, it does not stimulate insulin release from the pancreas. Because insulin inhibits food intake in people, this failure to stimulate insulin release could increase energy intake. In addition, fructose enters body cells via a transport protein not present in brain cells; thus, unlike glucose, fructose cannot enter brain cells and stimulate satiety signals. If we don't feel full, we are likely to continue eating or drinking.

The growing evidence linking the consumption of sugar-sweetened beverages with overweight and obesity in children has led to dramatic changes in soft drink availability in schools and at school-sponsored events. In 2006, the soft drink industry agreed to a voluntary ban on sales of all sweetened soft drinks in elementary and high schools. Despite these positive changes, there is still ample availability of foods and beverages containing added sugars in the marketplace.

Although the evidence pinpointing added sugars and HFCS as major contributors to the obesity epidemic may appear strong, other nutrition professionals disagree. It has been proposed that soft drinks would have contributed to the obesity epidemic whether the sweetener was sucrose or fructose, and that their contribution to obesity is due to increased consumption as a result of advertising, increases in serving sizes, and virtually unlimited access to soft drinks.[23] It is possible that the obesity epidemic has resulted from increased consumption of energy (from sweetened soft drinks and other high-energy foods) *and* a reduction in physical activity levels, and added sugars themselves are not to blame.

This issue is extremely complex, and more research needs to be done in humans before we can fully understand how added sugars contribute to our diet and our health.

CRITICAL THINKING QUESTIONS

1. After reading this, do you think added sugars should be banned from our food supply? Why or why not?
2. Should reducing sugar-sweetened beverages be up to individuals, or should it be mandatory for those at high risk for obesity? Why or why not?
3. Should families, schools, and our government play a central role in controlling the types of foods and beverages offered to young people throughout their day?

chapter **review**

test yourself | answers

1. **False.** At 4 kcal/g, carbohydrates have less than half the energy of a gram of fat. Eating a high-carbohydrate diet will not cause people to gain body fat unless their total diet contains more energy (kcal) than they expend. In fact, eating a diet high in complex, fiber-rich carbohydrates is associated with a lower risk for obesity.

2. **False.** There is no evidence that diets high in sugar cause hyperactivity in children.

3. **True.** Contrary to recent reports claiming harmful consequences related to the consumption of alternative sweeteners, major health agencies have determined that these products are safe for most of us to consume in limited quantities.

MasteringNutrition™

Check out these additional resources in the MasteringNutrition Study Area at www.masteringhealthandnutrition.pearson.com:

- Read It: Chapter Summary and RSS Feeds
- See It: ABC News videos and nutrition animations
- Hear It: MP3s
- Study It: Get Ready for Nutrition Math and Chemistry review
- Do It: NutriTools and "Find the Quack" feature
- Review It: Quizzes, flashcards, and glossary

review questions

1. Glucose, fructose, and galactose are
   a. monosaccharides.
   b. disaccharides.
   c. polysaccharides.
   d. complex carbohydrates.

2. Which of the following statements about carbohydrates is true?
   a. Carbohydrates are our main energy source during light activity and while we are at rest.
   b. Simple carbohydrates are higher in energy (kcals per gram) than complex carbohydrates.
   c. Excessive intake of carbohydrates can lead to ketoacidosis.
   d. Consuming a diet high in fiber-rich carbohydrates may reduce the level of cholesterol in the blood.

3. Glucose not immediately needed by the body
   a. is converted to cholesterol and stored in abdominal fat.
   b. is converted to glycogen and stored in the liver and muscles.
   c. passes into the large intestine and is fermented by bacteria.
   d. All of the above are possible fates of excess glucose.

4. The glycemic index rates
   a. the acceptable amount of alternative sweeteners to consume in 1 day.
   b. the potential of foods to raise blood glucose and insulin levels.
   c. the risk of a given food for causing diabetes.
   d. the ratio of soluble to insoluble fiber in a complex carbohydrate.

5. The Institute of Medicine recommends that adults consume
   a. up to 14 grams of fiber a day.
   b. at least 25% of our daily energy intake as added sugars.
   c. up to 65% of our daily energy intake as carbohydrate.
   d. at least half of all grains as whole grains.

6. The most common source of added sugar in the American diet is
   a. table sugar.
   b. white flour.
   c. alcohol.
   d. sweetened soft drinks.

7. Which of the following is a reliable source of fiber-rich carbohydrate?
   a. wheat bread
   b. unbleached flour
   c. whole-oat cereal
   d. enriched grains

8. Aspartame should not be consumed by people who have
   a. phenylketonuria.
   b. type 1 diabetes.
   c. lactose intolerance.
   d. diverticulosis.

9. **True or false?** In the process of photosynthesis, plants produce carbohydrate and store it as fiber.

10. **True or false?** Both insulin and glucagon are pancreatic hormones.

math review

11. Simon is trying to determine the minimum amount of carbohydrate he should consume in his diet to meet the AMDR for health. His total energy intake needed to maintain his current weight is 3,500 kcal per day. How many a) kcal, and b) grams, of carbohydrate should Simon consume each day?

Answers to Review Questions and Math Review are located at the back of this text and in the MasteringNutrition Study Area.

web resources

www.foodinsight.org
Food Insight—International Food Information Council Foundation

Search this site to find out more about sugars and low-Calorie sweeteners.

www.ada.org
American Dental Association

Go to this site to learn more about tooth decay as well as other oral health topics.

www.nidcr.nih.gov
National Institute of Dental and Craniofacial Research

Find out more about recent oral and dental health discoveries, and obtain statistics and data on the status of dental health in the United States.

www.caloriecontrol.org
Calorie Control Council

This site provides information about reducing energy and fat in the diet, achieving and maintaining a healthy weight, and eating various low-Calorie, reduced-fat foods and beverages.

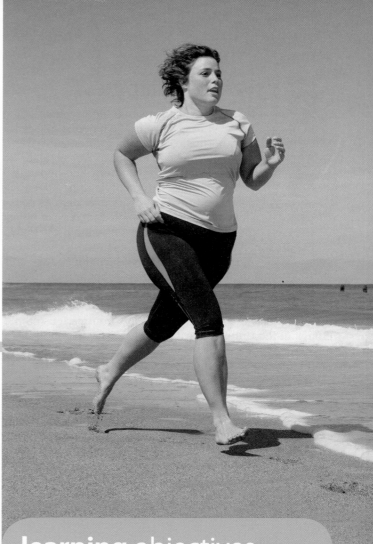

in depth
4.5

Diabetes

It was a typical day at a large medical center in the Bronx, New York: two patients were having toes amputated, another had nerve damage, one was being treated for kidney failure, another for infection, and another was blind. Despite their variety, these problems were due to just one disease: diabetes. On an average day, nearly half of the inpatients at the medical center have diabetes.[1] And the problem isn't limited to the Bronx. Throughout the United States, patients with diabetes have two to four times the risk for heart disease and stroke seen in people without diabetes. Moreover, nearly half the cases of kidney failure as well as the majority of amputations and new cases of blindness occur among people with diabetes.[2] A little over a decade ago these complications, which typically develop about 10 to 15 years after the onset of the disease, were rarely seen in people younger than age 60. But now, as more and more children and adolescents are being diagnosed with diabetes, these complications are increasingly seen in young adults.[2]

What is diabetes? Does eating too much carbohydrate cause it? What's the role of obesity? In this **In Depth**, we explore the differences between type 1 and type 2 diabetes and the relationship between our diet and our risk for the disease. We'll also explore the link between diabetes, obesity, and other chronic diseases.

learning objectives

After studying this In Depth, you should be able to:

1 Distinguish between type 1 diabetes, type 2 diabetes, and prediabetes, pp. 140–143.

2 Describe the signs and symptoms and long-term effects of uncontrolled diabetes, pp. 140–142.

3 List the risk factors for type 2 diabetes, p. 142.

4 Describe the lifestyle behaviors that can prevent or control diabetes, pp. 143–145.

5 List dietary changes that promote healthful eating in people with diabetes, pp. 143–145.

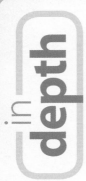

What is diabetes?

Hyperglycemia is a condition in which the level of glucose in the blood is higher than normal. **Diabetes** is a chronic disease in which the body can no longer regulate glucose within normal limits, and hyperglycemia becomes chronic. It is imperative to detect and treat the disease as soon as possible because, as just noted, excessive blood glucose injures tissues throughout the body.

Approximately 25.8 million people in the United States—8.3% of the total population, including adults and children—live with diabetes. Of these, 18.8 million have been diagnosed, and it is speculated that another 7 million have diabetes but do not know it.[2] **FIGURE 1** shows the percentage of adults with diabetes from various ethnic groups in the United States. As you can see, diabetes is much more common in American Indians/Alaska Natives than in members of other ethnic and racial groups.[2]

Diabetes Damages Blood Vessels

Diabetes causes disease when chronic exposure to elevated blood glucose levels damages the body's blood vessels, and this in turn damages other body tissues. As the concentration of glucose in the blood increases, a shift in the body's chemical balance allows glucose to attach to certain body proteins, including ones that make up blood

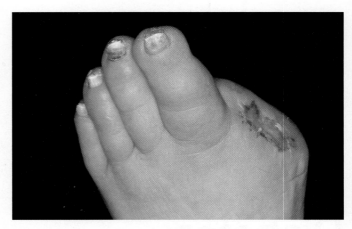

Amputations are a common complication of uncontrolled diabetes.

vessels.[3] Glucose coats these proteins like a sticky glaze, causing damage and dysfunction.[3]

Damage to large blood vessels results in problems referred to as *macrovascular complications*. These include cardiovascular disease, which occurs because damage to artery walls allows fatty plaque to accumulate and narrow or block the vessel.

Damage to small blood vessels results in problems referred to as *microvascular complications*. For example, the kidneys' microscopic blood vessels, which filter blood and produce urine, become thickened. This impairs their function and can lead to kidney failure. Blood vessels that serve the eyes can swell and leak, leading to blindness.

When blood vessels that supply nutrients and oxygen to nerves are affected, *neuropathy*, damage to the nerves, can also occur. This condition leads to a loss of sensation, most commonly in the hands and feet. At the same time, circulation to the limbs is reduced overall. Together, these changes increase the risk of injury, infection, and tissue death (necrosis), leading to a greatly increased number of toe, foot, and lower leg amputations in people with diabetes (see **FIGURE 2** for an overview of the processes involved in diabetes).

Because uncontrolled diabetes impairs carbohydrate metabolism, the body begins to break down stored fat, producing ketones for fuel. A build-up of excessive ketones can lead to ketoacidosis, a condition in which the brain cells do not get enough glucose to function properly. The

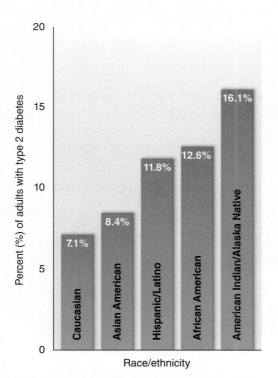

FIGURE 1 The percentage of adults from various ethnic and racial groups with type 2 diabetes.

Data from: The National Diabetes Information Clearinghouse (NDIC). 2011. National Diabetes Statistics, 2011. National Institutes of Health Publication No. 11–3892.

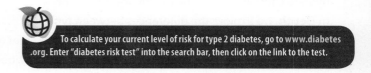

To calculate your current level of risk for type 2 diabetes, go to www.diabetes .org. Enter "diabetes risk test" into the search bar, then click on the link to the test.

hyperglycemia A condition in which blood glucose levels are higher than normal.

diabetes A chronic disease in which the body can no longer regulate glucose normally.

focus figure 2 | Diabetes

Diabetes is a chronic disease in which the body can no longer regulate glucose within normal limits, and blood glucose becomes dangerously high.

NORMAL

1 Liver releases glucose into bloodstream.

2 Beta cells of pancreas release insulin into bloodstream.

3 Insulin stimulates glucose transporters within cells to travel to the cell membrane and prompt the uptake of glucose into cells.

4 As glucose is taken into interior of cells, less glucose remains in bloodstream.

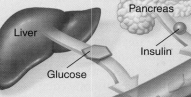

Pancreas

Liver

Insulin

Glucose

Insulin

Glucose transporter

Glucose

TYPE 1 DIABETES

1 Liver releases glucose into bloodstream.

2 Beta cells of pancreas are damaged or destroyed. Little or no insulin is released into bloodstream.

3 In the absence of insulin, glucose is not taken up by cells.

4 High levels of glucose remain in the bloodstream.

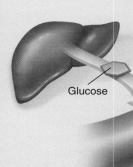

Glucose

TYPE 2 DIABETES

1 Liver releases glucose into bloodstream.

2 Beta cells of pancreas release insulin into bloodstream.

3 Insulin is present, but cells fail to respond adequately. Progressively higher amounts of insulin must be produced by the pancreas to stimulate cells to uptake glucose.

4 High levels of glucose remain in the bloodstream.

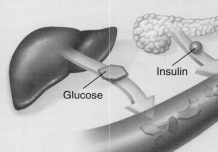

Insulin

Glucose

Insulin

person will become confused and lethargic and have trouble breathing. If left unchecked, ketoacidosis may result in coma and death. Indeed, as a result of cardiovascular disease, kidney failure, ketoacidosis, and other complications, diabetes is the seventh leading cause of death in the United States.[4]

The two main forms of diabetes are type 1 and type 2. Some women develop a third form, *gestational diabetes,* during pregnancy (see Chapter 14).

In Type 1 Diabetes, the Body Does Not Produce Enough Insulin

Approximately 5% of people with diabetes have **type 1 diabetes**, in which the body cannot produce enough insulin.[2] It is classified as an *autoimmune disease.* This means that the body's immune system attacks and destroys its own tissues—in this case, the insulin-producing cells of the pancreas. When people with type 1 diabetes eat a meal and their blood glucose rises, the pancreas is unable to secrete insulin in response. Glucose therefore cannot move into body cells and remains in the bloodstream. The kidneys try to expel the excess blood glucose by excreting it in the urine. In fact, the medical term for the disease is *diabetes mellitus* (from the Greek *diabainein,* "to pass through," and Latin *mellitus,* "sweetened with honey"), and frequent urination is one of its

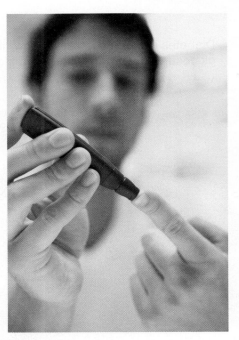

FIGURE 3 Monitoring blood glucose usually requires pricking the fingers and measuring the blood using a glucometer each day.

warning signs (see **TABLE 1** for other symptoms). If blood glucose levels are not controlled, a person with type 1 diabetes can develop ketoacidosis; left untreated, the ultimate result is death.

Most cases of type 1 diabetes are diagnosed in adolescents around 10 to 14 years of age, although the disease can appear in infants, young children, and adults. It has a genetic link, so siblings and children of those with type 1 diabetes are at greater risk.[5]

The only treatment for type 1 diabetes is the administration of insulin by injection or pump several times daily. Insulin is a hormone composed of protein, so it would be digested in the intestine if taken as a pill. Individuals with type 1 diabetes must also monitor their blood glucose levels closely to ensure that they remain within a healthful range (**FIGURE 3**). The **Hot Topic** box describes how technology helps one young man with type 1 diabetes to stay healthy.

In Type 2 Diabetes, Cells Become Less Responsive to Insulin

In **type 2 diabetes**, body cells become resistant (less responsive) to insulin. This type of diabetes develops progressively, meaning that the biological changes resulting in the disease occur over a long period. Approximately 90% to 95% of all cases of diabetes are classified as type 2.[2]

Obesity is the most common trigger for a cascade of changes that eventually results in this disorder. It is estimated that 80% to 90% of people with type 2 diabetes are overweight or obese. One factor linking obesity to diabetes is the inappropriate accumulation of lipids in muscle, the liver, and beta cells of the pancreas, which reduces the ability of body cells to respond to insulin.[6] As a result, the cells of many obese people begin to exhibit a condition called *insulin insensitivity* (insulin resistance).

The pancreas attempts to compensate for this insensitivity by secreting more insulin. At first, the increased secretion is sufficient to maintain normal blood glucose levels. However, over time, a person who is insulin insensitive will have to circulate very high levels of insulin to use glucose for energy. Eventually, this excessive production becomes insufficient for preventing a rise in fasting blood glucose. The resulting condition is referred

TABLE 1 Symptoms of Type 1 and Type 2 Diabetes

Type 1 Diabetes	Type 2 Diabetes*
Increased or frequent urination	Any of the type 1 signs and symptoms
Excessive thirst	Greater frequency of infections
Constant hunger	Sudden vision changes
Unexplained weight loss	Slow healing of wounds or sores
Extreme fatigue	Tingling or numbness in the hands or feet
Blurred vision	Very dry skin

*Some people with type 2 diabetes experience no symptoms.

Data adapted from: U.S. Dept. of Health and Human Services, National Diabetes Information Clearinghouse (NDIC). Available online at http://diabetes.niddk .nih.gov/dm/pubs/overview/index.aspx#what and from the Centers for Disease Control and Prevention, Basics about Diabetes.

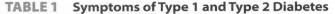

type 1 diabetes A disorder in which the body cannot produce enough insulin.

type 2 diabetes A progressive disorder in which body cells become less responsive to insulin.

HOT TOPIC

Diabetes Goes High-Tech

Vincent was diagnosed with type 1 diabetes when he was 10 years old. Now he's a college sophomore and has been living with the disease for 9 years. In that time, advances in diabetes monitoring and treatment have made Vincent's life a little easier.

For instance, all people with diabetes have to test their blood glucose level many times each day. Until recently, Vincent had to prick his fingers to do this, and they would get tender and develop calluses. Now, the FDA has approved several devices that measure blood glucose without pricking the finger. Some of them can read glucose levels through the skin, and others take readings from a small needle implanted in the body. Also, during his first few years with diabetes, Vincent had to give himself two to four shots of insulin each day. Now he uses an insulin infusion pump, which looks like a small pager and delivers insulin into the body through a thin tube gradually throughout the day.

Sure, Vincent still has to watch his diet carefully, eating three nutritious meals a day and limiting snacks. But with his new high-tech devices, it's easier to control his blood glucose, and he can play sports, travel, and do most of the things he wants to do, just like his friends.

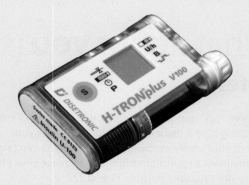

Insulin pumps can help people with diabetes eat a wider range of foods.

to as **impaired fasting glucose**, meaning glucose levels are higher than normal but not high enough to indicate a diagnosis of type 2 diabetes. Some health professionals refer to this condition as **prediabetes** because people with impaired fasting glucose are more likely to get type 2 diabetes than people with normal fasting blood glucose levels. Ultimately, the pancreas becomes incapable of secreting these excessive amounts of insulin and stops producing the hormone altogether.

In short, in type 2 diabetes, blood glucose levels may be elevated because 1) the person has developed insulin insensitivity, 2) the pancreas can no longer secrete enough

insulin, or 3) the pancreas has entirely stopped insulin production.

Diabetes is diagnosed when two or more tests of a person's fasting blood glucose indicate values in the clinically defined range. These values are:

- Normal = 70–99 mg/dL
- Prediabetes = 100–125 mg/dL
- Diabetes = 126 mg/dL

Who is at risk for type 2 diabetes?

As noted, obesity is the most common trigger for type 2 diabetes. But many other factors also play a role. For instance, relatives of people with type 2 diabetes are at increased risk, as are people with a sedentary lifestyle. A cluster of risk factors referred to as the *metabolic syndrome* is also known to increase the risk for type 2 diabetes. The criteria for metabolic syndrome include a waist circumference greater than 88 cm (35 in.) for women and 102 cm (40 in.) for men; elevated blood pressure; elevated blood glucose; and unhealthful levels of certain blood lipids.

Increased age is another risk factor for type 2 diabetes: most cases develop after age 45, and 27% of Americans 65 years and older have diabetes.[2] In fact, type 2 diabetes used to be referred to as *adult-onset diabetes* because it was virtually unheard of in children and adolescents until about 20 years ago. Unfortunately, the prevalence of the disease in young people has been increasing dramatically. In a 2012 study, more than 7% of college students were found to have prediabetes.[7] And each year, about 3,600 people under age 20 are newly diagnosed with full-blown type 2 diabetes.[2] So what's your risk? Try the **What About You?** risk calculator and find out.

Lifestyle choices can help prevent or control diabetes

Type 2 diabetes is thought to have become an epidemic in the United States because of a combination of our poor eating habits, sedentary lifestyles, increased obesity, and

To download a family history tree that you can fill out to determine your family history of diabetes, visit www.heart.org. Enter "my family health tree" into the search box, and then click on the link that appears.

---

impaired fasting glucose Fasting blood glucose levels that are higher than normal but not high enough to lead to a diagnosis of type 2 diabetes.

prediabetes A term used synonymously with *impaired fasting glucose*; it is a condition considered to be a major risk factor for both type 2 diabetes and heart disease.

an aging population. We can't control our age, but we can and do control how much and what types of foods we eat and how much physical activity we engage in—and that, in turn, influences our risk for obesity. Currently, over 34% of American college students are either overweight or obese.[8] Although adopting a healthful diet is important, moderate daily exercise may prevent the onset of type 2 diabetes more effectively than dietary changes alone. (See Chapter 12 for examples of moderate exercise programs.) Exercise will also assist in weight loss, and studies show that losing only 10 to 30 pounds can reduce or eliminate the symptoms of type 2 diabetes.[9] In summary, by eating a healthy diet, staying active, and maintaining a healthful body weight, you should be able to keep your risk for type 2 diabetes low.

What if you've already been diagnosed with type 2 diabetes? The Academy of Nutrition and Dietetics emphasizes that there is no *single* diet or eating plan for people with diabetes. You should follow guidelines to eat more healthfully in the same way you would to reduce your risk for heart disease, cancer, and overweight or obesity. One difference is that you may need to eat less carbohydrate and slightly more fat or protein to help regulate your blood glucose levels. Carbohydrates are still an important part of the diet, so, if you're eating less, make sure your choices are rich in nutrients and fiber. Because precise

nutri-case | JUDY

"My daughter, Hannah, has been pestering me about changing how we eat and getting more exercise. She says she's just trying to lose weight, but ever since we found out I have type 2 diabetes I know she's been worried about me. What I didn't get until last night is that she's worried about herself, too. All through dinner she was real quiet; then all of a sudden she says, 'Mom, I had my blood sugar tested at the health center, and guess what? They said I have prediabetes.' She said that's kind of like the first step toward diabetes and that, if she doesn't make some serious changes, she'll end up just like me. So I guess we both need to change some things. Trouble is, I don't really know where to start."

Are you surprised to learn that Hannah has prediabetes? What are her risk factors? Given what you know about Judy's and Hannah's lifestyle, what kind of small changes could both mother and daughter make immediately to start addressing their high blood glucose levels?

what about **you** ?

Calculate Your Risk for Type 2 Diabetes

To calculate your risk of developing type 2 diabetes, answer the following questions:

■ I am overweight or obese.	Yes/No
■ I am sedentary (I exercise fewer than three times a week).	Yes/No
■ I have a parent, brother, or sister with type 2 diabetes.	Yes/No
■ I am a member of one of the following groups: African American Hispanic American (Latino) American Indian or Alaska Native Pacific Islander	Yes/No
■ (For women) I have been diagnosed with gestational diabetes, or I gave birth to at least one baby weighing more than 9 pounds.	Yes/No
■ My blood pressure is 140/90 or higher, or I have been told that I have high blood pressure.	Yes/No
■ My cholesterol levels are not normal.	Yes/No

(See the discussion of cholesterol in Chapter 5.)

The more "yes" responses you give, the higher your risk of developing type 2 diabetes. You cannot change your ethnicity or your family members' health, but you can take steps to maintain a healthful weight and increase your physical activity (for tips, see Chapters 11 and 12).

Data from: The National Diabetes Information Clearinghouse (NDIC).

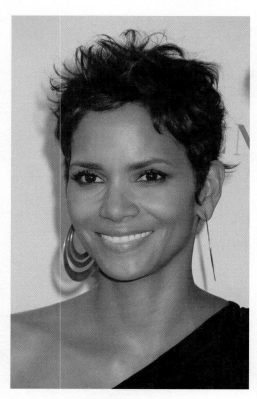

Actress Halle Berry has type 2 diabetes.

- Seek the expert advice of a registered dietitian/nutritionist to assist you with carbohydrate counting and using the exchange system.

In addition, people with diabetes should avoid alcoholic beverages, which can cause hypoglycemia, a drop in blood glucose that can cause confusion, clumsiness, and fainting. If left untreated, this can lead to seizures, coma, and death. The symptoms of alcohol intoxication and hypoglycemia are very similar. People with diabetes, their companions, and even healthcare providers may confuse these conditions; this can result in a potentially life-threatening situation.

When blood glucose levels can't be adequately controlled with lifestyle changes, oral medications may be required. These drugs work in either of two ways: they improve body cells' sensitivity to insulin or reduce the amount of glucose the liver produces. Interestingly, these drugs may not be as effective in treating young people. A 2012 study found that oral medications are not as effective in children and teens with type 2 diabetes as compared to adults.[11] Finally, if the pancreas can no longer secrete enough insulin, then people with type 2 diabetes must have daily insulin injections, just like people with type 1 diabetes.

nutritional recommendations vary according to each individual's responses to foods, consulting with a registered dietitian/nutritionist is essential.

The Academy of Nutrition and Dietetics identifies the following basic strategies for eating more healthfully while living with diabetes:[10]

- Eat meals and snacks regularly and at planned times throughout the day.
- Try to eat about the same amount and types of food at each meal or snack.
- Follow the Dietary Guidelines for Americans or the USDA Food Patterns to guide healthy food choices (see Chapter 2).

MasteringNutrition™

Check out these additional resources in the MasteringNutrition Study Area:

- Read It: Chapter Summary and RSS Feeds
- See It: ABC News videos and nutrition animations
- Hear It: MP3s
- Study It: Get Ready for Nutrition Math and Chemistry review
- Do It: NutriTools and "Find the Quack" feature
- Review It: Quizzes, flashcards, and glossary

web resources

www.eatright.org
Academy of Nutrition and Dietetics

Visit this website to learn more about diabetes, low- and high-carbohydrate diets, and healthy eating guidance for people with diabetes.

www.diabetes.org
American Diabetes Association

Find out more about the nutritional needs of people living with diabetes.

www2.niddk.nih.gov
National Institute of Diabetes and Digestive and Kidney Diseases (NIDDK)

Learn more about diabetes, including treatment, complications, U.S. statistics, clinical trials, and recent research.

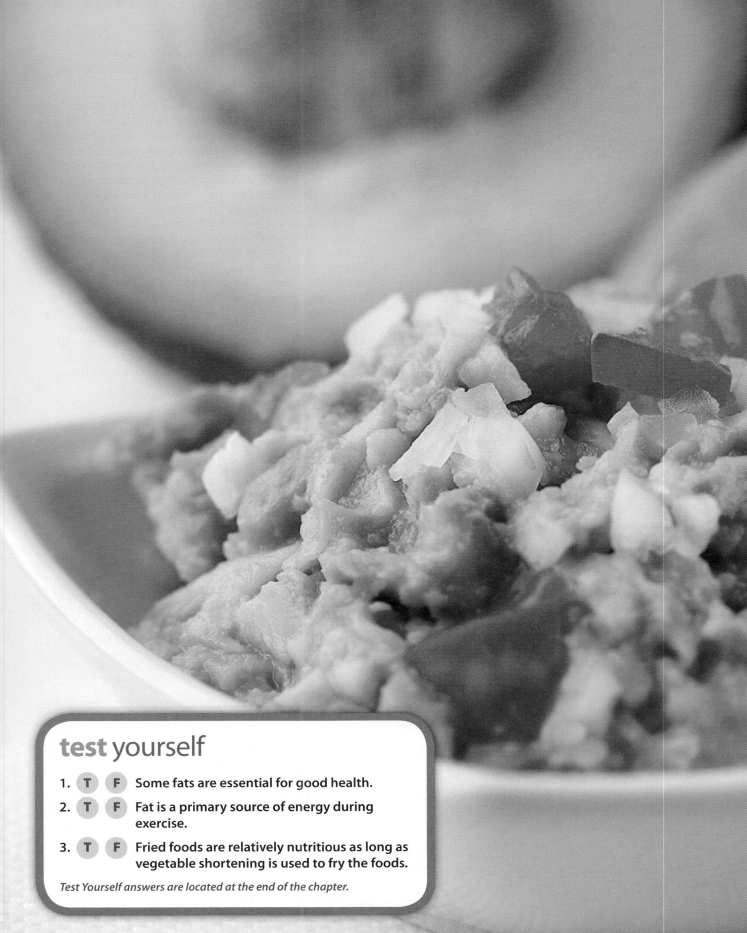

test yourself

1. **T** **F** Some fats are essential for good health.
2. **T** **F** Fat is a primary source of energy during exercise.
3. **T** **F** Fried foods are relatively nutritious as long as vegetable shortening is used to fry the foods.

Test Yourself answers are located at the end of the chapter.

Fats 5
Essential energy-supplying nutrients

How would you feel if you purchased a bag of potato **chips and were charged an extra 5% "fat tax"?** What if you ordered fish and chips in your favorite restaurant, only to be told that, in an effort to avoid lawsuits, fried foods were no longer being served? Sound surreal? Believe it or not, these and dozens of similar scenarios are being proposed, threatened, and defended in the current "obesity wars" raging around the globe. From Maine to California, from Iceland to New Zealand, local and national governments and healthcare policy advisors are scrambling to find effective methods for combating rising rates of obesity. Many of their proposals focus on limiting consumption of foods high in saturated fats—for instance, requiring food vendors to reduce the portion size of such foods; taxing them or increasing their purchase price; levying fines on manufacturers who produce them; removing them from vending machines; banning advertisements of these foods to children; or using food labels and public service announcements to warn consumers away from these foods. At the same time, "food litigation" lawsuits have been increasing, including allegations against restaurant chains and food companies for failing to warn consumers of the health dangers of eating their energy-dense, high-saturated-fat foods.

Is saturated fat really such a menace? If so, why? What is saturated fat, anyway? And are other fats just as bad?

Although some people think that all dietary fat should be avoided, a certain amount of fat is essential for life and health. In this chapter, we'll explore several types of dietary fat and discuss the critical functions of fat in the human body. We'll also identify changes you can make to shift your diet toward more healthful fats. The role of dietary fats in cardiovascular disease is discussed **In Depth** following this chapter.

learning objectives

After studying this chapter you should be able to:

1 List and describe the three types of lipids found in foods, pp. 148–156.

2 Discuss how the level of saturation of a fatty acid affects its shape and the form it takes, pp. 149–151.

3 Explain the health benefits and dietary sources of the essential fatty acids, pp. 152–154.

4 List five functions of fat, pp. 156–159.

5 Describe the steps involved in fat digestion, absorption, and transport, pp. 159–163.

6 Identify the dietary recommendations for intakes of total fat, saturated fat, *trans* fats, and the essential fatty acids, pp. 163–164 and pp. 167–168.

7 Identify at least three common food sources of unhealthful fats and three common sources of beneficial fats, pp. 167–170.

8 Summarize our current understanding of the relationship between a diet high in saturated fats and the development of cardiovascular disease and cancer, p. 173.

MasteringNutrition™

Go online for chapter quizzes, pre-tests, Interactive Activities, and more!

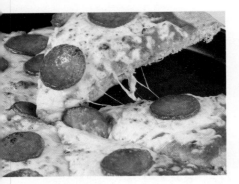

What are fats?

Fats are just one form of a much larger and more diverse group of organic substances called **lipids**, which are distinguished by the fact that they are insoluble in water. Think of a salad dressing made with vinegar, which is mostly water, and olive oil, which is a lipid. Shaking the bottle *disperses* the oil but doesn't *dissolve* it: that's why it separates back out again so quickly. Lipids are found in all sorts of living things, from bacteria to plants to human beings. In fact, their presence on your skin explains why you can't clean your face with water alone: you need some type of soap to break down the insoluble lipids before you can wash them away. In this chapter, we focus on the small group of lipids that are found in foods.

Fats and oils are two different types of lipids found in foods. Fats, such as butter, are solid at room temperature, whereas oils, such as olive oil, are liquid at room temperature. Because most people are familiar with the term *fats*, we will use that term generically throughout this book, including when we are referring to oils. Three types of fats are commonly found in foods: triglycerides, phospholipids, and sterols. Let's take a look at each.

Triglycerides Are the Most Common Food-Based Fat

About 95 % of the fat we eat is in the form of triglycerides (also called *triacylglycerols*). As reflected in the prefix *tri-*, a **triglyceride** is a molecule consisting of *three* fatty acids attached to a *three*-carbon glycerol backbone. **Fatty acids** are long chains of carbon atoms bound to each other as well as to hydrogen atoms. They are acids because they contain an acid group (carboxyl group) at one end of their chain. **Glycerol**, the backbone of a triglyceride molecule, is an alcohol composed of three carbon atoms. One fatty acid attaches to each of these three carbons to make the triglyceride (**FIGURE 5.1**).

Triglycerides are not only the most common form of fat in our diet, but also the form in which most of our body fat is stored. Body fat, clinically referred to as *adipose tissue* from the Latin root *adip-* meaning fat, is not inert. Rather, it is a metabolically active tissue that can contribute to or reduce our health. (We discuss the functions of fat later in this chapter.)

To understand why some triglycerides are better than others, we need to know more about their properties and how they work in our body. In general, triglycerides

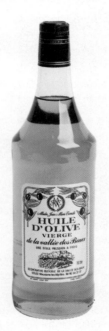

Some fats, such as olive oil, are liquid at room temperature.

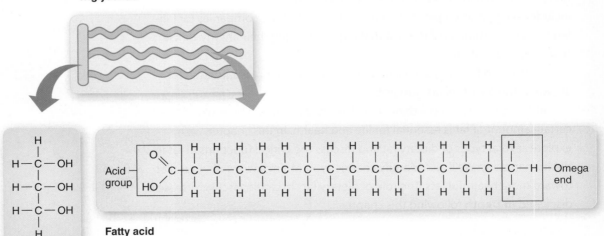

FIGURE 5.1 A triglyceride consists of three fatty acids attached to a three-carbon glycerol backbone.

can be classified by their chain length (number of carbons in each fatty acid), their level of saturation (how much hydrogen, H, is attached to each carbon atom in the fatty acid chain), and their shape, which is determined in some cases by how they are commercially processed. All of these factors influence how our body uses triglycerides.

Chain Length Affects Triglyceride Function

The fatty acids attached to the glycerol backbone can vary in the number of carbons they contain, referred to as their *chain length*.

- Short-chain fatty acids are usually fewer than six carbon atoms in length.
- Medium-chain fatty acids are six to twelve carbons in length.
- Long-chain fatty acids are fourteen or more carbons in length.

Fatty acid chain length is important because it determines the method of fat digestion and absorption and affects how fats function within the body. For example, short- and medium-chain fatty acids are digested and transported more quickly than long-chain fatty acids. We will discuss the digestion and absorption of fats in more detail shortly. In addition, chain length can determine saturation, as discussed in the next section.

Saturated Fats Contain the Maximum Amount of Hydrogen

Triglycerides can also vary by their level of saturation, which is determined by the types of bonds found in the fatty acid chains. If a fatty acid has no carbons bonded together with a double bond, it is referred to as a **saturated fatty acid (SFA)** (**FIGURES 5.2a** and **5.3a**). This is because every carbon atom in the chain is *saturated* with hydrogen: each has the maximum amount of hydrogen bound to it. Some foods that are high in saturated fatty acids are coconut oil, palm kernel oil, butter, cream, whole milk, and beef.

Unsaturated Fats Contain Less Hydrogen

If, within the chain of carbon atoms, two carbons are bound to each other with a double bond, then this double carbon bond excludes hydrogen. This lack of hydrogen at *one* part of the molecule results in a fat that is referred to as *monounsaturated* (recall from Chapter 4 that the prefix *mono-* means "one"). A **monounsaturated fatty acid (MUFA)** (shown in Figures 5.2b and 5.3a) is usually liquid at room temperature. Foods that are high in monounsaturated fatty acids are olive oil, canola oil, and cashew nuts.

If the fat molecule has *more than one* double bond, it contains even less hydrogen and is referred to as a **polyunsaturated fatty acid (PUFA)** (see Figure 5.3a). Polyunsaturated fatty acids are also liquid at room temperature and include cottonseed, canola, corn, and safflower oils.

Although foods vary in the types of fatty acids they contain, in general we can say that animal-based foods tend to be high in saturated fats and plant foods tend to be high in unsaturated fats. Specifically, animal fats provide approximately 40–60% of their energy from saturated fats, whereas plant fats provide 80–90% of their energy from monounsaturated and polyunsaturated fats. Most oils are a good source of both MUFAs and PUFAs. **FIGURE 5.4** (page 150) compares the percentages of the different types of fats in a variety of foods.

In general, saturated fats have a detrimental effect on our health, whereas unsaturated fats are protective. It makes sense, therefore, that diets high in plant foods— because they're low in saturated fats—are more healthful than diets high in animal products. We discuss the influence of various types of fatty acids on your risk for cardiovascular disease in the **In Depth** essay immediately following this chapter.

Carbon Bonding Affects Shape

Have you ever noticed how many toothpicks are packed into a small box? A hundred or more! But if you were to break a bunch of toothpicks into V shapes anywhere along their length, how many could you then fit into the same box? It would be very few because the bent toothpicks would jumble together, taking up much more space.

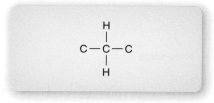

(a) Saturated fatty acid

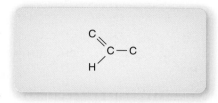

(b) Unsaturated fatty acid

FIGURE 5.2 An atom of carbon has four attachment sites. In fatty acid chains, two of these sites are filled by adjacent carbon atoms. **(a)** In saturated fatty acids, the other two sites are always filled by two hydrogen atoms. **(b)** In unsaturated fatty acids, at one or more points along the chain, a double bond to an adjacent carbon atom takes up one of the attachment sites that would otherwise be filled by hydrogen.

lipids A diverse group of organic substances that are insoluble in water; lipids include triglycerides, phospholipids, and sterols.

triglyceride A molecule consisting of three fatty acids attached to a three-carbon glycerol backbone.

fatty acids Long chains of carbon atoms bound to each other as well as to hydrogen atoms.

glycerol An alcohol composed of three carbon atoms; it is the backbone of a triglyceride molecule.

saturated fatty acid (SFA) A fatty acid that has no carbons joined together with a double bond; SFAs are generally solid at room temperature.

monounsaturated fatty acid (MUFA) A fatty acid that has two carbons in the chain bound to each other with one double bond; MUFAs are generally liquid at room temperature.

polyunsaturated fatty acid (PUFA) A fatty acid that has more than one double bond in the chain; PUFAs are generally liquid at room temperature.

Fatty acids

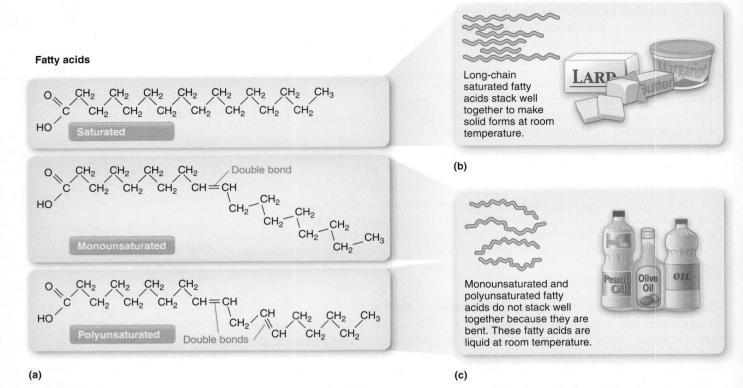

(a)

(b) Long-chain saturated fatty acids stack well together to make solid forms at room temperature.

(c) Monounsaturated and polyunsaturated fatty acids do not stack well together because they are bent. These fatty acids are liquid at room temperature.

⬧ **FIGURE 5.3** Examples of levels of saturation among fatty acids and how these levels of saturation affect the shape of fatty acids. **(a)** Saturated fatty acids are saturated with hydrogen, meaning they have no carbons bonded together with a double bond. Monounsaturated fatty acids contain two carbons bound by one double bond. Polyunsaturated fatty acids have more than one double bond linking carbon atoms. **(b)** Saturated fats have straight fatty acids packed tightly together and are solid at room temperature. **(c)** Unsaturated fats have "kinked" fatty acids at the area of the double bond, preventing them from packing tightly together; they are liquid at room temperature.

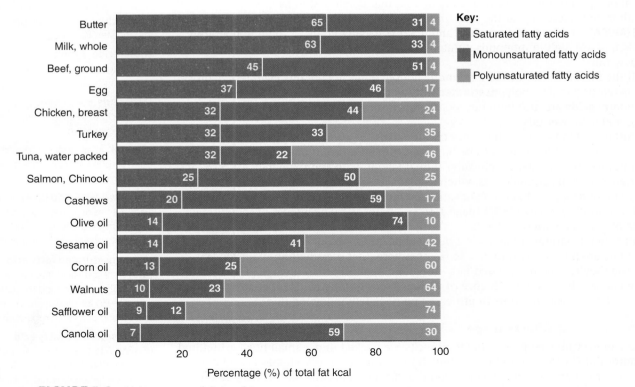

⬧ **FIGURE 5.4** Major sources of dietary fat.

Molecules of saturated fat are like straight toothpicks: they have no double carbon bonds and always form straight, rigid chains. Because they have no kinks, these chains can pack together tightly (see Figure 5.3b). That is why saturated fats, such as the fat in meats, are solid at room temperature.

In contrast, each double carbon bond of unsaturated fats gives them a kink along their length (see Figure 5.3c). This means that they are unable to pack together tightly—for example, to form a stick of butter—and instead are liquid at room temperature. In our body, unsaturated fatty acids are part of our cell membranes. They help keep the cell membranes flexible, allowing substances to move into and out of the cells.

We've just said that unsaturated fatty acids are kinked. That's true when they occur naturally as plant and fish oils. But unsaturated fatty acids can be manipulated by food manufacturers to create a type of straight, rigid fatty acid called a *trans* fat. Recall (from Chapter 2) that the Dietary Guidelines for Americans suggest that you keep your *trans* fat intake as low as possible. In fact, *trans* fats are considered at least as harmful to your health as saturated fats. We'll explain why in a moment. For now, let's make sure we know what *trans* fats really are.

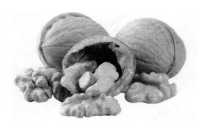

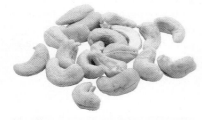

Walnuts and cashews are high in monounsaturated fatty acids.

Trans Fatty Acids Have Hydrogen Atoms on Opposite Sides

Unsaturated fatty acids can occur in either a *cis* or a *trans* shape. The prefix *cis* means things are located on the same side or near each other, whereas *trans* is a prefix that denotes across or opposite. These terms describe the positioning of the hydrogen atoms around the double carbon bond as follows:

- A *cis fatty acid* has both hydrogen atoms located on the same side of the double bond **(FIGURE 5.5a)**. This positioning gives the *cis* molecule a pronounced kink at the double carbon bond. We typically find the *cis* fatty acids in nature and, thus, in whole foods.

cis arrangement

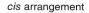

(a) *cis* polyunsaturated fatty acid

trans arrangement

(b) *trans* polyunsaturated fatty acid

FIGURE 5.5 Structure of **(a)** a *cis* and **(b)** a *trans* polyunsaturated fatty acid. Notice that *cis* fatty acids have both hydrogen atoms located on the same side of the double bond. This positioning makes the molecule kinked. In the *trans* fatty acids, the hydrogen atoms are attached on diagonally opposite sides of the double carbon bond. This positioning makes them straighter and more rigid.

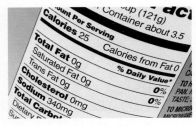

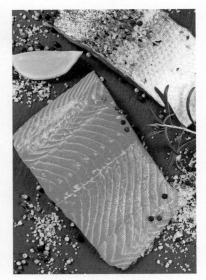

The U.S. FDA ruled that as of 2006, *trans* fatty acids, or *trans* fat, must be listed as a separate line item on the Nutrition Facts Panels for conventional foods and some dietary supplements.

Salmon is high in omega-3 fatty acid content.

hydrogenation The process of adding hydrogen to unsaturated fatty acids, making them more saturated and thereby more solid at room temperature.

essential fatty acids (EFAs) Fatty acids that must be consumed in the diet because they cannot be made by our body.

linoleic acid An essential fatty acid found in vegetable and nut oils; one of the omega-6 fatty acids.

alpha-linolenic acid (ALA) An essential fatty acid found in leafy green vegetables, flaxseed oil, soy oil, and other plant foods; an omega-3 fatty acid.

■ In a *trans fatty acid*, the hydrogen atoms are attached on diagonally opposite sides of the double carbon bond (see Figure 5.5b). This positioning makes *trans* fatty acid fats straighter and more rigid, just like saturated fats. Thus, "*trans* fats" is a collective term used to define fats with *trans* double bonds. Although a limited amount of natural *trans* fatty acids are found in cow's milk and meat, the majority of *trans* fatty acids in foods are produced by manipulating the fatty acids during food processing.

This process, called **hydrogenation**, was developed in the early 1900s in order to produce a type of cheap fat that could be stored in a solid form and would resist rancidity. During hydrogenation, pressurized hydrogen molecules are added directly to unsaturated fatty acids such as those found in corn and safflower oils. This causes the double bonds of the unsaturated fatty acids in the oil to be partially or totally removed. As a result, the fatty acid becomes more saturated and straighter.

The hydrogenation process can be controlled to make the oil more or less saturated: if only some of the double bonds are broken, the fat produced is called *partially hydrogenated,* a term you will see frequently on food labels. For example, corn oil margarine is a partially hydrogenated form of corn oil. Unless labeled as containing zero *trans* fatty acids, most margarines have more *trans* fatty acids than butter. So which is the more healthful choice—butter or margarine? Check out the **Nutrition Myth or Fact?** box to find out.

Incidentally, even when a product *is* labeled as having "zero" *trans* fats, there can still be *trans* fatty acids in the product! That's because the U.S. Food and Drug Administration (FDA) allows products that have less than 1 g of *trans* fat per serving to claim that they are *trans* fat-free. So, even if the Nutrition Facts Panel states 0 g *trans* fats, the product can still have 1/2 g of *trans* fat per serving. If the ingredients list states that the product contains partially hydrogenated oils, it contains *trans* fats.

For a period of several decades in the 20th century, processed foods made with partially hydrogenated oil were in demand. Americans were being urged to reduce their intake of saturated fats and switched to partially hydrogenated oils, including margarines, assuming that these products were more healthful and could reduce the risk for cardiovascular disease. But as we discuss later in this chapter, this assumption did not turn out to be true.

Some Triglycerides Contain Essential Fatty Acids

There has been a lot of press lately about "omega" fatty acids, so you might be wondering what they are and why they're so important. First, let's explain the Greek name. As illustrated in **FIGURE 5.6** (page 154), one end of a fatty acid chain (where it attaches to glycerol in a triglyceride) is designated the α (alpha) end (α is the first letter in the Greek alphabet). The other end of a fatty acid chain is called the ω (omega) end (ω is the last letter in the Greek alphabet). When synthesizing fatty acids, the body has no mechanism for inserting double bonds before the ninth carbon from the omega end.[1] This means that, when our body needs types of fatty acids having a double bond close to the omega end, it has to obtain them from the foods we eat. These are considered **essential fatty acids (EFAs)** because the body cannot make them, yet it requires them for healthy functioning. The EFAs are classified into two groups.

Omega-6 Fatty Acids. Fatty acids that have a double bond six carbons from the omega end (at ω-6) are known as *omega-6 fatty acids*. One omega-6 fatty acid, **linoleic acid**, is essential to human health. It is found in vegetable and nut oils, such as sunflower, safflower, corn, soy, and peanut oil. If you eat lots of vegetables or use vegetable-oil-based margarines or vegetable oils, you are probably getting adequate amounts of this EFA in your diet.

Omega-3 Fatty Acids. Fatty acids with a double bond three carbons from the omega end (at ω-3) are known as *omega-3 fatty acids*. The most common omega-3 fatty acid in our diet is **alpha-linolenic acid (ALA)**. It is derived primarily from plants, especially dark green, leafy vegetables, flaxseeds and flaxseed oil, soybeans and soybean oil, walnuts and walnut oil, and canola oil.[2]

nutrition myth or fact?

Is Margarine More Healthful Than Butter?

Your toast just popped up! Which will it be: butter or margarine? As you've just learned, butter is 65% saturated fat: 1 tablespoon provides 30 grams of cholesterol! In contrast, corn oil margarine is just 2% saturated fat, with no cholesterol. But how much *trans* fat does that margarine contain? And which is better—the more natural and more saturated butter or the more processed and less saturated margarine?

You're not the only one asking this question. Until recently, vegetable-based oils were hydrogenated to make margarines. These products were filled with *trans* fats that could increase the consumer's risk for cardiovascular disease as well as harm cell membranes, weaken immune function, and inhibit the body's natural anti-inflammatory hormones. Some margarines also contained harmful amounts of toxic metals, such as nickel and aluminum, as by-products of the hydrogenation process. These are among some of the reasons researchers began warning consumers against using margarines several years ago.

So does that mean that the saturated-fat, cholesterol-rich butter is the better choice? A decade ago, that may have been the case, but, over the last 10 years, food manufacturers have introduced "*trans* fat free margarines and spreads" that contain no cholesterol or *trans* fats and low amounts of saturated fats. The American Heart Association[3] advises that consumers choose these *trans* fat free margarines over butter. Others point out that such manufactured products are still "non-foods" and recommend that those who prefer whole foods choose unprocessed nut butters (peanut, walnut, cashew, and almond butters). These natural alternatives are rich in essential fatty acids and other heart-healthy unsaturated fats but are still as energy-dense as butter.

Remember, a label claiming that a margarine has zero *trans* fatty acids doesn't guarantee that the product is *trans* fatty acid-free (see the accompanying table). You have to look for margarines with no "partially hydrogenated" oil in them. That is the only way you will know your spread is entirely free of *trans* fatty acids. Check out the spreads listed in the table to help you decide which you're going to include in your diet.

Spreads for Your Bread*

Brand Name	Energy (kcal)	Sat fat (g)	*Trans* fat (g)	Sodium (mg)
Tubs and Squeezes Made without Partially Hydrogenated Oil				
Promise Fat Free; I Can't Believe It's Not Butter (fat free)	5	0	0	90
Country Crock Omega Plus Light	50	1	0	80
Smart Balance Omega Light	50	1.5	0	80
Parkay Squeeze	70	1.5	0	110
Canola Harvest Original	100	1.5	0	100
Tubs and Sticks Made with Partially Hydrogenated Oil				
Fleischmann's Light (tub)	50	0.5	NA	70
Fleischmann's Original (stick)	100	2	2.5	120
Blue Bonnet (tub)	60	1	0.4	130
Blue Bonnet Light (stick)	50	1	1	80
I Can't Believe It's Not Butter! Original (tub)	80	2	0.3	90
Butter				
Butter, any brand, stick	100	7.5	0.4	80
Land O'Lakes Light with Canola Oil	50	2	0	90
Nut Butters				
Peanut butter	95	1.5	0	78
Almond butter	99	1	0	70

*All portion sizes are 1 tablespoon.
Data from: Hurley, J., and B. Liebman. 2009, September. Covering the spreads: tracking down the butters and margarines. *Nutrition Action Healthletter,* 13–15. Food Processor-SQL, Version 10.3, ESHA Research, Salem, OR.

CRITICAL THINKING QUESTIONS

1. Which of the spreads (margarines, butter, and nut butters) listed in the table would you buy? What factors (for example, health, price, convenience, taste) would be most important to you when making this decision?
2. Which spread has the highest level of *trans* fatty acids? Which has the highest level of saturated fat? How do these two products compare in terms of Calories? Assume both products are available at the same price. Which one would you buy, and why?

FIGURE 5.6 Two essential fatty acids: linoleic acid (an omega-6 fatty acid) and alpha-linolenic acid (an omega-3 fatty acid).

FIGURE 5.6 Two essential fatty acids: linoleic acid (an omega-6 fatty acid) and alpha-linolenic acid (an omega-3 fatty acid).

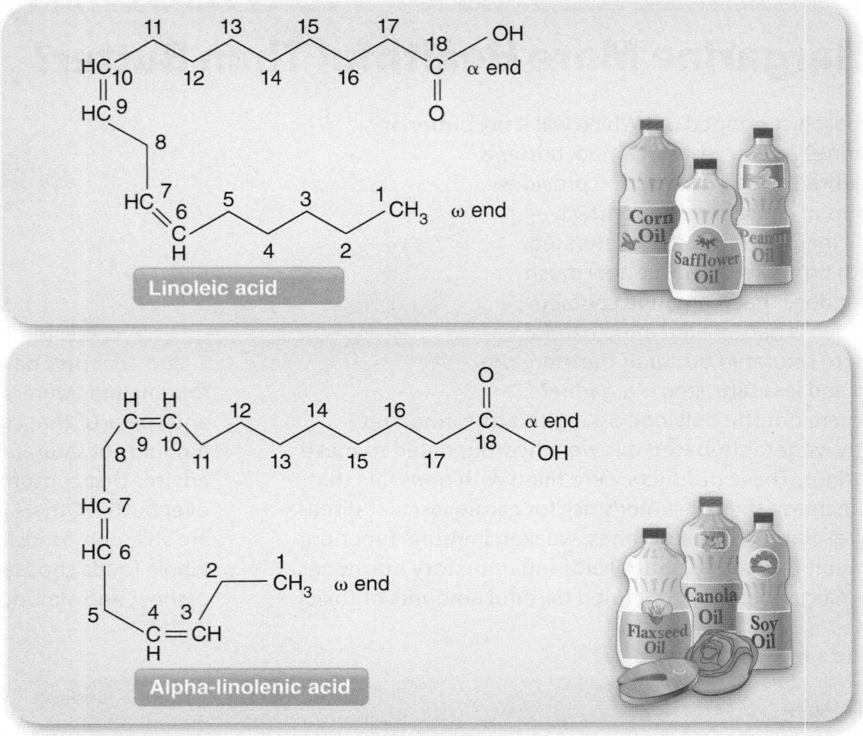

You may also have read news reports of the health benefits of the two omega-3 fatty acids found in many fish. These are **eicosapentaenoic acid (EPA)** and **docosahexaenoic acid (DHA)**. Although our body can use ALA to assemble the chains of EPA and DHA, the amount that can be converted is limited[2]; therefore, it is important to consume them directly from marine sources. They are found in fish, shellfish, and fish oils. Fish that naturally contain more oil, such as salmon and tuna, are higher in EPA and DHA than lean fish, such as cod or flounder.

Functions of EFAs. As a group, EFAs are essential to growth and health because they are precursors to important biological compounds called *eicosanoids,* which are produced in nearly every cell in the body.[3] Eicosanoids get their name from the Greek word *eicosa,* which means "twenty," because they are synthesized from fatty acids with twenty carbon atoms. In the body, eicosanoids are potent regulators of cellular function. For example, they help regulate gastrointestinal tract motility, blood clotting, blood pressure, the permeability of our blood vessels to fluid and large molecules, and the regulation of inflammation and gene expression.[4]

These fatty acids also have unique roles. For example, linoleic acid is metabolized in the body to arachidonic acid, which is a precursor to a number of eicosanoids. Linoleic acid is also needed for cell membrane structure and is required for the lipoproteins—lipid-protein compounds—that transport fats in our blood. In contrast, research indicates that diets high in the omega-3 fatty acids stimulate the production of eicosanoids that reduce inflammation, improve blood lipid profiles, and otherwise reduce an individual's risk for cardiovascular disease and cardiac death.[4,5]

Phospholipids Combine Lipids with Phosphate

Along with the triglycerides just discussed, we also find phospholipids and sterols in the foods we eat. **Phospholipids** consist of two fatty acids and a glycerol backbone with another compound that contains phosphate (**FIGURE 5.7**). This addition of a phosphate compound makes phospholipids soluble in water, a property that enables

eicosapentaenoic acid (EPA) An omega-3 fatty acid available from marine foods and as a metabolic derivative of alpha-linolenic acid.

docosahexaenoic acid (DHA) An omega-3 fatty acid available from marine foods and as a metabolic derivative of alpha-linolenic acid.

phospholipid A type of lipid in which a fatty acid is combined with another compound that contains phosphate; unlike other lipids, phospholipids are soluble in water.

HOT TOPIC

The Nuts and Bolts on Nuts

Nuts are rich in plant sterols, healthful unsaturated fats, protein, several minerals, and fiber. But they're also high in energy: 160–180 kcal for a 1-ounce serving (about 4 tablespoons, depending on the nut). So why are nuts the popular "new" food in so many diet plans?

Well, in several studies, when researchers fed people an ounce or two of nuts every day, the participants failed to gain the expected weight. And, in general, people who eat nuts are typically leaner than people who don't. No one has a definitive explanation for these findings. Some researchers speculate that people find nuts satiating and therefore eat less later on. Others propose that the energy in nuts may not be fully absorbed in the GI tract.

Will nuts help you control your weight? Maybe—if you can limit yourself to an ounce or two a day. Trouble is, they taste so good, it's easy to overdo it.

phospholipids to assist in transporting fats in our bloodstream. We discuss this concept in more detail later in this chapter (page 162). Also, phospholipids in our cell membranes regulate the transport of substances into and out of the cell. Phospholipids also help with the digestion of dietary fats: the liver uses phospholipids called *lecithins* to make bile. Note that our body manufactures phospholipids, so they are not essential for us to include in our diets. What *is* essential is phosphorus, a mineral that combines with oxygen to make phosphate.

Sterols Have a Ring Structure

Sterols are also a type of lipid found in foods and in the body, but their multiple-ring structure is quite different from that of triglycerides (**FIGURE 5.8a**). Sterols are found in both animal and plant foods and are produced in the body.

Cholesterol is the most commonly occurring sterol in the diet (see Figure 5.8b). It is found only in the fatty part of animal products such as butter, egg yolks, whole milk, meats, and poultry. Low- or reduced-fat animal products, such as lean meats and skim milk, have little cholesterol.

We don't need to consume cholesterol in our diet because our body continually synthesizes it, mostly in the liver and intestines. This continuous production is essential because cholesterol is part of every cell membrane, where it works in conjunction with fatty acids to help maintain cell membrane integrity. It is particularly plentiful in the neural cells that make up our brain, spinal cord, and nerves. The body also uses cholesterol to synthesize several important compounds, including sex hormones (estrogen, androgen, and progesterone), bile, adrenal hormones, and vitamin D. Given these important functions of cholesterol, you might be wondering why it has such a bad reputation. The answer is that a high level of cholesterol circulating in the blood is associated with cardiovascular disease, the subject of the **In Depth** following this chapter.

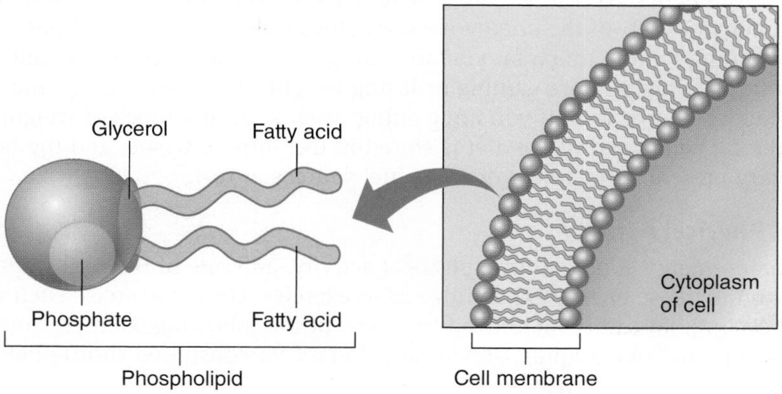

sterol A type of lipid found in foods and the body that has a ring structure; cholesterol is the most common sterol in our diets.

FIGURE 5.7 Structure of a phospholipid. Phospholipids consist of a glycerol backbone with two fatty acids and a compound that contains phosphate.

▶ FIGURE 5.8 Sterol structure. **(a)** Sterols are lipids that contain multiple-ring structures. **(b)** Cholesterol is the most commonly occurring sterol in our diets.

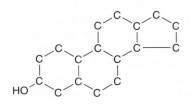

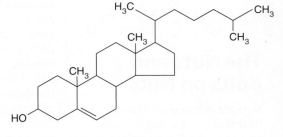

(a) Sterol ring structure

(b) Cholesterol

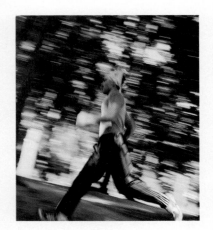

Learn more about plant sterols and how to incorporate them into your diet at www.webmd.com. Go to "cholesterol management", then "features", and then "low cholesterol diet plant sterols" to get underway.

As just noted, plants also contain some sterols. Plant sterols are not very well absorbed; nevertheless, they may confer a health benefit, because they appear to block the absorption of dietary cholesterol. Nuts are especially rich in plant sterols, but that's not the only reason you should eat them. See the **Hot Topic** for the nuts and bolts on nuts.

recap Fat is essential for health. Three types of fat are found in foods: triglycerides, phospholipids, and sterols. Triglycerides are the most common. A triglyceride is made up of glycerol and three fatty acids. These fatty acids can be classified based on chain length, level of saturation, and shape. Saturated and *trans* fatty acids increase our risk for cardiovascular disease, whereas unsaturated fatty acids, including the essential fatty acids, are protective. Phospholipids combine two fatty acids and a glycerol backbone with a phosphate-containing compound, making them soluble in water. Sterols have a multiple-ring structure; cholesterol is the most commonly occurring sterol in our diet.

Why do we need fats?

Dietary fat provides energy and helps our body perform some essential physiologic functions.

Fats Provide Energy

Dietary fat is a primary source of energy because fat has more than twice the energy per gram of carbohydrate or protein. Fat provides 9 kilocalories (kcal) per gram, whereas carbohydrate and protein provide only 4 kilocalories (kcal) per gram. This means that fat is much more energy dense. For example, 1 tbsp. of butter or oil contains approximately 100 kcal, whereas it takes 2.5 cups of steamed broccoli or 1 slice of whole-wheat bread to provide 100 kcal.

Fats Are a Major Fuel Source When We Are at Rest

Just as a candle needs oxygen for the flame to burn the tallow, our cells need oxygen to burn fat for energy. At rest, we are able to deliver plenty of oxygen to our cells, and approximately 30–70% of the energy we use comes from fat.[6] The exact percentage varies, according to how much fat you are eating in your diet, how physically active you are, and whether you are gaining or losing weight. If you are dieting, more fat will be used for energy than if you are gaining weight. During times of weight gain, more of the fat consumed in the diet is stored in the adipose tissue, and the body uses more dietary protein and carbohydrate as fuel sources at rest.

Fats Fuel Physical Activity

Fat is a major energy source during physical activity, and one of the best ways to lose body fat and increase energy expenditure is to exercise. During exercise such as running and cycling, fat can be mobilized from any of the following sources: muscle tissue, adipose tissue, blood lipids, and/or any dietary fat consumed shortly before or during exercise.

⬥ Dietary fat provides energy.

A number of hormonal changes signal the body to break down stored energy to fuel the working muscles. The hormonal responses, and the amount and source of the fat used, depend on your level of fitness; the type, intensity, and duration of the exercise; and how well fed you are before you exercise. For example, the hormone adrenaline strongly stimulates the breakdown of stored fat. Blood levels of adrenaline rise dramatically within seconds of beginning exercise.

This in turn activates additional hormones within the fat cell to begin breaking down fat. Adrenaline also signals the pancreas to *decrease* insulin production. This is important because insulin inhibits fat breakdown. Thus, when the need for fat as an energy source is high, blood insulin levels are typically low. As you might guess, blood insulin levels are high after eating, when our need for getting energy from stored fat is low and the need for fat storage is high.

Once fatty acids are released from the adipose cell, they travel in the blood attached to a protein, *albumin,* to the muscles, where they enter the mitochondria and use oxygen to produce ATP, which is the cell's energy source. Becoming more physically fit means you can deliver more oxygen to the muscle to use the fat that is delivered there. In addition, you can exercise longer when you are fit. Since the body has only a limited supply of stored carbohydrate as glycogen in muscle tissue, the longer you exercise, the more fat you use for energy. This point is illustrated in **FIGURE 5.9**. In this example, an individual is running for 4 hours at a moderate intensity. The longer the individual runs, the more depleted the muscle glycogen levels become and the more fat from adipose tissue is used as a fuel source for exercise.

Body Fat Stores Energy for Later Use

Our adipose tissue gives us ready access to energy even when we choose not to eat (or are unable to eat), when we are exercising, and while we are sleeping. The body has little stored carbohydrate—only enough to last about 1 to 2 days—and there is no place where our body can store extra protein. We cannot consider our muscles and organs as a place where "extra" protein is stored! For these reasons, the fat stored in our adipose tissue is necessary to keep the body going. Although we do not want too much stored adipose tissue, some fat storage is essential to good health. Incidentally, muscle tissue also stores some triglycerides; however, the amount is much less than in body fat. This fat is readily used during exercise to fuel the working muscle.

Fats Enable the Transport of Fat-Soluble Vitamins

Dietary fat enables the transport of the fat-soluble vitamins (A, D, E, and K) our body needs for many essential metabolic functions. For example, vitamin A is essential for

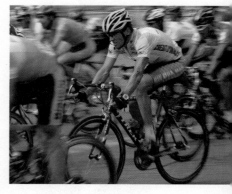

The longer you exercise, the more fat you use for energy. Cyclists in long-distance races use fat stores for energy.

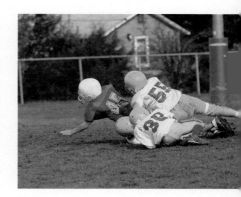

Adipose tissue pads our body and protects our organs when we fall or are bruised.

FIGURE 5.9 Various sources of energy used during exercise. As a person exercises for a prolonged period, fatty acids from adipose cells contribute relatively more energy than do carbohydrates stored in the muscle or circulating in our blood. Data adapted from: Substrate utilization during exercise in active people. *Am. J. Clin. Nutr.* 6(suppl):958S–979S.

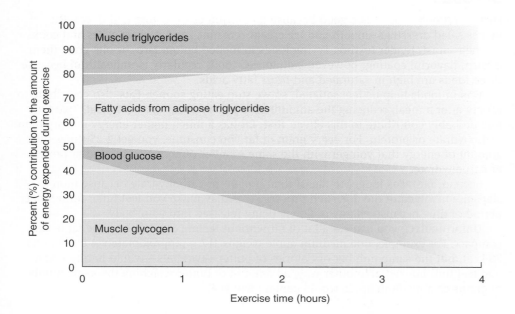

vision. Vitamin D is important for regulating blood calcium and phosphorus concentrations within normal ranges, which indirectly helps maintain bone health. Vitamin E protects cell membranes from potentially harmful by-products of metabolism. Finally, vitamin K is important for proteins involved in blood clotting and bone health. (These vitamins are discussed in detail in Chapters 8 and 9.)

Fats Help Maintain Cell Function

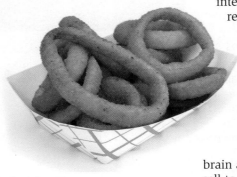

Fats, especially phospholipids, cholesterol, and PUFAs, are a critical part of every cell membrane. The various types of fats in cell membranes help maintain membrane integrity, determine what substances are transported into and out of the cell, and regulate what substances can bind to the cell; thus, fats strongly influence the function of the cell. In addition, fats help maintain cell fluidity and other physical properties of the cell membrane. For example, wild salmon live in very cold water and have high levels of omega-3 fatty acids in their cell membranes. These fats stay fluid and flexible even in very cold environments, allowing the fish to swim in extremely cold water. In the same way, fats help our membranes stay fluid and flexible. For example, they enable our red blood cells to bend and move through the smallest capillaries in our body, delivering oxygen to all our cells.

Fats, especially PUFAs, are also primary components of the tissues of the brain and spinal cord, where they facilitate the transmission of information from one cell to another. We also need fats for the development, growth, and maintenance of these tissues.

⬆ Fat adds texture and flavor to foods.

Some Stored Fat Is Essential

Many people think of body fat as "bad," but it helps keep us healthy. Besides being the primary site of stored energy, adipose tissue pads our body and protects our organs, such as the kidneys and liver, when we fall or are bruised. The fat under our skin also acts as insulation to help us retain body heat.

Although some stored fat is essential to life, too much increases our risk for chronic diseases, including cardiovascular disease and metabolic disorders such as type 2 diabetes. That's because adipose cells overloaded with triglycerides can malfunction, secreting proteins and other compounds that promote inflammation and insulin resistance. (Obesity is discussed in detail in Chapter 11.)

Fats Contribute to the Flavor, Texture, and Satiety of Foods

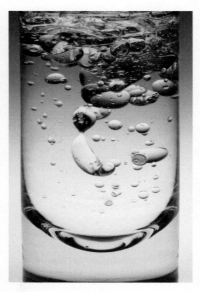

Dietary fat helps food taste good because it contributes to texture and flavor. Fat makes salad dressings smooth and ice cream "creamy," and it gives cakes and cookies their moist, tender texture. Frying foods in melted butter, lard, or oils gives them a crisp, flavorful coating; however, eating fried foods regularly is unhealthful because these foods are high in saturated and *trans* fatty acids.

Fats in foods help us feel satiated, so we stop eating sooner. Fats also contribute to satiety after a meal, reducing the amount of food you eat at the next meal. Two factors probably contribute to this effect: first, fat has a much higher energy density than carbohydrate or protein. For every gram of fat you consume, you get 2.25 times the amount of energy that you get with the same number of grams consumed in protein or carbohydrate.

Second, fat takes longer to digest than protein or carbohydrate because more steps are involved in the digestion process. This may make you feel fuller for a longer period of time because energy is slowly being released into your body.

Unfortunately, you can eat a lot of fat without feeling overfull because fat is so compact. For example, one medium apple weighs 117 g (approximately 4 oz) and has 70 kcal, but the same number of Calories of butter—two pats—would hardly make you feel full! Looked at another way, an amount of butter weighing the same number of grams as a medium apple would contain 840 kcal.

⬆ Fats and oils do not dissolve readily in water.

recap Dietary fats provide more than twice the energy of protein and carbohydrate, at 9 kcal per gram, and provide the majority of the energy required at rest. Fats are also a major fuel source during exercise, especially endurance exercise. Dietary fats help transport the fat-soluble vitamins into the body and help regulate cell function and maintain membrane integrity. Stored body fat in the adipose tissue helps protect vital organs and pad the body. Fats contribute to the flavor and texture of foods and the satiety we feel after a meal.

How does our body process fats?

Because fats are not soluble in water, they cannot enter our bloodstream easily from the digestive tract. Thus, fats must be digested, absorbed, and transported within the body differently than carbohydrates and proteins, which are water-soluble substances. The digestion and absorption of fat were discussed in Chapter 3, but we review the process here, and the steps are illustrated in **FIGURE 5.10** (page 160).

Salivary enzymes released during chewing have a limited role in the breakdown of fats, so most fat reaches the stomach intact. The primary role of the stomach in fat digestion is to mix and break up the fat into small droplets. Because they are not soluble in water, these fat droplets typically float on top of the watery digestive juices in the stomach until they are passed into the small intestine.

The Gallbladder, Liver, and Pancreas Assist in Fat Digestion

Because fat is not soluble in water, its digestion requires the help of bile from the gall-bladder and digestive enzymes from the pancreas. The gallbladder is a sac attached to the underside of the liver, and the pancreas is an oblong-shaped organ sitting below the stomach. Both have a duct connecting them to the small intestine.

As fat enters the small intestine from the stomach, the gallbladder contracts and releases bile, a compound synthesized in the liver and stored in the gallbladder until needed. Bile contains cholesterol, certain amino acids, and the mineral sodium in compounds referred to as *bile salts*. As shown in **FIGURE 5.11A** (page 161), bile salts act somewhat like soap, emulsifying large fat droplets into smaller and smaller drop-lets. At the same time, pancreatic lipases—lipid-digesting enzymes produced in the pancreas—travel through the pancreatic duct into the small intestine. By emulsifying the fat into small droplets, bile has exposed more surface area to the action of pancre-atic lipases, which now begin digesting the triglycerides. Each triglyceride molecule is broken down into two free fatty acids and one *monoglyceride*, a glycerol backbone with one fatty acid still attached.

Absorption of Fat Occurs Primarily in the Small Intestine

The majority of fat absorption occurs in the enterocytes with the help of micelles (see Figures 5.10 and 5.11b). A *micelle* is a spherical compound made up of bile and phos-pholipids that can trap the free fatty acids and monoglycerides, as well as cholesterol and phospholipids, and transport these products to the enterocytes for absorption.

Because fats do not mix with water, how does the absorbed fat get into the bloodstream? As the micelle nears the surface of the enterocytes, the fatty acids, monoglycerides, phospholipids, and cholesterol are released and absorbed. At this point the micelle itself is not absorbed; instead, it is absorbed later in the ileum of the small intestine, at which point it can be recycled back to the liver.

Once inside the enterocytes, the free fatty acids and monoglycerides are refor-mulated back into triglycerides, and then packaged into lipoproteins. A **lipoprotein** is a spherical compound in which the fat clusters in the center and phospholipids and proteins form the outside of the sphere (**FIGURE 5.12** on page 162). The spe-cific lipoprotein produced in the enterocyte to transport fat from a meal is called a

lipoprotein A spherical compound in which fat clusters in the center and phospholipids and proteins form the outside of the sphere.

focus figure 5.10 | Lipid Digestion Overview

The majority of lipid digestion takes place in the small intestine, with the help of bile from the liver and digestive enzymes from the pancreas. Micelles transport the end products of lipid digestion to the enterocytes for absorption and eventual transport via the blood or lymph.

ORGANS OF THE GI TRACT

MOUTH

Lingual lipase secreted by tongue cells and mixed with saliva digests some triglycerides.

Little lipid digestion occurs here.

STOMACH

Most fat arrives intact at the stomach, where it is mixed and broken into droplets.

Gastric lipase digests some triglycerides.

SMALL INTESTINE

Bile from the gallbladder breaks fat into smaller droplets.

Lipid-digesting enzymes from the pancreas break triglycerides into monoacylglycerides and fatty acids.

Lipid-digesting enzymes from the pancreas break dietary cholesterol esters and phospholipids into their components.

Products of fat digestion combine with bile salts to form micelles.

Micelles transport lipid digestion products to the enterocytes.

Within enterocytes, components from micelles reform triglycerides and are repackaged as chylomicrons for transport into the lymphatic system.

Shorter fatty acids can be absorbed directly into the bloodstream.

ACCESSORY ORGANS

SALIVARY GLANDS
Produce saliva.

LIVER
Produces bile, which is stored in the gallbladder.

GALLBLADDER
Contracts and releases bile into the small intestine.

PANCREAS
Produces lipid-digesting enzymes, which are released into the small intestine.

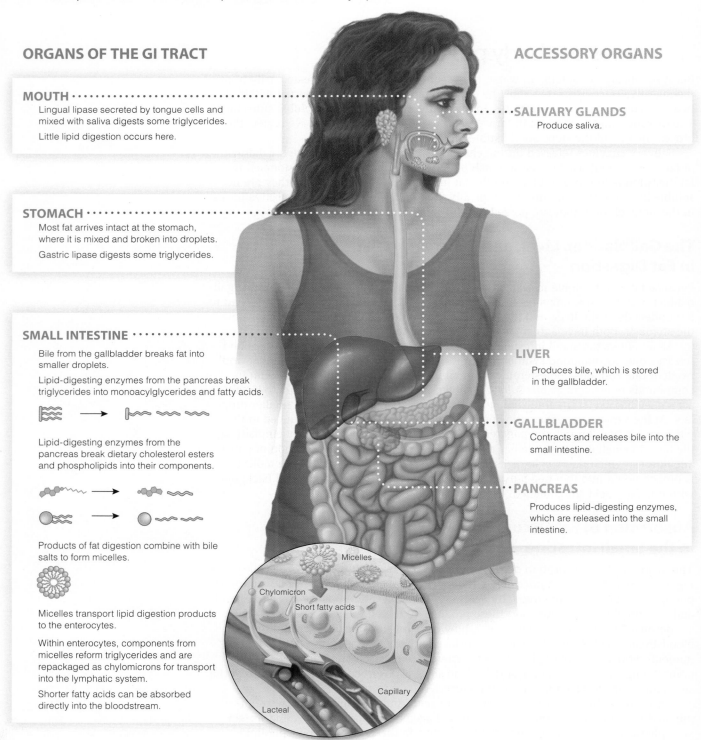

Micelles

Chylomicron

Short fatty acids

Capillary

Lacteal

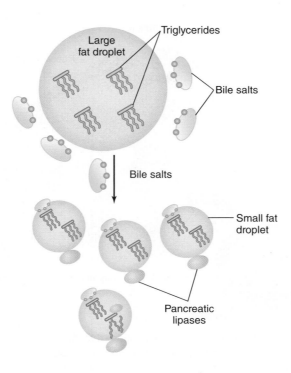

(a) Fat is emulsified by bile salts, then triglycerides are broken apart by pancreatic lipase.

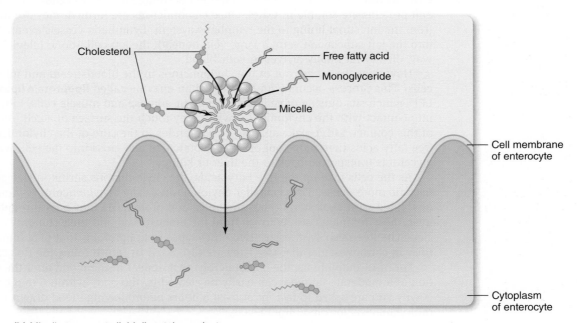

(b) Micelle transports lipid digestoin products to the enterocyte for absorption.

🔶 **FIGURE 5.11** Action of bile salts, pancreatic lipase, and micelles in fat emulsification, digestion, and absorption. **(a)** Large fat droplets filled with triglycerides are emulsified by bile into smaller and smaller droplets. Pancreatic lipase can then access the triglycerides and break them apart into free fatty acids and monoglycerides. **(b)** These products, along with cholesterol, are trapped in micelles, spherical compounds made up of bile salts and phospholipids. Micelles transport lipid digestion products to the enterocytes. Bile salts are taken up in the lower intestine and recycled by the liver.

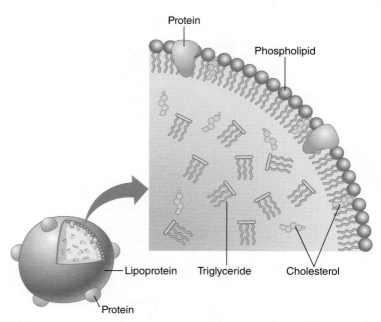

FIGURE 5.12 Structure of a lipoprotein. Notice that the fat clusters in the center of the molecule and the phospholipids and proteins, which are water soluble, form the outside of the sphere. This enables lipoproteins to transport fats in the bloodstream.

chylomicron. Again, this unique compound is soluble in water because phospholipids and proteins are soluble in water. Once chylomicrons are formed, they are transported from the intestinal lining to the lymphatic system. Lymphatic vessels eventually drain into the left subclavian vein, a large vein beneath the left collarbone (clavicle). In this way, dietary fat finally arrives in your blood.

How does the fat get out of the chylomicrons in the bloodstream and into body cells? This process occurs with the help of an enzyme called **lipoprotein lipase**, or LPL, which sits outside of cells, including our adipose and muscle cells. LPL comes into contact with the chylomicrons when they touch the surface of a cell. As a result of this contact, LPL breaks apart the triglycerides in the core of the chylomicrons. The free fatty acids then move out of the chylomicrons and cross into the cell, whereas the glycerol is transported back to the liver or kidney.[3]

As the cells take up the free fatty acids, the chylomicrons shrink in size and become more dense. These smaller chylomicrons, called *chylomicron remnants*, are now filled with cholesterol, phospholipids, and protein. As they pass through the liver, these remnants are removed from the bloodstream and their contents are recycled. The liver also synthesizes two other types of lipoproteins that play important roles in cardiovascular disease. They are discussed **In Depth** following this chapter.

For most individuals, the chylomicrons that appear in the blood after the consumption of a moderate fat meal can easily be cleared by the body within 6 to 8 hours. This is why you are asked to fast for at least 8 hours before having blood drawn for a laboratory analysis for blood lipid levels.

As mentioned earlier, short- and medium-chain fatty acids (those fewer than fourteen carbons in length) can be transported in the body more readily than the long-chain fatty acids. When short- and medium-chain fatty acids are digested and transported to the enterocytes, they do not have to be incorporated into chylomicrons. Instead, they can travel bound to either a transport protein, such as albumin, or a phospholipid. For this reason, shorter-chain fatty acids can get into the bloodstream more quickly than long-chain fatty acids.

Imagine a "magic pill" that would block your body's absorption of fat, allowing you to eat all the fat you wanted without any effects on your weight or your heart. Does such a pill exist? Check out the **Nutrition Debate** at the end of this chapter to find out.

chylomicron A lipoprotein produced in the enterocyte; transports dietary fat out of the intestinal tract.

lipoprotein lipase (LPL) An enzyme that sits on the outside of cells and breaks apart triglycerides, so that their fatty acids can be removed and taken up by the cell.

Fat Is Stored in Adipose Tissues for Later Use

As described earlier, with the help of LPL, the chylomicrons deliver their load of fatty acids to body cells. There are three primary fates of these fatty acids:

1. Cells can take them up immediately for use as a source of energy.
2. Cells can use them to make lipid-containing compounds needed by the body.
3. If the body doesn't need the fatty acids for immediate energy, muscle and adipose cells can re-create the triglycerides (using glucose for the glycerol backbone) and store them for later use.

Although the primary storage site for this extra energy is the adipose cell (**FIGURE 5.13**), if you are physically active, your body will preferentially store this extra fat in muscle cells first, so, the next time you work out, the fat is readily available to the cells for energy. Thus, people who engage in regular physical activity are likely to store fat in the muscle tissue after a meal and less likely to store the fat in adipose tissue—something many of us would prefer. Of course, fat stored in the adipose tissue can also be used for energy during exercise, but it must be broken down first and then transported to the muscle cells.

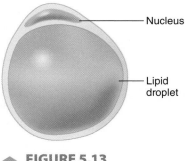

◆ FIGURE 5.13
Diagram of an adipose cell.

recap Before fat can be digested, it is emulsified into droplets by bile. Pancreatic lipases then digest the triglycerides into two free fatty acids and one mono-glyceride. These are transported into the enterocytes with the help of micelles. Once inside, triglycerides are re-formed and packaged into lipoproteins called chylomicrons. These enter the lymph, then the bloodstream, in which they travel to body cells that need energy. Fat stored in the muscle tissue is used as a source of energy during physical activity. Excess fat is stored in the adipose tissue and can be used whenever the body needs energy.

How much fat should we eat?

Without a doubt, Americans think dietary fat is bad! Yet, because fat plays such an important role in keeping our body healthy, we do need to include a moderate amount in our diet. But what, exactly, is a moderate amount? And what foods contain the most healthful fats? We'll explore these questions here.

Dietary Reference Intake for Total Fat

The Acceptable Macronutrient Distribution Range (AMDR) for fat is 20–35% of total energy.[7] This recommendation is based on evidence indicating that higher intakes of fat increase the risk for obesity and its complications, especially cardiovascular disease, but that diets too low in fat and too high in carbohydrate can also increase the risk for cardiovascular disease if they cause blood triglycerides to increase.[7] Within this range of fat intake, it is also recommended that we minimize our intake of saturated and *trans* fatty acids as much as possible.

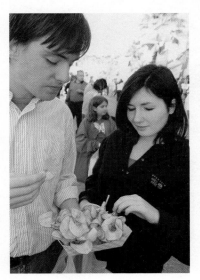

◆ In the United States, we eat too many saturated and *trans* fats.

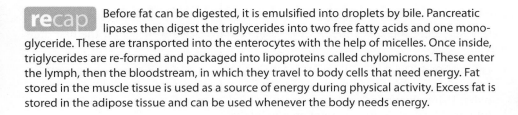

nutri-case | LIZ

"Lately I'm hungry all the time. I read online that if I limit my total fat intake to no more than 10% of my total Calories, I can eat all the carbs and protein that I want, and I won't gain weight. So, when I felt hungry after my last class, I stopped at the yogurt shop in the Student Union and ordered a sundae with nonfat vanilla yogurt and fat-free chocolate syrup. I have to admit, though, that about an hour after I ate it I was hungry again. Maybe it's stress."

What do you think of Liz's approach to her persistent hunger? What have you learned in this chapter about the role of fats that would be important information to share with her?

If you're an athlete, you've probably been advised to consume less fat and more carbohydrate to replenish your glycogen stores, especially if you participate in endurance activities. Specifically, you should consume 20–25% of your total energy from fat, 55–60% of energy from carbohydrate, and 12–15% of energy from protein.[8,9] This percentage of fat intake is still within the AMDR and represents approximately 45 to 55 g of fat per day for an athlete consuming 2,000 kcal per day, and 78 to 97 g of fat per day for an athlete consuming 3,500 kcal per day.

Although many people trying to lose weight consume less than 20% of their energy from fat, this practice may do more harm than good, especially if they are also limiting energy intake (eating fewer than 1,500 kcal per day). Research suggests that very-low-fat diets, those with less than 15% of energy from fat, do not provide additional health or performance benefits over moderate-fat diets and are usually very difficult to follow.[10] In fact, most people find they feel better, are more successful in weight maintenance, and are less preoccupied with food if they keep their fat intake at 20–25% of energy intake. Additionally, people attempting to reduce their dietary fat frequently eliminate foods such as meats, dairy, eggs, and nuts, which are sources of protein and many essential vitamins and minerals. Diets extremely low in fat may also be deficient in EFAs.

Dietary Reference Intakes for Essential Fatty Acids

Dietary Reference Intakes (DRIs) for the essential fatty acids were set for the first time in 2005.[7]

- **Linoleic acid.** The Adequate Intake (AI) for linoleic acid (an omega-6 fatty acid) is 14 to 17 g per day for adult men and 11 to 12 g per day for women 19 years and older. Using the typical energy intakes for adult men and women, this translates into an AMDR of 5–10% of total energy intake.
- **Alpha-linolenic acid (ALA).** The AI for ALA (an omega-3 fatty acid) is 1.6 g per day for adult men and 1.1 g per day for adult women. This translates into an AMDR of 0.6–1.2% of total energy. These DRIs are for omega-3 fatty acids as a group. No DRIs have been set for DHA or EPA specifically; however, because the AMDR for ALA was set in 2005, new research has supported a recommended intake of at least 250 mg per day of EPA+DHA.[4] So how do you know if you're getting enough in your diet? See **TABLE 5.1**.

Following these recommendations, an individual consuming 2,000 kcal per day should consume about 11 to 22 g per day of linoleic acid and about 1.3 to 2.6 g per day of ALA. Notice that the recommended intake of linoleic acid is close to ten times higher than the recommended intake of ALA. Because these EFAs compete for the same enzymes to produce various eicosanoids, this ratio helps keep eicosanoid production in balance; that is, one isn't overproduced at the expense of the other.

However, it is unrealistic for most Americans to keep track of the number of grams of linoleic acid and ALA they consume each day. Overall, we appear to get adequate amounts of linoleic acid in our diets because of the salad dressings, vegetable oils, margarines, and mayonnaise that we eat. In contrast, our consumption of ALA, EPA, and DHA is likely to be low, especially if we don't regularly consume dark green, leafy vegetables, walnuts, flax seeds, and fish or fish oils. Thus, it is more important to pay attention to including these foods in our diet (see Table 5.1.)

recap The Acceptable Macronutrient Distribution Range (AMDR) for total fat is 20–35% of total energy. The Adequate Intake (AI) for linoleic acid is 14 to 17 g per day for adult men and 11 to 12 g per day for adult women. The AI for alpha-linolenic acid (ALA) is 1.6 g per day for adult men and 1.1 g per day for adult women. No DRIs have been set for DHA or EPA.

Don't Let the Fats Fool You!

We know that unsaturated fat is necessary for good health, but too much fat, regardless of type, can be harmful. That's one reason nutritionists have been recommending the reduction of dietary fat for over a decade. To make the switch to more healthful

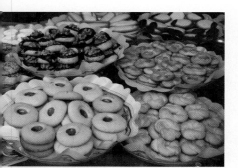

◆ Baked goods are often high in hidden fats and may contain *trans* fats.

Exactly how much fat should you eat per day? Find out with the fat intake calculator at www.healthcalculators.org; go to "calculators" and then "fat" in the search box.

visible fats Fats that are clearly present and visible in our food, or visibly added to food, such as butter, margarine, cream, shortening, salad dressings, chicken skin, and untrimmed fat on meat.

TABLE 5.1 **Omega-3 Fatty Acid Content of Selected Foods**

Food Item	Total Omega-3	DHA g/Serving	EPA
Flaxseed oil, 1 tbsp.	7.25	0.00	0.00
Salmon oil (fish oil), 1 tbsp.	4.39	2.48	1.77
Sardine oil, 1 tbsp.	3.01	1.45	1.38
Flaxseed, whole, 1 tbsp.	2.50	0.00	0.00
Herring, Atlantic, broiled, 3 oz	1.83	0.94	0.77
Salmon, Coho, steamed, 3 oz	1.34	0.71	0.46
Canola oil, 1 tbsp.	1.28	0.00	0.00
Sardines, Atlantic, w/ bones & oil, 3 oz	1.26	0.43	0.40
Trout, rainbow fillet, baked, 3 oz	1.05	0.70	0.28
Walnuts, English, 1 tbsp.	0.66	0.00	0.00
Halibut, fillet, baked, 3 oz	0.53	0.31	0.21
Shrimp, Canned, 3 oz	0.47	0.21	0.25
Tuna, white, in oil, 3 oz	0.38	0.19	0.04
Crab, Alaska King, steamed, 3 oz	0.36	0.10	0.25
Scallops, broiled, 3 oz	0.31	0.14	0.17
Smart Balance Omega-3 Buttery Spread (1 tbps.)	0.32	0.01	0.01
Tuna, light, in water, 3 oz	0.23	0.19	0.04
Avocado, Calif, fresh, whole	0.22	0.00	0.00
Spinach, ckd, 1 cup	0.17	0.00	0.00
Egglands Best, 1 large egg, with omega-3	0.12	0.06	0.03

EPA, Eicosapentaenoic acid; DHA, docosahexaenoic acid.

Data from: Food Processor SQL, Version 10.3, ESHA Research, Salem, OR, and manufacturer labels.

fats and reduce your total fat intake, you need to know where the fat in your diet is coming from.

Recognize the Fat in Foods

It is easy to eat a high-fat diet. First, we add fats, such as oils, butter, cream, shortening, margarine, mayonnaise, and salad dressings, to foods because they make food taste good. This type of fat is called **visible fat** because we can easily see that we are adding it to our food. When we add fat to foods ourselves, we generally know how much we are adding. Still, we may not be aware of the type of fat we're using and the number of Calories it adds to our meal. For instance, it's easy to make a salad into a high-fat meal by adding two or three tablespoons of full-fat salad dressing. Doing so also transforms the salad into a high-Calorie meal: concentrated fats, such as butter, oil, and salad dressings, have 100 kcal per tablespoon. When adding visible fats, use moderation and, when possible, select oils, such as canola oil, soybean oil, or olive oil, over solid fats such as butter or margarine. When selecting butter or margarine, use those made with or mixed with healthy oils.[11]

Also be on the lookout for **hidden fats**—that is, fats added to processed and pre-pared foods to improve taste and texture. Their invisibility often tricks us into choosing them over more healthful foods. For example, a blueberry scone is much higher in fat (43% of energy) than a blueberry bagel (6% of energy from fat), yet consumers assume that the fat content of these foods is the same because they are both bread products. The majority of the fat in the average American diet is invisible. Foods that can be high in invisible fats are baked goods, regular-fat dairy products, processed meats or meats that are highly marbled or not trimmed, and most convenience and fast foods, such as hamburgers, hot dogs, chips, ice cream, and French fries and other fried foods. When purchasing packaged foods, read the Nutrition Facts Panel and find

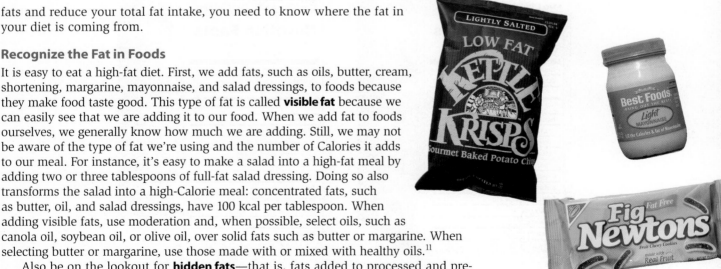

hidden fats Fats that are not apparent, or "hidden" in foods, such as the fats found in baked goods, regular-fat dairy products, marbling in meat, and fried foods.

nutrition label activity

How Much Fat Is in This Food?

How can you figure out how much fat is in a food you buy? One way is to read the Nutrition Facts Panel on the label. Two cracker labels are shown in **FIGURE 5.14**; one cracker is higher in fat than the other. Let's use the label to find out what percentage of energy is coming from fat in each product. The calculations are relatively simple.

1. Divide the total Calories from fat by the total Calories per serving, and multiply the answer by 100.
   - For the regular wheat crackers: 50 kcal/150 kcal = 0.33 × 100 = 33%.
   Thus, for the regular crackers, the total energy coming from fat is 33%.
   - For the reduced-fat wheat crackers: 35 kcal/130 kcal = 0.269 × 100 = 27%.
   Thus, for the reduced-fat crackers, the total energy coming from fat is 27%.

Although the energy per serving is not very different between these two crackers, the percentage from fat is quite different.

2. If the total Calories per serving from fat are not given on the label, you can quickly calculate this value by multiplying the grams of total fat per serving by 9 (because there are 9 kcal per gram of fat).
   - For the regular wheat crackers: 6 g fat × 9 kcal/gram = 54 kcal of fat.
   - To calculate the percentage of Calories from fat: 54 kcal/150 kcal = 0.36 × 100 = 36%.

This value is not exactly the same as the 50 kcal reported on the label or the 33% of Calories from fat calculated in example 1. That's because the values on food labels are rounded off. In summary, you can quickly calculate the percentage of fat per serving for any packaged food in three steps: 1) multiply the grams of fat per serving by 9 kcal per gram; 2) divide this number by the total kcal per serving; 3) multiply by 100.

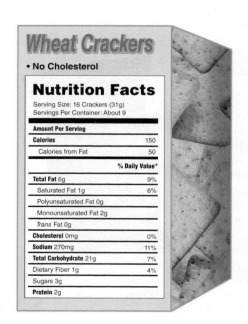

(a)

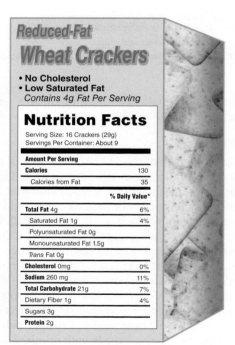

(b)

FIGURE 5.14 Labels for two types of wheat crackers. **(a)** Regular wheat crackers. **(b)** Reduced-fat wheat crackers.

out whether or not the product is high in hidden fats and what type of fat is in the product! The **Nutrition Label Activity** shows you how to calculate the amount of fat hidden in packaged foods.

Decipher Label Claims

Because high-fat diets have been associated with obesity, many Americans are trying to reduce their total fat intake. Because of this concern, food manufacturers have been more than happy to provide consumers with low-fat alternatives to their favorite foods—so you can have your cake and eat it, too! The FDA and the U.S. Department of Agriculture (USDA) have set specific regulations on allowable label claims for reduced-fat products. The following claims are defined for 1 serving:

- Fat-free = less than 0.5 g of fat
- Low-fat = 3 g or less of fat
- Reduced or less fat: at least 25% less fat as compared to a standard serving
- Light: one-third fewer Calories or 50% less fat as compared with a standard serving amount

There are now thousands of fat-modified foods in the market. However, if you're choosing such foods because of a concern about your weight, let the buyer beware! Lower-fat versions of foods may not always be lower in Calories. The reduced fat is often replaced with added simple carbohydrate, resulting in a very similar total energy intake.

You can see this for yourself by studying TABLE 5.2, where we list a number of full-fat foods with their lower-fat alternatives. If you were to incorporate such foods into your diet on a regular basis, you could significantly reduce the amount of fat you consume. Still, your choices may or may not reduce the amount of energy you consume. For example, as you can see in the table, drinking nonfat milk instead of whole milk would dramatically reduce both your fat and your energy intake. However, eating fat-free instead of regular Fig Newton cookies would not significantly reduce your energy intake. Thus, if you want to reduce both the amount of fat and energy you consume, read the Nutrition Facts Panel of modified-fat foods carefully before you buy.

Limit Saturated and *Trans* Fats

Research over the last two decades has shown that diets high in saturated and *trans* fatty acids negatively influence blood lipid levels, change cell membrane function,

TABLE 5.2 **Comparison of Full-Fat, Reduced-Fat, and Low-Fat Foods**

Product and Serving Size	Version	Energy (kcal)	Protein (g)	Carbohydrate (g)	Fat (g)
Milk, 8 oz	Whole, 3.3% fat	150	8.0	11.4	8.2
	2% fat	121	8.1	11.7	4.7
	Skim (nonfat)	86	8.4	11.9	0.5
Mayonnaise, 1 tbsp.	Regular	100	0.0	0.0	11.0
	Light	50	0.0	1.0	5.0
Margarine, corn oil, 1 tbsp.	Regular	100	0.0	0.0	11.0
	Reduced-fat	60	0.0	0.0	7.0
Peanut butter, 1 tbsp.	Regular	95	4.1	3.1	8.2
	Reduced-fat	81	4.4	5.2	5.4
Wheat Thins, 18 crackers	Regular	158	2.3	21.4	6.8
	Reduced- fat	120	2.0	21.0	4.0
Cookies, Oreo, 3 cookies	Regular	160	2.0	23.0	7.0
	Reduced- fat	130	2.0	25.0	3.5
Cookies, Fig Newton, 3 cookies	Regular	210	3.0	30.0	4.5
	Fat-free	204	2.4	26.8	0.0

Data from: Food Processor-SQL, Version 9.9, ESHA Research, Salem, OR.

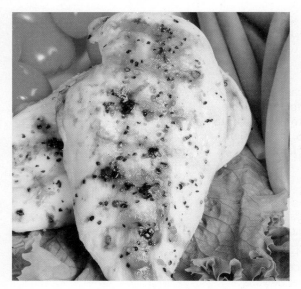

This skinless roasted chicken breast provides less than 1 g saturated fat and 131 kcal; with the skin, it would provide 3 g saturated fat and 235 kcal.

Concerned about the saturated fat and cholesterol in the meat you eat? Use the guide to choosing the leanest cuts of beef at www.mayoclinic.com; go to "health" and then "cuts of beef" in the search box to get started.

and alter the way cholesterol is removed from the blood. For these reasons, researchers believe that diets high in saturated and *trans* fatty acids can increase the risk for cardiovascular disease.

Reduce Your Intake of Saturated Fats

The recommended intake of saturated fats is less than 7–10% of our total energy; unfortunately, our average intake is between 11% and 12% of energy.[12] According to data from the National Health and Nutrition Examination Survey (NHANES), about 64% of adults in the United States exceed the dietary recommendation for saturated fats.[13] Let's look at the primary sources of saturated fats in the American diet.

- **Animal products.** Meats contain a mixture of fatty acids, including saturated fats. The precise amount of saturated fat will depend on the cut of the meat and how it is prepared. For example, red meats, such as beef, pork, and lamb, typically have more fat than skinless chicken or fish. Thus, lean meats are lower in saturated fat than regular cuts. In addition, broiled, grilled, or baked meats have less saturated fat than fried meats. Dairy products may also be high in saturated fat. Whole-fat milk has three times the saturated fat as low-fat milk, and nearly twice the energy. Whole eggs have just over a gram of saturated fat and are high in cholesterol.
- **Grain products.** Baked goods and snack foods are the main culprits in this food group. Pastries, cookies, and muffins may be filled with saturated fats. Tortilla chips, microwave and movie-theatre popcorn, snack crackers, and packaged rice and pasta mixes may also be high in saturated fat.
- **Vegetables and vegetable spreads/dressings.** We often don't think of plant foods as having high amounts of saturated fats, but if these foods are fried, breaded, or drenched in sauces they can become a source of saturated fat. For example, a small baked potato (138 g) has no fat and 134 kcal, whereas a medium serving (134 g) of french fries cooked in vegetable oil has 427 kcal, 23 g of fat, and 5.3 g of saturated fat. This is one-third of the saturated fat recommended for an entire day for a person on a 2,000-kcal/day diet.

You can significantly reduce your intake of saturated fats by making smart choices when you prepare and cook foods. The **Quick Tips** feature will help.

Avoid *Trans* Fatty Acids

The Institute of Medicine recommends that we keep our intake of *trans* fatty acids to an absolute minimum.[7] Currently, the average consumption of industrially produced *trans* fatty acids is only about 2–3% of total energy intake with the majority coming from deep-fried fast or frozen foods, some tub margarines, and bakery products.[7,14,15] So, if our current consumption is already so low, why the advice to reduce it even further?

Although *trans* fatty acids make up only a small fraction of the average American diet, their negative effect on our health appears to be dramatic. Many health professionals feel that diets high in *trans* fatty acids increase the risk for cardiovascular disease even more than diets high in saturated fats.[16] A research review that involved over 140,000 individuals showed that for every 2% increase in energy intake from *trans* fatty acids, there was a 23% increase in incidence of cardiovascular disease.[16] Next time you're at the grocery store, how can you limit the level of saturated and *trans* fats in the foods you buy? Let the **Quick Tips** feature (page 170) can help guide your choices.

What About Dietary Cholesterol?

Consumers are confused about whether they should avoid dietary cholesterol. This confusion is understandable given that health experts have changed their message over the years as they have learned more about saturated fat and cholesterol metabolism and their relationship to cardiovascular disease.[11,17] Here are three points to keep in mind:

- First, our body can make cholesterol with the majority being produced in the liver and intestine. Thus, we never have to worry about getting enough in our diet.

QuickTips

Reducing Saturated Fats When Cooking

✓ Trim visible fat from meats before cooking.

✓ Remove the skin from poultry before cooking.

✓ Instead of frying meats, poultry, fish, or potatoes or other vegetables, bake or broil them.

✓ If you normally eat two eggs for breakfast, discard the yolk from one for half the cholesterol. Do the same in recipes calling for two eggs.

✓ Cook with olive oil or canola oil instead of butter.

✓ Use cooking spray instead of butter or oils for stir-frying and baking.

✓ Substitute hard cheeses (such as parmesan), which are naturally lower in fat, for softer cheeses that are higher in fat (such as cheddar).

✓ Substitute low-fat or nonfat yogurt for cream, cream cheese, mayonnaise, or sour cream in recipes; on baked potatoes, tacos, and salads; and in dips.

When we consume cholesterol, our body typically reduces our internal production, which keeps our total cholesterol pool constant. However, the amount of cholesterol we make can be influenced by various factors such as the amount of saturated fat and cholesterol in the diet, amount of cholesterol absorbed, and body size.

■ Second, we absorb only about 40–60% of the cholesterol we consume.[18] The amount absorbed can vary between individuals, depending on body size, presence of type 2 diabetes, and the other foods consumed in the diet.[17,19] These variations in cholesterol absorptions mean that people can have different responses to alterations in their dietary cholesterol intake. For example, obese individuals will be less responsive to changes in dietary saturated fat and cholesterol intake than people of normal weight.[19]

■ Third, our body recycles cholesterol, so we always have enough. However, the recycling of cholesterol can be altered by a number of factors including your intake of various foods such as fiber, plant sterols, and medications.

Saturated fats can influence cholesterol metabolism in the liver as well as cholesterol uptake by body cells.[20] Thus, by keeping our intake of saturated fat low, we in turn can avoid excessive levels of cholesterol in our blood. Because saturated fat and cholesterol are typically found in the same foods, namely, fatty animal products, following the recommendation from the Institute of Medicine[7] to limit your intake of dietary cholesterol to less than 300 mg/day will also help keep your intake of saturated fats low.

Select Beneficial Fats

As mentioned earlier, it's best to switch to healthful fats without increasing your total fat intake. Americans appear to get adequate amounts of linoleic acid, probably because of the large amount of salad dressings, vegetable oils, margarine, and mayonnaise we eat. Our consumption of the omega-3 fatty acids is more variable and can be low in the diet. The following suggestions will help you find foods rich in the beneficial fats you need.

■ **Plants and plant oils.** Leafy green vegetables, avocados, soybeans, soybean oil, and soy milk, canola oil, and flaxseed oil are good sources of ALA. Consider using canola or soybean oil for cooking.

■ **Nuts and seeds.** Walnuts, almonds, flax seeds, and chia seeds are also a rich source of ALA. Consider adding ground flaxseeds to your cereal or walnuts to your salad, or try almond milk on your cereal.

QuickTips

Shopping for Foods Low in Saturated and *Trans* Fats

Read food labels. Look for foods with no hydrogenated oils and low amounts of saturated fats per serving.

Select liquid or tub margarine/butters over hard stick forms. Fats that are solid at room temperature are usually high in *trans* or saturated fatty acids. Also, select margarines made from healthful fats, such as canola oil.

Buy naturally occurring oils, such as olive and canola oil. These types of oils have not been hydrogenated and contain healthful unsaturated fatty acids and no *trans* fatty acids.

Select reduced-fat baked products, such as crackers, chips, cookies, and muffins, over full-fat versions. If you are watching your weight, choose products with fewer Calories per serving as well.

Cut back on packaged pastries, such as Danish, croissants, donuts, cakes, tarts, pies, and brownies. These baked goods are typically high in saturated and *trans* fatty acids.

Select reduced-fat salad dressing and mayonnaise or select those made with healthful fats, such as olive oil and vinegar. If you select the full-fat versions, remember that a tablespoon of oil or full-fat mayonnaise contains 100 kcal.

Add fish, especially those high in omega-3 fatty acids, to your shopping list. For example, select salmon, line-caught tuna, herring, and sardines. Many specialty markets now carry line-caught canned tuna, which is low in mercury. These tuna are smaller, usually less than 20 pounds, and have had less exposure to mercury in their lifetime.

For other healthful sources of protein, select lean cuts of meat and skinless poultry, meat substitutes made with soy, or beans or lentils.

Select low-fat or nonfat versions of milk, cheese, cottage cheese, yogurt, sour cream, cream cheese, and ice cream.

■ **Fish and fish oils.** To increase your intake of EPA and DHA, select fish, fish oil, or processed foods enriched with these fatty acids. Consider including fish in your diet at least twice a week or consider taking a fish oil supplement.

How can you specifically increase your intake of omega-3 fatty acids? Use Table 5.1 (page 165) to help you identify foods and supplements rich in these healthful fats. You can also buy food products enriched with EPA and DHA. Read the labels of such products carefully, however, to determine if the omega-3 fatty acid level in the product is worth the extra cost.

It is important to recognize that there can be some risks associated with eating large amounts of certain fish on a regular basis. Depending on the species and the level of pollution in the water in which it is caught, the fish may contain mercury, polychlorinated biphenyls (PCBs), and other environmental contaminants. Types of fish that are currently considered safe to consume include salmon (except from the Great Lakes region), farmed trout, flounder, sole, *mahi mahi*, and cooked shellfish. Line-caught tuna, either fresh or canned, is low in mercury. These tuna are smaller, usually less than 20 pounds, and have had less exposure to mercury in their lifetime. Fish more likely to be contaminated are shark, swordfish, golden bass, golden snapper, marlin, bluefish, and largemouth and smallmouth bass. Women who are pregnant or breastfeeding, women who may become pregnant, and small children should avoid these fish species entirely. (For more information on seafood safety, see Chapter 13.)

Of course, healthful fats include not only the EFAs but also polyunsaturated and monounsaturated fats in general. Plant oils are excellent sources of unsaturated fats, as are avocados, olives, nuts and nut butters, and seeds. Substituting beneficial fats for saturated or *trans* fats isn't difficult. See the **Eating Right All Day** feature for some sample menu choices.

Watch Out When You're Eating Out

Many college students eat most of their meals in dining halls and fast-food restaurants or buy to-go foods from the grocery delicatessen. If that describes you, watch out! The menu items you choose each day may be increasing the amount of fat in your diet, including your intake of saturated and *trans* fats. A recent national study found that fast-food consumers have higher total energy, total fat, and saturated fat intake than those who eat fast food infrequently.[21] And although many fast-food restaurants have eliminated *trans* fatty acids from certain menu items, some burgers, breakfast sandwiches, desserts, and shakes still contain them. The **Quick Tips** (page 172) are specific strategies for limiting fat in your menu choices.

Be Aware of Fat Replacers

One way to lower the fat content of processed foods is by using a *fat replacer*. Snack foods have been the primary target for fat replacers because it is difficult to simply reduce or eliminate the fat in these foods without dramatically changing their taste. In the mid-1990s, the food industry promoted fat replacers as the answer to the growing obesity problem. They claimed that substituting fat replacers for traditional fats in snack and fast foods might reduce both energy and fat intake and help Americans manage their weight better.

Products such as olestra (brand name *Olean*) hit the market in 1996 with a lot of fanfare, but the hype was short-lived. Initially, foods containing olestra had to bear a label warning of potential gastrointestinal side effects. In 2003, the FDA announced that this warning was no longer necessary because research showed that olestra causes only mild, infrequent discomfort. However, even with the new labeling, only a limited number of foods in the marketplace contain olestra. It is also evident from our growing obesity problem that fat replacers, such as olestra, do not help Americans lose weight or even maintain their current weight.

eating right all day

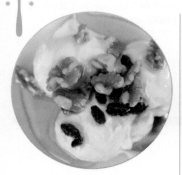

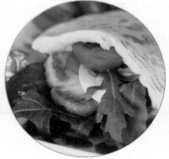

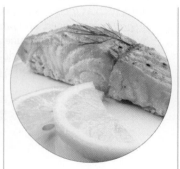

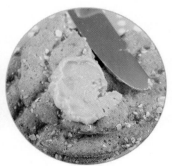

Breakfast
Non fat yogurt with walnuts instead of bacon and eggs!

Lunch
Veggie pita instead of a ham and cheese sandwich!

Dinner
Grilled salmon instead of steak!

Snack
Whole-grain crackers with peanut butter instead of potato chips!

QuickTips

Limiting Fat When You're Eating Out

When deciding where to eat out, choose a restaurant that allows you to order alternatives to the usual menu items. For instance, if you like burgers, look for a restaurant that will grill your burger instead of frying it and will let you substitute a salad for french fries.

Before you order, look for or ask about the saturated fat and Calorie content of the menu items you're considering.

Ask about the types of fats used in salad dressing, baked goods, and cooking processes. Many establishments are working to replace saturated and *trans* fatty acids with healthful fats in their menu items.

Select healthful appetizers, such as salads, broth-based soups, vegetables, or fruit, over white bread with butter, nachos, or fried foods such as chicken wings.

Select broth-based soups, which are lower in fat and Calories than cream-based soups, which are typically made with cream, cheese, and/or butter.

Ask that all visible fat be trimmed from meats and that poultry be served without the skin.

Select menu items that use cooking methods that add little or no additional fat, such as broiling, grilling, steaming, and sautéing. Be alert to menu descriptions such as *fried, crispy, creamed, buttered, au gratin, escalloped,* and *parmesan.* Also avoid foods served in sauces such as butter sauce, alfredo, and hollandaise. All of these types of food preparation typically add more fat to a meal.

Avoid meat and vegetable pot pies, quiches, and other items with a pastry crust because these may be high in *trans* fats.

Ask for spreads and condiments, such as butter, salad dressings, sauces, and sour cream, to be served on the side instead of added in the kitchen.

Request low-fat spreads on your sandwiches, such as mustards or chutneys, over full-fat mayonnaise or butter.

Substitute a salad, veggies, or fruit for the chips or french fries that come with the meal.

Select lower-fat desserts, such as sorbet or a small cookie, over full-fat ice cream or a brownie. Alternatively, share a full-fat dessert with friends or family members, which will reduce both the Calories and fat you consume.

Keep counting at your favorite cafe! Consider that a Starbucks tall cafe latte (12 oz) made with whole milk contains 200 kcal and 11 g of fat (7 g from saturated fat). Whipped cream can add 80–130 kcal and 8–12 g of fat. The same drink made with nonfat milk and no whipped cream contains 120 kcal and no fat. So ask for your coffee, hot chocolate, tea, or chai with nonfat milk and eliminate the whipped cream.

Select lower-fat options to accompany your coffee drink. For example, choose a biscotti or a small piece of dark chocolate instead of a croissant, a scone, a muffin, coffee cake, or a large cookie.

recap Visible fats are those foods that can be easily recognized as containing fat. Hidden fats are those fats added to our food during the manufacturing or cooking process, so we are not aware of how much fat has been added. By making simple substitutions when shopping, cooking, and eating out, you can reduce the quantity of saturated and *trans* fatty acids in your diet and increase your intake of healthful fats. Fat replacers are substances used to replace the typical fats found in foods.

What role do fats play in chronic disease?

There appears to be a generally held assumption that if you eat fat-free or low-fat foods you will lose weight and prevent chronic diseases. Certainly, we know that diets high in saturated and *trans* fatty acids can contribute to chronic diseases, including cardiovascular disease and cancer; however, as we have explored in this chapter, unsaturated fatty acids do not have this negative effect and are essential to good health. We also know that all forms of fat are high in energy, so a sensible health goal is to eat appropriate amounts of healthful types of fat.

The chronic disease most closely associated with diets high in saturated and *trans* fats is cardiovascular disease. This complex disorder is discussed **In Depth** following this chapter. In addition, high-fat diets have been linked to cancer. Is such a link supported by evidence?

Cancer develops as a result of a poorly understood interaction between the environment and genetic factors. In addition, most cancers take years to develop, so examining the impact of diet on cancer development can be a long and difficult process. Nevertheless, research does suggest that diet is one of several important environmental factors that influence the development of cancer.[22]

Of the many dietary factors that have been studied, the influence of dietary fat intake on the development of cancers of the breast, colon, and prostate has been extensively researched. The relationship between type and amount of fat consumed and increased risk for breast cancer is controversial.[22,23] Early research suggested an association between animal fat intake and increased risk for colon cancer, but more recent research indicates that the association involves factors other than fat that are found in red meat. Because we now know that physical activity can reduce the risk for colon cancer, earlier diet and colon cancer studies that did not control for this factor are now being questioned. The strongest association between dietary fat intake and cancer is for prostate cancer. Research shows that there is a consistent link between prostate cancer risk and consumption of animal fat, but not fat from plant sources. The exact mechanism by which animal fats may contribute to prostate cancer has not yet been identified.

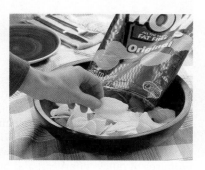

▲ Snack foods have been the primary target for fat replacers, such as Olean, because it is more difficult to eliminate the fat from these types of foods without dramatically changing the taste.

recap The types of fats we eat can significantly affect our health and risk for disease. Diets high in saturated and *trans* fatty acids increase our risk for cardiovascular disease. Selecting appropriate types of fat in the diet may also reduce your risk for some cancers, especially prostate cancer.

✳behavior change . . . getting started!

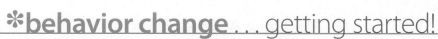

Now that you've read this chapter, try making these changes:

For yourself:

- Try tuna in your sandwich instead of lunch meat.
- Select a meatless meal this week.
- Opt for a baked potato instead of French fries.
- If you drink whole milk, switch to low-fat or skim.
- Get 30 minutes of physical activity today, and see how it makes you feel.

For your community:

- Talk to the manager of your campus dining hall and the fast-food restaurants where you eat about replacing the saturated fats in their foods with plant oils.
- Try fixing a meatless meal for yourself and friends. If you like it, post the recipes—with photos—on your Facebook page.

Fat Blockers—Help or Hype?

In the last 30 years, the rate of obesity has steadily increased among Americans. And growing right alongside our waistlines is the market for weight-loss supplements. It's a multibillion-dollar industry with new products continually tempting us with promises of quick, effortless, and dramatic results. Currently, there's no regulation of weight-loss supplements, so consumers have no way of knowing if the product they're considering is effective, or safe.

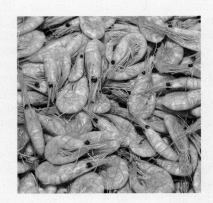

One popular group of weight-loss supplements are the so-called fat blockers. Do these products really "block" fat? Can they truly help you to lose weight?

What Are the Claims?

One way to reduce energy intake and body weight would be to block the absorption of energy-containing macronutrients—such as fat, which contains 9 kcal/gram. If we could block fat absorption, then we could eat large portions of our favorite high-fat foods, including fast foods, snacks, and desserts, without worrying about gaining weight. Fat blockers are said to decrease the amount of fat absorbed in the small intestine, leaving more to be excreted from the body.

The main ingredient in many of these supplements is chitosan, a nondigestible substance extracted mainly from the exoskeletons of marine crustaceans.[24] Chitosan is said to bind up to four to six times its weight in fat. Thus, for every gram of chitosan consumed, 4–6 g of fat should be "blocked." If this were true, then consuming 3 g of chitosan a day would block 12–18 g of fat a day, or 108–162 kcal/day. Chitosan is also thought to block the reabsorption of bile. (Recall that bile is delivered to the small intestine to emulsify fats.) If bile reabsorption is blocked, then the liver must produce new supplies. Because the liver takes cholesterol from the blood to make bile, fat blockers might reduce serum cholesterol as well.[24]

It all sounds good, but is there any evidence that fat blockers work? Let's review the research.

What Does the Research Say?

Chitosan has been studied extensively as a weight-loss aid. Two recent meta-analyses reviewing the efficacy of chitosan for weight loss from fourteen double-blind randomized controlled trials (RCTs) involving over 1,000 participants concluded that there is some limited evidence that chitosan reduces body weight in humans.[25,26,27] The authors found that chitosan used with other weight-loss supplements produced a small, but significant, greater average weight loss (1.7 kg, or 3.7 lb) over an average of 8.6 weeks compared to the placebo group (the group with no supplements). However, when the trials were limited to those who only used chitosan without other weight loss supplements, the weight loss was only 0.9 kg (1.9 lb). In considering these results, ask yourself, is such a small weight loss what you would expect from a weight-loss supplement?

In another study, researchers reported a slightly greater weight loss.[28] Overweight adults taking 3 grams of chitosan per day experienced a weight loss of 2.8 kg (6 lb.) in 8 weeks compared to the placebo group that gained weight (+0.8 kg, or +1.8 lb). The average weight loss of less than a pound a week was still meager, but many people struggling with obesity might consider it significant—especially if, as indicated in this study, chitosan could help prevent further weight gain over time. However, this study, too, is less than reliable: Participants were not consuming a controlled diet but were only asked to record their food intake and physical activity.

To learn more about the specific effects of chitosan, researchers at the University of California at Davis[29] studied its fat-trapping capacity in college students. They fed twelve men and twelve women a controlled diet for 4 days, followed by the same diet plus chitosan for 4 days. Fecal samples were collected to determine the amount of fat trapped by chitosan. They found that, with the control diet plus chitosan, fecal fat excretion increased by 1.8 g/day (16 kcal/day) for the men but not at all for the women. They concluded that the amount of fat trapped by chitosan was clinically insignificant. Based on the data from the men, 7 weeks of supplementation (at 2.5 g/day) would be required for a 1-pound weight loss.

Are There Any Side Effects?

The most common side effects experienced by individuals using chitosan are gastrointestinal distress and flatulence. Also, some product formulations contain ingredients such as caffeine, herbs, and other substances that may cause problems in some people.

CRITICAL THINKING QUESTIONS

1. A quick Internet search reveals that chitosan-containing products range widely in price from $5 to $40 or more for a one-month supply. Would you want to try this product to prevent weight gain? How much is a potential weight loss of less than a pound a week worth to you?
2. What would motivate you to try a weight-loss supplement you see on the drug store shelf or advertised on TV or the Internet? How would you research the product to determine if it was effective and safe?

chapter **review**

test yourself | answers

1. **True.** Although eating too much fat, or too much of unhealthful fats (such as saturated and *trans* fatty acids), can increase our risk for diseases such as cardiovascular disease and obesity, some fats are essential to good health. We need to consume a certain minimum amount to provide adequate levels of essential fatty acids and fat-soluble vitamins.

2. **True.** Fat is our primary source of energy when we are at rest and engaging in low- and moderate-intensity exercise. Fat is also an important fuel source during prolonged exercise. During periods of high-intensity exercise, carbohydrate becomes the dominant fuel source.

3. **False.** Even foods fried in vegetable shortening can be unhealthful because they are high in *trans* fatty acids, in total fat, and in energy and can contribute to overweight and obesity.

MasteringNutrition™

Check out these additional resources in the MasteringNutrition Study Area at www.masteringhealthandnutrition.pearson.com:

- Read It: Chapter Summary and RSS Feeds
- See It: ABC News videos and nutrition animations
- Hear It: MP3s
- Study It: Get Ready for Nutrition Math and Chemistry review
- Do It: NutriTools and "Find the Quack" feature
- Review It: Quizzes, flashcards, and glossary

review questions

1. Triglycerides with a double bond at one part of the molecule are referred to as
   a. monounsaturated fats.
   b. polyunsaturated fats.
   c. saturated fats.
   d. sterols.

2. Most plant oils contain
   a. only unsaturated fats.
   b. saturated and unsaturated fats.
   c. some EPA and DHA.
   d. small amounts of saturated fats and cholesterol.

3. Alpha-linolenic acid is
   a. converted by the body to linoleic acid.
   b. metabolized in the body to arachidonic acid.
   c. synthesized in the liver and small intestine.
   d. found in leafy green vegetables, flaxseeds, soy milk, walnuts, and almonds.

4. Fats
   a. do not provide as much energy, gram for gram, as carbohydrates.
   b. are a major source of fuel for the body at rest.
   c. enable the emulsification and digestion of fat-soluble vitamins.
   d. keep foods from turning rancid.

5. Fatty acids in chylomicrons are taken up by body cells with the help of
   a. lipoprotein lipase.
   b. micelles.
   c. bile salts.
   d. pancreatic lipase.

6. The DRI for EPA and DHA is
   a. about ten times higher than the DRI for ALA.
   b. 5–10% of total energy intake.
   c. 1.6 g per day for adult men and 1.1 g per day for adult women.
   d. none of the above.

7. Three healthful food sources of beneficial fats are
   a. skim milk, lean meats, and fruits.
   b. fruits, vegetables, and grains.
   c. vegetables, fish, and nuts.
   d. whole milk, egg whites, and stick margarine.

8. The risk for cardiovascular disease is increased in people who
   a. consume a diet high in saturated fats.
   b. consume a diet high in *trans* fats.
   c. consume a diet high in animal fats.
   d. all of the above.

9. **True or false?** Triglycerides are the same as fatty acids.

10. **True or false?** The Acceptable Macronutrient Distribution Range (AMDR) for fat is 20–35% of total energy.

math review

11. Getting adequate amounts of the omega-3 fatty acids can be tricky. Study Table 5.1. What food or combination of foods would you need to eat today to reach 250 mg of EPA and DHA?

12. Your friend Maria has determined that she needs to consume about 2,000 kcal per day to maintain her healthful weight. Create a chart for Maria showing the recommended maximum number of Calories she should consume in each of the following forms: unsaturated fat, saturated fat, linoleic acid, alpha-linolenic acid, and *trans* fatty acids.

Answers to Review Questions and Math Review are located at the back of this text, and in the MasteringNutrition Study Area.

web resources

www.americanheart.org
American Heart Association

Learn the best way to help lower your blood cholesterol level. Access the AHA's online cookbook for healthy-heart recipes and cooking methods.

www.caloriecontrol.org
Calorie Control Council

Go to this site to find out more about fat replacers.

www.nhlbi.nih.gov
National Heart, Lung, and Blood Institute

Learn how a healthful diet can lower your cholesterol levels. Use the online risk assessment tool to estimate your 10-year risk of having a heart attack.

www.nih.gov
The National Institutes of Health, U.S. Department of Health and Human Services

Search this site to learn more about dietary fats.

www.medlineplus.gov
MEDLINE Plus Health Information

Search for "fats" or "lipids" to obtain additional resources and the latest news on dietary lipids, cardiovascular disease, and cholesterol.

www.hsph.harvard.edu
The Nutrition Source: Knowledge for Healthy Eating
Harvard School of Public Health

Search under "nutrition source" on this site and click on "Fats & Cholesterol" to find out how selective fat intake can be part of a healthful diet.

www.ific.org
International Food Information Council Foundation

Access this site to learn more about fats and dietary fat replacers.

in depth

5.5

Cardiovascular Disease

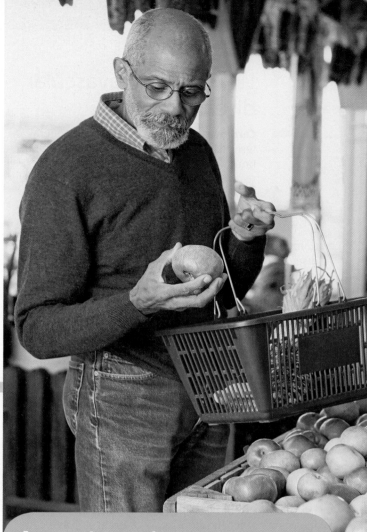

Only couch potatoes develop heart disease . . . or so we like to think. That's why the world was stunned in the summer of 2002 when Darryl Kile, a 33-year-old major league baseball pitcher for the St. Louis Cardinals, died of a heart attack in his Chicago hotel room the night before a scheduled game. An autopsy revealed a 90% blockage in two of Kile's coronary arteries—the vessels that supply blood to the heart. Although cardiovascular disease in an athlete is rare, Kile's family history revealed one very important risk factor: his father died of a heart attack at age 44.

What causes a heart attack? Are genetics always to blame? If you have a family history of cardiovascular disease, is there anything you can do to reduce your risk? We explore these questions **In Depth** here.

learning objectives

After studying this In Depth, you should be able to:

1 Identify four common forms of cariovascular disease, pp. 178–180.

2 Explain the role of atherosclerosis in the development of cardiovascular disease, p. 178.

3 Discuss the role of dietary fats in cardiovascular disease, pp. 181–184.

4 Specify several lifestyle choices that can reduce your risk for cardiovascular disease, pp. 184–188.

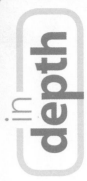

What is cardiovascular disease?

Cardiovascular disease (CVD) is a general term used to refer to any abnormal condition involving dysfunction of the heart (*cardio-* means "heart") and blood vessels (*vasculature*). There are many forms of this disease, but the most common are the following:

- *Coronary heart disease,* also known as *coronary artery disease,* occurs when blood vessels supplying the heart (the *coronary arteries*) become blocked or constricted; such blockage reduces the flow of blood—and the oxygen and nutrients it carries—to the heart muscle. This can result in chest pain, called *angina pectoris,* and lead to a heart attack.
- *Stroke* is caused by a blockage of one of the blood vessels supplying the brain (the *cerebral arteries*). When this occurs, the region of the brain that depends on that artery for oxygen and nutrients cannot function. As a result, the movement, speech, or other body functions controlled by that part of the brain suddenly stop.
- *Hypertension,* also called *high blood pressure,* is a condition that may not cause any symptoms, but it increases your risk for a heart attack or stroke. If your blood pressure is high, it means that the force of the blood flowing through your arteries is above normal.
- *Peripheral vascular disease* occurs when blood vessels in regions other than the heart or brain become constricted, causing a reduced blood flow to the periphery. It is especially common in the feet and legs, arms, stomach, or kidneys. Decreased blood flow to these areas can damage the tissues and organs.

To understand CVD, we need to look at a condition called *atherosclerosis,* which is responsible for the blockage of arteries underlying these four disorders.

Atherosclerosis Is Narrowing of Arteries

Atherosclerosis is a disease in which arterial walls accumulate deposits of lipids and scar tissue that build up to such a degree that they impair blood flow. It's a complex process that begins with injury to the cells that line the insides of all arteries **(FIGURE 1)**. Factors that commonly promote such injury are the forceful pounding of blood under high pressure and blood-vessel damage from irritants, such as the nicotine in tobacco, the excessive blood glucose in people with poorly controlled diabetes, increased levels of low-density lipoproteins (LDLs), which carry a high cholesterol load, or even chronic infection.

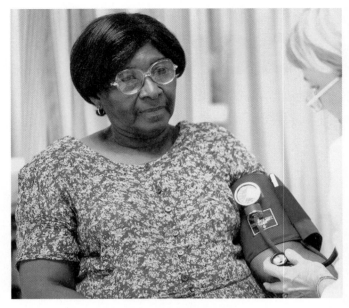

Hypertension is a major chronic disease in the United States, affecting more than 50% of adults over 65 years old.

Whatever the cause, the injury leads to vessel inflammation, which is increasingly being recognized as an important marker of CVD.[1] Inflamed lining cells release chemicals that cause blood lipids, mainly LDL cholesterol, to accumulate at the site. These lipids invade beneath the lining of the artery wall and become oxidized. As they do, they attract the attention of immune cells that move to the site, squeeze between the lining cells, and ingest the lipids beneath, becoming foam cells. Accumulated foam cells form *fatty streaks* that are the first visible sign of atherosclerosis.

Over time, these fat-filled cells, along with proteins, calcium, platelets (cell fragments found in blood), and other substances, form thick, grainy deposits called *plaque.* The term *atherosclerosis* reflects the presence of these deposits: *athere* is a Greek word meaning "a thick porridge." As plaques form, they narrow the interior of the blood vessel (see Figure 1). This slowly diminishes the blood supply to any tissues "downstream." As a result, these tissues—including heart muscle—wither, and gradually lose their ability to function. The person may experience angina, shortness of breath, and fatigue.

Alternatively, the blockage may occur suddenly; this happens when an enlarging plaque ruptures and the blood vessel tears. As a consequence, *platelets,* substances in blood that promote clotting, stick to the damaged area. This quickly obstructs the artery, causing the death of the

Knowing the warning signs of a heart attack could save your life. Download the wallet card from the National Institutes of Health at www.nhlbi.nih.gov; search on "public health" then "heart mi" and then "heart attack wallet card" to get going.

cardiovascular disease (CVD) A general term for abnormal conditions involving dysfunction of the heart and blood vessels, which can result in heart attack or stroke.

atherosclerosis A condition characterized by accumulation of cholesterol-rich plaque on artery walls; these deposits build up to such a degree that they impair blood flow.

FIGURE 1 | **Atherosclerosis**

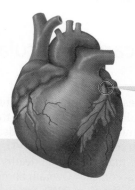

Plaque accumulation within coronary arteries narrows their interior and impedes the flow of oxygen-rich blood to the heart.

HEALTHY ARTERY

Blood flows unobstructed through normal, healthy artery.

ARTERIAL INJURY

The artery's lining is injured, attracting immune cells, and prompting inflammation.

LIPIDS ACCUMULATE IN WALL

Lipids, particulary cholesterol-containing LDLs, seep beneath the wall lining. The LDLs become oxidized. Immune cells, attracted to the site, engulf the oxidized LDLs and are transformed into foam cells.

FATTY STREAK

The foam cells accumulate to a form a fatty streak, which releases more toxic and inflammatory chemicals.

PLAQUE FORMATION

The foam cells, along with platelets, calcium, protein fibers, and other substances, form thick deposits of plaque, stiffening and narrowing the artery. Blood flow through the artery is reduced or obstructed.

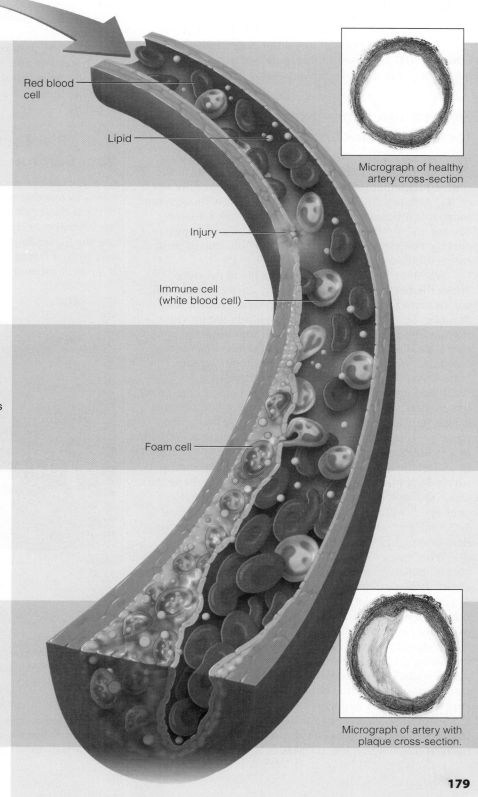

Red blood cell

Lipid

Injury

Immune cell (white blood cell)

Foam cell

Micrograph of healthy artery cross-section

Micrograph of artery with plaque cross-section.

tissue it supplies. As a result, the person experiences a heart attack or stroke.

Arteries damaged by atherosclerosis become not only narrow, but also stiff; that is, they lose their ability to stretch and spring back with each heartbeat. This characteristic is often referred to as "hardening of the arteries." As you can imagine, atherosclerosis strains the heart, because it is forced to exert increased pressure to eject each burst of blood into narrowed, stiffened vessels. Physicians refer to this increased pressure as *systolic hypertension*, as we explain next.

Hypertension Increases the Risk for Heart Attack and Stroke

Hypertension is one of the major chronic diseases in the United States. It affects over 29% of all adults in the United States and more than 67% of people over the age of 60.[2] Although hypertension itself is often without symptoms, it is a warning sign that a person's risk for heart disease and stroke is increased. Hypertension can also damage the kidneys, reduce brain function, impair physical mobility, and cause death.

When we define hypertension as blood pressure above the normal range, what exactly do we mean? Well, we measure blood pressure in two phases, systolic and diastolic. *Systolic blood pressure* represents the pressure exerted in our arteries at the moment that the heart contracts, sending blood into our blood vessels. *Diastolic blood pressure* represents the pressure in our arteries between contractions, when our heart is relaxed.

Blood pressure measurements are recorded in millimeters of mercury (mmHg). Optimal systolic blood pressure is *less than* 120 mmHg, whereas optimal diastolic blood pressure is *less than* 80 mmHg. *Prehypertension* is defined as a systolic blood pressure between 120 and 139 mmHg, or a diastolic blood pressure between 80 and 89 mmHg. About 28% of adults in the United States are prehypertensive.[2] You would be diagnosed with true hypertension if your systolic blood pressure were greater than or equal to 140 mmHg or your diastolic blood pressure were greater than or equal to 90 mmHg.

What causes hypertension? For about 45–55% of people, hypertension is hereditary. This type is referred to as *primary* or *essential hypertension*. For the other 45% of people with hypertension, a variety of factors may contribute. In addition to underlying atherosclerosis, as just explained, anything that increases the volume or viscosity (thickness) of blood forces the heart to beat harder, increasing the pressure of the ejected blood against the vessel walls. Because salt draws water, high blood sodium can increase the volume of blood and, thus, blood pressure. Other factors implicated in hypertension include kidney disease, sleep apnea (a sleep disorder that affects breathing), certain medications, psychosocial stressors, tobacco use, obesity, low physical activity, excessive alcohol intake, and dietary factors, including sensitivity to salt and low potassium intake.[3]

Who is at risk for cardiovascular disease?

According to the Centers for Disease Control and Prevention, coronary heart disease is the leading cause of death in the United States, and stroke is the third leading cause of death.[4] Hypertension contributes to both of these types of CVD, which together account for more than 35% of all deaths annually, or one death every 38 seconds.[3,5] Overall, about 80 million Americans of all ages suffer from CVD. So—who's at risk?

Many Risk Factors Are Within Your Control

Over the last two decades, researchers have identified a number of factors that contribute to an increased risk for CVD. Some of these risk factors are nonmodifiable, meaning they are beyond your control. These include age—the older you are, the higher your risk—male gender, and family history. Like pitcher Darryl Kile, you have an increased risk for CVD if a parent suffered a heart attack, especially at a young age.

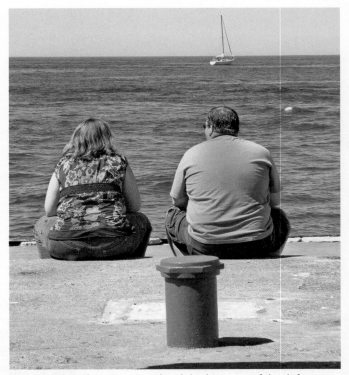

Being overweight is associated with higher rates of death from cardiovascular disease.

hypertension A chronic condition characterized by above-average blood pressure levels—specifically, systolic blood pressure over 140 mmHg, or diastolic blood pressure over 90 mmHg.

Other risk factors are modifiable—meaning they are at least partly within your control. Following is a brief description of each of these modifiable risk factors. Notice that many of them have a dietary component.[6, 7, 8]

Overweight   Being overweight is associated with CVD and higher rates of death from CVD. The risk is due primarily to a greater occurrence of high blood pressure, inflammation, abnormal blood lipids (discussed in more detail shortly), and higher rates of type 2 diabetes in people who are overweight. In general, an overweight condition develops from an energy imbalance from eating too much and exercising too little (see Chapter 11) for more details).

Physical Inactivity   A sedentary lifestyle increases the risk of CVD. On the other hand, numerous research studies have shown that regular physical activity can reduce your risk by improving several risk factors associated with the disease, including improved blood lipid levels, lower resting blood pressure, lower body fat and weight, and improved blood glucose levels both at rest and after eating. Physical activity can also significantly reduce the risk for type 2 diabetes, a major CVD risk factor in itself.[8] According to the 2008 U.S. Physical Activity Guidelines,[9] physical activity can reduce your risk for heart disease by 20–30%, stroke by 25–30%, and type 2 diabetes by 25–35%.

Smoking   There is strong evidence that smoking increases your risk for blood-vessel injury and atherosclerosis. Research indicates that smokers have a two- to sixfold greater chance of developing CVD than nonsmokers, depending on age and gender.[10] If you smoke, quitting is one of the best ways to reduce your risk for CVD. People who stop smoking live longer than those who continue to smoke, and smokers who quit by age 30 reduce their chances of dying from a smoking-related disease by more than 90%[11].

Type 2 Diabetes Mellitus   For many people with type 2 diabetes, the condition is directly related to being overweight or obese, which is also associated with abnormal blood lipids and high blood pressure. The risk for CVD is three times higher in women with diabetes and two times higher in men with diabetes compared to individuals without diabetes.

Inflammation   We noted earlier that when injury occurs in a blood vessel, the resulting inflammatory

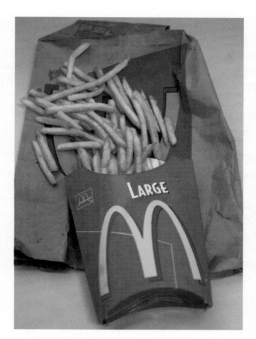

Because foods fried in hydrogenated vegetable oils, such as french fries, are high in *trans* fatty acids, these types of foods should be limited in our diet.

response eventually leads to the deposition of plaque in the vessel wall. Plaque buildup increases the risk for a heart attack or stroke. C-reactive protein (CRP) is a nonspecific marker of inflammation somewhere in the body. Its level can be measured with a simple blood test. Risk for CVD appears to be higher in individuals who have an elevated CRP level in addition to other risk factors, such as high blood lipids.[12] Thus, reducing the factors that promote inflammation, such as obesity and a diet low in omega-3 fatty acids and high in saturated fats, can lower your risk for CVD.

Abnormal Blood Lipids   As we explain next, abnormal levels of cholesterol and triglycerides in the blood are associated with an increased risk for CVD. Making lifestyle changes, such as lowering your intake of saturated and *trans* fat, increasing your physical activity and soluble fiber intake, and achieving a healthful body weight, can help improve your blood lipid profile.

The Role of Blood Lipids in Cardiovascular Disease

Recall that lipids are transported in the blood by lipoproteins made up of a lipid center and a protein outer coat. The names of lipoproteins reflect their proportion of lipid, which is less dense, to protein, which is very dense. For example, very-low-density lipoproteins (VLDLs) are only 10% protein, whereas high-density lipoproteins (HDLs) are 50% protein (**FIGURE 2** on page 182). Because lipoproteins are soluble in blood, they are commonly called *blood lipids*.

Research indicates that high intakes of saturated and *trans* fatty acids increase the blood's level of those lipids associated with CVD—namely, total blood cholesterol and the cholesterol found in VLDLs and low-density lipoproteins (LDLs). Conversely, omega-3 fatty acids decrease our CVD risk in a number of ways, such as by opposing inflammation, reducing blood triglycerides, and increasing HDLs, which protect the health of blood vessels.[13,14] Let's look at each of these blood lipids in more detail to determine how they are linked to your risk for cardiovascular disease (**FIGURE 3** on page 183).

Use this online risk assessment tool to estimate your 10-year risk of having a heart attack: www.hp2010.nhlbihin.net; serach on "atpii" and then "calculator" to find the estimator tool.

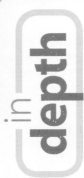

Chylomicrons

Only after consuming a meal does your blood contain chylomicrons, which we learned (in Chapter 5) are produced in the small intestine to transport dietary fat into the lymphatic vessels and from there into the bloodstream. At 85% triglyceride, chylomicrons have the lowest density.

Very-Low-Density Lipoproteins

More than half of the substance of **very-low-density lipoproteins (VLDLs)** is triglyceride. The liver is the primary source of VLDLs, but they are also produced in the intestines. VLDLs are primarily transport vehicles ferrying triglycerides from their source to the body's cells, including to adipose tissues for storage. The enzyme lipoprotein lipase (LPL) frees most of the triglyceride

from the VLDL molecules, resulting in its uptake by the body's cells.

Diets high in fat, simple sugars, and extra Calories can increase the production of endogenous VLDLs, whereas diets high in omega-3 fatty acids can help reduce their production. In addition, exercise can reduce VLDLs because the fat produced in the body is quickly used for energy instead of remaining to circulate in the blood.

Low-Density Lipoproteins

The molecules resulting when VLDLs release their triglyceride load are much higher in cholesterol, phospholipids,

---

very-low-density lipoprotein (VLDL) A lipoprotein made in the liver and intestine that functions to transport lipids, especially triglycerides, to the tissues of the body.

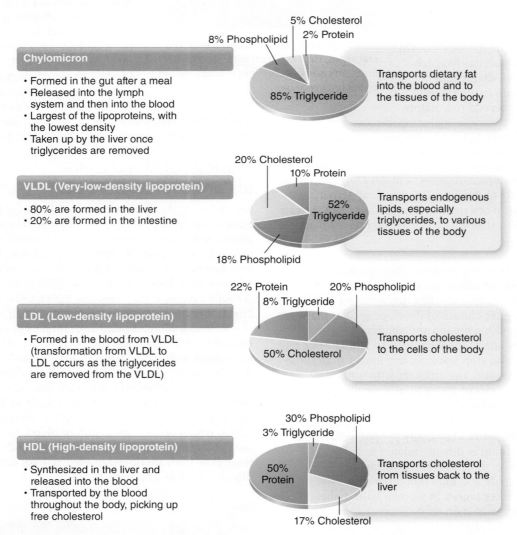

Chylomicron
- Formed in the gut after a meal
- Released into the lymph system and then into the blood
- Largest of the lipoproteins, with the lowest density
- Taken up by the liver once triglycerides are removed

8% Phospholipid · 5% Cholesterol · 2% Protein · 85% Triglyceride

Transports dietary fat into the blood and to the tissues of the body

VLDL (Very-low-density lipoprotein)
- 80% are formed in the liver
- 20% are formed in the intestine

20% Cholesterol · 10% Protein · 52% Triglyceride · 18% Phospholipid

Transports endogenous lipids, especially triglycerides, to various tissues of the body

LDL (Low-density lipoprotein)
- Formed in the blood from VLDL (transformation from VLDL to LDL occurs as the triglycerides are removed from the VLDL)

22% Protein · 20% Phospholipid · 8% Triglyceride · 50% Cholesterol

Transports cholesterol to the cells of the body

HDL (High-density lipoprotein)
- Synthesized in the liver and released into the blood
- Transported by the blood throughout the body, picking up free cholesterol

30% Phospholipid · 3% Triglyceride · 50% Protein · 17% Cholesterol

Transports cholesterol from tissues back to the liver

FIGURE 2 The chemical components of various lipoproteins. Notice that chylomicrons contain the highest proportion of triglycerides, making them the least dense, whereas high-density lipoproteins (HDLs) have the highest proportion of protein, making them the most dense.

FIGURE 3 | Lipoprotein Transport and Distribution

Lipids are transported in the body via several different lipoprotein compounds, such as chylomicrons, VLDLs, LDLs, and HDLs.

CHYLOMICRONS

Chylomicrons are produced in the enterocytes to transport dietary lipids. The enzyme lipoprotein lipase (LPL), found on the endothelial cells in the capillaries, hydrolyzes the triglycerides in the chylomicrons into fatty acids and glycerol, which enter body cells (such as muscle and adipose cells), leaving a chylomicron remnant. Chylomicron remnants are dismantled in the liver.

VLDLS

VLDLs (very-low-density lipoproteins) are produced primarily in the liver to transport endogenous fat in the form of triglycerides into the bloodstream. The enzyme lipoprotein lipase (LPL) found on the endothelial cells in the capillaries, breaks apart the triglycerides in the chylomicrons. The fatty acids can then enter the body cells, especially the muscle and adipose cells, leaving a chylomicron remnant. Glycerol is also released and is transported back to the liver.

LDLS

LDLs (low-density lipoproteins) are created with the removal of most of the VLDLs' triglyceride load. LDLs are rich in cholesterol, which they deliver to body cells with LDL receptors. LDLs not taken up by the cells are primarily taken up by the liver for degradation.

HDLS

HDLs (high-density lipoproteins) are produced in the liver and circulate in the blood, picking up cholesterol from dying cells, other lipoproteins, and arterial plaques. They return this cholesterol to the liver, where it can be recycled or eliminated from the body through bile.

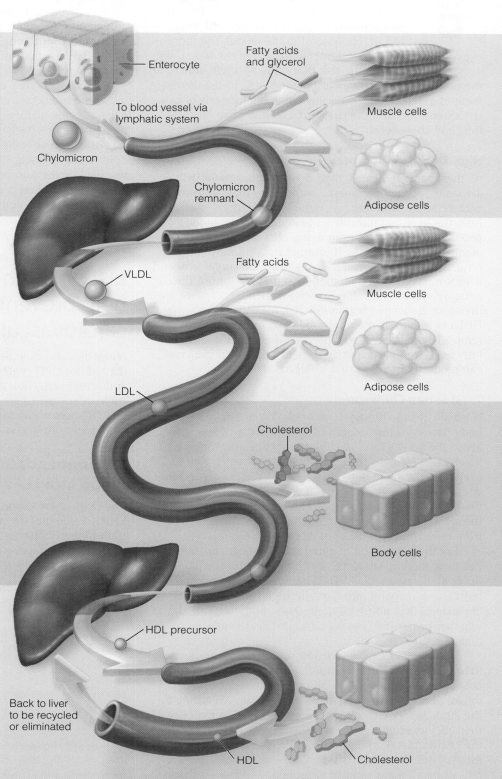

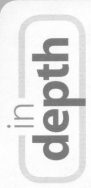

and protein and therefore somewhat more dense. These **low-density lipoproteins (LDLs)** circulate in the blood, delivering their cholesterol to cells. Diets high in saturated fat *decrease* the removal of LDLs by body cells.

What happens to LDLs not taken up by body cells? Failure to remove LDLs from the bloodstream results in an increased level of LDL-cholesterol in the blood. The more LDL-cholesterol circulating in the blood, the greater the risk that some of it will adhere to the walls of the blood vessels, contributing to the development of atherosclerosis. Because high blood levels of LDL-cholesterol increase the risk for CVD, it is often labeled the "bad cholesterol."

High-Density Lipoproteins

As their name indicates, **high-density lipoproteins (HDLs)** are small, dense lipoproteins with a very low cholesterol content and a high protein content. They are released from the liver and intestines to circulate in the blood, picking up cholesterol from dying cells and arterial plaques and transferring it to other lipoproteins, which return it to the liver. The liver takes up the cholesterol and uses it to synthesize bile, thereby removing it from the circulatory system. High blood levels of HDL-cholesterol are therefore associated with a low risk for CVD. That's why HDL-cholesterol is often referred to as the "good cholesterol." There is some evidence that diets high in omega-3 fatty acids and participation in regular physical exercise can modestly increase HDL-cholesterol levels.[15]

Total Serum Cholesterol

Normally, as the dietary level of cholesterol increases, the body decreases the amount of cholesterol it makes, which keeps the body's level of cholesterol constant. Unfortunately, this feedback mechanism does not work well in everyone. For some individuals, eating dietary cholesterol doesn't decrease the amount of cholesterol produced in the body, and their total body cholesterol level—including the level in their blood—rises. These individuals benefit from reducing their intake of dietary cholesterol.

For the population in general, researchers are still debating the impact of dietary cholesterol on the blood lipids associated with CVD. What we do know is that individuals respond differently to high levels of dietary cholesterol depending on their genes, body weight, and whether or not they have a chronic disease such as diabetes.[16]

Both dietary cholesterol and saturated fats are found in animal foods; thus, by limiting intake of animal products or selecting low-fat versions, people reduce their intake of both saturated fat and cholesterol. According to the 2010 Dietary Guidelines, Americans get the majority of their dietary cholesterol from eggs, chicken, beef (including beef burgers), and mixed dishes containing these foods. Thus, selecting fish, poultry without skin, lean cuts of meat, plant sources of protein, and low-fat dairy products, and consuming eggs in moderation can dramatically reduce the amount of cholesterol in the diet.

Calculating Your Risk for Cardiovascular Disease

Now that you know more about blood lipids, you're probably wondering what your levels look like. If so, check out the **What About You?** feature (page 186). It explains the simple lab test that can show you how your own blood lipids measure up.

To estimate your overall risk of developing CVD, you also need to know your blood pressure. Especially if you have a family history of CVD, it's important to have your blood pressure checked regularly.

After you've found out your blood pressure and blood lipid levels, the next step in assessing your CVD risk is to calculate the number of points for each risk factor in **FIGURE 4**, and then compare your total points to the points in the 10-year risk column. There is also an online version of this risk calculator. See Web Resources at the end of this chapter.

Lifestyle choices can help prevent or control cardiovascular disease

Many diet and exercise interventions aimed at reducing the risk for CVD center on reducing high levels of triglycerides and LDL-cholesterol while raising HDL-cholesterol. Approaches aimed specifically at reducing blood pressure include most of the same recommendations, along with strict monitoring of sodium intake.

Recommendations to Improve Blood Lipid Levels

The Centers for Disease Control and Prevention[17] and the Expert Panel on Detection, Evaluation, and Treatment of High Blood Cholesterol in Adults[18] have made the following recommendations to improve blood lipid levels and reduce the risk for CVD.[5,18,19,20,21,22]

■ Maintain total fat intake to within 20–35% of energy.[19] Polyunsaturated fats (for example, soy and canola oil) can comprise up to 10% of total energy intake, whereas monounsaturated fats (for example, olive oil) can

low-density lipoprotein (LDL) A lipoprotein formed in the blood from VLDLs that transports cholesterol to the cells of the body; often called "bad cholesterol."

high-density lipoprotein (HDL) A lipoprotein made in the liver and released into the blood. HDLs function to transport cholesterol from the tissues back to the liver; often called "good cholesterol."

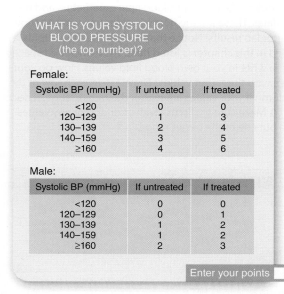
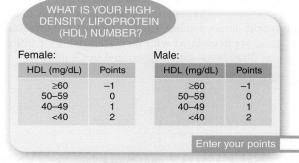

WHAT IS YOUR AGE?

Female:

Age	Points
20–34	–7
35–39	–3
40–44	0
45–49	3
50–54	6
55–59	8
60–64	10
65–69	12
70–74	14
75–79	16

Male:

Age	Points
20–34	–9
35–39	–4
40–44	0
45–49	3
50–54	6
55–59	8
60–64	10
65–69	11
70–74	12
75–79	13

Enter your points ▢

DO YOU SMOKE?

Nonsmoker, Female:

Age	Points
20–39	0
40–49	0
50–59	0
60–69	0
70–79	0

Nonsmoker, Male:

Age	Points
20–39	0
40–49	0
50–59	0
60–69	0
70–79	0

Smoker, Female:

Age	Points
20–39	9
40–49	7
50–59	4
60–69	2
70–79	1

Smoker, Male:

Age	Points
20–39	8
40–49	5
50–59	3
60–69	1
70–79	1

Enter your points ▢

WHAT IS YOUR SYSTOLIC BLOOD PRESSURE (the top number)?

Female:

Systolic BP (mmHg)	If untreated	If treated
<120	0	0
120–129	1	3
130–139	2	4
140–159	3	5
≥160	4	6

Male:

Systolic BP (mmHg)	If untreated	If treated
<120	0	0
120–129	0	1
130–139	1	2
140–159	1	2
≥160	2	3

Enter your points ▢

WHAT IS YOUR TOTAL CHOLESTEROL NUMBER?

Female:

Age	\<160	160–199	200–239	240–279	≥280	
			Total Cholesterol			
20–39	0	4	8	11	13	
40–49	0	3	6	8	10	Points
50–59	0	2	4	5	7	
60–69	0	1	2	3	4	
70–79	0	1	1	2	2	

Male:

Age	\<160	160–199	200–239	240–279	≥280	
			Total Cholesterol			
20–39	0	4	7	9	11	
40–49	0	3	5	6	8	Points
50–59	0	2	3	4	5	
60–69	0	1	1	2	3	
70–79	0	0	0	1	1	

Enter your points ▢

WHAT IS YOUR HIGH-DENSITY LIPOPROTEIN (HDL) NUMBER?

Female:

HDL (mg/dL)	Points
≥60	–1
50–59	0
40–49	1
<40	2

Male:

HDL (mg/dL)	Points
≥60	–1
50–59	0
40–49	1
<40	2

Enter your points ▢

WHAT IS YOUR TOTAL NUMBER OF POINTS (what is your 10-year risk)?

Female:

Point total	10-Year risk %
<9	<1
9	1
10	1
11	1
12	1
13	2
14	2
15	3
16	4
17	5
18	6
19	8
20	11
21	14
22	17
23	22
24	27
≥25	≥30

Male:

Point total	10-Year risk %
<0	<1
0	1
1	1
2	1
3	1
4	1
5	2
6	2
7	3
8	4
9	5
10	6
11	8
12	10
13	12
14	16
15	20
16	25
≥17	≥30

Enter your 10-year risk percentage ▢

FIGURE 4 Calculation matrix to estimate the 10-year risk for cardiovascular disease for men and women.

Data from: The National Institutes of Health, *Third Report of the National Cholesterol Education Program: Detection, Evaluation and Treatment of High Blood Cholesterol in Adults (ATP: III).* Bethesda, MD: National Cholesterol Education Program, National Heart, Lung, and Blood Institute, NIH, May 2001.

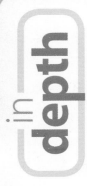

comprise up to 20% of total energy intake. For some people, a lower-fat intake may help them maintain a healthful body weight.

- Decrease dietary saturated fat to less than 7% of total energy intake. Decrease cholesterol intake to less than 300 mg per day, and keep *trans* fatty acid intake as low as possible (less than 1% of energy). Lowering the intakes of these fats will lower your LDL-cholesterol level. Replace saturated fat (for example, butter, margarine, vegetable shortening, or lard) with more healthful cooking oils, such as olive or canola oil. Select lean meats and meat alternatives and use fat-free or low-fat milk or soymilk.

- Increase intake of the omega-3 fatty acid ALA from dark green, leafy vegetables, soybeans or soybean oil, walnuts or walnut oil, flaxseed meal or oil, or canola oil. Also, consume fish, especially oily fish, at least twice a week to increase your intake of the omega-3 fatty acids EPA and DHA.

- Consume 400 μg/day of folate from dietary or supplemental sources to help maintain low blood levels of the amino acid homocysteine. High homocysteine levels in the blood are associated with increased risk for cardiovascular disease. (Folate is discussed in Chapter 10.)

- Increase dietary intakes of whole grains, fruits, and vegetables, so that total dietary fiber is 20 to 30 g per day with 10 to 25 g per day coming from fiber sources such as oat bran, beans, and fruits. Approximately 5–10 g/day of this type of fiber will reduce LDL-cholesterol by 5–10%. [18,23]

- Maintain blood glucose within normal ranges. High blood glucose levels are associated with high blood triglycerides. Dietary changes can help here as well: Consume foods whole (such as whole-wheat breads and cereals, whole fruits and vegetables, and beans and legumes), and select lean meats and low-fat dairy products, while limiting your intake of foods high in sugar and fat (for example, cookies, high-sugar drinks and snacks, candy, fried foods, and convenience and fast foods).

- Eat meals throughout the day instead of eating most of your Calories in the evening before bed. This approach decreases the load of fat entering the body at any one time. Exercising after a meal also helps keep blood lipids and glucose within normal ranges.

- Consume no more than two alcoholic drinks per day for men and one drink per day for women. Because heavy alcohol consumption can worsen high blood pressure, it is suggested that people with diagnosed hypertension abstain from drinking alcohol entirely. (Alcohol consumption is discussed **In Depth** following Chapter 7.)

what about **you**

Blood Lipid Levels: How Do Yours Measure Up?

One of the most important steps you can take to reduce your risk for CVD is to know your "numbers"—that is, your blood lipid values. The next time you go to a physician, ask to have your blood lipid levels measured. Record these numbers and have them checked every 1 to 2 years, or each time you visit your physician for a checkup. Many college and university health clinics, as well as community health fairs, offer a screening for total cholesterol as well. Based on your total cholesterol values, you can go to your physician to have a more complete testing of all your blood lipids. In this way,

you can know your own blood lipid levels and keep track of your CVD risk.

Let's look at the different blood lipid parameters and the target values. These are the normal values you want to show up on your lab results! Notice that each of the blood lipids discussed in this chapter is listed here. We've included space for you to write in your own blood lipid values. How do yours compare with the target values? Draw a ☺ in each row of the final column if your values are within the target range. If not, draw a ☹. Make sure to discuss with your doctor any values that are outside of the target range.

Blood Lipid Profile: Compare Your Values

Blood Lipid Parameter	Target Values*	Your Values	How Are You Doing? ☺/☹
Total blood cholesterol	<200 mg/dL	_____ mg/dL	
HDL-cholesterol	>40 mg/dL	_____ mg/dL	
LDL-cholesterol	<100 mg/dL	_____ mg/dL	
Triglycerides	<150 mg/dL	_____ mg/dL	

*Data from: The National Institutes of Health, *Third Report of the National Cholesterol Education Program: Detection, Evaluation and Treatment of High Blood Cholesterol in Adults (ATP: III)*. Bethesda, MD. National Cholesterol Education Program, National Heart, Lung, and Blood Institute, NIH, May 2001.

- If you smoke, stop. As noted earlier, smoking significantly increases the risk for CVD.
- Maintain an active lifestyle. Exercise most days of the week for 30 to 60 minutes if possible. Exercise will increase HDL-cholesterol while lowering blood triglyceride levels. Exercise also helps you maintain a healthful body weight and a lower blood pressure and reduces your risk for type 2 diabetes.
- Maintain a healthful body weight by balancing energy intake with physical activity. Blood lipids and glucose levels typically improve when overweight or obese individuals lose weight and engage in regular physical activity. Obesity promotes inflammation; thus, keeping body weight within a healthful range helps keep inflammation low.[24] In addition, blood pressure values have been shown to decrease three to four points in people who have lost several pounds of body weight.[25]

Recommendations to Reduce Blood Pressure

Again, hypertension is both a form of CVD and a risk factor in the development of atherosclerosis. Therefore, the lifestyle changes just identified are appropriate for anyone diagnosed with hypertension or prehypertension. In addition, recommendations for reducing blood pressure include limiting dietary sodium intake and following the DASH diet.

Limit Dietary Sodium

To help keep blood pressure normal, it is recommended that we reduce our intake of sodium. However, this recommendation is not without controversy.

For years it was believed that the high sodium intakes of the typical American diet led to hypertension. This is because people who live in countries where sodium intake is high have greater rates of hypertension than people from countries where sodium intake is low. We have recently learned, however, that not everyone with hypertension is sensitive to sodium. Unfortunately, it is impossible to know who is sensitive and who is not because there is no ready test for sodium sensitivity. Moreover, lowering sodium intake does not reduce blood pressure in all people with hypertension. Thus, there is significant debate over whether everyone can benefit from eating a lower-sodium diet.

Despite this debate, the leading health organizations, including the American Heart Association, the National

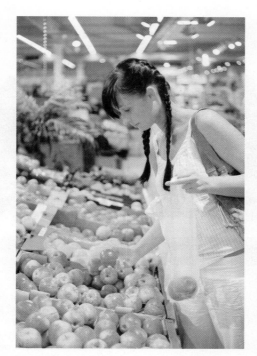

Consuming whole fruits and vegetables can reduce your risk for cardiovascular disease.

High Blood Pressure Education Program, and the National Heart, Lung, and Blood Institute of the National Institutes of Health (NIH), continue to support a reduction in dietary sodium to less than 2,300 mg/day, as recommended in the Dietary Guidelines for Americans.[26] Currently, the average sodium intake in the United States is about 3,300 mg/day.

Follow the DASH Diet

The impact of diet on reducing the risk for cardiovascular disease—including hypertension—was clearly demonstrated in a study from the NIH called Dietary Approaches to Stop Hypertension (DASH). The **DASH diet** is an eating plan that is high in several minerals that have been shown to help reduce hypertension, including calcium, magnesium, and potassium. At the same time, it is moderately low in sodium, low in saturated fat, and high in fiber, and it includes 10 servings of fruits and vegetables each day. **FIGURE 5** shows the DASH eating plan for a 2,000-kcal diet.

The results of the NIH study showed that eating the DASH diet can dramatically improve blood lipids and lower blood pressure.[25,27] For the study participants overall, systolic blood pressure decreased by an average of 5.5 mmHg, and diastolic blood pressure decreased by an average of 3.0 mmHg. For the study participants who had high blood pressure, systolic blood pressure dropped an average of 11.4 mmHg, and diastolic blood pressure dropped by an average of 5.5 mmHg. These decreases occurred within the first 2 weeks of eating the DASH diet and were maintained throughout the duration of the study. Researchers estimated that if all Americans followed the DASH diet plan and experienced reductions in blood pressure similar to this study, then coronary heart disease would be reduced by 15% and the number of strokes would be 27% lower.

Further study of the DASH diet has found that blood pressure decreases even more as sodium intake is reduced below 3,000 mg per day. In the subsequent study, participants ate a DASH diet that provided 3,300 mg (average U.S. intake), 2,300 mg (upper recommended intake), or 1,500 mg of sodium each day.[27] After 1 month on this diet, all people eating the DASH diet saw

---

DASH diet The diet developed in response to research into hypertension funded by the National Institutes of Health; DASH stands for "Dietary Approaches to Stop Hypertension."

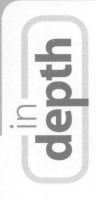

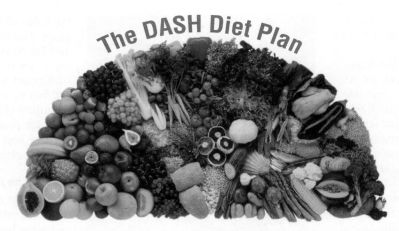

The DASH Diet Plan

Food Group	Daily Servings	Serving Size
Grains and grain products	7–8	1 slice bread 1 cup ready-to-eat cereal* ½ cup cooked rice, pasta, or cereal
Vegetables	4–5	1 cup raw leafy vegetables ½ cup cooked vegetable 6 fl. oz vegetable juice
Fruits	4–5	1 medium fruit ¼ cup dried fruit ½ cup fresh, frozen, or canned fruit 6 fl. oz fruit juice
Low-fat or fat-free dairy foods	2–3	8 fl. oz milk 1 cup yogurt 1½ oz cheese
Lean meats, poultry, and fish	2 or less	3 oz cooked lean meats, skinless poultry, or fish
Nuts, seeds, and dry beans	4–5 per week	⅓ cup or 1½ oz nuts 1 tbsp. or ½ oz seeds ½ cup cooked dry beans
Fats and oils†	2–3	1 tsp. soft margarine 1 tbsp. low-fat mayonnaise 2 tbsp. light salad dressing 1 tsp. vegetable oil
Sweets	5 per week	1 tbsp. sugar 1 tbsp. jelly or jam ½ oz jelly beans 8 fl. oz lemonade

*Serving sizes vary between ½ and 1¼ cups. Check the product's nutrition label.

†Fat content changes serving counts for fats and oils: for example, 1 tablespoon of regular salad dressing equals 1 serving; 1 tablespoon of a low-fat dressing equals ½ serving; 1 tablespoon of a fat-free dressing equals 0 servings.

FIGURE 5 **The DASH diet plan.** The plan is based on a 2,000 kcal/day diet. The number of servings in a food group may differ from the number listed here, depending on your individual energy needs.

Note: The plan is based on 2,000-kcal/day. The number of servings in a food group may differ from the number listed, depending on your own energy needs.
Data adapted from: Healthier Eating with DASH. The National Institutes of Health.

a significant decrease in their blood pressure; however, those who ate the lowest-sodium version of the DASH diet experienced the largest decrease. These results indicate that eating a diet low in sodium and high in fruits and vegetables reduces blood pressure and decreases your risk for heart attack and stroke.

> To download a free brochure describing the DASH diet plan, visit www.nhlbi .nih.gov, and search on "new dash pdf".

nutri-case | GUSTAVO

"Sometimes I wonder where doctors get their funny ideas. Yesterday I had my yearly checkup and my doctor says, 'You're doing great! Your weight is fine, your blood sugar's good. The only thing that concerns me is that your blood pressure is a little high, so I want you to watch your diet. Cut back on the red meats and eat fish instead. When you do eat red meat, trim off the fat. Use one of the new heart-healthy margarines instead of butter, and use olive oil instead of lard. And when you have eggs, don't eat the yolks.' I know he means well, but my wife's finally able to move around again after breaking her hip. How am I supposed to tell her she has to learn a whole new way to cook now?"

Do you think that Gustavo's objection to his doctor's advice is valid? Why or why not? Identify at least two alternatives or resources that might help Gustavo and his wife.

Prescription Medications Can Improve Blood Lipids and Blood Pressure

For some individuals, lifestyle changes are not completely effective in normalizing blood lipids and blood pressure. When this is the case, a variety of medications can be prescribed. Some inhibit the body's production of cholesterol. Others prevent the reabsorption of bile in the gastrointestinal (GI) tract. Because bile is made from cholesterol, blocking its reabsorption means the liver must draw on cholesterol stores to make more. Diuretics may be prescribed to flush excess water and sodium from the body, reducing blood volume and thus blood pressure. Other hypertension medications work to relax the blood vessel walls, allowing more room for blood flow. People taking such medications should also continue to practice the lifestyle changes listed earlier in this section because these changes will continue to benefit their long-term health.

MasteringNutrition™

Check out these additional resources in the MasteringNutrition Study Area:

- Read It: Chapter Summary and RSS Feeds
- See It: ABC News videos and nutrition animations
- Hear It: MP3s
- Study It: Get Ready for Nutrition Math and Chemistry review
- Do It: NutriTools and "Find the Quack" feature
- Review It: Quizzes, flashcards, and glossary

web resources

www.heart.org
American Heart Association

Learn the best way to help lower your blood cholesterol level. Access the AHA's online cookbook for healthy-heart recipes and cooking methods by searching on HEARTORG.

www.nhlbi.nih.gov
National Cholesterol Education Program

Search on "chd" for information on how to control your cholesterol.

www.nhlbi.nih.gov
National Heart, Lung, and Blood Institute

This site has news and information on a wide range of topics related to your heart health.

www.medlineplus.gov
MEDLINE Plus Health Information

Access this site to find the latest news on dietary lipids and cardiovascular disease.

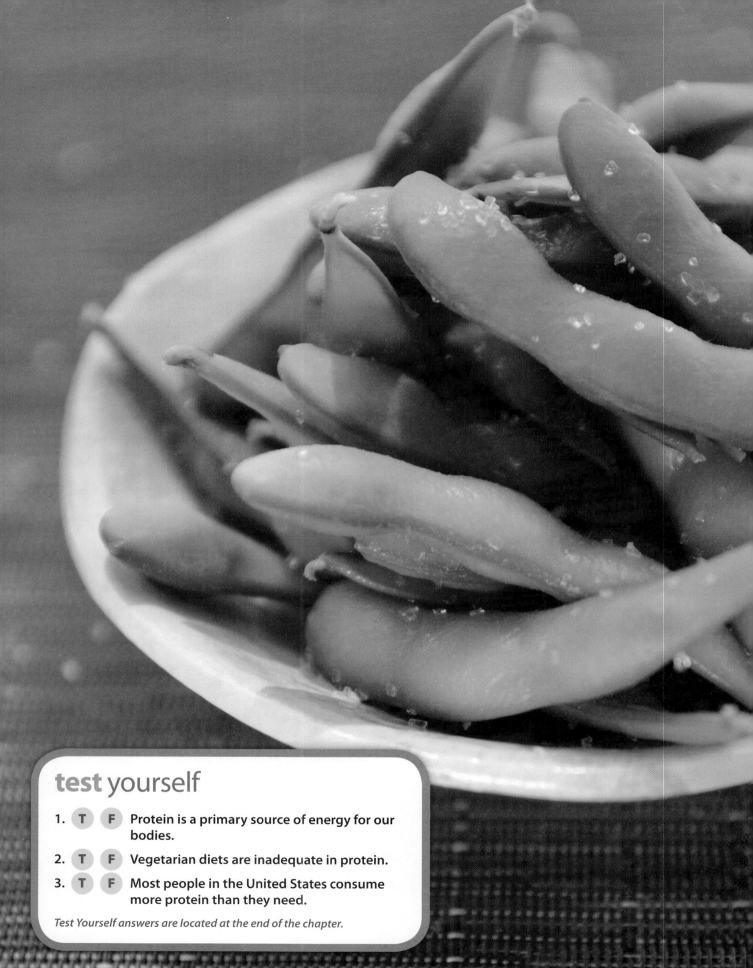

test yourself

1. **T** **F** Protein is a primary source of energy for our bodies.

2. **T** **F** Vegetarian diets are inadequate in protein.

3. **T** **F** Most people in the United States consume more protein than they need.

Test Yourself answers are located at the end of the chapter.

Proteins

Crucial components of all body tissues

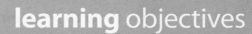

6

What do professional skateboarder Forrest Kirby, tennis pro Venus Williams, fitness guru Bob Harper, and hundreds of other athletes have in common?
They're all vegetarians! Boxing champ Mike Tyson says that his vegetarian diet "feels awesome . . . I wish I was born this way!"[1] Although statistics on the number of vegetarian athletes aren't available, in a 2012 poll nationwide, 4% of all U.S. adults reported that they are vegetarian (never eat meat, poultry, or fish), and another 14% said that more than half of their meals are vegetarian.[2]

What are proteins, and what makes them so different from carbohydrates or fats? How much protein do you really need, and do you get enough in your daily diet? What exactly is a vegetarian, anyway? Do you qualify? If so, how do you plan your diet to include sufficient protein, especially if you play competitive sports? Are there real advantages to eating meat, or is plant protein just as good?

It seems as if everybody has an opinion about protein, both how much you should consume and from what sources. In this chapter, we address these and other questions to clarify the importance of protein in the diet and dispel common myths about this crucial nutrient.

learning objectives

After studying this chapter you should be able to:

1 Describe how proteins differ from carbohydrates and fats, p. 192.

2 Describe the processes by which DNA directs protein synthesis and proteins organize into levels of structure, pp. 194–198.

3 Explain the significance of mutual supplementation and identify non-meat food combinations that are complete protein sources, pp. 199–200.

4 Describe four functions of proteins in our bodies, pp. 200–203.

5 Explain how proteins are digested, absorbed, and synthesized by our bodies, pp. 203–206.

6 Calculate your recommended daily allowance for protein, pp. 207–209, 212.

7 List the benefits and potential challenges of consuming a vegetarian diet, pp. 214–218.

8 Describe two disorders related to inadequate protein intake, pp. 218–220.

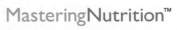

MasteringNutrition™
Go online for chapter quizzes, pre-tests, Interactive Activities, and more!

What are proteins?

Proteins are large, complex molecules found in the cells of all living things. Although proteins are best known as a part of our muscle mass, they are, in fact, critical components of all the tissues of the human body, including bones, blood, and skin. Proteins also function in metabolism, immunity, fluid balance, and nutrient transport, and in certain circumstances they can provide energy. The functions of proteins will be discussed in detail later in this chapter.

How Do Proteins Differ from Carbohydrates and Lipids?

Like carbohydrates and lipids, proteins are macronutrients found in a wide variety of foods. The human body is able to synthesize them, but unlike carbohydrates and lipids, proteins are made according to instructions provided by our genetic material, or DNA. We'll explore how DNA dictates the structure of proteins shortly.

Another key difference between proteins and the other macronutrients lies in their chemical makeup. In addition to the carbon, hydrogen, and oxygen also found in carbohydrates and lipids, proteins contain a special form of nitrogen that our bodies can readily use. Our bodies are able to break down the proteins in foods and utilize this nitrogen for many important processes. Carbohydrates and lipids do not provide nitrogen.

The Building Blocks of Proteins Are Amino Acids

The proteins in our bodies are made from a combination of building blocks called **amino acids**, molecules composed of a central carbon atom connected to four other groups: an amine group, an acid group, a hydrogen atom, and a side chain (**FIGURE 6.1a**). The word *amine* means "nitrogen-containing," and nitrogen is indeed the essential component of the amine portion of the molecule.

As shown in Figure 6.1b, the portion of the amino acid that makes each unique is its side chain. The amine group, acid group, and carbon and hydrogen atoms do not vary. Variations in the structure of the side chain give each amino acid its distinct properties.

The singular term *protein* is misleading because there are potentially an infinite number of unique types of proteins in living organisms. Most of the proteins in our bodies are made from combinations of just twenty amino acids, identified in **TABLE 6.1**. Two of the twenty amino acids listed in Table 6.1, cysteine and methionine,

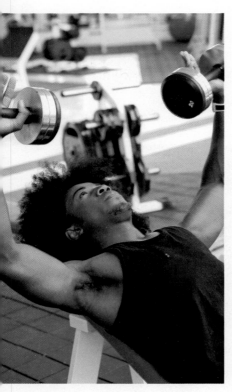

Proteins are an integral part of our body tissues, including our muscle tissue.

proteins Large, complex molecules made up of amino acids and found as essential components of all living cells.

amino acids Nitrogen-containing molecules that combine to form proteins.

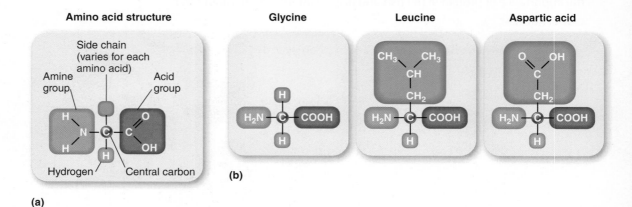

(a)
(b)

◀ **FIGURE 6.1** Structure of an amino acid. **(a)** All amino acids contain five parts: a central carbon atom; an amine group that contains nitrogen; an acid group; a hydrogen atom; and a side chain. **(b)** Only the side chain differs for each of the twenty amino acids, giving each its unique properties.

are unique in that, in addition to the components present in the other amino acids, they contain sulfur. By combining a few dozen to more than 300 of these twenty amino acids in various sequences, our bodies synthesize an estimated 10,000 to 50,000 unique proteins.

We Must Obtain Essential Amino Acids from Food

Of the twenty amino acids in our bodies, nine are classified as essential. This does not mean that they are more important than the others. Instead, an **essential amino acid** is one that our bodies cannot produce at all or cannot produce in sufficient quantities to meet our physiologic needs. Thus, we must obtain essential amino acids from food. Without an adequate supply of essential amino acids in our bodies, we lose our ability to make the proteins and other nitrogen-containing compounds we need.

The Body Can Make Nonessential Amino Acids

Nonessential amino acids are just as important to our bodies as essential amino acids, but our bodies can synthesize them in sufficient quantities, so we do not need to consume them in our diet. We make nonessential amino acids by transferring the amine group from other amino acids to a different acid group and side chain. This process is called **transamination**, and it is shown in **FIGURE 6.2**. The acid groups and side chains can be donated by amino acids, or they can be made from the breakdown products of carbohydrates and fats.

Under some conditions, a nonessential amino acid can become an essential amino acid. In this case, the amino acid is called a **conditionally essential amino acid**. Consider the disease known as phenylketonuria (PKU), in which the body cannot metabolize phenylalanine (an essential amino acid). In an infant with undiagnosed PKU, phenylalanine builds up in the blood to toxic levels that can cause irreversible brain damage. Moreover, because the body normally breaks down phenylalanine to produce the nonessential amino acid tyrosine, an inability to metabolize phenylalanine results in failure to make tyrosine, which then becomes a conditionally essential amino acid that must be provided by the diet. Other conditionally essential amino acids include arginine, cysteine, and glutamine.

recap Proteins are critical components of all the tissues of the human body. They contain carbon, hydrogen, oxygen, and nitrogen, and some contain sulfur. Their precise structure is dictated by DNA. The building blocks of proteins are amino acids. The amine group of the amino acid contains nitrogen. The portion of the amino acid that changes, giving each amino acid its distinct identity, is the side chain. Our bodies cannot make essential amino acids, so we must obtain them from our diet. Our bodies can make nonessential amino acids from parts of other amino acids, carbohydrates, and fats.

TABLE 6.1	**Amino Acids of the Human Body**
Essential Amino Acids	**Nonessential Amino Acids**
These amino acids must be consumed in the diet.	*These amino acids can be manufactured by the body.*
Histidine	Alanine
Isoleucine	Arginine
Leucine	Asparagine
Lysine	Aspartic acid
Methionine	Cysteine
Phenylalanine	Glutamic acid
Threonine	Glutamine
Tryptophan	Glycine
Valine	Proline
	Serine
	Tyrosine

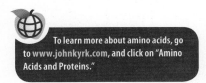 To learn more about amino acids, go to www.johnkyrk.com, and click on "Amino Acids and Proteins."

essential amino acids Amino acids not produced by the body that must be obtained from food.

nonessential amino acids Amino acids that can be manufactured by the body in sufficient quantities and therefore do not need to be consumed regularly in our diet.

transamination The process of transferring the amine group from one amino acid to another in order to manufacture a new amino acid.

conditionally essential amino acids Amino acids that are normally considered nonessential but become essential under certain circumstances when the body's need for them exceeds the ability to produce them.

Transamination

CH₃ CH₃ / CH / H₂N–C–COOH / H — Valine → O=C–COOH / Amine group is transferred to a different acid group and side chain → H₂N–C–COOH / H — Glycine

FIGURE 6.2 Transamination. Our bodies can make nonessential amino acids by transferring the amine group from an essential amino acid to a different acid group and side chain.

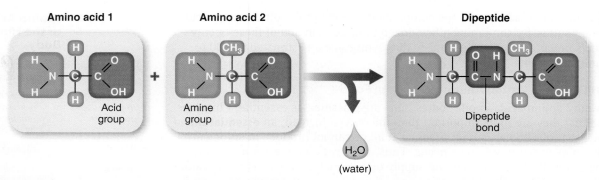

◆ FIGURE 6.3 Amino acid bonding. Two amino acids join together to form a dipeptide. By combining multiple amino acids, proteins are made.

How are proteins made?

As stated, our bodies can synthesize proteins by selecting the needed amino acids from the pool of all amino acids available at any given time. Let's look more closely at how this occurs.

Amino Acids Bond to Form a Variety of Peptides

FIGURE 6.3 shows that, when two amino acids join together, the amine group of one binds to the acid group of another in a unique type of chemical bond called a **peptide bond**. In the process, a molecule of water is released as a by-product.

Two amino acids joined together form a *dipeptide,* and three amino acids joined together are called a *tripeptide.* The term *oligopeptide* is used to identify a string of four to nine amino acids, whereas a *polypeptide* is ten or more amino acids bonded together. As a polypeptide chain grows longer, it begins to fold into any of a variety of complex shapes that give proteins their sophisticated structure.

Genes Regulate Amino Acid Binding

Each of us is unique because we inherited a specific "genetic code" that integrates the code from each of our parents. Each person's genetic code dictates minor differences in amino acid sequences, which in turn lead to differences in our bodies' individual proteins. These differences in proteins result in the unique physical and physiologic characteristics each one of us possesses.

A *gene* is a segment of deoxyribonucleic acid (DNA) that serves as a template for the synthesis—or expression—of a particular protein. That is, **gene expression** is the process by which cells use genes to make proteins.

Proteins are actually manufactured at the site of ribosomes in the cell's cytoplasm. But DNA never leaves the nucleus. So for gene expression to occur, a gene's DNA has to replicate itself—that is, it must make an exact copy of itself, which can then be carried out to the cytoplasm. DNA replication ensures that the genetic information in the original gene is identical to the genetic information used to build protein. Through the process of replication, DNA provides the instructions for building every protein in the body.

Cells use a special molecule to copy, or transcribe, the information from DNA and carry it to the ribosomes. This molecule is *messenger RNA* (*messenger ribonucleic acid,* or *mRNA*). During **transcription**, mRNA copies the genetic information from DNA in the nucleus (**FIGURE 6.4, STEP 1**). Then, mRNA detaches from the DNA and leaves the nucleus, carrying its genetic "message" to the ribosomes in the cytoplasm (Figure 6.4, step 2).

Once the genetic information reaches the ribosomes, **translation** occurs; that is, the language of the mRNA genetic information is translated into the language of amino acid sequences. At the ribosomes, mRNA binds with ribosomal RNA (rRNA) and its genetic information is distributed to molecules of transfer RNA (tRNA) (Figure 6.4, step 3). Now the tRNA molecules roam the cytoplasm until they succeed in binding

peptide bonds Unique types of chemical bonds in which the amine group of one amino acid binds to the acid group of another in order to manufacture dipeptides and all larger peptide molecules.

gene expression The process of using a gene to make a protein.

transcription The process through which messenger RNA copies genetic information from DNA in the nucleus.

translation The process that occurs when the genetic information carried by messenger RNA is translated into a chain of amino acids at the ribosome.

1 Part of the DNA unwinds, and a section of its genetic code is transcribed to the mRNA inside the nucleus.

2 The mRNA leaves the nucleus via a nuclear pore and travels to the cytoplasm.

3 Once the mRNA reaches the cytoplasm, it binds to a ribosome via ribosomal RNA (rRNA). The code on the mRNA is translated into the instructions for a specific order of amino acids.

4 The transfer RNA (tRNA) binds with specific amino acids in the cytoplasm and transfers the amino acids to the ribosome as dictated by the mRNA code.

5 The amino acid is added to the growing amino acid chain, and the tRNA returns to the cytoplasm.

6 Once the synthesis of the new protein is complete, the protein is released from the ribosome. The protein may go through further modifications in the cell or can be functional in its current state.

In the nucleus, genetic information from DNA is transcribed by messenger RNA (mRNA), which then carries it to ribosomes in the cytoplasm, where this genetic information is translated into a chain of amino acids that eventually make a protein.

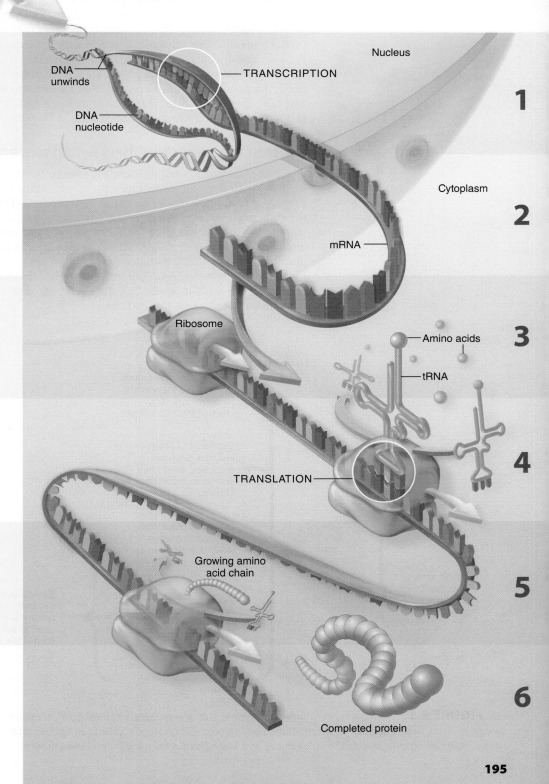

Cell

Nucleus

DNA unwinds

DNA nucleotide

TRANSCRIPTION

Nucleus

Cytoplasm

mRNA

Ribosome

Amino acids

tRNA

TRANSLATION

Growing amino acid chain

Completed protein

1

2

3

4

5

6

with the specific amino acid that matches their genetic information. They then transfer their amino acid to the ribosome, which assembles the amino acids into proteins (Figure 6.4, step 4).

Once the amino acids are loaded onto the ribosome, tRNA works to maneuver each amino acid into its proper position (Figure 6.4, step 5). When synthesis of the new protein is completed, it is released from the ribosome and can either go through further modification in the cell or can be functional in its current state (Figure 6.4, step 6).

Although the DNA for making every protein in our bodies is contained within each cell nucleus, not all genes are expressed and each cell does not make every type of protein. For example, each cell contains the DNA to manufacture the hormone insulin. However, only the beta cells of the pancreas *express* the insulin gene to produce insulin. Our physiologic needs alter gene expression, as do various nutrients. For instance, a cut in the skin that causes bleeding will prompt the production of various proteins that clot the blood. Or if we consume more dietary iron than we need, the gene for ferritin (a protein that stores iron) will be expressed, so that we can store this excess iron. Our genetic makeup and how appropriately we express our genes are important factors in our health.

Protein Turnover Involves Synthesis and Degradation

Our bodies constantly require new proteins to function properly. *Protein turnover* involves both the synthesis of new proteins and the degradation of existing proteins to provide the building blocks for those new proteins **(FIGURE 6.5)**. This process allows the cells to respond to the constantly changing demands of physiologic functions. For instance, skin cells live only for about 30 days and must continually be replaced. The amino acids needed to produce these new skin cells can be obtained from the body's *amino acid pool,* which includes those amino acids we consume in our diet as well as those that are released from the breakdown of other cells in our bodies. The body's pool of amino acids is used to produce not only new amino acids but also other products, including glucose, fat, and urea.

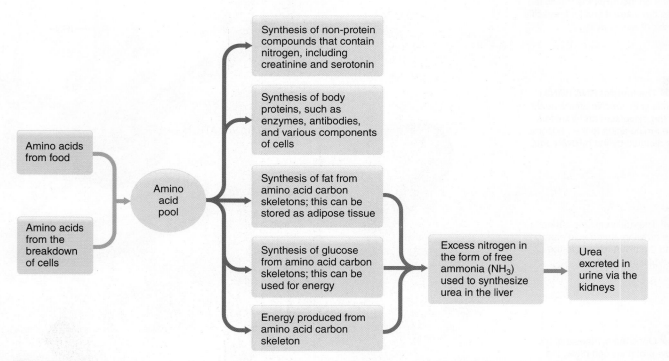

◆ **FIGURE 6.5** Protein turnover involves the synthesis of new proteins and breakdown of existing proteins to provide building blocks for new proteins. Amino acids are drawn from the body's amino acid pool and can be used to build proteins, fat, glucose, and non-protein nitrogen-containing compounds. Urea is produced as a waste product from any excess nitrogen, which is then excreted by the kidneys.

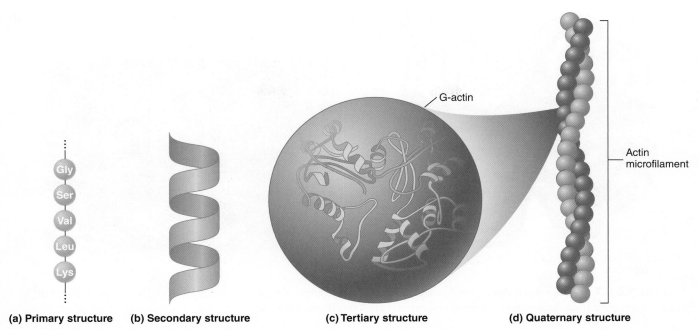

(a) Primary structure   **(b) Secondary structure**   **(c) Tertiary structure**   **(d) Quaternary structure**

FIGURE 6.6   Levels of protein structure. **(a)** The primary structure of a protein is the sequential order of amino acids. **(b)** The secondary structure of a protein is the twisting or folding of the amino acid chain. **(c)** The tertiary structure is a further folding that results in the three-dimensional shape of the protein. **(d)** In proteins with a quaternary structure, two or more polypeptides interact, forming a larger protein, such as the actin molecule illustrated here. In muscle tissue, strands of actin molecules intertwine to form contractile elements involved in generating muscle contractions.

Protein Organization Determines Function

Four levels of protein structure have been identified **(FIGURE 6.6)**. The sequential order of the amino acids in a protein is called the *primary structure* of the protein. The different amino acids in a polypeptide chain possess unique chemical characteristics that cause the chain to twist and turn into a characteristic spiral shape, or to fold into a so-called pleated sheet. These shapes are referred to as the protein's *secondary structure*. The stability of the secondary structure is achieved by hydrogen bonds that create a bridge between two protein strands or two parts of the same strand of protein. The spiral or pleated sheet of the secondary structure further folds into a unique three-dimensional shape, referred to as the protein's *tertiary structure.* Bonds between hydrogen atoms and between sulfur atoms, if any, maintain the tertiary shape, which is critical because it determines each protein's function in the body.

Many large proteins have a fourth level of organization. This *quaternary structure* forms when two or more identical or different polypeptides bond. The resulting larger protein may be *globular* or *fibrous*.

The importance of the shape of a protein to its function cannot be overemphasized. For example, the protein strands in muscle fibers are much longer than they are wide (see Figure 6.6d). This structure plays an essential role in enabling muscle contraction and relaxation. In contrast, the proteins that form red blood cells are globular in shape, and they result in the red blood cells being shaped like flattened discs with depressed centers, similar to a miniature doughnut **(FIGURE 6.7)**. This structure and the flexibility of the proteins in the red blood cells permit them to change shape and flow freely through even the tiniest capillaries to deliver oxygen and still return to their original shape.

Protein Denaturation Affects Shape and Function

Proteins can uncoil and lose their shape when they are exposed to heat, acids, bases, heavy metals, alcohol, and other damaging substances. The term used to

To view a video showing a protein developing from primary to quaternary structure, go to **www.dnatube.com**, click on "Videos," and then type "aminoacids" (as one word) into the search box. You'll see the video below, titled "How a bunch of aminoacids organize to form functional protein."

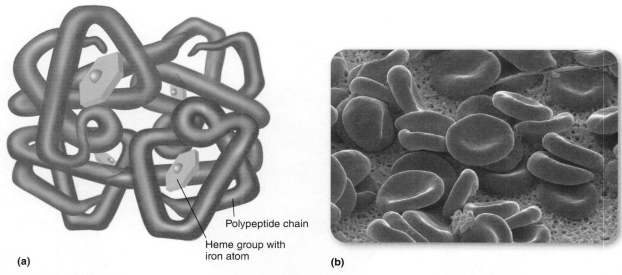

Polypeptide chain

Heme group with
iron atom

(a)   (b)

⬆ **FIGURE 6.7**   Protein shape determines function. **(a)** Hemoglobin, the protein that forms red blood cells, is globular in shape. **(b)** The globular shape of hemoglobin results in red blood cells being shaped like flattened discs.

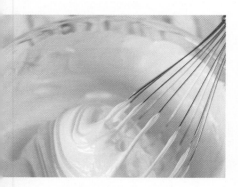

⬆ Stiffening egg whites adds air through the beating action, which denatures some of the proteins within them.

denaturation The process by which proteins uncoil and lose their shape and function when they are exposed to heat, acids, bases, heavy metals, alcohol, and other damaging substances.

limiting amino acid The essential amino acid that is missing or in the smallest supply in the amino acid pool and is thus responsible for slowing or halting protein synthesis.

describe this change in the shape of proteins is **denaturation**. Everyday examples of protein denaturation are the stiffening of egg whites when they are whipped, the curdling of milk when lemon juice or another acid is added, and the solidifying of eggs as they cook.

Denaturation does not affect the primary structure of proteins. However, when a protein is denatured, its function is lost. For instance, denaturation of critical body proteins on exposure to heat or acidity is harmful, because it prevents them from performing their functions. This type of denaturation can occur during times of high fever or when blood pH is out of the normal range. In some cases, however, denaturation is helpful. For instance, denaturation of proteins during the digestive process allows for their breakdown into amino acids and the absorption of these amino acids from the digestive tract into the bloodstream.

recap   Amino acids bind together to form proteins. Genes regulate the amino acid sequence, and thus the structure, of all proteins. The shape of a protein determines its function. When a protein is denatured by damaging substances, such as heat and acids, it loses its shape and its function.

Protein Synthesis Can Be Limited by Missing Amino Acids

For protein synthesis to occur, all essential amino acids must be available to the cell. If this is not the case, the amino acid that is missing or in the smallest supply is called the **limiting amino acid**. Without the proper combination and quantity of essential amino acids, protein synthesis slows to the point at which proteins cannot be generated. For instance, the protein hemoglobin contains the essential amino acid histidine. If we do not consume enough histidine, it becomes the limiting amino acid in hemoglobin production. Because no other amino acid can be substituted, our bodies become unable to make adequate hemoglobin, and we lose the ability to transport oxygen to our cells.

Inadequate energy consumption also limits protein synthesis. If there is not enough energy available from our diets, our bodies will use any accessible proteins for energy, thus preventing them from being used to build new proteins.

A protein that does not contain all of the essential amino acids in sufficient quantities to support growth and health is called an **incomplete** (*low-quality*) **protein**. Proteins that have all nine of the essential amino acids are considered **complete** (*high-quality*) **proteins**. The most complete protein sources are foods derived from animals and include egg whites, meat, poultry, fish, and milk. Soybeans and a pseudo-grain called quinoa (pronounced keen-wah) are the most complete sources of plant protein. In general, the typical American diet is very high in complete proteins because we consume proteins from a variety of food sources.

Protein Synthesis Can Be Enhanced by Mutual Supplementation

We also obtain complete proteins by combining foods. Consider a meal of red beans and rice. Red beans are low in the amino acids methionine and cysteine but have adequate amounts of isoleucine and lysine. Rice is low in isoleucine and lysine but contains sufficient methionine and cysteine. Combining red beans and rice creates a complete protein.

Mutual supplementation is the process of combining two or more incomplete protein sources to make a complete protein. The two foods involved are called complementary foods; these foods provide **complementary proteins** (FIGURE 6.8), which, when combined, provide all nine essential amino acids.

It is not necessary to eat complementary proteins at the same meal. Recall that we maintain a free pool of amino acids in the blood; these amino acids come from food and sloughed-off cells. When we eat one complementary protein, its amino acids join those in the free amino acid pool. These free amino acids can then combine to synthesize complete proteins. However, it is wise to eat complementary-protein foods during the same day because partially completed proteins cannot be stored and saved

incomplete proteins Foods that do not contain all of the essential amino acids in sufficient amounts to support growth and health.

complete proteins Foods that contain all nine essential amino acids.

mutual supplementation The process of combining two or more incomplete protein sources to make a complete protein.

complementary proteins Two or more foods that together contain all nine essential amino acids necessary for a complete protein. It is not necessary to eat complementary proteins at the same meal.

Combining Complementary Foods

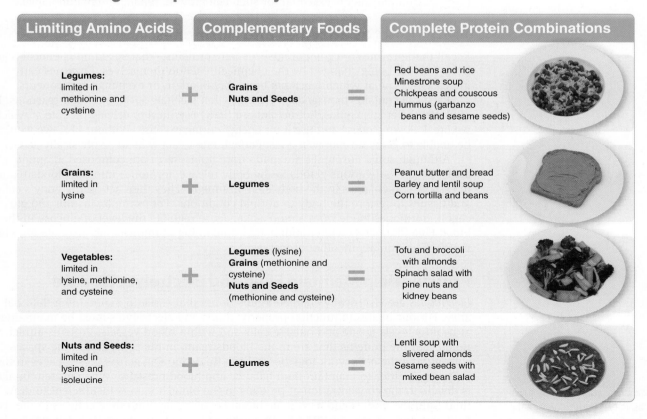

Limiting Amino Acids		Complementary Foods		Complete Protein Combinations
Legumes: limited in methionine and cysteine	+	**Grains** **Nuts and Seeds**	=	Red beans and rice Minestrone soup Chickpeas and couscous Hummus (garbanzo beans and sesame seeds)
Grains: limited in lysine	+	**Legumes**	=	Peanut butter and bread Barley and lentil soup Corn tortilla and beans
Vegetables: limited in lysine, methionine, and cysteine	+	**Legumes** (lysine) **Grains** (methionine and cysteine) **Nuts and Seeds** (methionine and cysteine)	=	Tofu and broccoli with almonds Spinach salad with pine nuts and kidney beans
Nuts and Seeds: limited in lysine and isoleucine	+	**Legumes**	=	Lentil soup with slivered almonds Sesame seeds with mixed bean salad

FIGURE 6.8 Complementary food combinations.

for a later time. Mutual supplementation is important for people eating a vegetarian diet, particularly if they consume no animal products whatsoever.

recap When a particular amino acid is limiting, protein synthesis cannot occur. A complete protein provides all nine essential amino acids. Mutual supplementation combines two complementary-protein sources to make a complete protein.

Why do we need proteins?

The functions of proteins in the body are so numerous that only a few can be described in detail in this chapter. Note that proteins function most effectively when we also consume adequate amounts of energy as carbohydrates and fat. When there is not enough energy available, the body uses proteins as an energy source, limiting their availability for the functions described in this section.

Proteins Contribute to Cell Growth, Repair, and Maintenance

The proteins in our bodies are dynamic, meaning that they are constantly being broken down, repaired, and replaced. When proteins are broken down, many amino acids are recycled into new proteins. Think about all of the new proteins that are needed to allow an embryo to develop and grow. In this case, an entirely new human body is being made! In fact, a newborn baby has more than 10 trillion body cells.

Even in adulthood, our cells are constantly turning over, as damaged or worn-out cells are broken down and their components are used to create new cells. Our red blood cells live for only 3 to 4 months and then are replaced by new cells that are produced in bone marrow. The cells lining our intestinal tract are replaced every 3 to 6 days. The "old" intestinal cells are treated just like the proteins in food; they are digested and the amino acids absorbed back into the body. The constant turnover of proteins from our diet is essential for such cell growth, repair, and maintenance.

Proteins Act as Enzymes and Hormones

Recall that enzymes are compounds—usually proteins—that speed up chemical reactions without being changed by the chemical reaction themselves. Enzymes can increase the rate at which reactants bond, break apart, or exchange components.

Each cell contains thousands of enzymes that facilitate specific cellular reactions. For example, the enzyme phosphofructokinase (PFK) is critical to driving the rate at which we break down glucose and use it for energy during exercise. Without PFK, we would be unable to generate energy at a fast enough rate to allow us to be physically active.

Although some hormones are made from lipids, most are composed of amino acids. Recall that various glands in the body release hormones into the bloodstream in response to changes in the body's environment. They then act on the body's cells and tissues to restore the body to normal conditions. For example, insulin and glucagon, hormones made from amino acids, act to regulate the level of glucose in the blood (see Chapter 4). Other amino acid–containing hormones help regulate growth, metabolism, and many other processes.

Proteins Help Maintain Fluid and Electrolyte Balance

Electrolytes are electrically charged atoms (ions) that assist in maintaining fluid balance. For our bodies to function properly, fluids and electrolytes must be maintained at healthy levels inside and outside cells and within blood vessels. Proteins attract fluids, and the proteins that are in the bloodstream, in the cells, and in the spaces surrounding the cells work together to keep fluids moving across these spaces in the proper quantities to maintain fluid balance and blood pressure. When protein intake is deficient, the concentration of proteins in the bloodstream is insufficient to draw fluid from the tissues and across the blood vessel walls; fluid then collects in the tissues, causing **edema** (FIGURE 6.9). In addition to being uncomfortable, edema can lead to serious medical problems.

edema A disorder in which fluids build up in the tissue spaces of the body, causing fluid imbalances and a swollen appearance.

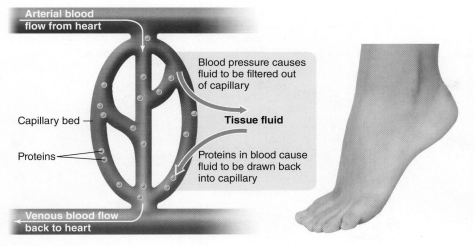

(a) Normal fluid balance

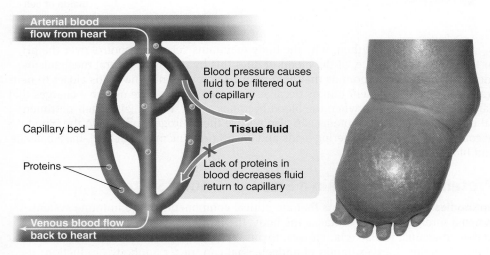

(b) Edema caused by insufficient protein in bloodstream

◀ **FIGURE 6.9** The role of proteins in maintaining fluid balance. The heartbeat exerts pressure that continually pushes fluids in the bloodstream through the arterial walls and out into the tissue spaces. By the time blood reaches the veins, the pressure of the heartbeat has greatly decreased. In this environment, proteins in the blood are able to draw fluids out of the tissues and back into the bloodstream. **(a)** This healthy (non-swollen) tissue suggests that body fluids in the bloodstream and in the tissue spaces are in balance. **(b)** When the level of proteins in the blood is insufficient to draw fluids out of the tissues, edema can result. This foot with edema is swollen due to fluid imbalance.

Sodium (Na^+) and potassium (K^+) are examples of common electrolytes. Under normal conditions, Na^+ is more concentrated outside the cell, and K^+ is more concentrated inside the cell. This proper balance of Na^+ and K^+ is accomplished by the action of **transport proteins** located within the cell membrane. **FIGURE 6.10** (page 202) shows how these transport proteins work to pump Na^+ outside and K^+ inside of the cell. The conduction of nerve signals and contraction of muscles depend on a proper balance of electrolytes. If protein intake is deficient, we lose our ability to maintain these functions, resulting in potentially fatal changes in the rhythm of the heart. Other consequences of chronically low protein intakes include muscle weakness and spasms, kidney failure, and, if conditions are severe enough, death.

Proteins Help Maintain Acid–Base Balance

The body's cellular processes result in the constant production of acids and bases. Recall that acids are fluids containing a level of hydrogen ions higher than that of pure water, whereas bases (alkaline fluids) have fewer hydrogen ions than pure water. Acids and bases are transported in the blood to be excreted through the kidneys and the lungs. The body goes into a state called **acidosis** when the blood becomes too acidic. **Alkalosis** results if the blood becomes too basic (alkaline). Both acidosis and alkalosis can be caused by respiratory or metabolic problems, and both can cause coma and death by denaturing body proteins.

transport proteins Protein molecules that help transport substances throughout the body and across cell membranes.

acidosis A disorder in which the blood becomes acidic; that is, the level of hydrogen in the blood is excessive. It can be caused by respiratory or metabolic problems.

alkalosis A disorder in which the blood becomes basic; that is, the level of hydrogen in the blood is deficient. It can be caused by respiratory or metabolic problems.

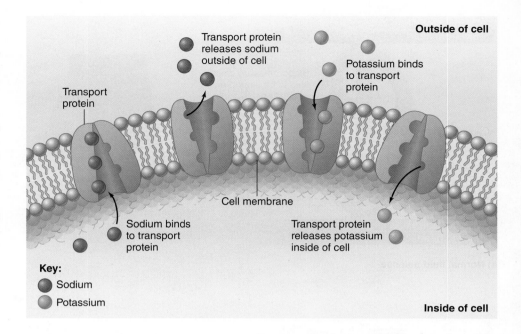

You can appreciate, then, why the body maintains very tight control over the pH, or the acid–base balance, of the blood. It does this by means of several mechanisms, including **buffers**, compounds that help return acidic and alkaline fluids closer to neutral. Proteins are excellent buffers because their side chains have negative charges that can bind hydrogen ions when the blood becomes acidic, neutralizing their detrimental effects on the body. Proteins can also release the hydrogen ions when the blood becomes too basic. By buffering acids and bases, proteins maintain acid–base balance and blood pH.

Proteins Help Maintain a Strong Immune System

Antibodies are special proteins that are critical components of the immune system. When a foreign substance attacks the body, the immune system produces antibodies to defend against it. Bacteria, viruses, toxins, and allergens (substances that cause allergic reactions) are examples of antigens that can trigger antibody production. (An *antigen* is any substance—but typically a protein—that our bodies recognize as foreign and that triggers an immune response.)

Each antibody is designed to destroy one specific invader. When that substance invades the body, antibodies are produced to neutralize or target the specific antigen so that it can be destroyed. Once antibodies have been made, the body "remembers" this process and can respond more quickly the next time that particular invader appears. *Immunity* refers to the development of the molecular memory to produce antibodies quickly upon subsequent invasions.

Adequate protein is necessary to support the increased production of antibodies that occurs in response to a cold, flu, or an allergic reaction. If we do not consume enough protein, our resistance to illnesses and disease is weakened. On the other hand, eating more protein than we need does not improve immune function.

Proteins Serve as an Energy Source

The body's primary energy sources are carbohydrate and fat. Remember that both carbohydrate and fat have specialized storage forms that can be used for energy—glycogen for carbohydrate and triglycerides for fat. Proteins do not have a specialized storage form for energy. This means that, when proteins need to be used for energy, they are taken from the blood and body tissues, such as the liver and skeletal muscle. In healthy people, proteins contribute very little to energy needs. Because we are efficient at recycling amino acids, protein needs are relatively low as compared to needs for carbohydrate and fat.

buffers Proteins that help maintain proper acid–base balance by attaching to, or releasing, hydrogen ions as conditions change in the body.

antibodies Defensive proteins of the immune system. Their production is prompted by the presence of bacteria, viruses, toxins, allergens, and other antigens.

To use proteins for energy, the liver removes the amine group from the amino acids in a process called **deamination**. The nitrogen bonds with hydrogen, creating ammonia, which is a toxic compound that can upset acid–base balance. To avoid this, the liver quickly converts ammonia to *urea*. The urea is then transported to the kidneys, where it is filtered out of the blood and is subsequently excreted in the urine. The remaining fragments of the amino acid contain carbon, hydrogen, and oxygen. The body can use these fragments to generate energy or to build carbohydrates. Certain amino acids can be converted into glucose via gluconeogenesis. This is a critical process during times of low carbohydrate intake or starvation. Fat cannot be converted into glucose, but body proteins can be broken down and converted into glucose to provide needed energy to the brain.

To protect the proteins in our body tissues, it is important that we regularly eat an adequate amount of carbohydrate and fat to provide energy. We also need to consume enough dietary protein to perform the required work without using up the proteins that already are playing an active role in our bodies. Unfortunately, our bodies cannot store excess dietary protein. As a consequence, eating too much protein results in the removal and excretion of the nitrogen in the urine and the use of the remaining components for energy. Any remaining components not used for energy can be converted and stored as body fat.

Proteins Assist in the Transport and Storage of Nutrients

Proteins act as carriers for many important nutrients in the body. As you've learned, lipoproteins contain lipids bound to proteins, which allows the transport of hydrophobic lipids through the watery medium of blood (see Chapter 5). Another example of a transport protein is transferrin, which carries iron in the blood. Ferritin, in contrast, is an example of a storage protein: it is the compound in which iron is stored in the liver.

We've also said that transport proteins located in cell membranes allow the proper transport of many nutrients into and out of the cell. These transport proteins also help in the maintenance of fluid and electrolyte balance and conduction of nerve impulses.

Other Roles of Proteins

The amino acids from proteins can also be used to make **neurotransmitters**, chemicals that transmit messages from one nerve cell to another. Examples of neurotransmitters include epinephrine and norepinephrine, both of which stimulate the sympathetic nervous system; *melatonin*, which plays a critical role in the regulation of sleep; and serotonin, which is important for the functioning of the central nervous system and the enteric nervous system of the gastrointestinal (GI) tract.

Proteins are also critical in blood clotting. The watery portion of blood, called plasma, contains clotting factors, proteins that initiate a chain of reactions that convert another plasma protein, fibrinogen, to a fibrous protein called *fibrin*. Strands of fibrin form a mesh that helps to temporarily seal a broken blood vessel. The scar tissue that is formed to heal wounds comprises another protein, *collagen*.

recap Proteins serve many important functions: (1) enabling growth, repair, and maintenance of body tissues; (2) acting as enzymes and hormones; (3) maintaining fluid and electrolyte balance; (4) maintaining acid–base balance; (5) making antibodies, which strengthen our immune system; (6) providing energy when carbohydrate and fat intake are inadequate; (7) transporting and storing nutrients; and (8) producing compounds such as neurotransmitters, fibrin, and collagen. Proteins function best when adequate amounts of energy, carbohydrate, and fat are consumed.

How do our bodies break down proteins?

Our bodies do not directly use proteins from the diet to make the proteins we need. Dietary proteins are first digested and broken into amino acids, so that they can be absorbed and transported to the cells. In this section, we will review how proteins are digested and absorbed. As you review each step in this process, refer to **FIGURE 6.11** for a visual overview of the process of protein digestion.

To learn more about how blood clots and wounds heal, go to www.medlineplus.gov, click on "Videos and Cool Tools," then click on "Anatomy Videos," and then click "blood clotting."

deamination The process by which an amine group is removed from an amino acid. The nitrogen is then transported to the kidneys for excretion in the urine, while the carbon and other components are metabolized for energy or used to make other compounds.

neurotransmitters Chemical compounds that transmit messages from one nerve cell to another.

Digestion of dietary proteins into single amino acids occurs primarily in the stomach and small intestine. The single amino acids are then transported to the liver, where they may be converted to glucose or fat, used for energy or to build new proteins, or transported to cells as needed.

ORGANS OF THE GI TRACT

MOUTH

Proteins in foods are crushed by chewing and moistened by saliva.

STOMACH

Proteins are denatured by hydrochloric acid.

Pepsin is activated to break proteins into single amino acids and smaller polypeptides.

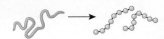

SMALL INTESTINE

Proteases are secreted to digest polypeptides into smaller units.

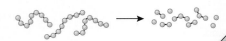

Cells in the wall of the small intestine complete the breakdown of dipeptides and tripeptides into single amino acids, which are absorbed into the bloodstream.

ACCESSORY ORGANS

PANCREAS

Produces proteases, which are released into the small intestine.

LIVER

Amino acids are transported to the liver, where they are converted to glucose or fat, used for energy or to build new proteins, or sent to the cells as needed.

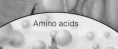

Amino acids

Enterocytes

Lacteal

Capillary

HOT TOPIC

Amino Acid Supplements: Necessity or Waste?

"Amino acid supplements—you can't gain without them!" This is just one of the headlines found in bodybuilding magazines and Internet sites touting amino acid supplements as the key to achieving power, strength, and performance "perfection." Many athletes who read these claims believe that taking amino acid supplements will boost their energy during events, replace proteins metabolized for energy during exercise, enhance muscle growth and strength, and hasten recovery from intense training or injury. Should you believe the hype?

As noted earlier in this chapter, we use very little protein for energy during exercise, and most Americans already consume more than they need. A diet providing adequate energy and meeting the athlete's RDA for protein will support either strength or endurance training and performance without the need for amino acid supplements. What about the claims related to muscle-building? Although some research has shown that intravenous infusions of various amino acids in the laboratory can stimulate certain hormones that enhance the building of muscle, there is little evidence that taking amino acid supplements orally can build muscle or improve strength. Because these supplements are relatively expensive, getting enough protein via your diet alone will put a lot less strain on your wallet!

Stomach Acids and Enzymes Break Proteins into Short Polypeptides

Virtually no enzymatic digestion of proteins occurs in the mouth. As shown in Figure 6.11, proteins in food are chewed, crushed, and moistened with saliva to ease swallowing and to increase the surface area of the protein for more efficient digestion. There is no further digestive action on proteins in the mouth.

When proteins reach the stomach, hydrochloric acid denatures the protein strands. It also converts the inactive enzyme, *pepsinogen,* into its active form, **pepsin,** which is a protein-digesting enzyme. Although pepsin is itself a protein, it is not denatured by the acid in the stomach because it has evolved to work optimally in an acidic environment. The hormone *gastrin* controls both the production of hydrochloric acid and the release of pepsin; thinking about food or actually chewing food stimulates the gastrin-producing cells located in the stomach. Pepsin begins breaking proteins into single amino acids and shorter polypeptides; these amino acids and polypeptides then travel to the small intestine for further digestion and absorption.

Enzymes in the Small Intestine Break Polypeptides into Single Amino Acids

As the polypeptides reach the small intestine, the pancreas and the small intestine secrete enzymes that digest them into oligopeptides, tripeptides, dipeptides, and single amino acids (see Figure 6.11). The enzymes that digest proteins in the small intestine are called **proteases.**

The cells in the wall of the small intestine then absorb the single amino acids, dipeptides, and tripeptides. Peptidases, enzymes located in the intestinal cells, break the dipeptides and tripeptides into single amino acids. The amino acids are then transported via the portal vein into the liver. Once in the liver, amino acids may be converted to glucose or fat, combined to build new proteins, used for energy, or released into the bloodstream and transported to other cells as needed.

The cells of the small intestine have different sites that specialize in transporting certain types of amino acids, dipeptides, and tripeptides. This fact has implications for users of amino acid supplements. When very large doses of supplements containing single amino acids are taken on an empty stomach, they typically compete for the same absorption sites. This competition can block the absorption of other amino acids and could in theory lead to deficiencies. In reality, people rarely take such large doses of single amino acids on an empty stomach. Refer to the **Hot Topic** to learn more about amino acid supplements.

pepsin An enzyme in the stomach that begins the breakdown of proteins into shorter polypeptide chains and single amino acids.

proteases Enzymes that continue the breakdown of polypeptides in the small intestine.

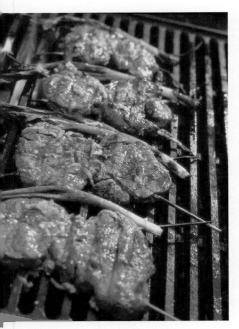

Meats are highly digestible sources of dietary protein.

Protein Digestibility Affects Protein Quality

Earlier in this chapter, we discussed how various protein sources differ in quality of protein. The quantity of essential amino acids in a protein determines its quality: higher-protein-quality foods are those that contain more of the essential amino acids in sufficient quantities needed to build proteins, and lower-quality-protein foods contain fewer essential amino acids. Another factor in protein quality is *digestibility*, or how well our bodies can digest a protein. Animal protein sources, such as meat and dairy products, are highly digestible, as are many soy products; we can absorb more than 90% of the amino acids in these protein sources. Legumes are also highly digestible (about 70% to 80%). Grains and many vegetable proteins are less digestible, ranging from 60% to 90%.

recap In the stomach, hydrochloric acid denatures proteins and converts pepsinogen to pepsin; pepsin breaks proteins into smaller polypeptides and individual amino acids. In the small intestine, proteases break polypeptides into smaller fragments and single amino acids. Enzymes in the cells in the wall of the small intestine break the smaller peptide fragments into single amino acids, which are then transported to the liver for distribution to our cells. Taking high doses of individual amino acid supplements can lead to deficiencies of other amino acids. Protein digestibility and the provision of essential amino acids influence protein quality.

How much protein should we eat?

Consuming adequate protein is a major concern of many people. In fact, one of the most common concerns among active people and athletes is that their diets are deficient in protein (see the **Nutrition Myth or Fact?** box (on page 208) for a discussion of this topic). This concern about dietary protein is generally unnecessary because we can easily consume the protein our bodies need by eating an adequate and varied diet.

Nitrogen Balance Is a Method Used to Determine Protein Needs

A highly specialized procedure referred to as *nitrogen balance* is used to determine a person's protein needs. Nitrogen is excreted through the body's processes of recycling or using proteins; thus, the balance can be used to estimate whether protein intake is adequate to meet protein needs.

Typically performed only in experimental laboratories, nitrogen balance involves measuring both nitrogen intake and nitrogen excretion over a 2-week period. A standardized diet, the nitrogen content of which has been measured and recorded, is fed to the study participant. The person is required to consume all of the foods provided. Because the majority of nitrogen is excreted in the urine and feces, laboratory technicians directly measure the nitrogen content of the subject's urine and fecal samples. Small amounts of nitrogen are excreted in the skin, hair, and body fluids such as mucus and semen, but, because of the complexity of collecting nitrogen excreted via these routes, the measurements are estimated. Then, technicians add the estimated nitrogen losses to the nitrogen measured in the subject's urine and feces. Nitrogen balance is then calculated as the difference between nitrogen intake and nitrogen excretion.

People who consume more nitrogen than is excreted are considered to be in positive nitrogen balance (**FIGURE 6.12**). This state indicates that the body is retaining or adding protein, and it occurs during periods of growth, pregnancy, or recovery from illness or a protein deficiency. People who excrete more nitrogen than they consume are in negative nitrogen balance. This situation indicates that the body is losing protein, and it occurs during starvation or when people are consuming very-low-energy diets. This is because, when energy intake is too low to meet energy demands over a prolonged period, the body metabolizes body proteins for energy. The nitrogen from these proteins is excreted in the urine and feces. Negative nitrogen balance also occurs during severe illness, infections, high fever, serious burns, or injuries

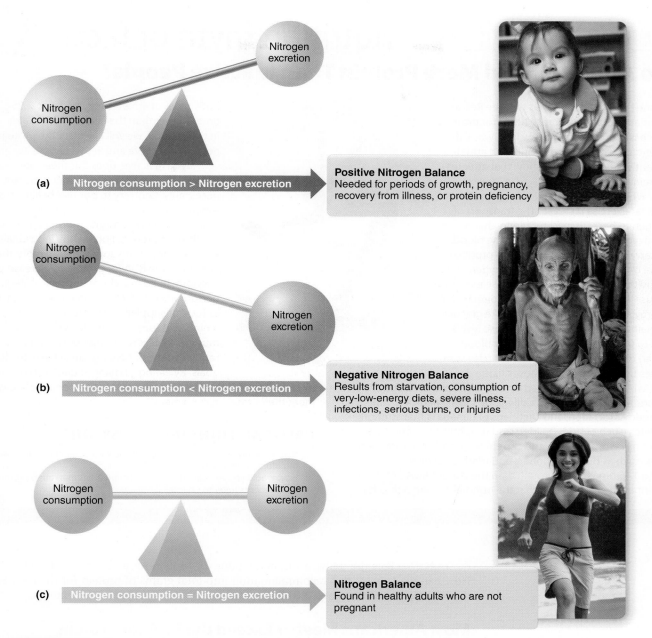

⬆ FIGURE 6.12 Nitrogen balance describes the relationship between how much nitrogen (protein) we consume and how much we excrete each day. **(a)** Positive nitrogen balance occurs when nitrogen consumption is greater than excretion. **(b)** Negative nitrogen balance occurs when nitrogen consumption is less than excretion. **(c)** Nitrogen balance is maintained when nitrogen consumption equals excretion.

that cause significant blood loss. People in these situations require increased dietary protein. A person is in nitrogen balance when nitrogen intake equals nitrogen excretion. This indicates that protein intake is sufficient to cover protein needs. Healthy adults who are not pregnant are in nitrogen balance.

Recommended Dietary Allowance for Protein

How much protein should we eat? The RDA for sedentary people is 0.8 g per kg body weight per day. The recommended percentage of energy that should come from protein is 10% to 35% of total energy intake. Protein needs are higher for children, adolescents, and pregnant/lactating women because more protein is needed during times of growth and development (see Chapters 14 and 15). Protein needs can also be higher for active people and for vegetarians.

nutrition myth or fact?

Do Athletes Need More Protein Than Inactive People?

At one time, it was believed that the Recommended Dietary Allowance (RDA) for protein, which is 0.8 g per kg body weight, was sufficient for both inactive people and athletes. Recent studies, however, show that athletes' protein needs are higher.

Why do athletes need more protein? Regular exercise increases the transport of oxygen to body tissues, requiring changes in the oxygen-carrying capacity of the blood. To carry more oxygen, we need to produce more of the protein that carries oxygen in the blood (hemoglobin). During intense exercise, we use a small amount of protein directly for energy. We also use protein to make glucose to maintain adequate blood glucose levels and to prevent hypoglycemia (low blood sugar) during exercise. Regular exercise stimulates tissue growth and causes tissue damage, which must be repaired by additional proteins. Current consensus from the American College of Sports Medicine, American Dietetic Association, and Dietitians of Canada is that strength athletes (such as bodybuilders and weightlifters) need 1.8 to 2 times more protein than the current RDA, and endurance athletes (such as distance runners and triathletes) need 1.5 to 1.75 times more protein than the current RDA.[3] More recent evidence suggests that the optimal protein needs for

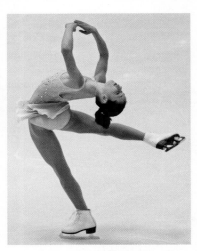

⬆ Some athletes who diet persistently are at risk for low protein intake.

both types of athletes may be 1.6 to 2.25 times higher than the current RDA.[4] Later in this chapter, we will calculate the protein needs for inactive and active people.

If you're active, does this mean you should add more protein to your diet? Not necessarily. Contrary to popular belief, most Americans, including inactive people *and* athletes, already consume more than twice the RDA for protein. For healthy individuals, evidence does not support eating more than two times the RDA for protein to increase strength, build muscle, or improve athletic performance. In fact, eating more protein as food or supplements or taking individual amino acid supplements does not cause muscles to become bigger or stronger. Only regular strength training can achieve these goals. By eating a balanced diet and consuming a variety of foods, both inactive and active people can easily meet their protein requirements.

CRITICAL THINKING QUESTIONS

1. Before taking this course, did you feel you would benefit from consuming more protein? Why or why not?
2. How would you evaluate the claims of companies marketing protein supplements (refer to Chapter 1)?

TABLE 6.2 lists the daily recommendations for protein for a variety of lifestyles. How can we convert this recommendation into total grams of protein for the day? See the **You Do the Math** (page 210) box to calculate Theo's protein requirements.

Most Americans Meet or Exceed the RDA for Protein

Surveys indicate that Americans eat 14–16% of their total daily energy intake as protein.[5] Men report eating about 73 to 104 g of protein per day, and women consume 59 to 72 g per day. Putting these values into perspective, let's assume that the average man weighs 75 kg (165 pounds) and the average woman weighs 65 kg (143 pounds). Their protein requirements (assuming they are not athletes or vegetarians) are 60 g and 52 g per day, respectively. As you can see, many adults in the United States eat more than the RDA for protein.

Research indicates that the protein intake of athletes participating in a variety of sports can also well exceed current recommendations.[6] For instance, the protein intake for some female distance runners is 1.2 g per kg of body weight per day, accounting for 15% of their total daily energy intake. In addition, some male bodybuilders consume 3 g per kg of body weight per day, accounting for almost 38% of their total daily intake! However, certain groups of athletes are at risk for low protein intakes. Athletes who consume inadequate energy and limit food choices, such as some distance runners, figure skaters, female gymnasts, and wrestlers who are dieting, are all at risk for low protein intakes. Unlike people who consume adequate energy, individuals who are restricting their total energy intake (kilocalories) need to pay close attention to their protein intake.

Can Too Much Dietary Protein Be Harmful?

High protein intakes have been identified with increased health risks. Three health conditions that have received particular attention are heart disease, bone loss, and kidney disease.

High Protein Intake and High Blood Cholesterol

High-protein diets composed of predominantly animal sources have been associated with higher blood cholesterol levels. This is probably due to the saturated fat in animal products, which is known to increase both blood cholesterol levels and the risk for heart disease. However, a review of studies examining this issue indicates that moderately high-protein diets, particularly those including protein sources low in saturated fat, are associated with a significantly healthier blood lipid profile, reduced blood pressure, and reduced risk for cardiovascular disease.[7] These experts state that the optimal amount and sources of protein to reduce the risk for cardiovascular disease are not yet known, and they encourage partially replacing refined carbohydrate foods in the diet with protein sources that are low in saturated fat. These sources do not necessarily have to come from animals because vegetarians have been shown to have a greatly reduced risk for heart disease.[8,9]

High Protein Intake May Contribute to Bone Loss

How might a high-protein diet lead to bone loss? Until recently, nutritionists have been concerned about high-protein diets because they increase calcium excretion. This may be because animal products contain more of the sulfur amino acids (methionine and cysteine). Metabolizing these amino acids makes the blood more acidic, and calcium is pulled from the bone to buffer these acids. Although eating more protein can cause an increased excretion of calcium, it is very controversial whether high protein intakes actually cause bone loss. In fact, we do know that eating too little protein causes bone loss, which increases the risk for fractures and osteoporosis. Higher intakes of animal and soy protein have been shown to protect bone in middle-aged and older women. A recent systematic review of the literature concluded that there is no evidence to support the contention that high-protein diets lead to bone loss, except in people consuming inadequate calcium.[10]

High Protein Intake Can Increase the Risk for Kidney Disease

A third risk associated with high protein intakes is kidney disease. A high-protein diet can increase the risk of acquiring kidney disease in people who are susceptible. People with diabetes have higher rates of kidney disease and may benefit from a lower-protein diet. The American Diabetes Association states that people with diabetes have a higher protein need than people without diabetes, but a protein intake of 15% to 20% of total energy is adequate to meet these increased needs.[11] This level of protein intake is deemed safe for people with diabetes who have normal renal function.

There is no evidence that eating more protein causes kidney disease in healthy people who are not susceptible to this condition.[12] In fact, a review of studies assessing the effect of high protein intakes on renal function in athletes found that regularly consuming over 2 g of protein per kg body weight per day does not appear to cause unhealthy changes in kidney function.[12] Thus, experts agree that eating no more than 2 g of protein per kg body weight each day is safe for healthy people.

It is important for people who consume a lot of protein to drink more water. This is because eating more protein increases protein metabolism and urea production. As mentioned earlier, urea is a waste product that forms when nitrogen is removed during amino acid metabolism. Adequate fluid is needed to flush excess urea from the kidneys. This is particularly important for athletes, who need more fluid to counterbalance higher sweat losses.

TABLE 6.2 Recommended Protein Intakes

Group	Protein Intake (grams per kilogram* body weight)
Sedentary adults[†]	0.8
Nonvegetarian endurance athletes[‡]	1.2 to 1.4
Nonvegetarian strength athletes[‡]	1.2 to 1.7
Vegetarian endurance athletes[‡]	1.3 to 1.5
Vegetarian strength athletes[‡]	1.3 to 1.8

Note: *To convert body weight to kilograms, divide weight in pounds by 2.2.
Weight (lb)/2.2 = Weight (kg)
Weight (kg) × protein recommendation (g/kg body weight/day) = protein intake (g/day)

[†]Data from: Food and Nutrition Board, Institute of Medicine. 2005. *Dietary Reference Intakes for Energy, Carbohydrate, Fiber, Fat, Fatty Acids, Cholesterol, Protein, and Amino Acids (Macronutrients).* Washington, DC: National Academies Press.

[‡]Data from: American College of Sports Medicine, American Dietetic Association, and Dietitians of Canada. 2009. Joint Position Statement. Nutrition and athletic performance. *Med. Sci. Sports Exerc.* 41(3):709–731.

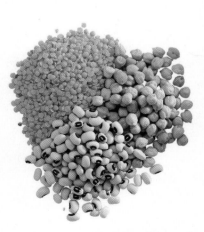

The quality of the protein in some legumes, such as these black-eyed peas, lentils, and garbanzo beans, is almost equal to that of meat.

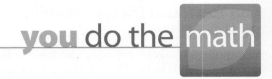

Calculating Your Protein Needs

Theo wants to know how much protein he needs each day. During the off-season, he works out three times a week at a gym and practices basketball with friends every Friday night. He is not a vegetarian. Although Theo exercises regularly, he would not be considered an endurance athlete or a strength athlete during the off-season. At this level of physical activity, Theo's requirement for protein probably ranges from the RDA of 0.8 up to 1.0 g per kg body weight per day. To calculate the total number of grams of protein Theo should eat each day:

1. Convert Theo's weight from pounds to kilograms. Theo presently weighs 200 pounds. To convert this value to kilograms, divide by 2.2:

$$200 \text{ pounds} \div 2.2 \text{ pounds/kg} = 91 \text{ kg}$$

2. Multiply Theo's weight in kilograms by his RDA for protein, like so:

$$91 \text{ kg} \times 0.8 \text{ g/kg} = 72.8 \text{ grams of protein per day}$$
$$91 \text{ kg} \times 1.0 \text{ g/kg} = 91 \text{ grams of protein per day}$$

What happens during basketball season, when Theo practices, lifts weights, and has games 5 or 6 days a week? This will probably raise his protein needs to approximately 1.2 to 1.7 g per kg body weight per day. How much more protein should he eat? See below:

$$91 \text{ kg} \times 1.2 \text{ g/kg} = 109.2 \text{ grams of protein per day}$$
$$91 \text{ kg} \times 1.7 \text{ g/kg} = 154.7 \text{ grams of protein per day}$$

Now calculate your own recommended protein intake based on your activity level.

Answers will vary depending upon body weight and individual activity levels.

Protein: Much More Than Meat!

TABLE 6.3 compares the protein content of a variety of foods. Although some people think that the only good sources of protein are meats (beef, pork, poultry, seafood), many other foods are rich in proteins. These include dairy products (milk, cheese, yogurt, and so on), eggs, legumes (including soy products), whole grains, and nuts. Fruits and many vegetables are not particularly high in protein; however, these foods are excellent sources of carbohydrates and energy, so eating them can enable your body to use proteins for building and maintaining tissues.

After reviewing Table 6.3, you might be wondering how much protein you typically eat. See the **What About You?** feature box (page 212) to find out.

Legumes

Legumes include foods such as soybeans, kidney beans, pinto beans, black beans, garbanzo beans (chickpeas), lentils, green peas, black-eyed peas, and lentils. Would you be surprised to learn that the quality of the protein in some of these legumes is almost equal to that of meat? It's true! The quality of soybean protein is almost identical to that of meat and is available as soy milk, tofu, textured vegetable protein, and tempeh, a firm cake that is made by cooking and fermenting whole soybeans. The protein quality of other legumes is also relatively high. In addition to being excellent sources of protein, legumes are high in fiber, iron, calcium, and many of the B-vitamins. They are also low in saturated fat and cholesterol.

Eating legumes regularly, including foods made from soybeans, may help reduce the risk for heart disease by lowering blood cholesterol levels. Diets high in legumes and soy products are also associated with lower rates of some cancers. Legumes are not nutritionally complete, however, because they do not contain vitamins B_{12}, C, or A. Most are also deficient in methionine, an essential amino acid; however, combining them with grains, nuts, or seeds gives you a complete protein.

Considering their nutrient profile, satiety value, and good taste, it's no wonder that many experts consider legumes an almost perfect food. From main dishes to snacks, the **Quick Tips** list (page 213) offers simple ways to add legumes to your daily diet.

TABLE 6.3 **Protein Content of Commonly Consumed Foods**

Food	Serving Amount	Protein (g)	Food	Serving Amount	Protein (g)
Beef:			**Beans:**		
Ground, lean, baked (15% fat)	3 oz	22	Refried	1/2 cup	6
Beef tenderloin steak, broiled (1/8-in. fat)	3 oz	22.5	Kidney, red	1/2 cup	8
Top sirloin, broiled (1/8-in. fat)	3 oz	23	Black	1/2 cup	7.6
Poultry:			**Nuts:**		
Chicken breast, broiled, no skin (bone removed)	1/2 breast	27	Peanuts, dry roasted	1 oz	6.7
Chicken thigh, bone and skin removed	1 thigh	28	Peanut butter, creamy	2 tbsp.	8
Turkey breast, roasted, Louis Rich	3 oz	13	Almonds, blanched	1 oz	6
Seafood:			**Cereals, Grains, and Breads:**		
Cod, cooked	3 oz	19	Oatmeal, quick instant	1 cup	6
Salmon, Chinook, baked	3 oz	22	Cheerios	1 cup	3.4
Shrimp, steamed	3 oz	19	Grape-Nuts	1/2 cup	7.2
Tuna, in water, drained	3 oz	16.5	Raisin Bran	1 cup	4.7
Pork:			Brown rice, cooked	1 cup	5
Pork loin chop, broiled	3 oz	22	Whole-wheat bread	1 slice	3.6
Ham, roasted, extra lean (5% fat)	3 oz	18	Bagel, 3-1/2-in.-diameter	1 each	10.5
Dairy:			**Vegetables:**		
Whole milk (3.25% fat)	8 fl. oz	7.7	Carrots, raw (7.25 to 8.5 in. long)	1 each	0.7
1% milk	8 fl. oz	8.2	Broccoli, raw, chopped	1 cup	2.6
Skim milk	8 fl. oz	8.3	Collards, cooked from frozen	1 cup	5
Low-fat, plain yogurt	8 fl. oz	13	Spinach, raw	1 cup	0.9
American cheese, processed	1 oz	5			
Cottage cheese, low-fat (2%)	1 cup	27			
Soy Products:					
Tofu, firm	1/2 cup	10			
Tempeh, cooked	3 oz	5.5			
Soy milk beverage	1 cup	8			

Data from: U.S. Department of Agriculture, Agricultural Research Service. 2012. USDA National Nutrient Database for Standard Reference, Release 25.

Nuts

Nuts are another healthful high-protein food. In the past, the high fat and energy content of nuts was assumed to be harmful, and people were advised to eat nuts only occasionally and in very small amounts. The results from recent epidemiological studies have helped to substantially change the way nutrition experts view nuts. These studies show that consuming about 2 to 5 oz of nuts per week significantly reduces people's risk for cardiovascular disease.[13,14] Additional evidence suggests that eating nuts, and in particular walnuts, is associated with a lower risk of type 2 diabetes.[15] Although the exact mechanism for the reduction in cardiovascular disease and type 2 diabetes risk with increased nut intake is not known, nuts contain many nutrients and other substances that are associated with health benefits, including fiber, unsaturated fatty acids, potassium, folate, plant sterols, and antioxidants.

"New" Foods

A new source of non-meat protein that is available on the market is *quorn*, a protein product derived from fermented fungus. It is mixed with a variety of other foods to produce various types of meat substitutes. Other "new" foods high in protein include

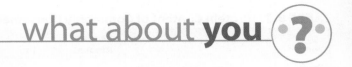

How Much Protein Do You Eat?

One way to find out if your diet contains enough protein is to keep a food diary. Record everything you eat and drink for at least 3 days, and the grams of protein each item provides. To determine the grams of protein, for packaged foods, use the Nutrition Facts panel, and make sure to adjust for the amount you actually consume. For products without labels, check Table 6.3 (on page 211), or use the diet analysis tools that accompany this text. There is also a U.S. Department of Agriculture website that lists the energy and nutrient content of thousands of foods (see **Web Resources**).

Below is an example, using Theo's food choices for 1 day. Do you think he's meeting his protein needs?

As calculated in the **You Do the Math** box (on page 210), Theo's RDA is 72.8 to 91 g of protein. He is consuming 2.3 to 2.8 times that amount! You can see that he does not need to use amino acid or protein supplements because he has more than adequate amounts of protein to build lean tissue.

Now calculate your own protein intake using food labels and a diet analysis program. Do you obtain more protein from animal or non-animal sources? If you consume mostly non-animal sources, are you eating soy products and complementary foods throughout the day? If you eat animal-based products on a regular basis, notice how much protein you consume from even small servings of meat and dairy products.

Foods Consumed	Protein Content (g)
Breakfast:	
Brewed coffee (2 cups) with 2 tbsp. cream	1.4
1 large bagel (5-in.-diameter)	13
Low-fat cream cheese (2 tbsp.)	1.6
Mid-morning snack:	
Cola beverage (32 fl. oz)	0
Low-fat strawberry yogurt (1 cup)	10
Fruit and nut granola bar (2; 37 g each)	5.7
Lunch:	
Ham and cheese sandwich:	
Whole-wheat bread (2 slices)	4
Mayonnaise (1.5 tbsp.)	0.2
Extra lean ham (4 oz)	24
Swiss cheese (2 oz)	15
Iceberg lettuce (2 leaves)	0.3
Sliced tomato (3 slices)	0.5
Banana (1 large)	1.5
Wheat Thin crackers (20)	3.6
Bottled water (20 fl. oz)	0.0

Foods Consumed	Protein Content (g)
Dinner:	
Cheeseburger:	
Broiled ground beef (1/2 lb cooked)	52
American cheese (1 oz)	5
Seeded bun (1 large)	8
Ketchup (2 tbsp.)	0.5
Mustard (1 tbsp.)	0.7
Shredded lettuce (1/2 cup)	0.3
Sliced tomato (3 slices)	0.5
French fries (30; 2- to 3-in. strips)	5
Baked beans (2 cups)	24
2% low-fat milk (2 cups)	16
Evening snack:	
Chocolate chip cookies (4; 3-in.-diameter)	3
2% low-fat milk (1 cup)	8
Total Protein Intake for the Day:	**203.8 g**

some very ancient grains! For instance, earlier we mentioned quinoa, a pseudo-grain that provides all nine essential amino acids. Quinoa is highly digestible and was so essential to the diet of the ancient Incas that they considered it sacred. Cooked much like rice, quinoa provides 8 g of protein in a 1-cup serving. A similar pseudo-grain, called amaranth, also provides complete protein. Teff, millet, and sorghum are grains long cultivated in Africa as rich sources of protein. They are now widely available

QuickTips

Adding Legumes to Your Daily Diet

Breakfast

Instead of cereal, eggs, or a doughnut, microwave a frozen bean burrito for a quick, portable breakfast.

Make your pancakes with soy milk, or pour soy milk on your cereal.

If you normally have a side of bacon, ham, or sausage with your eggs, have a side of black beans instead.

Lunch and Dinner

Try a sandwich made with hummus (a garbanzo bean spread), cucumbers, tomato, avocado, and/or lettuce on whole-wheat bread or in a whole-wheat pocket.

Use deli "meats" made with soy in your sandwich. Also try soy hot dogs, burgers, and "chicken" nuggets.

Add garbanzo beans, kidney beans, or fresh peas to tossed salads, or make a three-bean salad with kidney beans, green beans, and garbanzo beans.

Make a side dish using legumes such as peas with pearl onions; succotash (lima beans, corn, and tomatoes); or homemade chili with kidney beans and tofu instead of meat.

Make black bean soup, lentil soup, pea soup, minestrone soup, or a batch of dal (a type of yellow lentil used in Indian cuisine) and serve over brown rice. Top with plain yogurt, a traditional accompaniment in many Asian cuisines.

Use soy "crumbles" in any recipe calling for ground beef.

Make burritos with black or pinto beans instead of shredded meat.

To stir-fried vegetables, add cubes of tofu or strips of tempeh.

Make a "meatloaf" using cooked, mashed lentils instead of ground beef.

For fast food at home, keep canned beans on hand. Serve over rice with a salad for a complete and hearty meal.

Snacks

Instead of potato chips or pretzels, try one of the new bean chips.

Dip fresh vegetables in bean dip.

Serve hummus on wedges of pita bread.

Add roasted soy "nuts" to your trail mix.

Stock up on microwavable pouches of edamame (soybeans in pods). They're in the frozen foods section of most markets.

Keep frozen tofu desserts, such as tofu ice cream, in your freezer.

---

in the United States. Although these three grains are low in the essential amino acid lysine, combining them with legumes produces a complete-protein meal.

With such a wide variety of protein sources to choose from, it's easy to eat right all day! See the **Eating Right All Day** feature (page 214) for simple high-protein menu choices that are low in saturated fat and high in nutrients and phytochemicals.

recap   The RDA for protein for most nonpregnant, nonlactating, nonvegetarian adults is 0.8 g per kg body weight. Children, pregnant women, nursing mothers, vegetarians, and active people need slightly more. Most people who eat enough kilocalories and carbohydrates have no problem meeting their RDA for protein. Eating too much protein may increase a susceptible person's risk for kidney disease. Good sources of protein include meats, eggs, dairy products, legumes, nuts, quorn, and certain "ancient grains."

eating right all day

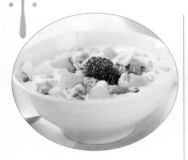

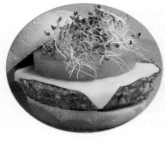

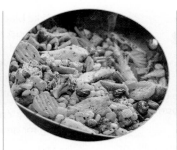

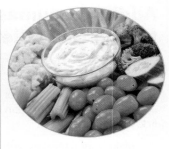

Breakfast
Whole-grain cereal with soymilk instead of a doughnut!

Lunch
Veggie burger instead of a ground beef burger!

Dinner
Stir fry chicken instead of fried chicken!

Snack
Raw veggies with low-fat dip instead of nachos!

Can a vegetarian diet provide adequate protein?

Vegetarianism is the practice of restricting the diet to food substances of plant origin, including vegetables, fruits, grains, and nuts. As stated in the chapter introduction, about 4% of American adults are vegetarians; of these, 25% are vegans—people who do not eat any kind of animal product, including dairy foods and eggs.[2] Many vegetarians are college students; moving away from home and taking responsibility for one's eating habits appears to influence some young adults to try vegetarianism as a lifestyle choice.

Types of Vegetarian Diets

There are almost as many types of vegetarian diets as there are vegetarians. Some people who consider themselves vegetarians regularly eat poultry and fish. Others avoid the flesh of animals but consume eggs, milk, and cheese liberally. Still others strictly avoid all products of animal origin, including milk and eggs, and even by-products such as candies and puddings made with gelatin. A type of "vegetarian" diet receiving significant media attention recently is the *flexitarian* diet: Flexitarians are considered semivegetarians who eat mostly plant foods, eggs, and dairy but occasionally eat red meat, poultry, and/or fish.

TABLE 6.4 identifies the various types of vegetarian diets, ranging from the most inclusive to the most restrictive. Notice that, the more restrictive the diet, the more challenging it becomes to achieve an adequate protein intake.

◀ Soy products are a good source of dietary protein.

Why Do People Become Vegetarians?

When discussing vegetarianism, one of the most often asked questions is why people would make this food choice. The most common responses are included here.

Religious, Ethical, and Food-Safety Reasons

Some make the choice for religious or spiritual reasons. Several religions prohibit or restrict the consumption of animal flesh; however, generalizations can be misleading. For example, whereas certain sects within Hinduism forbid the consumption of meat, perusing the menu at any Indian restaurant will reveal that many other Hindus regularly consume small quantities of meat, poultry, and fish. Many Buddhists are vegetarians, as are some Christians, including Seventh-Day Adventists.

vegetarianism The practice of restricting the diet to food substances of plant origin, including vegetables, fruits, grains, and nuts.

TABLE 6.4   Terms and Definitions of a Vegetarian Diet

Type of Diet	Foods Consumed	Comments
Semivegetarian (also called partial vegetarian or flexitarian)	Vegetables, grains, nuts, fruits, legumes; sometimes seafood, poultry, eggs, and dairy products	Typically exclude or limit red meat; may also avoid other meats
Pescovegetarian	Similar to semivegetarian but excludes poultry	*Pesco* means "fish," the only animal source of protein in this diet
Lacto-ovo-vegetarian	Vegetables, grains, nuts, fruits, legumes, dairy products (*lacto*), and eggs (*ovo*)	Excludes animal flesh and seafood
Lacto-vegetarian	Similar to lacto-ovo-vegetarian but excludes eggs	Relies on milk and cheese for animal sources of protein
Ovovegetarian	Vegetables, grains, nuts, fruits, legumes, and eggs	Excludes dairy, flesh, and seafood products
Vegan (also called strict vegetarian)	Only plant-based foods (vegetables, grains, nuts, seeds, fruits, legumes)	May not provide adequate vitamin B_{12}, zinc, iron, or calcium
Macrobiotic diet	Vegan-type diet; becomes progressively more strict until almost all foods are eliminated; at the extreme, only brown rice and small amounts of water or herbal tea	Taken to the extreme, can cause malnutrition and death
Fruitarian	Only raw or dried fruit, seeds, nuts, honey, and vegetable oil	Very restrictive diet; deficient in protein, calcium, zinc, iron, vitamin B_{12}, riboflavin, and other nutrients

Many vegetarians are guided by their personal philosophy to choose vegetarianism. These people feel that it is morally and ethically wrong to consume animals and any products from animals (such as dairy or egg products), usually because they view the practices in the modern animal industries as inhumane. They may consume milk and eggs but choose to purchase them only from family farms where animals are treated humanely.

There is also a great deal of concern about meat handling practices because contaminated meat has occasionally made its way into our food supply. For example, several outbreaks of severe illness, sometimes resulting in permanent disability and even death, have been traced to hamburgers served at fast-food restaurants as well as ground beef sold in markets and consumed at home. A concern surrounding beef is the potential for contracting the human variant of *mad cow disease*. (See the **Nutrition Myth or Fact?** box in Chapter 13 for a look at mad cow disease and its impact in the United States and other countries.)

Ecological Benefits

Many people choose vegetarianism because of their concerns about the effect of meat production on the global environment. Due to the high demand for meat in developed nations, meat production has evolved from small family farming operations to the larger system of agribusiness. Critics point to the environmental costs of agribusiness, including massive uses of water and grain to feed animals, methane gases and other wastes produced by animals themselves, and deforestation for land use to support livestock. For an in-depth discussion of this complex and often emotionally charged topic, refer to the **Nutrition Debate** at the end of this chapter.

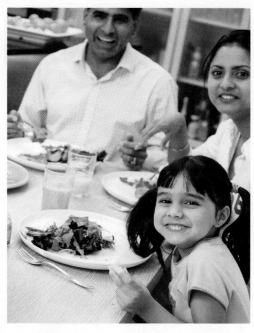

People who follow certain sects of Hinduism refrain from eating meat.

Health Benefits

Still others practice vegetarianism because of its health benefits. Research over several years has consistently shown that a varied and balanced vegetarian diet can reduce the risk for many chronic diseases. Health benefits of a vegetarian diet include:[16]

- Reduced intake of fat and total energy, which reduces the risk for obesity. This may in turn lower a person's risk for type 2 diabetes.
- Lower blood pressure, which may be due to a higher intake of fruits and vegetables. People who eat vegetarian diets tend to be nonsmokers, to drink little or no alcohol, and to exercise more regularly, which are also factors known to reduce blood pressure and help maintain a healthy body weight.

If you're interested in trying a vegetarian diet but don't know where to begin, check out the website of the Physicians Committee for Responsible Medicine at www.pcrm.org. Click on the Health and Nutrition button, and then scroll down the left-side margin until you see "Free Vegetarian Starter Kit." Open it up and get started!

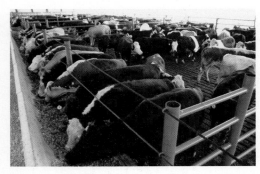

(a)

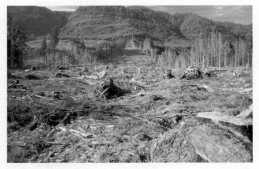

(b)

⬆ Some people choose vegetarianism out of concern for the environmental effects of meat production. For example, livestock production (a) and aggressive deforestation that clears land for grazing (b) both contribute to increased greenhouse gas emissions.

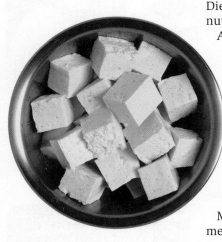

⬆ Vegetarians should eat two to three servings of beans, nuts, seeds, eggs, or meat substitutes (such as tofu) daily.

- Reduced risk for heart disease, which may be due to lower saturated fat intake and a higher consumption of *antioxidants,* substances that can protect our cells from damage. They are abundant in fruits and vegetables. (Antioxidants are discussed in detail in Chapter 8.)
- Fewer digestive problems such as constipation and diverticular disease, perhaps due to the higher fiber content of vegetarian diets.
- Reduced risk for some cancers. Research shows that vegetarians may have lower rates of cancer, particularly colon cancer. Many components of a vegetarian diet could contribute to reducing cancer risks, including higher fiber, no intake of red meats and processed meats (which increase the risk for colorectal cancer), and lower consumption of *carcinogens* (cancer-causing agents) that are formed when cooking meats.[17]
- Reduced risk for kidney disease, kidney stones, and gallstones. The lower protein contents of vegetarian diets, plus the higher intake of legumes and vegetable proteins such as soy, may be protective against these conditions.

What Are the Challenges of a Vegetarian Diet?

Although a vegetarian diet can be healthful, it also presents some challenges. Limiting the consumption of flesh and dairy products introduces the potential for inadequate intakes of certain nutrients, especially for people consuming a vegan, macrobiotic, or fruitarian diet. **TABLE 6.5** lists the nutrients that can be deficient in a vegan type of diet plan and describes good non-animal sources that can provide these nutrients. Vegetarians who consume dairy and/or egg products obtain these nutrients more easily.

Some female athletes at risk for disordered eating switch to a vegetarian diet.[18] As noted earlier, a balanced vegetarian diet can have significant health benefits; however, instead of eating a healthy variety of non-animal foods, people with disordered eating problems may use vegetarianism as an excuse to restrict many foods from their diets. Experts suggest that the possibility of disordered eating should be considered if the switch to a vegetarian diet is accompanied by unnecessary weight loss.[18]

Can a vegetarian diet provide enough protein? Because high-quality non-meat protein sources are quite easy to obtain in developed countries, a balanced vegetarian diet can provide adequate protein. In fact, the American Dietetic Association endorses an appropriately planned vegetarian diet as healthful, nutritionally adequate, and beneficial in reducing and preventing various diseases.[16] As you can see, the emphasis is on a *balanced* and *adequate* vegetarian diet; thus, it is important for vegetarians to consume soy products, eat complementary proteins, and obtain enough energy from other macronutrients to spare protein from being used as an energy source. Although the digestibility of a vegetarian diet is potentially lower than that of an animal-based diet, there is no separate protein recommendation for vegetarians who consume complementary plant proteins.[19]

Using MyPlate on a Vegetarian Diet

Although the USDA has not designed a version of MyPlate specifically for people following a vegetarian diet, healthy eating tips for vegetarians are available at MyPlate online (see **Web Resources** at the end of this chapter). For example, to meet their needs for protein and calcium, lacto-vegetarians can consume low-fat or nonfat dairy products. Vegans and ovovegetarians can consume calcium-fortified soy milk or one of the many protein bars fortified with calcium.

Vegans need to consume vitamin B$_{12}$ either from fortified foods or supplements because this vitamin is found naturally only in animal foods. They should also pay

TABLE 6.5   Nutrients of Concern in a Vegan Diet

Nutrient	Functions	Non-Meat/Non-Dairy Food Sources
Vitamin B_{12}	Assists with DNA synthesis; protection and growth of nerve fibers	Vitamin B_{12}–fortified cereals, yeast, soy products, and other meat analogs; vitamin B_{12} supplements
Vitamin D	Promotes bone growth	Vitamin D–fortified cereals, margarines, and soy products; adequate exposure to sunlight; supplementation may be necessary for those who do not get adequate exposure to sunlight
Riboflavin (vitamin B_2)	Promotes release of energy; supports normal vision and skin health	Whole and enriched grains, green leafy vegetables, mushrooms, beans, nuts, and seeds
Iron	Assists with oxygen transport; involved in making amino acids and hormones	Whole-grain products, prune juice, dried fruits, beans, nuts, seeds, and leafy vegetables (such as spinach)
Calcium	Maintains bone health; assists with muscle contraction, blood pressure, and nerve transmission	Fortified soy milk and tofu, almonds, dry beans, leafy vegetables, calcium-fortified juices, and fortified breakfast cereals
Zinc	Assists with DNA and RNA synthesis, immune function, and growth	Whole-grain products, wheat germ, beans, nuts, and seeds

special attention to consuming foods high in vitamin D, riboflavin (B$_2$), and the minerals zinc and iron. Supplementation of these micronutrients may be necessary for some people if they do not consume adequate amounts in their diet.

recap A balanced vegetarian diet may reduce the risk for obesity, type 2 diabetes, heart disease, digestive problems, some cancers, kidney disease, kidney stones, and gallstones. Whereas varied vegetarian diets can provide enough protein, vegetarians who consume no animal products need to make sure they consume adequate plant sources of protein and supplement their diet with good sources of vitamin B_{12}, vitamin D, riboflavin, iron, calcium, and zinc.

What disorders are related to protein intake or metabolism?

Consuming inadequate protein can result in severe illness and death. Typically, this occurs when people do not consume enough total energy, but a diet deficient specifically in protein can have similar effects.

The Vegetarian Resource Group offers a colorful, downloadable vegan MyPlate poster. Go to www.vrg.org, then click on "My Vegan Plate full color handout."

nutri-case | THEO

"No way would I ever become a vegetarian! The only way to build up muscle is to eat meat. I read in a bodybuilding magazine about some guy who doesn't eat anything from animals, not even milk or eggs, and he did look pretty buff . . . but I don't buy it. They can do anything to pictures these days. Besides, after a game I just crave red meat. If I don't have it, I feel sort of like my batteries don't get recharged. It's just not natural for a competitive athlete to go without meat!"

What claims does Theo make here about the role of red meat in his diet? Do you think his claims are valid? Why or why not? Without trying to convert Theo to vegetarianism, what facts might you offer him about the nature of plant and animal proteins?

Protein-Energy Malnutrition Can Lead to Debility and Death

When a person consumes too little protein and energy, the result is **protein-energy malnutrition** (also called *protein-Calorie malnutrition*). Two diseases that can follow are marasmus and kwashiorkor (**FIGURE 6.13**).

Marasmus Results from Grossly Inadequate Energy Intake

Marasmus is a disease that results from a grossly inadequate intake of total energy, especially protein. Essentially, marasmus is starvation. It is most common in young children (6 to 18 months of age) living in impoverished conditions who are severely undernourished. For example, the children may be fed diluted cereal drinks that are inadequate in energy, protein, and most nutrients.

People suffering from marasmus have a look of "skin and bones" because their body fat and tissues are wasting. The consequences of marasmus include:

- Wasting and weakening of muscles, including the heart muscle
- Stunted brain development and learning impairment
- Depressed metabolism and little insulation from body fat, causing a dangerously low body temperature
- Stunted physical growth and development
- Deterioration of the intestinal lining, which further inhibits the absorption of nutrients
- *Anemia* (abnormally low levels of hemoglobin in the blood)
- Severely weakened immune system
- Fluid and electrolyte imbalances

If marasmus is left untreated, death from dehydration, heart failure, or infection will result. Treatment begins with careful correction of fluid and electrolyte imbalances. Protein and carbohydrates are provided once the body's condition has stabilized. Fat is introduced much later because the protein levels in the blood must improve to the point at which the body can use them to carry fat so that it can be safely metabolized by the body.

Kwashiorkor Results from a Low-Protein Diet

Kwashiorkor often occurs in developing countries where infants are weaned early due to the arrival of a subsequent baby. This deficiency disease is typically seen in young

protein-energy malnutrition A disorder caused by inadequate consumption of protein. It is characterized by severe wasting.

marasmus A form of protein-energy malnutrition that results from grossly inadequate intake of energy and protein and other nutrients and is characterized by extreme tissue wasting and stunted growth and development.

kwashiorkor A form of protein-energy malnutrition that is typically seen in malnourished infants and toddlers and is characterized by wasting, edema, and other signs of protein deficiency.

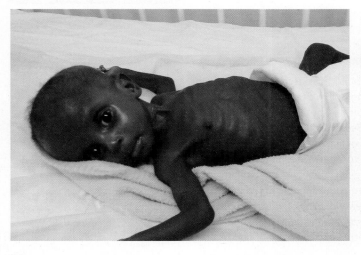

(a)

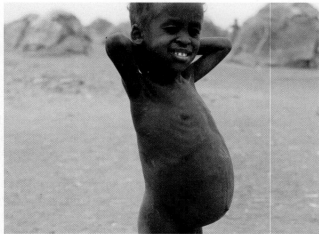

(b)

▲ **FIGURE 6.13** Two forms of protein-energy malnutrition: **(a)** marasmus and **(b)** kwashiorkor.

children (1 to 3 years of age) who no longer drink breast milk. Instead, they often are fed a low-protein, starchy cereal. Recent research suggests that dysfunctional GI bacteria combined with a low-protein diet interact to contribute to the development of kwashiorkor.[20] Unlike marasmus, kwashiorkor often develops quickly and causes the person to look swollen, particularly in the belly. This is because the low protein content of the blood is inadequate to keep fluids from seeping into the tissue spaces. These are other symptoms of kwashiorkor:

- Some weight loss and muscle wasting, with some retention of body fat
- Retarded growth and development but less severe than that seen with marasmus
- Edema, which results over time in extreme distention of the belly and is caused by fluid and electrolyte imbalances
- Fatty degeneration of the liver
- Loss of appetite, sadness, irritability, apathy
- Development of sores and other skin problems; skin pigmentation changes
- Dry, brittle hair that changes color, straightens, and falls out easily

Kwashiorkor can be reversed if adequate protein and energy are given in time. Because of their severely weakened immune systems, many individuals with kwashiorkor die from infectious diseases they contract in their weakened state. Of those who are treated, many return home to the same impoverished conditions, only to develop this deficiency once again.

Although children in developing countries are at highest risk for these diseases, protein-energy malnutrition occurs in all countries and affects both children and adults. In the United States, poor people living in inner cities and isolated rural areas are especially affected. Others at risk include the elderly, the homeless, people with eating disorders, those addicted to alcohol and other drugs, and individuals with wasting diseases, such as AIDS or cancer.

Disorders Related to Genetic Abnormalities

Numerous disorders are caused by defective DNA. These genetic disorders include *phenylketonuria* (PKU), sickle cell anemia, and cystic fibrosis.

As previously discussed, *phenylketonuria* is an inherited disease in which a person does not have the ability to break down the amino acid phenylalanine. As a result, phenylalanine and its metabolic by-products build up in tissues and can cause brain damage. Individuals with PKU must eat a diet that is severely limited in phenylalanine.

Sickle cell anemia is an inherited disorder of the red blood cells in which a single amino acid present in hemoglobin is changed. As shown in Figure 6.7, normal hemoglobin is globular, giving red blood cells a round, doughnut-like shape. Red blood cells do not have a nucleus; this allows them to easily change shape and ensure they can fit through various blood vessels in our bodies. The genetic alteration that occurs with sickle cell anemia causes the red blood cells to be shaped like a sickle or a crescent **(FIGURE 6.14)**. Because sickled red blood cells are stiff and sticky, they cannot flow smoothly through the smallest blood vessels. Instead, they block the vessels, depriving nearby tissues of their oxygen supply and eventually damaging vulnerable organs, particularly the spleen. Sickled cells also have a life span of only about 10 to 20 days, as opposed to the 120-day average for globular red blood cells. The body's greatly increased demand for new red blood cells leads to severe anemia. Other signs and symptoms of sickle cell anemia include impaired vision, headaches, convulsions, bone degeneration, and decreased function of various organs. This disease occurs in any person who inherits the sickle cell gene from both parents.

Cystic fibrosis is an inherited disease that primarily affects the respiratory system and digestive tract. It is caused by a defective gene that causes cells to build and then reject an abnormal version of a protein that, formed normally, would allow the passage of chloride into and out of certain cells. This alteration in chloride transport causes cells to secrete thick, sticky mucus. The linings of the lungs and pancreas are particularly affected, causing breathing difficulties, lung infections, and digestion

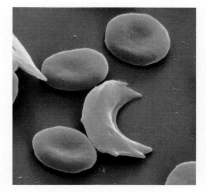

FIGURE 6.14 A sickled red blood cell.

sickle cell anemia A genetic disorder that causes red blood cells to be shaped like a sickle or crescent, impeding their transport to body tissues.

cystic fibrosis A genetic disorder that causes an alteration in chloride transport, leading to the production of thick, sticky mucus that causes life-threatening respiratory and digestive problems.

problems that lead to nutrient deficiencies. Symptoms include wheezing, coughing, and stunted growth. The severity of this disease varies greatly; some individuals with cystic fibrosis live relatively normal lives, whereas others are seriously debilitated and die in childhood.

recap Protein-energy malnutrition can lead to marasmus and kwashiorkor. These diseases primarily affect impoverished children in developing nations. However, residents of developed countries are also at risk, especially the elderly, the homeless, people struggling with substance abuse, and people with AIDS, cancer, and other wasting diseases. Genetic disorders involving abnormal proteins include phenylketonuria, sickle cell anemia, and cystic fibrosis.

*behavior change ... getting started!

Now that you've read this chapter, try making these changes:

For yourself:

- Try adding soy milk to your breakfast cereal.
- Make it a goal today to consume meals that provide adequate protein from sources low in saturated fats and cholesterol, such as fish, poultry without the skin, lean beef, egg whites, legumes, nuts and nut butters, and tofu.
- If you eat meat daily, try replacing one or two of your meat choices during the next week with a meat substitute, such as quorn, veggie burgers/sausages, or tofu.

For your community:

- Encourage the manager of your campus dining hall to support the Meatless Monday campaign (see **Web Resources** for a link to its website).
- Work with your friends to raise funds for an international hunger-relief agency. Check out options at www.charitynavigator.org.

Meat Consumption and Climate Change: Tofu to the Rescue?

Which causes more greenhouse gas emissions: livestock production or traffic? The answer may surprise you: according to the Food and Agriculture Organization of the United Nations (FAO), livestock production generates more of the gases responsible for global warming—18%—than transportation.[21] In a landmark 2006 report called *Livestock's Long Shadow*, the FAO estimated that livestock production accounts for the emission of

- 9% of all carbon dioxide (CO_2) production derived from human activity
- 37% of all human-induced methane
- 64% of ammonia, and
- 65% of human-related nitrous oxide.

The report generated considerable concern internationally. For example, in 2008, Dr. Rajendra Pachauri, chair of the United Nations Intergovernmental Panel on Climate Change, released a statement calling upon individuals to have one meat-free day a week and to progressively reduce their meat consumption even further.[22] Pachauri noted that reducing meat consumption is an action that anyone can take immediately, and one that can have a significant impact on climate change in a short period.

In addition to being a major source of greenhouse gas emissions, livestock production contributes to land degradation, using 30% of the earth's land surface for pasture or feed production. Aggressive deforestation has cleared about 70% of former forests in the Amazon region for grazing.[21] This loss of plant mass reduces the capture of greenhouse gases because plants use carbon dioxide to synthesize glucose. In addition, the production of feed crops for livestock uses 33% of global arable land. Livestock's presence in vast tracts of land and its demand for feed crops also have contributed significantly to a reduction in biodiversity and a decline in ecosystems.[21]

Another environmental concern is the effect of livestock production on the global water supply. The Water Footprint Network project explains that, whereas the production of a soy burger requires an investment of about 150 liters of water, the production of a beef burger of the same size requires 1,000 liters.[23] Moreover, animal waste, antibiotics, hormones, and fertilizers and pesticides used on feed crops can run off into neighboring streams, rivers, and lakes and into nearly irrigation fields used to produce crops for human consumption.

In response to many of these claims of environmental degradation due to livestock production, the Cattlemen's Beef Board and National Cattlemen's Beef Association website disputes many of the claims made by

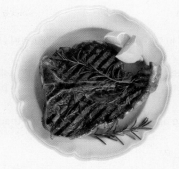

(a)

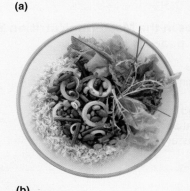

(b)

The difference in greenhouse gas emissions associated with (a) meat-based meals versus (b) vegetarian meals is similar to the difference between driving a large SUV and driving an average sedan.

environmental impact scientific experts and critics. They state the following:[24]

- The waste produced by cattle is very minor, accounting for only 2.6% of the country's greenhouse gas emissions, compared to 25% for transportation.
- Approximately 85% of all land is not suitable for growing vegetable or grain crops. Double the land area can be used to produce food by grazing animals on this land.
- Beef production is significantly more environmentally sustainable than 30 years ago. As compared to 1977, each pound of beef today produces 18% less carbon emissions, takes 30% less land, and requires 14% less water.

Although some people choose vegetarianism to protect the environment, it is not practical or realistic to expect every human around the world to adopt this lifestyle. Animal products provide important nutrients, and many people on the brink of starvation cannot survive without small amounts of milk and meat.

Still, if people were to reduce their consumption of meat even modestly, the change would have a powerful collective impact. The Environmental Working Group found that, if every American ate only plant foods just 1 day a week, the reduction in greenhouse gas emissions would be the equivalent of taking 7.6 million cars off the road.[25] If we were to reduce our intake more significantly, we could return to the system of small family farming, which is more environmentally friendly. When animals are raised on smaller farms and/or allowed to range freely, they consume grass, crop wastes, and scraps recycled from the kitchen, which is an efficient means of utilizing food sources that humans do not consume. What's more, the waste produced by these animals can be used for fertilizer and fuel.

CRITICAL THINKING QUESTIONS

1. Given the accelerated pace of climate change, as well as land and water degradation, is it our ethical responsibility as citizens of the planet to reduce our meat consumption?
2. What adverse impacts might reducing meat consumption have on farmers and ranchers? Would this be greater or worse than the impacts of climate change?
3. Would eating less meat be practical for you? What other actions could you take to reduce the "carbon footprint" of your diet?

chapter **review**

test yourself | answers

1. **False.** Although protein can be used for energy in certain circumstances, fats and carbohydrates are the primary sources of energy for our bodies.

2. **False.** Vegetarian diets can meet and even exceed an individual's protein needs, assuming that adequate energy-yielding macronutrients, a variety of protein sources, and complementary protein sources are consumed.

3. **True.** Most people in the United States consume up to two times more protein than they need.

MasteringNutrition™

Check out these additional resources in the MasteringNutrition Study Area at www.masteringhealthandnutrition.pearson.com:

- Read It: Chapter Summary and RSS Feeds
- See It: ABC News videos and nutrition animations
- Hear It: MP3s
- Study It: Get Ready for Nutrition Math and Chemistry review
- Do It: NutriTools and "Find the Quack" feature
- Review It: Quizzes, flashcards, and glossary

review questions

1. Proteins contain
   a. carbon, nitrogen, and aluminum.
   b. hydrogen, oxygen, and sulfur.
   c. hydrogen, carbon, oxygen, and nitrogen.
   d. helium, carbon, oxygen, and ammonia.

2. Which of the following statements about protein synthesis is true?
   a. Protein synthesis occurs in the nucleus of the cell.
   b. Messenger RNA carries amino acids to ribosomes for assembly into proteins.
   c. In the process of transcription, transfer RNA transfers its DNA onto a ribosome.
   d. None of the above is true.

3. The process of combining peanut butter and whole-wheat bread to make a complete protein is called
   a. deamination.
   b. vegetarianism.
   c. transamination.
   d. mutual supplementation.

4. Proteins in the blood
   a. exert pressure that draws fluid out of tissue spaces, preventing edema.
   b. can bind to excessive hydrogen ions, preventing alkalosis.
   c. can be converted to urea, which can then be used as energy.
   d. all of the above.

5. The enzyme that helps break down polypeptides in the small intestine is called
   a. hydrochloric acid.
   b. pepsin.
   c. protease.
   d. bile.

6. Which of the following statements about the RDA for protein is true?
   a. Vegetarian athletes typically require about three times as much protein as nonvegetarians who are not athletes.
   b. The RDA for protein is higher for men than for women.
   c. The RDA for protein is higher for children and adolescents than for adults.
   d. Most Americans eat about three times the RDA for protein.

7. Which of the following meals is typical of a vegan diet?
   a. rice, pinto beans, acorn squash, soy butter, and almond milk
   b. veggie dog, bun, and a banana blended with yogurt
   c. brown rice and green tea
   d. egg salad on whole-wheat toast, broccoli, carrot sticks, and soy milk

8. In treating protein-energy malnutrition, why is protein intake restored before feeding the patient fats?
   a. Protein is a more readily available source of energy than fats.
   b. Protein levels in the blood must be adequate to transport fat.
   c. Protein is made up of DNA, which directs the metabolism of fats.
   d. Protein is the primary component of bile, which is required to emulsify fats.

9. **True or false?** After leaving the small intestine, amino acids are transported to the liver and stored for later use.

10. **True or false?** When a protein is denatured, its shape is lost but its function is retained.

math review

11. Barry is concerned he is not eating enough protein. After reading this chapter, he recorded his diet each day for 1 week to calculate how much protein he is eating. Barry's average protein intake for the week is equal to 190 g, his body weight is 75 kg, and his daily energy intake averages 3,000 kcal. Based on your calculations, is Barry (a) meeting or exceeding the AMDR for protein and (b) meeting or exceeding the RDA for protein?

Answers to Review Questions and Math Review are located at the back of this text and in the MasteringNutrition Study Area.

web resources

www.eatright.org
Academy of Nutrition and Dietetics

Search for "vegetarian diets" to learn how to plan healthful meat-free meals.

www.fnic.nal.usda.gov
USDA Food and Nutrition Information Center

Click on "food consumption" in the left navigation bar to find a searchable database of the nutrient values of many foods.

www.who.int
World Health Organization Nutrition

Visit this site to find out more about the worldwide scope of protein–deficiency diseases and related topics, in their nutrition topics.

www.medlineplus.gov
MEDLINE Plus Health Information

Search for "sickle cell anemia" and "cystic fibrosis" to obtain additional information and resources and the latest developments for these inherited diseases.

www.vrg.org
The Vegetarian Resource Group

Visit this site for additional information on how to build a balanced vegetarian diet.

www.choosemyplate.gov
The USDA's MyPlate Website

The MyPlate website contains useful, healthy eating tips for vegetarians. Enter "vegetarian" in the search box, then enter "tips."

www.meatlessmonday.com
Meatless Monday Campaign

Find out how to start going meatless one day a week with this innovative campaign's website.

in depth
6.5

Vitamins and Minerals: Micronutrients with Macro Powers

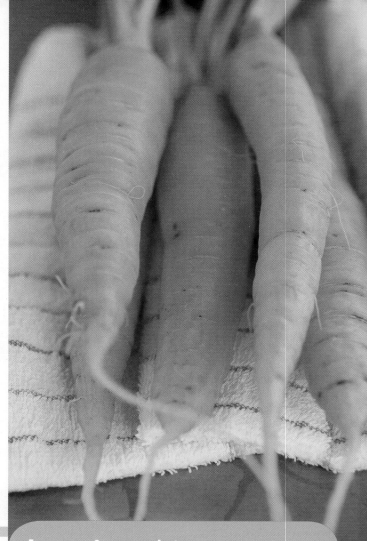

Have you heard about the college student on the junk-food diet who developed scurvy, a disease caused by inadequate intake of vitamin C? This urban legend seems to circulate on college campuses every year, but that may be because there's at least some truth behind it. Away from their families for the first time, many college students adopt diets that are deficient in one or more micronutrients. For instance, some students adopt a vegan diet that is low in iron, while others cut back on foods rich in calcium. Why is it important to consume adequate levels of micronutrients, and exactly what constitutes a micronutrient, anyway? This **In Depth** explores the discovery of micronutrients, their classification and naming, and their impact on our health.

Discovering the "hidden" nutrients

As you'll recall (from Chapter 1), there are three general classes of nutrients. Fluids provide water, which is essential for our survival and helps regulate many body functions. Macronutrients—which include carbohydrates, fats, and proteins—provide energy; thus, we need to consume them in relatively large amounts. **Micronutrients**, which include vitamins and minerals, are needed in much smaller amounts. They assist body functions such as energy metabolism and the formation and maintenance of healthy cells and tissues.

Much of our knowledge of vitamins and minerals comes from accidental observations of animals and humans. For instance, in the 1890s, a Dutch physician named C. Eijkman noticed that chickens fed polished rice developed paralysis, which could be reversed by feeding them whole-grain rice. Noting the high incidence of *beriberi*—a disease that results in extensive nerve damage—among hospital patients fed polished rice, Eijkman hypothesized that a highly refined diet was the primary cause of beriberi. We now know that whole-grain rice, with its nutrient-rich bran layer, contains the vitamin thiamin and that thiamin deficiency results in beriberi.

Similarly, in the early 1900s, it was observed that Japanese children living in fishing villages rarely developed a type of blindness common among Japanese children who did not eat fish. Experiments soon showed that cod liver oil, chicken liver, and eel fat prevented the disorder. We now know that each of these foods contains vitamin A, which is essential for healthy vision.

Such observations were followed by years of laboratory research before nutritionists came to fully accept the idea that very small amounts of substances present in food are critical to good health. In 1906, English scientist F. G. Hopkins coined the term *accessory factors* for those substances; we now call them vitamins and minerals.

How are vitamins classified?

Vitamins are organic compounds that regulate a wide range of body processes. Of the thirteen vitamins recognized as essential, humans can synthesize only small amounts of vitamins D and K, so we must consume virtually all of the vitamins in our diet. Most people who eat a varied and healthful diet can readily meet their vitamin needs from foods alone. The exceptions to this will be discussed shortly.

Fat-Soluble Vitamins

Vitamins A, D, E, and K are **fat-soluble vitamins** (TABLE 1 on page 226). They are found in the fatty portions of foods (butterfat, cod liver oil, corn oil, and so on) and are absorbed along with dietary fat. Fat-containing meats, dairy products, nuts, seeds, vegetable oils, and avocados are all sources of one or more fat-soluble vitamins.

In general, the fat-soluble vitamins are readily stored in the body's adipose tissue; thus, we don't need to consume them every day. While this may simplify day-to-day menu planning, there is also a disadvantage to our ability to store these nutrients. When we consume more of them than we can use, they build up in the adipose tissue, liver, and other tissues and can reach toxic levels. Symptoms of fat-soluble vitamin toxicity, described in Table 1, include damage to our hair, skin, bones, eyes, and nervous system. Overconsumption of vitamin supplements is the most common cause of vitamin toxicity in the United States; rarely do our food choices lead to toxicity. Of the four fat-soluble vitamins, vitamins A and D are the most toxic; **megadosing** with ten or more times the recommended intake of either can result in irreversible organ damage and even death.

Even though we can store the fat-soluble vitamins, deficiencies can occur, especially in people who have a malabsorption disorder, such as celiac disease, that

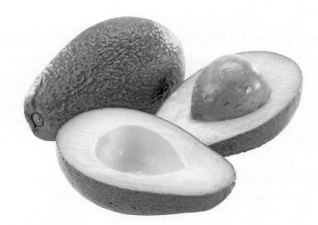

Avocados are a source of fat-soluble vitamins.

micronutrients Nutrients needed in the daily diet in relatively small amounts; vitamins and minerals are micronutrients.

vitamins Organic compounds that assist in regulating body processes.

fat-soluble vitamins Vitamins that are not soluble in water but are soluble in fat, including vitamins A, D, E, and K.

megadosing Consuming nutrients in amounts that are ten or more times higher than recommended levels.

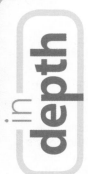

reduces their ability to absorb dietary fat. In addition, people who are "fat phobic," or eat very small amounts of dietary fat, are at risk for a deficiency. The consequences of fat-soluble vitamin deficiencies, described in Table 1, include osteoporosis, the loss of night vision, and even death in the most severe cases.

Water-Soluble Vitamins

Vitamin C (ascorbic acid) and the B-vitamins (thiamin, riboflavin, niacin, vitamin B_6, vitamin B_{12}, folate, pantothenic acid, and biotin) are all **water-soluble vitamins** (TABLE 2). They are found in a wide variety of foods, including whole grains, fruits, vegetables, meats, and dairy products. They are easily absorbed through the intestinal tract directly into the bloodstream, where they then travel to target cells.

With the exception of vitamin B_{12}, our bodies do not store large amounts of water-soluble vitamins. Instead, our kidneys filter from our bloodstream any excess

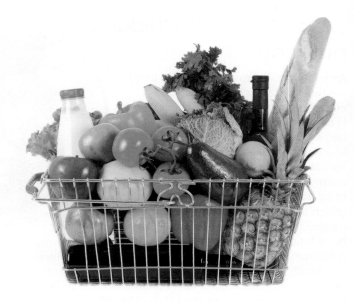

Water-soluble vitamins can be found in a variety of foods.

amounts, and they are excreted in urine. Because we do not maintain stores of these vitamins in our tissues, toxicity is rare. When it does occur, however, it is often from the overuse of high-potency vitamin supplements. Toxicity can cause nerve damage and skin lesions.

water-soluble vitamins Vitamins that are soluble in water, including vitamin C and the B-vitamins.

TABLE 1 Fat-Soluble Vitamins

Vitamin Name	Primary Functions	Recommended Intake*	Reliable Food Sources	Toxicity/Deficiency Symptoms
A (retinol, retinal, retinoic acid)	Required for ability of eyes to adjust to changes in light Protects color vision Assists cell differentiation Required for sperm production in men and fertilization in women Contributes to healthy bone Contributes to healthy immune system	RDA: Men: 900 µg Women: 700 µg UL: 3,000 µg/day	Preformed retinol: beef and chicken liver, egg yolks, milk Carotenoid precursors: spinach, carrots, mango, apricots, cantaloupe, pumpkin, yams	*Toxicity:* fatigue; bone and joint pain; spontaneous abortion and birth defects of fetuses in pregnant women; nausea and diarrhea; liver damage; nervous system damage; blurred vision; hair loss; skin disorders *Deficiency:* night blindness and xerophthalmia; impaired growth, immunity, and reproductive function
D (cholecalciferol)	Regulates blood calcium levels Maintains bone health Assists cell differentiation	RDA: Adult aged 19–70: 600 IU/day Adult aged >70: 800 IU/day UL: 4,000 IU/day	Canned salmon and mackerel, fortified milk and milk alternatives, fortified cereals	*Toxicity:* hypercalcemia *Deficiency:* rickets in children; osteomalacia and/or osteoporosis in adults
E (tocopherol)	As a powerful antioxidant, protects cell membranes, polyunsaturated fatty acids, and vitamin A from oxidation Protects white blood cells Enhances immune function Improves absorption of vitamin A	RDA: Men: 15 mg/day Women: 15 mg/day UL: 1,000 mg/day	Sunflower seeds, almonds, vegetable oils, fortified cereals	*Toxicity:* rare *Deficiency:* hemolytic anemia; impairment of nerve, muscle, and immune function
K (phylloquinone, menaquinone, menadione)	Serves as a coenzyme during production of specific proteins that assist in blood coagulation and bone metabolism	AI: Men: 120 µg/day Women: 90 µg/day	Kale, spinach, turnip greens, brussels sprouts	*Toxicity:* none known *Deficiency:* impaired blood clotting; possible effect on bone health

*Note: RDA, Recommended Dietary Allowance; UL, upper limit; AI, Adequate Intake.

TABLE 2 Water-Soluble Vitamins

Vitamin Name	Primary Functions	Recommended Intake[*]	Reliable Food Sources	Toxicity/Deficiency Symptoms
Thiamin (vitamin B$_1$)	Required as enzyme cofactor for carbohydrate and amino acid metabolism	RDA: Men: 1.2 mg/day Women: 1.1 mg/day	Pork, fortified cereals, enriched rice and pasta, peas, tuna, legumes	*Toxicity:* none known *Deficiency:* beriberi; fatigue, apathy, decreased memory, confusion, irritability, muscle weakness
Riboflavin (vitamin B$_2$)	Required as enzyme cofactor for carbohydrate and fat metabolism	RDA: Men: 1.3 mg/day Women: 1.1 mg/day	Beef liver, shrimp, milk and other dairy foods, fortified cereals, enriched breads and grains	*Toxicity:* none known *Deficiency:* ariboflavinosis; swollen mouth and throat; seborrheic dermatitis; anemia
Niacin, nicotinamide, nicotinic acid	Required for carbohydrate and fat metabolism Plays role in DNA replication and repair and cell differentiation	RDA: Men: 16 mg/day Women: 14 mg/day UL: 35 mg/day	Beef liver, most cuts of meat/fish/poultry, fortified cereals, enriched breads and grains, canned tomato products	*Toxicity:* flushing, liver damage, glucose intolerance, blurred vision differentiation *Deficiency:* pellagra; vomiting, constipation, or diarrhea; apathy
Pyridoxine, pyridoxal, pyridoxamine (vitamin B$_6$)	Required as enzyme cofactor for carbohydrate and amino acid metabolism Assists synthesis of blood cells	RDA: Men and women aged 19–50: 1.3 mg/day Men aged >50: 1.7 mg/day Women aged >50: 1.5 mg/day UL: 100 mg/day	Chickpeas (garbanzo beans), most cuts of meat/fish/poultry, fortified cereals, white potatoes	*Toxicity:* nerve damage, skin lesions *Deficiency:* anemia; seborrheic dermatitis; depression, confusion, and convulsions
Folate (folic acid)	Required as enzyme cofactor for amino acid metabolism Required for DNA synthesis Involved in metabolism of homocysteine	RDA: Men: 400 µg/day Women: 400 µg/day UL: 1,000 µg/day	Fortified cereals, enriched breads and grains, spinach, legumes (lentils, chickpeas, pinto beans), greens (spinach, romaine lettuce), liver	*Toxicity:* masks symptoms of vitamin B$_{12}$ deficiency, specifically signs of nerve damage *Deficiency:* macrocytic anemia; neural tube defects in a developing fetus; elevated homocysteine levels
Cobalamin (vitamin B$_{12}$)	Assists with formation of blood Required for healthy nervous system function Involved as enzyme cofactor in metabolism of homocysteine	RDA: Men: 2.4 µg/day Women: 2.4 µg/day	Shellfish, all cuts of meat/fish/poultry, milk and other dairy foods, fortified cereals and other fortified foods	*Toxicity:* none known *Deficiency:* pernicious anemia; tingling and numbness of extremities; nerve damage; memory loss, disorientation, and dementia
Pantothenic acid	Assists with fat metabolism	AI: Men: 5 mg/day Women: 5 mg/day	Meat/fish/poultry, shiitake mushrooms, fortified cereals, egg yolk	*Toxicity:* none known *Deficiency:* rare
Biotin	Involved as enzyme cofactor in carbohydrate, fat, and protein metabolism	RDA: Men: 30 µg/day Women: 30 µg/day	Nuts, egg yolk	*Toxicity:* none known *Deficiency:* rare
Ascorbic acid (vitamin C)	Antioxidant in extracellular fluid and lungs Regenerates oxidized vitamin E Assists with collagen synthesis Enhances immune function Assists in synthesis of hormones, neurotransmitters, and DNA Enhances iron absorption	RDA: Men: 90 mg/day Women: 75 mg/day Smokers: 35 mg more per day than RDA UL: 2,000 mg	Sweet peppers, citrus fruits and juices, broccoli, strawberries, kiwi	*Toxicity:* nausea and diarrhea, nosebleeds, increased oxidative damage, increased formation of kidney stones in people with kidney disease *Deficiency:* scurvy; bone pain and fractures, depression, and anemia

[*]*Note:* RDA, Recommended Dietary Allowance; UL, upper limit; AI, Adequate Intake.

Because most water-soluble vitamins are not stored in large amounts, they need to be consumed on a daily or weekly basis. Deficiency symptoms, including diseases or syndromes, can arise fairly quickly, especially during fetal development and in growing infants and children. The signs of water-soluble vitamin deficiency vary widely and are identified in Table 2.

Same Vitamin, Different Names and Forms

Food and supplement labels, magazine articles, and even nutrition textbooks such as this often use simplified alphabetic (A, D, E, K) names for the fat-soluble vitamins. The letters reflect their order of discovery: vitamin A was discovered in 1916, whereas vitamin K was not isolated until 1939. These lay terms, however, are more appropriately viewed as "umbrellas" that unify a small cluster of chemically related compounds. For example, the term *vitamin A* refers to the specific compounds retinol, retinal, and retinoic acid. Similarly, *vitamin E* occurs naturally in eight forms, known as tocopherols, of which the primary form is alpha-tocopherol. Compounds with *vitamin D* activity include cholecalciferol and ergocalciferol, and the *vitamin K* "umbrella" includes phylloquinone and menaquinone. As you can see, most of the individual compounds making up a fat-soluble vitamin cluster have similar chemical designations (tocopherols, calciferols, and so on). Table 1 lists both the alphabetic and chemical terms for the fat-soluble vitamins.

Similarly, there are both alphabetic and chemical designations for water-soluble vitamins. In some cases, such as *vitamin C* and *ascorbic acid*, you may be familiar with both terms. But few people would recognize *cobalamin* as designating the same micronutrient as *vitamin B$_{12}$*. Some of the water-soluble vitamins, such as niacin and vitamin B$_6$, mimic the "umbrella" clustering seen with vitamins A, E, D, and K: the term *vitamin B$_6$* includes pyridoxal, pyridoxine, and pyridoxamine. If you read any of these three terms on a supplement label, you'll know it refers to vitamin B$_6$.

Some vitamins exist in only one form. For example, thiamin is the only chemical compound known as *vitamin B$_1$*. There are no other related chemical compounds. Table 2 lists both the alphabetic and chemical terms for the water-soluble vitamins.

Because all vitamins are organic compounds, they are all more or less vulnerable to decay from exposure to heat, oxygen, or other factors. For tips

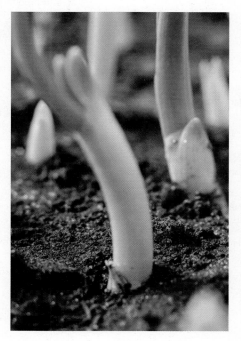

Plants absorb minerals from soil and water.

on preserving the vitamins in the foods you eat, see the **Quick Tips** box for details.

How are minerals classified?

Minerals—naturally occurring inorganic substances, such as calcium, iron, and zinc—are solid, crystalline substances that do not contain carbon. All minerals are elements; that is, they are already in the simplest chemical form possible, and the body does not digest or break them down prior to absorption. For the same reason, they cannot be degraded on exposure to heat or any other natural process, so the minerals in foods remain intact during storage and cooking. Furthermore, unlike vitamins, they cannot be

TABLE 3   Major Minerals

Mineral Name	Primary Functions	Recommended Intake*	Reliable Food Sources	Toxicity/Deficiency Symptoms
Sodium	Fluid balance Acid–base balance Transmission of nerve impulses Muscle contraction	AI: Adults: 1.5 g/day (1,500 mg/day)	Table salt, pickles, most canned soups, snack foods, cured luncheon meats, canned tomato products	*Toxicity:* water retention, high blood pressure, loss of calcium *Deficiency:* muscle cramps, dizziness, fatigue, nausea, vomiting, mental confusion
Potassium	Fluid balance Transmission of nerve impulses Muscle contraction	AI: Adults: 4.7 g/day (4,700 mg/day)	Most fresh fruits and vegetables: potatoes, bananas, tomato juice, orange juice, melons	*Toxicity:* muscle weakness, vomiting, irregular heartbeat *Deficiency:* muscle weakness, paralysis, mental confusion, irregular heartbeat
Phosphorus	Fluid balance Bone formation Component of ATP, which provides energy for our bodies	RDA: Adults: 700 mg/day	Milk/cheese/yogurt, soy milk and tofu, legumes (lentils, black beans), nuts (almonds, peanuts and peanut butter), poultry	*Toxicity:* muscle spasms, convulsions, low blood calcium *Deficiency:* muscle weakness, muscle damage, bone pain, dizziness
Chloride	Fluid balance Transmission of nerve impulses Component of stomach acid (HCl) Antibacterial	AI: Adults: 2.3 g/day (2,300 mg/day)	Table salt	*Toxicity:* none known *Deficiency:* dangerous blood acid–base imbalances, irregular heartbeat
Calcium	Primary component of bone Acid–base balance Transmission of nerve impulses Muscle contraction	RDA: Adults aged 19 to 50 and men aged 51–70: 1,000 mg/day Women aged 51–70 and adults aged >70: 1,200 mg/day UL for adults 19–50: 2,500 mg/day UL for adults aged 51 and above: 2,000 mg/day	Milk/yogurt/cheese (best-absorbed form of calcium), sardines, collard greens and spinach, calcium-fortified juices and milk alternatives	*Toxicity:* mineral imbalances, shock, kidney failure, fatigue, mental confusion *Deficiency:* osteoporosis, convulsions, heart failure
Magnesium	Component of bone Muscle contraction Assists more than 300 enzyme systems	RDA: Men aged 19–30: 400 mg/day Men aged >30: 420 mg/day Women aged 19–30: 310 mg/day Women aged >30: 320 mg/day UL: 350 mg/day	Greens (spinach, kale, collard greens), whole grains, seeds, nuts, legumes (navy and black beans)	*Toxicity:* none known *Deficiency:* low blood calcium, muscle spasms or seizures, nausea, weakness, increased risk for chronic diseases, such as heart disease, hypertension, osteoporosis, and type 2 diabetes
Sulfur	Component of certain B-vitamins and amino acids Acid–base balance Detoxification in liver	No DRI	Protein-rich foods	*Toxicity:* none known *Deficiency:* none known

Note: RDA, Recommended Dietary Allowance; UL, upper limit; AI, Adequate Intake; DRI, Dietary Reference Intake.

synthesized in the laboratory or by any plant or animal, including humans. Minerals are the same wherever they are found—in soil, a car part, or the human body. The minerals in our foods ultimately come from the environment; for example, the selenium in soil and water is taken up into plants and then incorporated into the animals that eat the plants. Whether humans eat the plant foods directly or eat the animal products, all of the minerals in our food supply originate from Mother Earth!

Major Minerals

Major minerals are those the body requires in amounts of at least 100 mg per day. In addition, these minerals are found in the human body in amounts of 5 g (5,000 mg) or higher. There are seven major minerals: sodium, potassium, phosphorus, chloride, calcium, magnesium, and sulfur. **TABLE 3** summarizes the primary functions, recommended intakes, food sources, and toxicity/deficiency symptoms of these minerals.

minerals Inorganic substances that are not broken down during digestion or absorption; they assist in regulating body processes.

major minerals Minerals that must be consumed in amounts of 100 mg/day or more and that are present in the body at the level of 5 g or more.

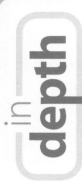
Trace Minerals

Trace minerals are those we need to consume in amounts of less than 100 mg per day. They are found in the human body in amounts of less than 5 g (5,000 mg). Currently, the Dietary Reference Intake (DRI) Committee recognizes eight trace minerals as essential for human health: selenium, fluoride, iodine, chromium, manganese, iron, zinc, and copper.[1] **TABLE 4** identifies the primary functions, recommended intakes, food sources, and toxicity/deficiency symptoms of these minerals.

Same Mineral, Different Forms

Unlike most vitamins, which can be identified by either alphabetic designations or the more complicated chemical

trace minerals Minerals that must be consumed in amounts of less than 100 mg/day and that are present in the body at the level of less than 5 g.

TABLE 4 Trace Minerals

Mineral Name	Primary Functions	Recommended Intake*	Reliable Food Sources	Toxicity/Deficiency Symptoms
Selenium	Required for carbohydrate and fat metabolism	RDA: Adults: 55 µg/day UL: 400 µg/day	Nuts, shellfish, meat/fish/poultry, whole grains	*Toxicity:* brittle hair and nails, skin rashes, nausea and vomiting, weakness, liver disease *Deficiency:* specific forms of heart disease and arthritis, impaired immune function, muscle pain and wasting, depression, hostility
Fluoride	Development and maintenance of healthy teeth and bones	RDA: Men: 4 mg/day Women: 3 mg/day UL: 2.2 mg/day for children aged 4–8; 10 mg/day for children aged >8	Fish, seafood, legumes, whole grains, drinking water (variable)	*Toxicity:* fluorosis of teeth and bones *Deficiency:* dental caries, low bone density
Iodine	Synthesis of thyroid hormones Temperature regulation Reproduction and growth	RDA: Adults: 150 µg/day UL: 1,100 µg/day	Iodized salt, saltwater seafood	*Toxicity:* goiter *Deficiency:* goiter, hypothyroidism, cretinism in infant of mother who is iodine deficient
Chromium	Glucose transport Metabolism of DNA and RNA Immune function and growth	AI: Men aged 19–50: 35 µg/day Men aged >50: 30 µg/day Women aged 19–50: 25 µg/day Women aged >50: 20 µg/day	Whole grains, brewer's yeast	*Toxicity:* none known *Deficiency:* elevated blood glucose and blood lipids, damage to brain and nervous system
Manganese	Assists many enzyme systems Synthesis of protein found in bone and cartilage	AI: Men: 2.3 mg/day Women: 1.8 mg/day UL: 11 mg/day for adults	Whole grains, nuts, leafy vegetables, tea	*Toxicity:* impairment of neuromuscular system *Deficiency:* impaired growth and reproductive function, reduced bone density, impaired glucose and lipid metabolism, skin rash
Iron	Component of hemoglobin in blood cells Component of myoglobin in muscle cells Assists many enzyme systems	RDA: Adult men: 8 mg/day Women aged 19–50: 18 mg/day Women aged >50: 8 mg/day	Meat/fish/poultry (best-absorbed form of iron), fortified cereals, legumes, spinach	*Toxicity:* nausea, vomiting, and diarrhea; dizziness, confusion; rapid heartbeat, organ damage, death *Deficiency:* iron-deficiency microcytic (small red blood cells), hypochromic anemia
Zinc	Assists more than 100 enzyme systems Immune system function Growth and sexual maturation Gene regulation	RDA: Men: 11 mg/day Women: 8 mg/day UL: 40 mg/day	Meat/fish/poultry (best-absorbed form of zinc), fortified cereals, legumes	*Toxicity:* nausea, vomiting, and diarrhea; headaches, depressed immune function, reduced absorption of copper *Deficiency:* growth retardation, delayed sexual maturation, eye and skin lesions, hair loss, increased incidence of illness and infection
Copper	Assists many enzyme systems Iron transport	RDA: Adults: 900 µg/day UL: 10 mg/day	Shellfish, organ meats, nuts, legumes	*Toxicity:* nausea, vomiting, and diarrhea; liver damage *Deficiency:* anemia, reduced levels of white blood cells, osteoporosis in infants and growing children

*Note: RDA, Recommended Dietary Allowance; UL, upper limit; AI, Adequate Intake.

terms, minerals are known by one name only. Iron, calcium, sodium, and all other minerals are simply referred to by their chemical name. That said, minerals do often exist within different chemical compounds; for example, a supplement label might identify calcium as calcium lactate, calcium gluconate, or calcium citrate. As we will discuss shortly, these different chemical compounds, although all containing the same elemental mineral, may differ in their ability to be absorbed by the body.

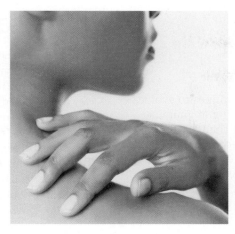
Minerals help maintain healthy skin and nails.

How do our bodies use micronutrients?

Our bodies must alter the composition of food in order to utilize the vitamins and minerals it contains. This is because the micronutrients found in foods and supplements are not always in a chemical form that can be readily used. This discussion will highlight some of the ways in which our bodies modify the food forms of vitamins and minerals in order to maximize their absorption and utilization.

What We Eat Differs from What We Absorb

The most healthful diet is of no value to our bodies unless the nutrients can be absorbed and transported to the cells that need them. Unlike carbohydrates, fats, and proteins, which are efficiently absorbed (85–99% of what is eaten makes it into the blood), some micronutrients are so poorly absorbed that only 3% to 10% of what is eaten ever enters the bloodstream.

The absorption of many vitamins and minerals depends on their chemical form. Dietary iron, for example, can be in the form of *heme iron* (found only in meats, fish, and poultry) or *non-heme iron* (found in plant and animal foods, as well as iron-fortified foods and supplements). Healthy adults absorb about 25% of heme iron but as little as 3% to 5% of non-heme iron.

In addition, the presence of other factors within the same food influences mineral absorption. For example, approximately 30% to 45% of the calcium found in milk and dairy products is absorbed, but the calcium in spinach, Swiss chard, seeds, and nuts is absorbed at a much lower rate

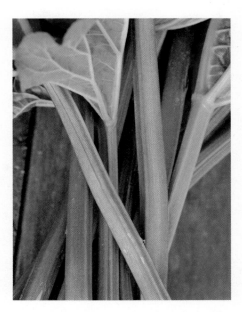
Foods high in oxalic acid, such as rhubarb, can decrease zinc and iron absorption.

because factors in these foods bind the calcium and prevent its absorption. Non-heme iron, zinc, vitamin E, and vitamin B_6 are other micronutrients whose absorption can be reduced by various binding factors in foods.

The absorption of many vitamins and minerals is also influenced by other foods within the meal. For example, the fat-soluble vitamins are much better absorbed when the meal contains some dietary fat. Calcium absorption is increased by the presence of lactose, found in milk, and non-heme iron absorption can be doubled if the meal includes vitamin C–rich foods, such as red peppers, oranges, or tomatoes. On the other hand, high-fiber foods, such as whole grains, and foods high in oxalic acid, such as tea, spinach, and rhubarb, can decrease the absorption of zinc and iron.

Finally, the absorption of micronutrients varies according to range of factors such as our age, and how much we consume of a given micronutrient throughout the day or at any one time. It may seem an impossible task to correctly balance your food choices to optimize micronutrient absorption, but the best approach, as always, is to eat a variety of healthful foods every day.

What We Eat Differs from What Our Cells Use

Many vitamins undergo one or more chemical transformations after they are eaten and absorbed into our bodies. For example, before they can go to work for our bodies, the B-vitamins must combine with other substances. For thiamin and vitamin B_6, a phosphate group is added. Vitamin D is another example: before cells can use it, the food form of vitamin D must have two hydroxyl (OH) groups added to its structure. These transformations activate the vitamin; because they don't occur randomly, but only when the active vitamin is needed, they help the body maintain control over its metabolic pathways.

Although the basic nature of minerals does not change, they can undergo minor modifications that change their atomic structure. Iron (Fe) may alternate between Fe^{2+} (ferrous) and Fe^{3+} (ferric); copper (Cu) may exist as Cu^{1+} or Cu^{2+}. These are just two examples of how the body modifies micronutrients to help the body make the best use of them.

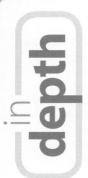

Controversies in micronutrient metabolism

The science of nutrition continues to evolve, and our current understanding of vitamins and minerals will no doubt change over the next several years or decades. Although some people interpret the term *controversy* in negative terms, nutrition controversies are exciting developments, proof of new information, and a sign of continued growth in the field.

Are Supplements Healthful Sources of Micronutrients?

For millions of years, humans relied solely on natural foodstuffs as their source of nutrients. Only within the past 60 years or so has a second option become available: nutrient supplements, including those added to fortified foods. Are the micronutrients in supplements any better or worse than those in foods? Do our bodies use the nutrients from these two sources any differently? These are issues that nutrition scientists and consumers continue to discuss.

As previously noted, the availability, or "usefulness," of micronutrients in foods depends in part on the food itself. The iron and calcium in spinach are poorly absorbed, whereas the iron in beef and the calcium in milk are absorbed efficiently. Because of these and other differences in the availability of micronutrients from different sources, it is difficult to generalize about the usefulness of supplements. Nevertheless, we can say a few things about this issue:

- In general, it is much easier to develop a toxic overload of nutrients from supplements than it is from foods. It is very difficult, if not impossible, to develop a vitamin or mineral toxicity through diet (food) alone.
- Some micronutrients consumed as supplements appear to be harmful to the health of certain subgroups of consumers. For example, recent research has shown that the use of common supplements, particularly iron, may actually increase rates of death in older women.[2] Earlier, it was shown that high-potency beta-carotene supplements increased death rates among male smokers. Alcoholics are more susceptible to the potentially toxic effects of vitamin A supplements and should avoid their use unless prescribed by a healthcare provider. There is also some evidence

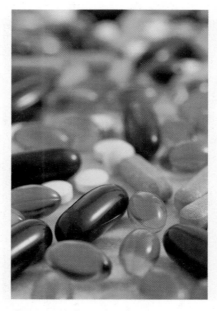

Thousands of supplements are marketed to consumers.

that high intake of vitamin A, including supplement use, increases the risk for osteoporosis and bone fractures in older women with low intakes of vitamin D.[3]

- Most minerals are better absorbed from animal food sources than they are from supplements. The one exception might be calcium citrate-malate, used in calcium-fortified juices. The body uses this form as effectively as the calcium from milk or yogurt.
- Enriching a low-nutrient food with a few vitamins and/or minerals does not turn it into a healthful food. For example, a soft drink that has been fortified with selected micronutrients is still basically a soft drink.
- Eating a variety of healthful foods provides you with many more nutrients, phytochemicals, and other dietary factors than supplements alone. Nutritionists are not even sure they have identified all the essential nutrients; it is possible that the list of essential micronutrients will expand in the future. Supplements provide only those nutrients that the manufacturer puts in; foods provide the nutrients that have been identified as well as yet-unknown factors.
- Many foods provide a balance of micronutrients and other factors, which work in concert with one another. The whole food is more healthful than its individual nutrients, providing benefits not always seen with purified supplements or highly refined, highly enriched food products. Two useful guidelines are "Eat food. Don't eat anything your great-great-grandmother wouldn't recognize as food"[4] and "Eat food, not too much, mostly plants."[5]

- A healthful diet, built from a wide variety of foods, offers social, emotional, and other benefits that are absent from supplements. Humans eat food, not nutrients.

On the other hand, micronutrient supplements can play an important role in promoting good health in some populations, such as pregnant women, children with poor eating habits, and people with certain illnesses. The risks and benefits of specific supplements versus whole foods are discussed later in this text (see Chapters 7–10).

Can Micronutrients Prevent or Treat Chronic Disease?

Nutritionists and other healthcare professionals clearly accept the role that dietary fat plays in the prevention and treatment of heart disease. The relationship between total carbohydrate intake and the management of diabetes is also firmly established. Less clear, however, are the links between individual vitamins and minerals and certain chronic diseases.

A number of research studies have suggested, but not proven, links between the following micronutrients and disease states. In each case, adequate intake of a given nutrient has been associated with lowered disease risk for, specifically:

- Vitamin D and colon cancer
- Vitamin E and complications of diabetes
- Vitamin K and osteoporosis
- Calcium and high blood pressure (hypertension)
- Chromium and type 2 diabetes in older adults
- Magnesium and muscle wasting (sarcopenia) in older adults
- Selenium and certain types of cancer

As consumers, it is important to critically evaluate any claims about the protective or disease-preventing ability of a specific vitamin or mineral. Supplements that provide megadoses of micronutrients are potentially harmful, and vitamin/mineral therapies should never replace more traditional, proven methods of disease treatment. Current, reputable information can provide updates as the research into micronutrients continues.

Do More Essential Micronutrients Exist?

Nutrition researchers continue to explore the potential of a variety of substances to qualify as essential micronutrients. Vitamin-like factors, such as carnitine and trace minerals, such as boron, nickel, and silicon, seem to have beneficial roles in human health, yet additional information is needed to fully define their metabolic roles. Until more research is done, such substances can't be classified as essential micronutrients.

Another subject of controversy is the question "What is the appropriate intake of each micronutrient?" Contemporary research suggests that the answer to this question is to be found in each individual's genetic profile. That is, some individuals require much higher or lower intakes of micronutrients to achieve optimal health. For example, researchers have identified a genetic variation in a subset of the population that increases their need for dietary folate.[6] Future studies may identify other examples of how a person's genetic profile influences his or her unique need for vitamins and minerals. As the science of nutrition continues to evolve, the next 50 years will be an exciting time for micronutrient research.

MasteringNutrition™

Check out these additional resources in the MasteringNutrition Study Area:

- Read It: Chapter Summary and RSS Feeds
- See It: ABC News videos and nutrition animations
- Hear It: MP3s
- Study It: Get Ready for Nutrition Math and Chemistry review
- Do It: NutriTools and "Find the Quack" feature
- Review It: Quizzes, flashcards, and glossary

web resources

www.fda.gov
U.S. Food and Drug Administration

Select "Food" and then "Dietary Supplements" for information on how to evaluate dietary supplements.

www.nal.usda.gov
Food and Nutrition Information Center

First, enter "food and nutrition information center" into search box, than click on "Dietary Supplements" to obtain information on vitamin and mineral supplements.

www.dietary-supplements.info.nih.gov
Office of Dietary Supplements

This site provides summaries of current research results and helpful information about the use of dietary supplements.

lpi.oregonstate.edu
Linus Pauling Institute of Oregon State University

This site provides information on vitamins and minerals that promote health and lower disease risk. You can search for individual nutrients (for example, vitamin C) as well as types of nutrients (for example, antioxidants).

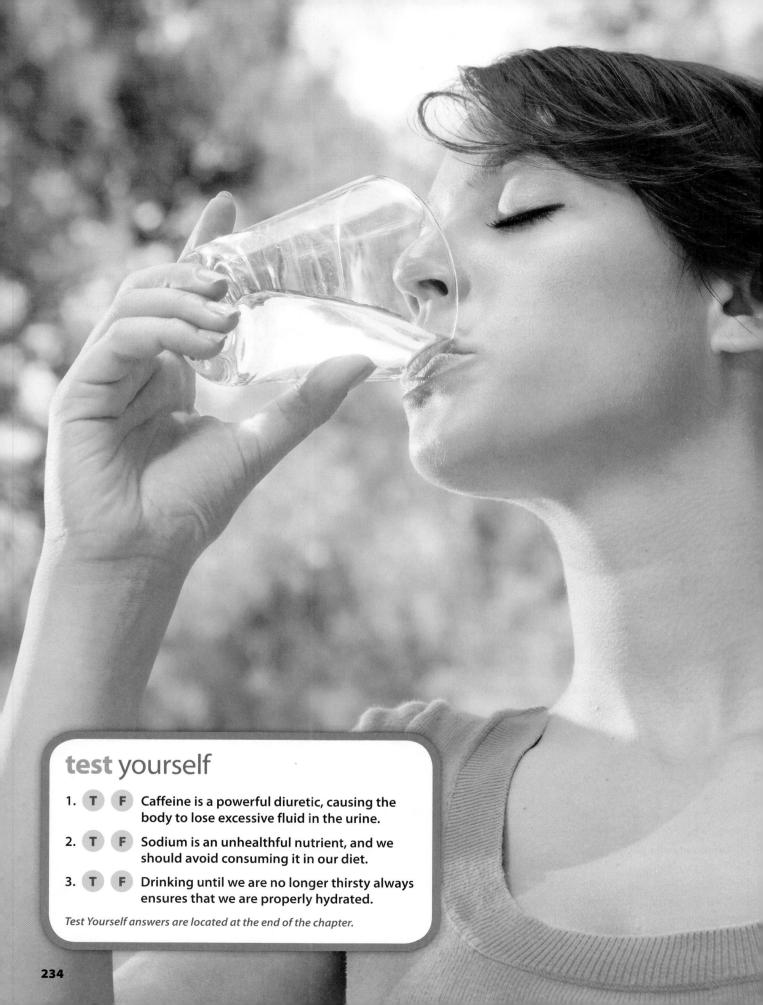

test yourself

1. (T) (F) Caffeine is a powerful diuretic, causing the body to lose excessive fluid in the urine.

2. (T) (F) Sodium is an unhealthful nutrient, and we should avoid consuming it in our diet.

3. (T) (F) Drinking until we are no longer thirsty always ensures that we are properly hydrated.

Test Yourself answers are located at the end of the chapter.

Nutrients Involved in Fluid and Electrolyte Balance

7

learning objectives

After studying this chapter you should be able to:

1 Describe the composition and location of body fluid, pp. 236–237.

2 List three functions of water in our body, pp. 237–239.

3 Describe how electrolytes assist in the regulation of healthful fluid balance, pp. 239–242.

4 Discuss the physical mechanisms that cause us to gain or lose fluids, pp. 242–244.

5 Identify the DRIs for water for adult men and women and the most healthful sources of fluids, pp. 245–247.

6 Identify the AI for sodium intake and the most common sources of sodium in our diet, pp. 244, 251–252.

7 Explain the importance of potassium, chloride, and phosphorus to human health, pp. 254–257.

8 Summarize the factors that most commonly contribute to dehydration and heat illnesses, pp. 258–260.

When hearing that someone has died from "drinking too much," most of us immediately think of alcohol. Over the past decade, however, several people have died after drinking too much water. That's right—pure, "wholesome" water. In 2005, for example, a fraternity hazing at California State University, Chico, left 21-year-old Matthew Carrington dead after he was forced to consume gallons of water while performing calisthenics in a cold basement. More recently, people have died after drinking too much water while following a fad diet, while participating in a radio contest, and while hiking. The official cause of these deaths is hyponatremia, or "low blood sodium." This condition is also known as water intoxication or water poisoning.

Are you at risk for either water intoxication or dehydration? Do sport beverages offer any protection against these types of fluid imbalances? If at the start of football practice on a hot, humid afternoon, a friend confided to you that he had been on a drinking binge the night before, what would you say to him? Would you urge him to tell his coach, and if so, why?

In this chapter, we'll explore the role of fluids and electrolytes in keeping the body properly hydrated and maintaining the functions of nerves and muscles. Immediately following this chapter, we take an **In Depth** look at the health benefits and concerns related to alcohol intake.

MasteringNutrition™

Go online for chapter quizzes, pre-tests, Interactive Activities, and more!

What are fluids and electrolytes, and what are their functions?

Of course, you know that orange juice, blood, and shampoo are all fluids, but what makes them so? A **fluid** is characterized by its ability to move freely, adapting to the shape of the container that holds it. This might not seem very important, but as you'll learn in this chapter, the fluid composition of your cells and tissues is critical to your body's ability to function.

Body Fluid Is the Liquid Portion of Our Cells and Tissues

Between 50% and 70% of a healthy adult's body weight is fluid. When we cut a finger, we can see some of this fluid dripping out as blood, but the fluid in the blood-stream can't account for such a large percentage. So where is all this fluid hiding?

About two-thirds of an adult's body fluid is held within the walls of cells and is therefore called **intracellular fluid** (**FIGURE 7.1a**). Every cell in our body contains fluid.

fluid A substance composed of molecules that move past one another freely. Fluids are characterized by their ability to conform to the shape of whatever container holds them.

intracellular fluid The fluid held at any given time within the walls of the body's cells.

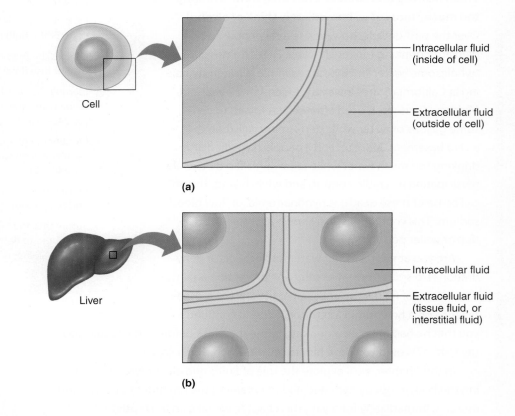

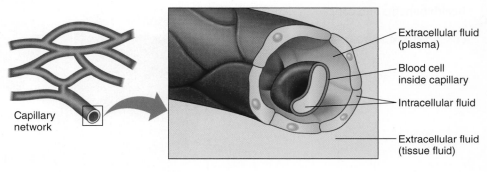

▶ **FIGURE 7.1** The components of body fluid. **(a)** Intracellular fluid is contained inside the cells that make up our body tissues. **(b)** Extracellular fluid is external to cells. Tissue fluid is external to tissue cells. **(c)** Another form of extracellular fluid is intravascular fluid—that is, fluid contained within vessels. Plasma is the fluid in blood vessels and is external to blood cells.

When our cells lose their fluid, they quickly shrink and die. On the other hand, when cells take in too much fluid, they swell and burst apart. This is why appropriate fluid balance—which we'll discuss throughout this chapter—is so critical to life.

The remaining third of body fluid is referred to as **extracellular fluid** because it flows outside our cells (Figure 7.1a). There are two types of extracellular fluid:

1. *Tissue fluid* (sometimes called *interstitial fluid*) flows between the cells that make up a particular tissue or organ, such as muscle fibers or the liver (Figure 7.1b). Other extracellular fluids, such as cerebrospinal fluid, mucus, and synovial fluid within joints, are also considered tissue fluid.
2. *Intravascular fluid* is found within blood and lymphatic vessels. Plasma is the fluid portion of blood that transports blood cells through blood vessels. Plasma also contains proteins that are too large to leak out of blood vessels into the surrounding tissue fluid. As you learned (in Chapter 6), protein concentration plays a major role in regulating the movement of fluids into and out of the bloodstream (Figure 7.1c).

Not every tissue in our body contains the same amount of fluid. Lean tissues, such as muscle, are more than 70% fluid by weight, whereas fat tissue is only between 10% and 20% fluid. This is not surprising, considering the water-repellant nature of lipids (see Chapter 5).

Body fluid levels also vary according to gender and age. Compared to females, males have more lean tissue and thus a higher percentage of body weight as fluid. The amount of body fluid as a percentage of total weight decreases with age. About 75% of an infant's body weight is water, whereas the total body water of an elderly person is generally less than 50% of body weight. This decrease in total body water is the result of the loss of lean tissue that typically occurs as people age.

Body Fluid Is Composed of Water and Electrolytes

Water is made up of molecules consisting of two hydrogen atoms bound to one oxygen atom (H_2O). You might think that pure water would be healthful, but we would quickly die if our cell and tissue fluids contained only pure water. Instead, within the body fluids are a variety of dissolved substances (called *solutes*) critical to life. These include four major minerals: sodium, potassium, chloride, and phosphorus. We consume these minerals in compounds called *salts*, including table salt, which is made of sodium and chloride.

These mineral salts are called **electrolytes** because when they dissolve in water, the two component minerals separate and form charged particles called **ions**, which can carry an electrical current and themselves are also commonly referred to as electrolytes. An ion's electrical charge, which can be positive or negative, is the "spark" that stimulates nerves and causes muscles to contract, making electrolytes critical to body functioning.

Of the four major minerals just mentioned, sodium (Na^+) and potassium (K^+) are positively charged, whereas chloride (Cl^-) and phosphorus (in the form of hydrogen phosphate, or HPO_4^{2-}) are negatively charged. In the intracellular fluid, potassium and phosphate are the predominant ions. In the extracellular fluid, sodium and chloride predominate. There is a slight difference in electrical charge on either side of the cell's membrane that is needed in order for the cell to perform its normal functions.

Fluids Serve Many Critical Functions

Water not only quenches our thirst; it also performs a number of functions that are critical to life.

Fluids Dissolve and Transport Substances

Water is an excellent **solvent**; that is, it's capable of dissolving a wide variety of substances. Because blood is mostly water, it's able to transport a variety of solutes—such as amino acids, glucose, water-soluble vitamins, minerals, and medications—to body cells. In contrast, fats do not dissolve in water. To overcome

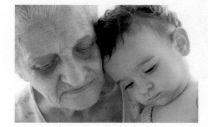

As we age, our body water content decreases: approximately 75% of an infant's body weight is composed of water, whereas an elderly adult's body weight is only 50% water (or less).

extracellular fluid The fluid outside the body's cells, either in the body's tissues or as the liquid portion of blood, called *plasma*.

electrolyte A substance that disassociates in solution into positively and negatively charged ions and is thus capable of carrying an electrical current.

ion Any electrically charged particle, either positively or negatively charged.

solvent A substance that is capable of mixing with and breaking apart a variety of compounds. Water is an excellent solvent.

this chemical incompatibility, lipids and fat-soluble vitamins are either attached to or surrounded by water-soluble proteins, so that they, too, can be transported in the blood to the cells.

Fluids Account for Blood Volume

Blood volume is the amount of fluid in blood; thus, appropriate fluid levels are essential to maintaining healthful blood volume. When blood volume rises inappropriately, blood pressure increases; when blood volume decreases inappropriately, blood pressure decreases. Hypertension (high blood pressure) is an important risk factor for heart attacks and strokes. (For more information, see the **In Depth** following Chapter 5). In contrast, low blood pressure can cause people to feel tired, confused, or dizzy.

Fluids Help Maintain Body Temperature

Just as overheating is disastrous to a car engine, a high internal temperature can cause our body to stop functioning. Fluids are vital to the body's ability to maintain its temperature within a safe range. Two factors account for the ability of fluids to keep us cool. First, water has a relatively high capacity for heat: in other words, it takes a lot of energy to raise its temperature. Because the body contains a lot of water, only prolonged exposure to high heat can increase body temperature.

Second, body fluids are our primary coolant. When heat needs to be released from the body, there is an increase in the flow of blood from the warm body core to the vessels lying just under the skin. This action transports heat from the body core out to the periphery, where it can be released from the skin. At the same time, sweat glands secrete more sweat from the skin. As this sweat evaporates off the skin's surface, heat is released and the skin and underlying blood are cooled **(FIGURE 7.2)**. This cooler blood flows back to the body's core and reduces internal body temperature.

Fluids Protect and Lubricate Our Tissues

Water is a major part of the fluids that protect and lubricate tissues. The cerebrospinal fluid that surrounds the brain and spinal cord protects them from damage, and a fetus in a mother's womb is protected by amniotic fluid. Synovial fluid lubricates joints, and tears cleanse and lubricate the eyes. Saliva moistens the food we eat and the mucus lining the walls of the gastrointestinal (GI) tract eases the movement of food. Finally, pleural fluid covering the lungs allows their friction-free expansion and retraction within the chest cavity.

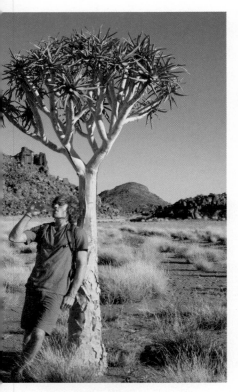

A hiker must consume adequate amounts of water to prevent heat illness in hot and dry environments.

Would the proteins in your body tissues "cook" at the same temperature that would fry an egg? For a short video on an experiment that answered this question, go to www.youtube.com and type in "NPR Science: How Much Heat Can You Take?"

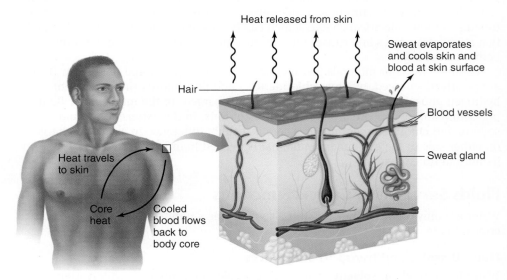

Heat released from skin

Sweat evaporates and cools skin and blood at skin surface

Hair

Blood vessels

Sweat gland

Heat travels to skin

Core heat

Cooled blood flows back to body core

FIGURE 7.2 Evaporative cooling occurs when heat is transported from the body core through the bloodstream to the surface of the skin. The water evaporates into the air and carries away heat. This cools the blood, which circulates back to the body core, reducing body temperature.

blood volume The amount of fluid in blood.

recap Our body fluids consist of water plus a variety of dissolved substances, including electrically charged minerals called electrolytes. Water serves many important functions in our body, including dissolving and transporting substances, accounting for blood volume, regulating body temperature, and protecting and lubricating body tissues.

Electrolytes Support Many Body Functions

Now that you know why fluid is so essential to the body's functioning, we're ready to explore the critical roles of electrolytes.

Electrolytes Help Regulate Fluid Balance

Cell membranes are *permeable* to water, meaning water flows easily through them. Cells cannot voluntarily regulate this flow of water and thus have no active control over the balance of fluid between the intracellular and extracellular environments. In contrast, cell membranes are *not* freely permeable to electrolytes. Sodium, potassium, and the other electrolytes stay where they are, either inside or outside a cell, unless they are actively transported across the cell membrane by special transport proteins. So how do electrolytes help cells maintain their fluid balance? To answer this question, a short review of chemistry is needed.

Imagine that you have a special filter with the same properties as cell membranes; in other words, this filter is freely permeable to water but not permeable to electrolytes. Now imagine that you insert this filter into a glass of dilute salt water to divide the glass into two separate chambers (**FIGURE 7.3a**). Of course, the water levels on both sides of the filter would be identical because the filter is freely permeable to water. Now imagine that you add a teaspoon of salt (which would immediately dissolve into sodium and chloride ions) to the water on only one side of the filter (Figure 7.3b). Immediately, you would see the water on the "dilute salt water" side of the glass begin to flow through the filter to the "saltier" side of the glass (Figure 7.3c).

Why would this movement of water occur? It is because water always moves from areas where solutes, such as sodium and chloride, are low in concentration (or completely absent) to areas where they are high in concentration. To put it another way, solutes *attract* water toward areas where they are more concentrated. This movement of water toward solutes, called **osmosis**, continues until the concentration of solutes is equal on both sides of the cell membrane.

Osmosis provides the body a mechanism for controlling the movement of fluid into and out of cells. Recall that cells can regulate the balance of fluids between their cytoplasm and the extracellular environment by using special transport proteins to

osmosis The movement of water (or any solvent) through a semipermeable membrane from an area where solutes are less concentrated to areas where solutes are highly concentrated.

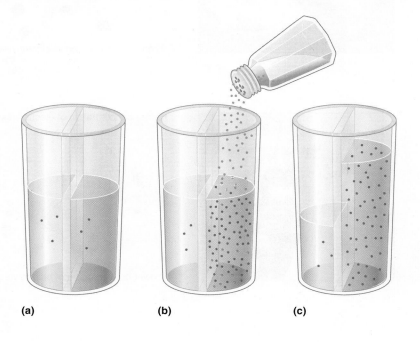

(a) (b) (c)

◀ **FIGURE 7.3** Osmosis. **(a)** A filter that is freely permeable to water but not permeable to solutes is placed in a glass of dilute salt water. **(b)** Additional salt is sprinkled on one side of the glass only. **(c)** Drawn by the high concentration of electrolytes, water flows to the "saltier" side of the filter. This flow of water into the more concentrated solution will continue until the concentration of electrolytes on both sides of the membrane is equal.

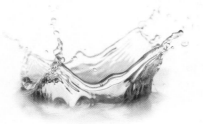

The health of our body's cells depends on maintaining the proper balance of fluids and electrolytes on both sides of the cell membrane, both at rest and during exercise. Let's examine how this balance can be altered under various conditions of exercise and fluid intake.

MODERATE EXERCISE

When you are appropriately hydrated, engaged in moderate exercise, and not too hot, the concentration of electrolytes is likely to be the same on both sides of cell membranes. You will be in fluid balance.

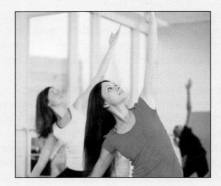

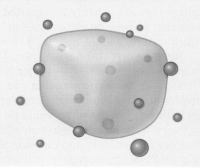

Concentration of electrolytes about equal inside and outside cell

STRENUOUS EXERCISE WITH RAPID AND HIGH WATER INTAKE

If a person drinks a great deal of water quickly during intense, prolonged exercise, the extracellular fluid becomes diluted. This results in the concentration of electrolytes being greater inside the cells, which causes water to enter the cells, making them swell. Drinking moderate amounts of water or sports drinks more slowly will replace lost fluids and restore fluid balance.

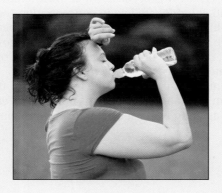

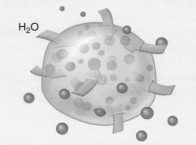

Lower concentration of electrolytes outside

H_2O

Higher concentration of electrolytes inside

STRENUOUS EXERCISE WITH INADEQUATE FLUID INTAKE

If a person does not consume adequate amounts of fluid during strenuous exercise of long duration, the concentration of electrolytes becomes greater outside the cells, drawing water away from the inside of the cells and making them shrink. Consuming sports drinks will replace lost fluids and electrolytes.

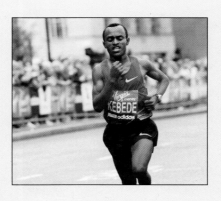

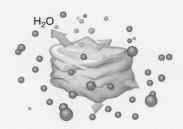

Higher concentration of electrolytes outside

H_2O

Lower concentration of electrolytes inside

actively pump electrolytes across the cell membrane (see Chapter 6). The health of the body's cells depends on maintaining an appropriate balance of fluid and electrolytes between the intracellular and extracellular environments. If the concentration of electrolytes is much higher inside cells as compared to outside, water will flow into the cells in such large amounts that the cells can burst. On the other hand, if the extracellular environment contains too high a concentration of electrolytes, water flows out of the cells, and they can dry up. **FIGURE 7.4** (on facing page) provides an illustration of how an imbalance between fluid and electrolyte intake during strenuous exercise can affect the balance of fluid and electrolytes between the intracellular and extracellular environments. Keep in mind that when you exercise, what and how much you should drink depends on multiple factors, including how strenuously you are exercising, how long the exercise session is, and how warm or humid the environment is.

Electrolytes Enable Our Nerves to Respond to Stimuli

In addition to their role in maintaining fluid balance, electrolytes are critical in allowing our nerves to respond to stimuli **(FIGURE 7.5)**. Nerve impulses are initiated at the membrane of a nerve cell in response to a stimulus—for example, the touch of a hand or the clanging of a bell. Stimuli prompt changes in membranes that allow an influx of sodium into the nerve cell, causing the cell to become slightly less negatively charged. This is called *depolarization*. If enough sodium enters the cell, an electrical impulse is generated along the cell membrane (Figure 7.5b).

Once this impulse has been transmitted, the cell membrane returns to its normal electrical state through the release of potassium to the outside of the cell (Figure 7.5c). This return to the initial electrical state is termed *repolarization*. Thus, both sodium and potassium play critical roles in ensuring that nerve impulses are generated, transmitted, and completed.

Electrolytes Signal Our Muscles to Contract

Muscles contract in response to a series of complex physiological changes that we will not describe in detail here. Simply stated, muscle contraction occurs in response to stimulation of nerve cells. As described earlier, sodium and potassium play a key role in the generation of nerve impulses, or electrical signals. When a muscle fiber is stimulated by an electrical signal, changes occur in the cell membrane that lead to an increased flow of calcium into the muscle from the extracellular space. This movement of calcium into the muscle provides the stimulus for muscle contraction. The muscles

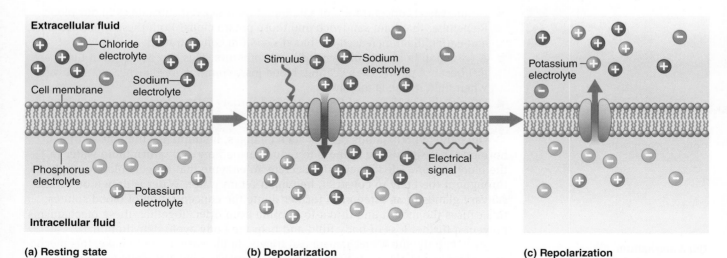

(a) Resting state   **(b) Depolarization**   **(c) Repolarization**

FIGURE 7.5 The role of electrolytes in conduction of a nerve impulse. **(a)** In the resting state, the intracellular fluid has slightly more electrolytes with a negative charge. **(b)** A stimulus causes changes to occur that prompt the influx of sodium into the interior of the cell. Sodium has a positive charge so when this happens, the charge inside the cell becomes slightly positive. This is called depolarization. If enough sodium enters the cell, an electrical signal is transmitted to adjacent regions of the cell membrane. **(c)** Release of potassium to the exterior of the cell allows the first portion of the membrane almost immediately to return to the resting state. This is called repolarization.

can relax after a contraction once the electrical signal is complete and calcium has been pumped out of the muscle cell.

Certain illnesses can threaten the delicate balance of fluid inside and outside the cells and impair the function of nerves and muscles. You may have heard of someone being hospitalized because of excessive diarrhea and/or vomiting. When this happens, the body loses a great deal of fluid from the intestinal tract and extracellular environment. This large fluid loss causes the extracellular electrolyte concentration to become very high. In response, a great deal of intracellular fluid flows out of the cells (see Figure 7.4c). This imbalance in fluid and electrolytes changes the flow of electrical impulses through the nerve and muscle cells of the heart, causing an irregular heart rate, which can eventually lead to death if left untreated. Food poisoning and eating disorders involving repeated vomiting and diarrhea can also result in death from life-threatening fluid and electrolyte imbalances.

> **recap** Electrolytes help regulate fluid balance by controlling the movement of fluid into and out of cells. Electrolytes, specifically sodium and potassium, play a key role in generating nerve impulses in response to stimuli. Calcium is an electrolyte that stimulates muscle contraction.

How does our body maintain fluid balance?

The proper balance of fluid is maintained in the body by a series of mechanisms that prompt us to drink and retain fluid when we are dehydrated and to excrete fluid as urine when we consume more than we need.

The Thirst Mechanism Prompts Us to Drink Fluids

Imagine that, at lunch, you ate a ham sandwich and a bag of salted potato chips. Now it's almost time for your afternoon seminar to end and you are very thirsty. The last 5 minutes of class are a torment, and when the instructor ends the session you dash to the nearest drinking fountain. What prompted you to suddenly feel so thirsty?

The body's command center for fluid intake is a cluster of nerve cells in the same part of the brain we studied in relation to food intake; that is, the *hypothalamus*. Within the hypothalamus is a group of cells, collectively referred to as the **thirst mechanism**, that causes you to consciously desire fluids. The thirst mechanism prompts us to feel thirsty whenever it is stimulated by the following:

- An increased concentration of salt and other dissolved substances in our blood. Remember that ham sandwich and those potato chips? Both these foods are salty, and eating them increased the blood's sodium concentration.
- A reduction in blood volume and blood pressure. This can occur when fluids are lost because of profuse sweating, blood loss, vomiting, or diarrhea, or simply when fluid intake is too low.
- Dryness in the tissues of the mouth and throat. Tissue dryness reflects a lower amount of fluid in the bloodstream, which causes a reduced production of saliva.

Once the hypothalamus detects such changes, it stimulates the release of a hormone that signals the kidneys to reduce urine flow and return more water to the bloodstream. The kidneys also secrete an enzyme that triggers blood vessels throughout the body to constrict, helping it retain water. Water is drawn out of the salivary glands in an attempt to further dilute the concentration of blood solutes; this causes the mouth and throat to become even drier. Together, these mechanisms prevent a further loss of body fluid and help the body avoid dehydration.

Although the thirst mechanism can trigger an increase in fluid intake, this mechanism alone is not always sufficient to fully normalize fluid status: People tend to drink until they are no longer thirsty, but the amount of fluid they consume may not be enough to achieve fluid balance. This is particularly true when body water is lost rapidly, such as during intense exercise in the heat. Because the thirst mechanism has some limitations, it is important to drink regularly throughout the day and not wait to drink until you become thirsty, especially if you are active.

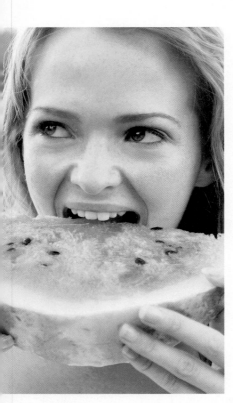

Fruits and vegetables are delicious sources of water.

thirst mechanism A cluster of nerve cells in the hypothalamus that stimulate our conscious desire to drink fluids in response to an increase in the concentration of salt in our blood or a decrease in blood pressure and blood volume.

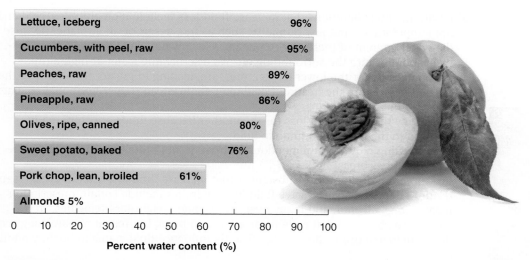

FIGURE 7.6 Water content of different foods. Much of your daily water intake comes from the foods you eat.

Data from: U.S. Department of Agriculture, Agricultural Research Service. 2011. USDA Nutrient Database for Standard Reference, Release 24. Nutrient Data Laboratory.

We Gain Fluids Through Intake and Metabolism

We obtain the fluid we need each day from two primary sources: dietary intake from beverages and foods and the production of metabolic water by the body. Of course, you know that beverages are mostly water, but it isn't as easy to see the water content in the foods we eat. For example, iceberg lettuce is almost 99% water, and even almonds contain a small amount of water (**FIGURE 7.6**).

Metabolic water is the water formed from the body's metabolic reactions such as the breakdown of carbohydrates, fats, and proteins. This water contributes about 10–14% of the water the body needs each day.

We Lose Fluids Through Urine, Sweat, Evaporation, Exhalation, and Feces

We can perceive—or sense—water loss through urine output and sweating, so we refer to this as **sensible water loss**. Most of the water we consume is excreted through the kidneys in the form of urine. When we consume more water than we need, the kidneys process and excrete the excess in the form of dilute urine.

The second type of sensible water loss is via sweat. Our sweat glands produce more sweat during exercise or when we are in a hot environment. The evaporation of sweat from the skin releases heat, which cools the skin and reduces the body's core temperature.

Water is continuously evaporated from the skin, even when a person is not visibly sweating, and water is continuously exhaled from the lungs during breathing. Water loss through these routes is known as **insensible water loss** because we do not perceive it. Under normal resting conditions, insensible water loss is less than 1 liter (L) of fluid each day; during heavy exercise or in hot weather, a person can lose up to 2 L of water per hour from insensible water loss. Under normal conditions, only about 150 to 200 ml of water is lost each day in feces. The gastrointestinal tract typically absorbs much of the fluid that passes through it each day.

In addition to these five common routes of fluid loss, certain situations can cause a significant loss of fluid from our body:

- Illnesses that involve fever, coughing, vomiting, diarrhea, and a runny nose significantly increase fluid loss. This is one reason that doctors advise people to drink plenty of fluids when they are ill.
- Traumatic injury, internal bleeding, blood donation, and surgery also increase loss of fluid because of the blood loss involved.
- Exercise increases fluid loss via sweat and respiration; although urine production typically decreases during exercise, fluid losses increase through the skin and lungs.

metabolic water The water formed as a by-product of our body's metabolic reactions.

sensible water loss Water loss that is noticed by a person, such as through urine output and visible sweating.

insensible water loss The loss of water not noticeable by a person, such as through evaporation from the skin and exhalation from the lungs during breathing.

■ Environmental conditions that increase fluid loss include high altitudes, cold and hot temperatures, and low humidity, such as in a desert or an airplane. Because the water content of these environments is low, water from the body more easily evaporates into the surrounding air. We also breathe faster at high altitudes to compensate for the lower oxygen pressure, leading to greater fluid loss via the lungs. We sweat in the heat, but cold temperatures can trigger hormonal changes that also increase fluid loss.

■ Pregnancy increases fluid loss for the mother because fluids are continually diverted to the fetus and amniotic fluid.

■ Breastfeeding requires a tremendous increase in fluid intake to make up for the loss of fluid as breast milk.

■ Consumption of **diuretics**—substances that increase fluid loss via the urine—can result in dangerously excessive fluid loss. Diuretics include certain prescription medications, alcohol, and many over-the-counter weight-loss remedies. In the past, it was believed that caffeine acted as a diuretic, but recent research suggests that caffeinated drinks do not significantly influence fluid status in healthy adults.[1]

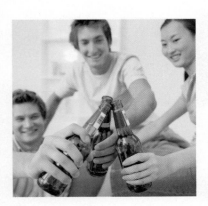

⬅ Drinking beverages that contain alcohol causes an increase in water loss because alcohol is a diuretic.

recap A healthy fluid level is maintained by balancing intake and excretion. The primary sources of fluids are water and other beverages, foods, and the production of metabolic water in the body. Fluid losses occur through urination, sweating, the feces, exhalation from the lungs, and insensible evaporation from the skin.

A profile of nutrients involved in hydration and neuromuscular function

The nutrients involved in maintaining hydration and neuromuscular function are water and the major minerals sodium, potassium, chloride, and phosphorus (TABLE 7.1). Calcium and magnesium also function as electrolytes and influence our body's fluid balance and neuromuscular function. (However, because of their critical importance to bone health, they are discussed in Chapter 9.)

Water

Water is essential for life. Although we can live weeks without food, we can survive only a few days without water, depending on the environmental temperature. The human body does not have the capacity to store water, so we must continuously replace the water lost each day.

How Much Water Should We Drink?

Our need for water varies greatly, depending on our age, body size, health status, physical activity level, and exposure to environmental conditions. It is important to pay attention to how much our need for water changes under various conditions so that we can avoid dehydration.

TABLE 7.1 **Overview of Minerals Involved in Hydration and Neuromuscular Function**

To see the full profile of these major minerals, see Chapter 6.5, **In Depth,** Vitamins and Minerals: Micronutrients with Macro Powers (pages 224–233).

Nutrient	Recommended Intake
Sodium	1.5 g/day*
Potassium	4.7 g/day*
Chloride	2.3 g/day*
Phosphorus	700 mg/day[†]

*Adequate Intake (AI).
[†]Recommended Dietary Allowance (RDA).

diuretic A substance that increases fluid loss via the urine. Common diuretics include alcohol, some prescription medications, and many over-the-counter weight-loss pills.

Fluid requirements are very individualized. For example, a highly active male athlete training in a hot environment may require up to 10 liters (L) of fluid per day to maintain a healthy fluid balance, whereas an inactive, petite woman who lives in a mild climate and works in a temperature-controlled office building may only require about 3 L of fluid per day.

The DRI for adult men aged 19 to 50 years is 3.7 L of total water per day. This includes approximately 3.0 L (13 cups) as beverages, including water. The DRI for adult women aged 19 to 50 years is 2.7 L of total water per day, including about 2.2 L (9 cups) as beverages.[2]

FIGURE 7.7 shows the amount and sources of water intake and output for a woman expending 2,500 kcal per day. Based on current recommendations, this woman needs about 3,000 ml (3 L) of fluid per day:

- Water from metabolism provides 300 ml of water.
- The foods she eats provide her with an additional 500 ml of water each day.
- The beverages she drinks provide the remainder of the water she needs, which is equal to 2,200 ml.

An 8-oz glass of fluid is equal to 240 ml. In this example, the woman would need to drink nine glasses of fluid to meet her needs. You may have read or heard that drinking eight glasses of fluid each day is recommended for most people. Remember, however, that this recommendation is a general guideline. You may need to drink a different amount to meet your individual fluid needs.

Athletes and other people who are active, especially those working in very hot environments, may require more fluid than the current recommendations. The amount of sweat lost during exercise is very individualized and depends on body size, exercise intensity, level of personal fitness, environmental temperature, and humidity. A recent study reported that professional and collegiate football players can lose up to 10 liters of sweat per day.[3] Thus, these individuals need to drink more to replace the fluid they lose. Sodium is the major electrolyte lost in sweat; we also lose some potassium and small amounts of iron and calcium in sweat.

Because of their high fluid and electrolyte losses during exercise, some athletes drink sports beverages instead of plain water to help them maintain fluid balance. Recently, sports beverages have also become popular with recreationally active people and non-athletes. Is it really necessary for people to consume these beverages if they are not highly active? See the **Nutrition Debate** on sports beverages at the end of this chapter to learn whether they are beneficial for recreationally active people and non-athletes.

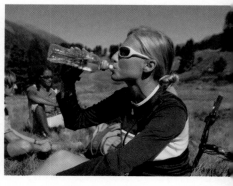

Vigorous exercise causes significant water loss, which must be replenished to optimize performance and health.

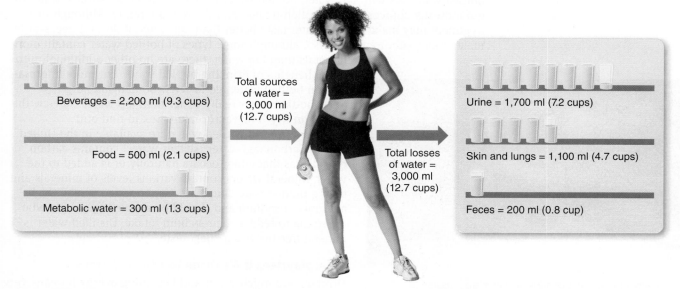

Beverages = 2,200 ml (9.3 cups)

Food = 500 ml (2.1 cups)

Metabolic water = 300 ml (1.3 cups)

Total sources of water = 3,000 ml (12.7 cups)

Total losses of water = 3,000 ml (12.7 cups)

Urine = 1,700 ml (7.2 cups)

Skin and lungs = 1,100 ml (4.7 cups)

Feces = 200 ml (0.8 cup)

FIGURE 7.7 Amount and sources of water intake and output for a woman expending 2,500 kcal/day.

Sources of Drinking Water

There are now many types of drinking water to choose from: how can we distinguish among them? Millions of Americans routinely consume the tap water found in homes and public places, which generally comes from two sources: surface water and groundwater. *Surface water* comes from lakes, rivers, and reservoirs. *Groundwater* comes from underground rock formations called *aquifers*. Many people who live in rural areas depend on groundwater pumped from a well as their water source.

In some areas, surface water and groundwater can be relatively high in calcium, which tends to contribute to the formation of white calcium salts, thus the term "hard water." In homes with hard water, there is often scaling around sinks, tubs, and showers. Many people living in hard water areas complain that their laundry does not come as clean as they like and their hair doesn't feel as soft as it once did. To ease this problem, many homeowners install water softeners, most of which make a simple chemical exchange in order to lower the calcium content: salt (sodium chloride) is added to the water softener and the sodium is exchanged for the calcium. Calcium levels drop; sodium levels go up. The soft water is then used for bathing, laundry, dishwashing, and other chores but not as the main source of drinking water.

The Environmental Protection Agency (EPA) sets and monitors the standards for public water systems. The most common chemical used to treat and purify public water supplies is *chlorine*, which is effective in killing many microorganisms. Water treatment plants also routinely check water supplies for hazardous chemicals, minerals, and other contaminants. Because of these efforts, the United States has one of the safest water systems in the world. Local water regulatory agencies, such as cities and counties, must provide an annual report on specific water contaminants to all households served by that agency. The EPA does not monitor water from private wells, but it publishes recommendations for well owners to help them maintain a safe water supply. For more information on drinking water safety, go to the EPA website (see **Web Resources** at the end of this chapter).

Over the past 20 years, there has been a major shift away from the use of tap water to the consumption of bottled water. Americans now drink about 29 gallons of bottled water per person, per year, totaling more than 9 billion gallons![4] The meteoric rise in bottled water production and consumption is most likely due to the convenience of drinking bottled water, the health messages related to drinking more water, and the public's fears related to the safety of tap water. Recent environmental concerns related to the disposal of water bottles has begun to limit the growth of bottled water, and the industry has responded by using smaller bottle caps, thinner bottles, and a higher proportion of recyclable materials.[5]

The Food and Drug Administration (FDA) is responsible for the regulation of bottled water. As with tap water, bottled water is taken from either surface water or groundwater sources. But it is often treated and filtered differently. Although this treatment may make bottled water taste better than tap water, it doesn't necessarily make it any safer to drink. Also, although some types of bottled water contain more minerals than tap water, there are no other additional nutritional benefits of drinking bottled water. For more information on bottled water, go to www.bottledwater.org.

Is bottled water really better than tap water? Review the **Nutrition Myth or Fact?** feature box to find out!

Many types of bottled water are available in the United States. Carbonated water (seltzer water) contains carbon dioxide gas that either occurs naturally or is added to the water. Mineral waters contain various levels of minerals and offer a unique taste. Some brands, however, contain high amounts of sodium and should be avoided by people who are trying to reduce their sodium intake. Distilled water is mineral-free but has a "flat" taste.

What Happens If We Drink Too Much Water?

Drinking too much water and becoming overhydrated is very rare, but as we said at the beginning of this chapter, it can

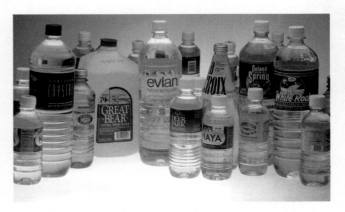

Numerous varieties of drinking water are available to consumers.

nutrition myth or fact?

Is Bottled Water Better Than Tap?

The next time you reach for a bottle of water, consider these little-known facts. If the label does not identify a specific location, the bottle may actually contain tap water with minerals added to improve the taste. To avoid paying a high price for bottled tap water, look for the phrase "Bottled at the source." Water that comes from a protected groundwater source is less likely to have contaminants, such as disease-causing microbes. If the label doesn't identify the water's source, it should at least provide contact information, such as a phone number or website of the bottled water company, so that you can track down the source.

Although many labels lack information about treatment methods, you might use the company's website to find out how their bottled water was treated. There are several ways of treating water, but what you're looking for is either of the following two methods, which have been proven to be most effective against the most common waterborne disease-causing microorganisms:

- *Micron filtration*, which is a process whereby water is filtered through screens with various-sized microscopic holes. High-quality micron filtration can eliminate most chemical contaminants and microbes.

- *Reverse osmosis*, which is a process often referred to as *ultrafiltration* because it uses a membrane with microscopic openings that allow water to pass through but not larger compounds. Reverse osmosis membranes also utilize electrical charges to reject harmful chemicals.

If the label on your bottle of water says that the water was purified using any of the following methods, you might want to consider switching brands: filtered, carbon-filtered, particle-filtered, ozonated or ozone-treated, ultraviolet light, ion exchange, or deionized. These methods have not been proven to be effective against the most common waterborne disease-causing microorganisms.

It is also a good idea to check the nutrient content on the water bottle label. Ideally, water should be high in magnesium (at least 20 mg per 8 fl. oz serving) and calcium but low in sodium (less than 5 mg per 8 fl. oz serving). Avoid bottled waters

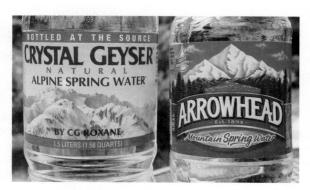

Can you tell where the water in each bottle comes from?

with sweeteners because their "empty Calories" can contribute significantly to your energy intake. These products are often promoted as healthful beverage choices with names including words such as *vitamins*, *herbs*, *nature*, and *life*, but they are essentially "liquid candy." Check the Nutrition Facts Panel and don't be fooled!

CRITICAL THINKING QUESTIONS

1. How much money do you think you spend each year on bottled water? If the average American consumes about 30 gallons of bottled water per year, often in 1/2 or 1 liter bottles, and each bottle costs about $1.50 to $2.50, that brings the annual cost up to between $170 and $285! How might you use that money to improve the nutrient quality of your diet? Which "investment" in your health would produce the most benefits and why?

2. Many schools and businesses are replacing old-fashioned water fountains with "filling stations" designed specifically to refill reusable water bottles. What are some strategies your school or business could utilize to increase use of these filling stations and reduce the number of single-use bottles of water? Are there any barriers that might turn people away from reusable water bottles?

---

occur. This dangerously dilutes blood sodium concentration, causing *hyponatremia,* which is discussed in more detail shortly. Certain illnesses also can cause excessive reabsorption, or retention, of water by the kidneys. They, too, lead to overhydration and dilution of blood sodium.

What Happens If We Don't Drink Enough Water?

Dehydration results when we do not drink enough water or are unable to retain the water we consume. It is one of the leading causes of death around the world. Dehydration is generally due to some form of illness or gastrointestinal infection that causes diarrhea and vomiting. The impact of dehydration on health is discussed in more detail shortly.

All Beverages Are Not Created Equal

Many commercial beverages contain several important nutrients in addition to their water content, whereas others provide water and refined sugar but very little else. Let's review the health benefits and potential concerns of some of the most popular beverages on the market.

Milk and Milk Substitutes

Low-fat and skim milk are healthful beverage choices because they provide protein, calcium, phosphorus, vitamin D, and, usually, vitamin A. Many brands of fluid milk are now "specialized" and provide additional calcium, vitamin E, essential fatty acids, and/or plant sterols (to lower serum cholesterol). Kefir, a blended yogurt drink, is also a good source of most of these nutrients. Calcium-fortified soy milk provides protein and calcium, and many brands provide vitamin D. In contrast, almond and rice milks are low in protein, with only 1 gram per cup.

When purchasing flavored milk, kefir, or milk substitutes, check the Nutrition Facts panel for the sugar content. Some brands of chocolate milk, for example, can contain 6 or more teaspoons of refined sugar in a single cup!

Beverages Containing Caffeine

Coffee made without cream or non-dairy creamer can be a healthful beverage choice if consumed in moderation. As mentioned earlier, recent research suggests that its caffeine content does not significantly decrease the body's hydration status, and the calcium in coffee drinks made with milk, such as café con leche and café latte, can be significant. Coffee is known to provide several types of phytochemicals that may lower risk of certain chronic diseases such as type 2 diabetes.[6] There is also growing evidence that people who drink coffee have a lower risk of stroke, although not all research supports that theory.[7] Although some people are sensitive to the caffeine in coffee, moderate consumption is safe and potentially healthful.

Tea is second only to water as the most commonly consumed beverage in the world. With the exception of red tea and herbal teas, which do not contain caffeine, all forms of tea come from the same plant, *Camellia sinesis*, and all contain caffeine. Black tea is the most highly processed (the tea leaves are fully fermented) and contains the highest level of caffeine, about half the amount in most brewed coffee. Oolong tea leaves are only partially fermented and have less caffeine. Both green and white tea leaves have been dried but not fermented. As compared to black and oolong teas, green and white teas are lower in caffeine and much higher in phytochemicals thought to decrease the risk of cardiovascular disease, diabetes, and certain cancers.[8] Some research suggests that green and white teas may have antibacterial and antiviral effects.[9] If consumed without added sugar, tea is an excellent source of fluid that may have unexpected long-term health benefits.

Chocolate and cocoa-based beverages also provide small amounts of caffeine, although the levels are much lower than those found in coffee, tea, or colas. Dark chocolate is rich in phytochemicals known as flavanols, which may lower risk of heart attacks and stroke.[10] Hot chocolate made with dark cocoa powder and skim or low-fat milk is a nutritious and satisfying drink.

Beverages with Added Sugars

Most soft drinks, juice drinks, flavored waters, and bottled teas and coffee drinks are loaded with added sugars. The current debate about the potential health consequences of widespread use of high fructose corn syrup (HFCS) has led many beverage manufacturers to switch to honey or "pure cane sugar" to sweeten their products; however, sugars provide the same number of Calories per gram, no matter their molecular structure. Similarly, some beverage producers have begun to use "fruit juice concentrate" as a source of added sugar. Although it sounds like a healthy option, the concentrate is little more than pure sugar, with none of the fiber or other nutrients that make fruit a nutritious food.

As package sizes continue to increase, the calorie count for these sweetened drinks can be unexpectedly high. Even 100% fruit juice with no added sugar is high

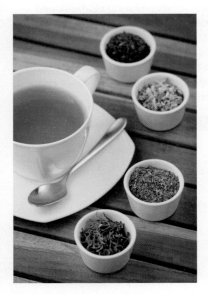

▲ After water, tea is the most commonly consumed beverage in the world.

HOT TOPIC

Can Fluids Make You Fat?

Until about 50 years ago, beverage choices were limited. But the introduction of a new, cheap sweetener derived from corn, *high-fructose corn syrup* (see Chapter 4), caused soda and other sweetened beverages to flood the market. Today, Americans take in approximately 21% of their Calories from beverages, mostly in the form of sweetened soft drinks and fruit juices. Recently, sweetened bottled waters, bottled teas, and specialty coffee drinks have contributed to the problem: a coffee mocha at one national chain of cafes provides 350 Calories, which is 17.5% of an average adult's total daily Calorie needs.

It's not surprising, then, that many (although not all!) researchers believe that Calories from such beverages have contributed significantly to the rise in caloric intake among Americans since the late 1970s. That's because beverages with a high Calorie content appear to do little to curb appetite, so people may not compensate for the extra Calories they drink by eating less.

in Calories. For instance, an 8-ounce carton of a popular brand of premium orange juice provides 110 Calories.

In the past, very few people realized how many Calories were in the beverages they drank, or how these Calories could be contributing to their increasing body weight. Recently, however, pubic health agencies have been raising awareness of the empty Calorie content of sweetened beverages. Some are advocating that a first step in any weight loss program should be to entirely eliminate these products from the diet. Some municipalities have proposed taxing sugary beverages; famously in early 2012, the New York City Board of Health approved a ban—since rescinded—on the sale of all sugary drinks larger than 16 ounces at city restaurants, food carts, movie theatres, and stadiums. In addition, the American Beverage Association has launched a "Clear on Calories" campaign, which puts Calorie information on the front of the product. All beverages sold in containers 20 fl. oz or smaller will display the total Calories per package, not just per serving. Now, when a consumer buys a 20-oz bottle of sweetened tea, he will know he'll be consuming, for example, 250 Calories if he drinks the whole bottle. Some beverage companies have reduced the average Calorie content of their products by introducing a variety of smaller sized containers. Most consumer advocates, however, view these efforts simply as a marketing ploy.

Designer Waters

So-called designer waters are made with added nutrients and/or herbs that supposedly enhance memory, delay aging, boost energy levels, or strengthen the immune response. Many of these products are labeled with disclaimers such as, "This statement has not been evaluated by the FDA. This product is not intended to diagnose, treat, cure, or prevent any disease." This disclaimer is required by the FDA whenever a food manufacturer makes a structure-function claim (see Chapter 2). It acknowledges that the statement made on the label is not based on research!

In fact, the amounts of nutrients, phytochemicals, or other substances added to these waters are usually so low, compared to what can be obtained from foods, that they rarely make much of an impact on the consumer's health or well-being. In contrast, some of these designer waters can add more than 300 Calories to the day's intake.

Energy Drinks

Energy drinks represent another popular beverage option, with over $10 billion in sales in 2012. These products advertise their ability to provide a boost, jump start, buzz, punch, or rocket-powered blast! About 30% of teenagers drink them on a regular basis, even though physicians, nutrition experts, and consumer groups have raised significant concerns.[11] Many of these beverages contain more than three times the amount of caffeine in a comparable serving of cola, and a few contain up to ten times the caffeine in cola. Also, many energy drinks contain guarana seed extract: guarana seeds contain more caffeine than coffee beans, so their "extract" is simply a potent

> To watch a video of the American Beverage Association's Clear on Calories ad, go to www.ameribev.org, and type in "nutrition," and then "ads clear on calories" to connect to a link to the video.

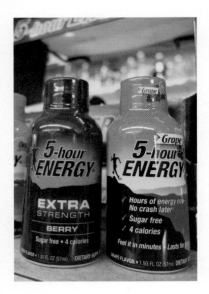

source of additional caffeine. Some also contain taurine, an amino acid associated with muscle contraction.

Unlike hot coffee, which is sipped slowly, the drinks are typically downed in a few minutes. Some are even packaged as a "shot." This sudden surge of caffeine can cause a dramatic rise in blood pressure and heart rate. Seizures, miscarriage, mood swings, insomnia, dehydration, and other health problems, as well as over 20,000 emergency department visits, have also been linked to consumption of energy drinks. The FDA has received information linking at least 18 deaths between 2009 and 2012 to two top-selling energy drinks. Although the FDA limits the amount of caffeine in soft drinks, it has no legal authority to regulate the ingredients, including caffeine, in energy drinks because they are classified as dietary supplements, not food. In contrast, Canada now caps caffeine levels in energy drinks, whereas Mexico is proposing to ban their sale to adolescents.

Energy drinks are also a source of significant added sugar. For example, a 16-ounce bottle of Rockstar Original contains 62 grams—more than 15 teaspoons—of sugar and 248 empty Calories. In short, as a source of fluid, energy drinks have a high potential for undesirable side-effects and should be avoided by children and adolescents and used sparingly by adults.

Sports Beverages and Coconut Water

Because of the potential for fluid and electrolyte imbalances during rigorous exercise, many endurance athletes drink sports beverages, which provide water, electrolytes, and a source of carbohydrate, before, during, and after workouts. Others are turning to coconut water, marketed as a good source of electrolytes and "natural sugars." Recently, sports beverages have also become popular with nonathletes, including children and adolescents.[12] Coconut water, although increasingly popular, is still regarded primarily as a specialty product. How necessary or helpful is it to consume such beverages? See the **Nutrition Debate** at the end of this chapter.

As you can see, American consumers have a wide range of beverage choices available to them. Poor choices can increase total caloric intake and lower daily nutrient intake. Over the past 40 years, the caloric contribution of beverages to our total energy intake has almost doubled. Plain drinking water is available free of charge, contributes no Calories, contains no additives, is highly effective in quenching thirst and maintaining hydration status, and poses no health threat. For most of us, most of the time, water really is the perfect beverage choice.

recap Fluid intake needs are highly variable and depend on body size, age, physical activity, health status, and environmental conditions. Drinking too much water can lead to overhydration and dilution of blood sodium. Drinking too little water leads to dehydration, one of the leading causes of death around the world. Many beverages contain added sugars and can contribute substantially to weight gain.

Sodium

Over the last 20 years, researchers have linked high sodium intake to an increased risk for hypertension among some groups of individuals. Because of this link, many people have come to believe that sodium is harmful to the body. This oversimplification, however, is just not true: sodium is a valuable nutrient that is essential for survival.

Functions of Sodium

Sodium has a variety of functions. As discussed earlier in this chapter, it is the major positively charged electrolyte in the extracellular fluid. Its exchange with potassium across cell membranes allows cells to maintain proper fluid balance, blood pressure, and acid–base balance.

Sodium also assists with the transmission of nerve signals and aids in muscle contraction. To review, the release of sodium from inside to outside the cell stimulates the spread of nerve signals within nervous tissue. The stimulation of muscles by nerve impulses provides the impetus for muscle contraction.

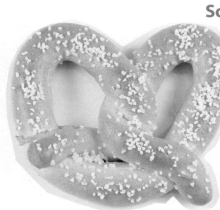

◆ Many popular snack foods are high in sodium.

what about **you** (?)

How Much Sodium Is in Your Diet?

About 90% of Americans eat too much sodium, virtually all in the form of salt. Although it isn't always easy to estimate the exact amount of sodium in your diet, there are some easy ways to judge if you are consuming too much sodium. Here are three quick questions for you:

1. *How much processed food is in my diet?* Foods that are canned, boxed, frozen, or otherwise processed are much higher in sodium than whole and account for as much as 80% of the sodium in the American diet. If you rely heavily on packaged dinners, cold cuts and cured meats/poultry, canned soups, frozen vegetables in sauce, pickled foods, and snack foods, you are probably consuming too much sodium. Each of these is in the "top ten" sources of sodium in the U.S. diet. See the **Quick Tips** (page 253) for better choices.

2. *How often do I eat foods naturally high in sodium?* Although not playing major roles in the typical American diet, there are several unprocessed foods that are surprisingly high in sodium. One serving of crab meat, for example, provides over 1,000 mg of sodium, more than half the

recommended Daily Value (DV)! Shellfish including clams, oysters, scallops, and mussels are two to three times higher in sodium than most other seafood. Cheese (which is technically processed milk but is rarely classified as a "processed" food) is often high in sodium. Three ounces of the following cheeses provide more than half the Daily Value: roquefort, parmesan, cheddar, swiss, and blue.

3. *Do I salt foods out of habit?* Many people pick up the salt shaker without even thinking about it. This unconscious habit quickly increases sodium intake: one teaspoon of salt contains about 2,000 mg of sodium, which is 87% of the recommended amount per day. And half of Americans should drop to 1,500 milligrams a day. Automatically reaching for the salt shaker is a habit that is sure to bring your sodium intake up into the unacceptably high range. A better plan is to avoid adding salt to foods until you've tasted what's on your plate. It does take time to adjust to using less table salt in your food, but most people quickly come to appreciate the natural flavor of foods once they break the salt shaker habit.

How Much Sodium Should We Consume?

The AI for sodium is listed in Table 7.1 (page 244). Most people in the United States consume two to four times the AI daily. Several health organizations recommend a daily sodium intake of no more than 2.3 g per day. The 2010 Dietary Guidelines for Americans specifically recommend that African Americans (who have a higher risk of hypertension, especially when consuming too much sodium) and all persons who already have hypertension limit their daily sodium intake to no more than 1.5 g.[13]

Do you have any idea of how much sodium you consume in an average day? If not, follow the steps in the **What About You?** feature to see if you might be getting too much.

Beyond Table Salt: Sneaky Sources of Sodium

Sodium is found naturally in many whole foods, but most dietary sodium comes from processed foods and restaurant foods, which typically contain large amounts of added sodium. Try to guess which of the following foods contains the most sodium: 1 cup of tomato juice, 1 oz of potato chips, or 4 saltine crackers. Now look at **TABLE 7.2** to find the answer. This table shows foods that are high in sodium and gives lower-sodium alternatives. Are you surprised to find out that, of all of these food items, the tomato juice has the most sodium?

Because sodium is so abundant, it's easy to overdo it. See the **Quick Tips** feature (on page 253) for ways to reduce your sodium intake. To help you curb your sodium intake, see the **Eating Right All Day** menu choices (page 254), which offer lower sodium options. Incidentally, each of these choices would be appropriate on the DASH diet (see the **In Depth** on cardiovascular disease following Chapter 5).

What Happens If We Consume Too Much Sodium?

Hypertension is typically more common in people who consume high-sodium diets, especially if potassium intake is low. This strong relationship has prompted many

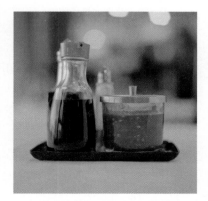

▲ Condiments can add sodium to your diet.

TABLE 7.2 **High-Sodium Foods and Lower-Sodium Alternatives**

High-Sodium Food	Sodium (mg)	Lower-Sodium Food	Sodium (mg)
Dill pickle (1 large, 4 in.)	1,731	Low-sodium dill pickle (1 large, 4 in.)	23
Ham, cured, roasted (3 oz)	1,023	Pork, loin roast (3 oz)	54
Turkey pastrami (3 oz)	915	Roasted turkey, cooked (3 oz)	54
Tomato juice, regular (1 cup)	877	Tomato juice, lower sodium (1 cup)	24
Macaroni and cheese (1 cup)	800	Spanish rice (1 cup)	5
Ramen noodle soup (chicken flavor) (1 package [85 g])	1,960	Ramen noodle soup made with sodium-free chicken bouillon (1 cup)	0
Teriyaki chicken (1 cup)	3,210	Stir-fried pork/rice/vegetables (1 cup)	575
Tomato sauce, canned (1/2 cup)	741	Fresh tomato (1 medium)	11
Creamed corn, canned (1 cup)	730	Cooked corn, fresh (1 cup)	28
Tomato soup, canned (1 cup)	695	Lower-sodium tomato soup, canned (1 cup)	480
Potato chips, salted (1 oz)	168	Baked potato, unsalted (1 medium)	14
Saltine crackers (4 crackers)	156	Saltine crackers, unsalted (4 crackers)	100

Data from: U.S. Department of Agriculture. 2011. USDA Nutrient Database for Standard Reference, Release 24.

health organizations to recommend lowering sodium intakes. Whether high-sodium diets actually cause hypertension is a matter of continuing debate; many researchers believe that a high-sodium/low-potassium dietary pattern is the greatest risk factor. Researchers also debate the effect of high-sodium intake on bone loss: some studies suggest high-sodium intakes have a negative effect on bone density, whereas other research has shown no impact on bone density.

Hypernatremia refers to an abnormally high blood sodium concentration. Although theoretically it could be caused by a rapid intake of high amounts of sodium—for instance, if a shipwrecked sailor resorted to drinking seawater—consuming too much sodium does not usually cause hypernatremia in a healthy person because the kidneys are able to excrete excess sodium in the urine. But people with congestive heart failure or kidney disease are not able to excrete sodium effectively, making them more prone to the condition. Hypernatremia is dangerous because it causes an abnormally high blood volume, again, by pulling water from the intracellular environment to dilute the sodium in the extracellular tissue spaces and vessels. This leads to edema (swelling) of tissues and elevation of blood pressure to unhealthy levels.

What Happens If We Don't Consume Enough Sodium?

Because the dietary intake of sodium is so high among Americans, deficiencies of sodium are extremely rare. Nevertheless, certain conditions can cause **hyponatremia**, abnormally low blood sodium levels.

Exercise-associated hyponatremia (EAH) can occur in people engaged in strenuous physical activity who drink large volumes of water or other beverages and fail to replace sodium.[14] This has actually led to the deaths of several highly fit marathon runners. Risk for EAH increases with longer race times, slower pace of running, and consumption of large amounts of water or other fluids during the event; thus, inexperienced runners are at greater risk. In addition, as many as one in five triathletes, who sequentially compete in swimming, cycling, and running events, are at risk for EAH.

Severe diarrhea, vomiting, or excessive, prolonged sweating can also cause hyponatremia. Symptoms include headaches, dizziness, fatigue, nausea, vomiting, and muscle cramps.

If hyponatremia is left untreated, it can progress to seizures, coma, and death. Treatment for hyponatremia includes replacement of the lost minerals by consuming

hypernatremia A condition in which blood sodium levels are dangerously high.

hyponatremia A condition in which blood sodium levels are dangerously low.

QuickTips

Reducing the Sodium in Your Diet

Put away the salt shaker—keep it off the table and train your taste buds to prefer foods with less salt.

Follow the DASH diet plan (see page 188), which is high in fruits, vegetables, whole grains, and lean protein foods. The more you include fresh, whole foods in your diet, the less sodium you will be eating.

Look for the words *low sodium* or *no added salt* when buying processed foods. Use the Nutrition Facts Panel to find foods that contain 5% or less of the daily value for sodium or less than 200 mg per serving.

Look for *hidden* salt content on food labels; for example, both monosodium glutamate and sodium benzoate are forms of sodium.

Compare the labels of various name brands of the same food because products can vary greatly in their sodium content.

Choose fresh or frozen vegetables (without added sauces) because they are usually much lower in sodium than canned vegetables. Alternatively, choose salt-free canned vegetables.

Stay away from prepared stews, canned and dried soups, gravies, and pasta sauces as well as packaged pasta, rice, and potato dishes that are high in sodium.

Choose low-sodium versions of pickles, olives, three-bean salad, and salad dressings.

Choose low-sodium versions of cheese, smoked meats and fish, and nuts.

Snack on fruits and vegetables instead of salty snack foods. If you do buy pretzels, chips, and other snack items, choose low-sodium versions.

When cooking, experiment with commercial salt substitutes, herbs, spices, salt-free rubs, lemon juice, chutneys, salsas, and possibly cooking wine to flavor your food. Products that end in the word *salt,* such as garlic salt or celery salt, are high in sodium and should be avoided.

Rinse canned legumes, such as black, navy, garbanzo, or kidney beans, with cold water to lower the sodium content before heating and consuming them.

Reduce the amounts of condiments you use. Condiments such as ketchup, mustard, pickle relish, and soy sauce can add a considerable amount of sodium to your foods. Again, check the labels of these items.

When eating out, look for entrées labeled "heart healthy" or "lower in sodium"; if nutrition information is provided, compare foods to select those with lower amounts of sodium.

Check the labels on your medications. Many medications, including aspirin, are high in sodium.

Check the labels of the beverages you consume as well; fluids are often a "hidden" source of dietary sodium.

---

liquids and foods high in sodium and other minerals. Hospitalization and/or the intravenous administration of an electrolyte-rich solution may be necessary in order to prevent life-threatening complications.

Potassium

As we discussed previously, potassium is the major positively charged electrolyte in the intracellular fluid. It is a major constituent of all living cells and is found in both plants and animals.

eating right all day

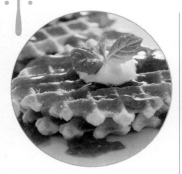

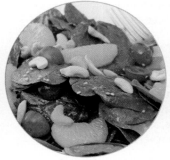

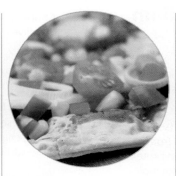

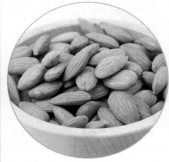

Breakfast
Whole-grain waffle with jam instead of a ham & cheese omlette!

Lunch
Spinach salad instead of canned spinach!

Dinner
Veggie pizza instead of pepperoni!

Snack
Unsalted almonds instead of corn chips!

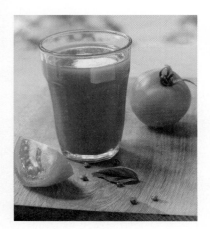

▲ Tomato juice is an excellent source of potassium. Make sure you choose the low-sodium variety!

hyperkalemia A condition in which blood potassium levels are dangerously high.

Functions of Potassium

Potassium and sodium work together to maintain proper fluid balance and regulate the transmission of nerve impulses and the contraction of muscles. And in contrast to a high-sodium diet, a diet high in potassium actually helps maintain a lower blood pressure.

How Much Potassium Should We Consume?

Potassium is found in abundance in many fresh foods, especially fresh fruits and vegetables. Processed foods generally have less potassium than fresh foods.

The AI for potassium is listed in Table 7.1. According to a recent report, the usual potassium intake of American adults falls well below the recommended amount.[15] By avoiding processed foods and eating more fresh fruits, vegetables, legumes, whole grains, and dairy foods, you'll increase your potassium intake and decrease your sodium intake, achieving a more healthful diet.

Sources of Potassium: Potatoes, Bananas, and More

As more and more people rely on processed foods, their sodium intake increases and their potassium intake decreases. Many researchers think that this sodium–potassium imbalance is a major factor contributing to the increased incidence of hypertension in the United States. Thus, fresh foods, particularly fresh fruits and vegetables, should be included in every meal. **FIGURE 7.8** identifies foods that are high in potassium. See the **Quick Tips** feature (page 255) on how to increase your dietary potassium.

What Happens If We Consume Too Much Potassium?

People with healthy kidneys are able to excrete excess potassium effectively. However, people with kidney disease are not able to regulate their blood potassium levels. **Hyperkalemia**, or high blood potassium levels, occurs when potassium is not excreted efficiently from the body. Because of potassium's role in cardiac muscle contraction, severe hyperkalemia can alter the normal rhythm of the heart, resulting in heart

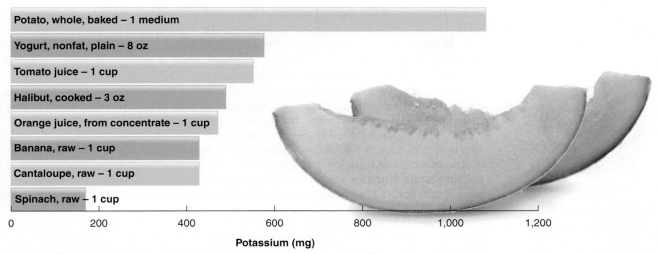

FIGURE 7.8 Common food sources of potassium. The AI for potassium is 4.7 g (or 4,700 mg) per day.
Data from: U.S. Department of Agriculture, Agricultural Research Service. 2011. USDA Nutrient Database for Standard Reference, Release 24.

QuickTips

Increasing Your Potassium Intake

✔ Avoid processed foods that are high in sodium and low in potassium. Check the Nutrition Facts Panel of the food before you buy it!

✔ For breakfast, look for cereals containing bran and/or wheat germ.

✔ Sprinkle wheat germ on yogurt and top with banana slices.

✔ Add wheat germ to baked goods, such as homemade pancakes and muffins.

✔ Drink milk! If you don't like milk, try one of the new drinkable yogurts. Many brands of soy milk are also good sources of potassium.

✔ Make a smoothie by blending ice cubes and low-fat vanilla ice cream or yogurt with a banana.

✔ Pack a can of low-sodium vegetable or tomato juice in your lunch in place of a soft drink.

✔ Serve avocado or bean dip with veggie slices.

✔ Replace the meat in your sandwich with thin slices of avocado or marinated tofu.

✔ Replace the meat in tacos and burritos with black or pinto beans.

✔ For a healthful alternative to french fries, toss slices of sweet potato in olive oil, place on a cookie sheet, and oven bake at 400° for 10–15 minutes.

✔ Toss a banana, some dried apricots, or a bag of sunflower seeds into your lunch bag.

✔ Make a fruit salad with apricots, bananas, cantaloupe, honeydew melon, mango, or papaya.

✔ Bake and enjoy a fresh pumpkin pie!

attack and death. People with kidney failure must monitor their potassium intake very carefully to prevent complications from hyperkalemia. Individuals at risk for hyperkalemia should avoid consuming salt substitutes because these products are high in potassium.

What Happens If We Don't Consume Enough Potassium?

Because potassium is widespread in many foods, a dietary potassium deficiency is rare. However, potassium deficiency is not uncommon among people who have serious medical disorders. Kidney disease, a complication of poorly controlled diabetes known as diabetic acidosis, and other illnesses can lead to potassium deficiency.

In addition, people with hypertension who are prescribed diuretic medications are at risk for potassium deficiency. Diuretics promote the excretion of fluid as urine through the kidneys and some also increase the excretion of potassium. People who are taking diuretic medications should have their blood potassium monitored regularly and should eat foods that are high in potassium to prevent **hypokalemia**, or low blood potassium levels. This is not a universal recommendation, however, because some diuretics are specially formulated to spare potassium; therefore, people taking this type of diuretic should not increase their dietary potassium above recommended levels.

Extreme dehydration, vomiting, and diarrhea can also cause hypokalemia. People who abuse alcohol or laxatives are also at risk for hypokalemia. Symptoms include confusion, loss of appetite, and muscle weakness. Severe cases of hypokalemia result in fatal changes in heart rate; many deaths attributed to extreme dehydration or eating disorders are caused by abnormal heart rhythms due to hypokalemia.

Chloride

Chloride should not be confused with *chlorine*, which is a poisonous gas used to kill bacteria and other germs in our water supply. Chloride is a negatively charged ion that is obtained almost exclusively in our diet from sodium chloride, or table salt.

Functions of Chloride

Coupled with sodium in the extracellular fluid, chloride assists with the maintenance of fluid balance. Chloride is also a part of hydrochloric acid (HCl) in the stomach, which aids in preparing food for further digestion (see Chapter 3). Chloride works with the white blood cells of our body during an immune response to help kill bacteria, and it assists in the transmission of nerve impulses.

How Much Chloride Should We Consume?

The AI for chloride is listed in Table 7.1 (page 244). Our primary dietary source of chloride is salt in our foods. Chloride is also found in some fruits and vegetables.

Virtually all dietary chloride is in the form of sodium chloride. As you've learned, consuming excess amounts of salt over a prolonged period leads to hypertension in salt-sensitive individuals. There is no other known toxicity symptom for chloride.[2]

Because of the relatively high dietary salt intake in the United States, most people consume more than enough chloride. Even when a person consumes a low-sodium diet, chloride intake is usually adequate. A chloride deficiency can occur, however, during conditions of severe dehydration and frequent vomiting. For example, it can develop in people with eating disorders who regularly vomit to rid their bodies of unwanted Calories.

Phosphorus

Phosphorus is the major intracellular negatively charged electrolyte. In the body, phosphorus is most commonly found in the form of phosphate, PO_4^{2-}. Phosphorus is an essential constituent of all cells and is found in both plants and animals.

Functions of Phosphorus

Phosphorus works with potassium inside cells to maintain proper fluid balance. It also plays a critical role in bone formation because it is part of the mineral complex of bone. In fact, about 85% of our body's phosphorus is stored in our bones.

As a primary component of adenosine triphosphate (ATP), phosphorus plays a key role in creating energy for our body. It also helps regulate many biochemical reactions by activating and deactivating enzymes. Phosphorus is a part of deoxyribonucleic

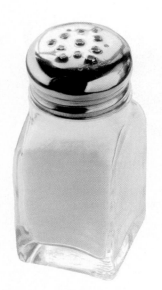

◀ Almost all chloride is consumed through table salt.

hypokalemia A condition in which blood potassium levels are dangerously low.

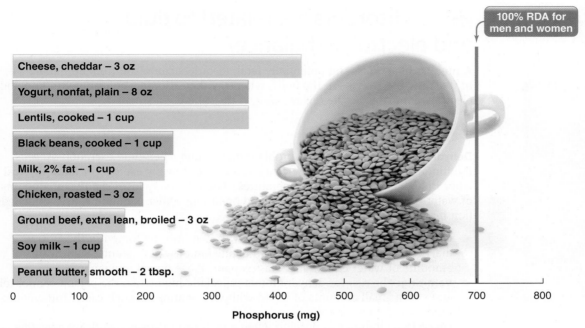

100% RDA for men and women

Cheese, cheddar – 3 oz

Yogurt, nonfat, plain – 8 oz

Lentils, cooked – 1 cup

Black beans, cooked – 1 cup

Milk, 2% fat – 1 cup

Chicken, roasted – 3 oz

Ground beef, extra lean, broiled – 3 oz

Soy milk – 1 cup

Peanut butter, smooth – 2 tbsp.

0   100   200   300   400   500   600   700   800

Phosphorus (mg)

FIGURE 7.9 Common food sources of phosphorus. The RDA for phosphorus is 700 mg/day.
Data from: U.S. Department of Agriculture, Agricultural Research Service. 2011. USDA Nutrient Database for Standard Reference, Release 24.

acid (DNA) and ribonucleic acid (RNA), and it is a component in cell membranes (as phospholipids) and lipoproteins.

How Much Phosphorus Should We Consume?

The RDA for phosphorus is listed in Table 7.1. The average U.S. adult consumes about twice this amount each day; thus, phosphorus deficiencies are rare. Phosphorus is widespread in many foods and is found in high amounts in foods that contain protein. Milk, meats, and eggs are good sources. **FIGURE 7.9** shows the phosphorus content of various foods.

It is important to note that phosphorus from animal sources is absorbed more readily than that from plant sources. The phosphorus in plant foods such as beans, cereals, and nuts is found in the form of **phytic acid**, a plant storage form of phosphorus. Our body does not produce enzymes that can break down phytic acid, but we are still able to absorb up to 50% of the phosphorus found in plant foods because other foods and the bacteria in our large intestine can help break down phytic acid.

People suffering from kidney disease, who cannot efficiently excrete phosphorus; people consuming excessive amounts of supplemental vitamin D, which tends to increase absorption and retention of phosphorus; and people taking too many phosphorus-containing antacids can suffer from high blood phosphorus levels. Severely high levels of blood phosphorus cause muscle spasms and convulsions.

As mentioned previously, deficiencies of phosphorus are rare. People who may suffer from low blood phosphorus levels include premature infants, elderly people with poor diets, and people who abuse alcohol. People with vitamin D deficiency, who poorly absorb phosphorus, those with hyperparathyroidism (oversecretion of parathyroid hormone), and those who overuse antacids that bind with phosphorus may also have low blood phosphorus levels.

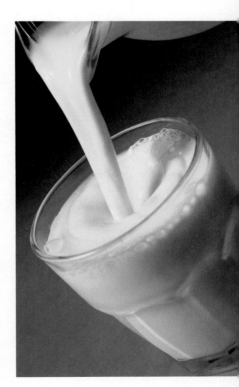

Milk is a good source of phosphorus.

recap The four electrolytes critical for hydration and neuromuscular function are sodium, potassium, chloride, and phosphorus. Most Americans consume too much sodium and often get too little potassium; intakes of chloride and phosphorus are almost always adequate but not excessive. Electrolyte imbalances can result in heart failure, seizures, and death.

phytic acid The form of phosphorus stored in plants.

What disorders are related to fluid and electrolyte balance?

A number of serious, and potentially fatal, disorders can result from an imbalance of fluid and electrolytes in the body, whereas other disorders contribute to fluid and electrolyte imbalance. We review some of these here.

Dehydration

Dehydration is a serious health problem that results when fluid excretion exceeds fluid intake. It most commonly occurs as a result of heavy exercise or hard physical labor in high environmental temperatures, when the body loses significant amounts of water through increased sweating and breathing. Other common causes of dehydration include the following:

- **Diarrhea:** When excess fluid is quickly drawn into the lumen of the GI tract, diarrhea develops, leading to rapid expulsion of watery stools. Significant amounts of water can be lost via frequent, loose bowel movements.
- **Vomiting:** The risk for dehydration is especially high when the person cannot tolerate even small amounts of liquid without vomiting. In such cases, intravenous fluids may be necessary.
- **Fever:** Dehydration can develop when a high fever causes significant sweating.
- **Burns (including sunburn):** Normal, intact skin keeps tissue fluid inside the body. In people with severe burns, including sunburns over a large surface area of the body, fluid loss through the skin can be extensive.
- **Poorly controlled diabetes:** When blood glucose levels are high, some of the glucose "spills" into the urine. The kidneys respond by increasing fluid output as well, diluting the urine but leaving the person dehydrated.
- **Abuse of diuretics or laxatives:** These products cause excessive loss of body fluid and should be used only under medical supervision because they significantly increase the risk for dehydration.

Older adults and infants are at a higher risk for dehydration than are healthy young and middle-aged adults. The elderly are at increased risk because they have a lower proportion of body water, thus a smaller "margin of error." Their thirst mechanism is less effective than that of a younger person, too, so they are less likely to meet their fluid needs. Infants, on the other hand, excrete urine at a higher rate, cannot tell us when they are thirsty, and have a greater ratio of body surface area to body core, causing them to respond more dramatically to heat and cold and to lose more body water than an older child.

Classifying Dehydration

Dehydration is classified in terms of the percentage of weight loss that is exclusively due to the loss of fluid (TABLE 7.3):

- Relatively small losses in body water, equal to a 1–2% change in body weight, result in symptoms such as thirst, dry mouth, discomfort, and loss of appetite. For a person weighing 160 pounds, these symptoms occur after a rapid loss of 1 to 4 pounds of body water.
- More severe water losses, equal to 3–5% of body weight, result in symptoms that include sleepiness, nausea, flushed skin, and inability to concentrate.
- Severe losses of body water, greater than 8% of body weight (about 13 pounds of water for someone weighing 160 pounds), can result in delirium, coma, and death because the rapid loss of body fluid leads to a dangerous increase in body temperature, which results in organ failure.

Preventing Dehydration During and After Physical Activity

Adequate fluid replacement is the most important factor in preventing dehydration. If you're physically active, how can you tell whether you are drinking enough fluid before, during, and after your exercise or training sessions? First, you can hop

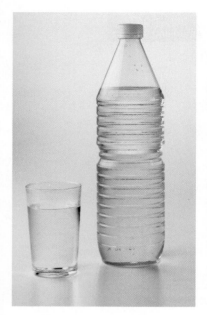

▲ Dehydration occurs when fluid excretion exceeds fluid intake.

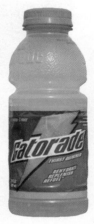

▲ Adequate fluid replacement during and after physical activity is critical in preventing dehydration.

dehydration The depletion of body fluid that results when fluid excretion exceeds fluid intake.

TABLE 7.3 **Percentages of Body Fluid Loss Correlated with Weight Loss and Symptoms**

Body Water Loss (%)	Weight Lost If You Weigh 160 lb	Weight Lost If You Weigh 130 lb	Symptoms
1–2	1.6–3.2 lb	1.3–2.6 lb	Strong thirst, loss of appetite, feeling uncomfortable
3–5	4.8–8.0 lb	3.9–6.5 lb	Dry mouth, reduced urine output, greater difficulty working and concentrating, flushed skin, tingling extremities, impatience, sleepiness, nausea, emotional instability
6–8	9.6–12.8 lb	7.8–10.4 lb	Increased body temperature that doesn't decrease, increased heart rate and breathing rate, dizziness, difficulty breathing, slurred speech, mental confusion, muscle weakness, blue lips
9–11	14.4–17.6 lb	11.7–14.3 lb	Muscle spasms, delirium, swollen tongue, poor balance and circulation, kidney failure, decreased blood volume and blood pressure

Data from: *Nutrition and Aerobic Exercise,* edited by D. K. Layman. © 1986 American Chemical Society.

on the scale before and after each session, ideally when unclothed or just wearing underclothes. If you weighed in at 160 pounds before basketball practice, and immediately afterwards you weighed 158 pounds, then you would have lost 2 pounds of body weight, virtually all as fluid. This is equal to 1.3% of your body weight prior to practice. As you can see in Table 7.3, you would most likely experience strong thirst and diminished appetite, and you might even feel generally uncomfortable.

If you find you have lost weight during a session of physical activity, what should you do about it? Your goal is to consume enough water and other fluids to replace one and one-half times as much fluid as was lost—and to do this prior to your next exercise session. Fortunately, this isn't difficult. For instance, a weight loss of 2 pounds would require an intake of about 6 cups of fluid because 2 lb of body weight loss is equivalent to a loss of just under 1 L of fluid, or about 4 cups. If you multiply that 4-cup loss by 1.5, your goal is about 6 cups of fluid. In general, by following the daily fluid intake recommendations discussed earlier, plus replacing fluids lost during sessions of physical activity, you should be able to avoid becoming dehydrated.

If you don't have time to weigh yourself before and after every workout, don't despair! A simpler method of monitoring your fluid levels is to observe the color of your urine. If you are properly hydrated, your urine should be clear to pale yellow in color, similar to diluted lemonade **(FIGURE 7.10)**. Urine that is medium to dark yellow in color, similar to apple juice, indicates an inadequate fluid intake. Very dark or brown urine, such as the color of a cola beverage, is a sign of severe dehydration and indicates potential muscle breakdown and kidney damage. Your goal should be to maintain a urine color that is clear or pale yellow.

Heat Illnesses

Three common types of heat illness are closely linked to dehydration: in order of severity, these are heat cramps, heat exhaustion, and heat stroke.

Heat Cramps

Heat cramps are painful muscle cramps, usually in the abdomen, arms, or legs, that develop during sessions of vigorous physical activity in the heat. The spasms can last for several seconds or even minutes and are caused by a fluid and electrolyte imbalance.

If you ever experience muscle cramps during a workout or athletic event, stop your activity immediately. Go to a cool place, rest, and sip a sports beverage, juice, or—if these are not available—plain water. You can also sprinkle a dash of salt into a full glass of water. If the cramps don't subside within an hour, seek medical attention.

Heat Exhaustion

Like heat cramps, **heat exhaustion** typically occurs when people are engaging in vigorous physical activity in a hot environment. It can also develop after several days in high temperatures when fluid intake is inadequate.

Signs and symptoms typically include increased thirst; weakness; muscle cramps; nausea and vomiting; dizziness and possibly fainting; and possibly elevated blood pressure and pulse. In a person with heat exhaustion, the sweat mechanism still

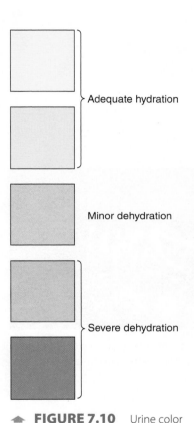

Adequate hydration

Minor dehydration

Severe dehydration

FIGURE 7.10 Urine color chart. Color variations indicate levels of hydration.

heat cramps Involuntary, spasmodic, and painful muscle contractions that are caused by electrolyte imbalances occurring as a result of strenuous physical activity in high environmental heat.

heat exhaustion A serious condition, characterized by heavy sweating, pallor, nausea and vomiting, dizziness, and moderately elevated body temperature, that develops from dehydration in high heat.

nutri-case | GUSTAVO

"Something is going on with me this week. Every day, at work, I've been feeling weak and like I'm going to be sick to my stomach. It's been really hot, over a hundred degrees out in the fields, but I'm used to that, and besides, I've been drinking lots of water. It's probably just my high blood pressure acting up again."

What do you think might be affecting Gustavo? If you learned that he was following a low-sodium diet to manage his hypertension, would this information argue for or against your assumptions about the source of his discomfort? Why or why not? What would you advise Gustavo to do differently at work tomorrow?

functions; in fact, the person is typically sweating heavily. Immediate cooling and fluid intake are essential to avoid heat stroke.

Heat Stroke

Heat stroke is a potentially fatal heat illness characterized by failure of the body's heat-regulating mechanisms. Thus, the person's skin is hot and dry, not sweaty. Other signs and symptoms include rapid pulse; high core body temperature; rapid, shallow breathing; and disorientation or loss of consciousness.

Recall that evaporative cooling is less efficient in a humid environment because the sweat is less able to evaporate. Therefore, athletes who work out in hot, humid weather are particularly vulnerable to heat stroke. Over a 1-week period in 2011, one coach and three high school football players died from heat-related complications.[16] Of course, heat-related deaths also occur among collegiate and professional athletes. The deaths are more common in overweight or obese athletes for two reasons: Significant muscle mass produces a lot of body heat, whereas excess body fat adds an extra layer of insulation that makes it more difficult to dissipate that heat. In football players, tight-fitting uniforms and helmets also trap warm air and blunt the ability of the body to cool itself.

If you are active in a hot environment and begin to feel dizzy, light-headed, disoriented, or nauseated, stop exercising at once. Get into a cool environment, such as a cool shower or a bath. Drink a sports beverage. If you are working out with someone who exhibits the symptoms of heat stroke, call 911 promptly.

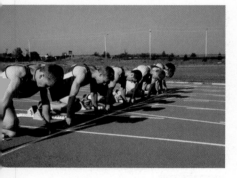

▲ Athletes who train or compete in hot weather are vulnerable to heat stroke.

✳behavior change . . . getting started!

Now that you've read this chapter, try making these changes:

For yourself:

- Try going for 1 week without soft drinks, energy drinks, juice drinks, or bottled coffees and teas. You'll save Calories and money, and you might find that you enjoy drinking plain water just as well.
- Make it a habit to taste your food before deciding whether or not to salt it.

For your community:

- If you don't already own one, buy a reusable water bottle and begin to use it instead of buying individual plastic bottles of water. Start a campaign on your campus to replace water fountains with water stations to encourage others to use reusable water bottles.
- Chat with the chef at your campus dining hall and find out whether salt is automatically added to foods during cooking. If it is, speak with the foodservice or dining hall manager or campus Health/Wellness Director to explore ways of lowering the use of salt across all campus dining outlets.

heat stroke A potentially fatal response to high temperature characterized by failure of the body's heat-regulating mechanisms; also commonly called *sunstroke*.

nutrition debate

Sports Beverages: Help or Hype?

Once considered specialty items used exclusively by elite athletes, sports beverages have become popular everyday beverage choices for both active and nonactive people. This surge in popularity leads us to ask four important questions:

- Do sport beverages benefit highly active athletes?
- Do sport beverages benefit recreationally active people?
- Do relatively inactive or sedentary adults benefit from the consumption of sports beverages?
- Are sports beverages necessary or appropriate for children and adolescents?

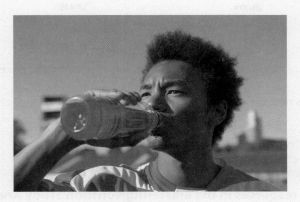

Sports beverages were originally designed to meet the needs of competitive athletes.

The first question is relatively easy to answer. Sports beverages were originally developed to meet the unique fluid, electrolyte, and carbohydrate needs of competitive athletes. Highly active people need to replenish both fluids and electrolytes to avoid either dehydration or hyponatremia. For example, endurance athletes are able to exercise longer, maintain a higher intensity, and improve performance times when they drink a sports beverage during exercise.[17] The carbohydrates in sports beverages may also help athletes consume more energy than they could by eating solid foods and water alone. Some competitive athletes regularly train or compete for 6 to 8 hours each day. With this schedule, it is virtually impossible for them to eat enough solid foods to meet their energy needs. For all these reasons, in response to the first question, the answer is "yes": endurance athletes are able to exercise longer, maintain a higher intensity, and improve performance times when they drink a sports beverage during exercise.

Do recreationally active people need to consume sports beverages? The short answer is that most probably do not. Those few who exercise for periods longer than 1 hour at an intense level of effort probably can benefit from consuming the carbohydrate and electrolytes in sports beverages during exercise.

If you're active, how do you know whether you should consume a sports beverage? The answer depends on the duration and intensity of exercise, the environmental conditions, and your unique characteristics. Here are some situations in which drinking a sports beverage is appropriate:[18]

- During exercise or physical work in high heat and/or high humidity or if you have recently experienced diarrhea or vomiting
- During exercise at high altitude and in cold environments
- After exercise if rapid rehydration is needed or desired
- Between exercise bouts, such as between multiple soccer matches during a tournament

- During exercise sessions that last longer than 60 minutes, when blood glucose levels get low and risk of dehydration increases
- During exercise sessions if glycogen stores are low due to illness or inability to eat enough solid food before exercising

Although sports beverages have become very popular with people who do little or no regular exercise, there is no evidence that these people derive any benefits from drinking them. Even if these individuals live in a hot environment, they should be able to replenish the fluid and electrolytes they lose during sweating by drinking water and other beverages and eating a normal diet.

In addition, inactive people who drink sports beverages are likely to gain weight. Although some manufacturers are producing "light" sports beverages that are lower in Calories than the traditional product, drinking 12 fl. oz (1.5 cups) of a traditionally formulated Gatorade adds 90 kcal to a person's daily energy intake. Many inactive people consume two to three times this amount each day.

Finally, are sports beverages beneficial for children and adolescents? They have been increasingly marketed to schools seeking alternatives to sweetened sodas, and their consumption is on the rise. However, consumption of sports beverages increases a child's risk for both weight gain and erosion of tooth enamel. Most sports drinks have a pH in the acidic range (pH 3 to 4) and many include citric acid, which rapidly demineralizes the tooth surface. Because of these risks, the American Academy of Pediatrics and the Institute of Medicine advise that sports drinks be used only by children engaging in prolonged, vigorous sports activities, and that, for children engaged in routine physical activity, plain water is appropriate.[19,20]

CRITICAL THINKING QUESTIONS

1. Why would some athletes find it easier to get some of their Calories from sports beverages instead of eating solid food? Consider it from the viewpoint of an endurance cyclist who might be on a 5-hour training ride.
2. What are three possible long-term consequences of providing children with sports beverages on a regular basis when they are engaged in brief, low-intensity activities? Consider their future health, future food/beverage choices, and ability to manage their weight as they grow as you formulate your answer.

chapter review

test yourself | answers

1. **False.** Recent research suggests that caffeine intake has virtually no effect on fluid balance.

2. **False.** Sodium is a nutrient necessary for human functioning, but we should not consume more than recommended amounts.

3. **False.** Our thirst mechanism signals that we need to replenish fluids, but it is not sufficient to ensure that we are completely hydrated.

MasteringNutrition™

Check out these additional resources in the MasteringNutrition Study Area at www.masteringhealthandnutrition.pearson.com:

- Read It: Chapter Summary and RSS Feeds
- See It: ABC News videos and nutrition animations
- Hear It: MP3s
- Study It: Get Ready for Nutrition Math and Chemistry review
- Do It: NutriTools and "Find the Quack" feature
- Review It: Quizzes, flashcards, and glossary

review questions

1. Plasma is one example of
   a. extracellular fluid.
   b. intracellular fluid.
   c. tissue fluid.
   d. metabolic water.

2. Which of the following is a critical function of fluids?
   a. They dissolve fat-soluble vitamins.
   b. Their relatively low heat capacity keeps the body warm.
   c. They provide protection for the brain and spinal cord.
   d. All of the above are true.

3. Which of the following is true of the cell membrane?
   a. It is freely permeable to electrolytes but not to water.
   b. It is freely permeable to water but not to electrolytes.
   c. It is freely permeable to both water and electrolytes.
   d. It is freely permeable to neither water nor electrolytes.

4. We lose fluids through
   a. sweat.
   b. breath.
   c. feces.
   d. all of the above.

5. Which of the following is the most healthful beverage for most people most of the time?
   a. tap water
   b. vitamin water sweetened with honey
   c. tomato or other vegetable juice
   d. energy drink made with non-Caloric sweetener

6. Which of the following statements about sodium is true?
   a. One serving of ramen noodle soup provides nearly half the AI for sodium.
   b. High-sodium diets are the primary cause of hypertension.
   c. Increased plasma (or serum) sodium draws water out of cells and into the extracellular fluid.
   d. All of the above statements are true.

7. Which of the following is a characteristic of potassium?
   a. It is the major positively charged electrolyte in the extracellular fluid.
   b. It can be found in fresh fruits and vegetables.
   c. It is a critical component of the mineral complex of bone.
   d. It is the major negatively charged electrolyte in the extracellular fluid.

8. Which of the following factors commonly contributes to dehydration?

   a. drinking too much plain water while active in a hot environment

   b. sweating and breathing heavily while active in a hot environment

   c. failure of the body's heat-regulating mechanisms

   d. failure to drink sports beverages during illnesses causing vomiting

9. **True or false?** Groundwater comes from lakes, rivers, and reservoirs.

10. **True or false?** Chloride's only important body function is to help maintain fluid balance.

math review

11. Your roommate comes home after basketball practice and tells you he has lost 3 lb. Knowing that 1 pound of body weight loss represents the loss of 2 cups of fluid, how much fluid should he consume over the next few hours in order to fully rehydrate?

Answers to Review Questions and Math Review are located at the back of this text and in the MasteringNutrition Study Area.

web resources

www.epa.gov
U.S. Environmental Protection Agency: Water

Go to the EPA's water website, by entering OW into the search box, for more information about drinking water quality, standards, and safety.

www.bottledwater.org
International Bottled Water Association

Find current information about bottled water from this trade association, which represents the bottled water industry.

www.mayoclinic.com
MayoClinic.com

Search for "hyponatremia" to learn more about this potentially fatal condition.

www.nih.gov
National Institutes of Health

Search this site to learn more about the Dietary Approaches to Stop Hypertension (DASH) diet.

www.nephrologychannel.com
Nephrologychannel.com: Electrolyte Imbalances

Visit this website and type "electrolytes" into the search field to learn more about hyponatremia, hypernatremia, hypokalemia, and hyperkalemia.

www.wqa.org
Water Quality Association

The website for the WQA, a trade association for the water treatment industry, lists recent news affecting municipal water supplies, home water testing, and water quality.

in depth 7.5

Alcohol

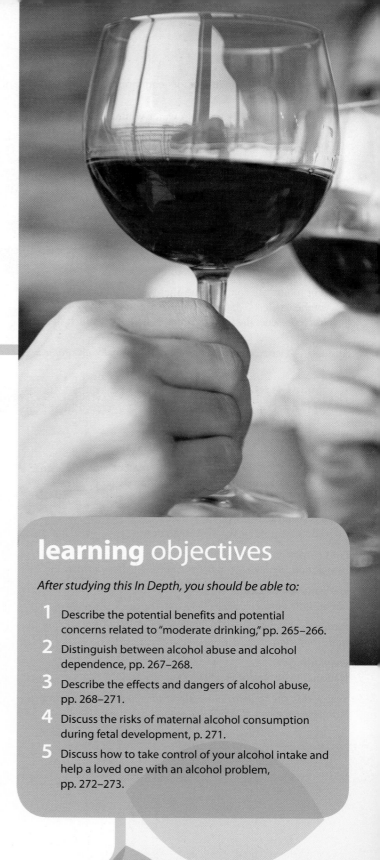

No one should have to spend his 21st birthday in an emergency department, but that's what happened to Todd the night he turned 21. His friends took him off campus to celebrate, and, with their encouragement, he attempted to drink 21 shots before the bar closed at 2:00 A.M. Fortunately for Todd, when he passed out and couldn't be roused, his best friend noticed his cold, clammy skin and erratic breathing and drove him to the local emergency department. There, his stomach was pumped and he was treated for alcohol poisoning. He regained consciousness but felt sick and shaky for several more hours. Not everyone is so lucky. Some people with alcohol poisoning never wake up.

What makes excessive alcohol intake so dangerous, and why is moderate alcohol consumption often considered healthful? How can you tell if someone is struggling with an alcohol problem, and what can you do to help? What if that someone is you? We explore these questions here.

Alcohols are chemical compounds structurally similar to carbohydrates. **Ethanol** is a specific type of alcohol found in beer, wine, and distilled spirits such as whiskey and vodka. Throughout this **In Depth** discussion, the common term *alcohol* will be used to represent the specific compound *ethanol*.

learning objectives

After studying this In Depth, you should be able to:

1 Describe the potential benefits and potential concerns related to "moderate drinking," pp. 265–266.

2 Distinguish between alcohol abuse and alcohol dependence, pp. 267–268.

3 Describe the effects and dangers of alcohol abuse, pp. 268–271.

4 Discuss the risks of maternal alcohol consumption during fetal development, p. 271.

5 Discuss how to take control of your alcohol intake and help a loved one with an alcohol problem, pp. 272–273.

What do we know about moderate alcohol intake?

Alcohol intake is usually described as "drinks per day." A **drink** is defined as the amount of a beverage that provides ½ fluid ounce of pure alcohol. For example, 12 oz of beer, 10 oz of a wine cooler, 4–5 oz of wine, and 1½ oz of 80-**proof** whiskey, scotch, gin, or vodka are each equivalent to one drink (FIGURE 1).

The 2010 Dietary Guidelines for Americans advise, "If alcohol is consumed, it should be consumed in moderation—up to one drink per day for women and two drinks per day for men – and only by adults of legal drinking age." Notice that this definition of **moderate drinking** is based on a maximal daily intake; a person who does not drink any alcohol on weekdays but downs a six-pack of beer most Saturday nights would *not* be classified as a "moderate drinker"!

The 2010 Dietary Guidelines for Americans also identify groups of individuals who should not consume alcohol at all, including women who are or may become pregnant and women who are breastfeeding. In addition, people who cannot restrict their drinking to moderate levels and those taking medications that interact with alcohol should not drink at all, nor should individuals driving, operating machinery, or engaged in other tasks that require attention and coordination. Finally, anyone younger than the legal drinking age should not consume alcohol.

As we discuss here, both health benefits and concerns are associated with moderate alcohol intake. When deciding whether or how much alcohol to drink, you need to weigh the pros and cons of alcohol consumption against your own personal health history.

Benefits of Moderate Alcohol Intake

In most people, moderate alcohol intake offers some psychological benefits; it can reduce stress and anxiety while improving self-confidence. It can also have nutritional benefits. Moderate use of alcohol can improve appetite and dietary intake, which can be of great value to the elderly and people with a chronic disease that suppresses appetite.[1]

In addition, moderate alcohol consumption has been linked to lower rates of heart disease, especially in older adults and those already at risk for heart disease, such as people with type 2 diabetes.[2] Alcohol increases levels of the "good" type of cholesterol (HDL) while lowering the concentration of "bad" cholesterol (LDL); it also reduces the risk of abnormal clot formation in the blood vessels.

Recently, there has been a lot of interest in **resveratrol**, a phytochemical found in red wines, grapes, and other plant foods.[3] Some researchers, based on experiments with mice, are proposing that resveratrol may be able to lower our risk for certain chronic diseases such as diabetes, heart disease, cancer, and liver disease as well as enhancing exercise tolerance. However, the amount in red wine is too minimal to provide a health benefit. Instead,

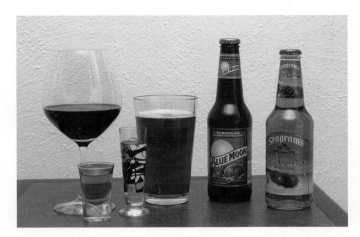

FIGURE 1 What does one drink look like? A drink is equivalent to 1-1/2 oz of distilled spirits, 4 to 5 oz of wine, 10 oz of wine cooler, or 12 oz of beer.

if resveratrol were found to be effective in promoting human health, it would have to be given as a purified supplement.

Concerns of Moderate Alcohol Intake

Not everyone responds to alcohol in the same manner. A person's age, genetic makeup, state of health, and use of medications can influence both immediate and long-term responses to alcohol intake, even at moderate levels. For example, some women appear to be at increased risk for breast cancer when consuming low to moderate amounts of alcohol. Also, consumption of less than 30 g alcohol per day (roughly equivalent to two drinks) has been shown to increase blood pressure in men over the age of 40 years.[4] In some studies, moderate use of alcohol has been linked

---

alcohol Chemically, a compound characterized by the presence of a hydroxyl group; in common usage, a beverage made from fermented fruits, vegetables, or grains and containing ethanol.

ethanol A specific alcohol compound (C_2H_5OH) formed from the fermentation of dietary carbohydrates and used in a variety of alcoholic beverages.

drink The amount of an alcoholic beverage that provides approximately 0.5 fl. oz of pure ethanol.

proof A measure of the alcohol content of a liquid; 100-proof liquor is 50% alcohol by volume, 80-proof liquor is 40% alcohol by volume, and so on.

moderate drinking Alcohol consumption of up to one drink per day for women and up to two drinks per day for men.

resveratrol A phytochemical known to play a role in limiting cell damage from the by-products of metabolic reactions. It is found in red wine and certain other plant-based foods.

to a higher rate of bleeding in the brain, resulting in what is termed *hemorrhagic stroke*; however, other research has found that light-to-moderate alcohol consumption does not increase risk of stroke.[5]

Another concern is the effect of alcohol on our waistlines. Although it provides virtually no nutritional value, alcohol does provide energy: at 7 kcal/g, alcohol has a relatively high Calorie content. Only fat (9 kcal/g) has more Calories per gram. Let's take a look at the Calorie counts of some common alcoholic beverages:

- A shot of whiskey, rum, vodka, or gin contains about 100 Calories.
- A 12-ounce can of beer and a 6-ounce glass of wine have the same Calorie count—about 150.
- A 12-ounce bottle of a wine cooler will cost you about 250 Calories.
- Many mixed drinks are loaded with Calories: a 6-ounce white Russian has about 320 Calories and a pineapple daiquiri packs 670 Calories into just 4 ounces!

As you can see, if you're watching your weight, it makes sense to strictly limit your consumption of alcohol to stay within your daily energy needs. Alcohol intake may also increase your food intake because alcoholic beverages enhance appetite, particularly during social events, leading some people to overeat. Both current and lifelong intakes of alcohol increase risk of obesity in males and females.[6]

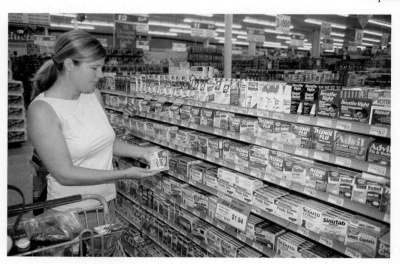

Alcohol can interfere with and increase the risks of using various over-the-counter and prescription medications.

To find out how many Calories your alcoholic beverages are costing you over a month and over a year, use the calculator at www.collegedrinkingprevention.gov. Enter "calculator" in the search box, which will take you to a page of links. Click on the top-most link to access this and two other alcohol-related calculators.

The potential for drug–alcohol interactions is well known; many medications carry a warning label advising consumers to avoid alcohol while taking the drug. Alcohol magnifies the effect of certain painkillers, sleeping pills, antidepressants, and antianxiety medications and can lead to loss of consciousness. It also increases the risk of gastrointestinal bleeding in people taking aspirin or ibuprofen as well as the risk of stomach bleeding and liver damage in people taking acetaminophen (Tylenol). In diabetics using insulin or oral medications to lower blood glucose, alcohol can exaggerate the drug's effect, leading to an inappropriately low level of blood glucose.

As you can see, there are both benefits and risks to moderate alcohol consumption. Experts agree that people who are currently consuming alcohol in moderation and who have low or no risk of alcohol addiction or medication interaction can safely continue their current level of use. Adults who abstain from alcohol, however, should not start drinking just for the possible health benefits. Individuals who have a personal or family history of alcoholism or fall into any other risk category should consider abstaining from alcohol use, even at a moderate level.

What happens to alcohol in the body?

Most of the alcohol someone drinks is readily absorbed from both the stomach and the small intestine; it does not require digestion prior to absorption. Consuming foods with some fat, protein, and fiber slows the absorption of alcohol and can reduce *blood alcohol concentration (BAC)* by as much as 50% compared to peak BAC when drinking on an empty stomach. Carbonated alcoholic beverages are absorbed very rapidly, which explains why champagne and sparkling wines are so quick to generate an alcoholic "buzz."

Women typically absorb 30% to 35% more of a given alcohol intake compared to a man of the same size, which may explain why women often show a greater response to alcohol compared to men.

Once absorbed, the alcohol moves through the bloodstream to the liver, where it is broken down at a fairly steady rate. As shown in **FIGURE 2**, two liver enzymes, known as alcohol dehydrogenase (ADH) and aldehyde dehydrogenase (ALDH), together break down alcohol. There are only two metabolic options for alcohol: it can be metabolized for energy or, if the body's energy needs are already met, it is converted to fatty acids. The fatty acids are then incorporated into triglycerides, which can accumulate in the liver (see the upcoming discussion on fatty liver) or be released into the bloodstream, increasing one's risk for heart disease and metabolic syndrome.

On average, a healthy adult metabolizes the equivalent of one drink per hour. If someone drinks more than that,

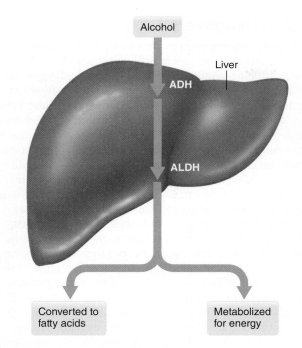

FIGURE 2 Metabolism of alcohol.

such as two or three alcoholic drinks in an hour, the excess alcohol is released from the liver back into the bloodstream, where it elevates BAC and triggers a variety of behavioral and metabolic reactions. The bloodstream efficiently and quickly distributes the alcohol throughout all body fluids and tissues, including the brain. Any time you consume more than one alcoholic beverage per hour, you are exposing every tissue in your body to the toxic effects of alcohol.

Despite what you may have heard, there is no effective intervention to speed up the breakdown of alcohol (TABLE 1). The key to keeping your BAC below the legal limit is to drink alcoholic beverages while eating a meal or large snack, to drink very slowly, no more than one drink per hour, and to limit your total consumption of alcohol on any one occasion.

TABLE 1   Myths About Alcohol Metabolism

The Claim	The Reality
Physical activity, such as walking around, will speed up the breakdown of alcohol.	Muscles don't metabolize alcohol; the liver does.
Drinking a lot of coffee will keep you from getting drunk.	Coffee does not cause alcohol to be excreted in the urine.
Using a sauna or steam room will force the alcohol out of your body.	Very little alcohol is lost in the sweat; the alcohol will remain in your bloodstream.
Herbal and nutritional products are available that speed up the breakdown of alcohol.	There is no scientific evidence that commercial supplements will increase the rate of alcohol metabolism; they will not lower blood alcohol levels.

A person who steadily increases his or her alcohol consumption over time becomes more tolerant of a given intake of alcohol. Chronic drinkers experience *metabolic tolerance*, a condition in which the liver becomes more efficient in its breakdown of alcohol. This means that the person's BAC rises more slowly after consuming a certain number of drinks. In addition, chronic drinkers develop what is called *functional tolerance*, meaning they show few, if any, signs of impairment or intoxication even at high BACs. As a result, these individuals may consume twice as much alcohol as when they first started drinking before they reach the same state of euphoria.

What are alcohol abuse and dependence?

The National Institute on Alcohol Abuse and Alcoholism (NIAAA) recognizes two general types of *alcohol use disorders*: alcohol abuse and alcohol dependence.[7] In the United States, about 18 million people have an alcohol use disorder.

Alcohol abuse is a pattern of alcohol consumption, whether chronic or occasional, that results in distress, danger, or harm to one's health, functioning, or interpersonal relationships. It can eventually lead to alcohol dependence. **Binge drinking**, the consumption of five or more alcoholic drinks on one occasion by a man (four or more drinks for a woman), is a form of alcohol abuse that occurs in about 15% of U.S. adults.[8] Males between the ages of 18 and 25 have the highest rate of binge drinking.[9] The effects of binge drinking include an increased risk of

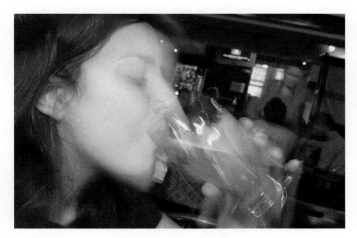

Alcohol abuse, such as binge drinking, can result in numerous negative consequences.

alcohol abuse A pattern of alcohol consumption, whether chronic or occasional, that results in harm to one's health, functioning, or interpersonal relationships.

binge drinking The consumption of five or more alcoholic drinks on one occasion.

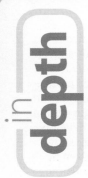

potentially fatal falls, drownings, automobile accidents, and acts of physical violence, including vandalism and physical and sexual assault. The consequences also carry over beyond the particular episode: binge drinking impairs planning, problem solving, memory, and inhibition, leading to social, academic, and employment problems and decreasing lifespan.[9]

Alcohol dependence, commonly known as *alcoholism*, is a disease characterized by:

- *Craving:* a strong need or urge to drink alcoholic beverages
- *Loss of control:* the inability to stop once drinking has begun
- *Physical dependence:* the presence of nausea, sweating, shakiness, and other signs of withdrawal after stopping alcohol intake
- *Tolerance:* the need to drink larger and larger amounts of alcohol to get the same "high" or pleasurable sensations associated with alcohol intake.

What are the effects of alcohol abuse?

Alcohol is a drug. It exerts a narcotic effect on virtually every part of the brain, acting as a sedative and depressant. Alcohol also has the potential to act as a direct toxin; in high concentrations, it can damage or destroy cell membranes and internal cell structures. As shown in **FIGURE 3**, an alcohol intake between 1/2 and 1 drink per day is associated with the lowest risk of mortality for both men and women. The risk of death increases sharply as alcohol intake increases above 2 drinks per day for women, and 3 1/2 drinks per day for men. These increased mortality risks are related to alcohol's damaging effects on the brain, the liver, and other organs as well as its role in motor vehicle accidents and other traumatic injuries.

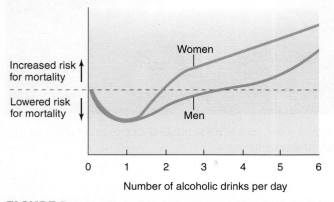

FIGURE 3 The effect of alcohol consumption on mortality risk. Consuming 1/2 to 1 drink per day is associated with the lowest mortality risk for all adults. The risk of death increases sharply at levels of alcohol intake above 2 drinks per day for women and above 3-1/2 drinks per day for men.

Alcohol Hangovers

An **alcohol hangover** is an extremely unpleasant consequence of drinking too much alcohol. It lasts up to 24 hours, and its symptoms include headache, fatigue, dizziness, muscle aches, nausea and vomiting, sensitivity to light and sound, and extreme thirst. Some people also experience depression, anxiety, irritability, and other mood disturbances. Some of the aftereffects of a binge may be due to simple dehydration, which is one reason why it is important to alternate the consumption of alcoholic beverages with other fluids as well as consuming water before going to bed and upon waking up. Other aspects of a hangover may be related to certain nonalcoholic compounds known as *congeners*. These chemicals are found in aged red wines, brandy, and whiskey and contribute to their characteristic flavors and odors. Some people believe that hangovers can be avoided by drinking alcoholic beverages with low or no congeners. In reality, however, most of the consequences seen in hangovers are directly related to the alcohol itself.

Although many folk remedies, including various herbal products, are claimed to prevent or reduce hangover effects, few have been proven effective. As previously noted, drinking water or other nonalcoholic beverages will minimize the risk of dehydration, whereas consumption of toast or dry cereal will bring blood glucose levels back to normal. Getting adequate sleep can counteract the fatigue, and use of antacids may reduce nausea and abdominal pain. Whereas aspirin, acetaminophen, and ibuprofen might be useful for headaches, they may worsen stomach pain and increase the risk of GI bleeding and liver damage.

Reduced Brain Function

Alcohol is well known for its ability to alter behavior, mainly through its effects on the brain. Even at low intakes, alcohol impairs reasoning and judgment **(TABLE 2)**. Alcohol also interferes with normal motor skills and sleep patterns and may prompt mood swings, irritation, intense anger, sadness, or lethargy. When teens or young adults chronically consume excessive amounts of alcohol, they may permanently damage brain structure and function.[10] Intellectual functioning, memory, and coordination can be reduced. In addition, early exposure to alcohol, particularly in those with a family history of alcohol abuse, increases risk of future alcohol addiction.[11]

Alcohol Poisoning

At very high intakes of alcohol, a person is at risk for **alcohol poisoning**, a metabolic state that occurs in

alcohol dependence A disease state characterized by chronic dependence on alcohol; commonly called *alcoholism*.

alcohol hangover A consequence of drinking too much alcohol; symptoms include headache, fatigue, dizziness, muscle aches, nausea and vomiting, sensitivity to light and sound, extreme thirst, and mood disturbances.

alcohol poisoning A potentially fatal metabolic state in which an overdose of alcohol results in cardiac and/or respiratory failure.

TABLE 2 Effects of Blood Alcohol Concentration (BAC) on Brain Activity

Blood Alcohol Concentration	Typical Response
0.02–0.05%	Feeling of relaxation, euphoria, relief
0.06–0.10%	Impaired judgment, fine motor control, and coordination; loss of normal emotional control; legally drunk in many states (at the upper end of the range)
0.11–0.15%	Impaired reflexes and gross motor control; staggered gait; legally drunk in all states; slurred speech
0.16–0.20%	Impaired vision; unpredictable behavior; further loss of muscle control
0.21–0.35%	Total loss of coordination; in a stupor
0.40% and above	Loss of consciousness; coma; suppression of respiratory response; death

storage, the synthesis of many essential compounds, and the detoxification of medications and other potential poisons. As noted earlier, it is the main site of alcohol metabolism. When an individual's rate of alcohol intake exceeds the rate at which the liver can break the alcohol down, liver cells are damaged or destroyed. The longer the alcohol abuse continues, the greater the damage to the liver.

Fatty liver, a condition in which abnormal amounts of fat build-up in the liver, is an early yet reversible sign of liver damage commonly linked to alcohol abuse. As shown in Figure 2, the synthesis of fatty acids is one of only two metabolic options for alcohol. Once alcohol intake stops and a healthful diet is maintained, the liver is able to rid itself of the excess fat, heal, and resume normal function.

Alcoholic hepatitis is a more severe condition, resulting in loss of appetite, nausea and vomiting, abdominal pain, and jaundice (a yellowing of the skin and eyes, reflecting reduced liver function). Mental confusion and impaired immune response often occur with alcoholic hepatitis. Avoidance of alcohol and a healthful diet often result in full recovery; however, many people experience lifelong complications.

Cirrhosis of the liver typically follows years of alcohol abuse; liver cells are permanently scarred, blood flow through the liver is impaired, and liver function declines (**FIGURE 4**). The damage is almost always irreversible. Blood pressure increases dramatically, large amounts of

response to binge drinking. At high BACs, the respiratory center of the brain is depressed. This reduces the level of oxygen reaching the brain and increases the individual's risk of death by respiratory or cardiac failure. Like Todd in our opening story, many binge drinkers lose consciousness before alcohol poisoning becomes fatal, but emergency care is often essential.

If someone passes out after a night of hard drinking, he or she should never be left alone to "sleep it off." Instead, the person should be placed on his or her side to prevent aspiration if vomiting occurs. The person should be watched carefully throughout the night for cold and clammy skin, a bluish tint to the skin, or slow, irregular breathing. If any of these signs become evident, if the person cannot be awakened, or there is any other reason to believe he or she has alcohol poisoning, seek emergency healthcare immediately.

Reduced Liver Function

The liver performs an astonishing number and variety of body functions, including nutrient metabolism, glycogen

fatty liver An early and reversible stage of liver disease often found in people who abuse alcohol and characterized by the abnormal accumulation of fat within liver cells.

alcoholic hepatitis Inflammation of the liver caused by alcohol; other forms of hepatitis can be caused by a virus or toxin.

cirrhosis of the liver End-stage liver disease characterized by significant abnormalities in liver structure and function; may lead to complete liver failure.

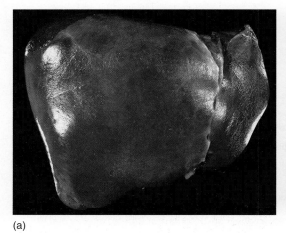
(a)

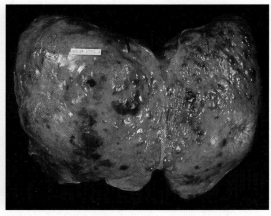
(b)

FIGURE 4 Cirrhosis of the liver is often caused by chronic alcohol abuse. **(a)** A healthy liver; **(b)** a liver damaged by cirrhosis.

fluid are retained in the abdominal cavity, and metabolic wastes accumulate. In some cases, liver function fails completely, resulting in the need for a liver transplant or the likelihood of death.

Increased Risk of Chronic Disease

Although moderate drinking may provide some health benefits, it is clear that chronically high intakes of alcohol damage a number of body organs and systems, increasing a person's risk of chronic disease and death:

- *Impaired bone health.* Men and women who are alcohol dependent experience a variety of metabolic changes that impair bone formation.[12]
- *Pancreatic injury and diabetes.* Alcohol damages the pancreas, which produces insulin, and decreases the body's ability to properly respond to insulin. The result is chronically elevated blood glucose levels and an increased risk of diabetes.
- *Cancer.* Research has most strongly linked excessive alcohol consumption to increased risk of cancers of the GI tract, liver, and female breast.[13,14]
- *Abdominal obesity.* Whereas the excess Caloric intake seen in some cases of chronic alcohol abuse contributes to increased risk of obesity, the risk of abdominal obesity is particularly high. As alcohol intake rises, and remains high, the liver produces and releases increasingly large amounts of triglycerides into the bloodstream. These triglycerides are readily stored in the

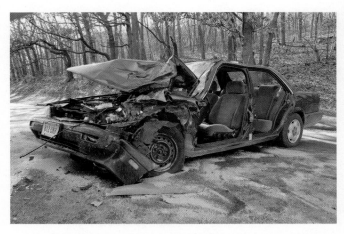

Excessive alcohol intake greatly increases the risks for car accidents and other traumatic injuries.

abdominal area, greatly increasing risk for metabolic syndrome, hypertension, type 2 diabetes, and stroke.

Malnutrition

As alcohol intake increases to 30% or more of total energy intake, appetite is lost and intake of healthful foods declines. Over time, the diet becomes deficient in protein, fats, carbohydrates, vitamins A and C, and minerals such as iron, zinc, and calcium (**FIGURE 5**). End-stage alcoholics may consume as much as 90% of their daily energy intake from alcohol, displacing virtually all foods. Even if food intake is maintained, the toxic effects of alcohol lead to

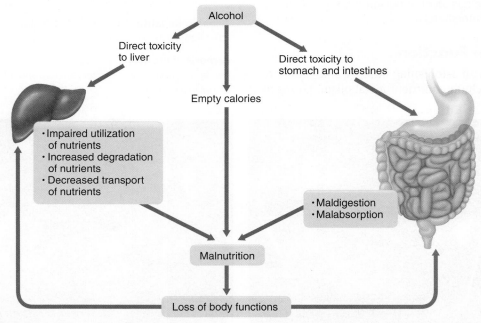

FIGURE 5 Alcohol-related malnutrition. Excess alcohol consumption contributes directly and indirectly to widespread nutrient deficiencies.

binge drinking during their pregnancy.[16] Alcohol is a known **teratogen** (a substance that causes fetal harm) that readily crosses the placenta into the fetal bloodstream. Because the immature fetal liver cannot effectively break down the alcohol, it accumulates in the fetal blood and tissues, increasing the risk for various birth defects. The effects of maternal alcohol intake are dose-related: the more the mother drirnks, the greater the potential harm to the fetus. Drinking early in pregnancy—even before the woman realizes she is pregnant—is particularly harmful.

Fetal alcohol syndrome (FAS) is the most severe consequence of maternal alcohol consumption and is characterized by malformations of the face, limbs, heart, and nervous system. The characteristic facial features of a child with FAS persist throughout life (**FIGURE 6**). Newborn and infant death rates are abnormally high and those who do survive may suffer from lifelong emotional, behavioral, social, learning, and developmental problems. FAS is one of the most common causes of mental retardation in the United States, despite the fact that it is completely preventable.

Fetal alcohol effects (FAE) are a more subtle set of consequences related to maternal alcohol intake. Although

impaired food digestion, nutrient absorption, and nutrient metabolism.

Long-term exposure to alcohol damages not only the liver but also the stomach, small intestine, and pancreas. As a result, the digestion of foods and absorption of nutrients such as the fat-soluble vitamins (A, D, E, and K), vitamin B_6, folate, and zinc become inadequate, leading to malnutrition and inappropriate weight loss.

Increased Risk of Traumatic Injury

Excessive alcohol intake is the third leading cause of preventable death for Americans, contributing to nearly 80,000 deaths per year.[15] It has been estimated that as many as 6,000 young Americans die each year from alcohol-related motor vehicle accidents, suicides, and homicides. Rates of fatal falls, drownings, and assaults also increase when people are under the influence of alcohol.

Fetal and Infant Health Problems

No level of alcohol consumption is considered safe for pregnant women. Women who are or think they may be pregnant should abstain from all alcoholic beverages. Despite the fact this advice is widely publicized, it is estimated that more than 40,000 U.S. infants are born each year with some type of alcohol-related defect. It is estimated that, among U.S. pregnant women, nearly 8% consumed alcohol and approximately 1.4% reported

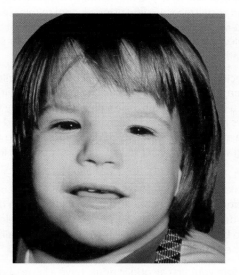

FIGURE 6 A child with fetal alcohol syndrome (FAS). The facial features typical of children with FAS include a short nose with a low, wide bridge; drooping eyes with an extra skinfold; and a flat, thin upper lip. These external traits are typically accompanied by behavioral problems and learning disorders. The effects of FAS are irreversible.

teratogen A compound known to cause fetal harm or danger.

fetal alcohol syndrome (FAS) A set of serious, irreversible alcohol-related birth defects characterized by certain physical and mental abnormalities, including malformations of the face, limbs, heart, and nervous system; impaired growth; and a spectrum of mild to severe cognitive, emotional, and physical problems.

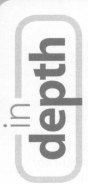

usually not diagnosed at birth, FAE often becomes evident when the child enters preschool or kindergarten. The child may exhibit hyperactivity, attention deficit disorders, or impaired learning abilities. It is estimated that the incidence of FAE may be ten times greater than that of FAS.

The only way to prevent these disorders is to abstain from all alcoholic beverages when trying to become pregnant and when pregnancy is suspected or confirmed. Women who are breastfeeding should also abstain from alcohol because it easily passes into the breast milk at levels equal to blood alcohol concentrations.

If consumed by the infant, the alcohol in breast milk can slow motor development, depress the central nervous system, and increase sleepiness in the child. Alcohol also reduces the mother's ability to produce milk, putting the infant at risk for malnutrition.

Knowing that a moderate intake of alcohol may provide some health benefits and that excessive intake results in a wide range of problems, what can you do to control your drinking? The **Quick Tips** feature shows practical strategies that can help you avoid the negative consequences of excessive alcohol consumption.

Should you be concerned about your alcohol intake?

You should be concerned about your alcohol intake if you engage in binge drinking or drink at inappropriate times (while pregnant, before or while driving a car, to deal with negative emotions, or while at work/school). (For a more detailed self-assessment, complete the **What About You** feature.)

If you recognize that you have an alcohol problem, it is important for you to speak with a trusted friend, coach, teacher, counselor, or healthcare provider, or the staff at your campus health services center. In addition, many campuses have support groups that can help.

QuickTips

Taking Control of Your Alcohol Intake

Think about WHY you are planning to drink. Is it to relax and socialize, or are you using alcohol to release stress? If the latter, try some stress-reduction techniques that don't involve alcohol, such as exercise, yoga, meditation, or simply talking with a friend.

Decide in advance what your alcohol intake will be, and plan some strategies for sticking to your limit. If you are going to a bar, for example, take only enough money to buy two beers and two sodas—and leave your credit card at home. If you are at a party, stay occupied dancing, sampling the food, or talking with friends, and stay as far away from the keg as you can.

Make sure you have a protein-containing meal or snack before your first alcoholic drink; having food in the stomach delays its emptying. This gives more of the alcohol a chance to be broken down and means that less is available to be absorbed into the bloodstream.

Before your first alcoholic drink, have a large glass of water, iced tea, or soda. Once your thirst has been satisfied, your rate of fluid intake will drop. After that, rotate between alcoholic and nonalcoholic drinks.

Dilute hard liquor with large amounts of diet soda, water, or juice. Remember, a glass of pure orange juice doesn't look any different from one laced with vodka. Diluted beverages are cheaper and lower in Calories, too.

Whether or not your drink is diluted, sip slowly to allow your liver time to keep up with your alcohol intake.

If your friends pressure you to drink and you'd rather not, volunteer to be the designated driver. You'll have a "free pass" for the night in terms of saying no to alcohol.

what about you

Do You Have a Problem with Alcohol Abuse?

Have you ever felt you should cut down on your drinking?	Yes/No
Have people annoyed you by criticizing your drinking?	Yes/No
Have you ever felt bad or guilty about your drinking?	Yes/No
Do you drink alone when you feel angry or sad?	Yes/No
Has your drinking ever made you late for school or work?	Yes/No
Have you ever had a drink first thing in the morning to steady your nerves or get rid of a hangover?	Yes/No
Do you ever drink after promising yourself you won't?	Yes/No

If you answered "yes" to one or more of these questions, provided by the National Institute on Alcohol Abuse and Alcoholism, you may have a problem with alcohol abuse and should consult your primary healthcare provider or a specialized counselor to explore it in more detail.

Talking to someone about an alcohol problem

You may suspect that a close friend or relative might be one of the nearly 18 million Americans with an alcohol use disorder. If you notice that your friend or relative uses alcohol to calm down, cheer up, or relax, that may be a sign of alcohol dependency. The appearance of tremors or other signs of withdrawal as well as the initiation of secretive behaviors when consuming alcohol are other indications that alcohol has become a serious problem.

Many people become defensive or hostile when asked about their use of alcohol; denial is very common. The single hardest step toward sobriety is often the first: accepting the fact that help is needed. Some people respond well when confronted by a single person, whereas others benefit more from a group intervention. There should be no blaming or shaming; alcohol use disorders are medical conditions with a genetic component. The National Institute on Alcoholism and Alcohol Abuse suggests the following approaches when trying to get a friend or relative into treatment:

- *Stop covering up and making excuses.* Many times, family and friends will make excuses to others to protect the person from the results of his or her drinking. It is important, however, to stop covering for that person so he or she can experience the full consequences of inappropriate alcohol consumption.
- *Intervene at a vulnerable time.* The best time to talk to someone about problem drinking is shortly after an alcohol-related incident such as a DUI arrest, an alcohol-related traffic accident, or a public scene. Wait until the person is sober and everyone is relatively calm.
- *Be specific.* Tell the person exactly why you are concerned; use examples of specific problems associated with his or her drinking habits (e.g., poor school or work performance; legal problems; inappropriate behaviors). Explain what will happen if the person chooses not to get help—for example, no longer going out with the person if alcohol will be available, no longer riding with him or her in motor vehicles, moving out of a shared home, and so on.
- *Get help.* Professional help is available from community agencies, healthcare providers, online sites, school or worksite wellness centers, and some religious organizations. Several contacts and websites are listed shortly. If the person indicates a willingness to get help, call immediately for an appointment and/or immediately bring him or her to a treatment center. The longer the delay, the more likely it is that the person will experience a change of heart.
- *Enlist the support of others.* Whether or not the person agrees to get help, calling on other friends and relatives can often be effective, especially if one of these people has battled alcohol abuse. Formal support groups such as Al-Anon and Alateen can provide additional information and guidance.

Treatment for alcohol use disorders works for many, but not all, individuals. "Success" is measured in small steps, and relapses are common. Most scientists agree that people who abuse alcohol cannot just "cut down." Complete avoidance of all alcoholic beverages is the only way for most people who abuse alcohol to achieve full and ongoing recovery.

MasteringNutrition™

Check out these additional resources in the MasteringNutrition Study Area:

- Read It: Chapter Summary and RSS Feeds
- See It: ABC News videos and nutrition animations
- Hear It: MP3s
- Study It: Get Ready for Nutrition Math and Chemistry review
- Do It: NutriTools and "Find the Quack" feature
- Review It: Quizzes, flashcards, and glossary

web resources

www.aa.org
Alcoholics Anonymous, Inc.

Go to this website for useful information on dealing with alcohol-related problems by this widely used organization.

www.al-anon.alateen.org
Al-Anon Family Group Headquarters, Inc.

Another helpful online source for a range of information on alcohol-related issues and concerns.

www.collegedrinkingprevention.gov
College Drinking: Changing the Culture

Check out this website for information on drinking issues within a college context.

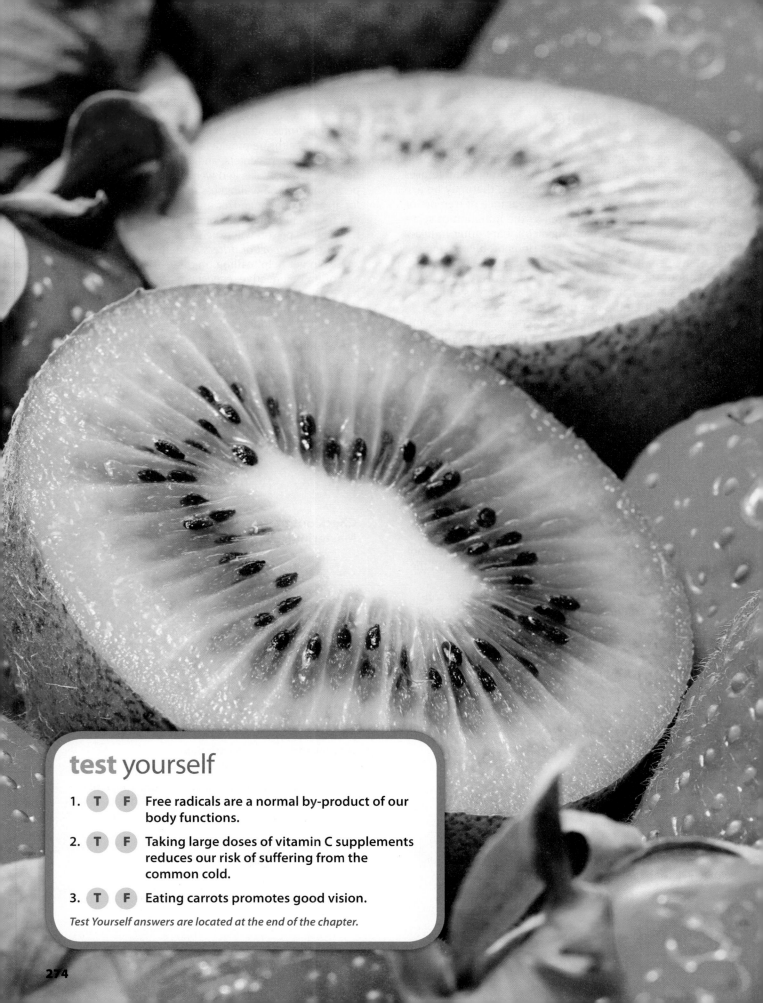

Nutrients Involved in Antioxidant Function and Vision

8

learning objectives

After studying this chapter you should be able to:

1 Describe the process of oxidation and explain how it can damage cells, pp. 276–278.

2 Define the term *antioxidant enzyme systems* and identify the minerals involved in these systems, pp. 278–279.

3 Discuss the interrelated roles of vitamins E and C in protecting cells from oxidative damage, pp. 279–280.

4 Explain how vitamin C helps maintain bone, skin, tendons, and other tissues, pp. 282–283.

5 Describe the relationship between beta-carotene and vitamin A, p. 289.

6 Discuss the role of vitamin A in vision, cell differentiation, growth, and reproduction pp. 291–295.

7 Identify the RDA, UL, and several food sources of vitamin A, pp. 295–296.

Mika, a first-year student at a university hundreds of miles from home, just opened another care package from her mom. As usual, it contained an assortment of healthful snacks, a box of chamomile tea, and several types of supplements: echinacea extract to ward off colds, powdered papaya for good digestion, and antioxidant vitamins. "Wow, Mika!" her roommate laughed. "Can you let your mom know I'm available for adoption?"

"I guess she just wants me to stay healthy," Mika sighed. She wondered what her mother would think if she found out how much junk food Mika had been eating since she'd started college, and had been binge drinking every weekend, and had been smoking since high school. "Still," Mika reminded herself, "at least I take the vitamins she sends."

What do you think of Mika's current lifestyle? Can a poor diet, binge drinking, and smoking cause cancer or other health problems, and can the use of dietary supplements provide some protection? What are antioxidant vitamins, and why do you think Mika's mom included a bottle of these in her care package? If your health food store were promoting an antioxidant supplement, would you buy it?

It isn't easy to sort fact from fiction when it comes to antioxidants— especially when they're in the form of supplements. Internet ads and magazine articles tout their benefits, yet some researchers claim they don't protect us from diseases and, in some cases, may even be harmful. In this chapter, you'll learn about antioxidants and how they work in the body. We'll also discuss the multiple roles of vitamin A in promoting healthy vision, cell differentiation, and other key functions.

MasteringNutrition™

Go online for chapter quizzes, pre-tests, Interactive Activities, and more!

What are antioxidants, and how does our body use them?

Antioxidants are compounds that protect our cells from the damage caused by oxidation. *Anti* means "against," and antioxidants work *against,* or *prevent,* oxidation. Before we can go further in our discussion of antioxidants, we need to learn what oxidation is and how it damages cells.

Oxidation Is a Chemical Reaction in Which Atoms Lose Electrons

A review of some basic chemistry will help you understand the process of oxidation. Earlier in this text (in Chapter 3), we said that our bodies are made up of atoms, tiny units of matter that cannot be broken down by natural means. Hydrogen, carbon, and iron are unique because their atoms are unique. Every atom of carbon, for example, is identical to every other atom of carbon, whether it is present in coal or in cheese. We also said that atoms join together to form molecules, such as saccharides and amino acids, which are the smallest *physical units* of a substance. Some molecules, such as hydrogen gas (H_2), contain only one type of atom—in this case, hydrogen. Most molecules, however, are *compounds*—they contain two or more different types of atoms (such as water, H_2O). Our body is constantly breaking down compounds of food, water, and air into their component atoms, then rearranging these freed atoms to build the different substances our body needs.

Atoms Are Composed of Particles

We just said that atoms cannot be broken down by natural means, but during the 20th century, physicists learned how to split atoms into their components, which they called *particles*. As you can see in **FIGURE 8.1**, this research revealed that all atoms have a central core, called a **nucleus**, which is positively charged. Orbiting around this nucleus at close to the speed of light are one or more **electrons**, which are negatively charged. The opposite attraction between the positive nucleus and the negative electrons keeps an atom together by making the atom stable, so that its electrons remain with it and do not veer off toward other atoms.

During Metabolism, Atoms Exchange Electrons

As you recall (from Chapter 1), the process by which our body breaks down and builds up molecules is called *metabolism*. During metabolism, atoms may lose electrons **(FIGURE 8.2a)**. We call this loss of electrons **oxidation**, because it is fueled by oxygen. Atoms are capable of gaining electrons during metabolism as well. We call this process *reduction* (Figure 8.2b). This loss and gain of electrons typically results in an even exchange of electrons. Scientists call this loss and gain of electrons an *exchange reaction*.

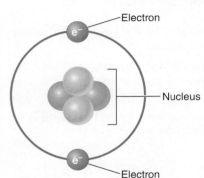

Electron

Nucleus

Electron

FIGURE 8.1 An atom consists of a central nucleus and orbiting electrons. The nucleus exerts a positive charge, which keeps the negatively charged electrons in its vicinity. Notice that this atom has an even number of electrons in orbit around the nucleus. This pairing of electrons results in the atom being chemically stable.

antioxidant A compound that has the ability to prevent or repair the damage caused by oxidation.

nucleus The positively charged, central core of an atom. It is made up of two types of particles—protons and neutrons—bound tightly together. The nucleus of an atom contains essentially all of its atomic mass.

electron A negatively charged particle orbiting the nucleus of an atom.

oxidation A chemical reaction in which molecules of a substance are broken down into their component atoms. During oxidation, the atoms involved lose electrons.

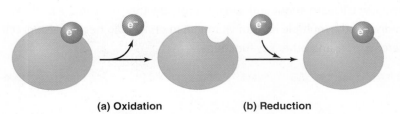

(a) Oxidation **(b) Reduction**

FIGURE 8.2 Exchange reactions consist of two parts. **(a)** During oxidation, atoms *lose* electrons. **(b)** In the second part of the reaction, atoms *gain* electrons, which is called reduction.

Oxidation Sometimes Results in the Formation of Free Radicals

Stable atoms have an even number of electrons orbiting in pairs at successive distances (called *shells* or *rings*) from the nucleus. When a stable atom loses an electron during oxidation, it is left with an odd number of electrons in its outermost shell. In other words, it now has an *unpaired electron*. In most exchange reactions, unpaired electrons immediately pair up with other unpaired electrons, making newly stabilized atoms, but in some cases, an atom's unpaired electrons remain unpaired. Such atoms are highly unstable and are called **free radicals**.

Free radicals are formed as a normal by-product of many of our body's fundamental physiologic processes. Still, excessive production of free radicals can cause serious damage to our cells and other body components. Let's look at the most common way they arise. Our body uses oxygen and hydrogen to generate the energy (ATP) it needs **(FIGURE 8.3)**. We are constantly inhaling air into our body, thereby providing the oxygen needed to fuel this reaction. At the same time, we generate the necessary hydrogen as a result of digesting food. As shown in **FIGURE 8.4** (page 278), occasionally during metabolism, oxygen accepts a single electron that was released during this process. When it does so, the oxygen atom becomes an unstable free radical because of the added unpaired electron.

Free radicals are also formed from other physiologic processes, such as when the immune system produces inflammation to fight allergens or infections. Other factors that cause free radical formation include exposure to air pollution, ultraviolet (UV) rays from the sun, other types of radiation, tobacco smoke, industrial chemicals, and asbestos. Continual exposure to these factors leads to uncontrollable free radical formation, cell damage, and disease, as discussed next.

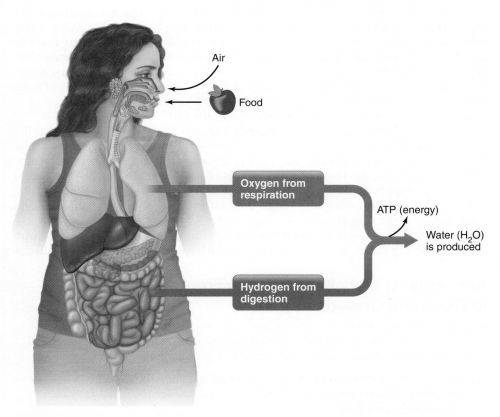

◆ **FIGURE 8.3** Oxygen (O) enters our body when we inhale air. Hydrogen (H) is released through the process of metabolizing food. As a result of exchange reactions during metabolism, electrons are freed to contribute to the production of the energy molecule ATP in body cells. The hydrogen and oxygen then recombine to form water (H_2O).

free radical A highly unstable atom with an unpaired electron in its outermost shell.

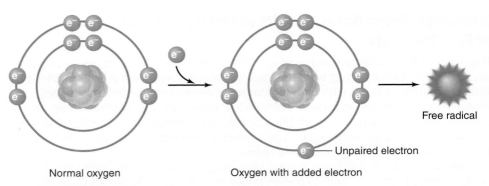

Normal oxygen   Oxygen with added electron

Free radical

Unpaired electron

◆ **FIGURE 8.4** Normally, an oxygen atom contains eight electrons. Occasionally, oxygen will accept an unpaired electron during the oxidation process. This acceptance of a single electron causes oxygen to become an unstable atom called a free radical.

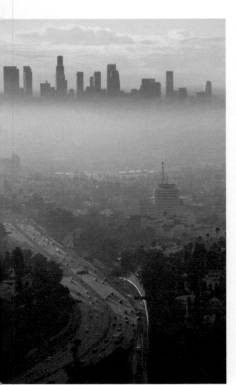

◆ Exposure to pollution from car exhaust and industrial waste increases our production of free radicals.

cofactor A mineral or other inorganic substance that is needed to allow enzymes to function properly.

Free Radicals Can Destabilize Other Molecules and Damage Our Cells

Why are we concerned with the formation of free radicals? Simply put, it is because of their destabilizing power. If you were to think of paired electrons as a married couple, a free radical would be an extremely seductive outsider. Its unpaired electron exerts a powerful attraction toward the stable molecules around it. In an attempt to stabilize itself, a free radical will "steal" an electron from these molecules, in turn generating more unstable free radicals. This is a dangerous chain reaction because the free radicals generated can damage or destroy cells.

One of the most significant sites of free radical damage is the cell membrane. As shown in **FIGURE 8.5a**, free radicals that form within the phospholipid bilayer of cell membranes steal electrons from the stable lipid heads. Recall that lipids are insoluble in water, so a stable line-up of lipid heads allows cell membranes to keep water out. When these lipid heads are destroyed, the cell membrane can no longer repel water. With the cell membrane's integrity lost, its ability to regulate the movement of fluids and nutrients into and out of the cell is also lost. This loss of cell integrity causes damage to the cell and to all systems affected by the cell.

Other sites of free radical damage include low-density lipoproteins (LDLs), cell proteins, and DNA. Damage to LDLs and cell proteins disrupts the transport of substances into and out of cells and alters cell function, whereas defective DNA results in faulty protein synthesis. These changes can also cause harmful changes (mutations) in cells or prompt cells to die prematurely. Free radicals also promote blood vessel inflammation and the formation of clots, both of which are risk factors for cardiovascular disease (see the **In Depth** following Chapter 5, starting page 177). Not surprisingly, many diseases are linked with free radical production, including cancer, heart disease, type 2 diabetes, arthritis, cataracts, and Alzheimer's and Parkinson's diseases.

Antioxidants Work by Stabilizing Free Radicals or Opposing Oxidation

How does our body fight free radicals and repair the damage they cause? These actions are performed by antioxidant vitamins, minerals, and phytochemicals and other compounds. These antioxidants perform their role in three ways:

1. Antioxidant vitamins work independently by donating their electrons or hydrogen atoms to free radicals to stabilize them and reduce the damage caused by oxidation (Figure 8.5b).
2. Antioxidant minerals, including selenium, copper, iron, zinc, and manganese, act as **cofactors**, inorganic substances required to activate enzymes so that they can do their work. These minerals function within complex *antioxidant enzyme systems* that convert free radicals to less damaging substances that are excreted by

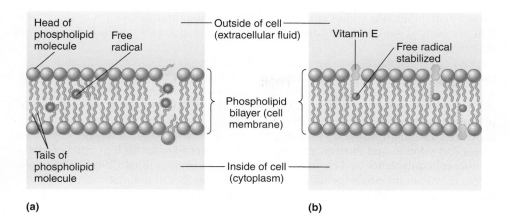

(a)   (b)

FIGURE 8.5 **(a)** The formation of free radicals in the lipid portion of our cell membranes can cause a dangerous chain reaction that damages the integrity of the membrane and can cause cell death. **(b)** Vitamin E is stored in the lipid portion of our cell membranes. By donating an electron to free radicals, it protects the lipid molecules in our cell membranes from being oxidized and stops the chain reaction of oxidative damage.

our bodies. They also work to break down fatty acids that have become oxidized, thereby destroying the free radicals associated with them. Antioxidant enzyme systems also make more vitamin antioxidants available to fight other free radicals. Examples of these antioxidant enzyme systems are superoxide dismutase, catalase, and glutathione peroxidase.

3. Phytochemicals (beneficial plant chemicals) such as beta-carotene and other compounds help stabilize free radicals and prevent damage to cells and tissues.

In summary, free radical formation is generally kept safely under control by certain vitamins, minerals working within antioxidant enzyme systems, and phytochemicals. Next, we take a look at the specific vitamins and minerals involved. (Phytochemicals are discussed in the **In Depth** on new frontiers in nutrition following Chapter 1.)

recap An atom is an infinitely small and unique unit of matter having a nucleus and orbiting electrons. Atoms join together to form molecules. During metabolism, molecules break apart and their atoms gain, lose, or exchange electrons; loss of electrons is called oxidation. Free radicals are highly unstable atoms with an unpaired electron in their outermost shell. A normal by-product of oxidation reactions, they can damage our LDLs, cell proteins, and DNA and are associated with many diseases. Antioxidant vitamins and phytochemicals donate electrons or hydrogen atoms to free radicals to stabilize them and reduce oxidative damage. Antioxidant minerals are part of antioxidant enzyme systems that convert free radicals to less damaging substances.

A profile of nutrients that function as antioxidants

Our bodies cannot form antioxidants spontaneously. Instead, we must consume them in our diets. Nutrients that appear to have antioxidant properties or are part of our protective antioxidant enzyme systems include vitamins E, C, and, possibly, A; the mineral selenium; and beta-carotene (a phytochemical that is a precursor to vitamin A) **(TABLE 8.1)**. The minerals copper, iron, zinc, and manganese play a peripheral role in fighting oxidation and are only mentioned in this chapter. Let's review each of these nutrients now and learn more about their functions in the body.

Vitamin E

Vitamin E is one of the fat-soluble vitamins; thus, dietary fats carry it from our intestines through the lymphatic system and eventually transport it to our cells.

TABLE 8.1 **Nutrients Involved in Antioxidant Function and Vision**

To see the full profile of all micronutrients, turn to Chapter 6.5, **In Depth**, Vitamins and Minerals: Micronutrients with Macro Powers (pages 224–233).

	Recommended Intake
Vitamin E (fat soluble)	RDA: Women and men = 15 mg alpha-tocopherol
Vitamin C (water soluble)	RDA: Women = 75 mg Men = 90 mg Smokers = 35 mg more per day than RDA
Selenium (trace mineral)	RDA: Women and men = 55 µg
Beta-carotene (fat soluble; provitamin for vitamin A)	None at this time
Vitamin A (fat soluble)	RDA: Women = 700 µg Men = 900 µg

As you remember, our bodies store the fat-soluble vitamins: about 90% of the vitamin E in our body is stored in our adipose tissue. The remaining vitamin E is found in cell membranes.

Vitamin E is actually two separate families of compounds, *tocotrienols* and **tocopherols**. None of the different tocotrienol compounds appears to play an active role in our body. The four tocopherol compounds—alpha, beta, gamma, and delta—are the biologically active forms. Of these, the most active, or potent, vitamin E compound found in food and supplements is *alpha-tocopherol*. The RDA for vitamin E is expressed as alpha-tocopherol in milligrams per day (α-tocopherol, mg per day). Food labels and vitamin and mineral supplements may express vitamin E in units of alpha-tocopherol equivalents (α-TE), in milligrams, and as International Units (IU). Supplements may contain either the natural form of vitamin E (call d-alpha-tocopherol) or the synthetic form (dl-alpha-tocopherol). The following can be used for conversion purposes:

- In food, 1 α-TE is equal to 1 mg of active vitamin E.
- In supplements containing the natural form of vitamin E, 1 IU is equal to 0.67 mg α-TE.
- In supplements containing the synthetic form of vitamin E, 1 IU is equal to 0.45 mg α-TE.

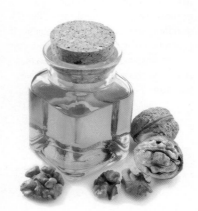

▲ Vegetable oils, nuts, and seeds are good sources of vitamin E.

Functions of Vitamin E

The primary function of vitamin E is as an antioxidant: it donates an electron to free radicals, stabilizing them and preventing them from destabilizing other molecules. Once vitamin E is oxidized, it is either excreted from the body or recycled back into active vitamin E through the help of other antioxidant nutrients, such as vitamin C.

Because vitamin E is prevalent in our adipose tissues and cell membranes, its action specifically protects polyunsaturated fatty acids (PUFAs) and other fatty components of our cells and cell membranes from being oxidized (see Figure 8.5b). Vitamin E also protects LDLs from being oxidized, thereby lowering our risk for heart disease. In addition to protecting PUFAs and LDLs, vitamin E protects the membranes of our red blood cells from oxidation and plays a critical role in protecting the cells of our lungs, which are constantly exposed to oxygen and the potentially damaging effects of oxidation. Vitamin E's role in protecting PUFAs and other fatty components also explains why it is added to many oil-based foods and skincare products—by preventing oxidation in these products, it reduces rancidity and spoilage.

Vitamin E serves many other roles essential to human health. It is critical for normal fetal and early childhood development of nerves and muscles as well as for maintenance of their functions. It protects white blood cells and other components of our immune system, thereby helping the body defend against illness and disease. It also improves the absorption of vitamin A if the dietary intake of vitamin A is low.

How Much Vitamin E Should We Consume?

Considering the importance of vitamin E to our health, you might think that you need to consume a huge amount daily. In fact, the RDA is modest: 15 mg alpha-tocopherol per day (see Table 8.1).[1] The Tolerable Upper Intake Level (UL) is 1,000 mg alpha-tocopherol per day. Remember that one of the primary roles of vitamin E is to protect PUFAs from oxidation. Thus, our need for vitamin E increases because we eat more oils and other foods that contain PUFAs. Fortunately, these foods also contain vitamin E, so we typically consume enough vitamin E within them to protect their PUFAs from oxidation.

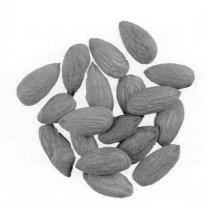

▲ Raw almonds are an appetizing way to help meet your vitamin E needs.

Vitamin E: The Vegetarian Vitamin

Vitamin E is widespread in foods from plant sources (**FIGURE 8.6**). Much of the vitamin E that we consume comes from products such as spreads, salad dressings, and mayonnaise made from vegetable oils, including safflower oil, sunflower oil, canola oil, and soybean oil. Nuts, seeds, soybeans, and some vegetables—including spinach, broccoli, and avocados—also contribute vitamin E to our diet. Although no single fruit or vegetable contains very high amounts of vitamin E, eating the recommended

tocopherol The active form of vitamin E in our body.

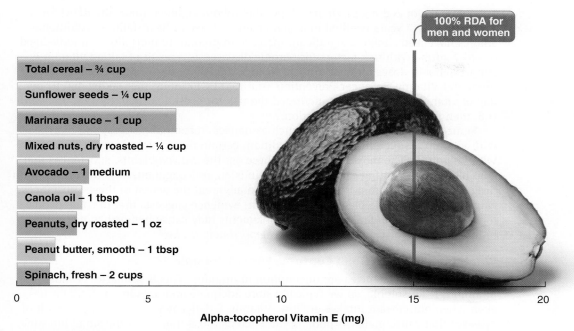

100% RDA for men and women

Total cereal – ¾ cup

Sunflower seeds – ¼ cup

Marinara sauce – 1 cup

Mixed nuts, dry roasted – ¼ cup

Avocado – 1 medium

Canola oil – 1 tbsp

Peanuts, dry roasted – 1 oz

Peanut butter, smooth – 1 tbsp

Spinach, fresh – 2 cups

0　　　　　5　　　　　10　　　　　15　　　　　20

Alpha-tocopherol Vitamin E (mg)

FIGURE 8.6　Common food sources of vitamin E. The RDA for vitamin E is 15 mg alpha-tocopherol per day for men and women.

Data from: U.S. Department of Agriculture, Agricultural Research Service, 2012. USDA Nutrient Database for Standard Reference, Release 25.

amounts of fruits and vegetables each day will help ensure adequate intake of this nutrient. Cereals are often fortified with vitamin E, and other grain products contribute modest amounts to our diet. Animal and dairy products are poor sources.

Vitamin E is destroyed by exposure to oxygen, metals, ultraviolet light, and heat. Although raw (uncooked) vegetable oils contain vitamin E, heating these oils destroys vitamin E. Thus, foods that are deep-fried and processed contain little vitamin E; this includes most fast foods. See the nearby **Quick Tips** for increasing your intake of vitamin E.

What Happens If We Consume Too Much Vitamin E?

Until recently, standard supplemental doses (one to eighteen times the RDA) of vitamin E were not associated with any adverse health effects. However, a 2005 study found that, among adults 55 years of age or older with vascular disease or diabetes,

QuickTips

Eating More Vitamin E

✓ Eat cereals high in vitamin E for breakfast or as a snack.

✓ Add sunflower seeds to salads and trail mixes, or just have them as a snack.

✓ Add sliced almonds to salads, granola, and trail mixes to boost vitamin E intake.

✓ Pack a peanut butter sandwich for lunch.

✓ Eat veggies throughout the day—for snacks, for sides, and in main dishes.

✓ When dressing a salad, use vitamin E–rich oils, such as sunflower, safflower, or canola.

✓ Enjoy some fresh, homemade guacamole: mash a ripe avocado with a squeeze of lime juice and a sprinkle of garlic salt.

a daily intake of 268 mg of vitamin E per day (about eighteen times the RDA) for approximately 7 years resulted in a significant increase in heart failure.[2] Additional studies have also shown a significant increase in premature mortality in middle-aged or older adults with risk factors for chronic diseases as a result of taking vitamin E supplements in doses ranging from 10 IU to 5,000 IU per day.[3,4] Moreover, the Selenium and Vitamin E Cancer Prevention Trial (SELECT) found that taking 400 IU per day of vitamin E supplements increased the risk for prostate cancer by 17% in healthy U.S. men from the general population.[5]

Some people report side effects such as nausea, intestinal distress, and diarrhea with vitamin E supplementation. In addition, certain medications interact negatively with vitamin E. The most important of these are the *anticoagulants,* substances that stop blood from clotting excessively. Aspirin is an anticoagulant, as is the prescription drug Coumadin. Vitamin E supplements can augment the action of these substances, causing uncontrollable bleeding. In addition, evidence suggests that in some people, long-term use of standard vitamin E supplements may cause hemorrhaging in the brain, leading to a type of stroke called *hemorrhagic stroke.*[6]

What Happens If We Don't Consume Enough Vitamin E?

True vitamin E deficiencies are uncommon in humans. This is primarily because vitamin E is fat soluble, so we typically store adequate amounts in our fatty tissues, even when our current intakes are low. Vitamin E deficiencies are usually a result of diseases that cause malabsorption of fat, such as those that affect the small intestine, liver, gallbladder, and pancreas. Recall that the liver makes bile, which is stored in the gallbladder and delivered to the small intestine, where it facilitates emulsification of fat. The pancreas makes fat-digesting enzymes. Thus, when the liver, gallbladder, or pancreas is not functioning properly, fat and the fat-soluble vitamins, including vitamin E, cannot be absorbed, leading to their deficiency.

Results from three national surveys suggest that the diets of most Americans do not provide the RDA for vitamin E.[7,8] However, these intake estimates may be low because the amounts and types of fat added during cooking are often not known and thus are not included in survey estimates.

Despite the rarity of true vitamin E deficiencies, they do occur. One vitamin E deficiency symptom is *erythrocyte hemolysis,* or the rupturing (*lysis*) of red blood cells (*erythrocytes*). This rupturing of red blood cells leads to *anemia,* a condition in which our red blood cells cannot carry and transport enough oxygen to our tissues, leading to fatigue, weakness, and a diminished ability to perform physical and mental work. (We discuss anemia in more detail in Chapter 10.) Vitamin E deficiency can also cause loss of muscle coordination and reflexes, leading to impairments in vision, speech, and movement. Vitamin E deficiency can also impair immune function, especially when body stores of the mineral selenium are low.

recap Vitamin E protects cell membranes from oxidation, enhances immune function, and improves our absorption of vitamin A if dietary intake is low. The RDA for vitamin E is 15 mg alpha-tocopherol per day for men and women. Vitamin E is found primarily in vegetable oils and nuts. Toxicity is uncommon, but taking very high doses can cause excessive bleeding. A genuine deficiency is rare, but symptoms include anemia and impaired vision, speech, and movement.

Vitamin C

Vitamin C is a water-soluble vitamin. We must therefore consume it on a regular basis because any excess is excreted (primarily in our urine) rather than stored. There are two active forms of vitamin C: ascorbic acid and dehydroascorbic acid. Interestingly, most animals can make their own vitamin C from glucose. Humans and guinea pigs are two groups that cannot synthesize their own vitamin C and must consume it in the diet.

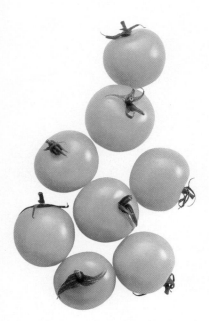

Many fruits, such as these yellow tomatoes, are high in vitamin C.

Functions of Vitamin C

Vitamin C is probably most well known for its role in preventing scurvy, a disease that ravaged sailors on long sea voyages centuries ago. In fact, the name *ascorbic acid* is derived from the combined Latin terms *a* (meaning "without") and *scorbic* (meaning "having scurvy"). Scurvy was characterized by bleeding tissues, especially of the gums, and is thought to have caused more than half of the deaths that occurred at sea. During these long voyages, the crew ate all of the fruits and vegetables early in the trip, then had only grain and animal products available until they reached land to resupply. In 1740 in England, Dr. James Lind discovered that citrus fruits can prevent scurvy. This is due to their high vitamin C content. Fifty years after the discovery of the link between citrus fruits and scurvy prevention, the British Navy finally required all ships to provide daily lemon juice rations for each sailor to prevent the onset of scurvy. A century later, sailors were given lime juice rations, earning them the nickname "limeys." It wasn't until 1930 that vitamin C was discovered and identified as a nutrient.

One reason that vitamin C prevents scurvy is that it assists in the synthesis of **collagen**. Collagen, a protein, is a critical component of all connective tissues in the body, including bone, teeth, skin, tendons, and blood vessels. Collagen assists in preventing bruises, and it ensures proper wound healing because it is a part of scar tissue and a component of the tissue that mends broken bones. Without adequate vitamin C, the body cannot form collagen, and tissue hemorrhage, or bleeding, occurs. Vitamin C may also be involved in the synthesis of other components of connective tissues, such as elastin and bone matrix.

In addition to connective tissues, vitamin C assists in the synthesis of DNA, bile, neurotransmitters such as serotonin (which helps regulate mood), and carnitine, which transports long-chain fatty acids from the cytosol into the mitochondria for energy production. Vitamin C also helps ensure appropriate levels of thyroxine, a hormone produced by the thyroid gland, to support basal metabolic rate and to maintain body temperature. Other hormones that are synthesized with assistance from vitamin C include epinephrine, norepinephrine, and steroid hormones.

Vitamin C also acts as an antioxidant. Because it is water soluble, it is an important antioxidant in the extracellular fluid. Like vitamin E, it donates electrons to free radicals, thus preventing the damage of cells and tissues. It also protects LDL-cholesterol from oxidation, which may reduce the risk for cardiovascular disease. Vitamin C acts as an important antioxidant in the lungs, helping protect us from the damage caused by ozone and cigarette smoke. It also enhances immune function by protecting white blood cells from the oxidative damage that occurs in response to fighting illness and infection. But contrary to popular belief, it is not a miracle cure (see the **Nutrition Myth or Fact?** box on page 284). In the stomach, vitamin C reduces the formation of *nitrosamines*, cancer-causing agents found in foods such as cured and processed meats. We discuss the role of vitamin C and other antioxidants in preventing some forms of cancer in the **In Depth** following this chapter (pages 301–309).

Vitamin C also regenerates vitamin E after it has been oxidized. This occurs when ascorbic acid donates electrons to vitamin E radicals, becoming dehydroascorbic acid. This enables vitamin E to continue to protect our cell membranes and other tissues.

Finally, vitamin C enhances the absorption of iron. It is recommended that people with low iron stores consume vitamin C-rich foods along with iron sources to improve absorption. For people with high iron stores, this practice can be dangerous and lead to iron toxicity (see Chapter 10).

How Much Vitamin C Should We Consume?

Although popular opinion suggests that our need for vitamin C is quite high, the RDA is easily obtained when we eat the recommended amounts of fruits and vegetables daily. The RDA for vitamin C is 90 mg per day for men and 75 mg per day for women (see Table 8.1).[1] The Tolerable Upper Intake Level (UL) is 2,000 mg per day for adults. Smoking increases a person's need for vitamin C; thus, the RDA for smokers is 35 mg more per day than for nonsmokers. This equals 125 mg per day for men and 110 mg per day for women. Other high-stress situations that may increase the need for vitamin C include healing from a traumatic injury, surgery, or burns and the use of oral contraceptives among women; there is no consensus on how much extra vitamin C is needed in these circumstances.

collagen A protein found in all the connective tissues in our body.

nutrition myth or fact?

Can Vitamin C Prevent the Common Cold?

What do you do when you feel a cold coming on? If you are like many people, you drink a lot of orange juice or take vitamin C supplements to ward it off. Do these tactics really help prevent a cold?

It is well known that vitamin C is important for a healthy immune system. A deficiency of vitamin C can seriously weaken the immune cells' ability to detect and destroy invading microbes, increasing susceptibility to many diseases and illnesses—including the common cold. Many people have taken vitamin C supplements to prevent the common cold, basing their behavior on its actions of enhancing our immune function. Nevertheless, scientific studies do not support this action. A recent review of many of the studies of vitamin C and the common cold found that people taking vitamin C regularly in an attempt to ward off the common cold experienced as many colds as people who took a placebo. However, the *duration* of their colds was reduced—by 8% in adults and 13.6% in children.[9] Timing appears to be important, though: taking vitamin C after the onset of cold symptoms did not reduce either the duration or the severity of the cold. Interestingly, taking vitamin C supplements regularly did reduce the number of colds experienced in marathon runners, skiers, and soldiers participating in exercises done under extreme environmental conditions.

The amount of vitamin C taken in these studies was at least 200 mg per day, with many using doses as high as 4,000 mg per day (more than forty times the RDA), with no harmful effects noted in those studies that reported adverse events.

In summary, it appears that, for most people, taking vitamin C supplements regularly will not prevent colds but may reduce their duration. Consuming a healthful diet that includes excellent sources of vitamin C will also help you maintain a strong immune system. Taking vitamin C after the onset of cold symptoms does not appear to help, so next time you feel a cold coming on, you may want to think twice before taking extra vitamin C.

CRITICAL THINKING QUESTIONS

1. Have you ever taken vitamin C to ward off colds? If so, what motivated you to do so?
2. Armed with this new information, what actions do you plan to take the next time you feel a cold coming on? What other behaviors might you change to reduce your risk of getting a cold?

Vitamin C: Citrus and More

Fruits and vegetables are the best sources of vitamin C (**FIGURE 8.7**). Because heat and oxygen destroy vitamin C, fresh sources of these foods have the highest content. Cooking foods, especially boiling them, leaches their vitamin C, which is then lost when we strain them. The forms of cooking that are least likely to compromise the vitamin C content of foods are steaming, microwaving, and stir-frying.

As shown in Figure 8.7, many fruits and vegetables are high in vitamin C. Citrus fruits (such as grapefruits, oranges, lemons, and limes), sweet potatoes, strawberries, tomatoes, kiwi fruit, broccoli, spinach and other leafy greens, cabbage, green and red peppers, and cauliflower are excellent sources of vitamin C. Fortified beverages and cereals are also good sources. Dairy foods, meats, and nonfortified cereals and grains provide little or no vitamin C. With such a wide variety of foods to choose from, it's easy to eat right all day! See **Eating Right All Day** for some simple menu choices that are high in vitamin C. In addition, the **Quick Tips** feature box (page 286) can help you increase your intake of vitamin C.

What Happens If We Consume Too Much Vitamin C?

Because vitamin C is water soluble, we usually excrete any excess. Consuming excess amounts in food sources does not lead to toxicity, and only supplements can lead to toxic doses. Taking a **megadose** of vitamin C is not fatally harmful. However, side effects of doses exceeding 2,000 mg/day for a prolonged period include nausea, diarrhea, nosebleeds, and abdominal cramps.

There are rare instances in which consuming even moderately excessive doses of vitamin C can be harmful. As mentioned earlier, vitamin C enhances the absorption of iron. This action is beneficial to people who need to increase iron absorption. It can

megadose A nutrient dose that is ten or more times greater than the recommended amount.

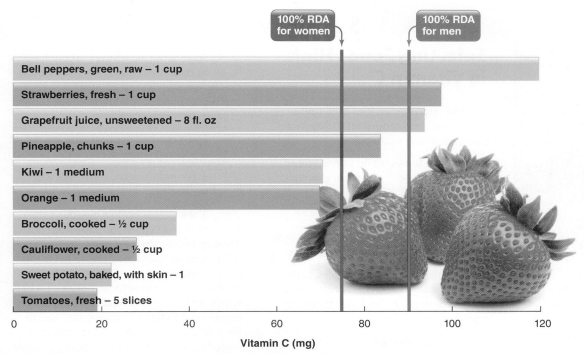

FIGURE 8.7 Common food sources of vitamin C. The RDA for vitamin C is 90 mg/day for men and 75 mg/day for women.

Data from: U.S. Department of Agriculture, Agricultural Research Service, 2012. USDA Nutrient Database for Standard Reference, Release 25.

be harmful, however, to people with a disease called *hemochromatosis,* which causes an excess accumulation of iron in the body. Such iron toxicity can damage tissues and lead to a heart attack. In people who have preexisting kidney disease, taking excess vitamin C can lead to the formation of kidney stones. This does not appear to occur in healthy individuals.

Critics of vitamin C supplementation claim that taking the supplemental form of the vitamin is "unbalanced" nutrition and leads vitamin C to act as a prooxidant. A **prooxidant**, as you might guess, is a nutrient that promotes oxidation. It does this by pushing the balance of exchange reactions toward oxidation, which promotes the production of free radicals. Although the results of a few older studies suggested that

prooxidant A nutrient that promotes oxidation and oxidative cell and tissue damage.

eating right all day

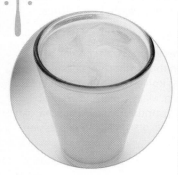

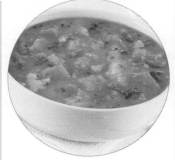

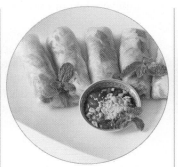

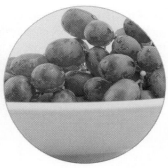

Breakfast
Grapefruit juice instead of sweetened coffee!

Lunch
Vegetable soup instead of chicken noodle!

Dinner
Spring rolls instead of sweet & sour pork!

Snack
Grapes instead of M&Ms!

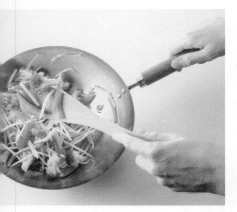

⬆ Fresh vegetables are good sources of vitamin C and beta-carotene.

QuickTips

Selecting Foods High in Vitamin C

✓ Mix strawberries, kiwi fruit, cantaloupe, and oranges for a tasty fruit salad loaded with vitamin C.

✓ Include tomatoes on salads, wraps, and sandwiches for more vitamin C.

✓ Make your own fresh-squeezed orange or grapefruit juice!

✓ Add your favorite vitamin C–rich fruits, such as strawberries, to smoothies.

✓ Buy ready-to-eat vegetables, such as baby carrots and cherry tomatoes, and toss some in a zip-lock bag to take to school or work.

✓ Put a few slices of romaine lettuce on your sandwich.

✓ Throw a small container of orange slices, fresh pineapple chunks, or berries into your backpack for an afternoon snack.

✓ Store some juice boxes in your freezer to pack with your lunch. They'll thaw slowly, keeping the rest of your lunch cool, and many brands contain a full day's supply of vitamin C in just 6 oz.

✓ Enjoy raw bell peppers with low-fat dip for a crunchy snack.

✓ Serve reduced-salt corn chips with fresh salsa.

✓ Make gazpacho! In a blender, combine 1–3 cups of tomato juice, chunks of green pepper and red onion, a cucumber with seeds removed (no need to peel), the juice of one lime, a garlic clove, a splash each of red-wine vinegar and olive oil, a half teaspoon each of basil and cumin, and salt and pepper to taste. Seed and dice two to three fresh tomatoes and add to blended ingredients. Chill for several hours and serve cold, topped with a dollop of low-fat sour cream or plain yogurt.

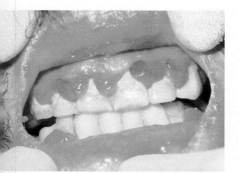

⬆ **FIGURE 8.8** Bleeding gums are one symptom of scurvy, the most common vitamin C–deficiency disease.

vitamin C acts as a prooxidant, these studies were found to be flawed or irrelevant for humans. At the present time, there appears to be no strong scientific evidence that vitamin C, from either food or dietary supplements, acts as a prooxidant in humans.

What Happens If We Don't Consume Enough Vitamin C?

Vitamin C deficiencies are rare in developed countries but can occur in developing countries. Scurvy is the most common vitamin C–deficiency disease. The symptoms of scurvy appear after about 1 month of a vitamin C–deficient diet and include bleeding gums (**FIGURE 8.8**), loose teeth, wounds that fail to heal, swollen ankles and wrists, bone pain and fractures, diarrhea, weakness, and depression. Anemia can also result from vitamin C deficiency. People most at risk are those who eat few fruits and vegetables, including impoverished or homebound individuals, and people who abuse alcohol and drugs.

recap Vitamin C scavenges free radicals and regenerates vitamin E after it has been oxidized. Vitamin C prevents scurvy and assists in the synthesis of collagen, hormones, neurotransmitters, and DNA. Vitamin C also enhances iron absorption. The RDA for vitamin C is 90 mg per day for men and 75 mg per day for women. Many fruits and vegetables are high in vitamin C. Toxicity is uncommon with dietary intake; symptoms include nausea, diarrhea, and nosebleeds. Deficiency symptoms include scurvy, anemia, diarrhea, and depression.

Selenium

Selenium is a trace mineral, and it is found in varying amounts in soil and thus in the food grown there. Keep in mind that although we need only minute amounts of trace minerals, they are just as important to our health as vitamins and the major minerals.

nutri-case | HANNAH

"Since I started college in September, I've had one cold after another. I guess it's being around so many different people every day, plus all the stress. Then a few weeks ago I found this cool orange-tasting vitamin C powder at the health food outlet on campus, and I started mixing it into my orange juice every morning. I guess it's working, because I haven't had a cold since I started using it! But this morning I woke up with stomach cramps and diarrhea, so now I guess I have to worry about a stomach flu. I wish there was a vitamin C powder for that!"

Given what you've learned about the effects of vitamin C supplementation, do you think it is possible that Hannah's vitamin C regimen is doing her more harm than good? Explain why or why not.

Functions of Selenium

It is only recently that we have learned about the critical role of selenium as a nutrient in human health. In 1979, Chinese scientists reported an association between a heart disorder called **Keshan disease** and selenium deficiency. This disease occurs in children in the Keshan province of China, where the soil is depleted of selenium. The scientists found that Keshan disease can be prevented with selenium supplementation.

Most of the selenium in our bodies is contained in amino acids: *selenomethionine* is the storage form for selenium, whereas *selenocysteine* is the active form of selenium. Selenocysteine is a critical component of the glutathione peroxidase antioxidant enzyme system noted earlier in this chapter (page 279). As shown in **FIGURE 8.9**, glutathione peroxidase breaks down peroxides (such as hydrogen peroxide) that are formed by the body, so that they cannot form free radicals. This decrease in the number of free radicals spares vitamin E and prevents oxidative damage to our cell membranes.

Like vitamin C, selenium is needed for the production of thyroxine, or thyroid hormone, which helps maintain our basal metabolism and body temperature. Selenium

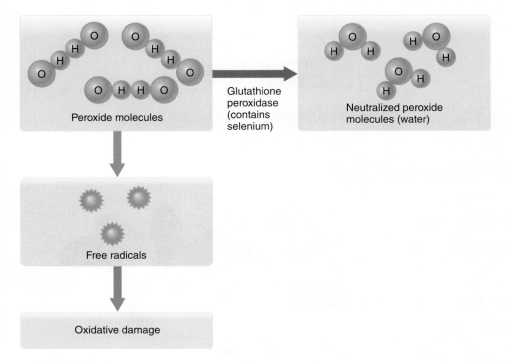

Peroxide molecules

Glutathione peroxidase (contains selenium)

Neutralized peroxide molecules (water)

Free radicals

Oxidative damage

◆ **FIGURE 8.9** Selenium is part of glutathione peroxidase, which neutralizes peroxide molecules (such as hydrogen peroxide, shown here) that are formed by the body. This prevents them from forming free radicals, spares vitamin E, and prevents oxidative damage.

Keshan disease A heart disorder caused by selenium deficiency. It was first identified in children in the Keshan province of China.

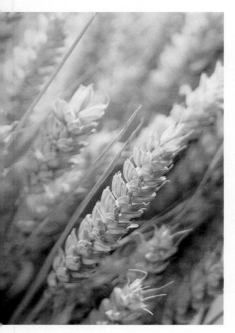

⬥ Wheat is a rich source of selenium.

also appears to play a role in immune function, and poor selenium status is associated with higher rates of some forms of cancer.

How Much Selenium Should We Consume?

The content of selenium in foods is highly variable. Because it is a trace mineral, we need only minute amounts to maintain health. The RDA for selenium is 55 µg per day for both men and women (see Table 8.1).[1] The UL is 400 µg per day.

Because it is stored in the tissues of animals, selenium is found in reliably consistent amounts in animal foods. Organ meats, such as liver and kidneys, as well as pork and fish, are particularly good sources **(FIGURE 8.10)**.

In contrast, the amount of selenium in plants varies according to the selenium content of the soil in which the plant is grown. Many companies marketing selenium supplements warn that the agricultural soils in the United States are depleted of selenium and inform us that we need to take selenium supplements. In reality, the selenium content of soil varies greatly across North America, and because we obtain our food from a variety of geographic locations, few people in the United States suffer from selenium deficiency. This is true for people who eat even small quantities of meat or fish.

What Happens If We Consume Too Much Selenium?

Selenium toxicity does not result from eating foods high in selenium. However, supplementation can cause toxicity. Toxicity symptoms include brittle hair and nails, which can eventually break and fall off. Other symptoms include skin rashes, nausea, vomiting, weakness, and cirrhosis of the liver.

What Happens If We Don't Consume Enough Selenium?

As discussed previously, selenium deficiency is associated with a form of heart disease called Keshan disease. Selenium deficiency does not cause the disease, but selenium is necessary to help the immune system effectively fight the viral infection that causes the disease. Selenium supplements significantly reduce the incidence of Keshan disease, but they cannot reduce the damage to the heart muscle once it occurs.

Another deficiency disease is *Kashin-Beck disease*, a disease of the cartilage that results in deforming arthritis **(FIGURE 8.11)**. Kashin-Beck disease is found in selenium-depleted areas in China and Tibet. Other deficiency symptoms include impaired

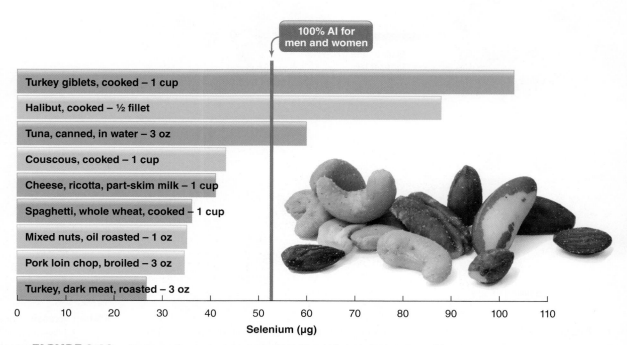

100% AI for men and women

Turkey giblets, cooked – 1 cup
Halibut, cooked – ½ fillet
Tuna, canned, in water – 3 oz
Couscous, cooked – 1 cup
Cheese, ricotta, part-skim milk – 1 cup
Spaghetti, whole wheat, cooked – 1 cup
Mixed nuts, oil roasted – 1 oz
Pork loin chop, broiled – 3 oz
Turkey, dark meat, roasted – 3 oz

0   10   20   30   40   50   60   70   80   90   100   110
Selenium (µg)

⬥ **FIGURE 8.10** Common food sources of selenium. The AI for selenium is 55 µg/day.
Data from: U.S. Department of Agriculture, Agricultural Research Service, 2012. USDA Nutrient Database for Standard Reference, Release 25.

immune responses, infertility, depression, hostility, impaired cognitive function, and muscle pain and wasting. Deficiencies of both selenium and iodine in pregnant women can cause a form of *cretinism* in the infant (discussed in Chapter 10).

Copper, Iron, Zinc, and Manganese Assist in Antioxidant Function

As discussed earlier, there are numerous antioxidant enzyme systems in our bodies. Copper, zinc, and manganese are a part of the superoxide dismutase antioxidant enzyme system. Iron is a part of the structure of catalase. In addition to their role in protecting against oxidative damage, these minerals play major roles in the optimal functioning of many other enzymes in our bodies. Copper, iron, and zinc help us maintain the health of our blood, and manganese is an important cofactor in carbohydrate metabolism (these nutrients are discussed in detail in Chapter 10).

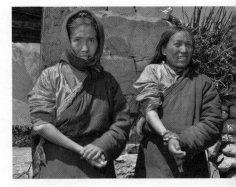

▲ **FIGURE 8.11** Selenium deficiency can lead to a deforming arthritis called Kashin-Beck disease.

recap Selenium is part of the glutathione peroxidase antioxidant enzyme system. It indirectly spares vitamin E from oxidative damage, and it assists with immune function and the production of thyroid hormone. Organ meats, pork, and seafood are good sources of selenium, as are nuts, wheat, and rice. The selenium content of plants varies according to the amount of selenium in the soil in which they are grown. Toxicity symptoms include brittle hair and nails, vomiting, nausea, and liver cirrhosis. Deficiency symptoms and side effects include Keshan disease, Kashin-Beck disease, impaired immune function, infertility, and muscle wasting. Copper, zinc, and manganese are cofactors for the superoxide dismutase antioxidant enzyme system. Iron is a cofactor for the catalase antioxidant enzyme. These minerals play critical roles in blood health and energy metabolism.

Learn more about enzymes and cofactors and their role in neutralizing peroxides at www.youtube.com. Enter "Biology Essentials 048" into the search bar, then click on the link to Enzymes by bozemanbiology.

Beta-Carotene

Although beta-carotene is considered a phytochemical, not an essential nutrient, it is a *provitamin* found in many fruits and vegetables. **Provitamins** are inactive forms of vitamins that the body cannot use until they are converted to their active form. Our body converts beta-carotene to the active form of vitamin A, *retinol;* thus, beta-carotene is a precursor of retinol.

Beta-carotene is classified as a **carotenoid**, one of a group of plant pigments that are the basis for the red, orange, and deep-yellow colors of many fruits and vegetables. (Even dark-green leafy vegetables contain plenty of carotenoids, but the green pigment, chlorophyll, masks their color.) Many carotenoids are known to have antioxidant properties, and researchers are beginning to explore other potential functions of carotenoids and how they might affect human health.

Although there are more than 600 carotenoids found in nature, only about 50 are found in the typical human diet. The six most common carotenoids found in human blood are alpha-carotene, beta-carotene, beta-cryptoxanthin, lutein, lycopene, and zeaxanthin (see Figure 1 in the **In Depth** Chapter 1.5, page 35). Of these, the body can convert only alpha-carotene, beta-carotene, and beta-cryptoxanthin to retinol. These are referred to as *provitamin A carotenoids.*

Although one molecule of beta-carotene splits to form two molecules of active vitamin A, twelve units of beta-carotene are considered equivalent to one unit of vitamin A. Several factors account for this. For example, our bodies don't convert to vitamin A all of the beta-carotene that we consume, and our absorption of beta-carotene is not as efficient as our absorption of vitamin A. Nutritionists express the units of beta-carotene in a food as Retinol Activity Equivalents, or RAE. This measurement indicates how much active vitamin A is available to the body after it has converted the beta-carotene in the food.

Functions of Beta-Carotene

Beta-carotene and some other carotenoids are recognized to have antioxidant properties. Like vitamin E, they are fat soluble and fight the harmful effects of oxidation in the lipid portions of our cell membranes and in LDLs; however, compared to

provitamin An inactive form of a vitamin that the body can convert to an active form. An example is beta-carotene.

carotenoid A fat-soluble plant pigment that the body stores in the liver and adipose tissues. The body is able to convert certain carotenoids to vitamin A.

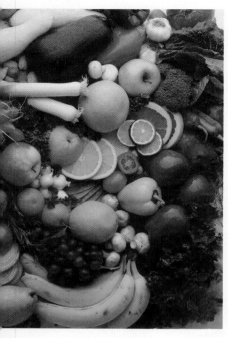

Foods that are high in carotenoids are easy to recognize by their bright colors.

vitamin E, beta-carotene is a relatively weak antioxidant. In fact, other carotenoids, such as lycopene and lutein, may be stronger antioxidants.

Through their antioxidant actions, carotenoids play other important roles in our body as well, such as:

- enhancing the immune system and boost the body's ability to fight illness and disease
- protecting skin from the damage caused by the sun's ultraviolet rays
- protecting our eyes from damage, preventing or delaying age-related vision impairment

Carotenoids are also associated with a decreased risk for certain types of cancer. (We discuss the roles of carotenoids and other antioxidants in cancer **In Depth** following this chapter.)

How Much Beta-Carotene Should We Consume?

Nutritional scientists do not consider beta-carotene and other carotenoids to be essential nutrients because they play no known essential roles in our bodies and are not associated with any deficiency symptoms. Thus, no RDA for these compounds has been established. Eating the recommended five servings of fruits and vegetables each day provide approximately 6 to 8 mg of beta-carotene.[10]

Supplements containing beta-carotene have become popular, but before you try one, read the **Nutrition Debate** located at the end of this chapter, where you'll learn about the risks of antioxidant supplementation.

Beyond Carrots: Food Sources of Beta-Carotene

Not only carrots, but fruits and vegetables that are red, orange, yellow, and deep green are generally high in beta-carotene and other carotenoids, such as lutein and lycopene. Tomatoes, sweet potatoes, leafy greens (such as kale and spinach), apricots, cantaloupe, and pumpkin are good sources. Eating the recommended amounts of fruits and vegetables each day ensures an adequate intake of carotenoids. Because of its color, beta-carotene is used as a natural coloring agent for many foods, including margarine, yellow cheddar cheese, cereal, cake mixes, gelatins, and soft drinks. However, these foods are not significant sources of beta-carotene. **FIGURE 8.12** identifies common foods that are high in beta-carotene.

We generally absorb only between 20% and 40% of the carotenoids present in the foods we eat. In contrast to vitamins E and C, carotenoids are better absorbed from cooked foods. Carotenoids are bound in the cells of plants, and the process of lightly cooking these plants breaks chemical bonds and can rupture cell walls, which humans don't digest. These actions result in more of the carotenoids being released from the plant. For instance, 1 cup of raw carrots contains approximately 9 mg of beta-carotene, whereas the same amount of cooked carrots contains approximately 13 mg.[11] The **Quick Tips** feature suggests ways to increase your intake of beta-carotene.

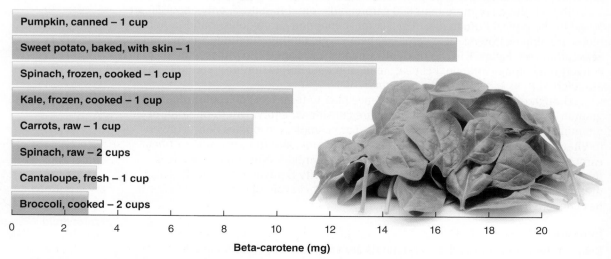

Pumpkin, canned – 1 cup
Sweet potato, baked, with skin – 1
Spinach, frozen, cooked – 1 cup
Kale, frozen, cooked – 1 cup
Carrots, raw – 1 cup
Spinach, raw – 2 cups
Cantaloupe, fresh – 1 cup
Broccoli, cooked – 2 cups

0   2   4   6   8   10   12   14   16   18   20

Beta-carotene (mg)

FIGURE 8.12 Common food sources of beta-carotene. There is no RDA for beta-carotene.

Data from: U.S. Department of Agriculture, Agricultural Research Service, 2012. USDA Nutrient Database for Standard Reference, Release 25.

QuickTips

Boosting Your Beta-Carotene

✓ Start your day with an orange, grapefruit, a pear, a banana, an apple, or a slice of cantaloupe. All are good sources of beta-carotene.

✓ Pack a zip-lock bag of carrot slices or dried apricots in your lunch.

✓ Instead of french fries, think orange! Slice raw sweet potatoes, toss the slices in olive or canola oil, and bake.

✓ Add veggies to homemade pizza.

✓ Add shredded carrots to cake and muffin batters.

✓ Taking dessert to a potluck? Make a pumpkin pie! It's easy if you use canned pumpkin and follow the recipe on the can.

✓ Go green, too! The next time you have a salad, go for the dark-green leafy vegetables instead of iceberg lettuce.

✓ Add raw spinach or other green leafy vegetables to wraps and sandwiches.

What Happens If We Consume Too Much Beta-Carotene?

Consuming large amounts of beta-carotene or other carotenoids in foods does not appear to cause toxic symptoms. However, your skin can turn yellow or orange if you consume large amounts of foods that are high in beta-carotene. This condition is referred to as *carotenosis* or *carotenoderma*, and it appears to be both reversible and harmless. Again, taking beta-carotene supplements is not recommended because we can get adequate amounts of this nutrient by eating more fruits and vegetables.

What Happens If We Don't Consume Enough Beta-Carotene?

There are no known deficiency symptoms for beta-carotene or other carotenoids apart from beta-carotene's function as a precursor for vitamin A.

recap Beta-carotene is a carotenoid and a provitamin of vitamin A. It protects the lipid portions of cell membranes and LDL-cholesterol from oxidative damage. It also enhances immune function and protects vision. There is no RDA for beta-carotene. Orange, red, and deep-green fruits and vegetables are good sources. There are no known toxicity or deficiency symptoms of beta-carotene when consumed from food, but yellowing of the skin can occur if too much beta-carotene is consumed.

What is the role of vitamin A in vision?

As early as AD 30, the Roman writer Aulus Cornelius Celsus described in his medical encyclopedia, *De Medicina*, a condition called night blindness and recommended as a cure the consumption of liver. We now know that night blindness is due to a deficiency of vitamin A, a fat-soluble vitamin stored primarily in the liver of animals. When we consume vitamin A, we store 90% in our liver, and the remainder in our adipose tissue, kidneys, and lungs.

Forms of Vitamin A

Because fat-soluble vitamins cannot dissolve in our blood, they require proteins that can bind with and transport them through the bloodstream to target tissues and cells. *Retinol-binding protein* is one such carrier protein for vitamin A. Retinol-binding protein carries one form of vitamin A, retinol, from the liver to the cells that require it.

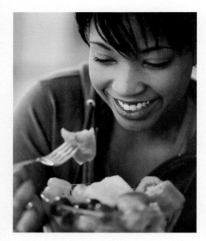

↞ Eating plenty of fruits and vegetables can help prevent vitamin A deficiency.

There are three active forms of vitamin A in our body: **retinol** is the alcohol form, **retinal** is the aldehyde form, and **retinoic acid** is the acid form. These three forms are collectively referred to as the *retinoids* (**FIGURE 8.13**). Of the three, retinol has the starring role in maintaining our body's physiologic functions. Remember from the previous section that beta-carotene is a precursor to vitamin A. When we eat foods that contain beta-carotene, it is converted to retinol in the wall of our small intestine.

The unit of expression for vitamin A is Retinol Activity Equivalents (RAE). You may still see the expression Retinol Equivalents (RE) or International Units (IU) for vitamin A on food labels and dietary supplements. The conversions to RAE from various forms of retinol are as follows:

- 1 RAE = 1 microgram (µg) retinol
- 1 RAE = 12 µg beta-carotene
- 1 RAE = 24 µg alpha-carotene or beta-cryptoxanthin
- 1 RAE = 1 RE
- 1 RAE = 3.3 IU

Conversion rates from IU to µg RAE are as follows:

- 1 IU retinol from food or supplements = 0.3 µg RAE
- 1 IU beta-carotene from supplements = 0.15 µg RAE
- 1 IU beta-carotene from food = 0.05 µg RAE
- 1 IU alpha-carotene or beta-cryptoxanthin = 0.025 µg RAE

Vitamin A Is Essential to Sight

Vitamin A affects our sight in two ways: it enables us to react to changes in the brightness of light, and it enables us to distinguish between various wavelengths of light—in other words, to see different colors. Let's take a closer look at this process.

Light enters our eyes through the cornea, travels through the lens, and then hits the **retina**, which is a delicate membrane lining the back of the inner eyeball (**FIGURE 8.14**). You might already have guessed how *retinal* got its name: it is found in—and is integral to—the retina. In the retina, retinal combines with a protein called *opsin* to form **rhodopsin**, a light-sensitive pigment. Rhodopsin is found in the *rod cells*, which are cells that react to dim light and interpret black-and-white images.

When light hits the retina, the rod cells go through a *bleaching process*. In this reaction, rhodopsin is split into retinal and opsin, and the rod cells lose their color. The retinal component also changes spatial orientation from a *cis* configuration, which is bent, into a *trans* configuration, which is straight. The opsin component also changes shape. These changes in retinal and opsin during the bleaching process generate a nerve impulse that travels to the brain, resulting in the perception of a black-and-white image. Most of the retinal is converted back to its original *cis* form and binds with opsin to regenerate rhodopsin, allowing the visual cycle to begin again. However, some of the retinal is lost with each cycle and must be replaced by retinol from the bloodstream. This visual cycle goes on continually, allowing our eyes to adjust moment to moment to subtle changes in our surroundings or in the level of light.

retinol An active, alcohol form of vitamin A that plays an important role in healthy vision and immune function.

retinal An active, aldehyde form of vitamin A that plays an important role in healthy vision and immune function.

retinoic acid An active, acid form of vitamin A that plays an important role in cell growth and immune function.

retina The delicate, light-sensitive membrane lining the inner eyeball and connected to the optic nerve. It contains retinal.

rhodopsin A light-sensitive pigment found in the rod cells that is formed by retinal and opsin.

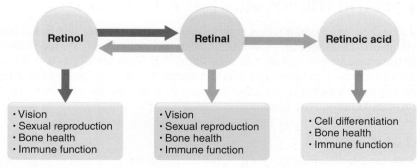

↞ **FIGURE 8.13** The three active forms of vitamin A in our body are retinol, retinal, and retinoic acid. Retinol and retinal can be converted interchangeably; retinoic acid is formed from retinal, and this process is irreversible. Each form of vitamin A contributes to many bodily processes.

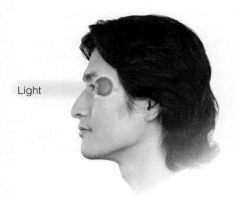

Light

Vitamin A is a component of two light-sensitive proteins, rhodopsin and iodopsin, that are essential for vision. Here we examine rhodopsin's role in vision. Although the breakdown of iodopsin is similar, rhodopsin is more sensitive to light than iodopsin and is more likely to become bleached.

EYE STRUCTURE

Eye cross-section

Cornea

Light

Retina

Macula

Optic nerve

Rod and cone cells in retina

Rod

Cone

Rhodopsin protein in rod cell membrane

Rhodopsin

Retinal (Vitamin A)

1 After light enters your eye through the cornea, it travels to the back of your eye to the macula, which is located in the retina. The macula allows you to see fine details and things that are straight in front of you.

2 Inside the retina are two types of light-absorbing cells, rods and cones. Rods contain the protein rhodopsin, while cones contain the protein iodopsin.

EFFECT OF LIGHT ON RHODOPSIN

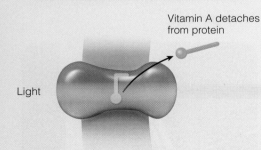

Vitamin A detaches from protein

Light

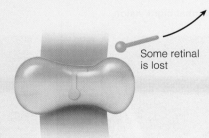

Some retinal is lost

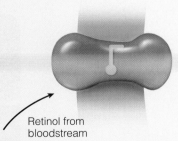

Retinol from bloodstream

1 As rhodopsin absorbs incoming light, the shape of vitamin A is altered, and it detaches from the rhodopsin.

2 This process, called bleaching, causes a cascade of events that transmits visual messages through your optic nerve to your brain. After bleaching, some retinal is lost.

3 Retinol from the blood is converted to retinal to replenish what is lost. The vitamin A returns to its original shape and becomes part of rhodopsin again, regenerating the eye's light-absorbing capabilities. This regeneration can take a few moments.

To learn more about the vision process visit www.youtube.com, and enter "anatomy and function of the eye" in the search box, then click on the video of the same name.

When levels of vitamin A are deficient, people suffer from a condition referred to as night blindness. **Night blindness** results in the inability of the eyes to adjust to dim light. It can also result in the failure to regain sight quickly after a bright flash of light (**FIGURE 8.15**).

At the same time we are interpreting black and white images, the *cone cells* of the retina, which are only effective in bright light, use retinal to interpret different wavelengths of light as different colors. The pigment involved in color vision is *iodopsin*. Iodopsin experiences similar changes during the color vision cycle as rhodopsin does during the black-and-white vision cycle. As with the rod cells, the cone cells can also be affected by a deficiency of vitamin A, resulting in color blindness.

In summary, our abilities to adjust to dim light, recover from a bright flash of light, and see in color are all critically dependent on adequate levels of retinal in our eyes.

Other Functions of Vitamin A

The known functions of vitamin A are numerous, and researchers speculate that many are still to be discovered.

Vitamin A Contributes to Cell Differentiation

Vitamin A contributes to **cell differentiation**, the process by which stem cells mature into highly specialized cells that perform unique functions. It begins when the retinoic acid form of vitamin A interacts with receptor sites on a cell's DNA. This interaction influences gene expression and the determination of the type of cells that the stem cells eventually become. Obviously, this process is critical to the development of healthy organs and effectively functioning body systems.

An example of cell differentiation is the development of epithelial cells, such as skin cells, and mucus-producing cells lining the lungs, vagina, intestines, stomach,

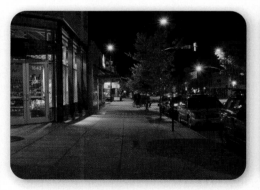 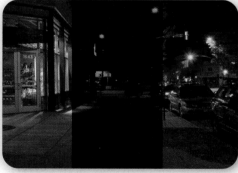

(a) Normal night vision   Poor night vision

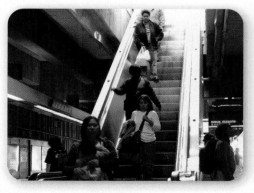 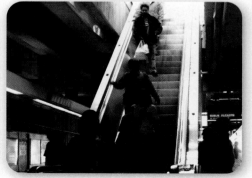

night blindness A vitamin A deficiency disorder that results in loss of the ability to see in dim light.

cell differentiation The process by which immature, undifferentiated stem cells develop into highly specialized functional cells of discrete organs and tissues.

(b) Normal light adjustment   Slow light adjustment

⬆ **FIGURE 8.15**   A deficiency of vitamin A can result in night blindness. This condition results in **(a)** diminished side vision and overall poor night vision and **(b)** difficulty in adjusting from bright light to dim light.

HOT TOPIC

Acne and Vitamin A—Is There a Link?

Search the Internet and you'll find plenty of sites claiming a direct link between vitamin A deficiency and acne and promising that vitamin A supplements can successfully treat acne. Should you believe the hype?

In 2006, a study reported an association between low blood levels of vitamin A and the presence of acne: the more severe the acne, the lower the levels of vitamin A.[12] Although these findings may seem suggestive, this study was conducted with a very small number of participants who were not randomly selected. Also, plasma levels of vitamin A were assessed to indicate vitamin A status; however, the Institute of Medicine states that plasma levels of vitamin A are not necessarily an indicator of vitamin A status.[13] To date, these results have not been replicated by other researchers, and there appears to be no evidence that vitamin A deficiency causes acne.

Interestingly, two effective treatments for acne are synthetic derivatives of vitamin A. Retin-A, or tretinoin, is applied to the skin. Accutane, or isotretinoin, is taken orally. These medications are available only by prescription and, because they are associated with an increased risk for severe birth defects, their use must be monitored by a licensed physician.

Contrary to what you might read on the Internet, vitamin A itself has no effect on acne; thus, vitamin A supplements are not recommended in its treatment.

bladder, urinary tract, and eyes. The mucus that epithelial cells produce lubricates the tissue and helps us propel microbes, dust particles, foods, and fluids out of our body tissues (for example, when we cough up secretions or empty our bladder). When vitamin A levels are insufficient, the epithelial cells fail to differentiate appropriately, and we lose these protective barriers against infectious microbes and irritants.

Vitamin A is also critical to the differentiation of specialized immune cells called *T-lymphocytes*, or *T-cells*, which assist in fighting infections. You can therefore see why vitamin A deficiency can lead to a breakdown of immune responses and to infections and other disorders of the lungs and respiratory tract, urinary tract, vagina, and eyes.

Vitamin A Contributes to Reproduction and Bone Growth

Vitamin A is involved in reproduction. Although its exact role is unclear, it appears necessary for sperm production in men and for fertilization to occur in women. It also contributes to healthy bone growth by assisting in breaking down old bone, so that new, longer, and stronger bone can develop. As a result of a vitamin A deficiency, children suffer from stunted growth and wasting.

Vitamin A May Act as an Antioxidant

Past limited research indicated that vitamin A may act as an antioxidant by scavenging free radicals and protecting LDLs from oxidation. However, in the absence of recent research confirming this view, we can only say that it is unclear if vitamin A makes some minimal contribution to antioxidant function.

Vitamin A in the Diet

Vitamin A can be obtained from both plant and animal sources. To calculate the total RAE in your diet, you must take into consideration both the amount of retinol and the amount of provitamin A carotenoids that are present in the foods eaten. For example, because 12 µg of beta-carotene yields 1 µg of RAE, if a person consumes 400 µg retinol and 1,200 µg of beta-carotene, the total RAE is equal to 400 µg + (1,200 µg ÷ 12), or 500 µg RAE.

How Much Vitamin A Should We Consume?

Vitamin A toxicity can occur readily because it is a fat-soluble vitamin, so it is important to consume only the amount recommended for your gender and age range. The RDA for vitamin A is 900 µg per day for men and 700 µg per day for women (see Table 8.1). The UL is 3,000 µg per day of preformed vitamin A in women (including those pregnant and lactating) and men.

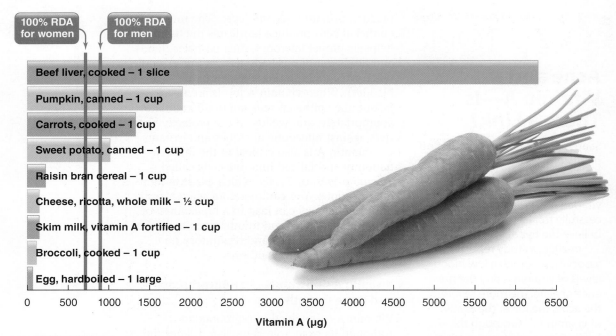

100% RDA for women

100% RDA for men

Beef liver, cooked – 1 slice

Pumpkin, canned – 1 cup

Carrots, cooked – 1 cup

Sweet potato, canned – 1 cup

Raisin bran cereal – 1 cup

Cheese, ricotta, whole milk – ½ cup

Skim milk, vitamin A fortified – 1 cup

Broccoli, cooked – 1 cup

Egg, hardboiled – 1 large

0   500   1000   1500   2000   2500   3000   3500   4000   4500   5000   5500   6000   6500

Vitamin A (µg)

FIGURE 8.16 Common food sources of vitamin A. The RDA for vitamin A is 900 µg/day for men and 700 µg/day for women.

Data from: U.S. Department of Agriculture, Agricultural Research Service, 2012. USDA Nutrient Database for Standard Reference, Release 25.

Food Sources of Preformed Vitamin A

The most abundant natural sources of dietary preformed vitamin A are animal foods, such as beef liver, chicken liver, eggs, and whole-fat dairy products. Vitamin A is also found in fortified reduced-fat milks, margarine, and some breakfast cereals (**FIGURE 8.16**).

Other good sources of vitamin A are foods high in beta-carotene and other carotenoids that can be converted to vitamin A. As discussed earlier in this chapter, dark-green, orange, and deep-yellow fruits and vegetables are good sources of beta-carotene and thus of vitamin A. Carrots, spinach, mango, cantaloupe, and tomato juice are examples.

What Happens If We Consume Too Much Vitamin A?

Vitamin A is highly toxic, and toxicity symptoms develop after consuming only three to four times the RDA. Toxicity rarely results from food sources, but vitamin A supplementation is known to have caused severe illness and even death. In pregnant women, it can cause serious birth defects and spontaneous abortion. Other toxicity symptoms include fatigue, loss of appetite, blurred vision, hair loss, skin disorders, bone and joint pain, abdominal pain, nausea, diarrhea, and damage to the liver and nervous system. If caught in time, many of these symptoms are reversible once vitamin A supplementation is stopped. However, permanent damage can occur to the liver, eyes, and other organs. Because liver contains such a high amount of vitamin A, children and pregnant women should not consume liver on a daily or weekly basis.

What Happens If We Don't Consume Enough Vitamin A?

As discussed earlier, night blindness and color blindness can result from vitamin A deficiency. How severe a problem is night blindness? Although much less common among people of developed nations, vitamin A deficiency is a severe public health concern in developing nations. According to the World Health Organization, approximately 250 million preschool children suffer from vitamin A deficiency.[14] Of the children affected, 250,000 to 500,000 become permanently blinded every year. Because of their risky health status, at least half of these children will die within 1 year of losing their sight. Death is due to infections and illnesses, including measles and diarrhea, which are easily treated in more affluent countries. Vitamin A deficiency is also a tragedy for pregnant women in many developing countries. They often suffer from

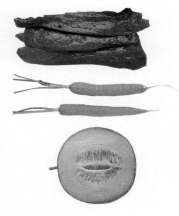

Liver, carrots, and cantaloupe all contain vitamin A.

night blindness, are more likely to transmit HIV to their child if HIV-positive, and run a greater risk for maternal mortality.

If vitamin A deficiency progresses, it can result in irreversible blindness due to hardening of the cornea (the transparent membrane covering the front of the eye), a condition called *xerophthalmia*. The prefix of this word, *xero-*, comes from a Greek word meaning "dry." Lack of vitamin A causes the epithelial cells of the cornea to lose their ability to produce mucus, causing the eye to become very dry. This leaves the cornea susceptible to damage, infection, and hardening. Once the cornea hardens in this way, the resulting blindness is irreversible. This is why it is critical to catch vitamin A deficiency in its early stages and treat it either with the regular consumption of fruits and vegetables that contain beta-carotene or with vitamin A supplementation.

Vitamin A deficiency can also lead to follicular *hyperkeratosis*, a condition characterized by the excess accumulation of the protein keratin in the hair follicles. Keratin is usually found only on the outermost surface of skin, hair, nails, and tooth enamel. With hyperkeratosis, keratin clogs hair follicles; makes skin rough and bumpy; prevents proper sweating through the sweat glands; and causes skin to become very dry and thick. Hyperkeratosis can also affect the epithelial cells of various tissues, including the mouth, urinary tract, vagina, and eyes, reducing the production of mucus by these tissues and leading to an increased risk for infection. Hyperkeratosis can be reversed with vitamin A supplementation.

Other deficiency symptoms include impaired immunity, increased risk for illness and infections, reproductive system disorders, and failure of normal growth. Individuals who are at risk for vitamin A deficiency include elderly people with poor diets, newborn or premature infants (due to low liver stores of vitamin A), young children with inadequate vegetable and fruit intakes, and alcoholics. Any condition that results in fat malabsorption can also lead to vitamin A deficiency. Children with cystic fibrosis; individuals with Crohn's disease, celiac disease, or diseases of the liver, pancreas, or gallbladder; and people who consume large amounts of the fat substitute Olestra are at risk for vitamin A deficiency.

recap Vitamin A is critical for maintaining our vision. It is also necessary for cell differentiation, reproduction, and growth. The role of vitamin A as an antioxidant is still under investigation. The RDA for vitamin A is 900 μg per day for men and 700 μg per day for women. Animal liver, dairy products, and eggs are good animal sources of vitamin A; fruits and vegetables are high in beta-carotene, which is used to synthesize vitamin A. Supplementation can be dangerous because toxicity is reached at levels of only three to four times the RDA. Toxicity symptoms include birth defects, spontaneous abortion, blurred vision, and liver damage. Deficiency symptoms include night blindness, impaired immune function, and growth failure.

*behavior change... getting started!

Now that you've read this chapter, try making these changes:

For yourself:

- Make it a goal to eat at least 5 servings of fruits and vegetables every day.
- Reduce your consumption of deep-fried foods—choose baked or stir-fried options instead.
- If you don't smoke, don't start. If you smoke, visit your campus health services center to find a smoking cessation program or method that fits your needs.

For your community:

- Exposure to air pollution, including secondhand tobacco smoke, promotes the formation of free radicals. More than 300 U.S. colleges and universities are now 100% tobacco-free. If your campus isn't one of them, visit the American Lung Association to find out how to lobby for clean air: www.lung.org.
- Work with your friends to raise funds for UNICEF, an international charity that is part of the Vitamin A Global Initiative working to end night blindness. Find out more at www.unicefusa.org.

Antioxidants: From Foods or Supplements?

As you've learned in this chapter, antioxidant nutrients play an important role in reducing free radical damage, which can, in turn, reduce the risk for chronic diseases such as cancer and cardiovascular disease (CVD). Despite this, data from research studies on the effects of antioxidant supplements on risks for cancer and CVD are troubling.

The results of large, randomized, controlled trials such as the Alpha-Tocopherol Beta-Carotene (ATBC) Cancer Prevention Study and the Beta-Carotene and Retinol Efficacy Trial (CARET) were particularly surprising.[15,16] The ATBC Cancer Prevention Study was conducted in Finland from 1985 to 1993 to determine the effects of beta-carotene and vitamin E supplements on lung and other forms of cancer among male smokers 50 to 69 years of age. Almost 30,000 men participated in the study for an average of 6 years and were given daily a beta-carotene supplement, a vitamin E supplement, a supplement containing both, or a placebo.

Contrary to expectations, the male smokers who took beta-carotene supplements experienced an *increased* number of deaths during the study. More men in this group died of lung cancer, and there were higher rates of prostate and stomach cancers. Also, more men died of heart disease and stroke.

CARET began as a pilot study in the United States in 1985 and included more than 18,000 men and women who were smokers, former smokers, or workers who had been exposed to asbestos. Participants were randomly assigned to take daily supplements of beta-carotene and retinol (vitamin A) or a placebo. After a 4-year follow-up period, the incidence of lung cancer was 28% higher among those taking the supplement. This significant finding, in addition to the results from the ATBC Cancer Prevention Study, prompted researchers to end the CARET study early and recommend that participants discontinue the supplements.[16]

A recent systematic review of the available published studies reports that beta-carotene supplementation has no effect on the incidence of all cancers combined, pancreatic cancer, colorectal cancer, prostate cancer, breast cancer, and skin cancer. However, the incidence of lung and stomach cancers was significantly increased in those taking higher doses (20–30 mg per day) as well as in smokers and asbestos workers.[17]

Studies of antioxidants and CVD also show inconsistent results. Two large-scale surveys conducted in the United States show that men and women who eat more fruits and vegetables have a significantly reduced risk of CVD.[18,19]

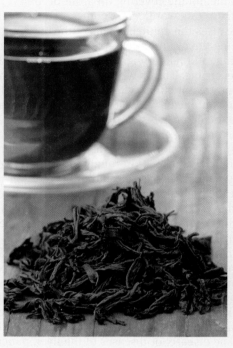

▲ The flavonoids in black tea might reduce the risk for CVD.

And in the ATBC Cancer Prevention Study, vitamin E was found to lower the number of deaths due to heart disease. However, it had no overall effect on the risk for stroke.[20] And, recently, other large intervention studies have shown no reductions in major cardiovascular events in adults taking vitamins E or C.[6,21] Thus, there is growing evidence that antioxidant supplements do not reduce our risk for CVD.

Why might foods high in antioxidants reduce our risks for cancer and CVD, whereas supplements are not beneficial and may even be harmful? First, as with any other chemicals, antioxidants may be beneficial at lower, appropriate doses—such as we consume in plant foods—but may become toxic at the higher doses present in a supplement. Second, other compounds (besides antioxidants) found in fruits, vegetables, and whole grains can reduce our risk for cancer and CVD. Here are just a few examples:

- Dietary fiber has been shown to reduce the risk for colorectal cancer, decrease blood pressure, lower total cholesterol levels, and improve blood glucose and insulin levels.
- Folate, a B-vitamin found in fortified cereals, green leafy vegetables, and some other plant foods, is known to reduce blood levels of the amino acid homocysteine, and a high concentration of homocysteine is a known risk factor for CVD.
- Flavonoids are a group of phytochemicals found in berries, nuts, soybeans, and many other plant foods, including black tea. A recent study has shown that individuals who drank more than three cups of black tea per day had a lower rate of heart attacks than non–tea drinkers.[22]

Thus, it appears that any number of nutrients and other components in fruits, vegetables, and whole-grain foods may be protective against cancer and CVD. As you can see, there is still much to learn about how people respond to foods high in antioxidants as compared to antioxidant supplements.

CRITICAL THINKING QUESTIONS

1. With everything you've learned in this chapter, do you still feel it is beneficial to take antioxidant supplements? Why or why not?
2. If a friend or family member decided to take antioxidant supplements as "health insurance," what advice might you give them about this decision?

chapter **review**

test yourself | answers

MasteringNutrition™

review questions

1. Oxidation is best described as a process in which
   a. radiation causes a mutation in a cell's DNA.
   b. an atom loses an electron.
   c. an element loses an atom of oxygen.
   d. a compound loses a molecule of water.

2. Which of the following disorders is linked to the production of free radicals?
   a. cardiovascular disease
   b. carotenosis
   c. ulcers
   d. all of the above

3. Which of the following function as a cofactor in antioxidant enzyme systems?
   a. iron
   b. zinc
   c. copper
   d. all of the above

4. Which of the following is a role of both vitamin E and vitamin C?
   a. Both vitamins spare vitamin A.
   b. Both vitamins donate electrons to free radicals.
   c. Both vitamins are critical cofactors in antioxidant enzyme systems.
   d. All of the above are true.

5. Which of the following is a function of vitamin C?
   a. promotes the differentiation of epithelial cells, such as skin cells and mucus-producing lining cells
   b. prevents the rupturing of blood cells in erythrocyte hemolysis
   c. promotes the synthesis of collagen in connective tissues in skin, bone, and other organs
   d. improves the absorption of vitamin A if dietary vitamin A intake is low

6. Which of the following statements about beta-carotene is true?
   a. Beta-carotene is a water-soluble form of vitamin A.
   b. Beta-carotene is a provitamin A carotenoid.
   c. The RDA for beta-carotene is twelve times the RDA for vitamin A.
   d. None of the above is true.

7. The light-sensitive pigment rhodopsin
   a. is composed of retinol and a lipid called opsin.
   b. is found in the cone cells of the retina.
   c. contains vitamin A in the form of retinal.
   d. both a and b are true.

8. Taking daily doses of three to four times the RDA of which of the following nutrients may cause death?
   a. vitamin A
   b. vitamin C
   c. vitamin E
   d. selenium

9. **True or false?** Free radical formation can occur as a result of normal cellular metabolism.

10. **True or false?** Pregnant women are advised to consume plenty of beef liver.

math review

11. Joey is home visiting his parents for the weekend, and he finds a bottle of vitamin E supplements in the medicine cabinet. He asks his parents about these, and his mother says that she is worried about having a weak immune system and read on the Internet that vitamin E can boost immunity. Because Joey's mother eats plenty of plant foods and oils that are good sources of vitamin E, he is worried she may be consuming too much by adding these supplements to her diet. Each supplement capsule contains 400 IU of dl-alpha-tocopherol, and she takes one capsule each day. Answer the following questions:

a. How much vitamin E in mg is Joey's mother consuming each day from these supplements?

b. What percentage of the RDA for vitamin E do these supplements provide?

c. Based on what you've learned in this chapter about vitamin E, should Joey's mother be worried about vitamin E toxicity? Would your answer be different if you learned that she is taking aspirin each day as prescribed by her doctor?

Answers to Review Questions and Math Review are located at the back of this text and in the MasteringNutrition Study Area.

web resources

www.who.int
World Health Organization

Click on "Health Topics" and select "nutrition disorders" and then "Nutrition: micronutrients" to find out more about vitamin A deficiency around the world.

www.americanheart.org
American Heart Association

Discover the best way to lower your risk for cardiovascular disease.

www.fda.gov
U.S. Food and Drug Administration

Select "Food" on the pull-down menu and then click on "Dietary Supplements" under the heading "Food Topics" for more information on how to make informed decisions and evaluate information related to dietary supplements.

www.fnic.nal.usda.gov
Food and Nutrition Information Center
USDA National Agricultural Library

Click on the "Dietary Supplements" link in the "Browse By Subject" box to obtain information on vitamin and mineral supplements, including consumer reports and industry regulations.

ods.od.nih.gov
Office of Dietary Supplements

Go to this site to obtain current research results and reliable information about dietary supplements.

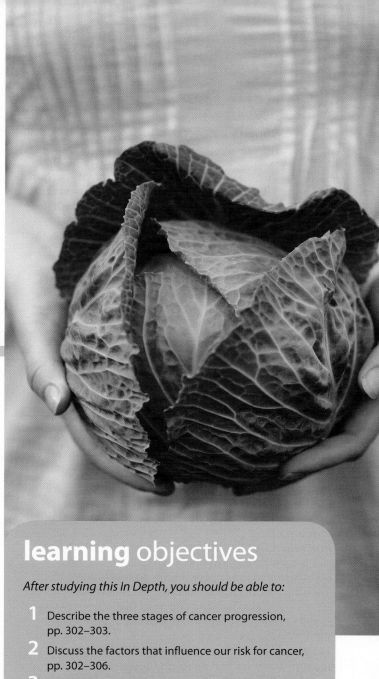

in depth 8.5

Cancer

The American Cancer Society (ACS) estimates that almost 1,600 Americans die of cancer every day. In the United States, cancer accounts for nearly one out of every four deaths, making it the second most common cause of death, exceeded only by heart disease.[1]

With such alarming statistics, it's not surprising that television commercials, Internet sites, and health and fitness publications are filled with product claims promising to reduce your risk of developing cancer. Many of these claims tout the benefits of antioxidants. In opposition to these claims, some research evidence suggests that taking antioxidant supplements may actually increase the risk of cancer for certain people (refer to the Nutrition Debate in Chapter 8, page 298). In this **In Depth**, we'll take a closer look at the group of diseases collectively known as cancer. We'll explore how it begins and spreads and identify the factors that most significantly increase our risk. We'll also review what is currently known about the role of antioxidant nutrients in cancer and identify other strategies for reducing your risk.

learning objectives

After studying this In Depth, you should be able to:

1 Describe the three stages of cancer progression, pp. 302–303.

2 Discuss the factors that influence our risk for cancer, pp. 302–306.

3 Describe the various cancer treatments currently available, p. 307.

4 Describe ways in which we can prevent, or reduce our risks for, cancer, pp. 307–309.

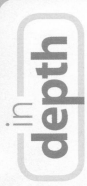

What is cancer?

Before we explore how antioxidants affect the risk for cancer, let's take a closer look at precisely what cancer is and how it spreads. **Cancer** is actually a group of diseases that are all characterized by cells that grow "out of control." By this we mean that cancer cells reproduce spontaneously and independently, and they are not inhibited by the boundaries of tissues and organs. Thus, they can aggressively invade tissues and organs far away from those in which they originally formed.

Most forms of cancer result in one or more **tumors**, which are newly formed masses of undifferentiated cells that are immature and have no physiologic function. Although the word *tumor* sounds frightening, it is important to note that not every tumor is *malignant,* or cancerous. Many are *benign* (not harmful to us) and are made up of cells that will not spread widely.

Cancer Progresses in Three Stages

FIGURE 1 shows how changes to normal cells prompt a series of other changes that can progress into cancer. There are three primary stages of cancer development: initiation, promotion, and progression. They occur as follows:

a. *Initiation.* The initiation of cancer occurs when a cell's DNA is *mutated* (changed). This mutation causes permanent changes in the cell that make it susceptible to promotion.

b. *Promotion.* During this phase, the genetically altered cell is stimulated to divide. A single mutated cell divides in two, and these double to four, and so on. The mutated DNA is locked into each new cell's genetic instructions. Because the enzymes that normally work to repair damaged cells cannot detect alterations in the DNA, the cells can continue to divide uninhibited. Moreover, mechanisms in the mutated cells allow them to avoid normal aging and *apoptosis,* a process by which old, worn cells normally die. Studies of the genes of cancer cells from a tumor suggest that it takes decades for a mutated cell to double repeatedly into a detectable tumor mass, and promotion is the longest

stage in cancer development.[2] Notice, however, that although a tumor is growing throughout the promotion phase, it is not yet exhibiting malignant behavior.[3]

c. *Progression.* During this phase, the mutated, proliferating cells engage in characteristically malignant behaviors.[3] They grow their own blood vessels, which supply them with blood and nutrients, and invade adjacent tissues. If not destroyed or removed surgically, the malignant tumor will disrupt body functioning at the primary site and may shed malignant cells that invade the circulatory and lymphatic systems to *metastasize* (spread) to distant sites in the body.

Although cancer is often fatal, a majority of people who develop cancer survive. In 2013 the American Cancer Society (ACS) reported that the 5-year survival rate for all cancers was 68%.[1] Of course, cancers can be more or less aggressive, some are more readily detectable than others, and some tissues and organs are more vulnerable to cancer. All these factors influence the overall mortality rate associated with different cancers. The type of cancer with the highest mortality rate is lung cancer, with almost 160,000 deaths in 2013. Cancer of the colon and/or rectum ranks second (more than 50,000 deaths in 2013), and breast cancer ranks third (just over 40,000 deaths).[1] Pancreatic cancer has received a great deal of attention in recent years because death rates from this form of cancer have increased slowly in men and women over the past decade, whereas death rates from other major cancers (such as female breast, lung, and prostate) have been slowly declining over this same period. Pancreatic cancer is one of the deadliest types, with most people dying within the first year of diagnosis and only 6% surviving 5 years following diagnosis.[1]

A Variety of Factors Influence Cancer Risk

Researchers estimate that about half of all men and one-third of all women will develop cancer during their lifetime.[1] But what factors cause cancer? Are you and your loved ones at risk? The answer depends on several factors,

Watch a video providing a basic overview of cancer on www.youtube.com. Enter "what is cancer?" into the search box, then click on the link to the video from the MD Anderson Cancer Center.

cancer A group of diseases characterized by cells that reproduce spontaneously and independently and may invade other tissues and organs.

tumor Any newly formed mass of undifferentiated cells.

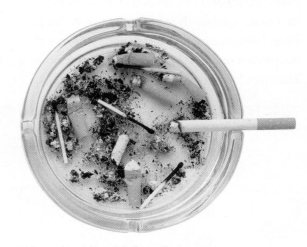

Using tobacco is a risk factor for cancer.

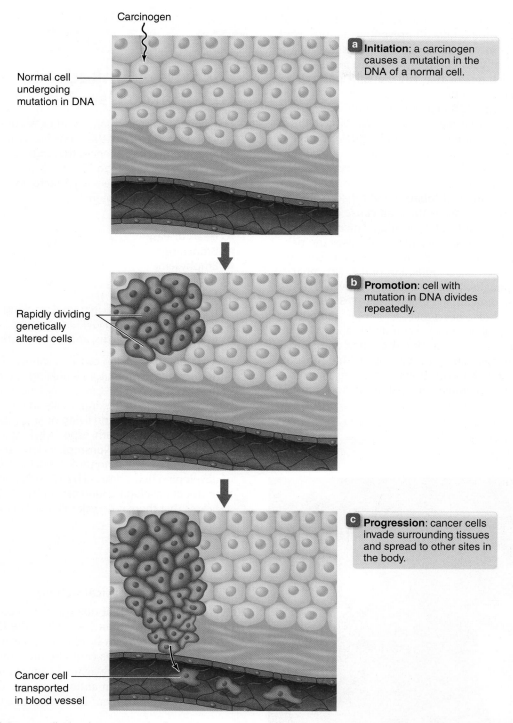

Carcinogen

Normal cell undergoing mutation in DNA

a **Initiation**: a carcinogen causes a mutation in the DNA of a normal cell.

Rapidly dividing genetically altered cells

b **Promotion**: cell with mutation in DNA divides repeatedly.

c **Progression**: cancer cells invade surrounding tissues and spread to other sites in the body.

Cancer cell transported in blood vessel

FIGURE 1 **(a)** Cancer cells develop as a result of a genetic mutation in the DNA of a normal cell. **(b)** The mutated cell replicates uncontrollably, eventually resulting in a tumor. **(c)** If not destroyed or removed, the cancerous tumor grows its own blood supply, invades nearby tissues, and metastasizes to other parts of the body.

including your family history of cancer, your exposure to environmental agents, and various lifestyle choices.

Heredity can play a role in the development of cancer. The presence of inherited "cancer genes," such as the defective variants of the *BRC1 and BRC2* genes for breast cancer, substantially increase the risk that an individual with those genes will develop cancer. However, only about 5% of all cancers are strongly hereditary.[1] In addition, it's important to bear in mind that a family history of cancer does not guarantee you will get cancer, too. It just means that you are at an increased risk and should take all preventive actions available to you. Although some risk factors are out of your control, others are modifiable, which means that you can take positive steps to reduce your risk.

The ACS identifies six modifiable risk factors that have been shown to have the greatest impact on an individual's cancer risk; each is discussed next.[1]

Tobacco Use

More than 40 compounds in tobacco and tobacco smoke are **carcinogens**, or substances that can cause cancer. Smoking accounts for at least 30% of all cancer deaths and 87% of lung cancer deaths, and it increases the risk for acute myeloid leukemia and cancers of the nasopharynx, nasal cavity, paranasal sinus, lip, oral cavity, pharynx, larynx, esophagus, pancreas, uterine cervix, ovaries, kidney, bladder, stomach, and colorectum (**FIGURE 2**).[1] Smoking can also cause heart disease, stroke, and emphysema. Overall, tobacco use accounts for about one in five deaths each year. (See the **Hot Topic** box on disorders linked to tobacco use.) The positive news is that tobacco use is a modifiable risk factor. If you smoke or use smokeless tobacco, you can reduce your risk for cancer considerably by quitting.

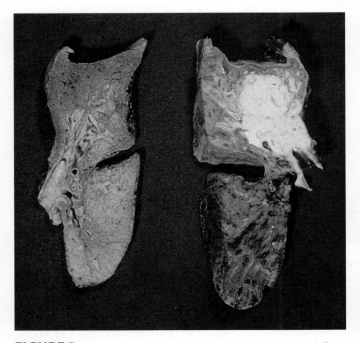

FIGURE 2 Cigarette smoking significantly increases our risk for lung and other types of cancer. The risk for lung cancer is 23 times higher in men who smoke and 12 times higher in women who smoke. **(a)** A normal, healthy lung; **(b)** the lung of a smoker. Notice the deposits of tar as well as the areas of tumor growth.

HOT TOPIC

Disorders Linked to Tobacco Use

Many people smoke cigarettes or cigars or use smokeless tobacco. The use of these products can lead to serious health consequences that together reduce life expectancy by more than 13 years in males and 14 years in females.[4] Tobacco use is a risk factor in the development of all of the following:

- Many cancers
- Heart disease
- Bronchitis
- Emphysema
- Stroke
- Erectile dysfunction
- Conditions related to maternal smoking
- Preterm delivery and low birth weight
- Miscarriages, stillbirths, and infant deaths

In addition, smoking causes a variety of other problems, such as the premature wrinkling and coarsening of the skin shown in **FIGURE 3**. Smoking also causes bad breath, yellowing of the fingernails and hair, and bad-smelling clothes, hair, and living quarters. Secondhand smoke is another concern, especially for those who live or work with smokers. Nonsmokers who are exposed to secondhand smoke at home or work increase their risk of developing heart disease by 25–30% and increase their risk of developing lung cancer by 20–30%. Research indicates that there is no risk-free level of exposure to secondhand smoke.[5]

Weight, Diet, and Physical Activity

Researchers estimate that one-quarter to one-third of cancers in high-income countries such as the United States are related to overweight or obesity, poor nutrition, and physical activity and thus could be prevented.[1] Nutritional factors that are protective against cancer include the consumption of foods rich in antioxidant micronutrients and phytochemicals, and fiber.[6] Diets high in saturated fats

Want to see how much money you or someone you know has spent on cigarettes in the past, and how much they could cost in the future? Check out the American Cancer Society's website at www.cancer.org, and enter "Smoking Cost Calculator" into the search box, then click on the link provided.

carcinogen Any substance capable of causing the cellular mutations that lead to cancer.

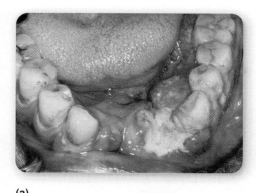

(a)

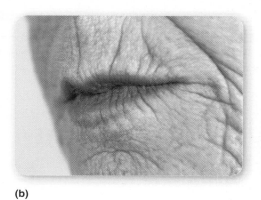

(b)

FIGURE 3 Effects of tobacco use. In addition to increasing your risk for lung cancer and cardiovascular disease, **(a)** using tobacco increases your risk for mouth cancer, and **(b)** smoking results in premature wrinkling of the skin, especially around the mouth.

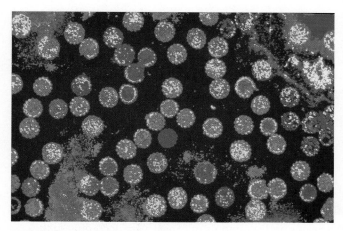

FIGURE 4 *Human papillomavirus (HPV)* is an infectious agent that can cause cancer.

and low in fruits and vegetables increase the risk for cancers of the esophagus, colon, breast, and prostate. Consumption of alcohol and compounds found in cured and charbroiled meats can also increase the risk for cancer.

A sedentary lifestyle increases the risk for colon cancer and possibly other forms of cancer. There is convincing evidence that regular physical activity decreases the risk for colon cancer as well as probable evidence of a protective effect for endometrial cancer and postmenopausal breast cancer.[7] There is limited evidence that suggests physical activity may also be protective against cancers of the lung, pancreas, and breast (premenopausal). At this time, we do not know how exercise reduces the overall risk for cancer or for certain types of cancers. However, these findings have prompted the ACS and the National Cancer Institute to promote increased physical activity as a way to reduce our risk for cancer.

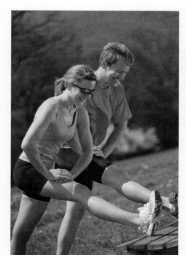

Staying physically active may help reduce the risk for some cancers.

What about you? Are you making dietary and physical activity choices that help reduce your risk for cancer and other chronic diseases? Check out the **What About You?** quiz (on page 306) and find out!

Infectious Agents

Infectious agents account for 18% of cancers worldwide. For example, persistent infection of the female cervix with certain strains of the sexually transmitted virus *Human papillomavirus* (HPV) is a known cause of cervical cancer (**FIGURE 4**), and infection with HIV (human immunodeficiency virus) can cause many cancers. The bacterium *Helicobacter pylori* is linked not only to ulcers but also to stomach cancer. Certain parasites are also linked to specific cancers. As microbial research advances, it is thought that more cancers will be linked to infectious agents.

Ultraviolet Radiation

Skin cancer is the most common form of cancer in the United States and accounts for over half of all cancers diagnosed each year. Most skin cancer cases are linked to exposure to ultraviolet (UV) rays from the sun and indoor tanning beds. UV rays damage the DNA of immature skin cells, which then reproduce uncontrollably. Research has shown that a person's risk for skin cancer doubles if he or she has had five or more sunburns; however, your risk for skin cancer still increases with UV exposure even if you do not get sunburned.[8] Exposure to tanning beds before age 35 increases by 75% your risk of developing the most invasive form of skin cancer.[9]

Skin cancer includes the nonmelanoma cancers (basal cell and squamous

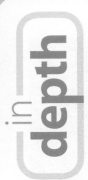

cell cancers), which are not typically invasive, and malignant melanoma, which is one of the most deadly of all types of cancer (FIGURE 5). Limiting exposure to sunlight to no more than 20 minutes between 10 AM and 4 PM can help reduce your risk for skin cancer while allowing your body to synthesize adequate vitamin D. After that, wear sun-protective clothing, a hat, and sunglasses, and use sunblock on exposed skin.

Cancer Prompts a Variety of Signs and Symptoms

The signs and symptoms of cancer vary according to the structures affected, how large the tumor is, and how widely it has metastasized. Here, we discuss the most common signs and symptoms that people diagnosed with cancer typically report. However, it's important to bear in mind that

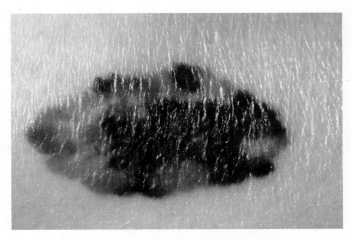

FIGURE 5   A lesion associated with malignant melanoma is characterized by asymmetry; uneven or blurred borders; mixed shades of tan, brown, black, and sometimes red or blue; and a diameter larger than a pencil eraser (6 mm).

what about **you**

Are You Living Smart?

Cancer often seems to strike apparently healthy people "out of the blue." Because genetic and certain environmental factors are beyond your control, you may be wondering how your diet and level of physical activity might be influencing your risk. If so, take the following quiz and see for yourself! Answer each question Yes or No. Then keep reading to see how you can keep living smart!

How Do You Rate?

Zero to 4 "Yes" answers: Diet Alert!
Your diet is probably too high in Calories and fat and too low in plant foods like vegetables, fruits, and grains. You may want to take a look at your eating habits and find ways to make some changes. Revisit the **Quick Tips** boxes in Chapters 5 and 8 for some ideas.

5 to 8 "Yes" answers: Not bad! You're Halfway There!
You still have a ways to go. Look at your "No" answers to help you decide which areas of your diet need to be improved, or whether your physical activity level should be increased. See Chapter 12 for ways to increase your level of physical activity.

9 to 12 "Yes" answers: Great Job! You're Living Smart!
Keep up the good habits and keep looking for ways to improve.

Data adapted from: *Living Smart*. The American Cancer Society.

■ I eat at least 2-1/2 cups of vegetables and fruits every day.	Yes/No
■ I eat whole-grain bread, pasta, and cereal every day.	Yes/No
■ I try to choose foods low in Calories and fat.	Yes/No
■ I rarely eat processed and red meat such as bacon, hot dogs, sausage, steak, ground beef, pork, or lamb.	Yes/No
■ I take it easy on high-Calorie baked goods such as pies, cakes, cookies, sweet rolls, and doughnuts.	Yes/No
■ I rarely add butter, margarine, oil, sour cream, or mayonnaise to foods when I'm cooking or at the table.	Yes/No
■ I rarely (less than twice a week) eat fried foods.	Yes/No
■ I try to maintain a healthful weight.	Yes/No
■ I get at least 150 minutes (2 hours and 30 minutes) of moderate or 75 minutes (1 hour and 15 minutes) of vigorous physical activity throughout each week.	Yes/No
■ I usually take the stairs instead of waiting for an elevator.	Yes/No
■ I try to spend most of my time being active, instead of watching television or sitting at the computer.	Yes/No
■ I never, or only occasionally, drink alcohol.	Yes/No

these also occur with many other illnesses and even non-illness conditions. Also, having just one or two of these symptoms rarely means that a person has cancer. Still, the ACS suggests that people who experience these symptoms for a long time see their primary healthcare provider.[10]

- *Unexplained weight loss.* Most people with cancer lose weight, so an unexplained weight loss of 10 pounds or more may be a first sign of cancer.
- *Fever.* Fever is very common with cancer, but it often happens when the cancer has metastasized or affects the blood.
- *Fatigue.* Extreme tiredness that isn't relieved with rest may be an important symptom of cancer. The blood loss that occurs with some cancers, such as colon and stomach cancers, can also cause fatigue.
- *Pain.* Headache, back pain, or bone pain that does not go away or respond to treatment can be an early symptom of certain types of cancer.
- *Skin changes.* Along with cancers of the skin, some other cancers can cause skin changes, including a darkened pigmentation, jaundice (yellowish skin tone), redness, excessive hair growth, and itching. Sores that don't heal and recent changes in a wart or mole should also be checked by a healthcare provider.
- *Change in bowel habits or bladder function.* Long-term constipation, diarrhea, painful urination, or the need to pass urine more or less frequently may signal cancer.
- *Indigestion or trouble swallowing.* Although these are most often caused by other disorders, if they persist, they should be evaluated by a healthcare provider.
- *White patches inside the mouth or on the tongue.* Especially in people who smoke or chew tobacco, these are important early signs of oral cancer.
- *Unusual bleeding or discharge.* Blood in the urine or stool, abnormal vaginal bleeding, a bloody discharge from the nipple, and bloody sputum (phlegm) can all occur in early or advanced cancer.
- *Any thickening or lump.* Many cancers can be felt through the skin, especially those involving the breast, testicle, or lymph nodes.
- *Nagging cough or hoarseness.* A cough that doesn't resolve can be a sign of lung cancer, whereas hoarseness can be a sign of cancer of the larynx (voice box) or thyroid gland.

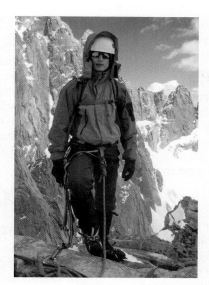

Arctic explorers wear special clothing to protect themselves from the cold as well as the high levels of ultraviolet rays from the sun.

How is cancer treated?

Physicians typically evaluate signs and symptoms of cancer using a variety of blood tests and diagnostic scans, such as ultrasound, computed tomography (CT), and magnetic resonance imaging (MRI) scans. Once a diagnosis is made, the patient is often referred to the care of an oncologist, a physician who specializes in cancer treatment (*onco-* means "tumor").

Cancer treatment varies according to the location of the cancer, the cell type, whether or not it has metastasized, and, if so, how much. Other factors, such as the patient's general health, extent of weight loss, age, and personal preferences, as well as the type, scope, and quality of healthcare insurance coverage, may also come into play. The three major types of cancer treatment are surgery, radiation, and chemotherapy. Surgery is most effective when it can entirely remove the mass. Radiation therapy delivers high-energy x-rays, gamma rays, electron beams, or photons to tumor cells to kill them outright or damage their DNA so that they can no longer reproduce. Chemotherapy is drug therapy, and any of more than 100 different drugs can be combined for different patient needs. For cancers that are localized—that is, confined to a limited area, with no metastasis—surgery may be the only treatment advised. Other cancers may require surgery followed by radiation and/or chemotherapy. Diffuse cancers, such as blood cancers, and tumors in locations that cannot be accessed safely with surgery, such as head and neck tumors, may be considered inoperable, and radiation and/or chemotherapy may be prescribed. In some cases, a large tumor is first radiated with the goal of shrinking it prior to surgery.

Can cancer be prevented?

Some types of cancer can be prevented. For instance, vaccines, the appropriate use of antibiotics, and behavioral changes can prevent certain cancers known to be caused by infectious agents. Most cancers, however, are multifactorial—we cannot link them to only one cause. This means that there is no way to guarantee that you—or anyone else—won't get cancer. Still, if you consider the population of the United States, more than half of all cancer deaths could be prevented if no one used tobacco and everyone took certain key steps to improve his or her health.[11] These steps can be summarized into four key cancer-prevention behaviors: check, quit, move, and nourish.

Check

Regular screening examinations can allow for the detection and removal of precancerous tissues. For instance, a test called a Pap smear can detect subtle changes in the cells lining a woman's cervix (the entrance to the uterus) that, if allowed to progress, could result in cervical cancer. Women with a Pap smear indicating these changes typically return to their physician for a quick outpatient

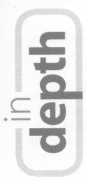
procedure in which the layer of precancerous cells is removed. Similarly, colonoscopies allow for the detection and removal of precancerous polyps. And regular skin checks allow for suspicious lesions to be removed—and cell samples sent to a lab—to evaluate for skin cancer. Screening can also allow for detection at an early stage, when cancer is most treatable. For example, a mammogram may be able to detect a breast mass that is too small for the woman to feel.

Quit

As noted earlier, tobacco use is a risk factor in the development of a wide variety of cancers, but all cancers caused by long-term tobacco use are entirely preventable. In fact, about one-third of all cancer deaths could be prevented if everyone followed the ACS recommendation to quit smoking.[1]

Alcohol abuse is also a factor in cancer. Excessive drinking is linked with an increased risk for cancers of the esophagus, pharynx, and mouth and may increase the risk for cancers of the liver, breast, colon, and rectum. Alcohol may also impair cells' ability to repair damaged DNA, increasing the possibility of cancer initiation.

Move

Regular physical activity can significantly lower your life-time risk for cancer. The ACS recommends that we engage in at least 150 minutes (2 hours and 30 minutes) of moderate or 75 minutes (1 hour and 15 minutes) of vigorous physical activity throughout each week. The amount of activity can be spread across the day and does not have to be done all at once. For example, on busy days, try to work in 10 minutes of activity three times a day. For instance, take a walk at lunch; then take a 10-minute exercise break between your afternoon classes. When you get home, cycle for 10 minutes. Short activity sessions like these can quickly add up to 30 minutes.[12]

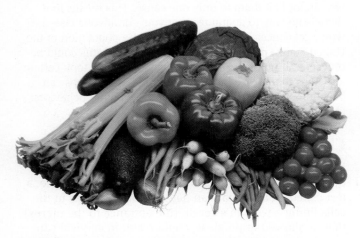

These vegetables provide antioxidant nutrients, fiber, and phytochemicals, all of which reduce the risk for some cancers.

Nourish

One of the smartest ways to reduce your risk for cancer is to maintain a healthful weight and a healthful diet. The ACS emphasizes reading food labels to increase your awareness around portion sizes and the Calorie content of food.[13] Consuming smaller portions of foods high in Calories and fat is suggested, as is reducing your intake of beverages high in added sugars such as soft drinks and fruit drinks. See the Quick Tips box for additional nutrition-related tips.

Quick Tips

Reducing Your Cancer Risk

✓ Lose weight or maintain your current healthful weight. Obesity appears to increase the risk for cancers of the breast, colon, prostate, endometrium (the lining of the uterus), cervix, ovary, kidney, gallbladder, liver, pancreas, rectum, and esophagus. The exact links between obesity and increased cancer risk are not clear but may involve hormonal changes associated with fat cells.

✓ Avoid heterocyclic amines in cooked meat. These carcinogenic chemicals are formed when meat is cooked at high temperatures, such as during broiling, barbecuing, and frying.

✓ Avoid nitrites and nitrates in cured meats. These compounds, which are found in some sausages, hams, bacon, and lunch meats, bind with amino acids to form nitrosamines, which are potent carcinogens.

✓ Eat a diet low in saturated fat. Diets high in saturated fat have been associated with increased risk for many cancers, including prostate and breast cancers. However, not all studies support this association.

✓ Eat a diet rich in vegetables and fruits. Consuming at least 2-1/2 cups of vegetables and fruit each day is recommended. These foods are high in antioxidants and in fiber, which some studies link to a reduced risk for certain cancers.

✓ When choosing fruits and vegetables, select versions that have more intense colors or flavors: purple potatoes instead of white, for example, and arugula instead of iceberg lettuce. These foods tend to be higher in antioxidant phytochemicals than lighter-colored or milder-tasting counterparts.

✓ Select foods containing phytoestrogens (plant estrogens). These compounds, found in soy-based foods and some vegetables and grains, may decrease the risk for breast, endometrial, and prostate cancers.

✓ Choose whole grain breads, cereals, pasta, and brown rice instead of products made from refined grains (see Chapter 4).

✓ Make sure to consume adequate omega-3 fatty acids (see Chapter 5). Consuming foods high in omega-3 fatty acids is associated with reduced rates of breast, colon, and rectal cancers.

Antioxidants Play a Role in Preventing Cancer

A large and growing body of evidence suggests that antioxidant micronutrients and phytochemicals consumed in food play an important role in cancer prevention, but how? The following are some proposed mechanisms:

- Enhancing the immune system, which assists in the destruction and removal of precancerous cells from the body
- Preventing oxidative damage to the cells' DNA by scavenging free radicals and stopping the formation and subsequent chain reaction of oxidized molecules
- Inhibiting the growth of cancer cells and tumors
- Inhibiting the capacity of cancer cells to avoid aging and apoptosis (programmed cell death)

Eating whole foods that are high in antioxidants—especially fruits, vegetables, and whole grains—is consistently shown to be associated with decreased risk for various cancers.[6] For example, several recent studies have suggested that consuming fruits, vegetables, spices, and teas high in a phytochemical called apigenin, a type of flavonoid, might alter gene regulation in cancer cells in a way that impairs their ability to avoid aging and apoptosis.[14,15] Another group of flavonoids, anthocyanins, are plant pigments thought to have antioxidant and anti-inflammatory properties. Produce with intense colors, such as blue corn and blackberries, has higher levels of anthocyanin pigments. Finally, glucosinolates, a group of phytochemicals found in cruciferous vegetables like Brussels sprouts and broccoli, as well as in bitter greens such as arugula, inhibit cell division and stimulate apoptosis in tumor cells.[16]

In addition, populations eating diets low in antioxidant micronutrients have a higher risk for cancer. These studies show varying levels of association between these factors, but they do not prove cause and effect. Nutrition experts agree that there are important interactions between antioxidant nutrients and phytochemicals, fiber, and other substances in foods, all of which may work together to reduce the risk for many types of cancers. Studies are now being conducted to determine whether eating foods high in antioxidants directly causes lower rates of cancer.

As noted previously, growing evidence over the past 20 years indicates that antioxidant supplementation does not reduce cancer risk; in fact, it may increase risks for various cancers and other chronic diseases. Why have antioxidant supplements failed to bring the health benefits one might expect? It has been speculated that antioxidants taken in supplement form may act as prooxidants in some

situations, whereas antioxidants consumed in foods may be more balanced.

Thus, it appears that the best way to try to reduce our risks for cancer is to eat a diet with ample fruits and vegetables, maintain a healthy body weight, stay regularly physically active, quit smoking if applicable, and avoid exposure to infectious agents and UV radiation. Many studies are currently examining the impact of whole foods on the risk for various forms of cancer. The results of these studies will provide important insights into the link between whole foods and cancer.

web resources

www.cancer.org
American Cancer Society

Get ACS recommendations for nutrition and physical activity for cancer prevention.

www.cancer.gov
The National Cancer Institute

Learn more about the nutritional factors that can influence your risk for cancer.

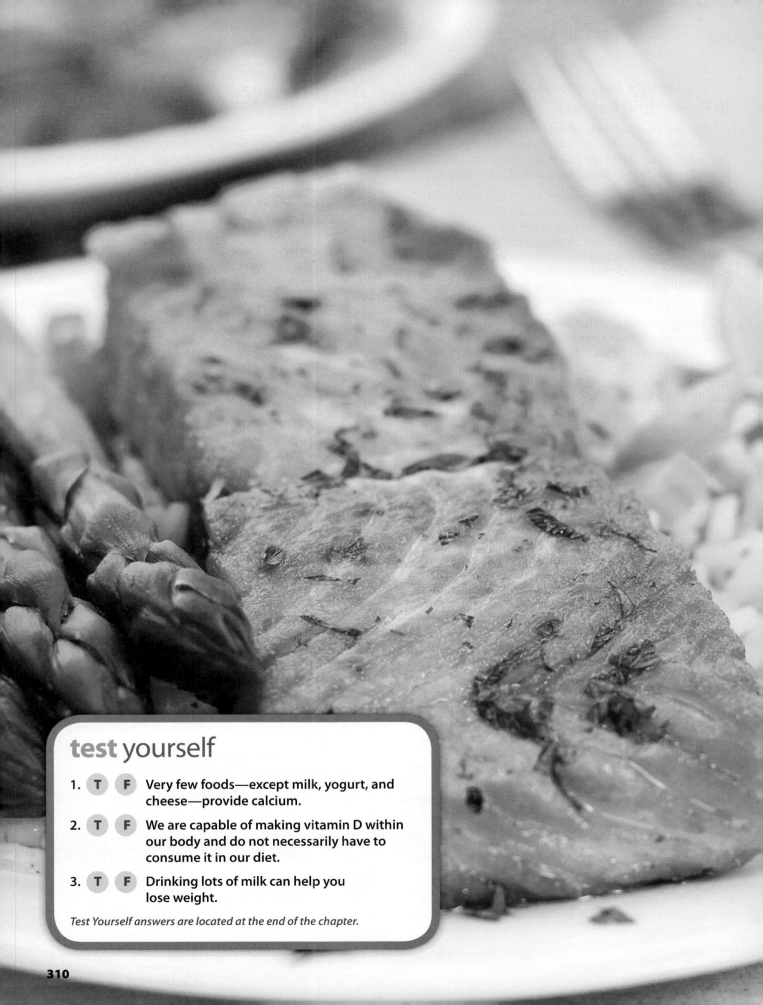

test yourself

1. **T** **F** Very few foods—except milk, yogurt, and cheese—provide calcium.

2. **T** **F** We are capable of making vitamin D within our body and do not necessarily have to consume it in our diet.

3. **T** **F** Drinking lots of milk can help you lose weight.

Test Yourself answers are located at the end of the chapter.

Nutrients Involved in Bone Health

9

Consumption of milk has plummeted from 31 gallons per person per year in 1970 to just 20.4 gallons in 2010, likely because of competition from other popular beverages. In 2010, the average American consumed less than 1 cup of milk each day, as opposed to more than 2.5 cups of carbonated soft drinks, fruit drinks, and sports beverages.[1] This trend concerns healthcare professionals because milk is a convenient source of a form of calcium that's easily absorbed by the body, and calcium is required for kids and teens to build dense, compact bones. What's more, milk is fortified with vitamin D and is a good source of phosphorus, two more nutrients critical to bone health.

Still, milk is hardly the only food source of these nutrients. What other foods build bone? And how does bone grow—and break down? We begin this chapter with a quick look at the components and activities of bone tissue. Then we'll discuss the nutrients, dietary choices, and other lifestyle factors that play a critical role in maintaining bone health.

learning objectives

After studying this chapter you should be able to:

1. Describe the differences between cortical bone and trabecular bone, pp. 312–313.

2. Discuss the processes of bone growth, modeling, and remodeling, pp. 313–314.

3. Describe how dual-energy x-ray absorptiometry (DEXA) is used to assess bone health and density, pp. 314–315.

4. Identify four key roles of calcium in human health, pp. 316–321.

5. Identify foods that are good sources of calcium, pp. 318–319.

6. Describe how vitamin D assists in regulating blood calcium levels, pp. 322–327.

7. Identify food sources of vitamin D and factors affecting skin synthesis, pp. 324–326.

8. Discuss the roles of vitamin K, phosphorus, magnesium, and fluoride in bone health, pp. 328–333.

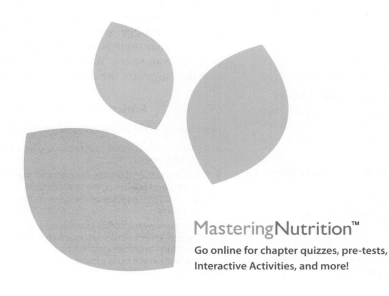

MasteringNutrition™

Go online for chapter quizzes, pre-tests, Interactive Activities, and more!

How do our bodies maintain bone health?

Contrary to what most people think, our skeleton is not an inactive collection of bones that simply holds our body together. Bones are living organs that contain several tissues, including two types of bone tissue, cartilage, and connective tissue. Nerves and blood vessels run within channels in bone tissue, supporting its activities. Bones have many important functions in our body, some of which might surprise you (TABLE 9.1). For instance, did you know that most of your blood cells are formed deep within your bones?

Given the importance of bones, it is critical that we maintain their health. Bone health is achieved through complex interactions among nutrients, hormones, and environmental factors. To better understand these interactions, we first need to learn about how bone structure and the constant activity of bone tissue influence bone health throughout our lifetime.

The Composition of Bone Provides Strength and Flexibility

We tend to think of bones as totally rigid, but if they were, how could we twist and jump our way through a basketball game or even carry an armload of books up a flight of stairs? Bones need to be both strong and flexible so that they can resist the compression, stretching, and twisting that occur throughout our daily activities. Fortunately, the composition of bone is ideally suited for its complex job: about 65% of bone tissue is made up of an assortment of minerals (mostly calcium and phosphorus) that provide hardness, but the remaining 35% is a mixture of organic substances that provide strength, durability, and flexibility. The most important of these substances is a fibrous protein called **collagen**. You might be surprised to learn that collagen fibers are actually stronger than steel fibers of similar size! Within our bones, the minerals form tiny crystals (called *hydroxyapatite*) that cluster around the collagen fibers. This design enables bones to bear weight while responding to our demands for movement.

If you examine a bone very closely, you will notice two distinct types of tissue (FIGURE 9.1): cortical bone and trabecular bone. **Cortical bone**, which is also called *compact bone*, is very dense. It constitutes approximately 80% of our skeleton. The outer surface of all bones is cortical; plus, many small bones of the body, such as the bones of the wrists, hands, and feet, are made entirely of cortical bone. Although cortical bone looks solid to the naked eye, it actually contains many microscopic openings, which serve as passageways for blood vessels and nerves.

In contrast, **trabecular bone** makes up only 20% of our skeleton. It is found within the ends of the long bones (such as the bones of the arms and legs), the spinal vertebrae, the sternum (breastbone), the ribs, most bones of the skull, and the pelvis. Trabecular bone is sometimes referred to as *spongy bone* because to the naked eye it looks like a sponge, with cavities and no clear organization. The microscope reveals that trabecular bone is, in fact, aligned in a precise network of columns that protects the bone from stress. You can think of trabecular bone as the scaffolding inside the bone that supports the outer cortical bone.

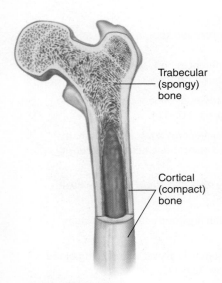

Trabecular (spongy) bone

Cortical (compact) bone

⬥ **FIGURE 9.1** The structure of bone. Notice the difference in density between the trabecular (spongy) bone and the cortical (compact) bone.

collagen A protein that forms strong fibers in bone and connective tissue.

cortical bone (compact bone) A dense bone tissue that makes up the outer surface of all bones as well as the entirety of most small bones of the body.

trabecular bone (spongy bone) A porous bone tissue that makes up only 20% of our skeleton and is found within the ends of the long bones, inside the spinal vertebrae, inside the flat bones (sternum, ribs, and most bones of the skull), and inside the bones of the pelvis.

TABLE 9.1   Functions of Bone in the Human Body

Functions Related to Structure and Support	Functions Related to Metabolic Processes
• Bones provide physical support for organs and body segments.	• Bone tissue acts as a storage reservoir for many minerals, including calcium, phosphorus, and fluoride. The body draws upon such deposits when these minerals are needed for various body processes; however, this can reduce bone mass.
• Bones protect vital organs; for example, the rib cage protects the lungs, the skull protects the brain, and the vertebrae of the spine protect the spinal cord.	• Most blood cells are produced in the bone marrow.
• Bones work with muscles and tendons to allow movement—muscles attach to bones via tendons, and their contraction produces movement at the body's joints.	

Cortical and trabecular bone also differ in their rate of turnover—that is, in how quickly the bone tissue is broken down and replenished. Trabecular bone has a faster turnover rate than cortical bone. This makes trabecular bone more sensitive to changes in hormones and nutritional deficiencies. It also accounts for the much higher rate of age-related fractures in the spine and pelvis (including the hip)—both of which contain a significant amount of trabecular bone. Let's investigate how bone turnover influences bone health.

The Constant Activity of Bone Tissue Promotes Bone Health

Bones develop through a series of three processes: bone growth, bone modeling, and bone remodeling (FIGURE 9.2). Bone growth and modeling begin during the early months of fetal life, when our skeleton is forming, and continue until early adulthood. Bone remodeling predominates during adulthood; this process helps us maintain a healthy skeleton as we age.

Bone Growth and Modeling Determine the Size and Shape of Our Bones

Through the process of *bone growth,* the size of bones increases. The first period of rapid bone growth is from birth to age 2, but growth continues in spurts throughout childhood and into adolescence. Although most girls reach their full adult height by about age 18, some continue to increase in height past age 19, although the rate of growth slows considerably. Most boys continue to grow up to the age of 21, although their rate of growth also slows over time. In the later decades of life, some loss in height usually occurs because of decreased bone density in the spine.[2]

Bone modeling is the process by which the shape of our bones is determined, from the round "pebble" bones that make up our wrists, to the uniquely shaped bones of our face, to the long bones of our arms and legs. Even after bones stop growing in length, they can still increase in thickness if they are stressed by engaging in repetitive exercise, such as weight training, or by being overweight or obese.

Although the size and shape of our bones do not change significantly after puberty, our **bone density**, or the compactness of our bones, continues to develop into early adulthood. *Peak bone density* is the point at which our bones are strongest because they are at their highest density. The following factors are associated with a lower peak bone density:[3–5]

- Late pubertal age in boys and late onset of menstruation in girls
- Inadequate calcium intake
- Low body weight
- Physical inactivity during adolescence

About 90% of a woman's bone density has been built by 17 years of age, whereas the majority of a man's has been built by his twenties. However, male or female, before we reach the age of 30 years, our bodies have reached peak bone mass, and we can no longer significantly add to our bone density. In our thirties, our bone density remains relatively stable, but by age 40, it has begun its irreversible decline.

Bone Remodeling Maintains a Balance Between Breakdown and Repair

Although our bones cannot increase their peak density after our twenties, bone tissue still remains very active throughout adulthood, balancing the breakdown of older bone tissue and the formation of new bone tissue. This bone recycling process is

bone density The degree of compactness of bone tissue, reflecting the strength of the bones. *Peak bone density* is the point at which a bone is strongest.

Bone growth	Bone modeling	Bone remodeling
· Determines bone size · Begins in the womb · Continues until early adulthood	· Determines bone shape · Begins in the womb · Continues until early adulthood	· Maintains integrity of bone · Replaces old bone with new bone to maintain mineral balance · Involves bone resorption and formation · Occurs predominantly during adulthood

◄ **FIGURE 9.2** Bone develops through three processes: bone growth, bone modeling, and bone remodeling.

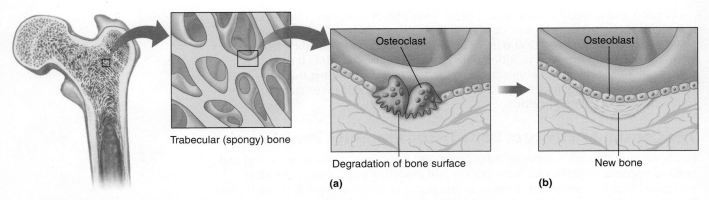

Trabecular (spongy) bone

Osteoclast

Degradation of bone surface

(a)

Osteoblast

New bone

(b)

FIGURE 9.3 Bone remodeling involves resorption and formation. **(a)** Osteoclasts erode the bone surface by degrading its components, including calcium, other minerals, and collagen; these components are then transported to the bloodstream. **(b)** Osteoblasts work to build new bone by filling the pit formed by the resorption process with new bone.

To see how bone modeling and remodeling work, watch the video at www.youtube.com. Type "amgen bone modeling" into the search bar, then click on the top link.

called **remodeling**. Remodeling is also used to repair fractures and to strengthen bone regions that are exposed to higher physical stress. The process of remodeling involves two steps: resorption and formation.

Bone is broken down through a process referred to as **resorption** (FIGURE 9.3a). During resorption, cells called **osteoclasts** erode the bone surface by secreting enzymes and acids that dig grooves into the bone matrix. One of the primary reasons the body regularly breaks down bone is to release calcium into the bloodstream. As discussed in more detail later in this chapter, calcium is critical for many physiologic processes, and bone is an important calcium reservoir. The body also breaks down bone that is fractured and needs to be repaired. Resorption at the injury site smooths the rough edges created by the break. Bone may also be broken down in areas away from the fracture site to obtain the minerals that are needed to repair the damage. Regardless of the reason, once bone is broken down, the resulting products are transported into the bloodstream and used for various body functions.

New bone is formed through the action of cells called **osteoblasts**, or "bone builders" (see Figure 9.3b). These cells work to synthesize new bone matrix by laying down the collagen-containing organic component of bone. Within this substance, the hydroxyapatite crystallizes and packs together to create new bone where it is needed.

In young, healthy adults, the processes of bone resorption and formation are equal so that just as much bone is broken down as is built, maintaining bone mass. Around 40 years of age, bone resorption begins to occur more rapidly than bone formation, and this imbalance results in an overall loss in bone density. Because this affects the vertebrae of the spine, people tend to lose height as they age. As discussed shortly, achieving a high peak bone mass through proper nutrition and exercise when we are young provides us with a stronger skeleton before the loss of bone begins. It can therefore reduce our risk for *osteoporosis*, a disorder characterized by low-density bones that fracture easily. Osteoporosis is discussed **In Depth** (on pages 338–345).

remodeling The two-step process by which bone tissue is recycled; includes the breakdown of existing bone and the formation of new bone.

resorption The process by which the surface of bone is broken down by cells called osteoclasts.

osteoclasts Cells that erode the surface of bones by secreting enzymes and acids that dig grooves into the bone matrix.

osteoblasts Cells that prompt the formation of new bone matrix by laying down the collagen-containing component of bone, which is then mineralized.

dual energy x-ray absorptiometry (DXA or DEXA) Currently, the most accurate tool for measuring bone density.

recap Bones are organs that contain metabolically active tissues composed primarily of minerals and a fibrous protein called collagen. Of the two types of bone, cortical bone is more dense and trabecular bone is more porous. Trabecular bone is also more sensitive to hormonal and nutritional factors and turns over more rapidly than cortical bone. The three types of bone activity are growth, modeling, and remodeling. Bones reach their peak bone mass by the late teenage years into the twenties; bone mass begins to decline around age 40.

How do we assess bone health?

Over the past 40 years, technological advancements have led to the development of a number of affordable methods for measuring bone health. **Dual energy x-ray absorptiometry (DXA or DEXA)** is considered the most accurate assessment tool for measuring

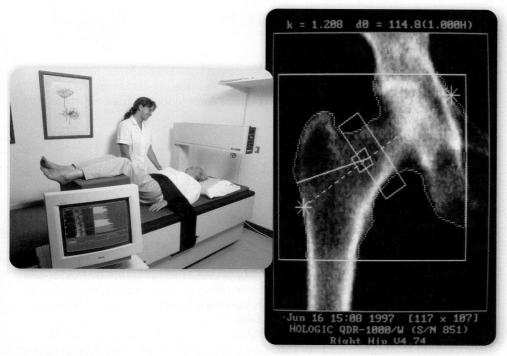

Take a closer look at a DXA scan at www.webmd.com. Type "dr. siris bone density test video" into the search bar to get started.

FIGURE 9.4 Dual energy x-ray absorptiometry is a safe and simple procedure that assesses bone density.

bone density. This method can measure the density of the bone mass over the entire body. Software is also available that provides an estimation of percentage body fat.

The DXA procedure is simple, painless, and noninvasive, and it is considered to be of minimal risk. It takes just 15 to 30 minutes to complete. The person participating in the test remains fully clothed but must remove all jewelry and other metal objects. The participant lies quietly on a table, and bone density is assessed through the use of a very low level of x-ray (**FIGURE 9.4**).

DXA is a very important tool in determining a person's risk for osteoporosis. It generates a bone density score, which is compared to the average peak bone density of a healthy 30-year-old. Doctors use this comparison, which is known as a **T-score**, to assess the risk for fracture and determine whether the person has osteoporosis. T-scores are interpreted as follows:

- A T-score between +1 and −1 means that the individual's bone density is normal.
- A T-score between −1 and −2.5 indicates low bone mass and an increased risk for fractures.
- A T-score more negative than −2.5 indicates that the person has osteoporosis.

DXA tests are generally recommended for postmenopausal women because they are at highest risk for osteoporosis and fracture. Men and younger women may also be recommended for a DXA test if they have significant risk factors for osteoporosis (see the **In Depth** on osteoporosis immediately following this chapter).

Other technologies have been developed to measure bone density. These use ultrasound or different forms of x-ray technology to measure the density of bone in the heel or another more peripheral part of the body. These technologies are frequently used at health fairs because the machines are portable and provide scores faster than the traditional DXA.

recap Dual energy x-ray absorptiometry (DXA or DEXA) is the gold standard measurement of bone mass. It is a simple, painless, and minimal-risk procedure. The result of a DXA is a T-score, which is a comparison of a person's bone density with that of a healthy 30-year-old. A T-score between +1 and −1 is normal; a score between −1 and −2.5 indicates poor bone density; and a score more negative than −2.5 indicates osteoporosis.

T-score A comparison of an individual's bone density to the average peak bone density of a 30-year-old healthy adult.

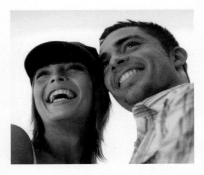

⬥ One major role of calcium is to form and maintain bones and teeth.

A profile of nutrients that maintain bone health

Calcium is the most recognized nutrient associated with bone health; however, vitamins D and K, phosphorus, magnesium, and fluoride are also essential for strong bones, and the roles of other vitamins, minerals, and phytochemicals are currently being researched.

Calcium

Recall from Chapter 1 that the major minerals are those required in our diets in amounts greater than 100 mg per day. Calcium is by far the most abundant major mineral in our bodies, comprising about 2% of our entire body weight! Not surprisingly, it plays many critical roles in maintaining overall function and health.

Functions of Calcium

One of the primary functions of calcium is to provide structure to our bones and teeth. About 99% of the calcium found in our bodies is stored in the hydroxyapatite crystals built up on the collagen foundation of bone. As noted earlier, the combination of crystals and collagen provides both the characteristic hardness of bone and the flexibility needed to support various activities.

The remaining 1% of calcium in our bodies is found in the blood and soft tissues. Calcium is alkaline, or basic, and plays a critical role in assisting with acid–base balance. We cannot survive for long if our blood calcium level rises above or falls below a very narrow range; therefore, our bodies maintain the appropriate blood calcium level at all costs.

FIGURE 9.5 illustrates how various organ systems and hormones work together to maintain blood calcium levels. When blood calcium levels fall (see Figure 9.5a), the

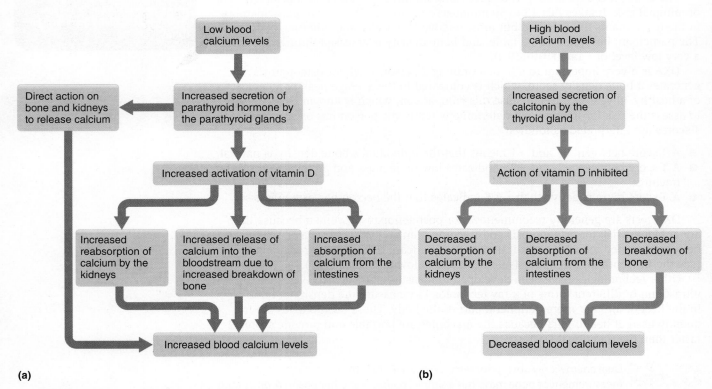

(a)

(b)

⬥ **FIGURE 9.5** Regulation of blood calcium levels by various organs and hormones. **(a)** Low blood calcium levels stimulate the production of parathyroid hormone, which not only acts directly on bone and kidneys to increase blood calcium levels, but also activates vitamin D. The actions of vitamin D further increase blood calcium levels. **(b)** High blood calcium levels stimulate the secretion of calcitonin, which inhibits the activities of vitamin D. This in turn causes a decrease in blood calcium levels.

parathyroid glands are stimulated to produce **parathyroid hormone (PTH)**. Also known as parathormone, PTH acts directly on bone and kidneys to increase blood calcium levels. PTH also stimulates the activation of vitamin D. Together, PTH and vitamin D stimulate the kidneys to reabsorb calcium from the bloodstream. They also stimulate osteoclasts to break down bone, releasing more calcium into the bloodstream. In addition, vitamin D increases the absorption of calcium from the intestines. Through these four mechanisms, blood calcium levels increase.

When blood calcium levels are too high, the thyroid gland secretes a hormone called **calcitonin**, which inhibits the actions of vitamin D (see Figure 9.5b). Thus, calcitonin prevents the reabsorption of calcium in the kidneys, limits calcium absorption in the intestines, and inhibits the osteoclasts from breaking down bone.

As just noted, the body must maintain blood calcium levels within a very narrow range. Thus, when an individual does not consume or absorb enough calcium from the diet, osteoclasts erode bone so that calcium can be released into the blood. To maintain healthy bone density, we need to consume and absorb enough calcium to balance the calcium taken from our bones.

Calcium is also critical for the normal transmission of nerve impulses. Calcium flows into nerve cells and stimulates the release of molecules called neurotransmitters, which transfer the nerve impulses from one nerve cell (neuron) to another. Without adequate calcium, our nerves' ability to transmit messages is inhibited. Not surprisingly, when blood calcium levels fall dangerously low, a person can experience convulsions.

A fourth role of calcium is to assist in muscle contraction, which is initiated when calcium flows into muscle cells. Conversely, muscles relax when calcium is pumped back outside of muscle cells. If calcium levels are inadequate, normal muscle contraction and relaxation are inhibited, and the person may suffer from twitching and spasms. This is referred to as **calcium tetany**. High levels of blood calcium can cause **calcium rigor**, an inability of muscles to relax, which leads to a hardening or stiffening of the muscles. These problems affect the function not only of skeletal muscles but also of heart muscle and can cause heart failure.

Other functions of calcium include the maintenance of healthy blood pressure, the initiation of blood clotting, and the regulation of various hormones and enzymes.

How Much Calcium Should We Consume?

The RDA for adult men aged 19 to 70 years and women aged 19 to 50 years is 1,000 mg per day. For men older than 70 years of age and women older than 50 years of age, the RDA increased to 1,200 mg of calcium per day. At 1,300 mg per day, the RDA for boys and girls aged 9 to 18 years is even higher, reflecting their developing bone mass. The Upper Limit (UL) for calcium is 2,500 mg for all age groups (TABLE 9.2).

Bioavailability is the degree to which our bodies can absorb and use any given nutrient. The bioavailability of calcium depends in part on our age and our calcium need. For example, infants, children, and adolescents can absorb more than 60% of the calcium they consume because calcium needs are very high during these stages of life. In addition, pregnant and lactating women can absorb about 50% of dietary calcium. In contrast, healthy young adults absorb only about 30% of the calcium consumed in the diet. When our calcium needs are high, the body can generally increase its absorption of calcium from the small intestine. Although older adults have a high need for calcium, their ability to absorb calcium from the small intestine diminishes with age and can be as low as 25%. These variations in bioavailability and absorption capacity were taken into account when calcium recommendations were determined.

The bioavailability of calcium also depends on how much calcium we consume throughout the day or at any one time. When our diet is generally high in calcium, absorption of calcium is reduced. In addition, our bodies cannot absorb more than 500 mg of calcium at any one time, and as the amount of calcium in a single meal or supplement goes up, the fraction that is absorbed goes down. This explains why it is critical to consume calcium-rich foods throughout the day rather than relying on a single, high-dose supplement. Conversely, when dietary intake of calcium is low, the absorption of calcium is increased.

parathyroid hormone (PTH) A hormone secreted by the parathyroid gland when blood calcium levels fall. Also known as parathormone, it increases blood calcium levels by stimulating the activation of vitamin D, increasing reabsorption of calcium from the kidneys, and stimulating osteoclasts to break down bone, which releases more calcium into the bloodstream.

calcitonin A hormone secreted by the thyroid gland when blood calcium levels are too high. Calcitonin inhibits the actions of vitamin D, preventing reabsorption of calcium in the kidneys, limiting calcium absorption in the small intestine, and inhibiting the osteoclasts from breaking down bone.

calcium tetany A condition in which muscles experience twitching and spasms as a result of inadequate blood calcium levels.

calcium rigor A failure of muscles to relax, which leads to a hardening or stiffening of the muscles; caused by high levels of blood calcium.

bioavailability The degree to which our body can absorb and utilize any given nutrient.

TABLE 9.2 **Overview of Nutrients Essential to Bone Health**

To see the full profile of micronutrients, turn to Chapter 6.5, **In Depth,** Vitamins and Minerals: Micronutrients with Macro Powers (pages 224–233).

Nutrient	Recommended Intake
Calcium (major mineral)	RDA: Adults aged 19 to 50 years = 1,000 mg/day Men aged 51 to 70 = 1,000 mg/day; men aged >70 = 1,200 mg/day Women aged >50 = 1,200 mg/day UL = 2,500 mg/day
Vitamin D (fat-soluble vitamin)	RDA:* Adults aged 19 to 50 years = 600 IU/day Adults aged 50 to 70 years = 600 IU/day Adults aged >70 years = 800 IU/day
Vitamin K (fat-soluble vitamin)	AI: Women: 90 µg/day Men: 120 µg/day
Phosphorus (major mineral)	RDA: Adults = 700 mg/day
Magnesium (major mineral)	RDA: Women aged 19 to 30 years = 310 mg/day Women aged >30 years = 320 mg/day Men aged 19 to 30 years = 400 mg/day Men aged >30 years = 420 mg/day
Fluoride (trace mineral)	RDA: Women = 3 mg/day Men = 4 mg/day UL = 2.2 mg/day for children aged 4 to 8; children >8 = 10 mg/day

*Note: * Based on the assumption that a person does not get adequate sun exposure.*

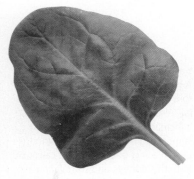

Although spinach contains high levels of calcium, binding factors in the plant prevent much of its absorption in the body.

Dietary factors can also affect our absorption of calcium. Binding factors, such as phytates and oxalates, occur naturally in some calcium-rich seeds, nuts, grains, and vegetables, such as spinach and Swiss chard. Such factors bind to the calcium in these foods and prevent its absorption from the small intestine. Additionally, consuming calcium with iron, zinc, magnesium, or phosphorus can interfere with the absorption and utilization of all these minerals. Despite these potential interactions, the Institute of Medicine has concluded that there is not sufficient evidence to suggest that these interactions cause deficiencies of calcium or other minerals in healthy individuals.[6]

Finally, because vitamin D is necessary for the absorption of calcium, a lack of vitamin D severely limits the bioavailability of calcium. We'll discuss this and other contributions of vitamin D to bone health shortly.

When you are selecting foods that are sources of calcium, remember that you don't absorb 100% of the calcium they contain. To learn more about how calcium absorption rates vary for select foods, see the **Nutrition Label Activity** (page 321).

Foods Rich in Calcium: Dairy, Greens, and More

Dairy products are among the most common sources of calcium in the U.S. diet. Skim milk, low-fat cheeses, and nonfat yogurt are nutritious sources of calcium (**FIGURE 9.6**). Greek yogurts have also become very popular and are a good source of calcium. However, it is important to remember that the calcium content of Greek yogurts is lower than that of regular yogurt (1 cup of Greek yogurt has about 270 mg calcium, compared to 448 mg in a cup of regular yogurt). Ice cream, regular cheese, and whole milk also contain a relatively high amount of calcium, but these foods should be eaten in moderation because of their high fat and energy content. Cottage cheese is one dairy product that is a relatively poor source of calcium because the processing of this food removes a great deal of the calcium. One cup of low-fat cottage cheese contains approximately 150 mg of calcium, whereas the same serving of low-fat milk contains almost 300 mg. However, calcium-fortified cottage cheese contains 400 mg of calcium.

Other good sources of calcium are green leafy vegetables, such as kale, collard greens, turnip greens, broccoli, cauliflower, green cabbage, brussels sprouts, and Chinese cabbage (bok choy). The bioavailability of the calcium in these vegetables is relatively high compared to spinach because these vegetables contain low levels of oxalates. Many packaged foods fortified with calcium are now available. For example, you can buy calcium-fortified orange juice, soy milk and other milk alternatives, and

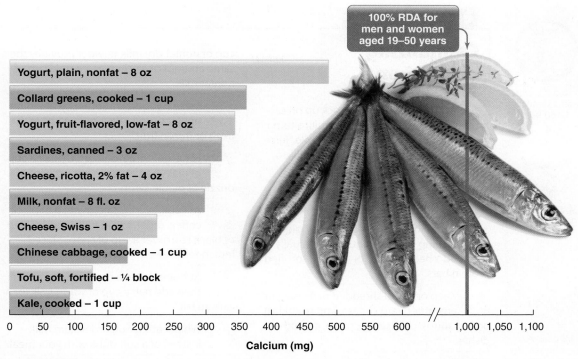

100% RDA for
men and women
aged 19–50 years

Yogurt, plain, nonfat – 8 oz

Collard greens, cooked – 1 cup

Yogurt, fruit-flavored, low-fat – 8 oz

Sardines, canned – 3 oz

Cheese, ricotta, 2% fat – 4 oz

Milk, nonfat – 8 fl. oz

Cheese, Swiss – 1 oz

Chinese cabbage, cooked – 1 cup

Tofu, soft, fortified – ¼ block

Kale, cooked – 1 cup

0   50   100   150   200   250   300   350   400   450   500   550   600   1,000 1,050 1,100

Calcium (mg)

FIGURE 9.6 Common food sources of calcium. The RDA for calcium is 1,000 mg of calcium per day for men and women aged 19 to 50.
Data from: U.S. Department of Agriculture, Agricultural Research Service. 2012. USDA Nutrient Database for Standard Reference, Release 25.

tofu processed with calcium. Some dairies have even boosted the amount of calcium in their brand of milk!

FIGURE 9.7 on page 320 illustrates serving sizes of various calcium-rich foods that contain the same amount of calcium as one glass (8 fl. oz) of skim milk. As you can see from this figure, a wide variety of foods can be consumed each day to contribute to adequate calcium intakes.

In general, meats and fish are not good sources of calcium. An exception is canned fish with bones (for example, sardines or salmon), providing you eat the bones. Fruits (except dried figs) and nonfortified grain products are also poor sources of calcium.

As you can see, many foods are good sources of calcium. Nevertheless, many Americans do not have adequate intakes because they consume very few dairy-based foods and calcium-rich vegetables. At particular risk are women and young girls. For example, a large national survey conducted by the U.S. Department of Agriculture found that teenage girls consume less than 60% of the recommended amount of calcium.[7]

A variety of quick, simple tools are available on the Internet to help you determine your daily calcium intake. Most of these tools are designed to provide you with an estimated calcium intake score based on the types and amounts of calcium-rich foods you consume. For more help in capitalizing on calcium, see the **Quick Tips** box (page 320).

As you can see, it's easy to increase your calcium intake by making smart menu choices throughout the day. **Eating Right All Day** (page 322) shows menu choices high in calcium. Notice that these are also low in fat and Calories.

What Happens If We Consume Too Much Calcium?

In general, consuming too much calcium from foods does not lead to significant toxicity symptoms in healthy individuals. Much of the excess calcium we consume is excreted in the feces. However, an excessive intake of calcium from supplements can lead to health problems. As mentioned earlier, one concern with consuming too much calcium is that it can lead to various mineral imbalances because calcium interferes with the absorption of other minerals, including iron, zinc, and magnesium. This interference may only be of major concern in individuals vulnerable to mineral

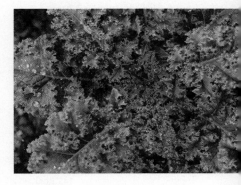

Kale is a good source of bioavailable calcium.

To find out if you are getting enough calcium in your diet, take the calcium quiz at **www.healthyeating.org**. Type "healthy eating tools calcium quiz" into the search box, then click on the top link.

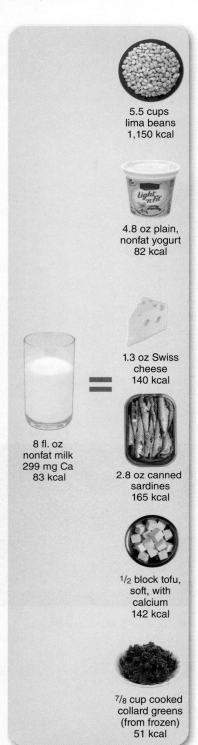

5.5 cups
lima beans
1,150 kcal

4.8 oz plain,
nonfat yogurt
82 kcal

1.3 oz Swiss
cheese
140 kcal

8 fl. oz
nonfat milk
299 mg Ca
83 kcal

2.8 oz canned
sardines
165 kcal

½ block tofu,
soft, with
calcium
142 kcal

⅞ cup cooked
collard greens
(from frozen)
51 kcal

FIGURE 9.7 Serving sizes and energy content of various foods that contain the same amount of calcium as an 8-fl. oz glass of skim milk.

hypercalcemia A condition marked by an abnormally high concentration of calcium in the blood.

QuickTips

Capitalizing on Calcium

At the grocery store, stock up on calcium-fortified juices and milk alternatives. Look for single-serving portable "juice boxes" with calcium-fortified juice, milk, or chocolate milk.

Purchase breakfast cereals and breads that are fortified with calcium.

For quick snacks, purchase single-serving cups of yogurt, individually wrapped "cheese sticks," or calcium-fortified protein bars.

Keep on hand shredded parmesan or any other hard cheese, and sprinkle it on hot soups, chili, salads, pasta, and other dishes.

In any recipe, replace sour cream or mayonnaise with nonfat plain yogurt.

Add nonfat dry milk powder to hot cereals, soups, chili, recipes for baked goods, coffee, and hot cocoa. One-third of a cup of nonfat dry milk powder provides the same amount of calcium as a whole cup of nonfat milk.

Make a yogurt smoothie by blending nonfat plain or flavored yogurt with fresh or frozen fruit.

For a "guilt-free" dessert, try half a cup of plain nonfat Greek yogurt with a drizzle of maple syrup.

At your favorite cafe, instead of black coffee, order a skim milk latte. Instead of black tea, order a cup of chai—spiced Indian tea brewed with milk.

At home, brew a cup of strong coffee; then add half a cup of warm milk for a café au lait.

When eating out, order skim milk instead of a soft drink with your meal.

If you do not consume enough dietary calcium, consider taking a calcium supplement. Refer to the **In Depth** on osteoporosis, Chapter 9.5, to learn how to choose a calcium supplement that is right for you.

imbalance, such as the elderly and people who consume very low amounts of minerals in their diets. Another potential problem is kidney stone formation: calcium from foods does not increase the risk for kidney stones, but some studies suggest that taking calcium supplements can.[8]

Various diseases and metabolic disorders can alter our ability to regulate blood calcium. **Hypercalcemia** is a condition in which our blood calcium levels reach abnormally high concentrations. Hypercalcemia can be caused by cancer and by the overproduction of PTH. Recall that PTH stimulates osteoclasts to break down bone and release more calcium into the bloodstream. Symptoms of hypercalcemia include fatigue, loss of appetite, constipation, and mental confusion, and it can lead to coma and possibly death. Hypercalcemia can also result in an accumulation of calcium deposits in the soft tissues, such as the liver and kidneys, causing failure of these organs.

What Happens If We Don't Consume Enough Calcium?

There are no short-term symptoms associated with consuming too little calcium. Even when we do not consume enough dietary calcium, our body continues to tightly regulate blood calcium levels by taking the calcium from bone. A long-term repercussion of inadequate calcium intake is osteoporosis. This disease is discussed **In Depth** immediately following this chapter.

Hypocalcemia is an abnormally low level of calcium in the blood. Hypocalcemia does not result from consuming too little dietary calcium but is caused by various diseases, including kidney disease, vitamin D deficiency, and diseases that inhibit the production of PTH. Symptoms of hypocalcemia include muscle spasms and convulsions.

nutrition label activity

How Much Calcium Am I Really Consuming?

As you've learned in this chapter, we do not absorb 100% of the calcium contained in our foods. This is particularly true for individuals who eat a diet rich in foods high in fiber, oxalates, and phytates, such as whole grains and certain vegetables. So if you want to design an eating plan that contains adequate calcium, it's important to understand how the rate of calcium absorption differs for the foods you include.

Estimates of the rate of calcium absorption have been established for a variety of common foods that are considered good sources of calcium. The following table shows some of these foods, their calcium content per serving, the calcium absorption rate, and the estimated amount of calcium absorbed from each food.

As you can see from this table, many dairy products have a similar calcium absorption rate, just over 30%. Interestingly, many green leafy vegetables have a higher absorption rate of around 60%; however, because a typical serving of these foods contains less calcium than dairy foods, you would have to eat more vegetables to get the same calcium as you would from a standard serving of dairy foods. Note the relatively low calcium absorption rate for spinach, even though it contains a relatively high amount of calcium. This is due to the high levels of oxalates in spinach, which bind with calcium and reduce its bioavailability.

Remember that the RDA for calcium takes these differences in absorption rate into account. Thus, the 300 mg of calcium in a glass of milk counts as 300 mg toward your daily calcium goal. In general, you can trust that dairy products are good, absorbable sources of calcium, as are most dark green leafy vegetables. Other dietary sources of calcium with good absorption rates include calcium-fortified orange juice and milk alternatives; tofu processed with calcium; and fortified breakfast cereals. Armed with this knowledge, you will be better able to select foods that can optimize your calcium intake and support bone health.

Food	Serving Size	Calcium per Serving (mg)[*]	Absorption Rate (%)[†]	Estimated Amount of Calcium Absorbed (mg)
Yogurt, plain skim milk	8 fl. oz	488	32	156
Milk, skim	1 cup	299	32	96
Milk, 2%	1 cup	293	32	94
Kale, frozen, cooked	1 cup	179	59	106
Turnip greens, boiled	1 cup	197	52	103
Broccoli, frozen, chopped, cooked	1 cup	61	61	37
Cauliflower, boiled	1 cup	20	69	14
Spinach, frozen, cooked	1 cup	291	5	14

[*] Data from: U.S. Department of Agriculture, Agricultural Research Service. 2012. USDA National Nutrient Database for Standard Reference, Release 25.

[†] Data from: Weaver, C. M., W. R. Proulx, and R. Heaney. 1999. Choices for achieving adequate dietary calcium with a vegetarian diet. *Am. J. Clin. Nutr.* 70(suppl.):543S–548S; Weaver, C. M., and K. L. Plawecki. 1994. Dietary calcium: adequacy of a vegetarian diet. *Am. J. Clin. Nutr.* 59(suppl.):1238S–1241S.

recap Calcium is the most abundant mineral in the human body and a significant component of our bones. It is also necessary for normal nerve and muscle function. Blood calcium is maintained within a very narrow range, and bone calcium is used to maintain normal blood calcium if dietary intake is inadequate. The RDA for calcium is 1,000 mg per day for adults aged 19 to 50; the RDA increases to 1,200 mg per day for men older than 70 years of age and women older than 50 years of age, and goes up to 1,300 mg per day for adolescents. Dairy products, canned fish with bones, and some green leafy vegetables are good sources of calcium. The most common long-term effect of inadequate calcium consumption is osteoporosis.

hypocalcemia A condition characterized by an abnormally low concentration of calcium in the blood.

eating right all day

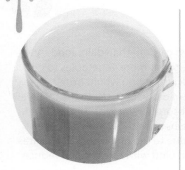

Breakfast

Skim-milk chai tea instead of a cola!

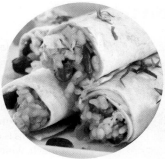

Lunch

Bean & cheese burrito instead of a beef burrito!

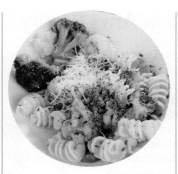

Dinner

Pasta with broccoli and grated cheese instead of meat sauce!

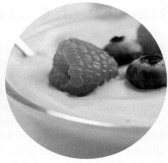

Snack

Nonfat fruit yogurt instead of Oreos!

Vitamin D

Vitamin D is like other fat-soluble vitamins in that we store excess amounts in our liver and adipose tissue. But vitamin D is different from other nutrients in two ways. First, vitamin D does not always need to come from the diet. This is because our bodies can synthesize vitamin D using energy from exposure to sunlight. However, when we do not get enough sunlight, we must consume vitamin D in our diets. Second, in addition to being a nutrient, vitamin D is considered a *hormone* because it is made in one part of the body yet regulates various activities in other parts of the body.

FIGURE 9.8 illustrates how our bodies make vitamin D by converting a cholesterol compound in our skin to the active form of vitamin D that we need to function

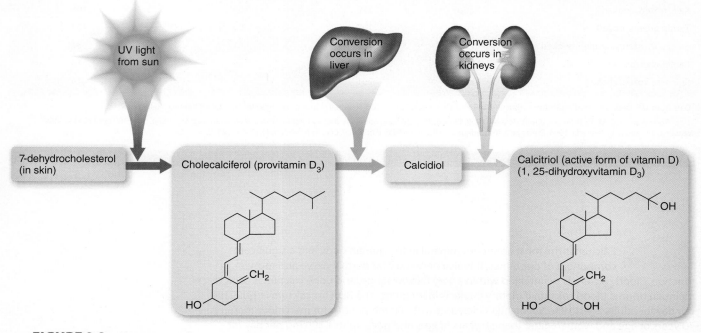

↞ **FIGURE 9.8** The process of converting sunlight into vitamin D in our skin. When the ultraviolet rays of the sun hit our skin, they react with 7-dehydrocholesterol. This compound is converted to cholecalciferol, an inactive form of vitamin D also called provitamin D_3. Cholecalciferol is then converted to calcidiol in the liver. Calcidiol travels to the kidneys, where it is converted into calcitriol, which is considered the primary active form of vitamin D in our body.

HOT TOPIC

Can Eating Dairy Foods Help You Lose Weight?

A 2004 research study suggested that a weight-loss diet high in calcium-rich foods may help people lose more weight than if they reduce their energy intake but do not consume enough dietary calcium.[9] This research led to a major advertising campaign by the dairy industry, called the "3-A-Day" campaign. This campaign encourages people who want to lose weight to eat at least 3 servings of dairy foods per day because study participants who ate calcium-rich foods experienced significantly more weight loss than those who consumed calcium supplements. Interestingly, subsequent studies have failed to replicate these findings.[10,11]

As a result of these conflicting findings, the United States Department of Agriculture funded research into this topic. This study found that some, but not all, overweight women consuming adequate dairy products during a weight loss program experienced a greater loss of body weight and fat than women consuming low levels of dairy; the variation in responses appears to be associated with complex interactions between the amount of calcium consumed prior to and during the study, and individual hormonal responses to energy restriction.[12] Thus it appears that consuming adequate dairy intake may be important in losing weight for some people, but more research is needed to better understand who might benefit and why.

properly. When the ultraviolet rays of the sun hit the skin, they react with 7-dehydrocholesterol. This cholesterol compound is converted into a precursor of vitamin D, **cholecalciferol**, which is also called provitamin D_3. This inactive form is then converted to calcidiol in the liver, where it is stored. When needed, calcidiol travels to the kidneys, where it is converted into **calcitriol**, which is considered the primary active form of vitamin D in our bodies. Calcitriol then circulates to various parts of the body, performing its many functions. Excess calcitriol can also be stored in adipose tissue for later use.

Functions of Vitamin D

As you've learned, vitamin D, PTH, and calcitonin all work together continuously to regulate blood calcium levels, which in turn maintains bone health. They do this by regulating the absorption of calcium and phosphorus from the small intestine, causing more to be absorbed when our needs for them are higher and less when our needs are lower. They also decrease or increase blood calcium levels by signaling the kidneys to excrete more or less calcium in our urine. Finally, PTH and vitamin D stimulate osteoclasts to break down bone when calcium is needed elsewhere in the body.

Vitamin D is also necessary for the normal calcification of bone; this means it assists the process by which minerals such as calcium and phosphorus are crystallized. Vitamin D may also play a role in decreasing the formation of some cancerous tumors because it can prevent certain types of cells from growing out of control. Like vitamin A, vitamin D appears to play a role in cell differentiation in various tissues.

How Much Vitamin D Should We Consume?

If your exposure to the sun is adequate, then you do not need to consume any vitamin D in your diet. But how do you know whether you are getting enough sun?

The RDA is based on the assumption that an individual does not get adequate sun exposure. Of the many factors that affect your ability to synthesize vitamin D from sunlight, latitude and time of year are the most significant (**TABLE 9.3**, page 324). People living in very sunny climates relatively close to the equator, such as the southern United States and Mexico, may synthesize enough vitamin D from the sun to meet their needs throughout the year—as long as they spend time outdoors. However, vitamin D synthesis from the sun is not possible during most of the winter months for people living in places located at a latitude of more than 37°N or more than 37°S. At these latitudes in winter the sun never rises high enough in the sky to provide the amount of direct sunlight needed. The 37°N latitude runs like a belt across the United States from northern

cholecalciferol Vitamin D_3, a form of vitamin D found in animal foods and the form we synthesize from the sun.

calcitriol The primary active form of vitamin D in the body.

TABLE 9.3   Factors Affecting Sunlight-Mediated Synthesis of Vitamin D in the Skin

Factors That Enhance Synthesis of Vitamin D	Factors That Inhibit Synthesis of Vitamin D
Season—summer months, particularly June and July, during which most vitamin D is produced	Season—winter months (October through February), resulting in little or no vitamin D production
Latitude—locations closer to the equator, which get more sunlight throughout the year	Latitude—regions north of 37°N and south of 37°S get inadequate sun during the winter
Time of day—generally, between the hours of 10:00 AM and 3:00 PM (depending on latitude and time of year)	Time of day—early morning, late afternoon, and evening hours
Age—Younger	Age—Older, due to reduced skin thickness with age
Limited or no use of sunscreen	Use of sunscreen with SPF 8 or greater
Sunny weather	Cloudy weather
Exposed skin	Protective clothing
Lighter skin pigmentation	Darker skin pigmentation
	Obesity—possible negative effect on metabolism and storage of vitamin D
	Glass and plastics—windows or other barriers made of glass or plastic (such as Plexiglas), which block the sun's rays

Virginia in the east to northern California in the west (**FIGURE 9.9**). In addition, entire countries, such as Canada and the United Kingdom, are affected, as are countries in the far southern hemisphere. Thus, many people around the world need to consume vitamin D in their diets, particularly during the winter months.

Other factors influencing vitamin D synthesis are time of day, skin color, age, and body weight status:

- More vitamin D can be synthesized during the time of day when the sun's rays are strongest, generally between 10 AM and 3 PM. Vitamin D synthesis is severely limited or may be nonexistent on overcast days.

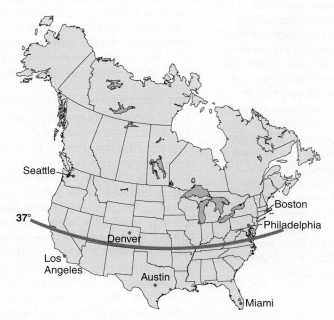

FIGURE 9.9   This map illustrates the geographical location of 37° latitude in the United States. In southern cities below 37° latitude, such as Los Angeles, Austin, and Miami, the sunlight is strong enough to allow for vitamin D synthesis throughout the year. In northern cities above 37° latitude, such as Seattle, Chicago, and Boston, the sunlight is too weak from about mid-October to mid-March to allow for adequate vitamin D synthesis.

- Darker skin contains more melanin pigment, which reduces the penetration of sunlight. Thus, people with dark skin have a more difficult time synthesizing vitamin D from the sun than do light-skinned people.
- People 65 years of age or older experience a fourfold decrease in their capacity to synthesize vitamin D from the sun; they are also more likely to spend more time indoors and may have inadequate dietary intakes.[13]
- Obesity is associated with lower levels of circulating vitamin D, possibly because of lower bioavailability of cholecalciferol from adipose tissue, decreased exposure to sunlight due to limited mobility or time spent outdoors with skin exposed, and alterations in vitamin D metabolism in the liver.[14,15]

Wearing protective clothing and sunscreen (with an SPF greater than 8) limits sun exposure, so it is suggested that we expose our hands, face, and arms to the sun two or three times per week for a period of time that is one-third to one-half of the amount needed to get sunburned.[16] This means that, if you normally sunburn in 1 hour, you should expose yourself to the sun for 20 to 30 minutes two or three times per week to synthesize adequate amounts of vitamin D. Again, this guideline does not apply to people living in more northern climates during the winter months; they can get enough vitamin D only by consuming it in their diet.

Because not everyone is able to get adequate sun exposure throughout the year, an RDA has been established for vitamin D. For men and women aged 19 to 70 years, the RDA is 600 IU, and for adults older than 70 years, it is 800 IU. The UL for vitamin D is 4,000 IU for everyone 9 years of age and older. Recent evidence suggests that the current RDA for vitamin D is not sufficient to maintain optimal bone health and reduce the risks for diseases such as cancer; the controversy surrounding the current recommendations for vitamin D are discussed in more detail in the **Nutrition Debate** at the end of this chapter. What about you? Do you think you're getting enough vitamin D each day? To find out, take the quiz in the **What About You?** feature box.

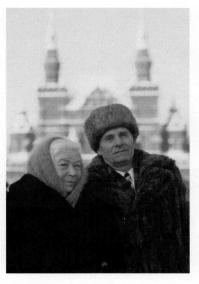

▲ Vitamin D synthesis from the sun is not possible during most of the winter months for people living in high latitudes. Therefore, many people need to consume vitamin D in their diet, particularly during the winter.

what about **you** (?)

Are You Getting Enough Vitamin D?

After reading this section, you may wonder whether you're getting enough vitamin D to keep your tissues healthy and strong. Take the following simple quiz to find out. For each question, circle either Yes or No:

I live south of 37° latitude (see Figure 9.9) and expose my bare arms and face to sunlight (without sunscreen) for at least a few minutes two or three times per week all year.	Yes/No
I consume a multivitamin supplement or vitamin D supplement that provides at least 5 μg or 200 IU per day.	Yes/No
I consume a diet high in fatty fish, fortified milk or milk alternatives, and/or fortified cereals that provides at least 5 μg or 200 IU per day.	Yes/No

If you answered No to all three of these questions, you are at high risk for vitamin D deficiency. You are probably getting enough vitamin D if you answered Yes to at least one of them. However, notice that, if you rely on sun exposure for your vitamin D, you must make sure that you expose your bare skin to sunlight for an adequate length of time. What's adequate varies for each person: the darker your skin tone, the more time you need in the sun. A general guideline is to expose your skin for a period that is one-third to one-half the amount of time in which you would get sunburned. This means that, if you normally sunburn in 1 hour, you should get 30 minutes of sun two or three times a week. Expose your skin when the sun is high in the sky (generally between the hours of 10 AM and 3 PM). Put on sunscreen only *after* your skin has had its daily dose of sunlight.[17]

Remember: if you live in the northern United States or Canada, you cannot get adequate sun exposure to synthesize vitamin D from approximately October through February, no matter how long you expose your bare skin to the sun. So, if you are not regularly consuming fortified foods, fatty fish, or cod liver oil, you need to supplement vitamin D during those months.

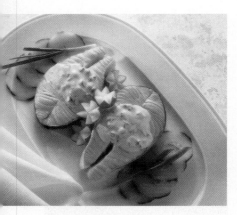

⬤ Fatty fish contain vitamin D.

ergocalciferol Vitamin D₂, a form of vitamin D found exclusively in plant foods.

Vitamin D: Fish, Fortified Foods, Supplements, or Sunlight

There are many forms of vitamin D, but only two can be converted into calcitriol. Vitamin D₂, also called **ergocalciferol**, is found exclusively in plant foods, whereas vitamin D₃, or cholecalciferol, is found in animal foods. As noted earlier, cholecalciferol is also the form of vitamin D we synthesize from the sun.

Most foods naturally contain very little vitamin D. The few exceptions are cod liver oil and fatty fish (such as salmon, mackerel, tuna, and sardines), foods that few Americans consume in adequate amounts. Eggs, butter, some margarines, and liver also provide small amounts of vitamin D, but we would have to eat very large amounts to consume enough vitamin D.

Thus, the primary source of vitamin D in the diet is from fortified foods such as milk (**FIGURE 9.10**). In the United States, milk is fortified with 100 IU of vitamin D per cup.[18] Additional foods fortified with vitamin D include some breakfast cereals, margarine, orange juice, and yogurt. Because plants contain very little vitamin D, vegetarians who consume no fortified dairy products need to obtain their vitamin D from sun exposure, fortified milk alternatives or cereal products, or supplements. When reading the labels of fortified foods and supplements, you will see the amount of vitamin D expressed in units of either µg or IU. For conversion purposes, 1 µg of vitamin D is equal to 40 IU of vitamin D.

What Happens If We Consume Too Much Vitamin D?

We cannot get too much vitamin D from sun exposure because our skin has the ability to limit its production. As just noted, foods contain little natural vitamin D. Thus, the only way we can consume too much vitamin D is through supplementation.

Consuming too much vitamin D causes hypercalcemia, or high blood calcium concentrations. As discussed in the section on calcium, symptoms of hypercalcemia include weakness, loss of appetite, constipation, mental confusion, vomiting, excessive urine output, and extreme thirst. Hypercalcemia also leads to the formation of calcium deposits in soft tissues, such as the kidneys, liver, and heart. In addition, toxic levels of vitamin D lead to increased bone loss because calcium is then pulled from the bones and excreted more readily from the kidneys.

What Happens If We Don't Consume Enough Vitamin D?

The primary deficiency associated with inadequate vitamin D is loss of bone mass. In fact, when vitamin D levels are inadequate, our small intestine can absorb only 10–15% of

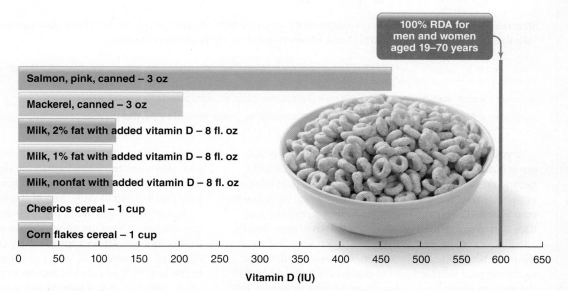

⬤ **FIGURE 9.10** Common food sources of vitamin D. For men and women aged 19 to 70 years, the RDA for vitamin D is 600 IU per day. The RDA increases to 800 IU per day for adults over the age of 70 years.

Data from: U.S. Department of Agriculture, Agricultural Research Service. 2012. USDA Nutrient Database for Standard Reference, Release 25.

the calcium we consume. Vitamin D deficiencies occur most often in individuals who have diseases that cause intestinal malabsorption of fat and thus the fat-soluble vitamins. People with liver disease, kidney disease, Crohn's disease, celiac disease, cystic fibrosis, or Whipple's disease may suffer from vitamin D deficiency and require supplements.

Vitamin D–deficiency disease in children, called **rickets**, is caused by inadequate mineralization or demineralization of the skeleton. The classic sign of rickets is deformity of the skeleton, such as bowed legs and knocked knees (**FIGURE 9.11**). However, severe cases can be fatal. Rickets is not common in the United States because of the fortification of milk products with vitamin D, but children with illnesses that cause fat malabsorption, or who drink no milk and get limited sun exposure, are at increased risk. There is no national surveillance program for rickets, and thus it is not clear what the prevalence of rickets is in the United States. However, a review of reported cases of rickets among children in the United States found that approximately 83% were African American, and that 95% had been breast-fed.[19,20] Breast milk contains very little vitamin D, and less than 5% of the breast-fed children were reported to have received vitamin D supplementation. Thus, rickets appears to occur more commonly in children with darker skin (their need for adequate sun exposure is higher than that of light-skinned children) and in breast-fed children who do not receive adequate vitamin D supplementation. In addition, rickets is still a significant nutritional problem for children outside of the United States.

Vitamin D–deficiency disease in adults is called **osteomalacia**, a term meaning "soft bones." With osteomalacia, bones become weak and prone to fractures. Osteoporosis (discussed **In Depth** on pages 338–345) can also result from a vitamin D deficiency.

Vitamin D deficiencies have recently been found to be more common among American adults than previously thought. This may be partly due to jobs and lifestyle choices that keep people indoors for most of the day. Not surprisingly, the population at greatest risk is older institutionalized individuals who get little or no sun exposure.

Various medications can also alter the metabolism and activity of vitamin D. For instance, glucocorticoids, which are medications used to reduce inflammation, can cause bone loss by inhibiting the ability to absorb calcium through the actions of vitamin D. Anti-seizure medications, such as phenobarbital and Dilantin, alter vitamin D metabolism. Thus, people who are taking such medications may need to increase their vitamin D intake.

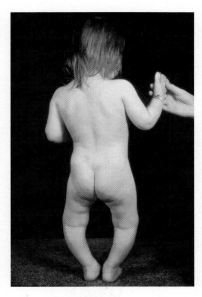

FIGURE 9.11 A vitamin D deficiency causes a bone-deforming disease in children called rickets.

recap   Vitamin D is a fat-soluble vitamin and a hormone. It can be made in the skin using energy from sunlight. Vitamin D regulates blood calcium levels and maintains bone health. The RDA for vitamin D is 600 IU per day for adult men and women aged 19 to 70 years; the RDA increases to 800 IU per day for adults over the age of 70 years. Foods contain little vitamin D, with fortified milk being the primary source. Vitamin D toxicity causes hypercalcemia. Vitamin D deficiency can result in osteoporosis; rickets is vitamin D deficiency in children, whereas osteomalacia is vitamin D deficiency in adults.

nutri-case | THEO

"The health center here on campus is running a study on vitamin D levels among students, and the instructor in my nutrition class encouraged everyone to participate. I don't think I need to be worried about it, though, 'cause I exercise outdoors a lot—at least, whenever Wisconsin weather allows it! It's true I don't drink much milk, and I hate fish, but otherwise I eat right, and besides, I'm a guy, so I don't have to worry about my bone density."

Should Theo have his vitamin D levels checked? Why or why not? Before you answer, take another look back at the information in this section. Also, consider Theo's assertion that because he is male he doesn't have to worry about his bone density. Is he right? And is calcium regulation the only significant role of vitamin D?

rickets A vitamin D–deficiency disease in children. Signs include deformities of the skeleton, such as bowed legs and knocked knees. Severe rickets can be fatal.

osteomalacia A vitamin D–deficiency disease in adults, in which bones become weak and prone to fractures.

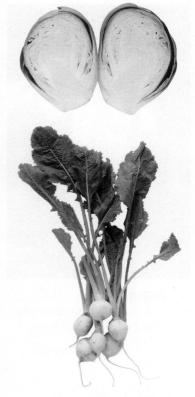

Green leafy vegetables, including brussels sprouts and turnip greens, are good sources of vitamin K.

Vitamin K

Vitamin K, a fat-soluble vitamin stored primarily in the liver, is actually a family of compounds known as quinones. *Phylloquinone,* which is the primary dietary form of vitamin K, is also the form found in plants; *menaquinone* is the animal form of vitamin K produced by bacteria in the large intestine.

The primary function of vitamin K is to assist in the production of *prothrombin,* a protein that plays a critical role in blood clotting (this is discussed in more detail in Chapter 10). Vitamin K also assists in the production of *osteocalcin,* a protein associated with bone turnover.

We can obtain vitamin K from our diets, and we absorb the vitamin K produced by bacteria in our large intestine. These two sources usually provide adequate amounts of this nutrient to maintain health, and there is no RDA or UL for vitamin K. AI recommendations are listed in Table 9.2.

Only a few foods contribute substantially to our dietary intake of vitamin K. Green leafy vegetables, including kale, spinach, collard greens, turnip greens, and lettuce, are good sources, as are broccoli, brussels sprouts, and cabbage. Vegetable oils, such as soybean oil and canola oil, are also good sources. **FIGURE 9.12** identifies the amount of vitamin K in micrograms per serving for these foods.

Based on our current knowledge, for healthy individuals there appear to be no side effects associated with consuming large amounts of vitamin K.[21] This appears to be true for both supplements and food sources.

Vitamin K deficiency is associated with a reduced ability to form blood clots, leading to excessive bleeding; however, primary vitamin K deficiency is rare in humans. People with diseases that cause malabsorption of fat, such as celiac disease, Crohn's disease, and cystic fibrosis, can suffer secondarily from a deficiency of vitamin K. Long-term use of antibiotics, which typically reduce bacterial populations in the colon, combined with limited dietary intake of vitamin K–rich food sources, can also lead to vitamin K deficiency. Newborns are typically given an injection of vitamin K at birth because they lack the intestinal bacteria necessary to produce this nutrient.

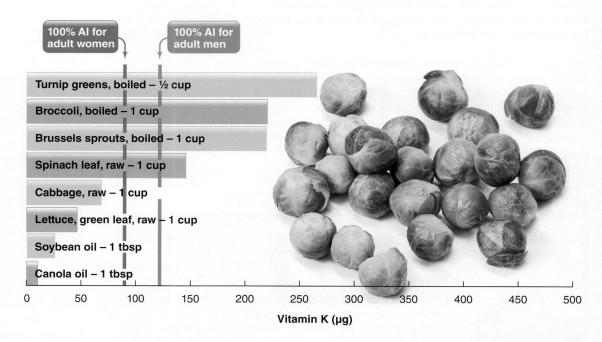

FIGURE 9.12 Common food sources of vitamin K. The AIs for adult men and women are 120 µg per day and 90 µg per day, respectively.

Data from: U.S. Department of Agriculture, Agricultural Research Service. 2012. USDA Nutrient Database for Standard Reference, Release 25.

The effect of vitamin K on bone mineral density appears to be modest, and studies report inconsistent results.[22] Thus, there is not enough scientific evidence to support the contention that vitamin K deficiency directly causes osteoporosis. In fact, there is no significant impact on overall bone density in people who take anticoagulant medications that result in a relative state of vitamin K deficiency.

recap · Vitamin K is a fat-soluble vitamin and coenzyme that is important for blood clotting and bone metabolism. We obtain vitamin K largely from bacteria in our large intestine. Green leafy vegetables and vegetable oils contain vitamin K. There are no known toxicity symptoms for vitamin K in healthy individuals. Vitamin K deficiency is rare and may lead to excessive bleeding.

Phosphorus

Phosphorus (as discussed in Chapter 7) is the major intracellular negatively charged electrolyte. In our body, phosphorus is most commonly found combined with oxygen in the form of phosphate (PO_4^{3-}). Phosphorus is an essential constituent of all cells and is found in both plants and animals.

Functions of Phosphorus

Phosphorus plays a critical role in bone formation because it is a part of the mineral complex of bone. As discussed earlier in this chapter, calcium and phosphorus crystallize to form hydroxyapatite crystals, which provide the hardness of bone. About 85% of our body's phosphorus is stored in our bones, with the rest stored in soft tissues, such as muscles and organs.

Phosphorus also helps activate and deactivate enzymes, and it is a component of lipoproteins, cell membranes, DNA and RNA, and several energy molecules, including adenosine triphosphate (ATP). (The role of phosphorus in maintaining proper fluid balance is examined in detail in Chapter 7.)

How Much Phosphorus Should We Consume?

The RDA for phosphorus is listed in Table 9.2. In general, phosphorus is widespread in many foods and is found in high amounts in foods that contain protein. Milk, meats, and eggs are good sources. (The details of phosphorus recommendations, food sources, and deficiency and toxicity symptoms are covered in Chapter 7.)

Phosphorus is also found in many processed foods as a food additive, where it enhances smoothness, binding, and moisture retention. Moreover, in the form of phosphoric acid, it is added to soft drinks to give them a sharper, or more tart, flavor and to slow the growth of molds and bacteria. Our society has increased its consumption of processed foods and soft drinks substantially over the past 30 years, resulting in an estimated 10–15% increase in phosphorus consumption.[6,23]

In the past, some studies associated consumption of soft drinks with reduced bone mass or an increased risk for fractures in youth and adults.[24–26] Some researchers proposed that the phosphoric acid content of soft drinks causes an increased loss of calcium because calcium is drawn from bone into the blood to neutralize the excess acid. More recent evidence suggests that, in older women, it is specifically the intake of cola beverages, not carbonated beverages in general, that is associated with low bone mineral density.[27] This has contributed to speculation that it is the caffeine in colas that causes increased calcium loss through the urine. However, experts in this area of research have concluded that the most likely explanation for the link between soft drink consumption and poor bone health is the *milk-displacement effect;* that is, soft drinks take the place of milk or calcium-fortified milk alternatives in our diets, depriving us of calcium and vitamin D.[28]

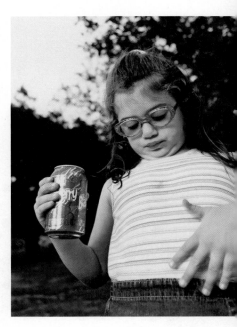

Phosphorus, in the form of phosphoric acid, is a major component of soft drinks.

What Happens If We Consume Too Much Phosphorus?

People with kidney disease and those who take too many vitamin D supplements or too many phosphorus-containing antacids can suffer from high blood phosphorus levels (as discussed in Chapter 7). Severely high levels of blood phosphorus can cause muscle spasms and convulsions.

What Happens If We Don't Consume Enough Phosphorus?

Phosphorus deficiencies are rare but can occur in people who abuse alcohol, in premature infants, and in elderly people with poor diets. People with vitamin D deficiency, people with hyperparathyroidism (oversecretion of parathyroid hormone), and those who overuse antacids that bind with phosphorus may also have low blood phosphorus levels.

recap Phosphorus is the major negatively charged electrolyte inside of the cell. It helps maintain fluid balance and bone health. It also assists in regulating chemical reactions, and it is a primary component of ATP, DNA, and RNA. Phosphorus is commonly found in high-protein foods. Excess phosphorus can lead to muscle spasms and convulsions, whereas phosphorus deficiencies are rare.

Magnesium

Magnesium is a major mineral. Our total body magnesium content is approximately 25 g. About 50–60% of our body's magnesium is found in our bones, with the rest located in our soft tissues.

Functions of Magnesium

Magnesium is one of the minerals that make up the structure of bone. It is also important in the regulation of bone and mineral status. Specifically, magnesium influences the formation of hydroxyapatite crystals through its regulation of calcium balance and its interactions with vitamin D and parathyroid hormone.

Magnesium is a critical *cofactor* for more than 300 enzyme systems. Recall from Chapter 8 that a cofactor is a compound that is needed for an enzyme to be active. Magnesium is necessary for the production of ATP, and it plays an important role in DNA and protein synthesis and repair. Magnesium supplementation has been shown to improve insulin sensitivity, and there is epidemiological evidence that a high magnesium intake is associated with a decrease in the risk for colorectal cancer.[29,30] Magnesium supports normal vitamin D metabolism and action and is necessary for normal muscle contraction and blood clotting.

How Much Magnesium Should We Consume?

Because magnesium is found in a wide variety of foods, people who are adequately nourished generally consume enough magnesium in their diets. The RDA for magnesium is identified in Table 9.2. There is no UL for magnesium consumed in food and water; the UL for magnesium from pharmacologic sources is 350 mg per day.

Magnesium is found in green leafy vegetables, such as spinach; whole grains; seeds; and nuts. Other good sources include seafood, beans, and some dairy products. Refined and processed foods are low in magnesium. **FIGURE 9.13** shows many foods that are good sources of magnesium.

The magnesium content of drinking water varies considerably. The "harder" the water, the higher its content of magnesium. This variability makes it impossible to estimate how much our drinking water may contribute to the magnesium content of our diet.

The ability of the small intestine to absorb magnesium is reduced when one consumes a diet that is extremely high in fiber and phytates because these

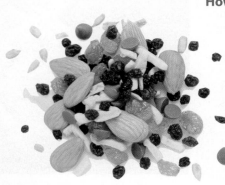

Trail mix with chocolate chips, nuts, and seeds is a common food source of magnesium.

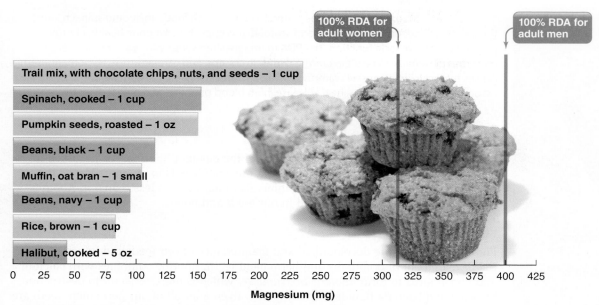

FIGURE 9.13 Common food sources of magnesium. For adult men 19 to 30 years of age, the RDA for magnesium is 400 mg per day; the RDA increases to 420 mg per day for men 31 years of age and older. For adult women 19 to 30 years of age, the RDA for magnesium is 310 mg per day; this value increases to 320 mg per day for women 31 years of age and older.
Data from: U.S. Department of Agriculture, Agricultural Research Service. 2012. USDA Nutrient Database for Standard Reference, Release 25.

substances bind with magnesium. Even though seeds and nuts are relatively high in fiber, they are excellent sources of absorbable magnesium. Overall, our absorption of magnesium should be sufficient if we consume the recommended amount of fiber each day (20 to 35 g per day). In contrast, higher dietary protein intakes enhance the absorption and retention of magnesium.

What Happens If We Consume Too Much Magnesium?

There are no known toxicity symptoms related to consuming excess magnesium in the diet. The toxicity symptoms that result from pharmacologic use of magnesium include diarrhea, nausea, and abdominal cramps. In extreme cases, large doses can result in acid–base imbalances, massive dehydration, cardiac arrest, and death. High blood magnesium levels, or **hypermagnesemia**, occur in individuals with impaired kidney function who consume large amounts of nondietary magnesium, such as antacids. Side effects include the impairment of nerve, muscle, and heart function.

What Happens If We Don't Consume Enough Magnesium?

Hypomagnesemia, or low blood magnesium, results from magnesium deficiency. This condition may develop secondary to kidney disease, chronic diarrhea, or chronic alcohol abuse. Elderly people seem to be at particularly high risk for low dietary intakes of magnesium because they have a reduced appetite and blunted senses of taste and smell. In addition, the elderly face challenges related to shopping and preparing micronutrient-dense meals, and their ability to absorb magnesium is reduced.

Low blood calcium levels are a side effect of hypomagnesemia. Other symptoms of magnesium deficiency include muscle cramps, spasms or seizures, nausea, weakness, irritability, and confusion. Considering magnesium's role in bone formation, it is not surprising that long-term magnesium deficiency is associated with osteoporosis. Magnesium deficiency is also associated with many other chronic diseases, including heart disease, high blood pressure, and type 2 diabetes.

hypermagnesemia A condition marked by an abnormally high concentration of magnesium in the blood.

hypomagnesemia A condition characterized by an abnormally low concentration of magnesium in the blood.

> **recap** Magnesium is a major mineral found in fresh foods, including spinach, nuts, seeds, whole grains, and seafood. It is important for bone health, energy production, and muscle function. The RDA for magnesium varies with age and gender. Hypermagnesemia can result in diarrhea, muscle cramps, and cardiac arrest. Hypomagnesemia causes hypocalcemia, muscle cramps, spasms, and weakness. Magnesium deficiencies are also associated with osteoporosis, heart disease, high blood pressure, and type 2 diabetes.

Fluoride

Fluoride, a trace mineral, is the ionic form of the element fluorine. As discussed in Chapter 1, trace minerals are minerals that our body needs in amounts less than 100 mg per day; the amount of trace minerals in our body is less than 5 g. About 99% of the fluoride in our body is stored in our teeth and bones.

Functions of Fluoride

Fluoride assists in the development and maintenance of our teeth and bones. During the development of both baby and permanent teeth, fluoride combines with calcium and phosphorus to form *fluorohydroxyapatite,* which is more resistant to destruction by acids and bacteria than is hydroxyapatite. Even after all of our permanent teeth are in, treating them with fluoride, whether at the dentist's office or by using fluoridated toothpaste, gives them more protection against dental caries (cavities) than teeth that have not been treated. That's because fluoride enhances tooth mineralization, decreases and reverses tooth demineralization, and inhibits the metabolism of the acid-producing bacteria that cause tooth decay.

Fluoride also stimulates new bone growth, and it is currently being researched as a potential treatment for osteoporosis, both alone and in combination with other medications. Although early results are promising, more research needs to be conducted to determine if fluoride is an effective treatment for osteoporosis.[31]

How Much Fluoride Should We Consume?

Our need for fluoride is relatively small. The AI for fluoride is listed in Table 9.2. The UL is 2.2 mg per day for children aged 4 to 8 years; the UL for everyone older than 8 years of age is 10 mg per day.

Fluoride is readily available in many communities in the United States through fluoridated water and dental products. In the mouth, fluoride is absorbed directly into the teeth and gums, and it can be absorbed from the gastrointestinal tract once it has been ingested. In the early 1990s, there was considerable concern that our intake of fluoride was too high due to the consumption of fluoridated water and fluoride-containing toothpastes and mouthwashes; it was speculated that this high intake could be contributing to an increased risk for cancer, bone fractures, kidney and other organ damage, infertility, and Alzheimer's disease. After reviewing the potential health hazards of fluoride, the U.S. Department of Health and Human Services and the National Cancer Institute found that there is no reliable scientific evidence available to indicate that fluoride increases our risk for these illnesses.[32,33]

There are concerns that individuals who consume bottled water exclusively may be getting too little fluoride and increasing their risk for dental caries because most bottled waters do not contain fluoride. However, these individuals may still consume fluoride through other beverages that contain fluoridated water and through fluoridated dental products. Toothpastes and mouthwashes that contain fluoride are widely marketed and used by the majority of consumers in the United States, and these products can contribute as much, if not more, fluoride to our diets than fluoridated water. Fluoride supplements are available only by prescription, and they are generally given only to children who do not have access to fluoridated water. Incidentally, tea is a good source of fluoride: one 8-oz cup provides about 20–25% of the AI.

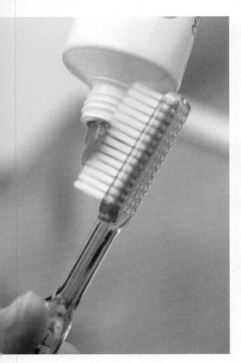

▲ Fluoride is readily available in many communities in the United States through fluoridated water and dental products.

What Happens If We Consume Too Much Fluoride?

Consuming too much fluoride increases the protein content of tooth enamel, resulting in a condition called **fluorosis**. Because increased protein makes the enamel more porous, the teeth become stained and pitted (**FIGURE 9.14**). Teeth seem to be at highest risk for fluorosis during the first 8 years of life, when the permanent teeth are developing. To reduce the risk for fluorosis, children should not swallow oral care products that are meant for topical use only, and children under the age of 6 years should be supervised while using fluoride-containing products. Mild fluorosis generally causes white patches on the teeth, but it has no effect on tooth function. Although moderate and severe fluorosis cause greater discoloration of the teeth, there appears to be no adverse effect on tooth function.[6]

Excess consumption of fluoride can also cause fluorosis of our skeleton. Mild skeletal fluorosis results in an increased bone mass and stiffness and pain in the joints. Moderate and severe skeletal fluorosis can be crippling, but it is extremely rare in the United States.[34]

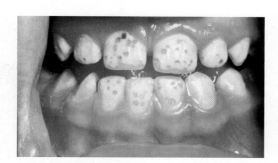

FIGURE 9.14 Consuming too much fluoride causes fluorosis, leading to staining and pitting of the teeth.

What Happens If We Don't Consume Enough Fluoride?

The primary result of fluoride deficiency is dental caries. Adequate fluoride intake appears necessary at an early age and throughout our adult life to reduce our risk for tooth decay. Inadequate fluoride intake may also be associated with lower bone density, but there is not enough research available to support the widespread use of fluoride to prevent osteoporosis. Studies are currently being done to determine the role fluoride might play in reducing our risk for osteoporosis and fractures.

recap Fluoride is a trace mineral whose primary function is to support the health of teeth and bones. Primary sources of fluoride are fluoridated dental products and fluoridated water. Fluoride toxicity causes fluorosis of the teeth and skeleton, whereas fluoride deficiency causes an increase in tooth decay.

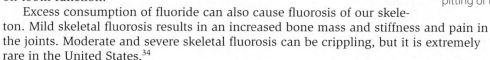

*behavior change . . . getting started!

Now that you've read this chapter, try making these changes:

For yourself:

- Make it a goal to eat at least 3 servings of foods every day that are high in calcium, such as low- or nonfat milk or yogurt, green, leafy vegetables, or calcium-fortified tofu.
- Use the Internet to find the latitude of the city in which you live—then set a plan for how you will get enough vitamin D from exposure to sun or from food and supplements all year round.

For your community:

- Write a blog for your college newsletter outlining a safe plan for sun exposure to optimize synthesis of vitamin D without increasing sunburn or skin cancer risk.
- Volunteer at a local senior center or assisted living facility to support participation of older adults in outdoor activities.

fluorosis A condition, marked by staining and pitting of the teeth, caused by an abnormally high intake of fluoride.

UV SAFETY

THE GLOBAL SOLAR ULTRAVIOLET INDEX

UV INDEX

Be extra careful outdoors!
Lighter skin will burn in minutes without protection. Avoid exposure from 10:00 to 4:00 and shield skin and eyes.

11+ EXTREME

UV levels are dangerous.
A change in skin color means UV radiation has damaged your skin. White sand and water increase your UV exposure.

10 9 8 VERY HIGH

Sunburn can happen quickly.
Children are especially sensitive to UV exposure. Cover up, use sunscreen, and play in the shade.

7 6 HIGH

It may *seem* safe but...
Up to 80% of solar UV radiation can penetrate light cloud cover. Use UV-blocking sunglasses and protect your skin.

5 4 3 MODERATE

Always protect yourself from the sun.
Even with a low index rating, you can be overexposed. On a sunny day, snow reflects enough UV radiation to damage eyes and skin.

2 1 LOW

EPA United States
Environmental Protection
Agency

EPA430-H-04-001
May 2004

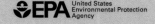

◆ **FIGURE 9.15** The Environmental Protection Agency is just one of many public health agencies that warn Americans about the danger of exposure to even low levels of sun.

Vitamin D Deficiency: Why the Surge, and What Can Be Done?

No doubt about it: unless you live at a latitude within 37° of the equator and spend time outdoors without sunscreen, it's tough to get enough vitamin D. That's because, as you learned in this chapter, there are very few natural food sources of vitamin D, and even fortified food sources are limited to milk and a handful of other products. But if meeting the Institute of Medicine's current RDA for vitamin D is already posing a challenge to many Americans, why are some researchers calling for an even higher intake recommendation?

Measurements of vitamin D status in a variety of population studies in recent years have led to a growing concern about widespread vitamin D deficiency and its associated diseases, including rickets in children and osteomalacia and osteoporosis in adults. Recent data from the National Health and Examination Survey (NHANES) indicate that, from 1994 to 2004, the prevalence of vitamin D deficiency in U.S. adults almost doubled, with over 90% of people with darker-pigmented skin (African Americans and Latinos) estimated to be vitamin D deficient.[35] In addition, since the Institute of Medicine set its vitamin D recommendations in 1997, new information has been published about vitamin D metabolism and its potential role in reducing the risks for diseases such as type 1 diabetes, some cancers, multiple sclerosis, and metabolic syndrome.[36,37] These discussions have resulted in a full review of the current research on vitamin D.[38]

First, what is contributing to the dramatic increase in vitamin D insufficiency among Americans, and what can we do about it? Researchers have proposed the following three causative factors:[37,39]

- A downward trend in the consumption of vitamin D–fortified milk products
- A significant increase in sun avoidance and the use of sun protection products, such as sunscreen
- An increased rate of obesity because obesity appears to alter the metabolism and storage of vitamin D such that vitamin D deficiency is more likely to occur

To address the first factor, people can increase their intake of vitamin D–fortified milk products; however, it is difficult to meet even the current RDA from consumption of milk alone. For instance, children and teens would have to drink a full quart each day to meet the recommendation![40] As a result, the use of vitamin D supplements is

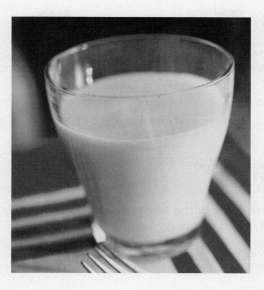

gaining wide support. Recently published clinical practice guidelines state that children and adolescents aged 1 to 18 years who are vitamin D deficient should be treated with 2,000 IU of vitamin D per day for at least 6 weeks, followed by a maintenance supplement of 600 to 1,000 IU per day.[38] Additionally, it is recommended that all adults who are vitamin D deficient should be treated with 6,000 IU of vitamin D per day for 8 weeks, followed by a maintenance supplement of 1,500 to 2,000 IU per day.[38] Supplementation with vitamin D is efficient, inexpensive, and effective. Used correctly, it is also very safe. Although vitamin D toxicity is rare, supplementation should be monitored to ensure both a safe and an adequate intake.

What about the second factor—lack of sufficient exposure to sunlight? Responsible, safe exposure to sunlight offers many advantages: it will never lead to vitamin D toxicity, it is easy and virtually cost-free, and sun exposure may offer benefits beyond that of improved vitamin D status.[41] That's why many healthcare professionals advocate moderate sun exposure. They suggest that public health authorities soften the "sun avoidance" campaigns of recent years (see **FIGURE 9.15**); they would like to see "well-balanced" recommendations that promote brief (15 minutes or so) periods of sun exposure without sunscreen or sun-blocking clothing two or three times a week, with avoidance of midday sun during summer months.[42]

To address the third factor in vitamin D deficiency—obesity—the only solution is to maintain a healthful weight. That means losing weight if you are overweight or obese. By doing so, you'll reduce your risk not only for vitamin D deficiency but also for cardiovascular disease, type 2 diabetes, and many forms of cancer.

Thus, although vitamin D deficiency is becoming a public health issue in the United States, there appear to be a number of strategies you can use to maintain a healthy vitamin D status.

CRITICAL THINKING QUESTIONS

1. Do you think you would benefit from vitamin D supplementation? Why or why not?
2. Would you prefer to try to increase your circulating levels of vitamin D through natural foods, fortified foods, supplements, or increased sun exposure? State your reasoning.

chapter **review**

test yourself | answers

1. **False.** There are many good sources of calcium besides milk, yogurt, and cheese, including calcium-fortified juices, soy milk, and other milk alternatives, as well as green, leafy vegetables, such as kale, broccoli, and collard greens.

2. **True.** When exposed to sunlight, our bodies can convert a cholesterol compound in our skin into vitamin D.

3. **False.** There is no clear, decisive evidence that consuming dairy products high in calcium, such as milk and yogurt, can result in weight loss.

MasteringNutrition™

Check out these additional resources in the MasteringNutrition Study Area at www.masteringhealthandnutrition.pearson.com:

- Read It: Chapter Summary and RSS Feeds
- See It: ABC News videos and nutrition animations
- Hear It: MP3s
- Study It: Get Ready for Nutrition Math and Chemistry review
- Do It: NutriTools and "Find the Quack" feature
- Review It: Quizzes, flashcards, and glossary

review questions

1. Which of the following statements about trabecular bone is true?
   a. It accounts for about 80% of our skeleton.
   b. It forms the core of almost all the bones of our skeleton.
   c. It is also called compact bone.
   d. It provides the scaffolding for cortical bone.

2. The process by which bone is formed through the action of osteoblasts and broken down through the action of osteoclasts is called
   a. resorption.
   b. remodeling.
   c. modeling.
   d. growth.

3. On a DXA test, a T-score of +1.0 indicates that the patient
   a. has osteoporosis.
   b. is at greater risk for fractures than an average, healthy 30-year-old.
   c. has normal bone density as compared to an average, healthy 30-year-old.
   d. has slightly lower bone density than an average, healthy person of the same age.

4. Calcium is necessary for several body functions, including
   a. demineralization of bone, nerve transmission, and immune responses.
   b. cartilage structure, nerve transmission, and muscle contraction.
   c. structure of bone, nerve, and muscle tissue; immune responses; and muscle contraction.
   d. structure of bone, nerve transmission, and muscle contraction.

5. Which of the following foods is rich in bioavailable calcium?
   a. broccoli
   b. spinach
   c. Swiss chard
   d. all of the above

6. Which of the following is a function of vitamin D?
   a. regulates the liver's reabsorption of calcium
   b. increases the activity of osteoclasts
   c. stimulates the release of parathyroid hormone (PTH) from the parathyroid glands
   d. stimulates the release of calcitonin by the thyroid gland

7. Which of the following individuals is most likely to require vitamin D supplements?

   a. a dark-skinned child living and playing outdoors in Hawaii

   b. a fair-skinned construction worker living in Florida

   c. a fair-skinned retired teacher living in a nursing home in Ohio

   d. None of the above individuals is likely to require vitamin D supplements.

8. Which of the following micronutrients assists in the production of osteocalcin?

   a. vitamin K

   b. phosphorus

   c. magnesium

   d. fluoride

9. True or false? Our bodies absorb vitamin D from sunlight.

10. True or false? Fluoride inhibits the reproduction of acid-producing bacteria in the mouth.

math review

11. Refer to the table in the Nutrition Label Activity (page 321) on calcium absorption rates for various food sources. How much broccoli would you need to consume to absorb the same amount of calcium as in 1 cup of skim milk?

Answers to Review Questions and Math Review are located at the back of this text and in the MasteringNutrition Study Area.

web resources

www.medlineplus.gov
MEDLINE Plus Health Information

Search for "rickets" or "osteomalacia" to learn more about these vitamin D–deficiency diseases.

www.ada.org
American Dental Association

Look under "Advocacy" and "Federal and State Issues" to learn more about the fluoridation of community water supplies and the use of fluoride-containing products.

ods.od.nih.gov
Office of Dietary Supplements, National Institutes of Health

Search for "calcium supplements" and "vitamin D supplements" to learn more about the supplementation in promoting bone health.

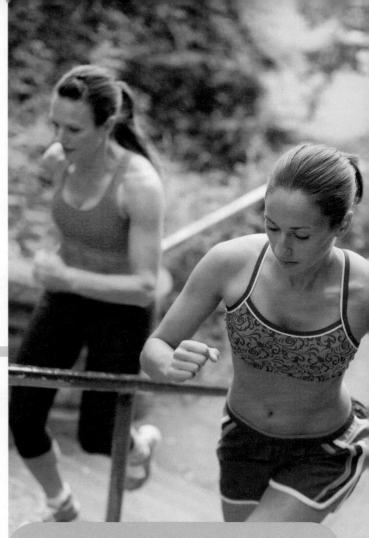

in depth
9.5

Osteoporosis

As a young woman, Erika Goodman leapt across the stage in leading roles with the Joffrey Ballet, one of the premier dance companies in the world. But at the age of 59, she died after falling in her Manhattan apartment. Goodman had a disease called *osteoporosis,* which means "porous bone." As noted previously (in Chapter 9), the less dense the bone, the more likely it is to break; in fact, osteoporosis can cause bones to break during even minor weight-bearing activities, such as carrying groceries. In advanced cases, bones in the hip and spine can fracture spontaneously, merely from the effort of holding the body erect.

In this **In Depth**, we'll take a closer look at the disease of osteoporosis. We'll explore its impact on a person's health and longevity and identify the factors that most significantly increase our risk. We'll also review what is currently known about the role of prescription medications in treating osteoporosis and identify other strategies for reducing your risk.

learning objectives

After studying this In Depth, you should be able to:

1 Define osteoporosis and discuss its impact on a person's health and longevity, p. 339.

2 Discuss the factors that influence our risk for osteoporosis, pp. 339–342.

3 Describe medical treatments and lifestyle changes used to manage osteoporosis, pp. 342–344.

4 Explain how we can prevent, or reduce our risks for, osteoporosis, pp. 344–345.

What is osteoporosis?

Of the many disorders associated with poor bone health, the most prevalent in the United States is **osteoporosis**, a disease characterized by low bone mass. The bone tissue of a person with osteoporosis deteriorates over time, becoming thinner and more porous than that of a person with healthy bone. These structural changes weaken the bone, leading to a significantly reduced ability of the bone to bear weight **(FIGURE 1)**. This greatly increases the person's risk for a fracture (a broken bone). In the United States, more than 2 million fractures each year are attributed to osteoporosis.[1]

Because the hip and the vertebrae of the spinal column are common sites of osteoporosis, it is not surprising that osteoporosis is the single most important cause of fractures of the hip and spine in older adults **(FIGURE 2)**. These fractures are extremely painful and can be debilitating, with many individuals requiring nursing home care. In addition, they increase the person's risk for infection and other related illnesses, which can lead to premature death. In fact, about 24% of adults 50 years and older who suffer a hip fracture die within 1 year after the fracture occurs, and because men are typically older at the time of fracture, death rates are higher for men than for women.[1,2]

Osteoporosis of the spine also causes a generalized loss of height and can be disfiguring and painful: gradual compression fractures in the vertebrae of the upper back lead to a shortening and hunching of the spine called *kyphosis*, commonly referred to as *dowager's hump* **(FIGURE 3**, page 340). The changes that kyphosis causes in the structure of the rib cage can impair breathing; moreover, back pain from collapsed or fractured vertebrae can be severe. However, especially in the early stages, osteoporosis can be a silent disease: the person may have no awareness of the condition until a fracture occurs.

Osteoporosis is a common disease: worldwide, one in three women and one in five men over the age of 50 are affected. In the United States, more than 10 million people have been diagnosed, and half of all women and one in four men over the age of 50 will suffer an osteoporosis-related fracture in their lifetime.[1,2]

What influences osteoporosis risk?

The factors that influence the risk for osteoporosis are age, gender, genetics, nutrition, and physical activity **(TABLE 1)**. Let's review these factors and identify lifestyle changes that reduce the risk for osteoporosis.

Aging Increases Osteoporosis Risk

Because bone density declines with age, low bone mass and osteoporosis are significant health concerns for older adults. The prevalence of osteoporosis and low bone mass are predicted to increase in the United States during the next 20 years, primarily because of increased longevity; as the U.S. population ages, more people will live long enough to suffer from osteoporosis.

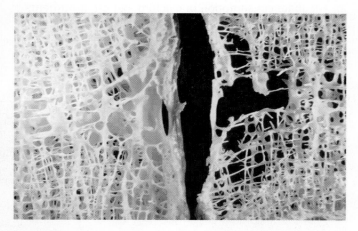

FIGURE 1 The vertebrae of a person with osteoporosis (right) are thinner and more collapsed than the vertebrae of a healthy person (left), in which the bone is more dense and uniform.

---

osteoporosis A disease characterized by low bone mass and deterioration of bone tissue, leading to increased bone fragility and fracture risk.

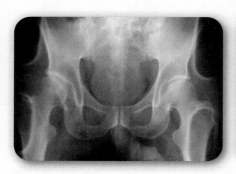

(a) Healthy hip bone

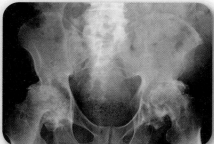

(b) Osteoporotic hip bone

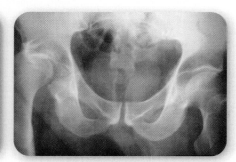

(c) Fractured hip bone

FIGURE 2 These x-rays reveal the progression of osteoporosis in hip bones. **(a)** Healthy bone. **(b)** A hip bone weakened by osteoporosis. **(c)** An osteoporotic bone that has fractured.

Hormonal changes that occur with aging have a significant impact on bone loss. Average bone loss is approximately 0.3–0.5% per year after 30 years of age; however, during menopause in women, levels of the hormone estrogen decrease dramatically and cause bone loss to increase to about 3% per year during the first 5 years of menopause. Both estrogen and testosterone play important roles in promoting the deposition of new bone and limiting the activity of osteoclasts. Thus, men can also suffer from osteoporosis, caused by age-related decreases in testosterone. In addition, reduced levels of physical activity in older people and a decreased ability to metabolize vitamin D with age exacerbate the hormone-related bone loss.

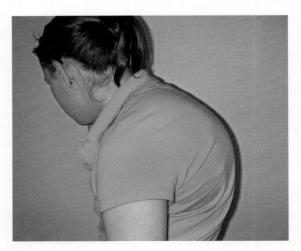

FIGURE 3 Gradual compression of the vertebrae in the upper back causes a shortening and rounding of the spine called *kyphosis*.

TABLE 1 Risk Factors for Osteoporosis

Modifiable Risk Factors	Nonmodifiable Risk Factors
Smoking	Older age (elderly)
Low body weight	Caucasian or Asian race
Low calcium intake	History of fractures as an adult
Low sun exposure	Family history of osteoporosis
Alcohol abuse	Gender (female)
History of amenorrhea (failure to menstruate) in women with inadequate nutrition	History of amenorrhea (failure to menstruate) in women with no recognizable cause
Estrogen deficiency (females)	
Testosterone deficiency (males)	
Repeated falls	
Sedentary lifestyle	

Data adapted from: "Osteoporosis: Evaluation and Treatment" in *Comprehensive Therapy*, Volume 26 (3), © November 3, 2000.

Gender and Genetics Affect Osteoporosis Risk

Approximately 80% of Americans with osteoporosis are women. There are three primary reasons for this:

- Women have a lower absolute bone density than men. From birth through puberty, bone mass is the same in girls as in boys. But during puberty, bone mass increases more in boys, probably because of their prolonged period of accelerated growth. This means that, when bone loss begins around age 40, women have less bone stored in their skeleton; thus, the loss of bone that occurs with aging causes osteoporosis sooner and to a greater extent in women.
- The hormonal changes that occur in men as they age do not have as dramatic an effect on bone density as those in women.
- On average, women live longer than men, and because risk increases with age, more elderly women suffer from this disease.

A secondary factor that is gender-specific is the social pressure on girls to be thin. Extreme dieting is particularly harmful in adolescence, when bone mass is building and an adequate consumption of calcium and other nutrients is critical. In many girls, weight loss causes both a loss of estrogen and reduced weight-bearing stress on the bones. In contrast, men experience pressure to "bulk up,"

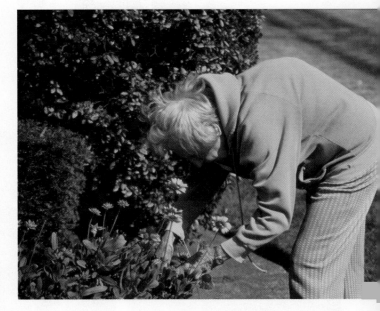

Approximately 80% of Americans with osteoporosis are women.

Think osteoporosis is just "an old woman's disease"? This video may change your mind: check out www.webmd.com. Type "osteoporosis prevention video" into the search bar, then click on the link to "Living with Osteoporosis-prevention videos."

typically by lifting weights. This puts healthful stress on the bones, resulting in increased density.

Some individuals have a family history of osteoporosis, which increases their risk for this disease. Particularly at risk are Caucasian women of low body weight who have a first-degree relative (such as a mother or sister) with osteoporosis. Asian women are at higher risk than other non-Caucasian groups. Although we cannot change our gender or genetics, we can modify the lifestyle factors that affect our risk for osteoporosis.

Tobacco, Alcohol, and Caffeine Influence Osteoporosis Risk

Cigarette smoking is known to decrease bone density because of its effects on the hormones that influence bone formation and resorption. For this reason, cigarette smoking increases the risk for osteoporosis and resulting fractures.

Chronic alcohol abuse is detrimental to bone health and is associated with high rates of fractures. In contrast, a meta-analysis of numerous research studies has shown that bone density is higher in people who are *moderate* drinkers.[3] Despite the fact that moderate alcohol intake may be protective for bone, the dangers of alcohol abuse for overall health warrant caution in considering any dietary recommendations. As is consistent with the alcohol intake recommendations related to heart disease, people should not start drinking if they are nondrinkers, and people who do drink should do so in moderation. That means no more than two drinks per day for men and one drink per day for women.

Some researchers consider excess caffeine consumption to be detrimental to bone health. Caffeine is known to increase calcium loss in the urine, at least over a brief period. Younger people are able to compensate for this calcium loss by increasing absorption of calcium from the intestine. However, older people are not always capable of compensating to the same degree. Although the findings have been inconsistent, recent research now indicates that the relative amounts of caffeine and calcium consumed are critical factors affecting bone health. In general, elderly women do not appear to be at risk for increased bone loss if they consume adequate amounts of calcium and moderate amounts of caffeine (equal to less than two cups of coffee, four cups of tea, or six 12-oz cans of caffeine-containing soft drinks per day).[4] Elderly women who consume high levels of caffeine (more than three cups of coffee per day) have much higher rates of bone loss than women with low intakes.[5] Thus, it appears important to bone health that we moderate our caffeine intake and consume an adequate amount of calcium.

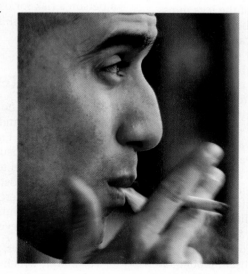
Smoking increases the risk for osteoporosis and resulting fractures.

Nutritional Factors Influence Osteoporosis Risk

In addition to their role in reducing the risk for heart disease and cancer, diets high in fruits and vegetables are also associated with improved bone health.[6,7] This is most likely due to the fact that fruits and vegetables are good sources of the nutrients that play a role in bone and collagen health, including magnesium, vitamin C, and vitamin K. The effects of protein, calcium, vitamin D, and sodium on bone health have been the subject of extensive research.

Protein

The effect of high dietary protein intake on bone health is controversial. High protein intakes have been shown to have both a negative and a positive impact on bone health. Although it is well established that high protein intakes increase calcium loss, protein is a critical component of bone tissue and is necessary for bone health. As with caffeine, the key to this mystery appears to be adequate calcium intake. In one study, older adults taking calcium and vitamin D supplements and eating higher-protein diets were able to significantly increase bone mass over a 3-year period, whereas those eating more protein and not taking supplements lost bone mass over the same time period.[8] Low protein intakes are also associated with bone loss and increased risk for osteoporosis and fractures in elderly people. Thus, it seems that adequate amounts of protein and calcium together support bone health.

Calcium and Vitamin D

Of the many nutrients that help maintain bone health, calcium and vitamin D have received the most attention for their role in the prevention of osteoporosis. It is clear that consuming adequate amounts of both nutrients in our diets is critical to optimize bone health because people who do not consume enough of these two nutrients over a prolonged period have a lower bone density and thus a higher risk for bone fractures. Whether taking calcium and vitamin D supplements is effective in preventing osteoporosis is somewhat controversial. Research studies conducted with older adults who are at increased risk for fractures have shown that taking calcium and vitamin D supplements reduces their risk of falls and subsequent fracture.[9] However, the evidence is less clear about the benefits of calcium and vitamin D supplementation in community-dwelling adults with no history of fractures.[9] Although a recent observational study has reported that women consuming up to 1,000 mg of calcium supplements per day and a higher dietary intake of calcium reduce their risk for premature death by about 22%,[10] there is emerging evidence that taking calcium supplements may increase a person's risk of a heart attack.[11,12]

Because bones reach peak density when people are young, it is very important that children and adolescents consume a high-quality diet that contains the proper balance of calcium, vitamin D, protein, and other nutrients to allow for optimal bone growth. Young adults also require a proper balance of these nutrients to maintain bone mass. In older adults, diets rich in calcium and vitamin D can help minimize bone loss.

Sodium

Higher intakes of sodium are known to increase the kidneys' excretion of calcium in the urine. One study found that diets moderately high in salt increased excretion of urinary calcium and had a negative impact on bone calcium balance in postmenopausal women, particularly when calcium intakes were low.[13] However, there is no direct evidence that a high-sodium diet causes osteoporosis. At this time, the Institute of Medicine states that there is insufficient evidence to warrant different calcium recommendations based on dietary salt intake.[14]

Regular Physical Activity Reduces Osteoporosis Risk

Regular exercise is highly protective against bone loss and osteoporosis. Athletes are consistently shown to have more dense bones than non-athletes, and regular participation in weight-bearing exercises (such as walking, jogging, skipping rope, tennis, and strength training) can help increase and maintain bone mass. When we exercise, our muscles contract and pull on our bones; this stresses bone tissue in a healthful way that stimulates increases in bone density. In addition, carrying weight during activities such as walking and jogging stresses the bones of the legs, hips, and lower back, resulting in a healthier bone mass in these areas. It appears that people of all ages can improve and maintain bone health through consistent physical activity.

Can exercise ever be detrimental to bone health? Yes, exercise can be harmful when the body is not receiving the nutrients it needs to rebuild the hydroxyapatite and collagen broken down in response to physical activity. Thus, active people who are chronically malnourished, including people who are impoverished and those who suffer from eating disorders, are at increased fracture risk. Research has confirmed this association among nutrition, physical activity, and bone loss in the *female athlete triad*, a potentially serious condition characterized by the coexistence of three (a *triad* of) clinical conditions in some physically active females: low energy availability (with or without eating disorders), menstrual dysfunction, and low bone density. In the female athlete triad, inadequate food intake and regular strenuous exercise together result in a state of severe energy drain that causes a multitude

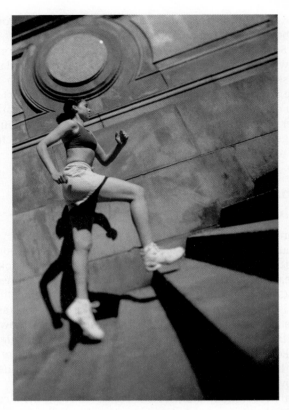

Regularly engaging in weight-bearing exercises, such as jogging, can help increase and maintain your bone mass.

of hormonal changes, including a reduction in estrogen production. Estrogen is important in maintaining healthy bone in women, so the loss of estrogen leads to low bone density and even osteoporosis in young women. The female athlete triad is discussed **In Depth** following chapter 11 (pages 429–439).

Now that we've identified the factors that influence a person's risk for osteoporosis, you may be wondering what your own risk is. If so, check out the **What About You?** feature box.

How is osteoporosis treated?

Although there is no cure for osteoporosis, a variety of lifestyle changes and medical therapies can slow and even reverse bone loss. First, individuals with osteoporosis are encouraged to consume a diet providing adequate calcium and vitamin D and to exercise regularly. Studies have shown that the most effective exercise programs include weight-bearing exercises, such as jogging, stair climbing, and resistance training.[15]

In addition, several medications are available:

- *Bisphosphonates*, such as alendronate (brand name Fosamax), which decrease bone loss and can increase bone density and reduce the risk for spinal and non-spinal fractures

what about **you** ?

Are You at Risk for Osteoporosis?

One in three women and one in five men will develop osteoporosis in their lifetime. But if you know you're at risk, you can take the steps identified in this **In Depth** chapter, such as increasing your amount of weight-bearing exercise and making sure you get enough calcium and vitamin D, to maintain the maximum amount of bone mass possible. That's why it's important to assess your risk. To the right is the International Osteoporosis Foundation's One-Minute Osteoporosis Risk Test. The more Yes answers you have, the greater the likelihood that you're in a higher-risk group than the general population.

If you answered Yes to any of these questions, it does not mean you have osteoporosis. Positive answers simply mean that you have clinically proven risk factors that may lead to osteoporosis and fractures. Discuss your results with your doctor, who can advise you on whether a fracture risk assessment and/or bone density test is recommended.

1. Has either of your parents been diagnosed with osteoporosis or broken a hip after a minor fall (a fall from standing height or less)?	Yes/No
2. Have you broken a bone after a minor fall as an adult?	Yes/No
3. Have you taken corticosteroid tablets (such as cortisone or prednisone) for more than 3 consecutive months?	Yes/No
4. After the age of 40, have you lost more than 3 cm (just over 1 in.) in height?	Yes/No
5. Do you regularly drink heavily (in excess of safe drinking limits)?	Yes/No
6. Do you currently, or have you ever, smoked cigarettes?	Yes/No
7. Do you suffer frequently from diarrhea (caused by problems such as celiac disease or Crohn's disease)?	Yes/No
For women:	
8. Did you undergo menopause before the age of 45?	Yes/No
9. Have your periods stopped for 12 months or more (other than because of pregnancy)?	Yes/No
For men:	
10. Have you ever suffered from impotence, lack of libido, or other symptoms related to low testosterone levels?	Yes/No

Data adapted from: *Are You at Risk of Osteoporosis? Take the One-Minute Osteoporosis Risk Test.* International Osteoporosis Foundation. 2013.

- *Selective estrogen receptor modulators*, such as raloxifene (brand name Evista), which have an estrogen-like effect on bone tissue, slowing the rate of bone loss and prompting some increase in bone mass
- *Calcitonin* (brand name Calcimar or Miacalcin), a pharmacologic preparation of the same thyroid hormone mentioned earlier, which can reduce the rate of bone loss
- *Hormone replacement therapy (HRT)*, which combines estrogen with a synthetic hormone called progestin, and can reduce bone loss, increase bone density, and reduce the risk for hip and spinal fractures

All of these drugs can prompt side effects. For example, bisphosphonates are associated with several gastrointestinal side effects, including abdominal pain, constipation, diarrhea, heartburn, irritation of the esophagus, and difficulty swallowing. Although there has been some evidence that long-term use of bisphosphonates may increase the risk for "atypical" fractures, two recent studies have found that these fractures are still quite rare and that the relative benefits of taking the medication outweigh the potential risks.[16,17] Side effects of HRT include breast tenderness, changes in mood, vaginal bleeding, and an increased risk for gallbladder disease.

The health benefits and risks of HRT are controversial based on current evidence. Until recently, it was believed that HRT protected women against heart disease. However, a landmark study published in 2002 found that one type of HRT actually increases a woman's risk for heart disease, stroke, and breast cancer.[18] The U.S. Preventive Services Task Force states that HRT does not affect one's risk for heart disease but increases the risk for stroke, blood clots in the legs, gallbladder disease, and urinary incontinence.[19]

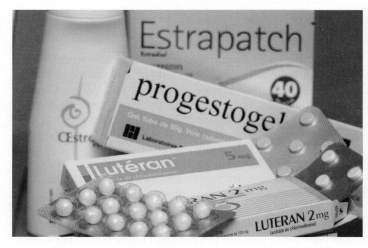

Hormone replacement medications come in a variety of forms.

343

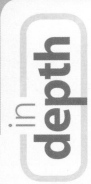

The type of HRT and the age and menopausal status of the woman appear to be important factors in affecting a person's risk of side effects; women over the age of 50 who are postmenopausal or who have had a hysterectomy (surgery to remove a woman's uterus) are advised against taking HRT to prevent chronic diseases.[19] As a result, hundreds of thousands of women in the United States have stopped taking HRT as a means to prevent or treat osteoporosis. However, HRT may still provide health benefits in managing symptoms of menopause and in women younger than 50 who have had a hysterectomy. Thus, women should work with their physician to discuss their individual circumstances and weigh these benefits against the increased risks for breast cancer, stroke, and heart disease when considering HRT as a treatment option for osteoporosis.

Can osteoporosis be prevented?

Although some risk factors for osteoporosis cannot be changed, such as age, gender, race, and family history, there is a great deal you can do to try to prevent osteoporosis.

Consider Supplements

Consuming adequate calcium and vitamin D throughout the life span is an essential first step. Now that so many products are fortified with these nutrients, from cereals and energy bars to orange juice and soy milk, it is not difficult for most people, even vegans, to get sufficient calcium and vitamin D from the diet. Still, small or inactive people who eat less to maintain a healthful weight may not be able to consume enough food to provide adequate amounts, and elderly people may need more than they can obtain in their normal diet. In these circumstances, supplements may be warranted; however, as already discussed, the benefits and risks of supplementation are controversial with more research needed in this area.

Calcium

Numerous calcium supplements are available to consumers, but which are best? Most supplements come in the form of calcium carbonate, calcium citrate, calcium lactate, or calcium phosphate. Our body is able to absorb about 30% of the calcium from these various forms. Calcium citrate malate, which is the form of calcium used in fortified juices, is slightly more absorbable, at 35%. Many antacids are also good sources of calcium, and it appears that they are safe to take, as long as you consume only enough to get the recommended level of calcium.

What is the most cost-effective form of calcium? In general, supplements that contain calcium carbonate tend to have more calcium per pill than other types. Thus, you are getting more calcium for your money when you buy

this type. However, be sure to read the label of any calcium supplement you are considering taking to determine just how much calcium it contains. Some very expensive calcium supplements do not contain a lot of calcium per pill, and you could be wasting your money.

The lead content of calcium supplements is an important public health concern. Those made from "natural" sources, such as oyster shell, bone meal, and dolomite, are known to be higher in lead, and some of these products can contain dangerously high levels. The Food and Drug Administration (FDA) has set an Upper Limit of 7.5 µg of lead per 1,000 mg calcium, but currently calcium supplements are not tested for lead content, and it is the manufacturer's responsibility to ensure that its supplements meet FDA standards. To avoid taking supplements that contain too much lead, look for supplements claiming to be lead-free, and make sure the word *purified* is on the label, in addition to the U.S. Pharmacopeia (USP) symbol.

If you decide to use a calcium supplement, how should you take it? Remember that the body cannot absorb more than 500 mg of calcium at one time. Thus, taking a supplement that contains 1,000 mg of calcium is no more effective than taking one that contains 500 mg. If at all possible, try to consume calcium supplements in small doses throughout the day. In addition, calcium is absorbed better with meals, because the calcium stays in the intestinal tract longer during a meal and more calcium can be absorbed.

By consuming foods high in calcium throughout the day, you can avoid the need for calcium supplements. But if you cannot consume enough calcium in your diet, many inexpensive, safe, and effective supplements are available. The best supplement for you is the one that you can tolerate and is affordable, lead-free, and readily available when you need it.

Vitamin D

Although an observational study in Canadian adults found no association between vitamin D supplementation and reduced risk for premature death, this study did not examine the impact of vitamin D on fracture risk.[10] A recent review study of twelve trials involving thousands of patients suggests that taking a daily vitamin D supplement reduces the risk for fractures in people age 65 and older.[20] The participants who took 482 to 770 IU per day of vitamin D cut their fracture risk by 18–20%. These effects weren't tied to participants also taking calcium supplements. So it seems that, at least for older adults, taking supplemental vitamin D is a smart preventive measure.

When it comes to vitamin D supplements, are some better than others? The Office of Dietary Supplements at the National Institutes of Health states that vitamin D_2 and D_3 appear to be equally effective in raising and maintaining blood levels of vitamin D.[21] Make sure the word *purified* is on the label, in addition to the U.S. Pharmacopeia (USP) symbol. Because vitamin D is a fat-soluble vitamin, it is important to stay below the UL of 4,000 IU (for adults) per day.

nutri-case | GUSTAVO

"When my wife, Antonia, fell and broke her hip, I was shocked. See, the same thing happened to her mother, but she was an old lady by then. Antonia's only 68, and she still seems young and beautiful—at least to me! As soon as she's better, her doctor wants to do some kind of scan to see how thick her bones are. But I don't think she has that disease everyone talks about. She's always watched her weight and keeps active with our kids and grandkids. It's true she likes her coffee and diet colas, and doesn't drink milk, but that's not enough to make a person's bones fall apart, is it?"

Take another look at Table 1 in this chapter. What risk factors do *not* apply to Antonia? What risk factors do? Given what Gustavo has said about his wife's nutrition and lifestyle, would you suggest he encourage her to have a bone density scan? Why or why not?

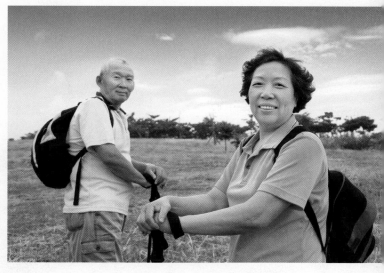

Because hiking requires your bones to bear your body weight plus the weight of your pack, it's a great form of exercise to reduce your risk for osteoporosis.

Other Preventive Measures

Another important strategy for preventing osteoporosis is engaging in regular physical activity throughout life. It's especially important to participate in weight-bearing activities. Examples include brisk walking, dancing, jogging, step-aerobics, hiking, tennis, tai chi, yoga, jumping rope, and resistance training. All of these activities help preserve bone density because they appropriately stress your bones and muscles.

It's also important to avoid becoming underweight. Remember Erika Goodman, the dancer we discussed at the beginning of this **In Depth** chapter? The factor that probably contributed most significantly to her early-onset osteoporosis was the drastic food restriction she practiced throughout her career. Appropriate body weight stresses the bones, and an adequate, balanced diet provides the nutrients to keep them healthy. In short, maintaining a healthy body weight is essential for preventing osteoporosis.

Other preventive measures include avoiding smoking and quitting if you are currently a smoker. It's also important to avoid alcohol abuse. Finally, increasing sun exposure safely will allow your body to synthesize adequate vitamin D and help prevent osteoporosis.

MasteringNutrition™

Check out these additional resources in the MasteringNutrition Study Area:

- Read It: Chapter Summary and RSS Feeds
- See It: ABC News videos and nutrition animations
- Hear It: MP3s
- Study It: Get Ready for Nutrition Math and Chemistry review
- Do It: NutriTools and "Find the Quack" feature
- Review It: Quizzes, flashcards, and glossary

web resources

www.nof.org
National Osteoporosis Foundation

Learn more about the causes, prevention, detection, and treatment of osteoporosis.

www.osteofound.org
International Osteoporosis Foundation

Find out more about this foundation and its mission to increase awareness and understanding of osteoporosis worldwide.

www.niams.nih.gov
National Institutes of Health: Osteoporosis and Related Bone Diseases—National Resource Center

Access this site for additional resources and information on metabolic bone diseases, including osteoporosis. Enter "bone health" into the search box, and then click on the top link to get started.

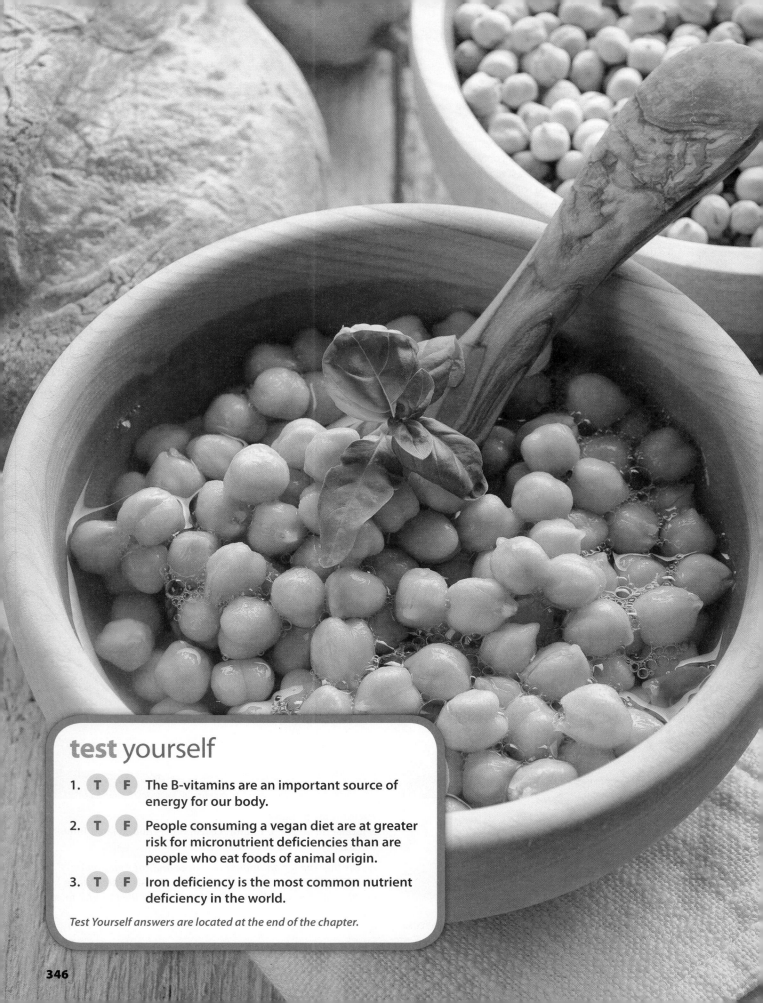

test yourself

1. **T** **F** The B-vitamins are an important source of energy for our body.

2. **T** **F** People consuming a vegan diet are at greater risk for micronutrient deficiencies than are people who eat foods of animal origin.

3. **T** **F** Iron deficiency is the most common nutrient deficiency in the world.

Test Yourself answers are located at the end of the chapter.

Nutrients Involved in Energy Metabolism and Blood Health

10

Dr. Bernstein looked in astonishment at the 80-year-old man in his office. A leading gastroenterologist and professor of medicine, he had admired Pop Katz for years as one of his most healthy patients, a vegan athlete who just weeks before had been going on 3-mile runs as if he were 40 years younger. Now he could barely stand. He was confused, cried easily, had wandered away from the house partially clothed, and had lost control of his bladder. Tests showed that he was not suffering from Alzheimer's disease, had not had a stroke, did not have a tumor or an infection, and had no evidence of exposure to pesticides, metals, drugs, or other toxins. Blood tests were normal, except that his red blood cells were slightly enlarged. Bernstein consulted with a neurologist, who diagnosed "rapidly progressive dementia of unknown origin."

Bernstein was unconvinced: "In a matter of weeks, a man who hadn't been sick for 80 years suddenly became demented. 'Holy smoke!' I thought, 'The man's been a vegetarian for 38 years. No meat. No fish. No eggs. No milk. He hasn't had any animal protein for decades. He has to be B_{12} deficient!'" Bernstein tested Katz's blood, then gave him an injection of B_{12}. The blood test confirmed that the level of B_{12} in Katz's blood was too low to measure. The morning after his injection, Katz could sit up without help. Within a week of treatment, he could read, play card games, and hold his own in conversations. Unfortunately, the delay in diagnosis left some permanent neurologic damage, including personality changes and an inability to concentrate.[1]

Continued next page

MasteringNutrition™
Go online for chapter quizzes, pre-tests, Interactive Activities, and more!

Continued—It was not until 1906—when the English biochemist F. G. Hopkins discovered what he called *accessory factors*—that scientists began to appreciate the many critical roles of micronutrients in maintaining human health. Vitamin B_{12}, for instance, was not isolated until 1948! In this chapter, we explore the micronutrients that contribute to the metabolism of carbohydrates, fats, and proteins and those that facilitate the formation and maintenance of our blood.

How do our bodies regulate energy metabolism?

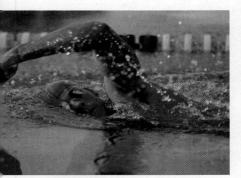

Several micronutrients we consume in our diet assist us in generating energy from the carbohydrates, fats, and proteins we eat along with them. Although vitamins and minerals do not directly provide energy, we are unable to generate energy from the macronutrients without them. The B-vitamins are particularly important in assisting us with energy metabolism. They include thiamin, riboflavin, vitamin B_6, niacin, folate, vitamin B_{12}, pantothenic acid, and biotin.

The primary role of the B-vitamins is to act as coenzymes. Recall that an *enzyme* is a protein that accelerates the rate of chemical reactions but is not used up or changed during the reaction. A **coenzyme** is a molecule that combines with an enzyme to activate it and help it do its job. **FIGURE 10.1** illustrates how coenzymes work. Without coenzymes, we would be unable to produce the energy necessary for sustaining life and supporting daily activities.

FIGURE 10.2 provides an overview of how some of the B-vitamins act as coenzymes to promote energy metabolism. For instance, thiamin is part of the coenzyme thiamin pyrophosphate, or TPP, which assists in the breakdown of glucose. Riboflavin is a part of two coenzymes, flavin mononucleotide (FMN) and flavin adenine dinucleotide (FAD), which help break down both glucose and fatty acids. The specific functions of each B-vitamin are described in detail shortly.

⬆ Vitamins do not provide energy directly, but the B-vitamins help our bodies create the energy we need from the foods we eat.

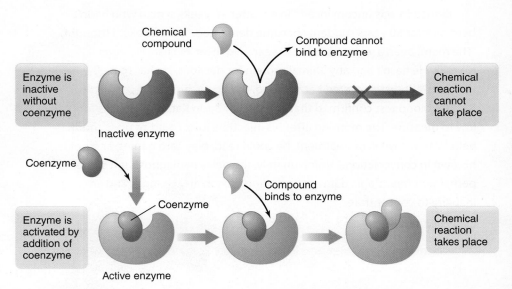

coenzyme A molecule that combines with an enzyme to activate it and help it do its job.

⬆ **FIGURE 10.1** Coenzymes combine with enzymes to activate them, ensuring that the chemical reactions that depend on these enzymes can occur.

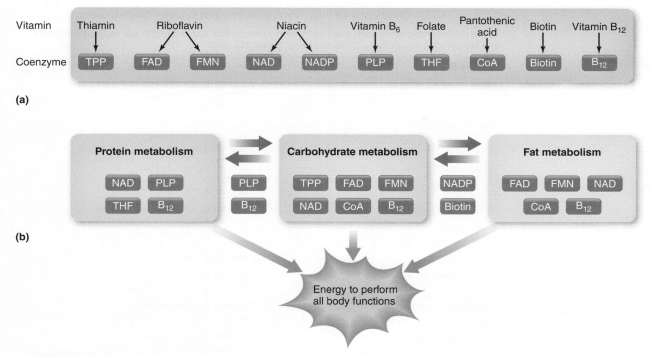

FIGURE 10.2 The B-vitamins play many important roles in the reactions involved in energy metabolism. **(a)** B-vitamins and the coenzymes they are a part of. **(b)** This chart illustrates many of the coenzymes essential for various metabolic functions; however, this is only a small sample of the thousands of roles that the B-vitamins serve in our body.

Some micronutrients promote energy metabolism by facilitating the transport of nutrients into the cells. For instance, the mineral chromium helps improve glucose uptake into cells. Other micronutrients assist in the production of hormones that regulate metabolic processes; the mineral iodine, for example, is necessary for the synthesis of thyroid hormones, which regulate our metabolic rate and promote growth and development. The details of these processes and their related nutrients are discussed in the following section.

recap Vitamins and minerals are not direct sources of energy, but they help generate energy from carbohydrates, fats, and proteins. Acting as coenzymes, nutrients such as the B-vitamins assist enzymes in metabolizing nutrients to produce energy. Minerals such as chromium and iodine assist with nutrient uptake into the cells and with regulating energy production and cell growth.

A profile of nutrients involved in energy metabolism

Thiamin (vitamin B_1), riboflavin (vitamin B_2), niacin (nicotinamide and nicotinic acid), vitamin B_6 (pyridoxine), folate (folic acid), vitamin B_{12} (cobalamin), pantothenic acid, and biotin are the nutrients identified as the B-vitamins. Other nutrients involved in energy metabolism include a vitamin-like substance called choline and the minerals iodine, chromium, manganese, and sulfur. In this section, we discuss the functions, food sources, toxicity, and deficiency symptoms for these vitamins and minerals. For a list of recommended intakes, see **TABLE 10.1**.

TABLE 10.1 **Overview of Nutrients Involved in Energy Metabolism**

To see the full profile of nutrients involved in energy metabolism, turn to Chapter 6.5, **In Depth,** Vitamins and Minerals: Micronutrients with Macro Powers (pages 224–233).

Nutrient	Recommended Intake
Thiamin (vitamin B_1)	RDA for 19 years and older: Women = 1.1 mg/day Men = 1.2 mg/day
Riboflavin (vitamin B_2)	RDA for 19 years and older: Women = 1.1 mg/day Men = 1.3 mg/day
Niacin (nicotinamide and nicotinic acid)	RDA for 19 years and older: Women = 14 mg/day Men = 16 mg/day
Vitamin B_6 (pyridoxine)	RDA for 19 to 50 years of age: Women and men = 1.3 mg/day RDA for 51 years and older: Women = 1.5 mg/day Men = 1.7 mg/day
Folate (folic acid)	RDA for 19 years and older: Women and men = 400 µg/day
Vitamin B_{12} (cobalamin)	RDA for 19 years and older: Women and men = 2.4 µg/day
Pantothenic acid	AI for 19 years and older: Women and men = 5 mg/day
Biotin	AI for 19 years and older: Women and men = 30 µg/day
Choline	AI for 19 years and older: Women = 425 mg/day Men = 550 mg/day
Iodine	RDA for 19 years and older: Women and men = 150 µg/day
Chromium	RDA for 19 to 50 years of age: Women = 25 µg/day Men = 35 µg/day RDA for 51 years and older: Women = 20 µg/day Men = 30 µg/day
Manganese	AI for 19 years and older: Women = 1.8 mg/day Men = 2.3 mg/day

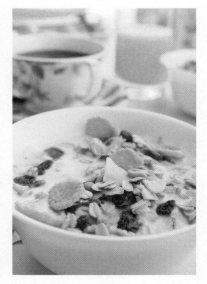

⬆ Ready-to-eat cereals are a good source of thiamin and other B-vitamins.

beriberi A disease of muscle wasting and nerve damage caused by thiamin deficiency.

Thiamin (Vitamin B_1)

Thiamin deficiency results in a disease called **beriberi**. The symptoms, which include paralysis of the lower limbs, have been described throughout recorded history. But it was not until the 19th century, when steam-powered mills began removing the outer shell of grains, especially rice, that the disease became widespread, especially in Southeast Asia. At the time, it was thought that milling grain improved the quality of the grain and made it more acceptable to consumers. What wasn't known was that the outer layer of the grain contained the highest concentrations of B-vitamins, especially thiamin.[2,3] Thus, most of the B-vitamins were being removed and discarded as the grain was milled or the rice polished. In 1884, Dr. Kanehiro Takaki, a Japanese naval surgeon, discovered that he could prevent beriberi by improving the quality of the diets of seamen. Then in 1890, Dr. Christiaan Eijkman, a Dutch physician living in Java, and his colleague, Dr. Gerrit Grijns, described how they could produce beriberi in chickens or pigeons by feeding them polished rice and could cure them by feeding back the rice bran that was removed during polishing.[3,4] In 1911, Polish chemist Casimir Funk was able to isolate the water-soluble nitrogen-containing compound in rice bran that was responsible for the cure. He referred to this compound as a "vital amine" and called it thiamin. Because it was the first B-vitamin discovered, it is designated vitamin B_1.[2]

Thiamin is part of the coenzyme thiamin pyrophosphate, or TPP. As a part of TPP, thiamin plays a critical role in the breakdown of glucose for energy and acts as a coenzyme in the metabolism of the essential amino acids leucine, isoleucine, and valine, also referred to as the *branched-chain amino acids*. These amino acids are metabolized primarily in the muscle and can be used to produce glucose if necessary. TPP also assists in producing DNA and RNA and plays a role in the synthesis of *neurotransmitters*, chemicals important in the transmission of messages throughout the nervous system.

Good food sources of thiamin include enriched cereals and grains, whole-grain products, wheat germ and yeast extracts, ready-to-eat cereals, ham and other pork products, organ meats of most animals, and some green vegetables, including peas, asparagus, and okra (**FIGURE 10.3**). Overall, whole grains are some of the best sources of thiamin, whereas more processed foods, such as refined sugars and fats, are the lowest sources. Unless milled grains are fortified (that is, the thiamin is added back), they are poor sources.

Because thiamin is involved in energy-generating processes, the symptoms of beriberi include a combination of fatigue, apathy, muscle weakness, and reduced cognitive function. The body's inability to metabolize energy or synthesize neurotransmitters also leads to muscle wasting, nerve damage, and the characteristic paralysis; in later stages, patients may be unable to move at all. The heart muscle may also be affected, and the patient may die of heart failure.

Beriberi is seen in countries where unenriched, processed grains are a primary food source; for instance, beriberi was widespread in China when rice was processed and refined, and it still occurs in refugee camps and other settlements dependent on poor-quality food supplies. Beriberi is also seen in industrialized countries in people with heavy alcohol consumption and limited food intake. Chronic alcohol abuse is associated with a host of neurologic symptoms, collectively called Wernicke-Korsakoff syndrome, in which thiamin intake is decreased and absorption and utilization impaired.[3] There are no known adverse effects from consuming excess amounts of thiamin; thus, the Institute of Medicine (IOM) has not been able to set a tolerable upper intake level (UL).[5]

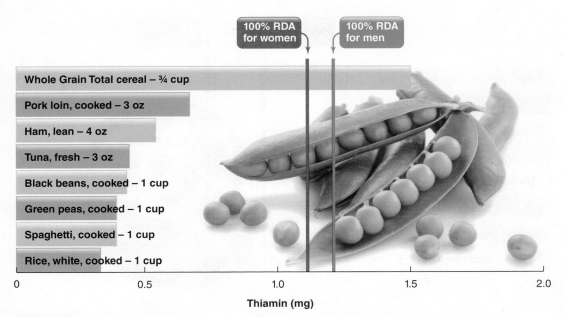

FIGURE 10.3 Common food sources of thiamin. The RDA for thiamin is 1.2 mg/day for men and 1.1 mg/day for women 19 years and older.

Data from: U.S. Department of Agriculture, Agricultural Research Service. 2011. USDA Nutrient Database for Standard Reference, Release 24.

Riboflavin (Vitamin B₂)

The theory that there might be more than one vitamin in rice bran was first proposed in the early 1900s after researchers noticed that rats fed diets of polished rice had poor growth.[4] Finally, in 1917 researchers found that there were at least two vitamins in the extracts of rice polishing, one that cured beriberi and another that stimulated growth. The latter substance was first called vitamin B₂ and then named riboflavin for its ribose-like side chain and the yellow color it produced in water (*flavus* means "yellow" in Latin).[6]

Riboflavin is an important component of coenzymes that are involved in chemical reactions occurring within the energy-producing metabolic pathways. These coenzymes, flavin mononucleotide (FMN) and flavin adenine dinucleotide (FAD), are involved in the metabolism of carbohydrates and fat. Riboflavin is also a part of the antioxidant enzyme glutathione peroxidase, thus assisting in the fight against oxidative damage.

Milk is a good source of riboflavin; however, riboflavin is destroyed when it is exposed to light. Thus, milk is generally stored in opaque containers to prevent the destruction of riboflavin. In the United States, meat and meat products, including poultry, fish, eggs, and milk and other dairy products, are the most significant sources of dietary riboflavin.[7] However, green vegetables, such as broccoli, asparagus, and spinach, are also good sources. Finally, although whole grains are relatively low in riboflavin, fortification and enrichment of grains have increased the intake of riboflavin from these sources, especially ready-to-eat cereals and energy bars, which can provide 25–100% of the Daily Value (DV) for riboflavin in 1 serving (**FIGURE 10.4**).

There are no known adverse effects from consuming excess amounts of riboflavin. Because coenzymes derived from riboflavin are so widely distributed in metabolism, riboflavin deficiency, referred to as **ariboflavinosis**, lacks the specificity seen with other vitamins. However, riboflavin deficiency can have profound effects on energy production, which result in "nondescript" symptoms such as fatigue and muscle weakness. More advanced riboflavin deficiency can result in lips that are dry and scaly, inflammation and ulcers of the mucous membranes of the mouth and throat, irritated patches on the skin, changes in the cornea, and anemia.[7] It is now known that cataract formation can be decreased by higher riboflavin intakes.[8] In addition, riboflavin is important in the metabolism of four other vitamins: folate, vitamin B₆,

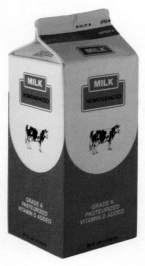

◄ Milk is a good source of riboflavin and is stored in opaque containers to prevent the destruction of riboflavin by light.

ariboflavinosis A condition caused by riboflavin deficiency.

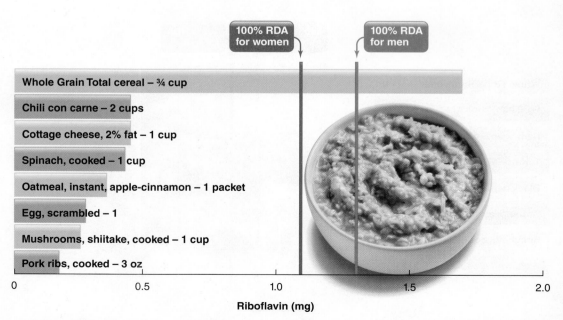

◄ **FIGURE 10.4** Common food sources of riboflavin. The RDA for riboflavin is 1.3 mg/day for men and 1.1 mg/day for women 19 years and older.

Data from: U.S. Department of Agriculture, Agricultural Research Service, 2011. USDA Nutrient Database for Standard Reference, Release 24.

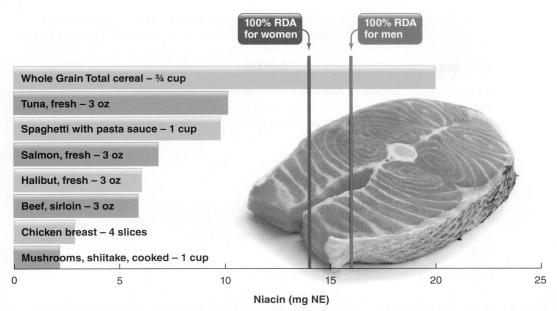

100% RDA for women

100% RDA for men

Whole Grain Total cereal – ¾ cup

Tuna, fresh – 3 oz

Spaghetti with pasta sauce – 1 cup

Salmon, fresh – 3 oz

Halibut, fresh – 3 oz

Beef, sirloin – 3 oz

Chicken breast – 4 slices

Mushrooms, shiitake, cooked – 1 cup

0   5   10   15   20   25

Niacin (mg NE)

◆ **FIGURE 10.5** Common food sources of niacin. The RDA for niacin is 16 mg niacin equivalents (NE)/day for men and 14 mg NE/day for women 19 years and older.
Data from: U.S. Department of Agriculture, Agricultural Research Service, 2011. USDA Nutrient Database for Standard Reference, Release 24.

vitamin K, and niacin.[9] Thus, a deficiency in riboflavin can affect a number of body systems.

Niacin

Pellagra, the deficiency of niacin, was first described in the 1700s in northern Spain but was also seen widely across the United States, Western and Eastern Europe, and the Middle East, where corn or maize was the dietary staple.[4] The term *pellagra* literally means "angry skin."[10] The four characteristic symptoms—dermatitis, diarrhea, dementia, and death—are referred to as the *four Ds*. Individuals who develop the disease first complain of inflammation and soreness in the mouth, followed by red, raw skin (dermatitis) on areas exposed to sunlight. The disease then progresses to the digestive and nervous systems. The symptoms of this stage of the disease are diarrhea, vomiting, and dementia. At the present time, pellagra is rarely seen in industrialized countries, except in cases of chronic alcoholism. Pellagra is still found in impoverished areas of some developing nations. (For more information on pellagra, see the **Nutrition Myth or Fact?** box, Chapter 1, page 5.)

Corn-based diets are low in niacin and the amino acid tryptophan, which can be converted to niacin in the body. The term *niacin* actually refers to two compounds, nicotinamide and nicotinic acid, which are converted to active coenzymes that assist in the metabolism of carbohydrates and fatty acids for energy. Niacin also plays an important role in DNA replication and repair and in the process of cell differentiation. Thus, it is not surprising that a deficiency of niacin can disrupt so many systems in the body.

Niacin is widely distributed in foods, with good sources being yeast, meats (including fish and poultry), cereals, legumes, and seeds **(FIGURE 10.5)**. Other foods such as milk, leafy vegetables, coffee, and some teas can also add appreciable amounts of niacin to the diet.[10,11] As with riboflavin, enriched or fortified breads, ready-to-eat cereals, and energy bars frequently provide 25–100% of the Daily Value for niacin.

Niacin can cause toxicity symptoms when taken in supplement form. These symptoms include *flushing*, which is defined as burning, tingling, and itching sensations accompanied by a reddened flush primarily on the face, arms, and chest. Liver damage, glucose intolerance, blurred vision, and edema of the eyes can be seen with very large doses of niacin taken over long periods.

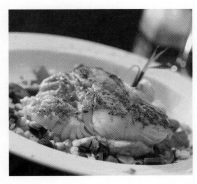

◆ Halibut is a good source of niacin.

pellagra A disease that results from severe niacin deficiency.

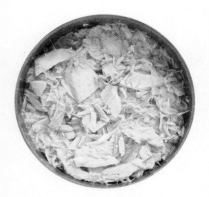

◀ Tuna is a good source of vitamin B_6.

homocysteine An amino acid that requires adequate levels of folate, vitamin B_6, and vitamin B_{12} for its metabolism. High levels of homocysteine in the blood are associated with an increased risk for vascular diseases, such as cardiovascular disease.

recap The B-vitamins include thiamin, riboflavin, niacin, vitamin B_6 (pyridoxine), folate, vitamin B_{12} (cobalamin), pantothenic acid, and biotin. Thiamin plays critical roles in the metabolism of glucose and the branched-chain amino acids. Whole grains are good sources. Thiamin-deficiency disease is called beriberi. Riboflavin is an important coenzyme involved in the metabolism of carbohydrates and fat. Milk, meats, and green vegetables are good sources. Riboflavin-deficiency disease is called ariboflavinosis. Niacin assists in the metabolism of carbohydrates and fatty acids. It also plays an important role in DNA replication and repair and in cell differentiation. Corn-based diets can be low in niacin and can result in the deficiency disease pellagra.

Vitamin B_6 (Pyridoxine)

Researchers discovered vitamin B_6 by ruling out a deficiency of other B-vitamins as the cause of a scaly dermatitis in rats.[4] They then discovered that B_6 deficiency was associated with convulsions in birds and later that infants fed formulas lacking B_6 also had convulsions and dermatitis.[12]

Functions of Vitamin B_6

The term *vitamin B_6* can actually refer to any of six related compounds: pyridoxine (PN), pyridoxal (PL), pyridoxamine (PM), and the phosphate forms of these three compounds. A coenzyme for more than 100 enzymes, vitamin B_6 is involved in many metabolic processes within the body, including the following:

- **Amino acid metabolism.** Vitamin B_6 is important for the metabolism of amino acids because it plays a critical role in transamination, which is a key process in making nonessential amino acids (see Chapter 6 for more details). Without adequate vitamin B_6, all amino acids become essential because our body cannot make them in sufficient quantities.
- **Neurotransmitter synthesis.** Vitamin B_6 is required for enzymes involved in the synthesis of several neurotransmitters, which is also a transamination process. Because of this, vitamin B_6 is important in cognitive function and normal brain activity. Abnormal brain waves have been observed in both infants and adults in vitamin B_6–deficient states.[13]
- **Carbohydrate metabolism.** Vitamin B_6 is required for an enzyme that breaks down stored glycogen to glucose. Thus, vitamin B_6 plays an important role in maintaining blood glucose during exercise. It is also important for the conversion of amino acids to glucose.
- **Heme synthesis.** Vitamin B_6 is necessary for the body to synthesize heme, a component of hemoglobin, the iron-containing protein that transports oxygen in our red blood cells. Chronic vitamin B_6 deficiency can lead to small red blood cells with inadequate amounts of hemoglobin.[13]
- **Immune function.** Vitamin B_6 plays a role in maintaining the health and activity of immune cells called lymphocytes and in producing adequate levels of antibodies in response to an immune challenge. The depression of immune function seen in vitamin B_6 deficiency may also be due to a reduction in the vitamin B_6–dependent enzymes involved in DNA synthesis.
- **Metabolism of other nutrients.** Vitamin B_6 also plays a role in the metabolism of other nutrients, including niacin and folate.[13]
- **Reduction in cardiovascular disease (CVD) risk.** Vitamin B_6, folate, and vitamin B_{12} are closely interrelated in some metabolic functions, including the metabolism of methionine, an essential amino acid. The body metabolizes methionine to another amino acid called **homocysteine**. In the presence of sufficient levels of vitamin B_6, homocysteine can then be converted to the nonessential amino acid cysteine **(FIGURE 10.6)**. In the presence of sufficient levels of folate and vitamin B_{12}, homocysteine can also be converted back to methionine if the body's level of methionine becomes deficient. If these nutrients are not available, these conversion reactions cannot occur and homocysteine will accumulate in the blood. High levels of homocysteine have been associated with an increased risk of cardiovascular disease and as a measure of poor dietary intakes of vitamin B_6, folate, and vitamin B_{12}.[14]

How Much Vitamin B_6 Should We Consume?

The recommended intakes for vitamin B_6 are listed in Table 10.1. Rich sources of vitamin B_6 are meats, fish, poultry, eggs, dairy products, and peanut butter (**FIGURE 10.7**). Many vegetables, such as asparagus, potatoes, and carrots; fruits, especially bananas; and whole-grain cereals are also good sources of vitamin B_6. As with the other B-vitamins discussed in this chapter, fortified or enriched grains, cereals, and energy bars can provide 25–100% of the Daily Value in 1 serving. Little vitamin B_6 is lost in the storage or handling of foods, except the milling of grains; however, vitamin B_6 is sensitive to both heat and light, so it can easily be lost in cooking.

Vitamin B_6 supplements have been used to treat conditions such as premenstrual syndrome (PMS) and carpal tunnel syndrome. You need to use caution, however, when using such supplements. Whereas consuming excess vitamin B_6 from food sources does not cause toxicity, excess B_6 from supplementing can result in nerve damage and lesions of the skin. A condition called *sensory neuropathy* (damage to the sensory nerves) has been documented in individuals taking high-dose B_6 supplements. The symptoms of sensory neuropathy include numbness and tingling involving the face, neck, hands, and feet, with difficulty manipulating objects and walking.

The symptoms of vitamin B_6 deficiency include anemia, convulsions, depression, confusion, and inflamed, irritated patches on the skin. As just discussed, deficiency of vitamin B_6 has also been associated with an increased risk for CVD. This also occurs with a deficiency of folate and vitamin B_{12}, as discussed in the next sections.

Folate

Reports of the symptoms we now recognize as folate deficiency go back two centuries.[15] By the late 1800s, a disorder associated with large red blood cells had been characterized, but it wasn't until the 1930s that researchers understood that the condition is related to diet. It took another 40 years before researchers more fully understood the relationship between this blood abnormality and a deficiency of folate, a substance found in many foods, especially leafy green vegetables. The name *folate* originated from the fact the vitamin is abundant in "foliage."[15]

FIGURE 10.6 The body metabolizes methionine, an essential amino acid, to homocysteine. Notice, however, that homocysteine can then be converted back to methionine through a vitamin B_{12}– and folate-dependent reaction or to cysteine through a vitamin B_6–dependent reaction. Cysteine is a nonessential amino acid important for making other biological compounds. Without these B-vitamins, blood levels of homocysteine can increase. High levels of homocysteine are a risk factor for cardiovascular disease.

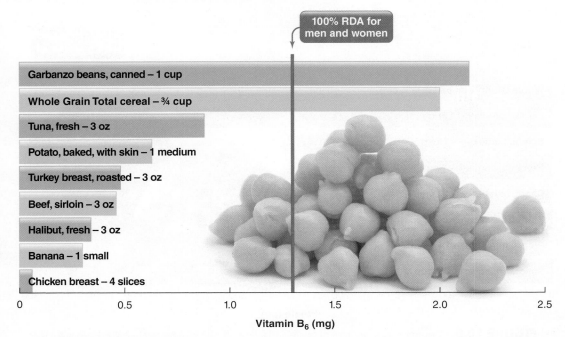

FIGURE 10.7 Common food sources of vitamin B_6. The RDA for vitamin B_6 is 1.3 mg/day for men and women 19–50 years.

Data from: U.S. Department of Agriculture, Agricultural Research Service, 2011. USDA Nutrient Database for Standard Reference, Release 24.

Functions of Folate

Folate-requiring reactions in the body are collectively called *1-C metabolism*. This means folate is involved in adding "one-carbon units" to other organic compounds during the synthesis of new compounds or the modification of existing ones. Thus, the most basic cellular functions require folate. The following are some of these functions:

- **Nucleotide synthesis.** Folate is required for the synthesis of nitrogen-containing compounds needed for DNA synthesis. For this reason folate is important for cell division. Adequate intake is especially critical during the first few weeks of pregnancy, when the combined sperm–egg cell multiplies rapidly to form the primitive tissues and structures of the human body. Folate continues to be important for tissue maintenance and repair throughout life. For example, low folate may predispose normal tissues to increased risk of transformation into cancer cells, whereas folate supplementation appears to suppress the development of tumors.[16]
- **Amino acid metabolism.** Folate is involved in the metabolism of many of the amino acids, including serine, glycine, histidine, and methionine. And as noted earlier, folate, vitamin B_{12}, and vitamin B_6 are required for the metabolism of methionine.
- **Red blood cell synthesis.** Without adequate folate, the synthesis of normal red blood cells is impaired.

How Much Folate Should We Consume?

The recommended intakes for folate are listed in Table 10.1 (page 350). The critical role of folate during the first few weeks of pregnancy and the fact that many women of childbearing age do not consume adequate amounts led to the mandatory fortification of enriched breads, flours, corn meals, rice, pasta, and other grain products with folic acid in 1998. Because of fortification, getting adequate folate in your diet is not difficult. The primary sources of folate in the American diet are ready-to-eat cereals, breads, and other grain products. Other good food sources include milk and eggs; oatmeal and whole grain foods; meats, especially liver; fruits, such as bananas, grapefruit, oranges, pears, pineapple, and strawberries; juices of these fruits; and vegetables, including asparagus, green beans, peas, beets, broccoli, cauliflower, corn, tomatoes, lentils, spinach, and romaine lettuce (**FIGURE 10.8**).

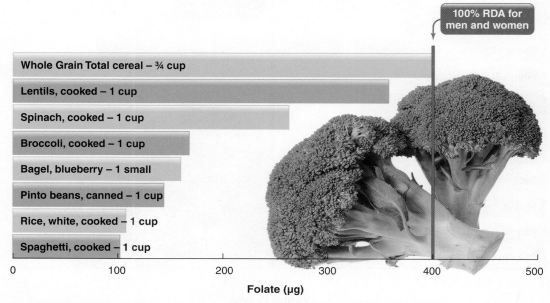

100% RDA for men and women

Whole Grain Total cereal – ¾ cup

Lentils, cooked – 1 cup

Spinach, cooked – 1 cup

Broccoli, cooked – 1 cup

Bagel, blueberry – 1 small

Pinto beans, canned – 1 cup

Rice, white, cooked – 1 cup

Spaghetti, cooked – 1 cup

0   100   200   300   400   500

Folate (μg)

FIGURE 10.8 Common food sources of folate and folic acid. The RDA for folate is 400 μg/day for men and women.

Data from: U.S. Department of Agriculture, Agricultural Research Service, 2011. USDA Nutrient Database for Standard Reference, Release 24.

HOT TOPIC

B₆ and Folic Acid for PMS? Think Twice!

An Internet search for treatments for premenstrual syndrome (PMS) is likely to elicit hundreds of ads for supplements, many of which contain 50 to 200 mg of vitamin B₆ and/or 400 μg of folic acid per capsule, with the recommendation to take at least two capsules per day. The UL of vitamin B₆ is 100 mg/day. Higher doses over time can cause neurologic disorders. The UL for folate is 1,000 μg per day. Higher doses can mask B₁₂ deficiency and may contribute to cancer, allergies, and other diseases.[18] Is there research to support consuming high levels of vitamin B₆ and folic acid for PMS?

A review of nine randomized clinical trials involving 940 subjects concluded that there is insufficient evidence to recommend using vitamin B₆ in the treatment of PMS.[19] One study showed that 58% of the individuals taking vitamin B₆ felt better, but so did 59% of those taking the placebo. Others showed improvement in certain symptoms of PMS, such as anxiety and food cravings, but not others. Finally, the level of treatment in the studies varied greatly, from just 50 mg/day of vitamin B₆ to 600 mg! However, one recent study did find that taking 80 mg/day of vitamin B₆ for 3 months reduced PMS symptoms.[20] As for folic acid, no studies have specifically examined its effect on PMS symptoms.

At this time, there is insufficient evidence to recommend vitamin B₆ or folic acid supplements for the treatment of PMS, especially at the high doses typically found in PMS supplements.

Because folate is sensitive to heat, it can be lost when foods are cooked. It can also leach out into cooking water, which may then be discarded.

What Happens If We Consume Too Much Folate?

There have been no studies suggesting toxic effects of consuming high amounts of folate in food; however, toxicity can occur when taking high amounts of supplemental folate.[17] One especially frustrating problem with folate toxicity is that it can mask a simultaneous vitamin B₁₂ deficiency. This often results in failure to detect the B₁₂ deficiency, and as you saw in the chapter-opening case, a delay in diagnosis of B₁₂ deficiency can contribute to severe damage to the nervous system. There do not appear to be any clear symptoms of folate toxicity independent from its interaction with vitamin B₁₂ deficiency.

What Happens If We Don't Consume Enough Folate?

Folate deficiency can cause many adverse health effects, the three most significant of which are discussed here.

Neural Tube Defects A woman's requirement for folate substantially increases during pregnancy. This is because of the high rates of cell reproduction needed for growth of the embryo and fetus, as well as enlargement of the uterus, development of the placenta, and expansion of the mother's red blood cells. Inadequate folate intake during pregnancy is associated with major birth defects.

Neural tube defects are the most common malformations of the central nervous system that occur during embryonic and fetal development. The neural tube is formed by the fourth week of pregnancy, and it eventually develops into the brain and the spinal cord of the fetus. In a folate-deficient environment, the tube will fail to fold and close properly. The resultant defect in the newborn depends on the degree of failure and can range from protrusion of the spinal cord outside of the spinal column to a partial absence of brain tissue. Some forms of neural tube defects are minor and can be surgically repaired, whereas other forms are fatal. (Neural tube defects are described in more detail in Chapter 14.)

The challenging aspect of neural tube defects is that they occur very early in a woman's pregnancy, almost always before she knows she is pregnant. Thus, adequate folate intake is extremely important for all sexually active women of childbearing age, whether or not they intend to become pregnant. To prevent neural tube defects, it is recommended that all women capable of becoming pregnant consume 400 μg of

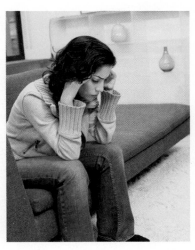

⬆ Headaches, anxiety, irritability, tension, and depression are common symptoms of PMS.

For a quick view of the importance of folic acid to the development of the neural tube, visit www.youtube.com. Enter "folic acid neural tube development" into the search bar; this takes you to a page with links to several related videos and animations.

neural tube defects The most common malformations of the central nervous system that occur during fetal development. A folate deficiency can cause neural tube defects.

folate daily from supplements or fortified foods, or both, in addition to the folate they consume in their standard diet.[5]

Vascular Disease and Homocysteine As noted earlier, folate, vitamin B_6, and vitamin B_{12} are necessary for the complete metabolism of the essential amino acid methionine. When intakes of these nutrients are insufficient, the blood level of homocysteine increases. High homocysteine levels have been associated with increased risk of heart attack and stroke.[21] The exact mechanism by which elevated homocysteine levels increase the risk for CVD is currently unknown. It has been speculated that homocysteine may damage the lining of blood vessels, prompting irregular vascular contractions and blood clotting abnormalities.[21] Thus, by consuming adequate amounts of vitamin B_6, folate, and vitamin B_{12}, we may decrease our risk for CVD, especially stroke. Although there is insufficient research to support a recommendation to consume B-vitamin supplements to reduce CVD risk, research does show that adequate levels of these B-vitamins are protective.[22,23]

Macrocytic Anemia The term *anemia* literally means "without blood"; it is used to refer to any condition in which hemoglobin levels are low. Some anemias are caused by genetic problems. For instance, *sickle cell anemia* is a genetic disorder in which the red blood cells have a sickle or "half-moon" shape. Another inherited anemia is *thalassemia,* a condition characterized by red blood cells that are small and short-lived. Other anemias are due to micronutrient deficiencies. These can be classified according to the general way they alter the size and shape of the red blood cells. Low iron, copper, and vitamin B_6 cause *microcytic anemia* (small red blood cells), whereas inadequate intakes of folate or vitamin B_{12} cause *macrocytic anemia* (large red blood cells) (**FIGURE 10.9**).

▶ FIGURE 10.9 Development of healthy red blood cells versus anemias. When folate or vitamin B_{12} is inadequate, macrocytic anemia develops because the red blood cells cannot mature and divide appropriately. When iron, copper, or vitamin B_6 is inadequate, microcytic anemia develops because there is not enough hemoglobin synthesis to make normal red blood cells.

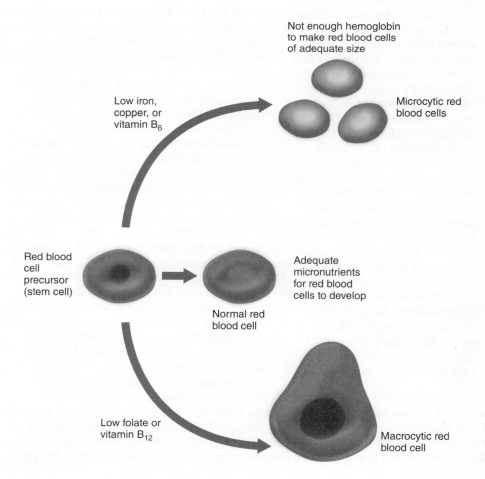

Deficiency of either folate or vitamin B_{12} can impair DNA synthesis, which decreases the ability of blood cells to divide. If they cannot divide, differentiate, and mature, the cells remain large and immature precursors to red blood cells, known as *megaloblasts* (from *megalo,* meaning "large," and *blast,* meaning "a precursor cell"). These immature cells contain inadequate hemoglobin; thus, their ability to transport oxygen is diminished. The resulting condition is sometimes referred to as *megaloblastic anemia* but is more commonly called **macrocytic anemia** (from *macro,* meaning "large," and *cyte,* meaning "cell"). Symptoms of macrocytic anemia are similar to those of other types of anemia, including weakness, fatigue, difficulty concentrating, irritability, headache, shortness of breath, and reduced exercise tolerance.

recap Vitamin B_6 is a coenzyme for more than 100 enzymes involved in processes such as the metabolism of amino acids and carbohydrates and the synthesis of neurotransmitters. It is widely found in animal-based foods and certain fruits and vegetables. The most basic cellular functions, such as the synthesis of DNA as well as cell differentiation, require folate. It is found in green leafy vegetables and is added to processed grain-based foods. Folate deficiency causes macrocytic anemia and can lead to neural tube defects in the developing fetus. Deficiency of vitamin B_6, folate, or vitamin B_{12} increase the risk for CVD.

Vitamin B_{12} (Cobalamin)

In 1855, a clinician named Thomas Addison described a strange form of anemia in patients that left them feeling weak and exhausted.[24,25] To our knowledge, this is the first report describing the often fatal course of vitamin B_{12} deficiency, later called **pernicious anemia** (the word *pernicious* means "causing great harm"). Several decades passed before an "animal protein factor" was associated with the cobalt-containing vitamin B_{12}. The first clinical experiments in humans were done by Drs. Minot and Murphy in the 1920s. They fed patients with pernicious anemia large doses of liver and documented the improvement in their red blood cells.[25] For this work they were awarded the Nobel Prize in 1934. This work was extended by others who identified that some special "extrinsic factor" in the liver or meat was combined with an "intrinsic factor" in the stomach. When both of these factors were present, patients with pernicious anemia recovered. The final step in the identification of vitamin B_{12} as the extrinsic factor and in determining its structure was done by Dr. Dorothy Crowfoot Hodgkin, who was awarded the Nobel Prize for Chemistry in 1964.[25]

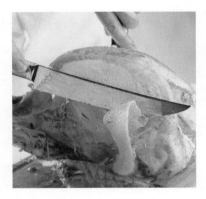

Turkey contains vitamin B_{12}.

Functions of Vitamin B_{12}

Vitamin B_{12} is part of coenzymes that assist with DNA synthesis, which is necessary for the proper formation of red blood cells. As noted earlier, adequate levels of folate, vitamin B_6, and vitamin B_{12} are also necessary to prevent the build-up of homocysteine and reduce the risk of CVD. Moreover, the metabolic pathway involved in the metabolism of methionine also converts folate to its active form, which is a vitamin B_{12}–dependent process. Without vitamin B_{12}, folate becomes "trapped" in an inactive form and folate deficiency symptoms develop, even though adequate amounts of folate may be present in the diet.

Vitamin B_{12} is also important for the metabolism of certain abnormal fatty acids. When vitamin B_{12} is deficient in the diet, these abnormal fatty acids accumulate in the blood and are incorporated into cell membranes, including those in the nervous system, where they cause neurologic problems. As you saw in the chapter-opening scenario, B_{12} also helps maintain the myelin sheath that coats nerve fibers. When this sheath is damaged or absent, the conduction of nervous signals is slowed, causing numerous neurologic problems.

How Much Vitamin B_{12} Should We Consume?

The recommended intakes for vitamin B_{12} are listed in Table 10.1. Vitamin B_{12} is found primarily in animal products, such as meats, fish, poultry, dairy products, and eggs, and in fortified cereal products, such as ready-to-eat cereals (**FIGURE 10.10**).

macrocytic anemia A form of anemia manifested as the production of larger than normal red blood cells containing insufficient hemoglobin, which inhibits adequate transport of oxygen; also called megaloblastic anemia. Macrocytic anemia can be caused by a severe folate deficiency.

pernicious anemia A form of anemia that is the primary cause of a vitamin B_{12} deficiency; occurs at the end stage of a disorder that causes the loss of certain cells in the stomach.

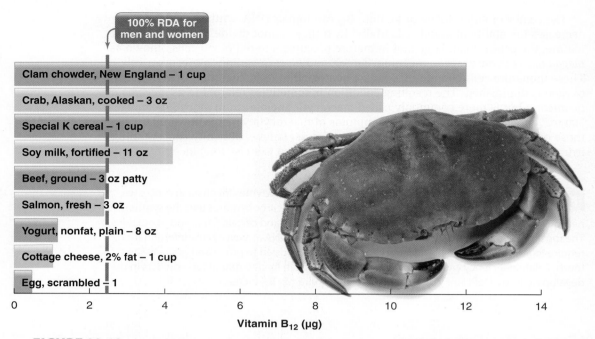

100% RDA for men and women

Clam chowder, New England – 1 cup
Crab, Alaskan, cooked – 3 oz
Special K cereal – 1 cup
Soy milk, fortified – 11 oz
Beef, ground – 3 oz patty
Salmon, fresh – 3 oz
Yogurt, nonfat, plain – 8 oz
Cottage cheese, 2% fat – 1 cup
Egg, scrambled – 1

Vitamin B$_{12}$ (µg)

↟ **FIGURE 10.10** Common food sources of vitamin B$_{12}$. The RDA for vitamin B$_{12}$ is 2.4 µg/day for men and women.

Data from: U.S. Department of Agriculture, Agricultural Research Service, 2011. USDA Nutrient Database for Standard Reference, Release 24.

Individuals consuming a vegan diet need to eat foods that are fortified with vitamin B$_{12}$ or take vitamin B$_{12}$ supplements or injections to ensure that they maintain adequate blood levels of this nutrient.

As we age, our sources of vitamin B$_{12}$ may need to change. People younger than 51 years are generally able to meet the RDA for vitamin B$_{12}$ by consuming it in foods. However, it is estimated that about 10–30% of adults older than 50 years have a condition referred to as **atrophic gastritis**, which results in low stomach acid secretion.[5] Because stomach acid separates food-bound vitamin B$_{12}$ from dietary proteins, if the acid content of the stomach is inadequate, then we cannot free up enough vitamin B$_{12}$ from food sources alone. Because atrophic gastritis can affect almost one-third of the older adult population, it is recommended that people older than 50 years of age consume foods fortified with vitamin B$_{12}$, take a vitamin B$_{12}$–containing supplement, or have periodic B$_{12}$ injections.

What Happens If We Consume Too Much Vitamin B$_{12}$?

There are no known adverse effects from consuming excess amounts of vitamin B$_{12}$ as either food or supplements.[5]

What Happens If We Don't Consume Enough Vitamin B$_{12}$?

The two primary causes of vitamin B$_{12}$ deficiency are insufficient intake and the inability to absorb the vitamin B$_{12}$ consumed. Insufficient vitamin B$_{12}$ intake typically occurs in people who follow a strict vegan diet and fail to take supplements or injections, or consume adequate amounts of fortified foods. The most common cause of malabsorption of vitamin B$_{12}$ is *pernicious anemia*, a condition arising from inadequate production of a protein called **intrinsic factor** that normally is secreted by certain cells in the stomach. Intrinsic factor binds to vitamin B$_{12}$ and aids its absorption in the small intestine. When not bound to intrinsic factor, vitamin B$_{12}$ is not recognized and absorbed by the enterocytes. Like atrophic gastritis, inadequate production of intrinsic factor occurs more commonly in older people. Individuals who lack intrinsic factor may receive periodic vitamin B$_{12}$ injections, thus bypassing the need for B$_{12}$ absorption in the intestines. Vitamin B$_{12}$ deficiency is also commonly seen in people with more generalized malabsorption disorders, such as celiac disease,

atrophic gastritis A condition that results in low stomach acid secretion; is estimated to occur in about 10–30% of adults older than 50 years.

intrinsic factor A protein secreted by cells of the stomach that binds to vitamin B$_{12}$ and aids its absorption in the small intestine.

as well as in people with tapeworm infestation of the gut because the worms take up the vitamin B_{12} before it can be absorbed by the intestines.

Symptoms of vitamin B_{12} deficiency, regardless of the cause, include pale skin, reduced energy and exercise tolerance, fatigue, and shortness of breath. In addition, because nerve cells are destroyed, patients with pernicious anemia lose the ability to perform coordinated movements and maintain their body's positioning. Central nervous system involvement can lead to irritability, confusion, depression, and even paranoia. As we saw in the case of Mr. Katz, after onset, such symptoms can only be partially reversed, even with prompt administration of vitamin B_{12} injections.

Pantothenic Acid

The path leading to the discovery of pantothenic acid was similar to that for the other water-soluble vitamins. First, researchers established that pantothenic acid was important for the growth of certain bacteria and yeasts. Then they identified it as important for growth and the prevention of dermatitis in chickens. Finally, it was identified as essential for other animals and humans. The vitamin was named after the Greek word meaning "from everywhere" because the vitamin is widespread in the food supply.[26]

Pantothenic acid is a component of an important coenzyme that is required for all the energy-producing metabolic pathways. It is especially important for the breakdown and synthesis of fatty acids within the body. Thus, pantothenic acid ensures that the foods we eat can be used for energy and that the excess energy we consume can be stored as fat.

The recommended intakes for pantothenic acid are listed in Table 10.1. Food sources include chicken, beef, egg yolks, potatoes, oat cereals, tomato products, whole grains, organ meats, and yeast **(FIGURE 10.11)**. There are no known adverse effects from consuming excess amounts of pantothenic acid. Deficiencies of pantothenic acid are very rare.

Biotin

Early in the 1900s, it was observed that rats could maintain normal growth while being fed a diet containing cooked egg whites as the sole source of protein. About the

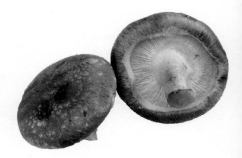

Shiitake mushrooms contain pantothenic acid.

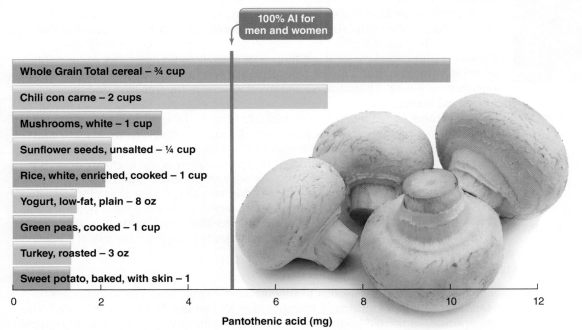

100% AI for men and women

- Whole Grain Total cereal – ¾ cup
- Chili con carne – 2 cups
- Mushrooms, white – 1 cup
- Sunflower seeds, unsalted – ¼ cup
- Rice, white, enriched, cooked – 1 cup
- Yogurt, low-fat, plain – 8 oz
- Green peas, cooked – 1 cup
- Turkey, roasted – 3 oz
- Sweet potato, baked, with skin – 1

Pantothenic acid (mg)

0   2   4   6   8   10   12

FIGURE 10.11 Common food sources of pantothenic acid. The AI for pantothenic acid is 5 mg/day for men and women.

Data from: U.S. Department of Agriculture, Agricultural Research Service. 2011. USDA Nutrient Database for Standard Reference, Release 24.

same time, other researchers observed that, if the egg whites were raw, rats developed diarrhea and skin problems.[4] The detrimental effects of feeding raw egg whites aroused great interest in the nutrition community. Could there be a toxic substance in raw egg whites that wasn't found in cooked egg whites? Experiments led to the discovery of biotin, a B-vitamin that prevented the diarrhea and skin problems that occurred when raw egg whites were fed to rats. Raw egg whites contain a protein called avidin, which binds biotin in the gastrointestinal (GI) tract and prevents its absorption.

Biotin is a coenzyme for five enzymes that are critical in the metabolism of carbohydrate, fat, and protein. It also plays an important role in gluconeogenesis. The recommended intakes for biotin are listed in Table 10.1. The biotin content has been determined for very few foods, and these values are not reported in food composition tables or dietary analysis programs. Biotin appears to be widespread in foods but is especially high in liver, egg yolks, and cooked cereals. Biotin is also produced by the GI flora, but its availability for absorption appears low.

There are no known adverse effects from consuming excess amounts of biotin. Biotin deficiencies are typically seen only in people who consume a large number of raw egg whites over long periods. Biotin deficiencies are also seen in people fed total parenteral nutrition (nutrients that are administered intravenously and bypass the gastrointestinal tract) that is not supplemented with biotin. Symptoms include thinning of hair; loss of hair color; development of a red, scaly rash around the eyes, nose, and mouth; depression; lethargy; and hallucinations.

recap Vitamin B$_{12}$ is essential for the metabolism of methionine and certain abnormal fatty acids. Deficiency leads to pernicious anemia, a type of macrocytic anemia, and nervous system damage. Low intakes of vitamin B$_6$, folate, and vitamin B$_{12}$ are associated with elevated blood homocysteine levels, which increase the risk for CVD. Pantothenic acid is especially important for the breakdown and synthesis of fatty acids, whereas biotin is a coenzyme for enzymes that are critical in the metabolism of carbohydrate, fat, and protein.

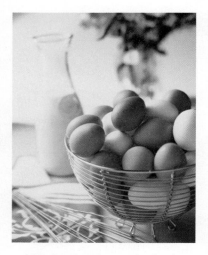

Choline is widespread in foods and can be found in eggs and milk.

Choline

Choline is a vitamin-like substance found in many foods. It is typically grouped with the B-vitamins because of its role in assisting homocysteine metabolism. Choline also accelerates the synthesis and release of **acetylcholine**, a neurotransmitter that is involved in many functions, including muscle movement and memory storage. Choline is also necessary for the synthesis of phospholipids and other components of cell membranes; thus, choline plays a critical role in the structural integrity of cell membranes. Finally, choline plays an important role in the transport and metabolism of fats and cholesterol.

The recommended intakes for choline are listed in Table 10.1. The choline content of foods is not typically reported in nutrient databases. However, we do know that choline is widespread in foods, especially milk, liver, eggs, and peanuts. Inadequate intakes of choline can lead to increased fat accumulation in the liver, which eventually leads to liver damage. Excessive intake of supplemental choline results in various toxicity symptoms, including a fishy body odor, vomiting, excess salivation, sweating, diarrhea, and low blood pressure. In addition, recent studies suggest a potential link between the digestion of choline (derived from lecithin) from consuming foods such as meat and egg yolks, and intestinal bacteria that may increase the risk of CVD.[27,28]

Iodine

Iodine is a trace mineral needed to support energy regulation. The heaviest metal required for human nutrition, it is responsible for just one function within the body, the synthesis of thyroid hormones.[29] Our body requires thyroid hormones to regulate body temperature, maintain resting metabolic rate, and support reproduction and growth. The form of iodine found in the earth's environment is predominantly inorganic iodide, whereas iodine, the oxidized form of iodide, is the form of the nutrient

acetylcholine A neurotransmitter that is involved in many functions, including muscle movement and memory storage.

most common in food. The iodine content of crops depends on the level of iodide in the soil. Iodide-deficient soils are common in mountainous areas and areas that have experienced frequent flooding. In general, the level naturally found in most foods and beverages is low.

Although our body needs relatively little iodine, adequate amounts are necessary to maintain health. The recommended intakes are listed in Table 10.1. Very few foods naturally contain iodine. Saltwater fish and shrimp tend to have higher amounts because marine animals concentrate iodine from seawater. Interestingly, iodine is added to dairy cattle feed and used in sanitizing solutions in the dairy industry, so milk and other dairy foods are an important source. In addition, iodized salt and white and whole-wheat breads made with iodized salt and bread conditioners are an important source of iodine. The United States began adding iodine to table salt in 1924. Today, a majority of households worldwide use iodized salt, and for many people, it is their only source of iodine. Approximately one-half teaspoon meets the full adult RDA for iodine. When you buy salt, look carefully at the package label because stores carry both iodized and non-iodized salt. Most specialty salts, such as kosher salt or sea salt, do not have iodine added. If iodine has been added to the salt, it will be clearly marked on the label.

Iodine toxicity, which generally occurs only with excessive supplementation, blocks the synthesis of thyroid hormones. As the thyroid attempts to produce more hormones, it may enlarge, a condition known as **goiter**. But because adequate levels of iodine are necessary for the synthesis of thyroid hormones, iodine deficiency also results in goiter. In fact, iodine deficiency is the primary cause of goiter worldwide. (Note that the term *goiter* refers only to the enlarged thyroid gland, regardless of its cause.)

A low level of circulating thyroid hormones is known as *hypothyroidism*. In addition to goiter, symptoms of hypothyroidism include decreased body temperature, inability to tolerate cold environmental temperatures, weight gain, fatigue, and sluggishness. If a woman experiences iodine deficiency during pregnancy, her infant has a high risk of being born with a form of mental impairment referred to as **cretinism**. In addition to mental impairment, these children may also suffer from stunted growth, deafness, and muteness. The World Health Organization (WHO) considers iodine deficiency the biggest single cause of preventable brain damage and mental retardation in the world.[30]

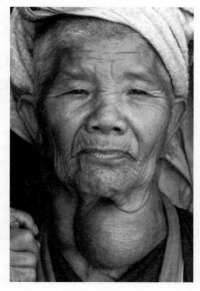

Goiter, or enlargement of the thyroid gland, most commonly develops as a result of iodine deficiency.

Chromium

Chromium is a trace mineral that plays an important role in carbohydrate metabolism. You may be interested to learn that the chromium in your body is the same metal used in the chrome plating for cars.

Chromium enhances the ability of insulin to transport glucose from the bloodstream into cells.[31] Chromium also plays important roles in the metabolism of RNA and DNA, in immune function, and in growth. Chromium supplements are marketed to reduce body fat and enhance muscle mass and have become popular with bodybuilders and other athletes interested in improving their body composition. The **Nutrition Myth or Fact?** box (page 364) investigates whether taking supplemental chromium is effective in improving body composition.

We have only very small amounts of chromium in our body. Whether the U.S. diet provides adequate chromium is controversial; our body appears to store less chromium as we age.

The recommended intakes for chromium are listed in Table 10.1. Foods that have been identified as good sources of chromium include mushrooms, prunes, dark chocolate, nuts, whole grains, cereals, asparagus, brewer's yeast, some beers, and red wine. Dairy products are typically poor sources of chromium.

There appears to be no toxicity related to consuming chromium naturally found in the diet or in most supplements. The chromium used for some industrial purposes can be toxic. Chromium deficiency appears to be uncommon in the United States. When induced in a research setting, chromium deficiency inhibits the uptake of glucose by the cells, causing a rise in blood glucose and insulin levels. Chromium deficiency can also result in elevated blood lipid levels and in damage to the brain and nervous system.

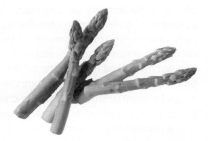

Our bodies contain very little chromium. Asparagus is a good dietary source of this trace mineral.

goiter Enlargement of the thyroid gland; can be caused by either iodine toxicity or deficiency.

cretinism A form of mental retardation that occurs in children whose mothers experienced iodine deficiency during pregnancy.

nutrition myth or fact?

Can Chromium Supplements Enhance Body Composition?

Because athletes are always looking for a competitive edge, a multitude of supplements are marketed and sold to enhance exercise performance and body composition. Chromium supplements, predominantly in the form of chromium picolinate, are popular with bodybuilders and weight lifters. This popularity stems from the claims that chromium increases muscle mass and muscle strength and decreases body fat.

An early study of chromium supplementation was promising in that chromium use in both untrained men and football players was found to decrease body fat and increase muscle mass.[32] These findings caused a surge in the popularity of chromium supplements and motivated many scientists across the United States to test the reproducibility of these early findings. The next study of chromium supplementation found no effects of chromium on muscle mass, body fat, or muscle strength.[33]

These contradictory reports led experts to closely examine the two studies and to design more sophisticated studies to assess the effect of chromium on body composition. There were a number of flaws in the methodology of these early studies. One major concern in the first study was that the chromium status of the research participants prior to the study was not measured or controlled.[32] It is possible that the participants were deficient in chromium; this deficiency could have caused a more positive reaction to chromium than would be expected in people with normal chromium status.

A second major concern was that body composition was measured in these studies using the skinfold technique, in which calipers are used to measure the thickness of the skin and fat at various sites on the body. Although this method gives a good general estimate of body fat in young, lean, healthy people, it is not sensitive to small changes in muscle mass. Thus,

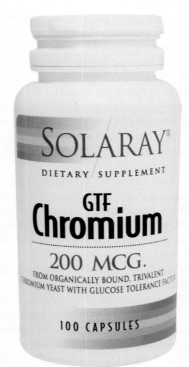

subsequent studies of chromium used more sophisticated methods of measuring body composition.

The results of research studies conducted over the past 15 years consistently show that chromium supplementation has no effect on muscle mass, body fat, or muscle strength in a variety of groups, including untrained college males and females, obese females, collegiate wrestlers, and older men and women.[34–41] Neither have scientists found an effect of chromium on body composition when different types of experimental designs have been used with varying energy intakes and exercise expenditures.[41,42]

Despite this overwhelming evidence to the contrary, many supplement companies still claim that chromium supplements enhance strength and muscle mass and reduce body fat.[43] These claims result in millions of dollars of sales of supplements to consumers each year. Before you decide to purchase a chromium supplement or a weight-loss product with chromium, read some of the studies cited here. The information they provide may help you avoid being one of the many consumers fooled by this costly nutrition myth.

CRITICAL THINKING QUESTIONS

1. If the science does not support using chromium for fat loss or changing body composition, why do you think supplement manufacturers still add chromium to their products?
2. Search the Internet for a weight-loss supplement with chromium. To whom is the product being marketed? Does the manufacturer cite any studies supporting the addition of chromium to the product?

Manganese

A trace mineral, manganese assists enzymes involved in energy metabolism and in the formation of urea, the primary component of urine. It also assists in the synthesis of the protein matrix found in bone tissue and in building cartilage, a tissue that supports joints. Manganese is also an integral component of superoxide dismutase, an antioxidant enzyme. Thus, manganese assists in the conversion of free radicals to less damaging substances, protecting our body from oxidative damage.

The recommended intakes for manganese are listed in Table 10.1. Manganese requirements are easily met because this mineral is widespread in foods and is readily available in a varied diet. Whole-grain foods, such as oat bran, wheat

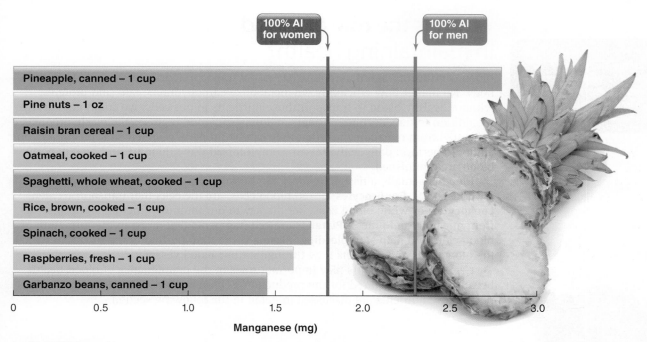

100% AI for women		100% AI for men

Pineapple, canned – 1 cup

Pine nuts – 1 oz

Raisin bran cereal – 1 cup

Oatmeal, cooked – 1 cup

Spaghetti, whole wheat, cooked – 1 cup

Rice, brown, cooked – 1 cup

Spinach, cooked – 1 cup

Raspberries, fresh – 1 cup

Garbanzo beans, canned – 1 cup

0   0.5   1.0   1.5   2.0   2.5   3.0

Manganese (mg)

🔶 **FIGURE 10.12** Common food sources of manganese. The AI for manganese is 2.3 mg/day for men and 1.8 mg/day for women.

Data from: U.S. Department of Agriculture, Agricultural Research Service, 2011. USDA Nutrient Database for Standard Reference, Release 24.

flour, whole-wheat spaghetti, and brown rice, are good sources of manganese **(FIGURE 10.12)**. Other good sources include pineapple, pine nuts, okra, spinach, and raspberries.

Manganese toxicity can occur in occupational environments in which people inhale manganese dust; it can also result from drinking water high in manganese. Toxicity results in impairment of the neuromuscular system, causing symptoms similar to those seen in Parkinson's disease, such as muscle spasms and tremors. Manganese deficiency is rare in humans. Symptoms of manganese deficiency include impaired growth and reproductive function, reduced bone density and impaired skeletal growth, impaired glucose and lipid metabolism, and skin rash.

Sulfur

Sulfur is a major mineral and a component of the B-vitamins thiamin and biotin. In addition, as part of the amino acids methionine and cysteine, sulfur helps stabilize the three-dimensional shapes of proteins. The liver requires sulfur to assist in the detoxification of alcohol and various drugs, and sulfur helps the body maintain acid–base balance.

The body is able to obtain ample amounts of sulfur from our consumption of protein-containing foods; as a result, there is no DRI specifically for sulfur. There are no known toxicity or deficiency symptoms associated with sulfur.

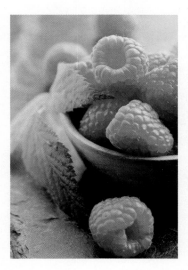

🔶 Raspberries are one of the many foods that contain manganese.

recap Choline is a vitamin-like substance that assists in homocysteine metabolism and the production of acetylcholine. Iodine is necessary for the synthesis of thyroid hormones, which regulate metabolic rate and body temperature. Chromium promotes glucose transport, metabolism of RNA and DNA, and immune function and growth. Manganese is involved in energy metabolism, urea formation, synthesis of bone and cartilage, and protection against free radicals. Sulfur is part of thiamin and biotin and the amino acids methionine and cysteine.

Watch a video of red blood cell production from the National Library of Medicine at www.medlineplus.gov. Search on "anatomy videos red blood cell production," then click on "Blood," and locate the video camera icon.

What is the role of blood in maintaining health?

Blood is critical to maintaining life because it transports virtually everything in our body. No matter how efficiently we metabolize carbohydrates, fats, and proteins, without healthy blood to transport those nutrients to our cells, we could not survive. In addition to transporting nutrients and oxygen, blood removes the waste products generated from metabolism so that they can be properly excreted. Our health and our ability to perform daily activities are compromised if the quantity and quality of our blood are diminished.

Blood is actually a tissue, the only fluid tissue in our body. It has four components (**FIGURE 10.13**). **Erythrocytes**, or red blood cells, are the cells that transport oxygen. **Leukocytes**, or white blood cells, are the key to our immune function and protect us from infection and illness. **Platelets** are cell fragments that assist in the formation of blood clots and help stop bleeding. **Plasma** is the fluid portion of the blood, in which the blood cells and platelets flow throughout our blood vessels.

Certain micronutrients play important roles in the maintenance of blood health because they are required for the production of proteins that regulate oxygen transport. These nutrients are discussed in detail in the following section.

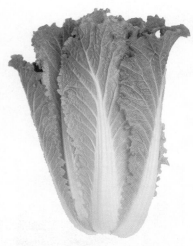

⬆ Green, leafy vegetables are a good source of vitamin K.

A profile of nutrients that maintain healthy blood

The nutrients recognized as playing a critical role in maintaining blood health are vitamin K, iron, zinc, and copper. Folate and vitamin B$_{12}$, as already discussed, are also essential for blood health. A list of recommended intakes of these nutrients is provided in **TABLE 10.2**.

Vitamin K

Vitamin K is a fat-soluble vitamin important for a number of metabolic functions, including bone and blood health.[44] It plays an important role in the synthesis of proteins involved in maintaining bone density (see Chapter 9). In addition, vitamin K acts

erythrocytes The red blood cells, which are the cells that transport oxygen in our blood.

leukocytes The white blood cells, which protect us from infection and illness.

platelets Cell fragments that assist in the formation of blood clots and help stop bleeding.

plasma The fluid portion of the blood; needed to maintain adequate blood volume so that the blood can flow easily throughout our body.

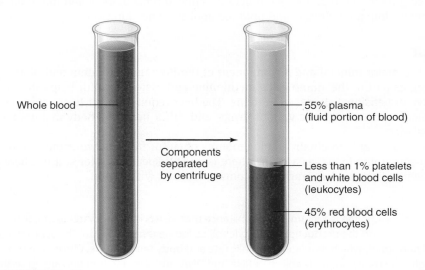

Whole blood

Components separated by centrifuge

55% plasma (fluid portion of blood)

Less than 1% platelets and white blood cells (leukocytes)

45% red blood cells (erythrocytes)

⬆ **FIGURE 10.13** Blood has four components, which are visible when the blood is drawn into a test tube and spun in a centrifuge. The bottom layer is the erythrocytes, or red blood cells. The milky layer above the erythrocytes contains the leukocytes and platelets. The yellow fluid on top is the plasma.

as a coenzyme that assists in the synthesis of a number of proteins that are involved in the coagulation (clotting) of blood, including *prothrombin* and several proteins called *procoagulants*, including *factors VII, IX,* and *X.* Without adequate vitamin K, blood does not clot properly: clotting time can be delayed or may even fail to occur. The failure of blood to clot can lead to increased bleeding from even minor wounds as well as internal hemorrhaging. More-over, research has revealed new roles for vitamin K in inflamma-tion, hormone regulation, and defense against cancer.[44]

Our need for vitamin K is relatively small, but intakes of this nutrient in the United States are highly variable because vitamin K is found in few foods.[44] Green, leafy vegetables contribute about 40–50% of our total vitamin K intake, followed by soybean and canola oils, which provide about 15% of our intake.[44] The recom-mended intakes for vitamin K are listed in Table 10.2. There is no upper limit (UL) established for vitamin K at this time.[31] Healthful intestinal bacteria produce vitamin K in our large intestine, pro-viding us with an important non-dietary source of vitamin K.

There are no known side effects associated with consuming large amounts of vitamin K from supplements or from food.[31] In the past, a synthetic form of vitamin K was used for therapeutic purposes and was shown to cause liver damage; this form is no longer used.

Vitamin K deficiency inhibits our ability to form blood clots, resulting in excessive bleeding and even severe hemorrhaging in some cases. Although vitamin K deficiency is rare in humans, people with diseases that cause malabsorption of fat, such as celiac disease, Crohn's disease, and cystic fibrosis, can suffer secondarily from a deficiency of vitamin K. Newborns are typically given an injection of vitamin K at birth because they lack the intestinal bacteria necessary to produce this nutrient.

The impact of vitamin K deficiency on bone health is controversial. Although a recent study found that poor intakes of vitamin K were associated with a higher risk for bone fractures in women, there is not enough scientific evidence to strongly illustrate that vitamin K deficiency causes osteoporosis or that supplementation will increase bone density.[31,44]

recap Blood is a fluid tissue composed of erythrocytes, leukocytes, plasma, and platelets. It transports nutrients and oxygen to our cells to support life and re-moves the waste products generated from metabolism. Vitamin K is a fat-soluble vitamin and coenzyme that is important for blood clotting and bone metabolism and may have other roles. Bacteria manufacture vitamin K in our large intestine.

Iron

Iron is essential to human survival, but it can be toxic in high doses. The body regulates iron levels within a narrow range that supplies adequate iron for essential biological processes without excess accumulation. Thus, iron is a trace mineral that is needed in very small amounts in our diets. Despite our relatively small need for iron, the World Health Organization lists iron deficiency as the most common nutrient deficiency in the world, including in industrialized countries.[45]

Functions of Iron

Iron is a component of numerous proteins in the body, including four primary iron-containing protein groups that carry out a number of important functions within the body. Two of these groups are oxygen-carrying proteins: hemoglobin and myoglobin. Almost two-thirds of all the iron in our body is found in **hemoglobin**, the oxygen-carrying protein in our red blood cells. As shown in **FIGURE 10.14**, the hemoglobin molecule consists of four polypeptide chains studded with four iron-containing

TABLE 10.2 Overview of Nutrients Essential to Blood Health

To see the full profile of nutrients essential to blood health, turn to Chapter 6.5, **In Depth,** Vitamins and Minerals: Micronutrients with Macro Powers (pages 224–233).

Nutrient	Recommended Intake (RDA or AI and UL)
Iron	RDA: Women 19 to 50 years = 18 mg/day Men 19 to 50 years = 8 mg/day UL = 45 mg/day
Zinc	RDA: Women 19 to 50 years = 8 mg/day Men 19 to 50 years =11 mg/day UL = 40 mg/day
Copper	RDA for all people 19 to 50 years = 90 µg/day UL = 10,000 µg/day
Vitamin K	AI: Women 19 to 50 years = 90 µg/day Men 19 to 50 years = 120 µg/day UL = none determined
Folate (folic acid)	RDA for all people 19 to 50 years = 400 µg/day UL = 1,000 µg/day
Vitamin B$_{12}$ (cobalamin)	RDA for all people 19 to 50 years = 2.4 µg/day UL = not determined (ND)

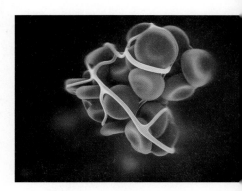

◄ Without enough vitamin K, our blood will not clot properly.

hemoglobin The oxygen-carrying protein found in our red blood cells; almost two-thirds of all the iron in our body is found in hemoglobin.

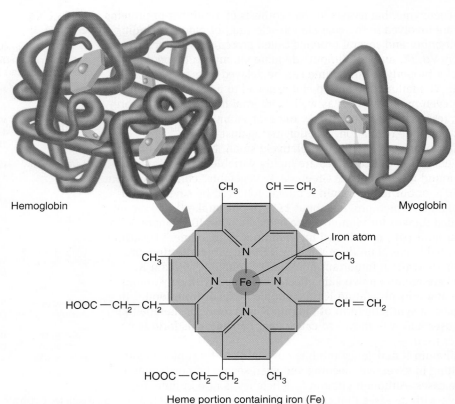

Heme portion containing iron (Fe)

FIGURE 10.14 Iron is contained in the heme portion of hemoglobin and myoglobin.

heme groups. You know that we cannot survive for more than a few minutes without oxygen. Thus, hemoglobin's ability to transport oxygen throughout the body is absolutely critical to life.

To transport oxygen, hemoglobin depends on the iron in its heme groups. Iron is able to bind with and release atoms such as oxygen, nitrogen, and sulfur very easily. It does this by transferring electrons to and from the other atoms as it moves between various oxidation states. In the bloodstream, iron acts as a shuttle, picking up oxygen from the environment, binding it during its transport in the bloodstream, and then dropping it off again in our tissues.

Iron is also a component of **myoglobin**, a protein similar to hemoglobin but found in muscle cells. As a part of myoglobin, iron assists in the transport of oxygen into muscle cells.

Iron is also found in a number of enzymes involved in energy production. Iron-requiring enzymes called *cytochromes* are electron carriers within the metabolic pathways that result in the production of energy from carbohydrates, fats, and proteins. In the mitochondria alone, there are more than twelve of these iron-requiring enzymes that help produce energy.[46] Iron is also critical to the function of certain enzymes important to some immune cells and their communication pathways; thus, iron is required for humans to mount an effective immune response to pathogens.[46] Finally, iron is a component of an antioxidant enzyme system that assists in fighting free radicals. Interestingly, excess iron can also act as a prooxidant and promote the production of free radicals.

Research over the last 30 years has also documented the importance of iron in neuromuscular functions. Like vitamin B_{12}, iron is required for maintenance of the myelin sheath covering nerve fibers; as noted earlier, without adequate myelin, conduction of nerve impulses is slowed. Iron is also needed for the production of neurotransmitters and for muscle function. Individuals who have poor iron status

heme The iron-containing molecule found in hemoglobin.

myoglobin An iron-containing protein similar to hemoglobin except that it is found in muscle cells.

complain of lethargy, apathy, and listlessness, which may be independent of iron's role in oxygen delivery. Some of these complaints might be due to the impact of iron deficiency on the brain or on fuel metabolism.

Iron Storage and Recycling

Our body contains relatively little iron; men have less than 4 g of iron in their body, while women have just over 2 g. Our body is capable of storing excess iron in two storage forms, **ferritin** and **hemosiderin**. The most common areas of iron storage in our body are the liver, bone marrow, intestinal mucosa, and spleen.

Because iron is so important for life, our body recycles the iron released from the breakdown of aging cells, especially cells high in iron, such as red blood cells. The liver and spleen are responsible for this iron-recycling program, which greatly reduces the body's reliance on dietary iron. Each day, about 85% of the iron released from hemoglobin breakdown is reused by the body.

How Is Iron Absorbed?

Our ability to absorb iron from the diet is influenced by the following factors.

Iron status. Typically, the amount of iron absorbed in the diet is low; however, if iron stores are low, absorption increases. Thus, people who have poor iron status, such as those with iron deficiency, pregnant women, and people who have recently experienced blood loss (including via menstruation), have the highest iron-absorption rates.

Stomach acid. Adequate amounts of stomach acid are necessary for iron absorption. People with low levels of stomach acid, including many older adults, have a decreased ability to absorb iron.

The amount of iron in the diet. The total amount of iron in your diet influences your absorption rate. People who consume low levels of dietary iron absorb more iron from their foods than those with higher dietary iron intakes. The body can also detect when iron stores are high; when this occurs, less iron is absorbed from food.

The type of iron in the diet. The type of iron in the foods you eat is a major factor influencing your iron absorption. Two types of iron are found in foods: heme iron and non-heme iron. **Heme iron** is a part of hemoglobin and myoglobin and is found only in animal-based foods, such as meat, fish, and poultry. **Non-heme iron** is the form of iron that is not a part of hemoglobin or myoglobin. It is found in both plant-based and animal-based foods. Heme iron is much more absorbable than non-heme iron. Since the iron in animal-based foods is about 40% heme iron and 60% non-heme iron, animal-based foods are good sources of absorbable iron. Meat, fish, and poultry also contain a special **meat factor**, which enhances the absorption of non-heme iron. In contrast, all of the iron found in plant-based foods is non-heme iron, and no absorption-enhancing factor is present. However, any vitamin C (ascorbic acid) in the food itself or in an accompanying food or beverage will enhance the absorption of non-heme iron.

Other dietary factors. Dietary factors that reduce iron absorption include phytates, polyphenols, vegetable proteins, and calcium. Phytates are found in legumes, rice, and whole grains. Polyphenols include tannins found in tea and coffee, and they are present in oregano and red wine. Soybean protein and calcium inhibit iron absorption. Because of the variability of iron absorption as a result of these dietary factors, it is estimated that the bioavailability of iron from a vegan diet is approximately 1–10%, whereas it averages 18% for a mixed Western diet.[47]

How Much Iron Should We Consume?

The range of iron availability from food sources was taken into consideration when estimating dietary recommendations for iron, which are listed in Table 10.2. Notice that the higher iron requirement for younger women is due to the excess iron and blood lost during menstruation. See the **You Do the Math** box (page 370) to learn how to calculate your iron intake.

A number of special circumstances can significantly affect iron requirements. These are identified in **TABLE 10.3**.

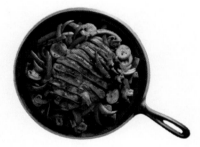

Cooking foods in cast-iron pans significantly increases their iron content.

ferritin A storage form of iron in our body, found primarily in the intestinal mucosa, spleen, bone marrow, and liver.

hemosiderin A storage form of iron in our body, found primarily in the intestinal mucosa, spleen, bone marrow, and liver.

heme iron Iron that is a part of hemoglobin and myoglobin; found only in animal-based foods, such as meat, fish, and poultry.

non-heme iron The form of iron that is not a part of hemoglobin or myoglobin; found in animal- and plant-based foods.

meat factor A special factor found in meat, fish, and poultry that enhances the absorption of non-heme iron.

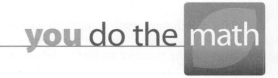

Calculating Daily Iron Intake

Determining whether or not you're getting the iron your body needs each day can be tricky because the amount you consume may not be the amount that is absorbed. Food combinations, fortified foods, and supplements all make a difference. Determine the amount of iron available for absorption in the following food choices for one day for Hannah, who is menstruating normally:

Foods with heme iron (15% available):

- Turkey, light meat (3 oz): 1.1 mg
- Tuna, light canned (3 oz): 1.3 mg

Foods with non-heme iron (5% available):

- Oatmeal, 1 instant packet: 11 mg
- Spinach, 1 cup raw: 6.4 mg
- Bread, whole wheat 2 slices: 1.4 mg

Multivitamin/mineral supplement with 18 mg of Fe (5% available). This is the amount of iron in a typical 1-day multivitamin/mineral supplement designed for menstruating women.

What is the total available iron for absorption (mg/d)? Does it cover the amount of iron lost each day? If Hannah were not taking a daily supplement, would she still be getting adequate iron?

Answers can be found in the MasteringNutrition Study Area.

TABLE 10.3 Special Circumstances Affecting Iron Status

Circumstances That Improve Iron Status	Circumstances That Diminish Iron Status
• Use of oral contraceptives—reduces menstrual blood loss in women. • Breastfeeding—delays resumption of menstruation in new mothers and thereby reduces menstrual blood loss. It is therefore an important health measure, especially in developing nations. • Consumption of iron-containing foods and supplements.	• Use of hormone replacement therapy—can cause uterine bleeding. • Eating a vegetarian diet—reduces or eliminates sources of heme iron. • Intestinal parasitic infection—causes intestinal bleeding. Iron-deficiency anemia is common in people with intestinal parasitic infection. • Blood donation—reduces iron stores; people who donate frequently, particularly premenopausal women, may require iron supplementation. • Intense endurance exercise training—appears to increase risk for poor iron status because of many factors, including inflammation, suboptimal iron intake, increased iron loss due to rupture of red blood cells, and losses in sweat and feces.

Data from: Dietary Reference Intakes for Vitamin A, Vitamin K, Arsenic, Boron, Chromium, Copper, Iodine, Manganese, Molybdenum, Nickel, Silicon, Vanadium, and Zinc © 2002 by the National Academy of Sciences, National Academies Press.

Finding Iron-Rich Foods

Good food sources of heme iron are meats, poultry, and fish **(FIGURE 10.15)**. Clams, oysters, and beef liver are particularly good sources. Many breakfast cereals and breads are enriched with iron; although this iron is the non-heme type and less absorbable, it is still significant because these foods are a major part of the U.S. diet. Some vegetables and legumes are also good sources of iron, and the absorption of their non-heme iron can be enhanced by eating them with even a small amount of meat, fish, or poultry, or with vitamin C–rich foods, such as citrus foods, red and green peppers, and broccoli.

Another way to increase your iron intake is to make smart menu choices throughout the day. See the **Quick Tips** feature for more iron food sources. The **Eating Right All Day** feature (page 372) shows menu choices high in iron. Some of these choices provide heme iron, whereas others are combination foods. For instance, the orange juice helps improve the absorption of the non-heme iron in the enriched bread.

What Happens If We Consume Too Much Iron?

Accidental iron overdose is the most common cause of poisoning deaths in children younger than 6 years of age in the United States.[48] It is important for parents to take

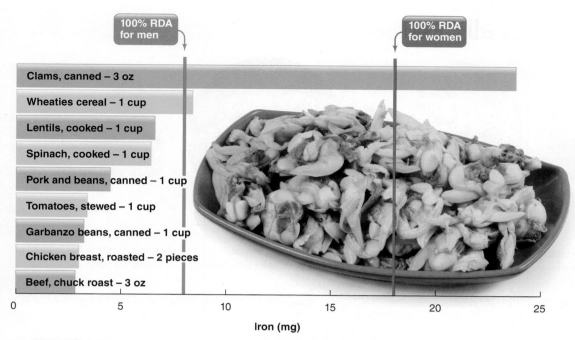

100% RDA for men

100% RDA for women

Clams, canned – 3 oz

Wheaties cereal – 1 cup

Lentils, cooked – 1 cup

Spinach, cooked – 1 cup

Pork and beans, canned – 1 cup

Tomatoes, stewed – 1 cup

Garbanzo beans, canned – 1 cup

Chicken breast, roasted – 2 pieces

Beef, chuck roast – 3 oz

0   5   10   15   20   25

Iron (mg)

⬆ **FIGURE 10.15**   Common food sources of iron. The RDA for iron is 8 mg/day for men and 18 mg/day for women aged 19 to 50 years.

Data from: U.S. Department of Agriculture, Agricultural Research Service, 2011. USDA Nutrient Database for Standard Reference, Release 24.

the same precautions with dietary supplements as they would with other drugs, keeping them in a locked cabinet or well out of reach of children. Symptoms of iron toxicity include nausea, vomiting, diarrhea, dizziness, confusion, and rapid heartbeat. If iron toxicity is not treated quickly, significant damage to the heart, central nervous system, liver, and kidneys can result in death.

QuickTips

Increasing Your Iron Intake

✅ Shop for iron-fortified breads and breakfast cereals. Check the Nutrition Facts panel!

✅ Consume a food or beverage that is high in vitamin C along with plant or animal sources of iron. For instance, drink a glass of orange juice with your morning toast to increase the absorption of the non-heme iron in the bread. Or add chopped tomatoes to beans or lentils. Or sprinkle lemon juice on fish.

✅ Add small amounts of meat, poultry, or fish to baked beans, vegetable soups, stir-fried vegetables, or salads to enhance the absorption of the non-heme iron in the plant-based foods.

✅ Cook foods in cast-iron pans to significantly increase their iron content. The iron in the pan will be absorbed into the food during the cooking process.

✅ Avoid drinking red wine, coffee, or tea when eating iron-rich foods because the polyphenols in these beverages will reduce iron absorption.

✅ Avoid drinking cow's milk or soy milk with iron-rich foods because both calcium and soybean protein inhibit iron absorption.

✅ Avoid taking calcium supplements or zinc supplements with iron-rich foods because these minerals decrease iron absorption.

eating right all day

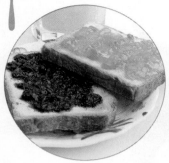

Breakfast
Whole-grain iron-fortified toast with orange juice instead of white toast with coffee!

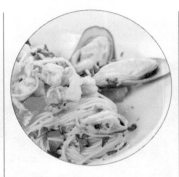

Lunch
Pasta with clams and tomatoes instead of mac & cheese!

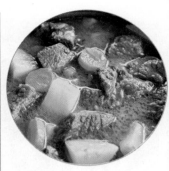

Dinner
Beef stew with vegetables instead of burgers with fries!

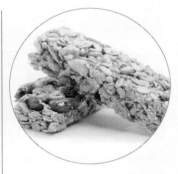

Snack
Low-cal nutrition bar instead of a chocolate bar!

Adults who take iron supplements even at prescribed doses commonly experience constipation and gastrointestinal distress, such as nausea, vomiting, and diarrhea.[31] Taking iron supplements with food can reduce these adverse effects in most, but not all, people.

Some people suffer from a hereditary disorder called hemochromatosis. This disorder affects as many as 1 in 200 individuals, mostly of northern European origin.[49] Hemochromatosis is characterized by excessive absorption of dietary iron and altered iron storage. Because the body has no mechanism for eliminating excess iron from the body, iron accumulates in body tissues over many years, causing organ damage and other diseases. Men are more at risk for this disease than women, who have higher losses of iron because of menstruation. Treatment includes reducing dietary intake of iron, avoiding high intakes of vitamin C, and occasionally withdrawing blood.

What Happens If We Don't Consume Enough Iron?

Iron deficiency is the most common nutrient deficiency in the world. People at particularly high risk for iron deficiency include infants and young children, adolescent girls, menstruating women, and pregnant women.

Iron deficiency progresses through three stages (**FIGURE 10.16**). The first stage, called iron depletion, is caused by a depletion of iron *stores*, resulting in reduced levels of ferritin in the blood. As discussed earlier, ferritin is one form of stored iron. Small amounts of ferritin circulate in the blood, and these concentrations are highly correlated with iron stores. During this first stage, there are generally no physical symptoms because hemoglobin levels are not yet affected. The second stage, called iron-deficiency erythropoiesis (meaning production of red blood cells), causes a decrease in the *transport* of iron. This manifests as a reduction in the transport protein for iron, called **transferrin**. The production of heme also starts to decline during this stage, leading to symptoms of reduced work capacity. During the third and final stage, **iron-deficiency anemia** results.

In iron-deficiency anemia, the production of normal, healthy red blood cells decreases. Red blood cells that are produced are smaller than normal and do not contain enough hemoglobin to transport adequate oxygen or to allow the proper transfer of electrons to produce energy. This type of anemia is often referred to as *microcytic anemia* (*micro*, meaning "small," and *cyte*, meaning "cell") (see Figure 10.9). As normal cellular death occurs over time, more and more healthy red blood cells are replaced by these deficient cells, and the classic symptoms of oxygen and energy

transferrin The transport protein for iron.

iron-deficiency anemia A form of anemia that results from severe iron deficiency.

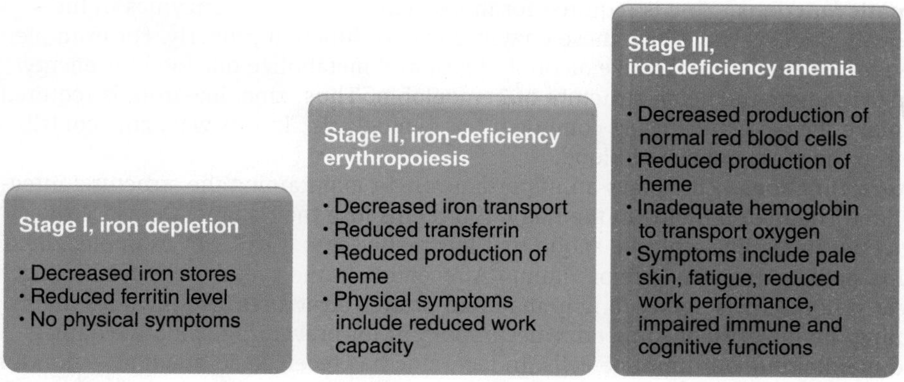

Stage I, iron depletion

- Decreased iron stores
- Reduced ferritin level
- No physical symptoms

Stage II, iron-deficiency erythropoiesis

- Decreased iron transport
- Reduced transferrin
- Reduced production of heme
- Physical symptoms include reduced work capacity

Stage III, iron-deficiency anemia

- Decreased production of normal red blood cells
- Reduced production of heme
- Inadequate hemoglobin to transport oxygen
- Symptoms include pale skin, fatigue, reduced work performance, impaired immune and cognitive functions

◀ FIGURE 10.16 Iron deficiency passes through three stages. The first stage is identified by decreased iron stores, or reduced ferritin levels. The second stage is identified by decreased iron transport, or a reduction in transferrin. The final stage of iron deficiency is iron-deficiency anemia, which is identified by decreased production of normal, healthy red blood cells and inadequate hemoglobin levels.

deprivation develop. These symptoms include impaired work performance, general fatigue, pale skin, depressed immune function, impaired cognitive and nerve function, and impaired memory. Pregnant women with severe anemia are at higher risk for low-birth-weight infants, premature delivery, and increased infant mortality. They are also at risk for postpartum hemorrhage (excessive bleeding immediately following childbirth), which further increases iron losses, and the risk for *postpartum anemia*.[50]

recap Iron is a trace mineral that, as part of the hemoglobin protein, plays a major role in the transportation of oxygen in our blood. Iron is also a coenzyme in many metabolic pathways involved in energy production. Meat, fish, and poultry are good sources of heme iron, which is more absorbable than non-heme iron. Toxicity symptoms for iron range from nausea and vomiting to organ damage and potentially death. If left untreated, iron deficiency eventually leads to iron-deficiency anemia.

nutri-case | LIZ

"It was really hard spending last summer with my parents, because we kept arguing over food! Even though I'd told them I'm a vegetarian, they kept serving meals with meat! Then they'd get mad when I'd fix myself a hummus sandwich! When it was my turn to cook, I made lentils with brown rice, whole-wheat pasta primavera, vegetarian curries, and lots of other yummy meals, but my dad kept insisting, "You have to eat meat or you won't get enough iron!" I told him that plant foods have lots of iron, but he wouldn't listen. Was I ever glad to get back to campus this fall!"

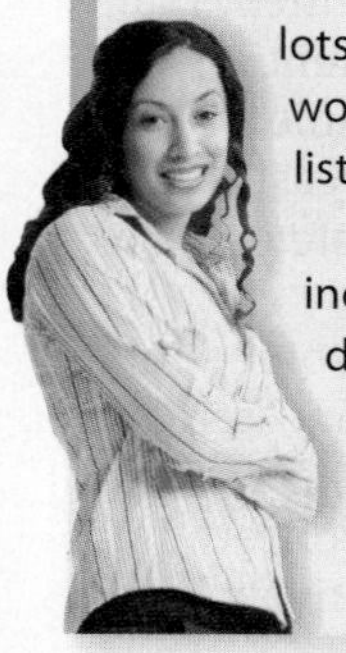

Recall that Liz is a ballet dancer who trains daily. If she eats a vegetarian diet including meals such as the ones she describes here, will she be at risk for iron deficiency? Why or why not? Are there any other micronutrients that might be low in Liz's diet because she avoids meat? If so, what are they? Overall, will Liz get enough energy to support her high level of physical activity on a vegetarian diet? How would she know if she were low energy?

Zinc

Zinc is a trace mineral that plays an important role in many physiologic processes in nearly every body system.

Functions of Zinc

The functions of zinc are easier to remember if we divide them into three categories: enzymatic, structural, and regulatory.

Enzymatic functions. Zinc is required for more than 100 different enzymes in the body. If zinc levels are low, these enzymes cannot function properly. For example, we require zinc to metabolize alcohol, digest and metabolize our food for energy, and synthesize the heme structure of hemoglobin. Thus, zinc, like iron, is required to make the oxygen-carrying component of hemoglobin. In this way, zinc contributes to the maintenance of blood.

Structural functions. Zinc plays an important role in maintaining the structural integrity and shape of proteins in the body. If proteins lose their shape, they lose their function, much like a plastic spoon that has melted into a ball. For example, zinc helps stabilize the structure of vitamin A receptors in the eye, thereby facilitating night vision. Zinc's ability to help maintain protein structures also includes maintaining the integrity of some enzymes important for preventing oxidative damage and maintaining our immune cells. In fact, zinc has received so much attention for its contribution to immune system health that zinc lozenges have been formulated to fight the common cold. The **Nutrition Debate** later in this chapter explores the question of whether or not these lozenges are effective.

Regulatory functions. Zinc helps regulate gene expression (that is, whether or not the cell actually uses a gene to build a protein). For example, without zinc, certain cells that help regulate cell growth during the development of the fetus are not activated. After the child is born, growth is stunted.

A number of biological actions require zinc in all three of the functions above. The major example of this is in reproduction. Zinc is critical for cell replication and normal growth. In fact, zinc deficiency was discovered in the early 1960s, when researchers were trying to determine the cause of severe growth retardation, anemia, and poorly developed testicles in a group of Middle Eastern men. These symptoms of zinc deficiency illustrate its critical role in normal growth and sexual maturation.

How Much Zinc Should We Consume?

As with iron, our need for zinc is relatively small, but our intakes are variable and absorption is influenced by a number of factors. Overall, zinc absorption is similar to that of iron, ranging from 10% to 35% of dietary zinc. People with poor zinc status absorb more zinc than individuals with optimal zinc status, and zinc absorption increases during times of growth, sexual development, and pregnancy.

Several dietary factors influence zinc absorption. High non-heme iron intakes can inhibit zinc absorption, which is a primary concern with iron supplements (which are non-heme), particularly during pregnancy and lactation. High intakes of heme iron appear to have no effect on zinc absorption. The phytates and fiber found in whole grains and beans strongly inhibit zinc absorption. In contrast, dietary protein, especially animal-based protein, enhances zinc absorption. It's not surprising, then, that the primary cause of the zinc deficiency in the Middle Eastern men just mentioned was their low consumption of meat and high consumption of beans and unleavened breads (also called *flat breads*). In leavening bread, the baker adds yeast to the dough. This not only makes the bread rise but also helps reduce the phytate content of the bread.

The recommended intakes for zinc are listed in Table 10.2. Good food sources of zinc include red meats, some seafood, whole grains, and enriched grains and cereals. The dark meat of poultry has a higher content of zinc than white meat. As zinc is significantly more absorbable from animal-based foods, zinc deficiency is a concern for people eating a vegan diet. **FIGURE 10.17** shows various foods that are relatively high in zinc.

What Happens If We Consume Too Much Zinc?

Eating high amounts of dietary zinc does not appear to lead to toxicity. Zinc toxicity can occur, however, from consuming high amounts of supplemental zinc. Toxicity symptoms include intestinal pain and cramps, nausea, vomiting, loss of appetite, diarrhea, and headaches. Excessive zinc supplementation has also been shown to depress immune function and decrease high-density lipoprotein concentrations. High intakes

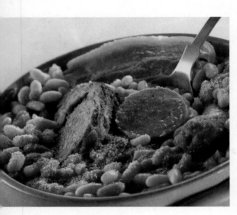
Zinc can be found in pork and beans.

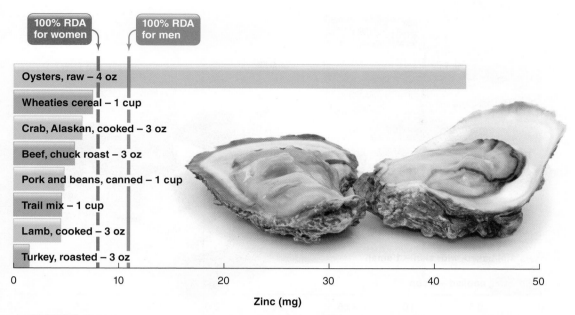

100% RDA for women

100% RDA for men

Oysters, raw – 4 oz

Wheaties cereal – 1 cup

Crab, Alaskan, cooked – 3 oz

Beef, chuck roast – 3 oz

Pork and beans, canned – 1 cup

Trail mix – 1 cup

Lamb, cooked – 3 oz

Turkey, roasted – 3 oz

0   10   20   30   40   50

Zinc (mg)

◆ **FIGURE 10.17**   Common food sources of zinc. The RDA for zinc is 11 mg/day for men and 8 mg/day for women.
Data from: U.S. Department of Agriculture, Agricultural Research Service, 2011. USDA Nutrient Database for Standard Reference, Release 24.

of zinc (five to six times the RDA) can also reduce copper status because zinc absorption interferes with the absorption of copper.

What Happens If We Don't Consume Enough Zinc?

Zinc deficiency is uncommon in the United States but occurs more often in countries in which people consume predominantly grain-based foods. Symptoms of zinc deficiency include growth retardation, diarrhea, delayed sexual maturation and impotence, eye and skin lesions, hair loss, and impaired appetite. As zinc is critical to a healthy immune system, zinc deficiency also results in increased incidence of infections and illnesses.

Copper

Copper is a trace mineral that functions in many enzymatic reactions. These include metabolic pathways that produce energy as well as those that produce the connective tissues collagen and elastin. Copper is also necessary for the regulation of certain neurotransmitters important to brain function, and it is part of the superoxide dismutase enzyme system that fights the damage caused by free radicals.

Copper plays an important role in blood health because it is a component of *ceruloplasmin,* a protein that is important for the oxidation of ferrous to ferric iron, which is necessary before iron can bind to transferrin and be transported in the plasma.[31] If ceruloplasmin levels are inadequate, iron accumulation results, causing symptoms similar to those described with the genetic disorder hemochromatosis.

As you can see in Table 10.2, our need for copper is small. Copper is widely distributed in foods, and people who eat a varied diet can easily meet their requirements. Good food sources of copper include organ meats, seafood, nuts, and seeds. Whole-grain foods are also relatively good sources. **FIGURE 10.18** identifies some foods relatively high in copper.

As with iron and zinc, people with low dietary copper intakes absorb more copper than people with high dietary intakes. Also recall that high zinc intakes can reduce copper absorption and, subsequently, copper status. In fact, zinc supplementation is used to treat a rare disorder called Wilson's disease, in which copper toxicity occurs. High iron intakes can also interfere with copper absorption in infants.

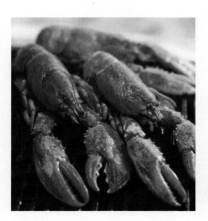

◆ Lobster is a food that contains copper.

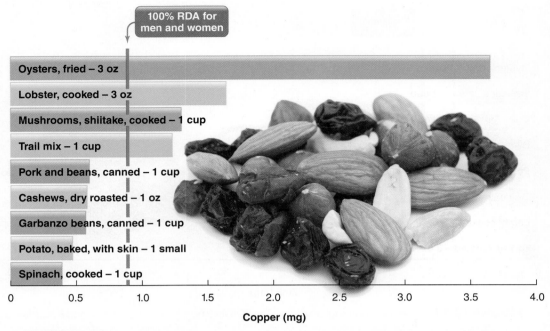

100% RDA for men and women

Oysters, fried – 3 oz

Lobster, cooked – 3 oz

Mushrooms, shiitake, cooked – 1 cup

Trail mix – 1 cup

Pork and beans, canned – 1 cup

Cashews, dry roasted – 1 oz

Garbanzo beans, canned – 1 cup

Potato, baked, with skin – 1 small

Spinach, cooked – 1 cup

0   0.5   1.0   1.5   2.0   2.5   3.0   3.5   4.0

Copper (mg)

FIGURE 10.18 Common food sources of copper. The RDA for copper is 900 µg/day for men and women.

Data from: U.S. Department of Agriculture, Agricultural Research Service, 2011. USDA Nutrient Database for Standard Reference, Release 24.

The long-term effects of copper toxicity are not well studied in humans. Toxicity symptoms include abdominal pain and cramps, nausea, diarrhea, and vomiting. Liver damage occurs in the extreme cases of copper toxicity that occur with Wilson's disease and other health conditions associated with excessive copper levels.

Copper deficiency is rare but can occur in premature infants fed milk-based formulas and in adults fed prolonged formulated diets that are deficient in copper. Deficiency symptoms include anemia, reduced levels of white blood cells, and osteoporosis in infants and growing children.

recap Zinc is a trace mineral that is a part of almost a hundred enzymes that impact virtually every body system. It plays a critical role in hemoglobin synthesis, physical growth and sexual maturation, and immune function and assists in fighting oxidative damage. Copper is a trace mineral that functions in the metabolic pathways that produce energy, in the production of connective tissues, and as part of an antioxidant enzyme system. It is also a component of ceruloplasmin, a protein that is critical for the transport of iron.

*behavior change . . . getting started!

Now that you've read this chapter, try making these changes:

For yourself:

■ Include more micronutrient-rich whole foods in each meal—including fruits, vegetables, legumes, and whole-grain cereals and breads.

■ Select more nutrient-dense foods high in blood-building nutrients such as low-fat meat, fish, poultry, eggs, beans, and whole grains.

For your community:

■ According to several surveys, more and more college students are adopting a vegan diet each year. Use your campus website or your social networking pages to spread the word about the importance of getting vitamin B_{12} from fortified foods or supplements if you're following a vegan diet.

Do Zinc Lozenges Help Fight the Common Cold?

Approximately 1 billion cases of the common cold occur in the United States each year.[51] Children suffer from six to ten colds each year, resulting in approximately 22 million school days lost each year.[52] Colds are also the most common reason people visit a medical professional, accounting for over 100 million primary care visits per year.[53] Thus, finding a cure for the common cold has been at the forefront of modern medicine for many years.

Although a group of viruses called rhinoviruses account for nearly half of all colds, it is estimated that more than 200 different viruses can be to blame.[51,52]

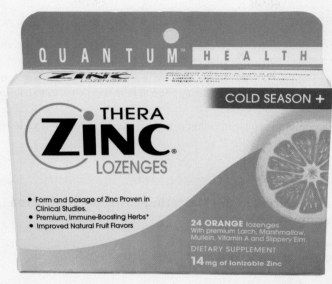

Zinc lozenges come in different formulations and dosages.

Because of this variety, developing vaccines or other preventive measures for colds is extremely challenging.

The role of zinc in the health of our immune system is well known, but zinc has also been shown specifically to inhibit the replication of viruses that cause the common cold. These findings have led to the formulation of zinc supplements to reduce the length and severity of colds.[54,55] These are readily found in a variety of formulations and dosages in most drugstores. The most common are zinc lozenges.

Does taking zinc lozenges actually reduce the length and severity of a cold? Two recent reviews examining thirteen randomized controlled trials with over 966 participants addressed this question.[56,57] The results were somewhat mixed. The first study found that if you take zinc lozenges (30–160 mg/day) within 24–48 hours of the onset of symptoms, there was a reduction in severity and duration by 1 day. The second review divided the research studies by the dose of zinc taken. They found that if 75 mg/day or less was taken, no effect occurred. However, three studies found that if more than 75 mg/day of zinc acetate was given there was a 42% reduction in cold duration.

Unfortunately, we will probably never know the true effect of zinc lozenges on colds for the following reasons:

- *It is difficult to truly 'blind' participants to the treatment*. Because zinc lozenges have a unique taste, it may be difficult to 'blind' the research participants as to whether or not they are getting zinc lozenges or a placebo. Knowing what they are taking could lead participants to report biased results.
- *Self-reported symptoms are subject to inaccuracy*. Many studies had the research participants self-report changes in cold symptoms. Self-reports are commonly influenced by mood and other emotional factors.
- *Subject compliance may be suspect*. Typically, participants are required to take the lozenges on a set schedule for 6–10 days. Unless carefully monitored, researchers must rely on participants to self-report their compliance. Differences in compliance could lead to different outcomes.
- *A wide variety of viruses can cause a cold*. It is highly unlikely that zinc can combat all of the over 200 different viruses capable of causing the common cold. It is possible that people whose symptoms do not improve are infected with a cold virus that does not respond to zinc.
- *Zinc dosages and formulations differ*. It is estimated that, for zinc to be effective, at least 80 mg/day of zinc should be consumed and that people should begin using zinc lozenges within 48 hours of the onset of cold symptoms, yet the studies followed a variety of dosing and timing protocols. Also, different sweeteners and flavorings found in different zinc lozenge formulations may bind the zinc and inhibit its ability to be absorbed into the body, limiting its effectiveness.

Because there is suggestive but not conclusive evidence supporting the effectiveness of zinc lozenges in treating the common cold, the debate over whether people should take them will most likely continue.

One word of caution: If you decide to use zinc lozenges, more is not better. Excessive or prolonged zinc supplementation can reduce immune function and cause other mineral imbalances. Check the label of the product you are using, and do not exceed its recommended dosage or duration of use.

CRITICAL THINKING QUESTIONS

1. Studies of zinc lozenges typically require participants to take several lozenges each day for 6–10 days. The best outcome shown was a 42% reduction in duration of symptoms. If taking zinc lozenges could reduce the length of your discomfort from effort of taking 10 to 6 days, would that be worth the effort of taking lozenges several times each day?

2. Why do you think it is that researchers can't simply develop a vaccine against the common cold?

chapter **review**

test yourself | answers

1. **False.** B-vitamins do not directly provide energy for our body. However, they play critical roles in ensuring that our body is able to generate energy from carbohydrates, fats, and proteins.

2. **True.** People who consume a vegan diet need to pay particularly close attention to consuming enough vitamin B$_{12}$, iron, and zinc. In some cases, these individuals may need to take supplements to consume adequate amounts of these nutrients.

3. **True.** This deficiency is particularly common in infants, children, and women of childbearing age.

MasteringNutrition™

Check out these additional resources in the MasteringNutrition Study Area at www.masteringhealthandnutrition.com:

- Read It: Chapter Summary and RSS Feeds
- See It: ABC News videos and nutrition animations
- Hear It: MP3s
- Study It: Get Ready for Nutrition Math and Chemistry review
- Do It: NutriTools and "Find the Quack" feature
- Review It: Quizzes, flashcards, and glossary

review questions

1. A coenzyme is
   a. an inactive enzyme.
   b. any enzyme containing a B vitamin.
   c. a molecule that combines with and activates an enzyme.
   d. a molecule such as a B-vitamin that is released as a by-product of enzymatic reactions.

2. The B-vitamins include
   a. niacin, folate, and iodine.
   b. cobalamin, choline, and chromium.
   c. manganese, riboflavin, and pyridoxine.
   d. thiamin, pantothenic acid, and biotin.

3. Adequate folate intake is critical for women of childbearing age because
   a. it reduces the risk for giving birth to an infant with a neural tube defect.
   b. it reduces the risk for giving birth to an infant with pernicious anemia.
   c. it reduces the woman's risk for microcytic anemia.
   d. it reduces the woman's risk for excessive blood loss during menstruation.

4. Homocysteine is
   a. a by-product of glycolysis.
   b. a trace mineral.
   c. an amino acid.
   d. a B-vitamin.

5. The components of blood are
   a. iron, zinc, copper, and vitamin K.
   b. erythrocytes, leukocytes, platelets, and plasma.
   c. four polypeptide chains with four heme groups.
   d. whole blood, serum, and plasma.

6. Which of the following statements about iron is true?
   a. Iron picks up oxygen in the lungs, binds it to cytochromes in red blood cells, and exchanges it for carbon dioxide in the liver.
   b. About two-thirds of the body's iron is found in hemoglobin, the oxygen-carrying compound in red blood cells.
   c. Iron transports oxygen in the bloodstream within a compound called ferritin.
   d. Excess iron is stored primarily in the form of myoglobin in muscle tissue.

7. The micronutrient most closely associated with blood clotting is

a. iron.

b. vitamin K.

c. zinc.

d. vitamin B_{12}.

8. A significantly decreased number and size of red blood cells is characteristic of

a. iron-deficiency anemia.

b. sickle cell anemia.

c. pernicious anemia.

d. megaloblastic anemia.

9. True or false? Iron is found only in foods of animal origin.

10. True or false? Copper deficiency can result in accumulation of iron in the body.

math review

11. About 2 g of zinc are stored in the body of an average adult. An adult male consumes 20 mg of zinc each day. He thereby replaces his total body store of zinc every 100 days. Is this statement true or false? Why?

Answers to Review Questions and Math Review are located at the back of this text and in the MasteringNutrition Study Area.

web resources

www.womenshealth.gov
National Women's Health Information Center
Premenstrual Syndrome Fact Sheet

To locate this fact sheet providing information about PMS and a form to help track symptoms, type "Premenstrual Syndrome Fact Sheet" into the search box on the home page.

www.cancer.org
American Cancer Society

Type "B-Vitamins" into the Search box for an overview of the B-vitamins as a group, with functions, food sources, and research into their use in disease prevention.

www.ars.usda.gov
Nutrient Data Laboratory Home Page

Start by entering "nutrient data laboratory home page" in the search box. Then, click on "Reports for Single Nutrients" to find reports listing food sources for selected nutrients.

www.anemia.com
Anemia Lifeline

Visit this site to learn about anemia and its various treatments.

www.medlineplus.gov
Medline Plus

Search this site for "neural tube defects" to find a wealth of information on the development and prevention of these conditions.

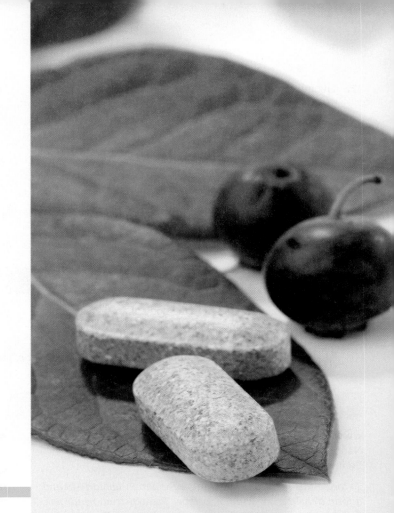

in depth 10.5

Dietary Supplements: Necessity or Waste?

Marcus has type 2 diabetes and high blood pressure, and is worried about his health. He attended a free "nutrition seminar" in which the health benefits of various dietary supplements were touted. After attending this seminar, sponsored by a health products company, Marcus was convinced that he needed to take a supplement providing 200–800% of the Daily Value for many vitamins and minerals as well as an herbal preparation for "heart health." After a few months of taking these supplements on a daily basis, Marcus started to experience headaches, nausea, diarrhea, and tingling in his hands and feet. Although Marcus was not an expert in nutrition, he suspected that he might be experiencing side effects related to nutrient toxicity. He decided to talk to his doctor about the supplements he was taking to determine whether they could be causing his symptoms.

Continued next page

learning objectives

After studying this In Depth, you should be able to:

1 Discuss the limitations in current regulation of dietary supplements sold in the United States, pp. 381–383.

2 Explain what constitutes an herbal supplement and what special precautions are indicated for its use, pp. 383–384.

3 Identify groups of people who might benefit from taking a dietary supplement as well as situations in which dietary supplements are not advised, pp. 384–386.

Continued—Marcus's story is not unique. The use of dietary supplements in the United States has skyrocketed in recent years. Annual sales of supplements in the United States were more than $30 billion in 2011 and continue to grow.[1] Currently about half of American adults report using one or more dietary supplements.[2] However, many say they don't report the use of these products to their physicians because they feel their physicians have little knowledge of supplements and may discourage their use. Interestingly, many supplement users state that they would continue to use these products even if scientific studies found them to be ineffective!

Why do so many people take dietary supplements? The most common reason that adults give is to improve or maintain overall health. The next most common reasons are to improve or maintain the health of bones or other specific organs such as the heart, bowels, eyes, or joints.[3] Many people also believe they cannot consume adequate nutrients in their diet, and they take a supplement as extra nutritional insurance. Others have been advised by their healthcare provider to take a supplement to address a given health concern. There are people, like Marcus, who believe that they can use certain supplements to treat or prevent disease. Others use supplements in the hope that they'll enhance their appearance or athletic performance.

Are such uses wise? A waste of money? Dangerous? Who *should* be taking supplements?

An overview of dietary supplements

According to the U.S. Food and Drug Administration (FDA), a **dietary supplement** is "a product taken by mouth that contains a 'dietary ingredient' intended to supplement the diet."[4] Supplements may contain vitamins, minerals, herbs or other botanicals, amino acids, enzymes, tissues from animal organs or glands, or a concentrate, a metabolite, a constituent, or an extract. Supplements come in many forms, including pills, capsules, liquids, and powders **(FIGURE 1)**.

The Dietary Supplement Health and Education Act (DSHEA) of 1994 classified dietary supplements within the general group of foods, not drugs. This means that the regulation of supplements is much less rigorous than the regulation of drugs. Currently, the FDA is reconsidering how it regulates foods and supplements that are marketed with health claims, but no changes have been finalized at this time. As an informed consumer, you should know that:

- Dietary supplements do not need approval from the FDA before they are marketed.
- The company that manufactures a supplement is responsible for determining that the supplement is safe; the FDA does not test any supplement for safety prior to marketing.

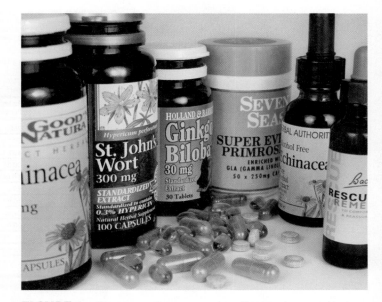

FIGURE 1 Dietary supplements can be pills, capsules, powders, or liquids and contain micronutrients, amino acids, herbs, or other substances.

---

dietary supplement A product taken by mouth that contains a "dietary ingredient" intended to supplement the diet.

- Supplement companies do not have to provide the FDA with any evidence that their supplements are safe unless the company is marketing a new dietary ingredient that was not sold in the United States prior to 1994.
- There are at present no federal guidelines on practices to ensure the purity, quality, safety, and composition of dietary supplements.
- There are no rules to limit the serving size or amount of a nutrient in any dietary supplement.
- Once a supplement is marketed, the FDA must prove it unsafe before the product will be removed from the market.

Despite these limitations in supplement regulation, supplement manufacturers are required to follow dietary supplement labeling guidelines. **FIGURE 2** shows a label from a multivitamin and mineral supplement. As you can see, there are specific requirements for the information that must be included on the supplement label. Federal advertising regulations also require that any claims on the label must be truthful and not misleading and that

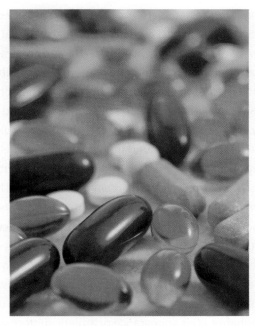

Always research a dietary supplement and its manufacturer before taking it.

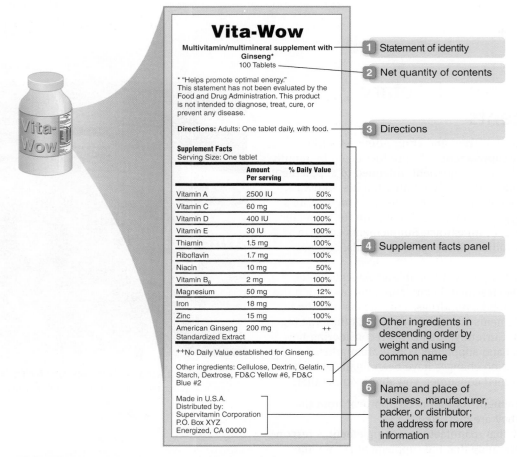

FIGURE 2 A multivitamin-mineral supplement label highlighting the dietary supplement labeling guidelines.

advertisers must be able to substantiate all label claims. In addition, labels bearing a claim must also include the disclaimer "This statement has not been evaluated by the FDA. This product is not intended to diagnose, cure, or prevent any disease." Any products not meeting these guidelines can be removed from the market.

Although many of the supplement products sold today are safe, some are not. In addition, some companies are less than forthright about the ingredients in their supplements. How can you avoid purchasing fraudulent or dangerous supplements, whether over the Internet or in a health food or grocery store? The FDA suggests that you keep in mind the **Quick Tips** feature points when evaluating dietary supplements.[5]

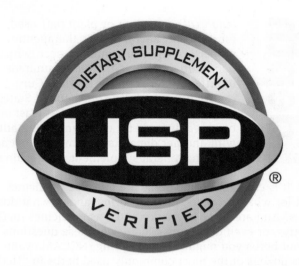

The USP Verified Mark indicates that the manufacturer has followed certain standards for features such as purity, strength, and quality.

QuickTips

Taking Precautions with Supplements

✓ Check with your healthcare provider or a registered dietician nutritionist about any nutrients you may need in addition to your regular diet.

✓ Ask your healthcare provider for help distinguishing between reliable and questionable information.

✓ Look for the Pharmacopeia (USP) Verified Mark on the label. This mark indicates that the manufacturer followed the standards that the USP has established for features such as purity, strength, quality, packaging, labeling, and acceptable length of storage.

✓ Consider buying recognized brands of supplements. Although not guaranteed, products made by nationally recognized companies more likely have well-established manufacturing standards.

✓ Do not assume that the word *natural* on the label means that the product is safe. Arsenic, lead, and mercury are all natural substances that can kill you if consumed in large enough quantities.

✓ Be skeptical of anecdotal information or personal "testimonials."

✓ Ask yourself if the claims for the supplement sound too good to be true. Warning signs include exaggerated, unrealistic, or extreme claims; for example, promising that the supplement will enable you to lose a large amount of weight in a short amount of time, or that it can cure a chronic disease.

✓ Do not hesitate to question a company about how it makes its products. Reputable companies have nothing to hide and are more than happy to inform their customers about the safety and quality of their products.

Special precautions for herbal supplements

A common saying in India cautions that "A house without ginger is a sick house." Indeed, ginger, echinacea, lavender, and many other herbs have been used by different cultures throughout the world for centuries to promote health and treat discomfort and disease. The National Center for Complementary and Alternative Medicine (NCCAM) defines an **herb** (also called a

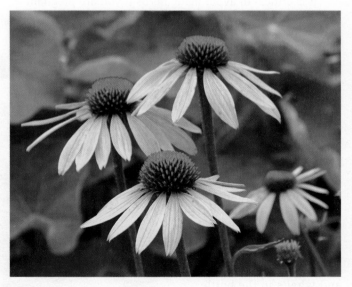

Echinacea, commonly known as purple coneflower, has been used for centuries to prevent colds, flu, and other infections.

herb A plant or plant part used for its scent, flavor, and/or therapeutic properties (also called a *botanical*).

botanical) as a plant or plant part used for its scent, flavor, and/or therapeutic properties.[6] As you would suspect, with a definition this broad there are hundreds of different herbs on the market. Currently, 20% of adults in the United States use a dietary supplement with at least one botanical ingredient, either in combination with another dietary supplement, such as a vitamin/mineral supplement with echinacea, or alone.[2]

It is clear that some herbs are effective medicines, but for what disorders, in what forms, and at what dosages? And are some herbs promoted as medicines ineffective, or even dangerous? To answer these questions about herbs you might be considering, NCCAM evaluates dozens of the most commonly used herbs in "Herbs at a Glance" fact sheets, available at its website (see **Web Resources** at the end of this chapter). In addition, NCCAM recommends that you practice the **Quick Tips** (p. 383) for all types of dietary supplements, as well as the following precautions, which are specific to the use of herbs.

Consult a healthcare provider before using any herbal supplement. Herbs can act the same way as drugs; therefore, they can cause medical problems if not used correctly or if taken in large amounts. In some cases, people have experienced negative effects even though they followed the instructions on a supplement label. It's especially important to check with your healthcare provider if you are taking any prescription medications. Some herbal supplements are known to interact with medications in ways that cause health problems.

It is critical to avoid using herbs if you are pregnant or nursing, unless your physician has approved their use. Some can promote miscarriage or birth defects or can enter breast milk. This caution also applies to treating children with herbal supplements.

Finally, be aware that the active ingredients in many herbs and herbal supplements are not known. There may be dozens, even hundreds, of unknown compounds in an herbal supplement. Also, published analyses of herbal supplements have found differences between what's listed on the label and what's in the bottle. This means you may be taking less—or more—of the supplement than what the label indicates or ingesting

substances not mentioned on the label. Some herbal supplements have been found to be contaminated with metals, unlabeled prescription drugs, microorganisms, and other substances. An investigation by the United States Government Accountability Office reported in 2010 that nearly all of the herbal supplements it had tested were found to contain traces of lead and other contaminants.[7] Be aware that the word *standardized, certified,* or *verified* on a label is no guarantee of product quality; in the United States, these terms have no legal definition for supplements.

Should you take a dietary supplement?

Contrary to what some people believe, the U.S. food supply is not void of nutrients, and all people do not need to supplement their diets all of the time. Foods contain a diverse combination of compounds that interact to maintain our health, whereas vitamin and mineral supplements contain just the micronutrients identified on the label. Thus, they are not substitutes for whole foods. However, nutritional needs change throughout the life span, so you may benefit from taking a supplement at certain times for certain reasons. For instance, if you were to adopt a vegan diet, your healthcare provider might prescribe a supplement providing micronutrients absent or less available from plant foods, including riboflavin, vitamin B_{12}, vitamin D, calcium, iron, and zinc. Or if you joined your college soccer team, your team's sport dietician might review your diet and advise taking a supplement formulated to provide micronutrients that support intense physical activity.

Dietary supplements include hundreds of thousands of products sold for many purposes, and it is impossible to discuss here all of the various situations in which their use may be advisable. So to simplify this discussion, **TABLE 1** identifies groups of people who may benefit from vitamin and/or mineral supplementation. Even if you fall within one of these groups, you might not need to take the supplement indicated. Taking an unnecessary supplement increases the probability that you could exceed the UL for that particular vitamin or mineral.[2] So check with your healthcare provider or a registered dietitian nutritionist (RDN) before taking any supplements.

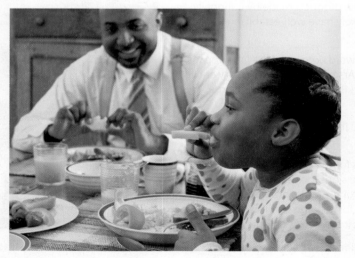

One of the best strategies for maintaining good health is to eat a diet that provides a rich variety of whole foods. If you do that, you probably won't need to take supplements.

TABLE 1 Individuals Who May Benefit from Dietary Supplementation

Type of Individual	Specific Supplements That May Help
Newborns	Routinely given a single dose of vitamin K at birth
Infants	Depends on age and nutrition; may need iron, vitamin D, or other nutrients
Children not drinking fluoridated water	Fluoride supplements
Children on strict vegetarian diets	Vitamin B_{12}, iron, zinc, vitamin D (if not exposed to sunlight)
Children with poor eating habits or overweight children on an energy-restricted diet	Multivitamin-multimineral supplement that does not exceed the RDA for the nutrients it contains
Pregnant teenagers	Iron and folic acid; other nutrients may be necessary if diet is very poor
Women who may become pregnant	Multivitamin or multivitamin-multimineral supplement that contains 0.4 mg of folic acid
Pregnant or lactating women	Multivitamin-multimineral supplement that contains iron, folic acid, zinc, copper, calcium, vitamin B_6, vitamin C, and vitamin D
People on prolonged weight-reduction diets	Multivitamin-multimineral supplement
People recovering from serious illness or surgery	Multivitamin-multimineral supplement
People with HIV/AIDS or other wasting diseases; people addicted to drugs or alcohol	Multivitamin-multimineral supplement or single-nutrient supplements
People who do not consume adequate calcium	Calcium supplements: for example, teens need to consume 1,300 mg of dietary calcium per day; thus, supplements may be necessary
People whose exposure to sunlight is inadequate to allow synthesis of adequate vitamin D	Vitamin D
People eating a vegan diet	Vitamin B_{12}, riboflavin, calcium, vitamin D, iron, and zinc
People who have had portions of their intestinal tract removed; people who have a malabsorptive disease	Depends on the exact condition; may include various fat-soluble and/or water-soluble vitamins and other nutrients
People with lactose intolerance	Calcium supplements
Elderly people	Multivitamin-multimineral supplement, vitamin B_{12}

Of course, many people who do not need to take supplements do so anyway. The following are instances in which taking vitamin and mineral supplements is unnecessary, or even harmful:

- Providing fluoride supplements to children who already drink fluoridated water.
- Taking supplements in the belief that they will cure a disease, such as cancer, diabetes, arthritis, or heart disease.
- Taking supplements with certain medications. For instance, people who take the blood-thinning drug Coumadin should not take vitamin E or K supplements, as this can cause excessive bleeding. People who take aspirin daily should check with their physician before taking vitamin E or K supplements because aspirin also thins the blood.[8]
- Taking nonprescribed supplements if you have liver or kidney disease. Physicians may prescribe vitamin and mineral supplements for their patients because many nutrients are lost during treatment for these diseases. However, these individuals cannot properly metabolize certain supplements and should not take any that are not prescribed by their physician because of a high risk for toxicity.
- Taking beta-carotene supplements if you are a smoker. There is evidence that beta-carotene supplementation increases the risk for lung and other cancers in smokers.
- Taking vitamins and minerals in an attempt to improve physical appearance or athletic performance. There is no evidence that vitamin and mineral supplements enhance appearance or athletic performance in healthy adults with good nutritional status and who consume a varied diet with adequate energy.
- Taking supplements to increase your energy level. Vitamin and mineral supplements do not provide energy because they do not contain fat, carbohydrate, or protein (sources of Calories). Although many vitamins and minerals are necessary for us to produce energy, taking dietary supplements in place of eating food will not provide us with the energy necessary to live a healthy and productive life.

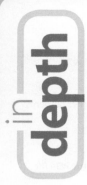

- Taking single-nutrient supplements, unless a qualified healthcare practitioner prescribes a single-nutrient supplement for a diagnosed medical condition (for example, prescribing iron supplements for someone with anemia). These products contain very high amounts of the given nutrient, and taking them can quickly lead to toxicity.

The Academy of Nutrition and Dietetics advises that the ideal nutritional strategy for optimizing health is to eat a healthful diet that contains a variety of whole foods.[9] This way, you probably will not need to take vitamin and mineral supplements. And if you do use a supplement, select one that contains no more than 100% of the recommended levels for the nutrients it contains. Avoid taking single-nutrient supplements unless advised to do so by your healthcare practitioner. Finally, avoid taking supplements that contain substances that are associated with illness and injuries. Some of these substances are listed in TABLE 2.

TABLE 2 Supplement Ingredients Associated with Illnesses and Injuries

Ingredient	Potential Risks
Herbal Ingredients	
Chaparral	Liver disease
Kava (also known as *kava kava*)	Severe liver toxicity
Comfrey	Obstruction of blood flow to liver, possible death
Slimming/dieter's teas	Nausea, diarrhea, vomiting, stomach cramps, constipation, fainting, possible death
Ephedra (also known as *ma huang*, Chinese ephedra, and epitonin)	High blood pressure, irregular heartbeat, nerve damage, insomnia, tremors, headaches, seizures, heart attack, stroke, possible death
Germander	Liver disease, possible death
Lobelia	Breathing problems, excessive sweating, rapid heartbeat, low blood pressure, coma, possible death
Magnolia-Stephania preparation	Kidney disease, can lead to permanent kidney failure
Willow bark	Reye's syndrome (a potentially fatal disease that may occur when children take aspirin), allergic reaction in adults
Wormwood	Numbness of legs and arms, loss of intellectual processing, delirium, paralysis
Vitamins and Essential Minerals	
Vitamin A (when taking 25,000 IU or more per day)	Birth defects, bone abnormalities, severe liver disease
Vitamin B_6 (when taking more than 100 mg per day)	Loss of balance, injuries to nerves that alter our touch sensation
Niacin (when taking slow-release doses of 500 mg or more per day, or when taking immediate-release doses of 750 mg or more per day)	Stomach pain; nausea; vomiting; bloating; cramping; diarrhea; liver disease; damage to the muscles, eye, and heart
Selenium (when taking 800 to 1,000 µg per day)	Tissue damage
Other Ingredients	
Germanium (a nonessential mineral)	Kidney damage
L-tryptophan (an amino acid)	Eosinophilia-myalgia syndrome (a potentially fatal blood disorder that causes high fever)

Data from: U.S. Food and Drug Administration. 2007. *Dietary supplements. Warnings and safety information.*

"You know, I never thought I needed to take a multivitamin-mineral supplement because I'm healthy and I eat all different kinds of foods. But now I've learned in my nutrition course about what these vitamins and minerals do in the body, and I'm thinking, heck, maybe I should take one just for insurance. I mean, I use up a lot of fuel playing basketball and working out. Maybe if I popped a pill every day, I'd have an easier time keeping my weight up!"

Do you think Theo should take a multivitamin-mineral supplement "just for insurance"? Why or why not? Would taking one be likely to have any effect on Theo's weight?

web resources

www.dietary-supplements.info.nih.gov
Office of Dietary Supplements

Search this website to find reports evaluating individual supplements you might be considering as well as general information about the health benefits, safety, and regulation of dietary supplements.

www.cfsan.fda.gov
U.S. Food and Drug Administration
Center for Food Safety and Applied Nutrition

This site provides information on how to make informed decisions and evaluate information related to dietary supplements.

www.nal.usda.gov
The Food and Nutrition Information Center

Enter FNIC into the search box. Then, click on the Dietary Supplements button to obtain information on vitamin and mineral supplements, including consumer reports and industry regulations.

www.nccam.nih.gov
National Center for Complementary and Alternative Medicine

Enter "herbs at a glance" in the search engine, then click on the name of an herb to find out how it has traditionally been used, the status of current research into its effectiveness and safety, and other information.

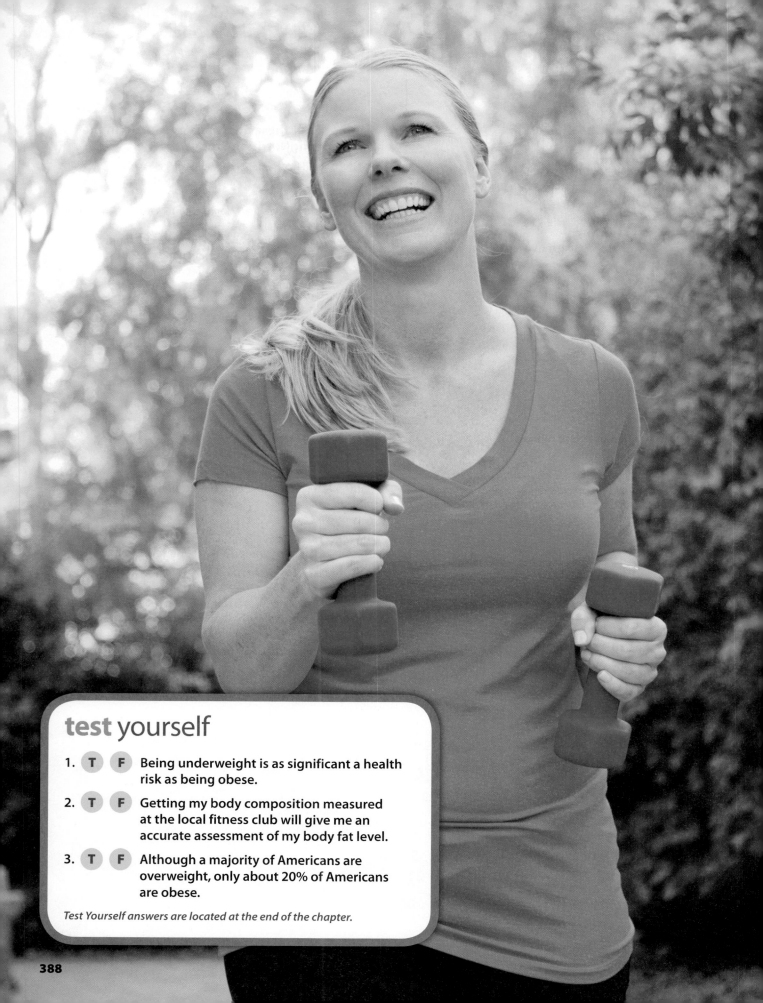

test yourself

1. **T** **F** Being underweight is as significant a health risk as being obese.

2. **T** **F** Getting my body composition measured at the local fitness club will give me an accurate assessment of my body fat level.

3. **T** **F** Although a majority of Americans are overweight, only about 20% of Americans are obese.

Test Yourself answers are located at the end of the chapter.

Achieving and Maintaining a Healthful Body Weight

11

learning objectives

After studying this chapter you should be able to:

1 Define what is meant by a healthful weight, p. 390.

2 Explain how to use each of three methods to assess your body weight and weight-related health risks, pp. 390–395.

3 Identify and discuss the three components of energy expenditure and explain the concept of energy balance, pp. 395–401.

4 Identify at least one example from each of the following factors that can influence body weight: genetic, metabolic, physiological, cultural, economic, psychological, and social, pp. 401–408.

5 Identify three key strategies for healthful weight loss, pp. 408, 411–417.

6 Define the terms *underweight*, *overweight*, *obesity*, and *morbid obesity* and discuss the potential health risks of each of these weight classifications, pp. 417–422.

7 Discuss three treatment options for obesity, pp. 422–425.

In February 2012, at age 23, British pop singer Adele became only the second woman in history to win six Grammy Awards in one night. She has won critical acclaim from musicians of various genres and the adoration of millions of fans worldwide. Still, some critics— most famously the fashion designer Karl Lagerfeld—have focused not on her big, soulful voice, but on her weight. Is Adele overweight? A size "14 to 16," she exudes supreme confidence in her large, curvy body and insists she's not interested in losing weight just because someone else thinks she should. Rather than worry about something as "petty" as what you look like, Adele suggests that, "The first thing to do is be happy with yourself and appreciate your body."[1]

Are you happy with your weight, shape, body composition, and fitness? If not, what needs to change—your diet, your level of physical activity, or maybe just your attitude? What role do diet and physical activity play in maintaining a healthful body weight? How much of your body size and shape is due to genetics? What influence does society— including food advertising—have on your weight? And if you decide that you do need to lose weight, what's the best way to do it? In this chapter, we will explore these questions and provide some answers.

MasteringNutrition™

Go online for chapter quizzes, pre-tests, Interactive Activities, and more!

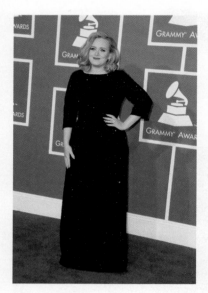

➤ British pop singer Adele, who came under some media scrutiny for her weight, states that she is comfortable with who she is and how she looks.

You can also calculate your BMI more precisely on the Internet using the BMI calculator found at the National Institutes of Health: Heart, Lung & Blood Institute. Go to www.nhlbi.nig.gov and click on "Public." Scroll down to "Health Assessment Tools," then click on "Body Mass Index Calculator."

How can you evaluate your body weight?

As you begin to think about achieving and maintaining a healthful weight, it's important to make sure you understand what a healthful body weight actually is and the various methods you can use to figure out if your own weight is healthful.

Understand What a Healthful Body Weight Really Is

We can define a healthful weight as all of the following:[2]

- A weight that is appropriate for your age and physical development
- A weight that you can achieve and sustain without severely curtailing your food intake or constantly dieting
- A weight that is compatible with normal blood pressure, lipid levels, and glucose tolerance
- A weight that is based on your genetic background and family history of body shape and weight
- A weight that promotes good eating habits and allows you to participate in regular physical activity
- A weight that is acceptable to you

As you can see, a healthful weight is one at which you don't have to be extremely thin or overly muscular. In addition, there is no one body type that can be defined as healthful. Thus, achieving a healthful body weight should not be dictated by the latest fad or current societal expectations of what is acceptable.

Various methods are available to help you determine whether you are currently maintaining a healthful body weight. Let's review a few of these methods.

Determine Your Body Mass Index (BMI)

Body mass index (BMI, or *Quetelet's index*) is a commonly used index representing the ratio of a person's body weight to the square of his or her height. You can calculate your BMI using the following equation:

$$\text{BMI (kg/m}^2) = \text{weight (kg)/height (m)}^2$$

For those less familiar with the metric system, there is an equation to calculate BMI using weight in pounds and height in inches:

$$\text{BMI (kg/m}^2) = [\text{weight (lb)/height (in.)}^2] \times 703$$

A less exact but practical method is to use the graph in **FIGURE 11.1**, which shows approximate BMIs for your height and weight and whether your BMI is in a healthful range.

Why Is BMI Important?

Your BMI provides an important clue to your overall health because it is associated with one of five weight categories, each of which involves a certain level of health risk:

- **Underweight.** A person having a BMI less than 18.5 kg/m² is considered underweight. Physicians, nutritionists, and other scientists define **underweight** as having too little body fat to maintain health, causing a person to have a weight that is below an acceptably defined standard for a given height. Being underweight is associated with an increased risk for many health problems.
- **Normal weight.** Normal weight ranges from 18.5 to 24.9 kg/m². This weight is associated with the lowest disease risk.
- **Overweight.** Having a BMI between 25 and 29.9 kg/m² indicates that a person is overweight. **Overweight** is defined as having a moderate amount of excess body fat, resulting in a person having a weight that is greater than some accepted standard for a given height but is not considered obese.
- **Obesity.** A BMI value between 30 and 39.9 kg/m² is consistent with obesity. Clinicians define **obesity** as having an excess of body fat that adversely affects health, resulting in a person having a weight that is substantially greater than

body mass index (BMI) A measurement representing the ratio of a person's body weight to his or her height.

underweight Having too little body fat to maintain health, causing a person to weigh less than an acceptably defined standard for a given height.

overweight Having a moderate amount of excess body fat, resulting in a person weighing more than an accepted standard for a given height but not considered obese.

obesity Having an excess of body fat that adversely affects health, resulting in a person weighing substantially more than an accepted standard for a given height.

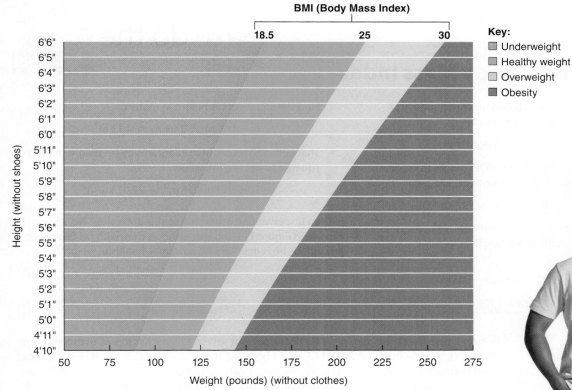

BMI (Body Mass Index)

Key:
- Underweight
- Healthy weight
- Overweight
- Obesity

FIGURE 11.1 Estimate your body mass index (BMI) using this graph. To determine your BMI, find the value for your height on the left and follow this line to the right until it intersects with the value for your weight on the bottom axis. The area on the graph where these two lines intersect is your BMI.

some accepted standard for a given height. Research studies show that a person's risk for type 2 diabetes, high blood pressure, heart disease, and many other diseases increases significantly when BMI is above a value of 30.

- **Morbid obesity.** People can also suffer from **morbid obesity**, defined as a BMI greater than or equal to 40 kg/m^2; in this case, the person's body weight exceeds 100% of normal, putting him or her at very high risk for serious health consequences.

In addition to the effect of body weight on disease risk, researchers study the relationship between body weight and risk for premature death. Until recently, data from national surveys have indicated that having a BMI value within the healthful range means that your risk of dying prematurely is within the expected average. Thus, if your BMI value fell outside this range, either higher or lower, your risk of dying prematurely was considered greater than the average risk. However, recent evidence suggests that having a BMI in the overweight category may actually be protective against dying prematurely.[3] (Refer to the **Hot Topic** (page 394) for more information.) In contrast, having a BMI in the obesity category increases a person's risk of dying prematurely 18% above that of people with a BMI value in the normal-weight range.

Theo always worries about being too thin, and he wonders if he is underweight. Theo calculates his BMI (see the calculations in the **You Do the Math** box, page 392) and is surprised to find that it is 22 kg/m^2 and falls within the healthy range.

Limitations of BMI

Although calculating your BMI can be very helpful in estimating your health risk, this method has a number of limitations that should be taken into consideration. BMI cannot tell us how much of a person's body mass is composed of fat, nor can it give us an indication of where on the body excess fat is stored. As we'll discuss shortly, upper-body fat stores increase the risk for chronic disease more than fat stores in the lower body. A

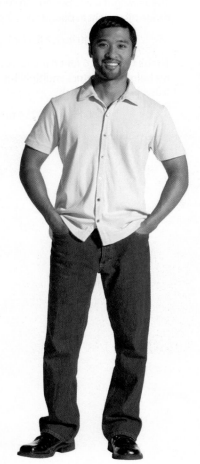

A healthful weight is one that is appropriate for your age, physical development, heredity, and other factors.

morbid obesity A condition in which a person's body weight exceeds 100% of normal, putting him or her at very high risk for serious health consequences.

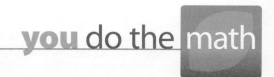

Calculating Your Body Mass Index

Calculate your personal BMI value based on your height and weight. Let's use Theo's values as an example:

$$BMI = weight\ (kg)/height\ (m)^2$$

1. Theo's weight is 200 pounds. To convert his weight to kilograms, divide his weight in pounds by 2.2 pounds per kilogram:

$$200\ lb/2.2\ lb\ per\ kg = 90.91\ kg$$

2. Theo's height is 6 feet 8 inches, or 80 inches. To convert his height to meters, multiply his height in inches by 0.0254 meter per inch:

$$80\ in. \times 0.0254\ m/in. = 2.03\ m$$

3. Find the square of his height in meters:

$$2.03\ m \times 2.03\ m = 4.13\ m^2$$

4. Then, divide his weight in kilograms by his height in meters squared to get his BMI value:

$$90.91\ kg/4.13\ m^2 = 22.01\ kg/m^2$$

Is Theo underweight, according to this BMI value? No. As you can see in Figure 11.1, this value shows that, with his BMI number around 22, he is maintaining a normal, healthful weight!

---

person's age affects his or her BMI; BMI does not give a fair indication of overweight or obesity in people over the age of 65 years because the BMI standards are based on data from younger people, and BMI does not accurately reflect the differential rates of bone and muscle loss in older people. BMI also cannot reflect differences in bone and muscle growth in children. Recent research indicates that BMI is more strongly associated with height in young people; thus, taller children are more likely to be identified as overweight or obese, even though they may not have higher levels of body fat.[4]

BMI also does not take into account physical and metabolic differences between people of different ethnic backgrounds. At the same BMI, people from different ethnic backgrounds will have different levels of body fat. For instance, African American and Polynesian people have less body fat than whites at the same BMI value, whereas Indonesians, Thais, and Ethiopians have more body fat than whites at the same BMI value.[5,6] There is also evidence that, even at the same BMI level, Asian, Hispanic, and African American women have a higher risk for diabetes than white women.[7] The same study also found that, when Asian and Hispanic women gained weight, their risk of developing diabetes over a 20-year period was approximately twice as high as it was for white and African American women who gained the same amount of weight.

Finally, BMI is limited when used with people who have a disproportionately higher muscle mass for a given height. People who fall into this category include some athletes and pregnant and lactating women. For example, one of Theo's friends, Randy, is a 23-year-old weight lifter who is 5'7" and weighs 210 pounds. According to our BMI calculations, Randy's BMI is 32.9, placing him in the obese category. Is Randy really obese? In cases such as his, an assessment of body composition is necessary.

Measure Your Body Composition

There are many methods available to assess your **body composition**, or the amount of body fat (or *adipose tissue*) and lean body mass (or *lean tissue*) you have. **FIGURE 11.2** lists and describes some of the more common methods. It is important to remember that measuring body composition provides only an *estimate* of your body fat and lean body mass; it cannot determine your exact level of these tissues. Because the range of error of these methods can be from 3% to more than 20%, body composition results should not be used as the only indicator of health status.

Let's return to Randy, whose BMI of 32.9 kg/m² places him in the obese category. But is he obese? Randy trains with weights 4 days per week, rides an exercise bike for about 30 minutes per session three times per week, and does not take drugs, smoke cigarettes, or drink alcohol. Through his local gym, Randy contacted a trained

body composition The ratio of a person's body fat to lean body mass.

Method	Limitations

Underwater weighing:
Considered the most accurate method. Estimates body fat within a 2–3% margin of error. This means that if your underwater weighing test shows you have 20% body fat, this value could be no lower than 17% and no higher than 23%. Used primarily for research purposes.

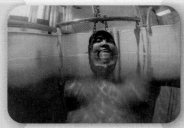

- Subject must be comfortable in water.
- Requires trained technician and specialized equipment.
- May not work well with extremely obese people.
- Must abstain from food for at least 8 hours and from exercise for at least 12 hours prior to testing.

Skinfolds:
Involves "pinching" a person's fold of skin (with its underlying layer of fat) at various locations of the body. The fold is measured using a specially designed caliper. When performed by a skilled technician, it can estimate body fat with an error of 3–4%. This means that if your skinfold test shows you have 20% body fat, your actual value could be as low as 16% or as high as 24%.

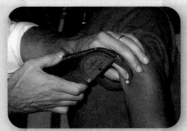

- Less accurate unless technician is well trained.
- Proper prediction equation must be used to improve accuracy.
- Person being measured may not want to be touched or to expose their skin.
- Cannot be used to measure obese people, as their skinfolds are too large for the caliper.

Bioelectrical impedance analysis (BIA):
Involves sending a very low level of electrical current through a person's body. As water is a good conductor of electricity and lean body mass is made up of mostly water, the rate at which the electricity is conducted gives an indication of a person's lean body mass and body fat. This method can be done while lying down, with electrodes attached to the feet, hands, and the BIA machine. Hand-held and standing models (which look like bathroom scales) are now available. Under the best of circumstances, BIA can estimate body fat with an error of 3–4%.

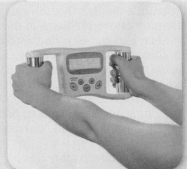

- Less accurate.
- Body fluid levels must be normal.
- Proper prediction equation must be used to improve accuracy.
- Should not eat for 4 hours and should not exercise for 12 hours prior to the test.
- No alcohol should be consumed within 48 hours of the test.
- Females should not be measured if they are retaining water due to menstrual cycle changes.

Dual-energy x-ray absorptiometry (DXA):
The technology is based on using very-low-level x-rays to differentiate among bone tissue, soft (or lean) tissue, and fat (or adipose) tissue. It involves lying for about 30 minutes on a specialized bed fully clothed, with all metal objects removed. The margin of error for predicting body fat ranges from 2% to 4%.

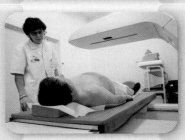

- Expensive; requires trained technician with specialized equipment.
- Cannot be used to measure extremely tall, short, or obese people, as they do not fit properly within the scanning area.

Bod Pod:
A machine that uses air displacement to measure body composition. This machine is a large, egg-shaped chamber made from fiberglass. The person being measured sits inside, wearing a swimsuit. The door is closed and the machine measures how much air is displaced. This value is used to calculate body composition. It appears promising as an easier and equally accurate alternative to underwater weighing in many populations, but it may overestimate body fat in some African American men.

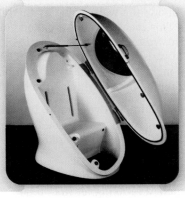

- Expensive.
- Less accurate in some populations.

FIGURE 11.2 Overview of various body composition assessment methods.

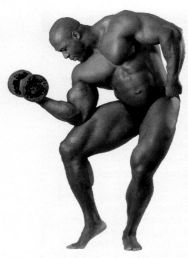

← BMI is not an accurate indicator of overweight for certain populations, including heavily muscled people.

technician who assesses body composition. The results of his skinfold measurements show that his body fat is 9%. This value is within the healthful range for men. Randy is an example of a person whose BMI appears to be very high but who is not actually obese.

Assess Your Fat Distribution Patterns

To evaluate the health of your current body weight, it is also helpful to consider the way fat is distributed throughout your body. This is because your fat distribution pattern is known to affect your risk for various diseases. **FIGURE 11.3** shows two types of fat patterning. *Apple-shaped fat patterning*, or upper-body obesity, is known to significantly increase a person's risk for many chronic diseases, such as type 2 diabetes, heart disease, and high blood pressure. It is thought that the apple-shaped patterning causes problems in the metabolism of fat and carbohydrate, leading to unhealthful changes in blood cholesterol, insulin, glucose, and blood pressure. In contrast, *pear-shaped fat patterning*, or lower-body obesity, does not seem to significantly increase your risk for chronic diseases. Women tend to store fat in their lower body, and men in their abdominal region.

You can use the following three-step method to determine your type of fat patterning:

1. Ask a friend to measure the circumference of your natural waist—that is, the narrowest part of your torso as observed from the front **(FIGURE 11.4A)**.
2. Then have that friend measure your hip circumference at the maximal width of the buttocks as observed from the side (Figure 11.4b).
3. Then divide the waist value by the hip value. This measurement is called your *waist-to-hip ratio*. For example, if your natural waist is 30 inches and your hips are 40 inches, then your waist-to-hip ratio is 30 divided by 40, which equals 0.75.

Once you figure out your ratio, how do you interpret it? An increased risk for chronic disease is associated with the following waist-to-hip ratios:

- In men, a ratio higher than 0.90
- In women, a ratio higher than 0.80

These ratios suggest an apple-shaped fat distribution pattern. In addition, waist circumference alone can indicate your risk for chronic disease. For males, your risk of chronic disease is increased if your waist circumference is above 40 inches (102 cm). For females, your risk is increased at measurements above 35 inches (88 cm).

HOT TOPIC

Can Being Overweight Be Good For You?

For decades numerous scientific research studies have supported the view that having a BMI above the normal range increases our risks for a range of chronic diseases and for dying prematurely. However, a 2013 analysis of 97 previously published studies[3] has challenged this view. It found that people who are overweight (BMI of 25 to 29.99 kg/m²) but not obese have a 6% *lower* risk of dying prematurely than those with a normal BMI.

These findings have created a firestorm of controversy among health professionals and prompted numerous scientists to question the study.[4] Most notably, Dr. Walter Willett of the Harvard School of Public Health has called the findings "rubbish" and warned that they will confuse health care providers and discourage overweight and obese people from losing weight. In contrast, an editorial published in the journal *Nature* has questioned the motives and views of these critics, emphasizing that the topic is highly complex, and concluding that "a bit of extra weight" does appear to be protective for people who are middle-aged or older or who are already sick.[5]

This controversy has drawn international attention to *how* research findings are reported in the media: Is it acceptable to reject major research findings when they don't agree? And should we oversimplify our public health messages when this requires that we ignore the complexity of an issue such as obesity? This will certainly be a Hot Topic for years to come.

recap Body mass index, body composition, and the waist-to-hip ratio and waist circumference are tools that can help you evaluate the health of your current body weight. None of these methods is completely accurate, but most may be used appropriately as general health indicators.

What makes us gain and lose weight?

Have you ever wondered why some people are thin but others are overweight, even though they seem to eat about the same diet? If so, you're not alone. For hundreds of years, researchers have puzzled over what makes us gain and lose weight. In this section, we'll explore some information and current theories that may shed some light on this question.

We Gain or Lose Weight When Energy Intake and Expenditure Are Out of Balance

Fluctuations in body weight are a result of changes in our **energy intake** (the food we eat) and our **energy expenditure** (the amount of energy we expend at rest and during physical activity). This relationship between what we eat and how we use food to fuel our bodies is defined by the energy balance equation:

Energy balance occurs when *energy intake = energy expenditure*

Although the concept of energy balance appears simple, it is a dynamic process.[8] This means that, over time, factors that impact the energy intake side of the equation (including total energy consumed and the macronutrient composition of this energy) need to balance with the factors that impact the energy expenditure side of the equation. **FIGURE 11.5** shows how our weight changes when either side of this equation is altered. From this figure, you can see that, in order to lose body weight, we must expend more energy than we consume. In contrast, to gain weight, we must consume more energy than we expend. Unless we purposefully change one side of the equation, weight change is typically gradual, occurring over an extended period. Finding the proper balance between energy intake and expenditure allows us to maintain a healthful body weight.

Energy Intake Is the Food We Eat Each Day

Energy intake is equal to the amount of energy in the food we eat each day. This value includes all foods and beverages. Daily energy intake is expressed as *kilocalories per day* (*kcal/day,* or *kcal/d*). The energy content of each food is a function of the amount of carbohydrate, fat, protein, and alcohol that each food contains; vitamins and minerals have no energy value, so they contribute zero kcal to our energy intake.

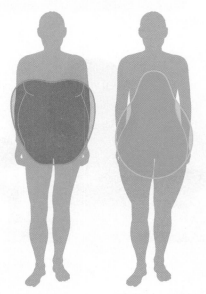

(a) Apple-shaped fat patterning   **(b) Pear-shaped fat patterning**

FIGURE 11.3 Fat distribution patterns. **(a)** An apple-shaped fat distribution pattern increases an individual's risk for many chronic diseases. **(b)** A pear-shaped fat distribution pattern does not seem to be associated with an increased risk for chronic disease.

To determine how much energy you consume in one meal or on 1 day, log onto ChooseMyPlate SuperTracker at www.choosemyplate.gov. Go to the tab for SuperTracker & Other Tools, then from the drop-down menu, choose SuperTracker.

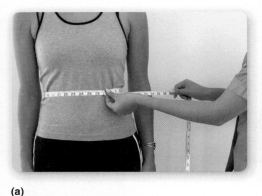
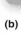

(a)   **(b)**

FIGURE 11.4 Determining your type of fat patterning. **(a)** Measure the circumference of your natural waist. **(b)** Measure the circumference of your hips at the maximal width of the buttocks as observed from the side. Dividing the waist value by the hip value gives you your waist-to-hip ratio.

energy intake The amount of food a person eats; in other words, it is the number of kilocalories consumed.

energy expenditure The energy the body expends to maintain its basic functions and to perform all levels of movement and activity.

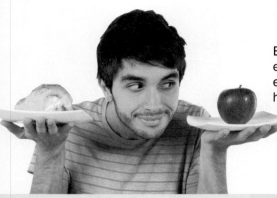

Energy balance is the relationship between the food we eat and the energy we expend each day. Finding the proper balance between energy intake and energy expenditure allows us to maintain a healthy body weight.

ENERGY INTAKE < ENERGY EXPENDITURE = WEIGHT LOSS

ENERGY DEFICIT

When you consume fewer Calories than you expend, your body will draw upon your stored energy to meet its needs. You will lose weight.

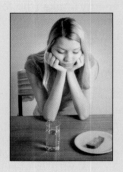

Calories in   Calories out

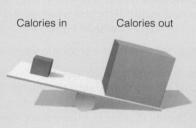

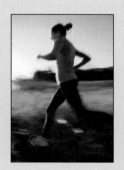

ENERGY INTAKE = ENERGY EXPENDITURE = WEIGHT MAINTENANCE

ENERGY BALANCE

When the Calories you consume meet your needs, you are in energy balance. Your weight will be stable.

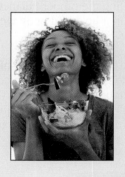

Calories in   Calories out

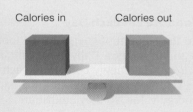

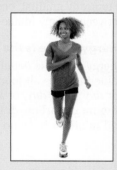

ENERGY INTAKE > ENERGY EXPENDITURE = WEIGHT GAIN

ENERGY EXCESS

When you take in more Calories than you need, the surplus Calories will be stored as fat. You will gain weight.

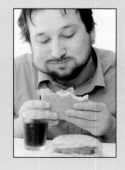

Calories in   Calories out

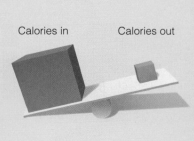

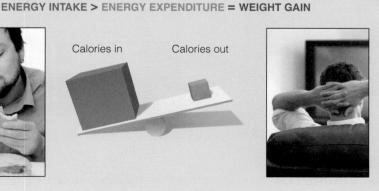

Remember that the energy value of carbohydrate and protein is 4 kcal/g and the energy value of fat is 9 kcal/g. The energy value of alcohol is 7 kcal/g. By multiplying the energy value (in kcal/g) by the amount of the nutrient (in grams), you can calculate how much energy is in a particular food. For instance, 1 cup of quick oatmeal has an energy value of 142 kcal. How is this energy value derived? One cup of oatmeal contains 6 g of protein, 25 g of carbohydrate, and 2 g of fat. Using the energy values for each nutrient, you can calculate the total energy content of oatmeal:

$$6 \text{ g protein} \times 4 \text{ kcal/g} = 24 \text{ kcal from protein}$$
$$25 \text{ g carbohydrate} \times 4 \text{ kcal/g} = 100 \text{ kcal from carbohydrate}$$
$$2 \text{ g fat} \times 9 \text{ kcal/g} = 18 \text{ kcal from fat}$$
$$\text{Total kcal for 1 cup oatmeal} = 24 \text{ kcal} + 100 \text{ kcal} + 18 \text{ kcal} = 142 \text{ kcal}$$

Over time, when someone's total daily energy intake exceeds the amount of energy that person expends, then weight gain results.

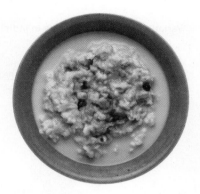

The energy provided by a bowl of oatmeal is derived from its protein, carbohydrate, and fat content.

Energy Expenditure Includes More Than Just Physical Activity

Energy expenditure (also known as energy output) is the energy the body expends to maintain its basic functions and to perform all levels of movement and activity. Total 24-hour energy expenditure is calculated by estimating the energy used during rest and as a result of physical activity. There are three components of energy expenditure: basal metabolic rate (BMR), thermic effect of food (TEF), and energy cost of physical activity (**FIGURE 11.6**).

Our Basal Metabolic Rate Is Our Energy Expenditure at Rest

Basal metabolic rate, or **BMR**, is the energy expended just to maintain the body's *basal,* or *resting,* functions. These functions include respiration, circulation, maintaining body temperature, synthesis of new cells and tissues, secretion of hormones, and nervous system activity. The majority of our energy output each day (about 60–75%) is a result of our BMR. This means that 60–75% of our energy output goes to fuel the basic activities of staying alive, aside from any physical activity.

BMR varies widely among people. The primary determinant of our BMR is the amount of lean body mass we have. People with a higher lean body mass have a higher BMR because lean body mass is more metabolically active than body fat. Thus, it takes more energy to support this active tissue. One common assumption is that obese people have a depressed BMR. This is usually not the case. Most studies of obese people show that the amount of energy they expend for every kilogram of lean body mass is similar to that of a non-obese person. Moreover, people who weigh more also have more lean body mass and consequently have a *higher* BMR. See **FIGURE 11.7** (page 398) for an example of how lean body mass can vary for people with different body weights and body fat levels.

BMR decreases with age, approximately 3–5% per decade after age 30. This age-related decrease results partly from hormonal changes, but much of this change is due to the loss of lean body mass resulting from physical inactivity. Thus, a large proportion of this decrease may be prevented with regular physical activity. There are other factors that can affect a person's BMR, and some of these are listed in **TABLE 11.1**.

How can you estimate the amount of energy you expend for your BMR? Of the many methods that can be used, one of the simplest is to multiply your body weight in kilograms by 1.0 kcal per kilogram of body weight per hour for men or by 0.9 kcal per kilogram of body weight per hour for women. A little later in this chapter, you will have an opportunity to calculate your BMR and determine your total daily energy needs.

The Thermic Effect of Food Is the Energy Expended to Process Food

The **thermic effect of food (TEF)** is the energy we expend to digest, absorb, transport, metabolize, and store the nutrients we need. The TEF is equal to about 5–10% of the energy content of a meal, a relatively small amount. Thus, if a meal contains 500 kcal, the thermic effect of processing that meal is about 25 to 50 kcal. These values apply to eating what is referred to as a mixed diet, or a diet containing carbohydrate, fat, and protein. Individually, the processing of each nutrient takes a different amount of energy. Whereas fat requires very little energy to digest, transport, and store in our cells, protein and carbohydrate require relatively more energy to process.

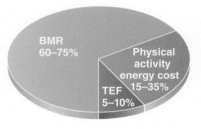

Components of energy expenditure

FIGURE 11.6 The components of energy expenditure are basal metabolic rate (BMR), the thermic effect of food (TEF), and the energy cost of physical activity. BMR accounts for 60–75% of our total energy output, whereas TEF and physical activity together account for 25–40%.

basal metabolic rate (BMR) The energy the body expends to maintain its fundamental physiologic functions.

thermic effect of food (TEF) The energy expended as a result of processing food consumed.

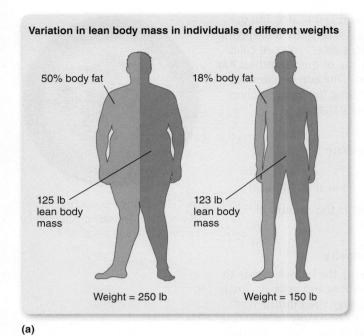

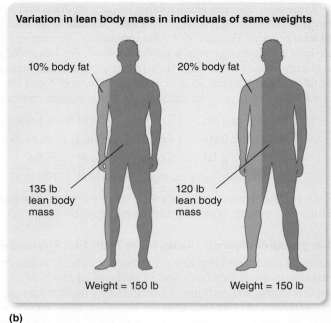

⬤ **FIGURE 11.7** Lean body mass varies in people with different body weights and body fat levels. **(a)** The person on the left has greater body weight, body fat, and lean body mass than the person on the right. **(b)** The two people are the same weight, but the person on the right has more body fat and less lean body mass than the person on the left.

TABLE 11.1 Factors Affecting Basal Metabolic Rate (BMR)

Factors That Increase BMR	Factors That Decrease BMR
Higher lean body mass	Lower lean body mass
Greater height (more surface area)	Lower height
Younger age	Older age
Elevated levels of thyroid hormone	Depressed levels of thyroid hormone
Stress, fever, illness	Starvation or fasting
Male gender	Female gender
Pregnancy and lactation	
Certain drugs, such as stimulants, caffeine, and tobacco	

The Energy Cost of Physical Activity Is Highly Variable The **energy cost of physical activity** represents about 15–35% of our total energy output each day. This is the energy we expend in any movement or work above basal levels. *Non-exercise activity thermogenesis (NEAT)* is a term used to refer to the energy we expend to do all activities above BMR and TEF, but excluding volitional sporting activities. This also includes *spontaneous physical activity*, which includes subconscious activities such as fidgeting and shifting in one's seat. The energy cost of physical activity also includes the energy we expend participating in higher-intensity activities such as running, skiing, and bicycling. One of the most obvious ways to increase how much energy we expend as a result of physical activity is to do more activities for a longer period.

    TABLE 11.2 lists the energy costs for certain activities. As you can see, activities such as running, swimming, and cross-country skiing that involve moving our larger muscle groups (or more parts of the body) require more energy. The amount of energy we expend during activities is also affected by our body size, the intensity of the activity, and how long we perform the activity. This is why the values in Table 11.2 are expressed as kcal of energy per kilogram of body weight per minute.

energy cost of physical activity
The energy that is expended on body movement and muscular work above basal levels.

TABLE 11.2   Energy Costs of Various Physical Activities

Activity	Intensity	Energy Cost (kcal/kg body weight/min)
Sitting, studying (including reading or writing)	Light	0.022
Cooking or food preparation (sitting or standing)	Light	0.033
Walking (e.g., to neighbor's house)	Light	0.042
Stretching—Hatha yoga	Moderate	0.042
Cleaning (dusting, straightening up, vacuuming, changing linen, carrying out trash)	Moderate	0.058
Weight lifting (free weights, Nautilus, or universal type)	Light or moderate	0.050
Bicycling, 10 mph	Leisure (work or pleasure)	0.067
Walking, 4 mph (brisk pace)	Moderate	0.083
Aerobics	Low impact	0.083
Weight lifting (free weights, Nautilus, or universal type)	Vigorous	0.100
Bicycling, 12 to 13.9 mph	Moderate	0.133
Running, 5 mph (12 minutes per mile)	Moderate	0.138
Running, 6 mph (10 minutes per mile)	Moderate	0.163
Running, 8.6 mph (7 minutes per mile)	Vigorous	0.205

Data from: The Compendium of Physical Activities Tracking Guide. Healthy Lifestyles Research Center, College of Nursing & Health Innovation, Arizona State University.

Using the energy value for running at 6 miles per hour (or a 10-minute-per-mile running pace) for 30 minutes, let's calculate how much energy Theo would expend doing this activity:

- Theo's body weight (in kg) = 200 lb/2.2 lb/kg = 90.91 kg
- Energy cost of running at 6 mph = 0.163 kcal/kg body weight/min
- At Theo's weight, the energy cost of running per minute = 0.163 kcal/kg body weight/min × 90.91 kg = 14.82 kcal/min
- If Theo runs at this pace for 30 minutes, his total energy output = 14.82 kcal/min × 30 min = 445 kcal

Given everything we've discussed so far, you're probably asking yourself, "How many kcal do I need each day to maintain my current weight?" This question is not always easy to answer because our energy needs fluctuate from day to day according to our activity level, environmental conditions, and other factors such as the amount and type of food we eat and our intake of caffeine, which temporarily increases our BMR. However, you can get a general estimate of how much energy your body needs to maintain your present weight. The **You Do the Math** box (page 400) shows you how.

Limitations of the Energy Balance Equation

As researchers have learned more about the factors that regulate body weight, the accuracy and usefulness of the classic energy balance equation illustrated in Figure 11.5 has been called into question. Many researchers point out that the equation in its current form is static—meaning it does not account for many factors that can alter energy intake and expenditure nor does it help explain why people gain and lose weight differently.

For example, if an individual were to consume an additional 100 kcal each day above the energy needed to maintain weight (the energy content of 8 fl. oz of a cola beverage) for 10 years, he or she would consume an extra intake of 365,000 kcal! Based on the static energy balance equation, and assuming that no other changes occur in energy expenditure, this individual should gain 104 pounds. However, the static energy balance calculation does not take into account the increase in energy

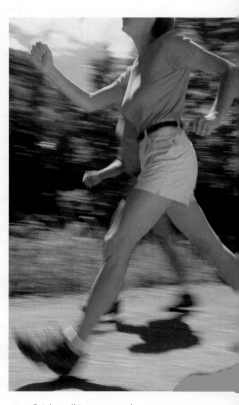

Brisk walking expends energy.

you do the math

Calculating BMR and Total Daily Energy Needs

One potential way to estimate how much energy you need each day is to record your total food and beverage intake for a defined period, such as 3 or 7 days. You can then use a food composition table or computer dietary assessment program to estimate the amount of energy you eat each day. Assuming that your body weight is stable over this period, your average daily energy intake should represent how much energy you need to maintain your present weight.

Unfortunately, many studies of energy intake in humans have shown that dietary records estimating energy needs are not very accurate. Most studies show that humans underestimate the amount of energy they eat by 10–30%. Overweight people tend to underestimate by an even higher margin, at the same time overestimating the amount of activity they do. This means that someone who really eats about 2,000 kcal/day may record eating only 1,400 to 1,800 kcal/day. So one reason many people are confused about their ability to lose weight is that they are eating more than they realize.

A simpler and more accurate way to estimate your total daily energy needs is to calculate your BMR, and then add the amount of energy you expend as a result of your activity level. Refer to the example below to learn how to do this. Because the energy cost for the thermic effect of food is very small, you don't need to include it in your calculations.

1. **Calculate your BMR:** If you are a man, you will need to multiply your body weight in kilograms by 1 kcal per kilogram body weight per hour. Assuming you weigh 175 pounds, your body weight in kilograms would be 175 lb/2.2 lb/kg = 79.5 kg. Next, multiply your weight in kilograms by 1 kcal per kilogram body weight per hour:

   1 kcal/kg body weight/hour × 79.5 kg = 79.5 kcal/hour

   Calculate your BMR for the total day (or 24 hours):

   79.5 kcal/hour × 24 hours/day = 1,909 kcal/day

   If you are a woman, multiply your body weight in kilogram by 0.9 kcal/kg body weight/hour.

2. **Estimate your activity level by selecting the description that most closely fits your general lifestyle.** The energy cost of activities is expressed as a percentage of your BMR. Refer to the values in the following table when estimating your own energy output.

3. **Multiply your BMR by the decimal equivalent of the lower and higher percentage values for your activity level.** Let's use the man referred to in step 1. He is a college student who lives on campus. He walks to classes located throughout campus, carries his book bag, and spends most of his time reading and writing. He does not exercise on a regular basis. His lifestyle would be defined as lightly active, meaning he expends 50–70% of his BMR each day in activities. You want to calculate how much energy he expends at both ends of this activity level. How many kcal does this equal?

   1,909 kcal/day × 0.50 (or 50%) = 955 kcal/day

   1,909 kcal/day × 0.70 (or 70%) = 1,336 kcal/day

   These calculations show that this man expends about 955 to 1,336 kcal/day doing daily activities.

4. **Calculate total daily energy output by adding together BMR and the energy needed to perform daily activities.** In this man's case, his total daily energy output is:

   1,909 kcal/day + 955 kcal/day = 2,864 kcal/day

   or

   1,909 kcal/day + 1,336 kcal/day = 3,245 kcal/day

   Assuming this man is maintaining his present weight, he requires between 2,864 and 3,245 kcal/day to stay in energy balance!

	Men	Women
Sedentary/Inactive Involves mostly sitting, driving, or very low levels of activity.	25–40%	25–35%
Lightly Active Involves a lot of sitting; may also involve some walking, moving around, and light lifting.	50–70%	40–60%
Moderately Active Involves work plus intentional exercise such as an hour of walking or walking 4 to 5 days per week; may have a job requiring some physical labor.	65–80%	50–70%
Heavily Active Involves a great deal of physical labor, such as roofing, carpentry work, and/or regular heavy lifting and digging.	90–120%	80–100%
Exceptionally Active Involves a lot of physical activities for work and intentional exercise. Also applies to athletes who train for many hours each day, such as triathletes and marathon runners or other competitive athletes performing heavy, regular training.	130–145%	110–130%

expenditure that would occur, including increased BMR and increased cost of moving a larger body, as weight increased. Thus, after a short period of positive energy balance, body weight would increase, resulting in an increase in energy expenditure that would eventually balance the increased energy intake. The individual would then achieve energy balance and become weight stable at a higher body weight. Thus, the extra 100 kcal/d would actually result in a more realistic weight gain of a few pounds. To maintain this larger body size the individual would need to continue to eat these additional kcals. Of course, the amount of weight an individual gains when overeating will depend on the number of extra kcals consumed, the macronutrient composition of these kcals (that is, the amount of fat, carbohydrate, protein, or alcohol), and overall energy expenditure.

The inadequacy of the classic energy balance equation has prompted experts to propose a dynamic equation of energy balance that takes into account the rates of energy intake and expenditure and their effect on rate of change of energy stores (including fat and lean tissues) in the body, not simply on body weight overall.[8]

> Predict a more realistic time course for weight loss or weight gain for yourself based on a dynamic simulation model of human metabolism by going to http://bwsimulator.niddk.nih.gov.

recap The energy balance equation relates food intake to energy expenditure. Eating more energy than you expend causes weight gain, whereas eating less energy than you expend causes weight loss. Energy expenditure can be measured using direct calorimetry, indirect calorimetry, and doubly labeled water. The three components of energy expenditure are basal metabolic rate, the thermic effect of food, and the energy cost of physical activity.

Genetic Factors Affect Body Weight

Our genetic background influences our height, weight, body shape, and metabolic rate. A classic study shows that the body weights of adults who were adopted as children are similar to the weights of their biological parents, not their adoptive parents.[9] How much of our BMI can be accounted for by genetic influences remains controversial, however, with proposed values ranging from 50% to 90%.[10] This means that 10–50% of our BMI is accounted for by nongenetic, environmental factors and lifestyle choices such as exposure to cheap, high-energy food and low levels of physical activity. Unfortunately, this message that a relatively large proportion of our BMI is accounted for by genetic influences could discourage people who want to lose weight from making helpful lifestyle changes. Bloss and colleagues found that individuals who were genetically tested and found to have higher genetic risk for obesity were more likely to report a higher fat intake and lower levels of physical activity 6 months after they received these results.[11]

Exactly how do genetic factors influence body weight? We discuss here some theories attempting to explain this link.

The FTO Gene

The existing evidence on genetics and obesity indicate that there is no one single "obesity gene." Instead, more than 120 genes currently are thought to be associated with an increased risk for obesity.[12] Nevertheless, one gene that has received a great deal of attention is the FTO (fat mass and obesity-associated) gene. This gene is relatively common: approximately 44–65% of people are estimated to have at least one copy. The gene appears to stimulate excessive food intake and may diminish feelings of satiety; thus, it's not surprising that people who carry the gene weigh more, on average, than people who do not. A recent study indicates that physical activity can attenuate the influence of the FTO gene on obesity risk in adults and children by 27%. These results highlight the importance of regular physical activity in reducing risk for obesity in people who are genetically predisposed.[13]

The Thrifty Gene Theory

The **thrifty gene theory** suggests that some people possess a gene (or genes) that causes them to be energetically thrifty. This means that at rest and even during active

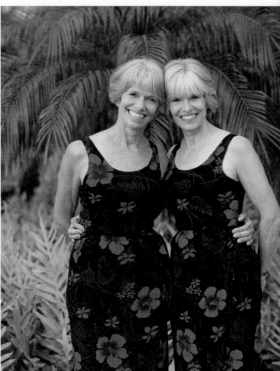

Identical twins tend to maintain a similar weight throughout life.

thrifty gene theory The theory that some people possess a gene (or genes) that causes them to be energetically thrifty, resulting in their expending less energy at rest and during physical activity.

times, these individuals expend less energy than people who do not possess this gene. The proposed purpose of this gene is to protect a person from starving to death during times of extreme food shortages. This theory has been applied to some Native American tribes because these societies were exposed to centuries of feast and famine. Those with a thrifty metabolism survived when little food was available, and this trait was passed on to future generations. Although an actual thrifty gene (or genes) has not yet been identified, researchers continue to study this explanation as a potential cause of obesity.

If this theory is true, think about how people who possess this thrifty gene might respond to today's environment. Low levels of physical activity, inexpensive food sources that are high in fat and energy, and excessively large serving sizes are the norm in our society. People with a thrifty metabolism would experience a great amount of weight gain, and their bodies would be more resistant to weight loss.

The Set-Point Theory

The **set-point theory** suggests that our bodies are designed to maintain our weight within a narrow range, or at a "set point." In many cases, the body appears to respond in such a way as to maintain a person's current weight. When we dramatically reduce energy intake (such as with fasting or strict diets), the body responds with physiologic changes that cause BMR to drop. This causes a significant slowing of our energy output. In addition, being physically active while fasting or starving is difficult because a person just doesn't have the energy for it. These two mechanisms of energy conservation may contribute to some of the rebound weight gain many dieters experience after they quit dieting.

Conversely, overeating in some people may cause an increase in BMR thought to be due to an increased thermic effect of food as well as an increase in spontaneous physical activity. This in turn increases energy output and prevents weight gain. These changes may explain the limitations of the classic energy balance equation mentioned earlier in predicting how much weight people will gain from eating excess food.

In addition, we don't eat exactly the same amount of food each day; some days we overeat, other days we eat less. When you think about how much our daily energy intake fluctuates (about 20% above and below our average monthly intake), our ability to maintain a certain weight over long periods suggests that there is some evidence to support the set-point theory.

Can we change our weight set point? It appears that when we maintain changes in our diet and activity level over a long period, weight change does occur. This is obvious in the case of obesity because many people who were normal weight as young adults become obese during middle adulthood. Also, many people do successfully lose weight and maintain that weight loss over long periods. Thus, the set-point theory cannot entirely account for the body's resistance to weight loss.

A classic study on weight gain in twins demonstrated how genetics may affect our tendency to maintain a set point.[14] Twelve pairs of male identical twins volunteered to stay in a dormitory, where they were supervised 24 hours a day for 120 consecutive days. Researchers measured how much energy each man needed to maintain his body weight at the beginning of the study. For 100 days, the subjects were fed 1,000 kcal more per day than they needed to maintain body weight. Daily physical activity was limited, but each person was allowed to walk outdoors for 30 minutes each day, read, watch television and videos, and play cards and video games. The research staff stayed with these men to ensure that they did not stray from the study protocol.

Although these men were all overfed enough energy to gain about 26 pounds, the average weight gain they experienced was only 18 pounds. They gained mostly fat but also about 6 pounds of lean body mass. Interestingly, although each twin gained an amount similar to that of his brother, there was a very wide range of weight gained overall: The lowest weight gain was 9.5 pounds, whereas the highest was more than 29 pounds! Keep in mind that the food these men ate and the activities they performed were tightly controlled.

This study shows that, when people overeat by the same amount of food, they can gain very different amounts of weight. Researchers theorize that those who are more

set-point theory The theory that the body raises or lowers energy expenditure in response to increased or decreased food intake and physical activity. This action maintains an individual's body weight within a narrow range.

resistant to weight gain when they overeat have the ability to increase BMR, store more excess energy as lean body mass instead of fat, and increase spontaneous physical activity. Thus, genetic differences may explain why some people are better able to maintain a certain weight set point.

recap Many factors affect our ability to gain and lose weight. Our genetic background influences our height, weight, body shape, and metabolic rate. The FTO gene variant appears to prompt overeating and weight gain. The thrifty gene theory suggests that some people possess a thrifty gene, or set of genes, that causes them to expend less energy at rest and during physical activity than people who do not have this gene (or genes). The set-point theory suggests that our body is designed to maintain weight within a narrow range, also called a set point.

Composition of the Diet Affects Fat Storage

As previously discussed, when we eat more energy than we expend, we gain weight. Most people eat a mixed diet made up of carbohydrate, fat, and protein. Scientists used to think that people would gain the same amount of weight if they ate too much food of any type, but now there is evidence to support the theory that, when we overeat, our bodies more readily store the extra energy that comes from dietary fat because this is the most efficient way to store excess energy. This may be due to the fact that eating fat doesn't cause much of an increase in metabolic rate, and the body stores fat in the form of adipose tissue quite easily. In contrast, when we consume excess energy by overeating protein or carbohydrate, the body's initial response is to use the energy from these macronutrients to fuel the body, with a smaller amount of the excess stored as fat. This does not mean, however, that you can eat as many low-fat foods as you want and not gain weight! Consistently overeating protein or carbohydrate will also lead to weight gain. Instead, maintain a balanced diet combining fat, carbohydrate, and protein, and reduce dietary fat to less than 35% of total energy. This strategy may help reduce your storage of fat energy as adipose tissue.

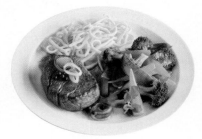

A balanced diet contains protein, carbohydrate, and fat.

Metabolic Factors Influence Weight Loss and Gain

Four metabolic factors are thought to be predictive of a person's risk for weight gain and resistance to weight loss.[8] These factors are:

- Relatively low metabolic rate. As discussed previously, obese individuals weigh more and have a higher amount of lean tissue than people of normal weight and thus will have a higher absolute BMR. However at any given size, people vary in their relative BMR—it can be high, normal, or low. People who have a relatively low BMR are more at risk for weight gain and are resistant to weight loss.
- Low level of spontaneous physical activity. People who exhibit less spontaneous physical activity are at increased risk for weight gain.
- Low sympathetic nervous system activity. The sympathetic nervous system plays an important role in regulating all components of energy expenditure, and people with lower rates of sympathetic nervous system activity are more prone to obesity and more resistant to weight loss.
- Low fat oxidation. Some people oxidize relatively more carbohydrate for energy, which means that less fat will be oxidized. Instead, it will be stored in adipose tissue. Thus, these people are at higher risk for gaining weight. People who oxidize relatively more fat for energy are more resistant to weight gain and are more successful at maintaining weight loss.

Physiologic Factors Influence Body Weight

Numerous physiologic factors affect body weight, including hypothalamic regulation of hunger and satiety, specific hormones, and other factors. Together, these contribute to the complexities of weight regulation.

Hunger and Satiety

As previously introduced (in Chapter 3), *hunger* is the innate, physiologic drive or need to eat. Physical signals such as a growling stomach and lightheadedness indicate when one is hungry. This drive for food is triggered by physiologic changes, such as low blood glucose, that affect cells in the hypothalamus. A group of hypothalamic cells referred to as the *feeding center* responds to conditions of low blood glucose, causing hunger and driving a person to eat. Once one has eaten and the body has responded accordingly, cells in the hypothalamus' satiety center are triggered, and the desire to eat is reduced. Some people may have an insufficient satiety mechanism, which prevents them from feeling full after a meal, allowing them to overeat. However, people with a sufficient satiety mechanism also can and do override satiety signals and overeat even when they are not hungry.

Energy-Regulating Hormones

Leptin is a protein produced by adipose cells that functions as a hormone. First discovered in mice, leptin acts to reduce food intake and cause a decrease in body weight and body fat.

When these findings were first published, a great deal of excitement was generated about the possibility of administering leptin injections to decrease obesity in humans. Unfortunately, studies have shown that, although obese mice respond positively to leptin injections, obese humans do not. Instead, they already tend to have high amounts of leptin in their bodies and are insensitive to its effects. In truth, we have just begun to learn about leptin and its role in the human body. Researchers are currently studying its role in starvation and overeating, and it appears it might play a role in cardiovascular and kidney complications that result from obesity and related diseases.

In addition to leptin, numerous proteins affect the regulation of appetite and storage of body fat. Primary among these is **ghrelin**, a protein synthesized in the stomach. It acts as a hormone and plays an important role in appetite regulation through its actions in the hypothalamus. Ghrelin stimulates appetite and increases the amount of food one eats. Ghrelin levels increase before a meal and fall within about 1 hour after a meal. This action indicates that ghrelin may be a primary contributor to both hunger and satiety. Ghrelin levels appear to increase after weight loss, and researchers speculate that this factor could help to explain why people who have lost weight have difficulty keeping it off.[15] We noted earlier that obese people seem to lose their sensitivity to leptin, but this is not true for ghrelin: obese people are just as sensitive to the effects of ghrelin as non-obese people.[16] For this reason, potential mechanisms that can block the actions of ghrelin are currently a prime target of research into the treatment of obesity.

Peptide YY, or **PYY**, is a protein produced in the gastrointestinal tract. It is released after a meal, in amounts proportional to the energy content of the meal. In contrast with ghrelin, PYY decreases appetite and inhibits food intake in animals and humans. Interestingly, obese individuals have lower levels of PYY when they are fasting and also show less of an increase in PYY after a meal as compared with non-obese individuals, which suggests that PYY may be important in the manifestation and maintenance of obesity.[17]

Uncoupling proteins have recently become the focus of research into body weight. These proteins are found in the inner membrane of the mitochondria, which you may recall (from Chapter 3) are organelles present within cells that generate adenine triphosphate (ATP), including skeletal muscle cells and adipose cells. Some research suggests that uncoupling proteins uncouple certain steps in ATP production; when this occurs, the process produces heat instead of ATP. This production of heat increases energy expenditure and results in less storage of excess energy. Thus, a person with more uncoupling proteins or a higher activity of these proteins would be more resistant to weight gain and obesity.

Three forms of uncoupling proteins (UCPs) have been identified: UCP1 is found exclusively in **brown adipose tissue**, a type of adipose tissue that has more mitochondria than white adipose tissue. It is found in significant amounts in animals and newborn humans. It was traditionally thought that adult humans have very little brown adipose tissue. However, recent evidence suggests that humans may have substantially more brown adipose tissue than previously assumed,[18] and that people with

leptin A hormone, produced by body fat, that acts to reduce food intake and to decrease body weight and body fat.

ghrelin A protein, synthesized in the stomach, that acts as a hormone and plays an important role in appetite regulation by stimulating appetite.

peptide YY (PYY) A protein, produced in the gastrointestinal tract, that is released after a meal in amounts proportional to the energy content of the meal; it decreases appetite and inhibits food intake.

brown adipose tissue A type of adipose tissue that has more mitochondria than white adipose tissue and which can increase energy expenditure by uncoupling oxidation from ATP production. It is found in significant amounts in animals and newborn humans.

higher BMI values have lower amounts of brown adipose tissue.[19] Two other uncoupling proteins, UCP2 and UCP3, are known to be important to energy expenditure and resistance to weight gain. These proteins are found in various tissues, including white adipose tissue and skeletal muscle.

Other Physiologic Factors

The following other physiologic factors are known to increase satiety (or decrease food intake):

- The hormones serotonin and cholecystokinin (CCK); serotonin is made from the amino acid tryptophan, and CCK is produced by the intestinal cells and stimulates the gallbladder to secrete bile.
- An increase in blood glucose levels, such as that normally seen after the consumption of a meal.
- Stomach expansion.
- Nutrient absorption from the small intestine.

The following other physiologic factors can decrease satiety (or increase food intake):

- Beta-endorphins, which are hormones that enhance a sense of pleasure while eating, increasing food intake.
- Neuropeptide Y, an amino-acid-containing compound produced in the hypothalamus; neuropeptide Y stimulates appetite.
- Decreased blood glucose levels, such as the decrease that occurs after an overnight fast.

Cultural and Economic Factors Affect Food Choices and Body Weight

Both cultural and economic factors can contribute to obesity. As discussed in the **In Depth** on Eating Wisely (pages 65–71), cultural factors (including religious beliefs and learned food preferences) affect our food choices and eating patterns. In addition, the customs of many cultures put food at the center of celebrations of festivals and holidays, and overeating is tacitly encouraged. In addition because both parents now work outside the home in most American families, more people are embracing the "fast-food culture," eating highly processed and highly Caloric fast foods from restaurants and grocery stores rather than lower-kcal, home-cooked meals.

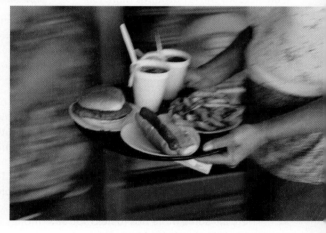

◀ Fast foods may be inexpensive and filling, but they're often high in saturated fat, salt, and sugar.

Coinciding with these cultural influences on food intake are cultural factors that promote inactivity. These include the shift from manual labor to more sedentary jobs and increased access to labor-saving devices in all areas of our lives. Even seemingly minor changes—such as walking through an automated door instead of pushing a door open—add up to a lower expenditure of energy by the end of the day. Research with sedentary ethnic minority women in the United States indicates that other common barriers to increasing physical activity include lack of personal motivation, no physically active role models to emulate, acceptance of larger body size, exercise being considered culturally unacceptable, and fear for personal safety in both rural and urban settings.[20,21] In short, cultural factors influence both food consumption and levels of physical activity and can contribute to weight gain.

Economic status is known to be related to health status, particularly in developed countries such as the United States: people of lower economic status have higher rates of obesity and related chronic diseases than people of higher incomes.[22] In addition to the impact of one's income on access to healthcare, economic factors strongly impact our food choices and eating behaviors. It is a common belief that healthful foods are expensive, and that only wealthy people can afford to purchase them. Although it is true that certain foods considered more healthful, such as organic foods, imported fruits and vegetables, many fish, and leaner selections of some meats, can be costly, does healthful eating always have to be expensive? Refer to the **Nutrition Myth or Fact?** box (page 406) to learn more about whether a healthful diet can also be affordable.

nutrition myth or fact?

Does It Cost More to Eat Right?

The shelves of American supermarkets are filled with an abundance of healthful food options: organic meats and produce, exotic fish, out-of-season fresh fruits and vegetables that are flown in from warmer climates, whole-grain breads and cereals, and low-fat and low-sodium options of traditional foods. With all of this choice, it would seem easy for anyone to consume healthful foods throughout the year. But a closer look at the prices of these foods suggests that for many they simply are not affordable. This raises the question: Does eating right have to be expensive?

It is a fact that organic foods are more expensive than non-organic options. However (as we'll explore in detail in Chapter 13), there is little evidence indicating that organic foods are actually more nutritious than non-organic foods. In addition, some of the lowest-cost foods currently available in stores are also some of the most nutritious: these include beans, lentils, and other legumes, seasonal fruits, root vegetables such as potatoes and winter squashes, frozen fruits and vegetables, and cooking oils high in mono- and polyunsaturated fats. In fact, frozen as well as canned fruits and vegetables are generally just as nutritious as fresh options and may be more so depending on how long the fresh produce has been transported and stored, and how long it has been sitting on the supermarket shelves. Thus, with some knowledge, skills, and focused attention, people can still eat healthfully on a tight budget.

Here are some more tips to help you save money when shopping for healthful foods:

- Buy whole grains such as cereals, brown rice, and pastas in bulk—they store well for longer periods and provide a good base for meals and snacks.
- Buy frozen vegetables on sale and stock up—these are just as healthful as fresh vegetables, require less preparation, and can be much cheaper.

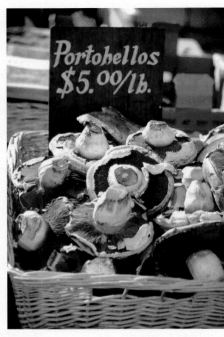

Some specialty foods (such as organic or imported products) can be expensive, and lower-cost alternatives can be just as nutritious.

- If lower-sodium options of canned vegetables are too expensive, buy the less expensive regular option and drain the juice from the vegetables before cooking.
- Consume smaller amounts of leaner meats—by eating less you'll not only save money but reduce your total intake of energy and fat while still providing nutrients that support good health.
- Choose frozen fish or canned salmon or tuna packed in water as an alternative to fresh fish.
- Avoid frozen or dehydrated prepared meals. These are usually expensive; high in sodium, saturated fats, and energy; and low in fiber and other important nutrients.
- Buy generic or store brands of foods—be careful to check the labels to ensure the foods are similar in nutrient value as the higher-priced options.
- Cut coupons from local newspapers and magazines, and watch the sale circulars so that you can stock up on healthful foods you can store.
- Consider cooking more meals at home; you'll have more control over what goes into your meals and will also be able to cook larger amounts and freeze leftovers for future meals.

As you can see, eating healthfully does not have to be expensive. However, it helps to become a savvy consumer by reading food labels, comparing prices, and gaining the skills and confidence to cook at home. The information shared throughout this text should help you acquire these skills so that you can eat healthfully, even on a limited budget!

CRITICAL THINKING QUESTIONS

1. What two changes can you make to your current food shopping habits to reduce your grocery bill?
2. How do the prices of fresh fruits and vegetables compare between your favorite supermarket and your local farmers' market? Which is the better option for choice, freshness, and cost?

Social Factors Influence Behavior and Body Weight

In the **In Depth** on Eating Wisely (following Chapter 2), we explored the concept that *appetite* can be experienced in the absence of hunger. Appetite may therefore be considered a psychological drive to eat and is stimulated by a variety of social factors, such as learned preferences for food, particular situations that promote eating, and social cues related to the timing and size of meals. Social factors also affect our level of activity. Thus, they strongly influence our body weight.

Some Social Factors Promote Overeating

Social factors—such as pressure from family and friends to eat the way they do—can encourage people to overeat. For example, the pressure to overeat on holidays is high because family members or friends offer extra servings of favorite holiday foods and follow a very large meal with a rich dessert.

Americans also have numerous opportunities to overeat because of easy access throughout the day to foods high in fat and energy. Vending machines selling junk foods are everywhere, shopping malls are filled with fast-food restaurants, and food manufacturers are producing products in ever-larger serving sizes: Hardee's Monster Thickburger packs 1,290 kcal—which is 65% of the Calorie intake recommended for an average adult for an entire day! Even some foods traditionally considered healthful, such as some brands of peanut butter, yogurt, chicken soup, and flavored milks, may be filled with added sugars and other ingredients that are high in energy. This easy access to high-energy meals and snacks leads many people to overeat.

> To test your understanding of a serving size, take an interactive quiz from the National Institutes of Health. Just enter "NIH Portion Distortion" into your Internet browser and it will take you to the main page; then click on the Portion Distortion links, and explore the other resources located there.

Some Social Factors Promote Inactivity

Social factors can also cause people to be less physically active. For instance, we don't have to expend much energy preparing food anymore because so many foods are ready to serve or require just microwave cooking. Other social factors restricting physical activity include living in an unsafe community; watching a lot of television; coping with family, community, and work responsibilities that do not involve physical activity; and living in an area with harsh weather conditions. Many overweight people identify such factors as major barriers to engaging in regular physical activity, and research seems to confirm their influence.

Certainly, social factors are contributing to decreased physical activity among children. There was a time when children played outdoors regularly and when physical education was offered daily in school. Today, many children cannot play outdoors due to safety concerns and lack of recreational facilities, and few schools have the resources to regularly offer physical education to children.

Another social factor promoting inactivity in both children and adults is the increasing dominance of technology in our choices of entertainment. Instead of participating in sports or gathering for a dance at the community hall, we go to the movies or stay at home watching television, surfing the Internet, and playing with video games and other hand-held devices. By reducing energy expenditure, these behaviors contribute to weight gain. For instance, a study of 11- to 13-year-old schoolchildren found that children who watched more than 2 hours of television per night were more likely to be overweight or obese than children who watched less than 2 hours of television per night. Similarly, television watching in adults has been shown to be associated with weight gain over a four-year period.[23]

Social Pressures Can Promote Underweight

On the other hand, social pressures to maintain a lean body are great enough to encourage many people to undereat or to avoid foods that are perceived as "bad," especially fats. Our society ridicules and often ostracizes overweight people, many of whom face discrimination in housing, employment, and other areas of their lives. A recent study found that children who are obese are 60% more likely to experience bullying than children of normal weight.[24] Moreover, media images of waiflike fashion models and men in tight jeans with muscular chests and abdomens encourage many people—especially adolescents and young adults—to skip meals, resort to crash diets, and exercise obsessively. Even some people of normal body weight push themselves to achieve an unrealistic and unattainable weight goal, in the process threatening their health and even their lives (see the **In Depth** immediately following this chapter for information on the consequences of disordered eating).

It should be clear that how a person gains, loses, and maintains body weight is a complex matter. Most people who are overweight have tried several diet programs but have been unsuccessful in losing weight or maintaining their weight loss.

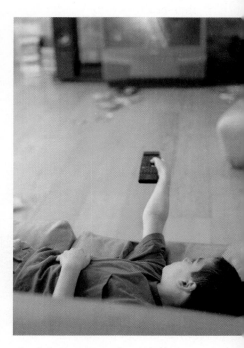

Behaviors learned as a child can affect weight and physical activity patterns.

A significant number of these people have consequently given up all weight-loss attempts. Some even suffer from severe depression related to their body weight. Should we condemn these people as failures and continue to pressure them to lose weight? Should people who are overweight but otherwise healthy (for example, low blood pressure, cholesterol, triglycerides, and glucose levels) be advised to lose weight? As we continue to search for ways to help people achieve and maintain a healthful body weight, our society must take measures to reduce the social pressures facing people who are overweight or obese.

recap The macronutrient composition of the diet influences the storage of body fat, and metabolic factors such as low relative resting metabolic rate, low spontaneous physical activity, low sympathetic nervous system activity, and low fat oxidation increase the risk for weight gain. Physiologic factors, such as various energy-regulating hormones, impact body weight by their effects on satiety, appetite, and energy expenditure. Cultural and economic factors can significantly influence the amounts and types of food we eat. Social factors influencing weight include the ready availability of large portions of high-energy foods and lack of physical activity. Social pressures on those who are overweight can drive people to use harmful methods to achieve an unrealistic body weight.

How can you achieve and maintain a healthful body weight?

Now that you understand what constitutes a healthful body weight, how are you feeling about yours? You might decide that you'd like to lose weight, but are you really committed to making the changes required? To find out, check out the **What About You?** box (pages 409–411). If your results suggest that you are, then take heart. Achieving and maintaining a healthful body weight involve three primary strategies:

- Gradual changes in energy intake
- Incorporation of regular and appropriate physical activity
- Application of behavior modification techniques

In this section, we first discuss popular weight-loss plans, which may or may not incorporate these strategies. We then explain how to design a personalized weight-loss plan that includes all three of them.

nutri-case | HANNAH

"I wonder what it would be like to be able to look in the mirror and not feel fat. Like my friend Kristi—she's been skinny since we were kids. I'm the opposite: I've felt bad about my weight ever since I can remember. One of my worst memories is from YMCA swim camp the summer I was 10 years old. Of course, we had to wear a swimsuit, and the other kids picked on me so bad I'll never forget it. One of the boys called me 'fatso,' and the girls were even meaner, especially when I was changing in the locker room. That was the last year I went to swim camp, and I haven't owned a swimsuit since."

Think back to your own childhood. Were you ever teased for some personal aspect that you felt unable to change? How might organizations that work with children—such as schools, YMCAs, scout troops, and church-based groups—increase their awareness of the social stigmatization that overweight children often experience, and reduce incidents of teasing, bullying, and other forms of insensitivity?

what about **you** ?

Are You Really Ready to Lose Weight?

Do you think you're ready for a weight-loss program? For each question, circle the answer that best describes your attitude. Tally your score as you go, and use the guides in sections 2 through 5 to see what your score means.

1. Diet History

A. How many times in the last year have you been on a diet?

0 times   1–2 times   3–5 times   6–12 times   More than 13

B. What is the most weight you lost on any of these diets?

0 lb   1–2 lb   3–5 lb   6–12 lb   More than 13 lb

C. How long did you stay at the new lower weight?

Less than 1 mo   2–5 mo   6–8 mo   9–11 mo   Over 1 yr

D. Why do you think you started to regain the weight?

E. Put a mark by each dieting method you've used previously:

_____ skipping breakfast

_____ skipping lunch or dinner

_____ taking over-the-counter appetite suppressants

_____ counting Calories

_____ cutting out fats

_____ cutting out carbohydrates

_____ increasing regular exercise

_____ taking weight-loss supplements

_____ cutting out snacks

_____ using meal replacements

_____ taking prescription appetite suppressants

_____ taking laxatives

_____ inducing vomiting

_____ other _____

2. Readiness to Start a Weight-Loss Program

A. How motivated are you to lose weight?

1 Not at all motivated   **2** Somewhat motivated   **3** Very motivated

B. How certain are you that you will stay committed to a weight-loss program long enough to reach your goal?

1 Not at all certain   **2** Somewhat certain   **3** Very certain

C. To what extent can you tolerate the effort required to stick to your diet plan?

1 Cannot commit   **2** Can commit   **3** Can readily commit

D. Have you allotted a realistic amount of time for weight loss?

1 Very unrealistic   **2** Somewhat realistic   **3** Extremely realistic

E. While dieting, do you fantasize about eating your favorite foods?

1 Always   **2** Sometimes   **3** Never

F. While dieting, do you feel deprived, angry, upset?

1 Always   **2** Sometimes   **3** Never

Total your scores from this section and circle your score category.

6 to 10: This may not be a good time for you to start a diet. Inadequate motivation and commitment and unrealistic goals could block your progress. Think about what contributes to your unreadiness.

(*continued*)

11 to 14: You may be almost ready to begin a program but should think about how to support your efforts.

15 to 18: You are ready to start safely losing weight.

3. Hunger, Appetite, and Eating

   A. Do you routinely experience food cravings and the sensation of hunger?

1	**2**	**3**
Never	Sometimes	Always

   B. How often do you eat for a reason other than physical hunger?

1	**2**	**3**
Never	Sometimes	Always

   C. Do you snack between meals?

1	**2**	**3**
Never	Sometimes	Always

   Total your scores from this section and circle your score category.

   3 to 5: You rarely indulge, largely as a result of your mindset and approach to eating.

   6 to 7: You may sometimes eat less carefully due to easy availability of snacks or treats.

   8 to 9: Work on reducing your exposure to less healthful foods that can tempt you.

4. Controlling Overeating

   A. When you eat out, or have meals not prepared by you at home, you tend to:

1	**2**	**3**
Eat less	Eat somewhat more	Eat a lot more

   B. When you "slip up" from more healthful eating habits, your usual response is to then:

1	**2**	**3**
Eat less	Eat somewhat more	Eat a lot more

   C. You often "reward" yourself for good eating behavior by:

1	**2**	**3**
Keeping up good efforts	Eating a small indulgence	Eating a big indulgence

   Total your scores from this section and circle your score category.

   3 to 5: You're able to maintain control but may have to watch your impulse to be too rigid.

   6 to 7: You have a sensible approach and are able to work through short-term set-backs.

   8 to 9: You should try to work on a more balanced approach that doesn't undermine your other good efforts.

5. Emotional Eating

   A. You eat whatever you feel like eating or crave when you're under stress or in an emotional state.

1	**2**	**3**
Never	Often	Always

   B. You reward yourself with food when you feel you deserve it or are in a good mood.

1	**2**	**3**
Never	Often	Always

C. You overindulge with food when you encounter difficulties or challenges.

1	**2**	**3**
Never	Often	Always

Total your scores from this section and circle your score category.

3 to 5: You are in control of your emotions and they don't drive you to eating behaviors you'll regret.

6 to 7: Your control over your emotional state in regard to food can waver at times. Think about how to anticipate problematic responses to stress.

8 to 9: You're often subject to food reactions that stem from your emotions. Work on dealing with your feelings in ways that don't negatively impact your health.

6. Exercise Patterns and Attitudes

A. You get moderate-to-vigorous exercise:

1	**2**	**3**
Never	Occasionally	Often

B. What level of confidence do you have about being able to really integrate regular exercise into your life?

1	**2**	**3**
Not at all confident	Somewhat confident	Very confident

C. What association with your self-image does exercise have for you?

1	**2**	**3**
Negative	Somewhat positive	Very positive

D. What level of certainty do you have about being truly ready to integrate regular exercise into your life?

1	**2**	**3**
Not at all certain	Somewhat certain	Very certain

Total your scores from this section and circle your score category.

4 to 6: You could benefit from getting more exercise than you currently are. Reflect on why you have feelings of resistance.

7 to 9: You're interested in exercise and may already be doing some exercises. Think about ways you could be even more receptive to increasing your activity level.

10 to 12: You're ready to start a regular exercise program. Find ways to support your motivation.

Data based on: "The Diet Readiness Test," in "When and How to Diet," *Psychology Today* (June 1989) 41–46. Copyright © 1989 Sussex Publishers, Inc.

If You Decide to Follow a Popular Weight-Loss Plan, Choose One Based on the Three Strategies

If you'd like to lose weight and feel more comfortable following an established plan, many are available. How can you know whether or not it is based on sound dietary principles, and whether its promise of long-term weight loss will prove true for *you*? Look to the three strategies just identified: Does the plan promote gradual reductions in energy intake? Does it advocate increased physical activity? Does it include strategies for modifying your eating and activity-related behaviors? Reputable diet plans incorporate all of these strategies. Unfortunately, many dieters are drawn to fad diets, which do not.

Avoid Fad Diets

Beware of fad diets! They are simply what their name implies—fads that do not result in long-term, healthful weight changes. To be precise, fad diets are programs that enjoy short-term popularity and are sold based on a marketing gimmick that appeals to the public's desires and fears. Of the hundreds of such diets on the market today, most will "die" within a year, only to be born again as a "new and improved" fad diet. The goal of the person or company designing and marketing a fad diet is to make money.

How can you tell if the program you are interested in qualifies as a fad diet? Here are some pointers to help you:

- The promoters of the diet claim that the program is new, improved, or based on some new discovery; however, no scientific data are available to support these claims.
- The program is touted for its ability to promote rapid weight loss or body fat loss, usually more than 2 pounds per week, and may include the claim that weight loss can be achieved with little or no physical exercise.
- The diet includes special foods and supplements, many of which are expensive and/or difficult to find or can be purchased only from the diet promoter. Common recommendations for these diets include avoiding certain foods, eating only a special combination of certain foods, or including "magic" foods in the diet that "burn fat" and "speed up metabolism."
- The diet may include a rigid menu that must be followed daily or may limit participants to eating a few select foods each day. Variety and balance are discouraged, and restriction of certain foods (such as fruits and vegetables) is encouraged.
- Many programs promote supplemental foods and/or nutritional supplements that are described as critical to the success of the diet. They usually include claims that these supplements can cure or prevent a variety of health ailments or that the diet can stop the aging process.

In a world where many of us feel we have to meet a certain physical standard to be attractive and "good enough," fad diets flourish, with millions of people trying one each year.[25] Unfortunately, the only people who usually benefit from them are their marketers, who can become very wealthy promoting programs that are highly ineffectual.

Diets Focusing on Macronutrient Composition May or May Not Work for You

It is well recognized that achieving a negative energy balance is the major factor in successful weight loss. The impact of the macronutrient composition of a diet is currently a topic of considerable debate. The three main types of weight-loss diets that have been most seriously and comprehensively researched all encourage increased consumption of certain macronutrients and restrict the consumption of others. Provided here is a brief review of these three main types and their general effects on weight loss and health parameters.

Diets High in Carbohydrate and Moderate in Fat and Protein   Nutritionally balanced high-carbohydrate, moderate-fat, and moderate-protein diets typically contain 55–60% of total energy intake as carbohydrate, 20–30% of total energy intake as fat, and 15–20% of energy intake as protein. These diets include Weight Watchers, Jenny Craig, and others that follow the general guidelines of the DASH diet and the USDA Food Guide. All of these diet plans emphasize that weight loss occurs when energy intake is lower than energy expenditure. The goal is gradual weight loss, or about 1 to 2 pounds of body weight per week. Typical energy deficits are between 500 and 1,000 kcal/day. It is recommended that women eat no less than 1,000 to 1,200 kcal/day and that men consume no less than 1,200 to 1,400 kcal/day. Regular physical activity is encouraged.

To date, these types of low-energy diets have been researched more than any others. A substantial amount of high-quality scientific evidence (from randomized controlled trials) indicates that they may be effective in decreasing body weight—at least initially. In addition, the people who lose weight on these diets may also decrease their LDL-cholesterol, reduce their blood triglyceride levels, and decrease their blood pressure. However, recently published results from a randomized controlled trial following almost 50,000 U.S. women for 7 years has caused considerable debate around whether these types of diets result in long-term weight loss or reduce the risk for chronic diseases. This study found that contrary to established beliefs, this type of diet did not result in significant long-term weight loss or reduce the risks for breast and colorectal cancers or cardiovascular disease.[26-29] Is it possible that diets high in carbohydrate and moderate in fat and protein are not as effective as we'd come to believe? Refer to the **Nutrition Debate** at the end of this chapter to learn more about this controversy.

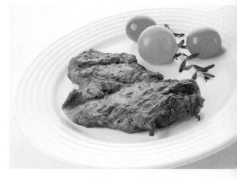

Diets Low in Carbohydrate and High in Fat and Protein   Low-carbohydrate, high-fat, and high-protein diets cycle in and out of popularity on a regular basis. By definition, these types of diets generally contain about 55–65% of total energy intake as fat and most of the remaining balance of daily energy intake as protein. Examples of these types of diets include Dr. Atkins' Diet Revolution, the Carbohydrate Addict's Diet, Life Without Bread, Sugar Busters, and Protein Power. These diets minimize the role of restricting total energy intake on weight loss. They instead advise participants to restrict carbohydrate intake, proposing that carbohydrates are addictive and that they cause significant overeating, insulin surges leading to excessive fat storage, and an overall metabolic imbalance that leads to obesity. The goal is to reduce carbohydrates enough to cause ketosis, which will decrease blood glucose and insulin levels and can reduce appetite.

"Low-carb" diets may lead to weight loss but can be nutritionally inadequate and have negative side effects.

Countless people claim to have lost substantial weight on these types of diets. Although quality scientific studies of these diets are just beginning to be conducted, the current limited evidence suggests that individuals following them, in both free-living and experimental conditions, do lose weight. In addition, it appears that those people who lose weight may also experience positive metabolic changes similar to those seen with higher-carbohydrate diets.

So are low-carb diets effective? A recent review of all of the published studies of these diets resulted in the conclusion that low-carb diets are just as effective, and possibly more effective, in promoting weight loss and reducing cardiovascular disease risk for a period of up to 1 year.[30] However, the authors conclude that long-term health benefits of this type of a diet are unknown at this time, and more research must be conducted in this area.

Low-Fat and Very-Low-Fat Diets   Low-fat diets contain 11–19% of total energy as fat, whereas very-low-fat diets contain less than 10% of total energy as fat. Both of these types of diets are high in carbohydrate and moderate in protein. Examples include Dr. Dean Ornish's Program for Reversing Heart Disease and the New Pritikin Program. Not originally designed for weight loss, these programs were developed to decrease or reverse heart disease. They do not focus on total energy intake but emphasize eating foods higher in complex carbohydrates and fiber. Consumption of sugar and white flour is very limited. The Ornish diet is vegetarian, whereas the Pritikin diet allows 3.5 oz of lean meat per day. Regular physical activity is a key component of both.

These diets are not popular with consumers, who view them as too restrictive and difficult to follow. Thus, there are limited data on their effects. However, high-quality evidence suggests that people following the diets do lose weight, and some data suggest that they also experience decreased LDL-cholesterol, blood triglyceride, glucose, and insulin levels as well as lower blood pressure. Few side effects have been reported on these diets; the most common is flatus, which typically decreases over time. Low-fat diets are low in vitamin B_{12}, and very-low-fat diets are low in essential fatty acids, vitamins B_{12} and E, and zinc. Thus, supplementation is needed. These types of diets are not considered safe for people with diabetes who are insulin dependent (either type 1 or type 2) or for people with carbohydrate-malabsorption illnesses.

If You Decide to Design Your Own Weight-Loss Plan, Include the Three Strategies

As we noted earlier, a healthful and effective weight-loss plan involves a modest reduction in energy intake, incorporating physical activity into each day, and practicing changes in behavior that can assist you in reducing your energy intake and increasing your energy expenditure. Following are some guidelines for designing your own personalized plan that incorporates these strategies.

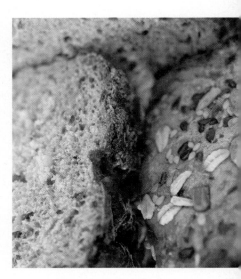

Low-fat and very-low-fat diets emphasize eating foods higher in complex carbohydrates and fiber.

Set Realistic Goals

The first key to safe and effective weight loss is setting realistic goals related to how much weight to lose and how quickly to lose it. Although making gradual changes in body weight is frustrating for most people, this slower change is much more effective in maintaining weight loss over the long term. Ask yourself the question, "How long did it take me to gain this extra weight?" If you are like most people, your answer is that it took 1 or more years, not just a few months. A fair expectation for weight loss is similarly gradual: experts recommend a pace of about 0.5 to 2 pounds per week. A weight-loss plan should never provide less that 1,200 kcal/day unless you are under a physician's supervision. Your weight-loss goals should also take into consideration any health-related concerns you have. After checking with your physician, you may decide initially to set a goal of simply maintaining your current weight and preventing additional weight gain. After your weight has remained stable for several weeks, you might then write down realistic goals for weight loss.

Goals that are more likely to be realistic and achievable share the following characteristics:

- **They are specific.** Telling yourself "I will eat less this week" is not helpful because the goal is not specific. An example of a specific goal is "I will eat only half of my restaurant entrée tonight and take the rest home and eat it tomorrow for lunch."
- **They are reasonable.** If you are not presently physically active, it would be unreasonable to set a goal of exercising for 30 minutes every day. A more reasonable goal would be to exercise for 15 minutes per day, 3 days per week. Once you've achieved that goal, you can increase the frequency, intensity, and time of exercise according to the improvements in fitness that you have experienced.
- **They are measurable.** Effective goals are ones you can measure. An example is "I will lose at least 1 pound by May 1st," or "I will substitute drinking water for my regular soft drink at lunch each day this week." Recording your specific, measurable goals will help you to better determine whether you are achieving them.

By monitoring your progress regularly you can determine whether you are meeting your goals or whether you need to revise them based on accomplishments or challenges that arise.

Eat Smaller Portions of Lower-Fat Foods

The portion sizes of foods offered and sold in restaurants and grocery stores have expanded considerably over the past 40 years. One of the most challenging issues related to food is understanding what a healthful portion size is and how to reduce the portion sizes of foods that we eat.

Studies indicate that when children and adults are presented with large portion sizes of foods and beverages, they eat more energy overall and do not respond to cues of fullness.[31,32] Thus, it has been suggested that effective weight-loss strategies include reducing both the portion size and energy density of foods consumed and replacing energy-dense beverages with low-Calorie or non-Calorie beverages.[32]

What specific changes can you make to reduce your energy intake and stay healthy? Refer to the **Quick Tips** box to learn more about how to control your portion sizes.

In addition to controlling portion sizes, try to increase the number of times each day that you choose foods that are relatively low in energy density. This includes salads (with low- or non-Calorie dressings), fruits, vegetables, low- and non-fat dairy products, and broth-based soups. Research indicates that eating a diet low in energy density results in greater weight loss than simply reducing portion sizes.[33,34] Because low–energy-dense foods are relatively higher in water and fiber than more–energy-dense foods, they have a greater volume and occupy more space in the stomach, helping a person to feel full. In addition, low–energy-dense foods are just as satiating as those higher in energy density but are lower in energy for every gram of food consumed. Thus, the energy content of an energy-dense eating plan is lower but equally as satisfying.

FIGURE 11.8 illustrates two sets of meals, one higher in energy density and one lower in energy density. You can see from this figure that simple changes to a meal, such as choosing lower-fat dairy products, skipping the high-fat condiments, and

QuickTips

Controlling Portion Sizes

To help increase your understanding of the portion sizes of packaged foods, measure out the amount of food that is identified as 1 serving on the Nutrition Facts panel, and eat it from a plate or bowl instead of straight out of the box or bag.

Try using smaller dishes, bowls, and glasses. This will make your portion appear larger, and you'll be eating or drinking less.

When cooking at home, put a serving of the entrée on your plate; then freeze any leftovers in single-serving containers. This way, you won't be tempted to eat the whole batch before the food goes

bad, and you'll have ready-made servings for future meals.

To fill up, take second helpings of plain vegetables. That way, dessert may not seem so tempting!

When buying snacks, go for single-serving, prepackaged items. If you buy larger bags or boxes, divide the snack into single-serving bags.

When you have a treat, such as ice cream, measure out ½ cup, eat it slowly, and enjoy it!

To test your understanding of what exactly constitutes a serving size, take the "Portion Distortion" interactive quiz from the National Institutes of Health. (See **Web Resources** at the end of this chapter.)

About 3,300 Calories (kcal)/day

Breakfast:
1½ cups Fruit Loops cereal
1 cup 2% milk
1 cup orange juice
2 slices white toast
1 tbsp. butter (on toast)

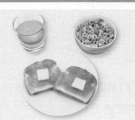

Lunch:
McDonald's Big Mac hamburger
French fries, extra large
3 tbsp. ketchup
Apple pie

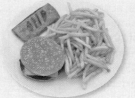

Dinner:
4.5 oz ground beef (80% lean, crumbled), cooked
2 medium taco shells
2 oz cheddar cheese
2 tbsp. sour cream
4 tbsp. store-bought salsa
1 cup shredded lettuce
½ cup refried beans
6 Oreos

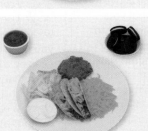

About 1,700 Calories (kcal)/day

Breakfast:
1½ cups Cheerios cereal
1 cup skim milk
½ fresh pink grapefruit

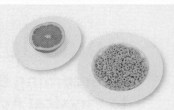

Lunch:
Subway cold-cut trio 6" sandwich
Granola bar, hard, with chocolate chips, 1 bar (24 g)
1 fresh medium apple

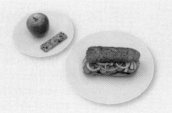

Dinner:
5 oz ground turkey, cooked
2 soft corn tortillas
3 oz low-fat cheddar cheese
4 tbsp. store-bought salsa
1 cup shredded lettuce
1 cup cooked mixed veggies
3 Oreos

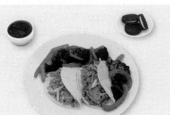

◆ **FIGURE 11.8** The energy density of two sets of meals. The set on the left is higher in energy density, whereas the set on the right is lower in energy density and the preferred choice for a person trying to lose weight.

eating fresh fruit for dessert, can reduce energy intake without sacrificing taste, pleasure, or nutritional quality!

Participate in Regular Physical Activity

The Dietary Guidelines for Americans emphasize the role of physical activity in maintaining a healthful weight. Why? Of course, we expend extra energy during physical activity, but there's more to it than that because exercise alone (without a reduction of energy intake) does not result in dramatic weight loss. Instead, one of the most important reasons for being regularly active is that it helps us maintain or increase our lean body mass and our BMR. In contrast, energy restriction alone causes us to lose lean body mass. As you've learned, the more lean body mass we have, the more energy we expend over the long term.

Although very few weight-loss studies have documented long-term maintenance of weight loss, those that have find that only people who are regularly active are able to maintain most of their weight loss. The National Weight Control Registry is an ongoing project documenting the habits of people who have lost at least 30 pounds and kept their weight off for at least 1 year. Of the more than 4,000 people studied thus far, the average weight loss was 73 pounds over 5.7 years.[35] Almost all of the people (89%) reported changing both physical activity and dietary intake to lose weight and maintain weight loss. No one form of exercise seems to be most effective, but many people report doing some form of aerobic exercise (walking is the most commonly reported form of activity) for approximately 1 hour per day most days of the week. In fact, on average, this group expended more than 2,600 kcal each week through physical activity!

In addition to expending energy and maintaining lean body mass and BMR, regular physical activity improves our mood, results in a higher quality of sleep, increases self-esteem, and gives us a sense of accomplishment. All of these changes enhance our ability to engage in long-term healthful lifestyle behaviors.

What specific changes can you make to your level of physical activity? Although plenty of practical suggestions will be offered later in this text (in Chapter 12), the nearby **Quick Tips** box provides some ideas that can help you to start identifying and overcoming your barriers to an active life.

QuickTips

Overcoming Barriers to Physical Activity

I don't have enough time! An active lifestyle doesn't have to consume all your free time. Try to do a minimum of 30 minutes of moderate activity most—preferably all—days of the week. If you can, do 45 minutes. But remember, you don't have to get in all of your daily activity in one go! Be active for a few minutes at a time throughout your day. Walk from your dorm or apartment to classes, if possible. Instead of meeting friends for lunch, meet them for a lunchtime walk, jog, or workout. Break up study sessions with 3 minutes of jumping jacks. Skip the elevator and take the stairs. When you're talking on the phone, pace instead of sitting still.

I can't manage the details! Bust this excuse by keeping clean clothes, shoes, water, and equipment for physical activity in a convenient place. If time management is an obstacle, enroll in a scheduled fitness class, yoga class, sports activity, walking group, or running club. Put it on your schedule of academic classes and make it part of your weekly routine.

I just don't like to work out! You don't have to! Try dancing, roller blading, walking, hiking, swimming, tennis, or any other activity you enjoy.

I can't stay motivated. Friends can help. Use the "buddy" system by exercising with a friend and calling each other when you need encouragement to stay motivated. Or keep a journal or log of your daily physical activity. Write your week's goal at the top of the page (such as "Walk to and from campus each day, and at least 10 minutes on campus at lunch"). Then track your progress. You can also use the form in **FIGURE 11.9**. If you achieve your goal for the week, reward yourself with a massage, a new song for your iPod, or some other nonfood treat.

My Weekly Activity Goals

Week 1 Goals

I commit to begin_____(type of

activity) for _____minutes on

❑ Monday   ❑ Tuesday   ❑ Wednesday
❑ Thursday   ❑ Friday   ❑ Saturday   ❑ Sunday

Week 2 Goals

I commit to begin_____(type of

activity) for _____minutes on

❑ Monday   ❑ Tuesday   ❑ Wednesday
❑ Thursday   ❑ Friday   ❑ Saturday   ❑ Sunday

Week 3 Goals

I commit to begin_____(type of

activity) for _____minutes on

❑ Monday   ❑ Tuesday   ❑ Wednesday
❑ Thursday   ❑ Friday   ❑ Saturday   ❑ Sunday

Week 4 and Beyond

I commit to begin_____(type of

activity) for _____minutes on

❑ Monday   ❑ Tuesday   ❑ Wednesday
❑ Thursday   ❑ Friday   ❑ Saturday   ❑ Sunday

FIGURE 11.9 Use this goal-setting card to help you set—and reach—weekly activity goals.
Data from: *Active at Any Size!* NIH Publication No. 10-4352. National Institute of Diabetes and Digestive and Kidney Diseases.

Incorporate Appropriate Behavior Modifications into Daily Life

Successful weight loss and long-term maintenance of a healthful weight require people to modify their behaviors. Some of the behavior modifications related to food and physical activity have been discussed in the previous sections. Here are a few more **Quick Tips** (page 418) on modifying behavior that will assist you in losing weight and maintaining a healthful weight.

recap Achieving and maintaining a healthful weight involve gradual reductions in energy intake, such as by eating smaller portions of foods lower in energy density; engaging in regular physical activity; and applying appropriate behavior modification techniques. Fad diets do not use these strategies and do not result in long-term, healthful weight change. A variety of diets based on macronutrient composition may promote weight loss but may or may not result in long-term maintenance of the lower body weight.

What disorders are related to energy intake?

At the beginning of this chapter, we provided definitions of underweight, overweight, obesity, and morbid obesity. Let's take a closer look at these disorders.

Underweight

As defined earlier in this chapter, underweight occurs when a person has too little body fat to maintain health. People with a BMI of less than 18.5 kg/m^2 are typically

QuickTips

Modifying Your Behaviors Related to Food

Shop for food only when you're not hungry.

Avoid buying problem foods—that is, foods that you may have difficulty eating in moderate amounts.

Avoid purchasing high-fat, high-sugar food from vending machines and convenience stores.

Avoid feelings of deprivation by eating small, regular meals throughout the day.

Eat only at set times in one location. Do not eat while studying, working, driving, watching television, and so forth.

Always use appropriate utensils.

Eat mindfully, savoring the aromas, tastes, and textures of each food.

Slow down while eating. Chew food slowly, taking at least 20 minutes to eat a full meal.

Stop at once if you begin to feel full. Leave food on your plate or store it for the next meal.

Keep a log of what you eat, when, and why. (See the **In Depth** on Eating Wisely on pages 65–71). Try to identify social or emotional cues that cause you to overeat, such as getting a poor grade on an exam or feeling lonely. Then strategize about nonfood-related ways to cope, such as phoning a sympathetic friend.

Save high-fat, high-kilocalorie snack foods (such as ice cream, doughnuts, and cakes) for occasional special treats.

Whether at home or dining out, share food with others.

Prepare healthful snacks to take along with you, so that you won't be tempted by foods from vending machines, fast-food restaurants, and so forth.

Don't punish yourself for deviating from your plan (and you will—everyone does). Ask others to avoid responding to any slips you make.

---

considered underweight. Being underweight can be just as unhealthful as being obese because it increases the risk for infections and illness and impairs the body's ability to recover. Some people are healthy but underweight because of their genetics and/or because they are very physically active and consume adequate energy to maintain their underweight status but not enough to gain weight. In others, underweight is due to heavy smoking, a malabsorption disorder, an underlying disease such as cancer or AIDS, or an eating disorder such as anorexia nervosa (see the **In Depth** on disordered eating on pages 429–439).

Safe and Effective Weight Gain

With so much emphasis in the United States on obesity and weight loss, some find it surprising that many people are actually trying to gain weight. People looking to gain weight include those who are underweight to an extent that it is compromising their health and many athletes who are attempting to increase strength and power for competition.

To gain weight, people must eat more energy than they expend. Although overeating large amounts of foods high in saturated fats (such as bacon, sausage, and cheese) can cause weight gain, doing this without exercising is not considered healthful because most of the weight gained is fat, and diets high in saturated fat increase our risks for cardiovascular and other diseases. However, as previously discussed (in Chapter 2), diets that are relatively higher in mono- and polyunsaturated fats, such as a

Mediterranean-style diet, can be a healthful approach to weight gain. Recommendations for weight gain include:

- Eat a diet that includes about 500 to 1,000 kcal/day more than is needed to maintain present body weight. Although we don't know exactly how much extra energy is needed to gain 1 pound, estimates range from 3,000 to 3,500 kcal. Thus, eating 500 to 1,000 kcal/day in excess should result in a gain of 1 to 2 pounds of weight each week.
- Eat frequently, including meals and numerous snacks throughout the day. Many underweight people do not take the time to eat often enough.
- Avoid the use of tobacco products because they depress appetite and increase metabolic rate, and both of these effects oppose weight gain. Tobacco use also causes lung, mouth, esophageal, and other cancers and is a factor in cardiovascular disease.
- Exercise regularly and incorporate weight lifting or some other form of resistance training into your exercise routine. This form of exercise is most effective in increasing muscle mass. Performing aerobic exercise (such as walking, running, bicycling, or swimming) at least 30 minutes for 3 days per week will help maintain a healthy cardiovascular system.

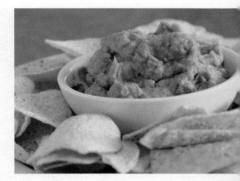

Eating frequent nutrient- and energy-dense snacks can help promote weight gain.

The key to gaining weight is to eat frequent meals throughout the day and to select healthful energy-dense foods. For instance, smoothies and milkshakes made with low-fat milk or yogurt are a great way to take in a lot of energy. Eating peanut butter with fruit or celery and including salad dressings on your salad are other ways to increase the energy density of foods. The biggest challenge to weight gain is setting aside time to eat; by packing a lot of foods to take with you throughout the day, you can enhance your opportunities to eat more.

Amino Acid and Protein Supplements Do Not Increase Muscle Mass

As with weight loss, there are many products marketed for weight gain. Many of these products are said to be *anabolic,* that is, to increase muscle mass. The most common of these include amino acid and protein supplements, often powders used to make protein "shakes." Do these substances really work?

A growing body of evidence exists showing that amino acid and protein supplements are not necessary to enhance muscle gain; adequate intake of energy, protein from high-quality food sources, and resistance training promote healthy increases in muscle mass.[36] The health consequences of using them are unknown. Moreover, although they are legal to sell in the United States, all potentially anabolic substances are banned by the National Football League, the National Collegiate Athletic Association, and the International Olympic Committee. We also know that buying these substances can have a substantial slenderizing effect—on your wallet!

Overweight

Overweight occurs when a person has a moderate amount of excess body fat. People with a BMI between 25 and 29.9 kg/m^2 are considered overweight. Being overweight does not appear to be as detrimental to our health as being obese; as discussed previously, recent evidence suggests that, as we age, having a BMI in the overweight category may actually be protective against dying prematurely.[3] However, some evidence suggests that being overweight can increase our risk for high blood pressure and osteoarthritis. Overweight people also have a higher risk of becoming obese than people of normal weight, and obesity confers an even higher risk for these diseases and for premature death. Because of these concerns, health professionals recommend that overweight individuals adopt a lifestyle that incorporates healthful eating and regular physical activity in an attempt to prevent additional weight gain, to reduce body weight to a normal level, and/or to support long-term health even if body weight is not significantly reduced.

Obesity and Morbid Obesity

Obesity is a weight category characterized by a significant amount of excess body fat that adversely affects health. People with a BMI between 30 and 39.9 kg/m^2 are considered obese. Morbid obesity occurs when a person's body weight exceeds 100% of normal; people who are morbidly obese have a BMI greater than or equal to 40 kg/m^2.

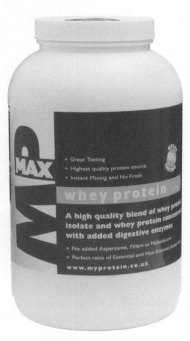

High-protein diets are a multimillion-dollar industry.

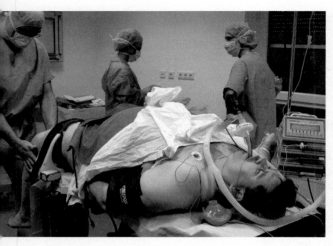

Obesity increases a person's risk of experiencing a heart attack, stroke, or other medical emergency.

Why Is Obesity Harmful?

Obesity rates in the United States have increased more than 50% during the past 20 years, and it is now estimated that about 35.7% of adults 20 years and older are obese.[37] This alarming rise in obesity is a major health concern because it is linked to many chronic diseases and complications:

- Hypertension
- Dyslipidemia, including elevated total cholesterol, triglycerides, and LDL-cholesterol and decreased HDL-cholesterol
- Type 2 diabetes
- Heart disease
- Stroke
- Gallbladder disease
- Osteoarthritis
- Sleep apnea
- Certain cancers such as colon, breast, endometrial, and gallbladder
- Menstrual irregularities and infertility
- Gestational diabetes, premature fetal deaths, neural tube defects, and complications during labor and delivery
- Depression
- Alzheimer's disease, dementia, and cognitive decline

Abdominal obesity, specifically a large amount of visceral fat that is stored deep within the abdomen (**FIGURE 11.10**), is one of five risk factors collectively referred to as the **metabolic syndrome**. A diagnosis of metabolic syndrome, which is typically made if a person has three or more of the factors, increases one's risk for heart disease, type 2 diabetes, and stroke. These risk factors include:

- Abdominal obesity (defined as a waist circumference greater than or equal to 40 inches for men and 35 inches for women)
- Higher than normal triglyceride levels (greater than or equal to 150 mg/dL)
- Lower than normal HDL-cholesterol levels (less than 40 mg/dL in men and 50 mg/dL in women)
- Higher than normal blood pressure (greater than or equal to 130/85 mm Hg)
- Fasting blood glucose levels greater than or equal to 100 mg/dL, including people with diabetes[38]

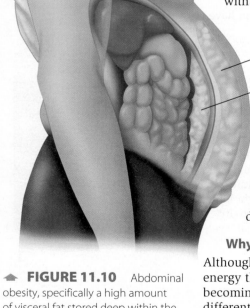

Subcutaneous fat

Visceral fat

FIGURE 11.10 Abdominal obesity, specifically a high amount of visceral fat stored deep within the abdomen, is one of the risk factors for metabolic syndrome.

The metabolic syndrome is a key component of global *cardiometabolic risk*, which also includes the risk factors of elevated LDL-cholesterol (≥130 mg/dL), smoking, inflammation, and insulin resistance.[39,40] People with metabolic syndrome are twice as likely to develop heart disease and five times as likely to develop type 2 diabetes than people without metabolic syndrome. About 34% of adults in the United States have metabolic syndrome, and rising obesity rates are contributing to increased rates.[41]

Obesity is also associated with an increased risk of premature death: As discussed previously, having a BMI equal to or greater than 30 kg/m² increases a person's risk of dying prematurely 18% above that of people with a BMI value in the range of 18.5–24.99 kg/m². Several of the obesity-related diseases just listed are leading causes of death in the United States.

Why Do People Become Obese?

Although it is certainly true that obesity, like overweight, is caused by eating more energy than is expended, it is also true that some people are more susceptible to becoming obese than others. As was seen with the twin study earlier in this chapter, different people consuming the same excessive energy and engaging in the same low level of physical activity will gain very different amounts of weight. Why? Research on the causes of obesity are ongoing, but let's explore some current theories.

Genetic and Physiologic Factors Influence Obesity Risk Because a person's genetic background influences his or her height, weight, body shape, metabolic rate, and propensity to oxidize relatively more fat or carbohydrate, it can also affect a person's risk for obesity. As discussed previously, three genetic factors that may increase a person's risk for obesity are the FTO gene variant, possessing a thrifty gene (or set of genes), and maintaining weight within a narrow range, or set point. As we learn more about genetics, we will gain a greater understanding of the role it plays in the development and treatment of obesity.

We also discussed earlier several physiologic factors that may influence an individual's experience of hunger and satiation. These include the proteins leptin, ghrelin, PYY, and uncoupling proteins. Other physiologic factors such as beta-endorphins, neuropeptide Y, and decreased blood glucose can reduce satiety or increase hunger, theoretically promoting overeating and weight gain.

An abnormally low level of thyroid hormone, or an elevated level of the hormone cortisol, can lead to weight gain and obesity. A physician can check your blood for levels of these hormones. Certain prescription medications, including steroids used for asthma and other disorders, seizure medications, and some antidepressants, can slow basal metabolic rate or stimulate appetite, leading to weight gain.[42]

Childhood Obesity Is Linked to Adult Obesity The prevalence of obesity in children and adolescents increased at an alarming rate in the United States over the last 50 years (**FIGURE 11.11**). There was a time when having extra "baby fat" was considered healthy and that the child would grow out of it. Although it is important for children to have a certain minimum level of body fat to maintain health and to grow properly, researchers are now concerned that obesity is harming children's health and increasing their risk of obesity in adulthood.

Health data demonstrate that obese children are already showing signs of chronic disease while they are young, including elevated blood pressure, high cholesterol levels, and changes in insulin and glucose metabolism that may increase the risk for type 2 diabetes (formerly known as *adult-onset diabetes*). In some communities, children as young as 5 years of age have been diagnosed with type 2 diabetes. Unfortunately, many of these

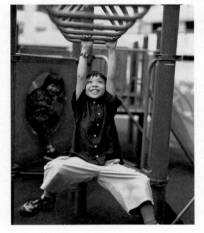

Adequate physical activity is instrumental in preventing childhood obesity.

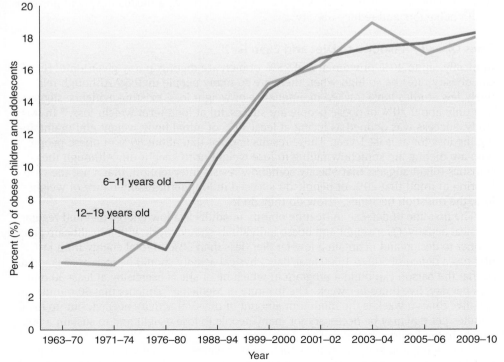

FIGURE 11.11 Increases in childhood and adolescent obesity from 1963 to 2010.
Data from: Prevalence of Obesity Among Children and Adolescents: United States, Trends 1963–1965 through 2009–2010. Centers for Disease Control and Prevention, National Center for Health Statistics, 2012.

metabolic syndrome A cluster of risk factors that increase one's risk for heart disease, type 2 diabetes, and stroke, including abdominal obesity, higher than normal triglyceride levels, lower than normal HDL-cholesterol levels, higher than normal blood pressure (greater than or equal to 130/85 mm Hg), and elevated fasting blood glucose levels.

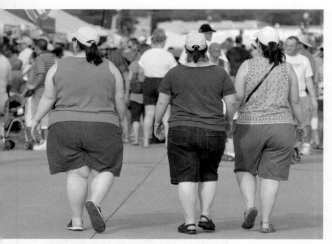

Having a spouse, sibling, or close friend who is obese may increase your risk for obesity.

children will maintain these disease risk factors into adulthood. Moreover, although some children who are obese grow up to have a normal body weight, it has been estimated that about 70% of children who are obese maintain their higher weight as adults.[43]

Having either one or two overweight parents increases the risk of obesity two to four times. This may be explained in part by genetics or by unhealthful eating patterns or lack of physical activity within the family. We know that children who eat healthful diets that do not contain a lot of empty Calories and are very physically active are unlikely to become obese. In contrast, children who consume a lot of empty Calories and spend most of their time on the computer or watching television are more likely to be obese. When these patterns are carried into adolescence and adulthood, the obesity is likely to persist.

Social Factors Appear to Influence Obesity Risk   We noted earlier that social factors influence body weight. In particular, poverty has been linked to obesity. One reason for this may be that high-Calorie processed foods cost less, are more satiating, and are easier to find and prepare than more healthful foods such as fresh fruits and vegetables. Also, people living in poverty may not have access to safe places to walk, hike, or engage in other forms of physical activity, or to afford the cost of membership in a health club or commercial weight-loss program.

Our social ties may also have a subtle influence on our risk for obesity. Although their data have been challenged, researchers from Harvard Medical School evaluated a social network of more than 12,000 people and concluded that an individual's risk of becoming obese increased by 37% if their spouse became obese, 40% higher if a sibling became obese, and 57% higher if a friend became obese.[44] There was no evidence that neighbors had any effect on a person's obesity risk. Social distance was found to be much more important than geographic distance, suggesting that it was not exposure to the same environmental factors that caused people in close social networks to become obese. It may be that a person's perceptions of the acceptability of obesity changes when those close to him or her become obese. The researchers also theorized that if social networks can increase obesity, they could be used as a means to spread positive health behaviors and reduce obesity.

Does Obesity Respond to Diet and Exercise?

Ironically, up to 40% of women and 25% of men are dieting at any given time. How can obesity rates be so high when there are so many people dieting? Although relatively few studies have tracked maintenance of weight loss, existing evidence suggests that only about 20% of obese people are successful at long-term weight loss.[35] In this study, success was defined as losing at least 10% of initial body weight and maintaining the loss for at least 1 year. These results suggest that about 80% of obese people who are dieting are somehow failing to lose weight or to keep it off. Although these statistics might suggest that obesity somehow resists intervention, that's not the case. Bearing in mind that 20% of people do succeed in long-term maintenance of weight loss, the question becomes, "How do they do it?"

The first line of defense in treating obesity in adults is a low-energy diet and regular physical activity. Overweight and obese individuals should work with a healthcare practitioner to design and maintain a low-fat diet (less than 30% of total energy from fat) that has a deficit of 500 to 1,000 kcal/day. Physical activity should be increased gradually so that the person can build a program in which he or she is exercising at least 30 minutes per day, five times per week. The Institute of Medicine[45] concurs that 30 minutes a day, five times a week is the minimum amount of physical activity needed, but up to 60 minutes per day may be necessary for many people to lose weight and to sustain a body weight in the healthy range over the long term.

Counseling and support groups such as Overeaters Anonymous (OA) can help people maintain these dietary and activity changes. Psychotherapy can be particularly helpful in challenging clients to examine the underlying thought patterns, situations, and stressors that may be undermining their efforts at weight loss.

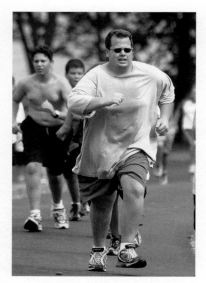

Increased physical activity can help many obese people succeed in losing weight and keeping it off.

Weight Loss Can Be Enhanced with Prescribed Medications

The biggest complaint about the lifestyle recommendations for healthful weight loss is that they are difficult to maintain. Many people have tried to follow them for years but have not been successful. In response to this challenge, prescription drugs have been developed to assist people with weight loss. These drugs typically act as appetite suppressants and may also increase satiety.

Weight-loss medications should be used only with proper supervision from a physician. Physician involvement is so critical because many drugs developed for weight loss have serious side effects. Some have even proven deadly. These life-threatening drugs have been banned, yet they still serve as examples illustrating that the treatment of obesity through pharmacological means is neither simple nor risk-free.

Seven prescription weight-loss drugs are currently available.[46] The long-term safety of many of these drugs is still being explored:

- Diethylpropion (brand name Tenuate), phentermine (brand name Adipex), benzphetamine (brand name Didrex), and phendimetrazine (brand name Bontril) are drugs that decrease appetite and increase feelings of fullness. These are approved for only short-term use (typically less than 12 weeks) because of their potential to be abused. Side effects include increased blood pressure and heart rate, nervousness, insomnia, dry mouth, and constipation.
- Lorcaserin (brand name Belviq) also works by decreasing appetite and increasing feelings of fullness. Side effects include increased heart rate, headache, dizziness, and nausea.
- Orlistat (brand name Xenical) is a drug that acts to inhibit the absorption of dietary fat from the intestinal tract. Orlistat is also available in a reduced-strength form (brand name Alli) that is available without a prescription. Side effects include intestinal cramps, gas, diarrhea, and oily spotting. Although rare, liver injury can occur; thus, people taking orlistat should be aware of symptoms of liver injury, which include itching, loss of appetite, yellow eyes or skin, light-colored stools, or brown urine.
- Combination phentermine-topiramate (brand name Qsymia) decreases appetite and increases feelings of fullness. Side effects include increased heart rate, tingling of hands and feet, dry mouth, constipation, anxiety, and birth defects. Because of this increased risk for birth defects, women of childbearing years must avoid getting pregnant while taking this medication. Although it has been approved for long-term use, Qsymia contains phentermine and thus has the potential for abuse.

Although the use of prescribed weight-loss medications is associated with side effects and a certain level of risk, they are justified for people who are obese. That's because the health risks of obesity override the risks of the medications. They are also advised for people who have a BMI greater than or equal to 27 kg/m^2 who also have other significant health risk factors such as heart disease, high blood pressure, and type 2 diabetes.

Many People Use Dietary Supplements for Weight Loss

Dietary supplements are also marketed for weight loss. It is important to remember that the Food and Drug Administration (FDA) requires prescription and over-the-counter medications to undergo rigorous testing for safety and effectiveness before they can be released onto the market, but the FDA does not have a similar level of control over the sale of dietary supplements. Moreover, the FDA can pull a dietary supplement from the shelves only if it can prove that the supplement is dangerous. It cannot force the makers of an ineffective but harmless supplement to stop selling it. Two reviews of various supplements and alternative treatments for weight loss[47, 48] have concluded that their use is common (20.6% among women and 9.7% among men) and that there is insufficient evidence of effectiveness: chromium, spirulina (or blue-green algae), ginseng, chitosan (derived from the exoskeleton of crustaceans), green tea, and psyllium (a source of fiber). Yet these products continue their brisk sales to people desperate to lose weight.

Many products marketed for weight loss do indeed increase metabolic rate and decrease appetite; however, they prompt these effects because they contain *stimulants*, substances that speed up physiologic processes. Use of these products may be dangerous because abnormal increases in heart rate and blood pressure can occur. Stimulants commonly found in weight loss supplements include caffeine, phenylpropanolamine (PPA), and ephedra:

- **Caffeine.** In addition to being a stimulant, caffeine is addictive; nevertheless, it is legal and unregulated in most countries and is considered safe when consumed in moderate amounts (up to the equivalent of 3 to 4 cups of coffee). Adverse effects of high doses of caffeine include nervousness, irritability, anxiety, muscle twitching and tremors, headaches, elevated blood pressure, and irregular or rapid heartbeat. Long-term overuse of high doses of caffeine can lead to sleep and anxiety disorders that require clinical attention. Deaths due to caffeine toxicity have occurred primarily as a result of taking caffeine tablets.
- **Phenylpropanolamine (PPA).** In the year 2000, in response to several deaths, the FDA banned over-the-counter medications containing PPA, an ingredient that had been used in many cough and cold medications as well as in weight-loss formulas. However, PPA may still be present in dietary supplements marketed for weight loss because these are beyond FDA control.
- **Ephedra.** The use of ephedra has been associated with dangerous elevations in heart rate, blood pressure, and death. The FDA has banned the manufacture and sale of ephedra in the United States; however, some weight-loss supplements still contain *ma huang,* the so-called herbal ephedra. *Ma huang* is simply the Chinese name for ephedra. Some weight-loss supplements contain a combination of *ma huang,* caffeine, and aspirin. As you can see, using weight-loss dietary supplements entails serious health risks.

Surgery Can Be Used to Treat Morbid Obesity

For people who are morbidly obese, surgery may be recommended. Generally, surgery is advised in people with a BMI greater than or equal to 40 kg/m^2 or in people with a BMI greater than or equal to 35 kg/m^2 who have other life-threatening conditions such as diabetes, hypertension, or elevated cholesterol levels. The three most common types of weight-loss surgery performed are sleeve gastrectomy, gastric bypass, and gastric banding (**FIGURE 11.12**).

Surgery is considered a last resort for morbidly obese people who have not been able to lose weight with energy restriction, exercise, and medications. This is because the risks of surgery in people with morbid obesity are extremely high. They include an increased rate of infections, formation of blood clots, and adverse reactions to anesthesia. After the surgery, many recipients face a lifetime of problems with chronic diarrhea, vomiting, intolerance to dairy products and other foods, dehydration, and nutritional deficiencies resulting from alterations in nutrient digestion and absorption

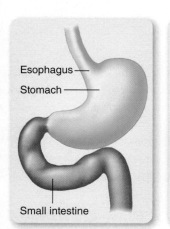

(a) Normal anatomy

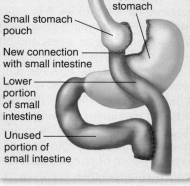

(b) Sleeve gastrectomy

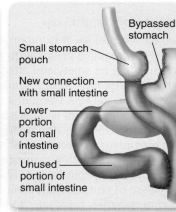

(c) Gastric bypass

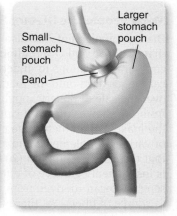

(d) Gastric banding

◆ **FIGURE 11.12** Various forms of surgery alter the normal anatomy **(a)** of the gastrointestinal tract to result in weight loss. Sleeve gastrectomy **(b)**, gastric bypass **(c)**, and gastric banding **(d)**, are three surgical procedures used to reduce morbid obesity.

that occur with bypass procedures. Thus, the potential benefits of the procedure must outweigh the risks. It is critical that each surgery candidate is carefully screened by a trained physician. If the immediate threat of serious disease and death is more dangerous than the risks associated with surgery, then the procedure is justified.

About one-third to one-half of people who receive obesity surgery lose significant amounts of weight and keep this weight off for up to 5 years.[49] They may also reduce their risk for type 2 diabetes and cardiovascular disease and may even improve their ability to stay physically active over a prolonged period.[50,51] Reasons that one-half to two-thirds do not experience long-term success include:

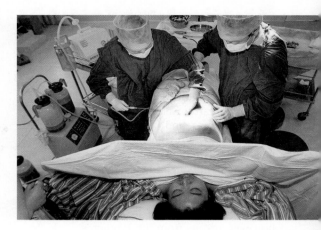

Liposuction surgery removes fat cells from specific areas of the body.

- Inability to eat less over time, even with a smaller stomach
- Loosening of staples and gastric bands and enlargement of stomach pouch
- Failure to survive the surgery or the postoperative recovery period

Liposuction is a cosmetic surgical procedure that removes fat cells from localized areas in the body. It is not recommended or typically used to treat obesity or morbid obesity. Instead, it is often used by normal or mildly overweight people to "spot reduce" fat from various areas of the body. This procedure is not without risks; blood clots, skin and nerve damage, adverse drug reactions, and perforation injuries can and do occur as a result of liposuction. It can also cause deformations in the area where the fat is removed. This procedure is not the solution to long-term weight loss because the millions of fat cells that remain in the body after liposuction enlarge if the person continues to overeat. In addition, although liposuction may reduce the fat content of a localized area, it does not reduce a person's risk for the diseases that are more common among overweight or obese people. Only traditional weight loss with diet and exercise can reduce body fat and the risks for chronic diseases.

recap Weight gain can be achieved by eating more and performing weight-lifting and aerobic exercise. Protein and amino acid supplements do not increase muscle mass, and their potential side effects are unknown. Obesity is a multifactorial disease, and genetics, physiology, and lifestyle choices are all thought to contribute. In addition, childhood obesity is strongly associated with adult obesity. Treatments for obesity include lifestyle changes and prescription weight-loss medications. Surgery is typically reserved for people who are morbidly obese.

*behavior change . . . getting started!

Now that you've read this chapter, try making these changes:

For yourself:

- Calculate your BMI and measure your waist-to-hip ratio to determine whether you are normal weight, overweight, or obese and to estimate if you have abdominal obesity.
- Set two specific, realistic goals for the coming week that will help you work toward achieving or maintaining a healthy body weight.

For your community:

- Join the international campaign promoting a Fat Talk Free week on your campus or in your community. Enter "fat talk free week" into your internet browser for links to multiple sites addressing this topic.
- Write a blog for your school newsletter highlighting the characteristics and ineffectiveness of fad diets.

High-Carbohydrate, Moderate-Fat Diets—Have They Been Oversold?

For the past 30 years, dietary fat has been demonized as the cause of obesity, cardiovascular disease, type 2 diabetes, and many types of cancers. As a result, nutrition professionals have emphasized the health benefits of eating a moderate-fat, high-carbohydrate diet, and national dietary guidelines have promoted this message. Recently, however, results from the Women's Health Initiative Randomized Controlled Dietary Modification Trial have caused experts to seriously question the existing beliefs that moderate-fat diets are the key to reducing our risks for many chronic diseases.

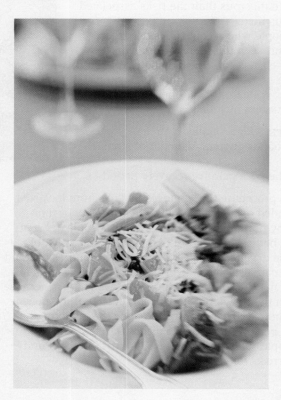

The trial involved 48,835 ethnically diverse postmenopausal women aged 50 to 79 years.[52] Women were randomized into either a control group that received a copy of the Dietary Guidelines for Americans and other health materials, or an intervention group that engaged in an intensive behavioral modification program involving 18 group sessions in the first year of the study, followed by quarterly maintenance sessions. The intervention promoted dietary changes to achieve a goal of 20% of energy intake from fat (7% of energy intake from saturated fat), an increase in fruit and vegetable intake to at least 5 servings per day, and an increase in whole grains to at least 6 servings per day. However, the diet was not intended to reduce energy intake or induce weight loss. The average length of time to follow-up participants was 8 years.

The results from this study surprised many experts. At the end of the follow-up period, there was no significant health benefit in the intervention group—no reduction in risk for cardiovascular disease, breast cancer, or colorectal cancer.[52–54] One benefit that was observed was that women in the intervention group lost weight during the first year (a loss of approximate 4.8 pounds), and they maintained a lower weight than women in the control group over 7.5 years.[55] Some women in the control group also lost weight, and the greatest amount of weight lost in both groups occurred in those who decreased their percentage of energy intake from fat.

What do these results mean? Should we no longer be concerned about the health risks of dietary fat? Should we eat however we choose? The study had a number of limitations, and an editorial published by the Harvard School of Public Health has helped to put these findings into perspective.[56] Although participants in the intervention reduced their fat intake from 38–29% of total energy intake, they did not reach the target goal of consuming no more than 20% of energy intake from fat. Thus it has been suggested that a lower-fat diet might be more effective in reducing the risk for chronic diseases. In addition, participants were postmenopausal women, and it might be that intervening at this age may be too late to prevent the development of cardiovascular disease and various cancers. Because dietary intake was self-reported, it might also be possible that the women did not improve their diet as much as they said they had. Another issue is that it may take longer than 8 years to see the health benefits of this type of diet, and thus a much longer study would be needed.

However, there is now a growing body of evidence that the key to reducing chronic disease risks is focusing on changing the *type* of dietary fat consumed, not the total amount.[56] The challenge with reducing the amount of dietary fat is that many people choose to substitute low-fiber, highly refined carbohydrate foods in place of fat. This leads to negative changes in blood lipids and blood glucose. Instead, replacing saturated and *trans* fats with poly- and monounsaturated fats appears to be the healthiest approach. Again, lowering total fat intake may not be important unless a person is trying to reduce total energy intake. Even under these circumstances, people should be encouraged to optimize their intake of healthy fats and avoid replacing fat with refined carbohydrates. Another take-home message is that too many Calories from any source will lead to weight gain.

CRITICAL THINKING QUESTIONS

1. Do you think that other diets are better or worse alternatives to higher-carbohydrate, lower-fat diets? Why or why not?
2. What diet do you think would work best to help you maintain a healthful weight and muscle mass and provide enough energy and nutrients to maintain your lifestyle and your long-term health?

chapter **review**

test yourself | answers

1. **True.** Being underweight increases the risk for illness and premature death and in many cases can be just as unhealthful as being obese.

2. **False.** Body composition assessments can help give you a general idea of your body fat level, but most methods are not highly accurate.

3. **False.** According to the Centers for Disease Control and Prevention, in 2009–2010, approximately 35.7% of all adults in the United States were considered obese.

MasteringNutrition™

review questions

1. A healthful weight is
   a. the lowest weight that an individual can achieve without constant dieting and excessive exercise.
   b. appropriate for your gender, age, genetics, physical development, and family history.
   c. characterized by an amount of body fat that meets accepted cultural standards.
   d. whatever the individual defines it to be.

2. The ratio of a person's body weight to height is represented as his or her
   a. body composition.
   b. basal metabolic rate.
   c. bioelectrical impedance.
   d. body mass index.

3. The body's total daily energy expenditure includes
   a. basal metabolic rate, thermal effect of food, and effect of physical activity.
   b. basal metabolic rate, standing, and sleeping.
   c. effect of physical activity, standing, and sleeping.
   d. body mass index, thermal effect of food, and effect of physical activity.

4. The set-point theory proposes that
   a. people who are overweight have a gene not found in slender people that causes them to overeat when their weight drops below a point higher than a normal healthful weight.
   b. people who are overweight have a gene that causes them to be energetically thrifty.
   c. the body raises or lowers energy expenditure in response to changes in food intake and physical activity.
   d. all people have a hormone that regulates their weight so that it always hovers near a given set point.

5. The three key strategies for healthful weight loss are
   a. reducing total fat consumption, engaging in vigorous physical activity daily, and eating mindfully.
   b. avoiding fad diets, setting realistic goals, and exercising at least 30 minutes a day.
   c. making gradual changes in energy intake, engaging in regular and appropriate physical activity, and applying behavioral modification techniques.
   d. adopting a diet low in energy density, engaging in physical activity equivalent to walking about 1 hour a day, and modifying food purchases and eating behaviors.

6. Which of the following statements about obesity is true?
   a. Obesity is clinically defined as a BMI greater than or equal to 40 kg/m².
   b. Obesity is associated with a risk of premature death that is 18% higher than that of someone of normal weight.
   c. Obesity is a risk factor for all forms of cardiovascular disease, diabetes, and cancer as well as osteoporosis, osteoarthritis, and dementia.
   d. All of the above are true.

7. Which of the following statements about obesity treatment is true?
   a. Obesity does respond to lifestyle interventions such as dieting and exercise.
   b. Prescription weight-loss medications are useful in treatment for obesity, but all have serious side effects.
   c. Weight-loss surgery is most commonly reserved for morbidly obese people who have not been able to lose weight with lifestyle changes and medications.
   d. All of the above are true.

8. **True or false?** Pear-shaped fat patterning is known to increase a person's risk for many chronic diseases, including diabetes and heart disease.

9. **True or false?** Almost all of the people in the National Weight Control Registry who lost weight and kept it off engaged in significant physical activity almost every day.

10. **True or false?** Underweight is associated with an increased risk for infections and illness, a reduced ability to recover from illness, and an increased risk of premature death.

math review

11. Your friend Misty joins you for lunch and confesses that she is discouraged about her weight. She says that she has been trying "really hard" for 3 months to lose weight but that no matter what she does, she cannot drop below 148 pounds. Based on her height of 5'8", calculate Misty's BMI. Is she overweight? You know Misty exercises regularly. What questions would you suggest she think about? How would you advise her?

12. Misty's level of physical activity would classify her as moderately active. Approximately how many kcal does she need each day to maintain her current body weight?

Answers to Review Questions and Math Review are located at the back of this text and in the MasteringNutrition Study Area.

web resources

www.ftc.gov
Federal Trade Commission

Click on "Consumer Resources" and then "Health and Fitness" to find how to avoid false weight-loss claims.

www.eatright.org
Academy of Nutrition and Dietetics

Go to this site to learn more about fad diets and nutrition facts.

www.niddk.nih.gov
National Institute of Diabetes and Digestive and Kidney Diseases

Find out more about healthy weight loss and how it pertains to diabetes and digestive and kidney diseases. Enter "Health" and "Nutrition" into the main page search box for deeper links.

www.nih.gov
The "Portion Distortion" interactive quiz from the National Institutes of Health.

Just enter "portion distortion quiz" into the main page search box, then click on the first link ("Quizzes") and you'll see the Portion Distortion link.

www.sne.org
Society for Nutrition Education

Click on "Resources" and then "Weight Realities Division Resource List" for additional resources related to positive attitudes about body image and healthful alternatives to dieting.

www.oa.org
Overeaters Anonymous

Visit this site to learn about ways to reduce compulsive overeating.

in depth
11.5

Disordered Eating

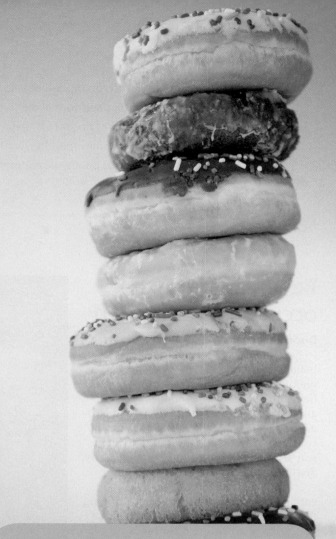

On August 2, 2006, Uruguayan fashion model Luisel Ramos collapsed during a fashion show. Just 22 years old, she was pronounced dead of heart failure brought on by anorexia nervosa, a condition of self-imposed starvation. Family members say that, in the months prior to her death, she had adopted a diet of lettuce leaves and diet cola, and at 5′9′ tall, her weight had dropped to just 98 pounds. The following month, Madrid's "Fashion Week" responded to Ramos' death by banning from its runway fashion models who could not meet a minimum body mass index (BMI, kg/m^2) of 18.0. The Milan fashion show quickly responded by imposing a minimum BMI of 18.5. In addition, several modeling agencies began to require prospective models to present medical records attesting to their health. Although promising, such measures alone were clearly inadequate, and at least four more models had died from self-starvation by the end of 2010. Early in 2012, the Council of Fashion Designers of America (CFDA) released new guidelines for the hiring of runway models, including measures such as educating staff to recognize the warning signs of an eating disorder. The CFDA imposed no sanctions, however, for noncompliance. Then, in March 2012, Israel took a major step forward in the fight against eating disorders. The government passed a law banning the use of underweight models in advertisements. The new law states that models with a BMI under 18.5 cannot be hired unless a doctor explicitly confirms that they are not underweight.

Continued next page

learning objectives

After studying this In Depth, you should be able to:

1 Discuss the observation that eating behaviors occur on a continuum, p. 430.

2 Identify several factors that contribute to the development of eating disorders, pp. 430–433.

3 Identify the most common characteristics and health risks of anorexia nervosa, bulimia nervosa, and binge-eating disorder, pp. 433–436.

4 Describe night-eating syndrome and the female athlete triad, pp. 436–438.

5 Compare treatment options for disordered eating behaviors, pp. 438–439.

6 Role-play a discussion with a friend about his or her disordered eating behaviors, p. 439.

Continued—Do only fashion models develop eating disorders, or can they occur in people like you? When does normal dieting cross the line into disordered eating? What early warning signs might tip you off that a friend was crossing that line? If you noticed the signs in a friend or family member, would you confront him or her? If so, what would you say? In the following pages, we explore **In Depth** some answers to these important questions.

Eating behaviors occur on a continuum

Disordered eating is a general term used to describe a variety of atypical eating behaviors that people use to achieve or maintain a lower body weight. These behaviors may be as simple as going on and off diets or as extreme as refusing to eat any fat. Such behaviors don't usually continue for long enough to make a person seriously ill, nor do they significantly disrupt the person's normal routine.

In contrast, some people alter their eating behaviors so much and for so long that they become dangerously ill. These people have an **eating disorder**, a psychiatric condition that involves extreme body dissatisfaction and long-term eating patterns that negatively affect body functioning. Three clinically diagnosed eating disorders are anorexia nervosa, bulimia nervosa, and binge-eating disorder. Whereas anorexia nervosa is characterized by severe food restriction, bulimia nervosa and binge-eating disorder involve extreme overeating. These disorders will be discussed in more detail shortly.

When does normal dieting cross the line into disordered eating? Eating behaviors occur on a *continuum*, a spectrum that can't be divided neatly into parts. An example is a rainbow—where exactly does the red end and the orange begin? Thinking about eating behaviors as a continuum makes it easier to understand how a person can progress from relatively normal eating behaviors to a pattern that is disordered. For instance, let's say that for several years you've skipped breakfast in favor of a midmorning snack, but now you find yourself avoiding the cafeteria until early afternoon. Is this normal? To answer that question, you'd need to consider your feelings about food and your **body image**—the way you perceive your body.

Take a moment to study the Eating Issues and Body Image Continuum (**FIGURE 1**). Which of the five columns

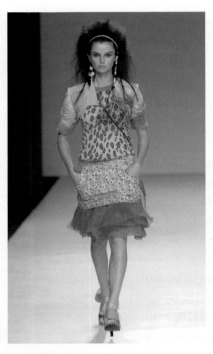

Brazilian model Ana Carolina Reston, who died in November of 2006 at the age of 21, was one of several models who have died in recent years as a result of eating disorders.

best describes your feelings about food and your body? If you find yourself identifying with the statements on the left side of the continuum, you probably have few issues with food or body image. Most likely you accept your body size and view food as a normal part of maintaining your health and fueling your daily physical activity. As you progress to the right side of the continuum, food and body image become bigger issues, with food restriction becoming the norm. If you identify with the statements on the far right, you are probably afraid of eating and dislike your body. If so, what can you do to begin to move toward the left side of the continuum? How can you begin to develop a more healthful approach to food selection and to view your body in a more positive light? Before you can begin to find solutions, you need to understand the many complex factors that contribute to eating disorders and disordered eating and the differences between these terms.

Many factors contribute to disordered eating behaviors

The factors that contribute to the development of disordered eating in any particular individual are very complex.

---

disordered eating A general term used to describe a variety of abnormal or atypical eating behaviors that are used to keep or maintain a lower body weight.

eating disorder A clinically diagnosed psychiatric disorder characterized by severe disturbances in body image and eating behaviors.

body image A person's perception of his or her body's appearance and functioning.

• I am not concerned about what others think regarding what and how much I eat. • When I am upset or depressed I eat whatever I am hungry for without any guilt or shame. • I feel no guilt or shame no matter how much I eat or what I eat. • Food is an important part of my life but only occupies a small part of my time. • I trust my body to tell me what and how much to eat.	• I pay attention to what I eat in order to maintain a healthy body. • I may weigh more than what I like, but I enjoy eating and balance my pleasure with eating with my concern for a healthy body. • I am moderate and flexible in goals for eating well. • I try to follow Dietary Guidelines for healthy eating.	• I think about food a lot. • I feel I don't eat well most of the time. • It's hard for me to enjoy eating with others. • I feel ashamed when I eat more than others or more than what I feel I should be eating. • I am afraid of getting fat. • I wish I could change how much I want to eat and what I am hungry for.	• I have tried diet pills, laxatives, vomiting, or extra time exercising in order to lose or maintain my weight. • I have fasted or avoided eating for long periods of time in order to lose or maintain my weight. • I feel strong when I can restrict how much I eat. • Eating more than I wanted to makes me feel out of control.	• I regularly stuff myself and then exercise, vomit, or use diet pills or laxatives to get rid of the food or Calories. • My friends/family tell me I am too thin. • I am terrified of eating fat. • When I let myself eat, I have a hard time controlling the amount of food I eat. • I am afraid to eat in front of others.
FOOD IS NOT AN ISSUE	**CONCERNED/WELL**	**FOOD PREOCCUPIED/ OBSESSED**	**DISRUPTIVE EATING PATTERNS**	**EATING DISORDERED**
BODY OWNERSHIP	**BODY ACCEPTANCE**	**BODY PREOCCUPIED/ OBSESSED**	**DISTORTED BODY IMAGE**	**BODY HATE/ DISASSOCIATION**
• Body image is not an issue for me. • My body is beautiful to me. • My feelings about my body are not influenced by society's concept of an ideal body shape. • I know that the significant others in my life will always find me attractive. • I trust my body to find the weight it needs to be at so I can move and feel confident about my physical body.	• I base my body image equally on social norms and my own self-concept. • I pay attention to my body and my appearance because it is important to me, but it only occupies a small part of my day. • I nourish my body so it has the strength and energy to achieve my physical goals. • I am able to assert myself and maintain a healthy body without losing my self-esteem.	• I spend a significant amount of time viewing my body in the mirror. • I spend a significant amount of time comparing my body to others. • I have days when I feel fat. • I am preoccupied with my body. • I accept society's ideal body shape and size as the best body shape and size. • I believe that I'd be more attractive if I were thinner, more muscular, etc.	• I spend a significant amount of time exercising and dieting to change my body. • My body shape and size keep me from dating or finding someone who will treat me the way I want to be treated. • I have considered changing or have changed my body shape and size through surgical means so I can accept myself. • I wish I could change the way I look in the mirror.	• I often feel separated and distant from my body—as if it belongs to someone else. • I hate my body and I often isolate myself from others. • I don't see anything positive or even neutral about my body shape and size. • I don't believe others when they tell me I look OK. • I hate the way I look in the mirror.

FIGURE 1 The Eating Issues and Body Image Continuum. The progression from normal eating (far left) to disordered eating (far right) occurs along a continuum.

Data adapted from: *Eating Issues and Body Image Continuum.* University of Arizona Campus Health Service. Arizona Board of Regents.

Influence of Genetic Factors

Overall, the diagnosis of an eating disorder is several times more common in siblings and other blood relatives who also have the diagnosis than in the general population.[1-3] Data from twin studies estimate that genetic factors account for 50–83% of the variance in eating disorders.[2] These observations might imply the existence of an "eating disorder gene"; however, it is difficult to separate the contribution of genetic and environmental factors within families.

Influence of Family

Research suggests that family conditioning, structure, and patterns of interaction can influence the development and maintenance of an eating disorder. Based on observational studies, compared to families without a member with an

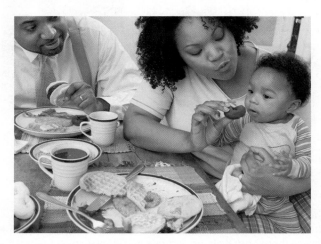

Genetic factors and family environment can influence when, what, and how much we eat.

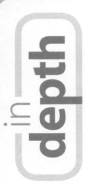

eating disorder, there are three traits that run within families of people with eating disorders: [4]

- *Anxiety.* Within families, anxiety can be contagious and can maintain or even exacerbate a pattern of disordered eating. For example, parents may display a high level of anxiety in response to a child's disordered eating behaviors. The child senses this anxiety and responds by intensifying the behavior.
- *Compulsivity.* The families of individuals who develop eating disorders are typically characterized by inflexibility, rigidity, and the need for order. Thus, when the family experiences an unpredictable event, the individual may turn to compulsive behaviors—such as refusing food or obsessively exercising—to adapt.
- *Abnormal eating behavior in one family member.* A pattern of disordered eating may already be present within the family, leading other family members to view this behavior as normal or acceptable.

Influence of Media

We now know media can play an important role in the formation of body image, especially in young females, and can create unrealistic expectations for body weight.[5] Every day, we are confronted with advertisements in which computer-enhanced images of very lean, beautiful women promote everything from beer to cars. Most adult men and women understand that these images are unrealistic, but adolescents, who are still developing a sense of their identity and body image, can lack the same ability to distance themselves from what they see.[6] Because body image influences eating behaviors, it is likely that the barrage of media models may be contributing to the increase in eating disorders. However, scientific evidence demonstrating that the media are *causing* increased eating disorders is difficult to obtain.

Influence of Social and Cultural Values

Eating disorders are significantly more common in white females in Western societies than in other women worldwide.[3] This may be due in part to the white Western culture's association of slenderness with attractiveness, wealth, and high fashion. In contrast, until recently, the prevailing view in developing societies has been that excess body fat is desirable as a sign of health and material abundance.

The members of society with whom we most often interact—our family members, friends, classmates, and co-workers—also influence the way we see ourselves. Their comments related to our body weight or shape can be particularly hurtful—enough so to cause some people to start down the path of disordered eating. For example, individuals with bulimia nervosa report that they perceived greater pressure from their peers to be thin, whereas research shows that peer teasing about weight increases both body dissatisfaction and eating disturbances.[7] Thus, our comments to others regarding their weight do count. Peer relationships also appear to be highly influential in the development of anorexia. A 2011 study from the London School of Economics concluded that anorexia is primarily socially induced. The higher the BMI of one's peers, the lower the risk of developing anorexia.[8]

Influence of Personality

A number of studies suggest that people with anorexia nervosa exhibit high negative emotionality and

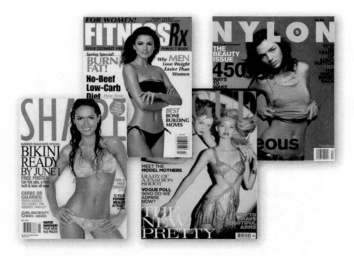

Photos of models and celebrities are routinely airbrushed or altered to "enhance" their appearance. Unfortunately, many people believe these portrayals are accurate and, hence, strive to meet unrealistic physical goals.

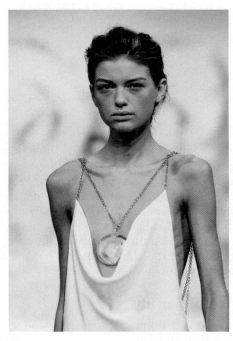

The preferred look among runway models can require extreme emaciation, often achieved by self-starvation and/or drug abuse.

perfectionism and tend to be socially inhibited and compliant.[9,10] Unfortunately, many studies observe these behaviors only in individuals who are very ill and in a state of starvation, which may affect personality. Thus, it is difficult to determine if personality is the cause or effect of the disorder.

In contrast to people with anorexia nervosa, people with bulimia nervosa tend to be more impulsive, have low self-esteem, and demonstrate an extroverted, erratic personality style that seeks attention and admiration. In these people, negative moods are more likely to cause overeating than food restriction.[9,10]

Eating disorders are psychiatric diagnoses

Recall that eating disorders are psychiatric conditions. The clinical manual of the American Psychiatric Association, which is the world's largest psychiatric organization, recognizes three such eating disorders. These are anorexia nervosa, bulimia nervosa, and binge-eating disorder.[1]

Anorexia Nervosa

Anorexia nervosa is a potentially life-threatening eating disorder that is characterized by an extremely low body weight achieved through self-starvation, which eventually leads to a severe nutrient deficiency. According to the Office of Women's Health, 85–95% of people with anorexia nervosa are young girls or women.[11] Approximately 0.5–3.7% of American females develop anorexia, and 20% of these women will die prematurely from complications related to their disorder, including suicide and heart problems.[12] These statistics make anorexia nervosa the most common and most deadly psychiatric disorder diagnosed in women and the leading cause of death in females between the ages of 15 and 24 years.[12] As the statistics indicate, anorexia nervosa also occurs in males, but the prevalence is much lower than in females.

Signs and Symptoms of Anorexia Nervosa

The classic sign of anorexia nervosa is an extremely restrictive eating pattern that leads to self-starvation. These individuals may fast completely, restrict energy intake to only a few kilocalories per day, or eliminate all but one or two food groups from their diet. They also have an intense fear of weight gain, and even small amounts (for example, 1–2 lb) trigger high stress and anxiety.

In females, **amenorrhea** (the condition of having no menstrual periods for at least 3 continuous months) is a common feature of anorexia nervosa. It occurs when a young woman consumes insufficient energy to maintain normal body functions.

The American Psychiatric Association identifies the following criteria for diagnosis of anorexia nervosa:[13]

- Refusal to maintain body weight at or above a minimally normal weight for age and height

- Intense fear of gaining weight or becoming fat, even though considered underweight by all medical criteria
- Disturbance in the way in which one's body weight or shape is experienced, undue influence of body weight or shape on self-evaluation, or denial of the seriousness of the current low body weight

The signs of an eating disorder such as anorexia nervosa may be somewhat different in males. Females report that they feel fat even though they typically are normal weight or even underweight before they develop the disorder. In contrast, males are more likely to have actually been overweight or even obese.[14,15] Thus, a male's fear of "getting fat again" is more often based on reality. In addition, males with disordered eating are less concerned with actual body weight (scale weight) than females but are more concerned with body composition (percentage of muscle mass compared to fat mass).

The methods that men and women use to achieve weight loss also appear to differ. Males are more likely to use excessive exercise as a means of weight control, whereas females tend to use severe energy restriction, vomiting, and laxative abuse. These weight-control differences may stem from sociocultural biases; that is, dieting is considered to be more acceptable for women, whereas

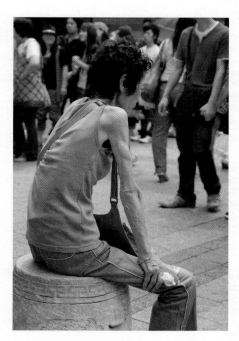

People with anorexia nervosa experience an extreme drive for thinness, resulting in potentially fatal weight loss.

---

anorexia nervosa A potentially life-threatening eating disorder that is characterized by self-starvation and leads to a deficiency in energy and essential nutrients.

amenorrhea The absence of menstruation. In females who had previously been menstruating, it is defined as the absence of menstrual periods for 3 or more continuous months.

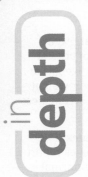

in depth

the overwhelming sociocultural belief is that "real men don't diet."[15] For more information on eating disorders in men, see the nearby **Hot Topic**.

Health Risks of Anorexia Nervosa

Left untreated, anorexia nervosa eventually leads to a deficiency in energy and other nutrients that are required by the body to function normally. The body will then use stored fat and lean tissue (for example, organ and muscle tissue) as an energy source to maintain brain tissue and vital body functions. The body will also shut down or reduce nonvital body functions to conserve energy. Electrolyte imbalances can lead to heart failure and death. **FIGURE 2** highlights many of the health problems that occur in people with anorexia nervosa. The best chance for recovery is when an individual receives intensive treatment early.

Bulimia Nervosa

Bulimia nervosa is characterized by recurrent episodes of binge eating and purging:

■ **Binge eating** is usually defined as consumption of a quantity of food that is large for the person and for the amount of time in which it is eaten. For example, a person may eat a dozen brownies with 2 quarts of ice cream in a period of just 30 minutes. While binge eating, the person feels a loss of self-control, including an

bulimia nervosa A serious eating disorder characterized by recurrent episodes of binge eating and recurrent inappropriate compensatory behaviors in order to prevent weight gain, such as self-induced vomiting, fasting, excessive exercise, or misuse of laxatives, diuretics, enemas, or other medications.

binge eating Consumption of a large amount of food in a short period of time, usually accompanied by a feeling of loss of self-control.

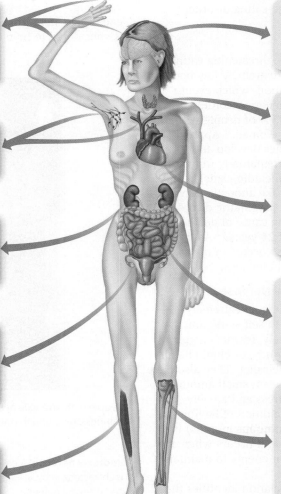

Skin/hair/nails:
· Hair becomes thin, dry, and brittle; hair loss occurs
· Skin is dry, easily bruised, and discolored
· Nails turn brittle

Blood and immune system:
· Anemia
· Compromised immune system increases risk of infection

Kidneys:
· Dehydration
· Electrolyte abnormalities that can be life-threatening
· Chronic renal failure

Reproductive function:
· Disruption of sex hormone production, resulting in menstrual dysfunction and amenorrhea in females
· Infertility

Muscle:
· Loss of muscle tissue as the body uses the muscles as an energy source

Brain:
· Altered levels of serotonin and other neurotransmitters
• Alteration in glucose metabolism
• Mood changes

Thyroid gland:
· Abnormal thyroid levels due to starvation

Heart:
· Low blood pressure and abnormal heart rate contribute to dizziness and fainting
· Abnormal electrocardiogram (ECG)
· Sudden death due to ventricular arrhythmias

Gastrointestinal system:
· Abdominal pain and bloating caused by slowed gastric emptying and intestinal motility
· Acute pancreatitis
· Constipation

Bone:
· Decreased bone mineral density (osteopenia)
· Decreased ability to absorb calcium due to low estrogen levels
· Decreased intake of bone-building nutrients due to starvation
· Increased loss of bone due to elevated cortisol levels

FIGURE 2   The impact of anorexia nervosa on the body.

HOT TOPIC

Muscle Dysmorphia: The Male Eating Disorder?

Is there a reverse form of anorexia nervosa unique to men? For decades, bodybuilders have recognized that some men view themselves as "puny" even when they are normal size or even very muscular; work out obsessively; and adhere to an extremely restrictive diet.

Recently, psychiatrists have confirmed that this disorder exists. They call it *muscle dysmorphia* (in medicine, a *dysmorphia* is an abnormality of structure). Some classify it as a body image disorder, because these patients perceive themselves as small and frail even though they may in reality be large and muscular. As a result, they are pathologically preoccupied with muscularity. They spend long hours lifting weights and follow a meticulous high-protein diet, but no matter how "buff" they become, their reflection in the mirror does not match their ideal.

Others classify muscle dysmorphia as an eating disorder, pointing out that the patients' pathological pursuit of muscle gain causes them to engage in behaviors similar to those of patients with anorexia. Patients also report "feeling fat," are not comfortable exposing their body to others, and have increased rates of other psychiatric illnesses.[16] Moreover, researchers note that the risk factors and treatment options for the two disorders are similar.[17]

Like anorexia nervosa, muscle dysmorphia can cause significant distress and may even be life-threatening. Men with the disorder are more likely to report substance abuse—including anabolic steroids—and are more likely to have attempted suicide. Therapy can help.

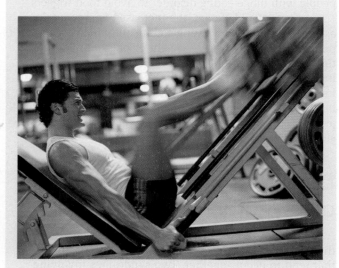

Men are more likely than women to exercise excessively in an effort to control their weight.

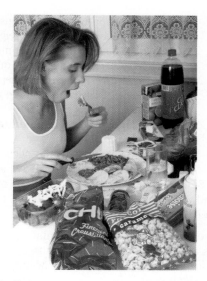

People with bulimia nervosa typically consume relatively large amounts of food in brief periods of time.

inability to end the binge once it has started.[1] At the same time, the person feels a sense of euphoria not unlike a drug-induced high.

■ **Purging** is a compensatory behavior used to prevent weight gain. Methods of purging include vomiting, laxative or diuretic abuse, enemas, fasting, and excessive exercise. For example, after a binge, a runner may increase her daily mileage to equal the "calculated" energy content of the binge.

The prevalence of bulimia nervosa is higher than that of anorexia nervosa, affecting an estimated 1–4% of women.[12] Like anorexia nervosa, bulimia nervosa is found predominantly in women: six to ten females are diagnosed for every one male. The mortality rate for bulimia nervosa is approximately 4%.[12]

Although the prevalence of bulimia nervosa is much higher in women, rates for men are significant in some predominantly "thin-build" sports in which participants are encouraged to maintain a low body weight (for example, horse racing, wrestling, crew, and gymnastics). Individuals in these sports typically do not have all the characteristics of bulimia nervosa, however, and the purging behaviors they practice typically stop once the sport is discontinued.

Symptoms of Bulimia Nervosa

The American Psychiatric Association has identified the following criteria for diagnosis of bulimia nervosa:[18]

■ Recurrent episodes of binge eating (for example, eating a large amount of food in a short period, such as within 2 hours).

purging An attempt to rid the body of unwanted food by vomiting or other compensatory means, such as excessive exercise, fasting, or laxative abuse.

- Recurrent inappropriate compensatory behavior in order to prevent weight gain, such as self-induced vomiting; misuse of laxatives, diuretics, enemas, or other medications; fasting; or excessive exercise.
- Binge eating occurs on average at least twice a week for 3 months.
- Body shape and weight unduly influence self-evaluation.
- The disturbance does not occur exclusively during episodes of anorexia nervosa. Some individuals will have periods of binge eating and then periods of starvation, which makes classification of their disorder difficult.

Moreover, an individual with bulimia nervosa typically purges after most episodes but not necessarily on every occasion. Weight gain as a result of binge eating can therefore be significant.

How can you tell if someone has bulimia nervosa? In addition to the recurrent and frequent binge eating and purging episodes, the National Institutes of Health have identified the following symptoms of bulimia nervosa:[19]

- Chronically inflamed and sore throat
- Swollen glands in the neck and below the jaw
- Worn tooth enamel and increasingly sensitive and decaying teeth as a result of exposure to stomach acids
- Gastroesophageal reflux disorder
- Intestinal distress and irritation from laxative abuse
- Kidney problems from diuretic abuse
- Severe dehydration from purging of fluids

Health Risks of Bulimia Nervosa

The destructive behaviors of bulimia nervosa can lead to illness and even death. The most common health consequences associated with bulimia nervosa are:

- Electrolyte imbalance typically caused by dehydration and the loss of potassium and sodium from the body with frequent vomiting. This can lead to irregular heartbeat and even heart failure and death.
- *Gastrointestinal problems*: inflammation, ulceration, and possible rupture of the esophagus and stomach from frequent bingeing and vomiting. Chronic irregular bowel movements and constipation may result in people with bulimia who chronically abuse laxatives.
- *Dental problems*: tooth decay and staining from stomach acids released during frequent vomiting.

As with anorexia nervosa, the chance of recovery from bulimia nervosa increases, and the negative effects on health decrease, if the disorder is detected at an early stage. Familiarity with the warning signs of bulimia nervosa can help you identify friends and family members who might be at risk.

Binge-Eating Disorder

When was the last time a friend or relative confessed to you about "going on an eating binge"? Most likely, he or she explained that the behavior followed some sort of

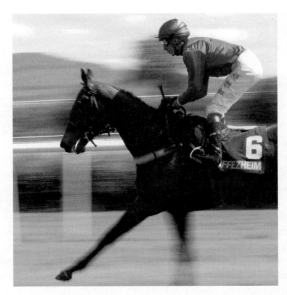

Men who participate in "thin-build" sports, such as jockeys, have a higher risk for bulimia nervosa.

stressful event, such as a problem at work, the breakup of a relationship, or a poor grade on an exam. Many people have one or two binge episodes every year or so in response to stress. But in people with **binge-eating disorder**, the behavior occurs frequently. Because it is not usually followed by purging, the person tends to gain a lot of weight. This lack of compensation for the binge distinguishes binge-eating disorder from bulimia nervosa.

The prevalence of binge-eating disorder is estimated to be 2–5% of the adult female population, and 8% of the obese population.[12,20] In contrast to anorexia and bulimia, binge-eating disorder is also common in men. Our current food environment, which offers an abundance of good-tasting, cheap food any time of the day, makes it difficult for people with binge-eating disorder to avoid food triggers.

As you would expect, the increased energy intake associated with binge eating significantly increases a person's risk of being overweight or obese. In addition, the types of foods individuals typically consume during a binge episode are high in fat and sugar, which can increase blood lipids. Finally, the stress associated with binge eating can have psychological consequences, such as low self-esteem, avoidance of social contact, depression, and negative thoughts related to body size.

Disordered eating can be part of a syndrome

A *syndrome* is a type of disorder characterized by the presence of two or more distinct health problems that tend to occur together. Two syndromes involving

binge-eating disorder A disorder characterized by binge eating an average of twice a week or more, typically without compensatory purging.

disordered eating behaviors are night-eating syndrome and the female athlete triad.

Night-Eating Syndrome

Night-eating syndrome was first described in a group of patients who were not hungry in the morning but spent the evening and night eating and reported insomnia. Like binge-eating disorder, it is associated with obesity because, although night eaters don't typically binge, they do consume significant energy in their frequent snacks, and they don't compensate for the excess energy intake.

The distinguishing characteristic of night-eating syndrome is the time during which most of the day's energy intake occurs. Night eaters have a daily pattern of significantly increasing their energy intake in the evening and/or at nighttime and not being hungry at breakfast time. Thus, night-eating syndrome is diagnosed by one or both of the following criteria:[21]

- Eating at least 25% of daily food intake after the evening meal
- Experiencing at least two episodes per week of night eating; that is, getting up to eat after going to bed

Night eating is also characterized by a depressed mood and insomnia.[22] In short, this syndrome combines three unique disorders: an eating disorder, a sleep disorder, and a mood disorder.[21] Many night eaters are obese, and many experience anxiety or engage in substance abuse. Some engage in other disordered eating behaviors.

Night-eating syndrome is important clinically because of its association with obesity, which increases the risk for several chronic diseases, including heart disease, high blood pressure, stroke, type 2 diabetes, and arthritis. Obesity also increases the risk for sleep apnea, which can further disrupt the night eater's already abnormal sleeping pattern.

The Female Athlete Triad

The **female athlete triad** (**FIGURE 3**) is a serious syndrome that consists of three clinical conditions in some physically active females:[23]

- Low energy availability (such as inadequate energy intake to maintain menstrual function or to cover energy expended in exercise) with or without eating disorders
- Menstrual dysfunction, such as amenorrhea (the absence of menstruation for 3 months or more)
- Low bone density

Certain sports that strongly emphasize leanness or a thin body build may place a young girl or a woman at risk for the female athlete triad. These sports typically

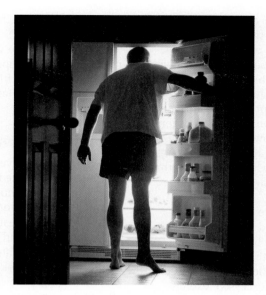

People with night-eating syndrome consume most of their daily energy between 8 PM and 6 AM.

include figure skating, gymnastics, and diving; classical ballet dancers are also at increased risk for the disorder.

Active women experience the general social and cultural demands placed on women to be thin, as well as pressure from their coach, teammates, judges, and/or spectators to meet weight standards or body-size expectations for their sport. Failure to meet these standards can result in severe consequences, such as being cut from the team, losing an athletic scholarship, or decreased participation with the team.

As the pressure to be thin mounts, active women may restrict their energy intake, typically by engaging in disordered eating behaviors. Combined with their high levels of physical activity, this energy restriction can disrupt the menstrual cycle and result in amenorrhea. Notice that these women do not necessarily have to have a clinical eating disorder

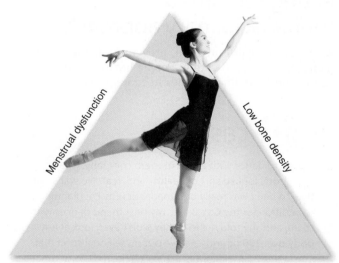

FIGURE 3 The *female athlete triad* is a syndrome composed of three coexisting disorders: low energy availability (with or without eating disorders), menstrual dysfunction (such as amenorrhea), and low bone density (such as osteoporosis). Energy availability is defined as dietary energy intake minus exercise energy expenditure.

night-eating syndrome Disorder characterized by intake of the majority of the day's energy between 8:00 PM and 6:00 AM. Individuals with this disorder also experience mood and sleep disorders.

female athlete triad A serious syndrome that consists of three clinical conditions in some physically active females: low energy availability (with or without eating disorders), menstrual dysfunction, and low bone density.

or even be dieting. They are just not eating enough to cover the energy costs of their exercise training as well as all the other energy demands of the body and daily living.

Female athletes with menstrual dysfunction, regardless of the cause, typically have reduced levels of the reproductive hormones estrogen and progesterone. When estrogen levels in the body are low, it is difficult for bone to retain calcium, and gradual loss of bone mass occurs. Thus, many female athletes develop premature bone loss (osteoporosis) and are at increased risk for fractures.

Recognition of an athlete with one or more of the components of the female athlete triad can be difficult, especially if the athlete is reluctant to be honest when questioned about the symptoms. For this reason, familiarity with the early warning signs is critical. These include excessive dieting and/or weight loss, excessive exercise, stress fractures, and self-esteem that appears to be dictated by body weight and shape.

Treatment for disordered eating requires a multidisciplinary approach

As with any health problem, prevention is the best treatment for disordered eating. People having trouble with eating and body image issues need help to deal with these issues before they develop into something more serious.

Treating anyone with disordered eating requires a multidisciplinary approach. In addition to a physician and psychologist, a nutritionist, the person's coach and trainer (if an athlete), and family members and friends all must work together.

Inpatient Nutritional Therapies

Patients who are severely underweight, display signs of malnutrition, are medically unstable, or are suicidal may require immediate hospitalization. The goals of nutritional therapies are to restore the individual to a healthy body weight, normalize eating patterns, learn to identify hunger and satiety cues, and resolve the nutrition-related health issues.[24] For stable hospitalized patients, the expected weight gain per week ranges from 2 to 3 pounds. For outpatient settings, the expected weight gain is much lower (0.5 to 1 pound/week). However, determining the energy intake needed to achieve these levels of weight gain can be difficult because energy estimates used for healthy individuals of normal weight may not be appropriate for people who are underweight.

Patients frequently try a variety of methods to avoid consuming the food presented to them. They may discard the food, vomit, exercise excessively, or engage in a high level of non-exercise motor activity to eliminate the Calories they have just consumed. For this reason, patients are carefully watched by hospital staff or family members. In addition to increasing amounts of food, patients may be given vitamin and mineral supplements to ensure that adequate micronutrients are consumed.

Nutrition counseling is an important aspect of inpatient treatment, especially to deal with the body image issues that occur as weight is regained. Once the patient reaches an acceptable body weight, nutrition counseling will address issues such as the acceptability of certain foods; dealing with food situations, such as family gatherings and eating out; and learning to put together a healthful food plan for weight maintenance.

Outpatient Nutrition Counseling

Patients with anorexia nervosa who are underweight but medically stable may be able to enter an outpatient program designed to meet their specific needs. Outpatient programs are also an option for patients with other forms of disordered eating who are of normal weight or overweight. Some outpatient programs are extremely intensive, requiring patients to come in each day for treatment, whereas others are less rigorous, requiring only weekly visits for counseling.

Nutrition counseling generally focuses on identifying and dealing with events and feelings that trigger food restriction or binge eating or purging. Another goal is to establish structured eating behaviors that can enable the patient to maintain a healthful body weight. In addition, nutrition counseling will address factors

nutri-case | LIZ

"I used to dance with a cool modern company, where everybody looked sort of healthy and 'real.' No waifs! After they folded I was really bummed, but now I'm planning to audition for the City Ballet. My best friend dances with them, and she told me that they won't even *look* at anybody over 100 pounds. So I've put myself on a strict diet. Most days I come in under 1,200 Calories, but sometimes I cheat a little and then I feel so out of control. Last week, my dance teacher stopped me after class and asked me if I was still getting my periods. I thought that was a pretty weird question, so I just said sure, but when I thought about it I realized I've been so focused and stressed lately that I really don't know! But my audition is only a week away, so I'm definitely going on a juice fast this weekend."

Which factors increase Liz's risk for the female athlete triad? What, if anything, do you think Liz's dance teacher should do? Is intervention even necessary because the audition is only a week away?

specific to the individual, such as negative feelings about foods or fears associated with uncontrolled binge eating.

Talking to someone about disordered eating

Discussing a friend's eating behaviors can be difficult. It is important to choose an appropriate time and place to raise your concerns and to listen closely and with great sensitivity to your friend's feelings. Here, we outline an approach you might use.

Before approaching a friend or family member you suspect of having an eating disorder, learn as much as you possibly can about it. Make sure you know the difference between the facts and myths about eating disorders. Locate a health professional specializing in eating disorders to whom you can refer your friend, and be ready to go with your friend if he or she does not want to go alone. If you are at a university or college, check with your campus health center to see if it has an eating disorder specialist or can recommend someone to you.

The National Eating Disorders Association recommends the following steps to take during your discussion:[25]

- *Schedule a time to talk.* Set aside a time and place for a private discussion in which you can share your concerns openly and honestly in a caring and supportive way. Make sure the setting is quiet and away from other distractions.
- *Communicate your concerns.* Share your memories of specific times when you felt concerned about your friend's eating or exercise behaviors. Explain that you think these things may indicate that there is a problem that needs professional attention.

- *Ask your friend to explore these concerns with a counselor, doctor, nutritionist, or other health professional* who is knowledgeable about eating issues. If you feel comfortable doing so, offer to help your friend make an appointment or accompany your friend on the first visit.
- *Avoid conflicts or a "battle of the wills" with your friend.* If your friend refuses to acknowledge that there is a problem, or any reason for you to be concerned, restate your feelings and the reasons for them and leave yourself open and available as a supportive listener.
- *Avoid placing shame, blame, or guilt on your friend regarding his or her actions or attitudes. Do not use accusatory "you" statements, such as "You just need to eat" or "You are acting irresponsibly." Instead, use "I" statements—for example, "I'm concerned about you because I never see you in the cafeteria anymore" or "It makes me afraid when I hear you vomit."
- *Avoid giving simple solutions*—for example, "If you would just stop, everything would be fine."
- *Express your continued support.* Remind your friend that you care and want your friend to be healthy and happy.

MasteringNutrition™

Check out these additional resources in the MasteringNutrition Study Area:

- Read It: Chapter Summary and RSS Feeds
- See It: ABC News videos and nutrition animations
- Hear It: MP3s
- Study It: Get Ready for Nutrition Math and Chemistry review
- Do It: NutriTools and "Find the Quack" feature
- Review It: Quizzes, flashcards, and glossary

web resources

www.massgeneral.org
Harris Center for Education and Advocacy in Eating Disorders, Massachusetts General Hospital

Enter "Harris Center" into the search box on the main page. This site provides information about current eating disorder research as well as sections on understanding eating disorders and resources for those with eating disorders.

www.nimh.nih.gov
National Institute of Mental Health (NIMH) Office of Communications and Public Liaison

Search this site for "disordered eating" or "eating disorders" to find numerous articles on the subject.

www.anad.org
National Association of Anorexia Nervosa and Associated Disorders

Visit this site for information and resources about eating disorders.

www.nationaleatingdisorders.org
National Eating Disorders Association

This site is dedicated to expanding public understanding of eating disorders and promoting access to treatment for those affected and support for their families.

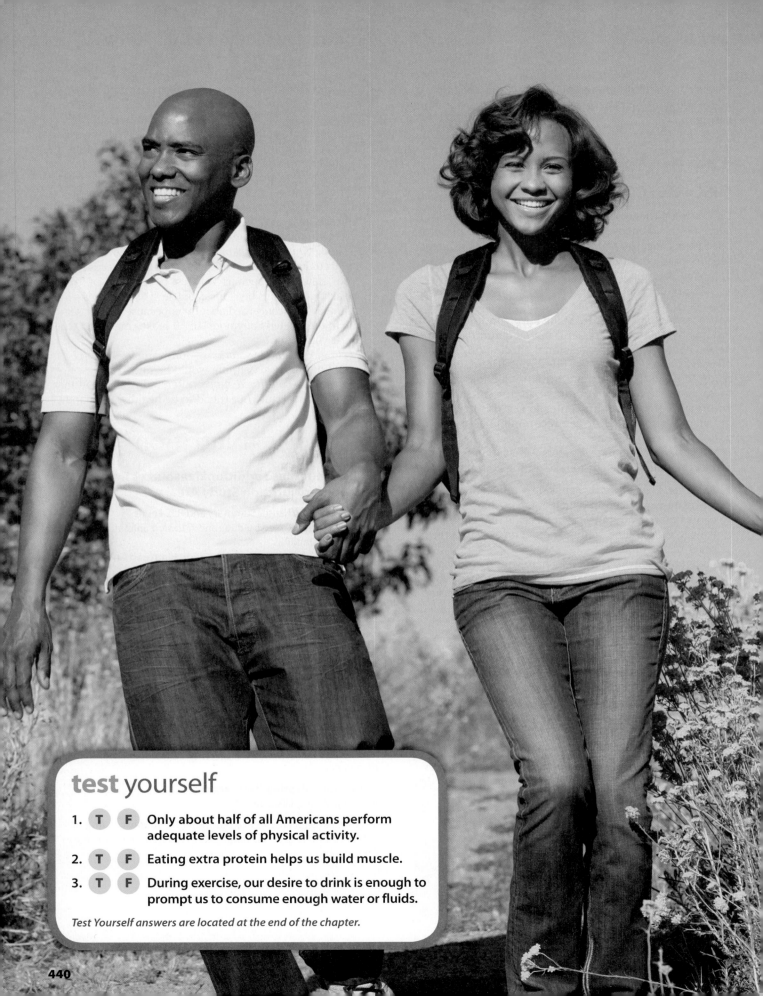

test yourself

1. **T** **F** Only about half of all Americans perform adequate levels of physical activity.

2. **T** **F** Eating extra protein helps us build muscle.

3. **T** **F** During exercise, our desire to drink is enough to prompt us to consume enough water or fluids.

Test Yourself answers are located at the end of the chapter.

Nutrition and Physical Activity
Keys to good health

12

learning objectives

After studying this chapter you should be able to:

1 Compare and contrast the concepts of physical activity, leisure-time physical activity, exercise, and physical fitness, pp. 442–443.

2 Identify the four components of physical fitness, p. 442.

3 List at least four health benefits of being physically active on a regular basis, p. 443.

4 Describe the FITT principle and calculate your maximal and training heart rate range, pp. 446–448.

5 List and describe at least three processes by which the body breaks down fuels to support physical activity, pp. 450–457.

6 Discuss at least three changes in nutrient needs that can occur in response to an increase in physical activity or vigorous exercise training, pp. 457–467.

7 Describe the concept of carbohydrate loading, and discuss situations in which this practice may be beneficial to athletic performance, pp. 462–463.

In the summer of 2013, Lillian Web of Florida and Harold Bach of North Dakota each took the gold medal for the 100-meter dash in track and field at the National Senior Games. Web did it in just over 38 seconds, and Bach's time was less than 22 seconds. If these performance times don't amaze you, perhaps they will when you consider these athletes' ages: Web was 99 years old, and Bach was 93!

There's no doubt about it: regular physical activity dramatically improves strength, stamina, health, and quality of life—throughout the life span. But what qualifies as "regular physical activity"? In other words, how much do we need to do to reap the benefits? And if we do become more active, does our diet have to change, too?

Healthy eating practices and regular physical activity are like two sides of the same coin, interacting in a variety of ways to improve our strength and stamina and increase our resistance to many acute illnesses and chronic diseases. In this chapter, we'll define physical activity, identify its many benefits, and discuss the nutrients needed to maintain an active life.

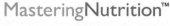

MasteringNutrition™

Go online for chapter quizzes, pre-tests, Interactive Activities, and more!

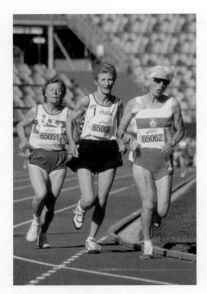

With the help of a nutritious diet, many people are able to remain physically active—and even competitive—throughout adult life.

What are the benefits of physical activity?

The term **physical activity** describes any movement produced by muscles that increases energy expenditure. Different categories of physical activity include occupational, household, leisure-time, and transportation.[1] **Leisure-time physical activity** is any activity not related to a person's occupation and includes competitive sports, planned exercise training, and recreational activities such as hiking, walking, and bicycling. **Exercise** is therefore considered a subcategory of leisure-time physical activity and refers to activity that is purposeful, planned, and structured.[2]

Physical Activity Increases Our Fitness

A lot of people are looking for a "magic pill" that will help them maintain weight loss, reduce their risk for diseases, make them feel better, and improve their quality of sleep. Although they may not be aware of it, regular physical activity is this "magic pill." That's because it promotes **physical fitness**: the ability to carry out daily tasks with vigor and alertness, without undue fatigue, and with ample energy to enjoy leisure-time pursuits and meet unforeseen emergencies.[1]

The four components of physical fitness are cardiorespiratory fitness, which is the ability of the heart, lungs, and circulatory system to efficiently supply oxygen and nutrients to working muscles; musculoskeletal fitness, which is fitness of the muscles and bones; flexibility; and body composition **(TABLE 12.1)**.[3] These are achieved through three types of exercise:

- **Aerobic exercise** involves the repetitive movement of large muscle groups, which increases the body's use of oxygen and promotes cardiovascular health. In your daily life, you get aerobic exercise when you walk to a bus stop or take the stairs to a third-floor classroom.
- **Resistance training** is a form of exercise in which our muscles work against resistance, such as against handheld weights. Carrying grocery bags or books and moving heavy objects are everyday activities that make our muscles work against resistance.
- **Stretching** exercises are those that increase flexibility, as they involve lengthening muscles using slow, controlled movements. You can perform stretching exercises even while you're sitting in a classroom by flexing, extending, and rotating your neck, limbs, and extremities.

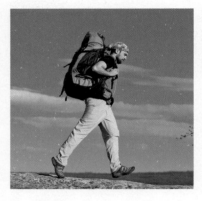

Hiking is a leisure-time physical activity that can contribute to your physical fitness.

Physical Activity Reduces Our Risk for Chronic Disease

In addition to contributing to our fitness, regular physical activity can improve our health right now, and reduce our risk for certain diseases. Specifically, the health benefits of physical activity include **(FIGURE 12.1)**:

- *Reduces our risks for, and complications of, heart disease, stroke, and high blood pressure.* Regular physical activity increases high-density lipoprotein (HDL) cholesterol and lowers triglycerides in the blood, improves the strength of the heart, helps maintain healthy blood pressure, and limits the progression of atherosclerosis.

physical activity Any movement produced by muscles that increases energy expenditure; includes occupational, household, leisure-time, and transportation activities.

leisure-time physical activity Any activity not related to a person's occupation; includes competitive sports, recreational activities, and planned exercise training.

exercise A subcategory of leisure-time physical activity; any activity that is purposeful, planned, and structured.

TABLE 12.1 The Components of Fitness

Fitness Component	Examples of Activities One Can Do to Achieve Fitness in Each Component
Cardiorespiratory	Aerobic-type activities, such as walking, running, swimming, cross-country skiing
Musculoskeletal fitness:	Resistance training, weight lifting, calisthenics, sit-ups, push-ups
Muscular strength	Weight lifting or related activities using heavier weights with few repetitions
Muscular endurance	Weight lifting or related activities using lighter weights with more repetitions
Flexibility	Stretching exercises, yoga
Body composition	Aerobic exercise, resistance training

Reduces risk of heart disease, strengthens heart, reduces risk of high blood pressure

Increases lung efficiency and capacity

Reduces risk of type 2 diabetes

Reduces risk of colon cancer

Strengthens immune system

Strengthens bones

Reduces risk of bone, muscle, and joint injuries

Promotes healthful body composition and weight management

Benefits psychological health and stress management

FIGURE 12.1 Health benefits of regular physical activity.

Sitting too long, studying for tomorrow's exam? Stretching can help! Learn some simple stretches by watching the how-to video collection from the Mayo Clinic at www.mayoclinic.com. Enter "health," and then "office stretches" into the search box.

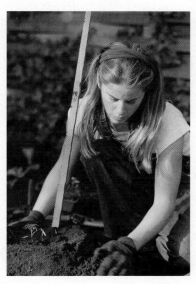

Moderate physical activity, such as gardening, helps maintain overall health.

- *Reduces our risk for obesity.* Regular physical activity maintains lean body mass and promotes more healthful levels of body fat, may help in appetite control, and increases energy expenditure and the use of fat as an energy source.
- *Reduces our risk for type 2 diabetes.* Regular physical activity enhances the action of insulin, which improves the cells' uptake of glucose from the blood, and it can improve blood glucose control in people with diabetes, which in turn reduces the risk for, or delays the onset of, diabetes-related complications.
- *May reduce our risk for colon cancer.* Although the exact role that physical activity may play in reducing colon cancer risk is still unknown, we do know that regular physical activity enhances gastric motility, which reduces transit time of potential cancer-causing agents through the gut.
- *Reduces our risk for osteoporosis.* Regular physical activity, especially weight-bearing exercise, increases bone density and enhances muscular strength and flexibility, thereby reducing the likelihood of falls and the incidence of fractures and other injuries when falls occur.

Regular physical activity is also known to improve our sleep patterns, reduce our risk for upper respiratory infections by improving immune function, and reduce anxiety and mental stress. It also can be effective in treating mild and moderate depression.

Most Americans Are Inactive

For most of our history, humans were very physically active. This was not by choice, but because their survival depended on it. Prior to the industrial age, humans expended a considerable amount of energy each day foraging and hunting for food, planting and harvesting food, preparing food once it was acquired, and securing shelter. In addition, their diet was composed primarily of small amounts of lean meats and naturally grown vegetables and fruits. This lifestyle pattern contrasts considerably with today's, which is characterized by sedentary jobs, easy access to an

physical fitness The ability to carry out daily tasks with vigor and alertness, without undue fatigue, and with ample energy to enjoy leisure-time pursuits and meet unforeseen emergencies.

aerobic exercise Exercise that involves the repetitive movement of large muscle groups, increasing the body's use of oxygen and promoting cardiovascular health.

resistance training Exercise in which our muscles act against resistance.

stretching Exercise in which muscles are gently lengthened using slow, controlled movements.

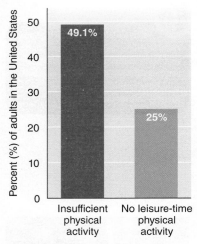

FIGURE 12.2 Rates of physical inactivity in the United States. Almost 50% of the U.S. population does not do enough physical activity to meet national health recommendations, and 25% report doing no leisure-time physical activity.

Data from: National Center for Health Statistics. 2012. Health, United States, 2011: With Special Feature on Socioeconomic Status and Health. Hyattsville, MD.; and Centers for Disease Control and Prevention, 2008. 1988–2007 No Leisure-Time Physical Activity Trend Chart.

overabundance of energy-dense foods, and few opportunities for or little interest in expending energy through occupational or recreational activities.

Given these changes, it isn't surprising that most people find the "magic pill" of physical activity hard to swallow. The Centers for Disease Control and Prevention report that almost 50% of people in the United States do not do enough physical activity to meet national health recommendations, and 25% admit to doing no leisure-time physical activity at all (**FIGURE 12.2**).[4,5] These statistics mirror the reported increases in obesity, heart disease, and type 2 diabetes in industrialized countries.

This trend toward inadequate physical activity levels is also occurring in young people. Among high school students, only 18.5% of girls and 38.3% of boys are meeting the recommended 60 minutes per day on 5 or more days per week.[6] Although physical education (PE) is part of the mandated curriculum in most states, only 27.2% of girls and 34.6% of boys participate in daily PE. Because our habits related to eating and physical activity are formed early in life, it is imperative that we provide opportunities for children and adolescents to engage in regular, enjoyable physical activity. An active lifestyle during childhood increases the likelihood of an active, healthier life as an adult.

recap Physical activity is any movement produced by muscles that increases energy expenditure. Physical fitness is the ability to carry out daily tasks with vigor and alertness, without undue fatigue, and with ample energy to enjoy leisure-time pursuits and meet unforeseen emergencies. Physical activity provides a multitude of health benefits, including reducing our risks for obesity and many chronic diseases and relieving anxiety and stress. Most people in the United States, including many children, are insufficiently active.

How can you improve your fitness?

Several widely recognized qualities of a sound fitness program, as well as guidelines to help you design one that is right for you, are explored in this section. Keep in mind that people with heart disease, high blood pressure, diabetes, obesity, osteoporosis, asthma, or arthritis should get approval to exercise from their healthcare practitioner prior to starting a fitness program. In addition, a medical evaluation should be conducted before starting an exercise program for an apparently healthy but currently inactive man 40 years or older or woman 50 years or older.

Assess Your Current Level of Fitness

Before beginning any fitness program, it is important to know your initial level of fitness. This information can then be used to help you design a fitness program that meets your goals and is appropriate for you. How can you go about estimating your current fitness level? The President's Council on Fitness, Sports and Nutrition can help! Check out the **What About You?** box (page 445) to take The President's Challenge Adult Fitness Test.

Identify Your Personal Fitness Goals

A fitness program that may be ideal for you is not necessarily right for everyone. Before designing or evaluating any program, it is important to define your personal fitness goals. Do you want to prevent osteoporosis, diabetes, or another chronic disease that runs in your family? Do you simply want to increase your energy and stamina? Or do you intend to compete in athletic events? Each of these scenarios requires a unique fitness program. This concept is referred to as the *specificity principle*: specific actions yield specific results.

Training is generally defined as activity leading to skilled behavior. Training is very specific to any activity or goal. For example, if you want to train for athletic competition, a traditional approach that includes planned, purposive exercise sessions under the guidance of a trainer or coach would be beneficial. If you wanted to achieve cardiorespiratory fitness, you might be advised to participate in an aerobics class at least three times per week or jog for at least 20 minutes three times per week.

what about **you**

Taking the President's Challenge Adult Fitness Test

The President's Challenge Adult Fitness test is designed for adults 18 years of age and older who are in good general health. The tests assess aerobic fitness, muscle strength and endurance, flexibility, and body composition. Detailed instructions for completing each test can be found at www.adultfitnesstest.org. Below is a form for recording your test results. It is suggested that you do these tests with a partner to assist you with keeping track of your time and scores on each test.

Before getting started, make sure you're healthy enough to take the test. Go to www.adultfitnesstest.org, and search under "risk questionaire," to complete the American Heart Association Physical Activity Readiness Questionnaire.

1. Aerobic Fitness – you must enter either a 1-mile walk time and heart rate or enter a 1.5-mile run time

Mile walk time: _____ minutes _____ seconds

Heart rate (after walk): _____ beats per minute

Weight: _____ lb (required for result calculation)

OR

1.5-mile run time: _____ minutes _____ seconds

2. Muscular Strength and Endurance

Half sit-ups: _____ (in 1 minute)

Push-ups: _____

3. Flexibility

Sit and Reach _____ inches

4. Body Composition

Body mass index: Height _____ feet _____ inches
Weight _____ lb

Waist measurement _____ inches

Once you complete the form, enter your data online to get your fitness score at www.adultfitnesstest.org and search under "data entry."

In contrast, if your goal is to transition from doing no regular physical activity to doing enough physical activity to maintain your overall health, you could follow the minimum recommendations put forth in the 2008 Physical Activity Guidelines for Americans.[7] To gain significant health benefits, including reducing the risk for chronic diseases, you can participate in at least 30 minutes per day of moderate-intensity aerobic physical activity (such as gardening, brisk walking, or basketball). The activity need not be completed in one session. You can divide the amount of physical activity into two or more shorter sessions throughout the day as long as the total cumulative time is achieved (for example, brisk walking for 10 minutes three times per day). Although these minimum guidelines are appropriate for achieving health benefits, performing physical activities at a higher intensity and for longer duration will confer even greater health benefits and more significant improvements in physical fitness.

The promotion of various physical activity guidelines in recent years has led to some confusion among consumers regarding exactly how much physical activity is enough to enhance health and fitness levels. For example, the Institute of Medicine published guidelines stating that the minimum amount of physical activity that should be done each day to maintain health and fitness is 60 minutes—not 30 minutes, as published in the 1996 report of the Surgeon General and the more recent 2008 Physical Activity guidelines.[1,7,8] Refer to the **Nutrition Debate** at the end of this chapter to learn more about this controversy.

Make Your Program Varied, Consistent, and Fun!

A number of factors motivate us to be active. Some are *intrinsic* factors, which are those done for the satisfaction a person gains from engaging in the activity. Others are *extrinsic*, which are those done to obtain rewards or outcomes that are separate from the behavior itself.[9] Examples of intrinsic factors that motivate us to engage in physical activity include the desire to gain competence, the desire to be challenged by the activity and enhance our skills, and enjoyment. Some of the most common extrinsic factors are desires to improve appearance and to increase fitness. Recently, some employers have been offering financial incentives to log in time at the company's fitness center. This would be another example of an extrinsic factor.

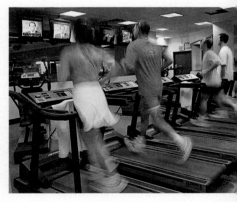

Watching television or reading can provide variety while running on a treadmill.

If we're going to reap the benefits of physical activity, we need to do it consistently. People who are regularly active tend to be more motivated by intrinsic factors, including enjoyment, whereas extrinsic factors appear to be more important to people who are not regularly active or are trying to engage in activity for the first time.[10]

Thus an important motivator in maintaining regular physical activity is enjoyment—or fun! What activities do you consider fun? If you enjoy the outdoors, hiking, camping, fishing, and rock climbing are potential activities for you. If you would rather exercise with friends between classes, walking, climbing stairs, jogging, roller-blading, or bicycle riding may be more appropriate. Or you may prefer to use the programs and equipment at your campus or community fitness center or purchase your own treadmill and free weights.

Variety is also important to maintaining your fitness and your interest in being regularly active. Although some people enjoy doing similar activities day after day, many get bored with the same fitness routine. Incorporating a variety of activities into your fitness program will help maintain your interest and increase your enjoyment while promoting different types of fitness identified in Table 12.1. Variety can be achieved by:

- Combining aerobic exercise, resistance training, and stretching
- Combining indoor and outdoor activities throughout the week
- Taking different routes when you walk or jog each day
- Watching a movie, reading a book, or listening to music while you ride a stationary bicycle or walk on a treadmill
- Participating in different activities each week, such as walking, dancing, bicycling, yoga, weight lifting, swimming, hiking, and gardening

This "smorgasbord" of activities can increase your fitness without leading to monotony and boredom.

Appropriately Overload Your Body

In order to improve your fitness, an extra physical demand must be placed on your body. This is referred to as the **overload principle**. A word of caution is in order here: *the overload principle does not advocate subjecting your body to inappropriately high stress*, because this can lead to exhaustion and injuries. In contrast, an appropriate overload on various body systems will result in healthy improvements in fitness. For example, a gain in muscle strength and size that results from repeated work that overloads the muscle is referred to as **hypertrophy**. When muscles are not worked adequately, they **atrophy**, or decrease in size and strength.

To achieve an appropriate overload, four factors should be considered, collectively known as the **FITT principle**: *f*requency, *i*ntensity, *t*ime, and *t*ype of activity. You can use the FITT principle to design either a general physical fitness program or a performance-based exercise program. **FIGURE 12.3** shows how the FITT principle applies to a cardiorespiratory and muscular fitness program. Let's consider each of the FITT principle's four factors in more detail.

Frequency

Frequency refers to the number of activity sessions per week. Depending on your goals for fitness, the frequency of your activities will vary. The Physical Activity Guidelines for Americans recommend engaging in aerobic (cardiorespiratory) activities for at least 150 minutes a week. To achieve cardiorespiratory fitness, training should be at least 3 to 5 days per week. On the other hand, training more than 6 days per week does not cause significant gains in fitness but can substantially increase the risks for injury. Training 3 to 6 days per week appears optimal to achieve and maintain cardiorespiratory fitness. In contrast, only 2 to 3 days of training are needed to achieve muscular fitness.

Intensity

Intensity refers to the amount of effort expended or to how difficult the activity is to perform. We describe the intensity of activity as being low, moderate, or vigorous:

- **Low-intensity activities** are those that cause very mild increases in breathing, sweating, and heart rate. Examples include walking at a leisurely pace, fishing, and light house-cleaning.

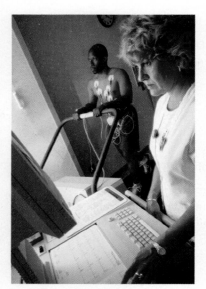

Testing in a fitness lab is the most accurate way to determine maximal heart rate.

overload principle Placing an extra physical demand on your body in order to improve your fitness level.

hypertrophy The increase in strength and size that results from repeated work to a specific muscle or muscle group.

atrophy A decrease in the size and strength of muscles that occurs when they are not worked adequately.

FITT principle The principle used to achieve an appropriate overload for physical training; FITT stands for *f*requency, *i*ntensity, *t*ime, and *t*ype of activity.

frequency Refers to the number of activity sessions per week you perform.

intensity The amount of effort expended during an activity, or how difficult the activity is to perform.

low-intensity activities Activities that cause very mild increases in breathing, sweating, and heart rate.

	Frequency	Intensity	Time and Type
Cardiorespiratory fitness	At least 30 minutes most days of the week	50–70% maximal heart rate for moderate intensity; 70–85% maximal heart rate for vigorous intensity	At least 30 consecutive minutes Choose swimming, walking, running, cycling, dancing, or other aerobic activities
Muscular fitness	2–3 days per week	70–85% maximal weight you can lift	1–3 sets of 8–12 lifts for each set A minimum of 8–10 exercises involving the major muscle groups such as arms, shoulders, chest, abdomen, back, hips, and legs, is recommended.
Flexibility	2–4 days per week	Stretching through full range of motion	For stretching, perform 2–4 repetitions per stretch. Hold each stretch for 15–30 seconds. Or try yoga, tai chi, or other flexibility programs.

FIGURE 12.3 Using the FITT principle to achieve cardiorespiratory and musculoskeletal fitness and flexibility. The recommendations in this figure follow the 2008 Physical Activity Guidelines for Americans (still in effect today).

- **Moderate-intensity activities** cause moderate increases in breathing, sweating, and heart rate. For instance, you can carry on a conversation, but not continuously. Examples include brisk walking, water aerobics, doubles tennis, ballroom dancing, and bicycling slower than 10 miles per hour.
- **Vigorous-intensity activities** produce significant increases in breathing, sweating, and heart rate, so that talking is difficult when exercising. Examples include jogging, running, racewalking, singles tennis, aerobics, bicycling 10 miles per hour or faster, jumping rope, and hiking uphill with a heavy backpack.

Traditionally, heart rate has been used to indicate level of intensity during aerobic activities. You can calculate the range of exercise intensity that is appropriate for you by estimating your **maximal heart rate**, which is the rate at which your heart beats during maximal-intensity exercise. Maximal heart rate is estimated by subtracting your age from 220.

FIGURE 12.4 shows an example of a heart rate training chart, which you can use to estimate the intensity of your own workout. The Centers for Disease Control and Prevention makes the following recommendations:[11]

- To achieve moderate-intensity physical activity, your target heart rate should be 50–70% of your estimated maximal heart rate. Older adults and anyone who has been inactive for a long time may want to exercise at the lower end of the moderate-intensity range.
- To achieve vigorous-intensity physical activity, your target heart rate should be 70–85% of your estimated heart rate. Those who are physically fit or are striving for a more rapid improvement in fitness may want to exercise at the higher end of the vigorous-intensity range.
- Competitive athletes generally train at a higher intensity, around 80–95% of their maximal heart rate.

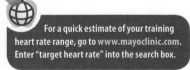
For a quick estimate of your training heart rate range, go to www.mayoclinic.com. Enter "target heart rate" into the search box.

moderate-intensity activities Activities that cause moderate increases in breathing, sweating, and heart rate.

vigorous-intensity activities Activities that produce significant increases in breathing, sweating, and heart rate; talking is difficult when exercising at a vigorous intensity.

maximal heart rate The rate at which your heart beats during maximal-intensity exercise.

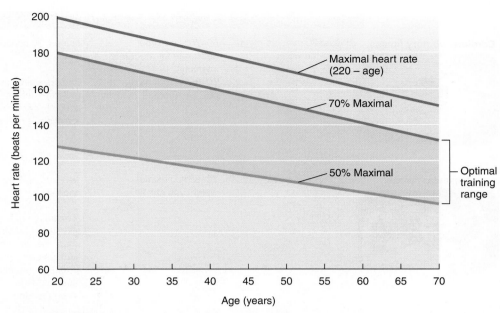

FIGURE 12.4 This heart rate training chart can be used to estimate aerobic exercise intensity. The top line indicates the predicted maximal heart rate value for a person's age (220 – age). The shaded area represents the heart rate values that fall between 50% and 70% of maximal heart rate, which is the range generally recommended to achieve aerobic fitness.

> Want to learn more about the various tools used to measure physical activity levels? Go to the University of Pittsburgh Physical Activity Resource Center for Public Health at www.parcph.org to find out more.

Although the calculation of *220 minus age* has been used extensively for years to predict maximal heart rate, it was never intended to accurately represent everyone's true maximal heart rate or to be used as the standard of aerobic training intensity. The most accurate way to determine your own maximal heart rate is to complete a maximal exercise test in a fitness laboratory; however, this test is not commonly conducted with the general public and can be very expensive. Although not completely accurate, the estimated maximal heart rate method can still be used to give you a general idea of your aerobic training range.

So what is your maximal heart rate and training range? To find out, try the easy calculation in the **You Do the Math** box (page 449).

Time of Activity

Time of activity refers to how long each session lasts. To achieve general health, you can do multiple short bouts of activity that add up to 30 minutes each day. However, to achieve higher levels of cardiovascular fitness, it is important that the activities be done for at least 30 consecutive minutes.

For example, let's say you want to compete in triathlons. To be successful during the running segment of the triathlon, you will need to be able to run quickly for at least 5 miles. Thus, it is appropriate for you to train so that you can complete 5 miles during one session and still have enough energy to swim and bicycle during the race. You will need to consistently train at a distance of 5 miles; you will also benefit from running longer distances.

Type of Activity

Type of activity refers to the range of physical activities a person can engage in to promote health and physical fitness. Many examples of types of physical activities one can engage in are illustrated in Table 12.1 and Figure 12.3. The types of activity you choose to engage in will depend on your goals for health and physical fitness, your personal preferences, and the range of activities available to you.

Include a Warm-Up and a Cool-Down Period

To properly prepare for and recover from an exercise session, warm-up and cool-down activities should be performed. **Warm-up**, also called preliminary exercise, includes

time of activity How long each exercise session lasts.

type of activity The range of physical activities a person can engage in to promote health and physical fitness.

warm-up Also called preliminary exercise; includes activities that prepare you for an exercise bout, including stretching, calisthenics, and movements specific to the exercise bout.

cool-down Activities done after an exercise session is completed; should be gradual and allow your body to slowly recover from exercise.

you do the math

Calculating Your Maximal and Training Heart Rate Range

Judy's healthcare provider has recommended she begin an exercise program. She plans to begin by either walking on the treadmill or riding the stationary bicycle at the fitness center during her lunch break.

Judy's doctor has recommended that she set her exercise intensity range at the low end of the currently recommended moderate intensity, or 50–70% estimated maximal heart rate.

Judy is 38 years old. Let's calculate her maximal heart rate values:

- Maximal heart rate: 220 – age = 220 – 38 = 182 beats per minute (bpm)
- Lower end of intensity range: 50% of 182 bpm = 0.50 × 182 bpm = 91 bpm
- Higher end of intensity range: 70% of 182 bpm = 0.70 × 182 bpm = 127 bpm

Because Judy is a trained nurse's aide, she is skilled at measuring a heart rate, or pulse. To measure your own pulse, take the following steps:

- Place your second (index) and third (middle) fingers on the inside of your wrist, just below the wrist crease and near the thumb. Press lightly to feel your pulse. Don't press too hard, or you will occlude the artery and be unable to feel its pulsation.

- If you can't feel your pulse at your wrist, try the carotid artery at your neck. This is located below your ear, on the side of your neck directly below your jaw. Press lightly against your neck under the jaw bone to find your pulse.

- Begin counting your pulse with the count of "zero;" then count each beat for 15 seconds.

- Multiply that value by 4 to estimate heart rate over 1 minute.

- Do not take your pulse with your thumb because it has its own pulse, which would prevent you from getting an accurate estimate of your heart rate.

As you can see from these calculations, when Judy walks on the treadmill or rides the bicycle, her heart rate should be between 91 and 127 bpm; this will put her in her aerobic training zone and allow her to achieve cardiorespiratory fitness. It will also help her lose weight, assuming she consumes less energy than she expends each day.

Now you do the math. Sam is a recreational runner who is 70 years old and wishes to train to compete in track and field events at the National Senior Games. His doctor has approved him for competition and has advised that Sam train at 75–80% of his maximal heart rate. (A) Calculate Sam's maximal heart rate. (B) What is Sam's heart rate training range in bpm?

Answers are located online in the MasteringNutrition Study Area.

general activities, such as gentle aerobics, calisthenics, and then stretching followed by specific activities that prepare you for the actual activity, such as jogging or swinging a golf club. The warm-up should be brief (5 to 10 minutes), gradual, and sufficient to increase muscle and body temperature. It should not cause fatigue or deplete energy stores.

Warming up prior to exercise is important because it properly prepares your muscles for exertion by increasing blood flow and body temperature. It enhances the body's flexibility and may also help prepare you psychologically for the exercise session or athletic event.

Cool-down activities are done after the exercise session. The cool-down should be gradual, allowing your body to recover slowly. The cool-down should include some of the same activities you performed during the exercise session, but at a low intensity, and should allow ample time for stretching. Cooling down after exercise assists in the prevention of injury and may help reduce muscle soreness.

Keep It Simple, Take It Slow

There are 1,440 minutes in every day. Spend just 30 of those minutes in physical activity, and you'll be taking an important step toward improving your health. See the **Quick Tips** (page 450) for working daily activity into your life.

If you have been inactive for a while, use a sensible approach by starting out slowly. The first month is an initiation phase, which is the time to start to incorporate relatively brief bouts of physical activity into your daily life and reduce the time you spend in sedentary activities. Gradually build up the time you spend doing the activity by adding a few minutes every few days until you reach 30 minutes a day.

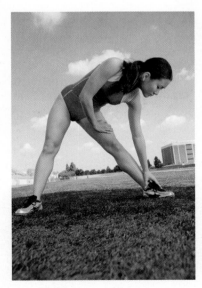

Stretching should be included in the warm-up before and the cool-down after exercise.

QuickTips

Increasing Your Physical Activity

✓ Walk as often and as far as possible: park your car farther away from your dorm, lecture hall, or shops; walk to school or work; go for a brisk walk between classes; get on or off the bus one stop away from your destination. And don't be in such a rush to reach your destination—take the long way and burn a few more Calories.

✓ At every opportunity, take the stairs instead of the escalator or elevator.

✓ When working on the computer for long periods, take a 3- to 5-minute break every hour to stretch, walk to another room, or make a cup of tea.

✓ Exercise while watching television—for example, by doing sit-ups, stretching, or using a treadmill or stationary bike.

✓ While talking on your cell phone, memorizing vocabulary terms, or practicing your choral part, don't stand still—pace!

✓ Turn on some music and dance!

✓ Get an exercise partner: join a friend for walks, hikes, cycling, skating, tennis, or a fitness class.

✓ Take up a group sport.

✓ Register for a class from the physical education department in an activity you've never tried before, maybe yoga or fencing.

✓ Register for a dance class, such as jazz, tap, or ballroom.

✓ Use the pool, track, rock-climbing wall, or other facilities at your campus fitness center or join a health club, gym, or YMCA/YWCA in your community.

✓ Join an activity-based club, such as a skating, tennis, or hiking club.

✓ Play golf without using a golf cart—choose to walk and carry your clubs instead.

✓ Choose a physically active vacation that provides daily activities combined with exploring new surroundings.

The next 4 to 6 months is the improvement phase, in which you can increase the intensity and duration of the activities you engage in. As you become more fit, the 30-minute minimum becomes easier and you'll need to gradually increase either the length of time you spend in activity or the intensity of the activities you choose, or both, to continue to progress toward your fitness goals. Once you've reached your goals and a plateau in your fitness gains, you've entered into the maintenance phase. At this point you can either maintain your current activity levels, or you may choose to re-evaluate your goals and alter your training accordingly.

Map your walking, running, or cycling route and share it with friends—or check out dozens of fitness loops right in your neighborhood at www.livestrong.com. Enter "loops" into the search box to get underway.

recap A sound fitness program must meet your personal fitness goals. It should be fun and include variety and consistency to help you maintain interest and achieve fitness in all components. It must also place an extra physical demand, or an overload, on your body. To achieve appropriate overload, follow the FITT principle: *frequency* refers to the number of activity sessions per week; *intensity* refers to how difficult the activity is to perform; *time* refers to how long each activity session lasts; *type* refers to the range of physical activities one can engage in. Warm-up exercises prepare the muscles for exertion by increasing blood flow and temperature. Cool-down activities help prevent injury and may help reduce muscle soreness.

What fuels our activities?

adenosine triphosphate (ATP) The common currency of energy for virtually all cells of the body.

In order to perform exercise, or muscular work, we must be able to generate energy. The common currency of energy for virtually all cells in the body is **adenosine triphosphate,** or **ATP**. As you might guess from its name, a molecule of ATP includes

nutri-case | JUDY

"I can't remember a time in my life when I wasn't trying to lose weight, but nothing ever works! Last week I had my annual check-up and my doctor confirmed what I already knew—I'm obese! The doctor also said my weight is contributing to my high blood sugar, and my blood pressure is high, too. As a nurse's aide, I see the health problems caused by obesity every day. But knowing how bad it is doesn't help me lose weight and keep it off. So we talked about some "slow and steady" strategies for losing weight: I promised I'd watch my diet, take my meds, and start working out at the new fitness center here at the hospital. It has a couple of treadmills and stationary bikes right in front of a big TV so you can watch the soaps while you work out. Still, I'm not really sure what I'm supposed to do, or how many times a week, or for how long. I mean, if I only had to lose 5 pounds that would be easy. But I've got to lose 50! And I only get half an hour for lunch!"

Imagine that you were a trainer at the Valley Hospital employee fitness center, and Judy told you about her weight-loss and health goals. Applying the FITT principle, recommend an initial physical activity program that can get Judy started on improving her health that includes an appropriate:

- number of times per 5-day work week
- intensity
- duration of activity
- variety of activities

an organic compound called adenosine and three phosphate groups (**FIGURE 12.5**). When one of the phosphates is cleaved, or broken away, from ATP, energy is released. The products remaining after this reaction are adenosine diphosphate (ADP) and an independent inorganic phosphate group (P_i). In a mirror image of this reaction, the body regenerates ATP by adding a phosphate group back to ADP. In this way, we continually provide energy to our cells.

The amount of ATP stored in a muscle cell is very limited; it can keep the muscle active for only about 1 to 3 seconds. Thus, we need to generate ATP from other sources to fuel activities for longer time periods. Fortunately, we are able to generate ATP from the breakdown of carbohydrate, fat, and protein, providing our cells with a variety of sources from which to receive energy. The primary energy systems that provide energy for physical activities are the adenosine triphosphate–creatine phosphate (ATP-CP) energy system and the anaerobic and aerobic breakdown of carbohydrates. Our bodies also generate energy from the breakdown of fats. As you will see, the type, intensity, and duration of the activities performed determine the amount of ATP needed and, therefore, the energy system that is used.

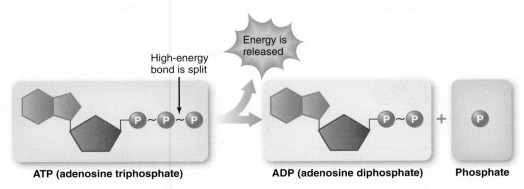

FIGURE 12.5 Structure of adenosine triphosphate (ATP). Energy is produced when ATP is split into adenosine diphosphate (ADP) and inorganic phosphate (P_i).

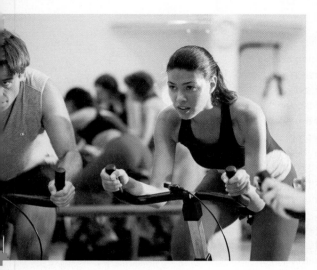

The amount of daily physical activity you should participate in is determined by your personal fitness goals.

The ATP-CP Energy System Uses Creatine Phosphate to Regenerate ATP

As previously mentioned, muscle cells store only enough ATP to maintain activity for 1 to 3 seconds. When more energy is needed, a high-energy compound called **creatine phosphate (CP)** (also called *phosphocreatine*, or *PCr*) can be broken down to support the regeneration of ATP **(FIGURE 12.6)**. Because this reaction can occur in the absence of oxygen, it is referred to as an **anaerobic** reaction (meaning "without oxygen").

Muscle tissue contains about four to six times as much CP as ATP, but there is still not enough CP available to fuel long-term activity. CP is used the most during very intense, short bouts of activity, such as lifting, jumping, and sprinting **(FIGURE 12.7)**. Together, our stores of ATP and CP can support a *maximal* physical effort for only about 3 to 15 seconds. We must rely on other energy sources, such as carbohydrate and fat, to support activities of longer duration.

The Breakdown of Carbohydrates Provides Energy for Exercise

During activities lasting about 30 seconds to 3 minutes, our body needs an energy source that can be used quickly to produce ATP. The breakdown of carbohydrates, specifically glucose, provides this quick energy in a process called **glycolysis**. The most common source of glucose during exercise comes from glycogen stored in the muscles and glucose found in the blood. As shown in **FIGURE 12.8**, for every glucose molecule that goes through glycolysis, two ATP molecules are produced. The primary end product of glycolysis is **pyruvic acid**.

When oxygen availability is limited in the cell, pyruvic acid is converted to **lactic acid**. For years it was assumed that lactic acid was a useless, even potentially toxic, by-product of high-intensity exercise. We now know that lactic acid is an important intermediate of glucose breakdown and that it plays a critical role in supplying fuel for working muscles, the heart, and resting tissues. But does lactic acid build-up cause muscle fatigue and soreness? See the **Nutrition Myth or Fact?** box (page 455) for the answer.

creatine phosphate (CP) A high-energy compound that can be broken down for energy and used to regenerate ATP.

anaerobic Means "without oxygen;" the term used to refer to metabolic reactions that occur in the absence of oxygen.

glycolysis The breakdown of glucose; yields two ATP molecules and two pyruvic acid molecules for each molecule of glucose.

pyruvic acid The primary end product of glycolysis.

lactic acid A compound that results when pyruvic acid is metabolized in the presence of insufficient oxygen.

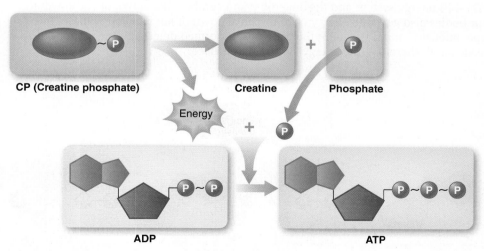

CP (Creatine phosphate)   Creatine   Phosphate

Energy

ADP

ATP

FIGURE 12.6 When the compound creatine phosphate (CP) is broken down into a molecule of creatine and an independent phosphate molecule, energy is released. This energy, along with the independent phosphate molecule, can then be used to regenerate ATP.

focus figure 12.7 | What Fuels Our Activities?

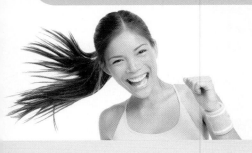

Depending on the duration and intensity of the activity, our bodies may use ATP-CP, carbohydrate, or fat in various combinations to fuel muscular work. Keep in mind that the amounts and sources shown below can vary based on the person's fitness level and health, how well fed the person is before the activity, and environmental temperatures and conditions.

SPRINT START (0–3 seconds)
A short, intense burst of activity like sprinting is fueled by ATP and creatine phosphate (CP) under anaerobic conditions.

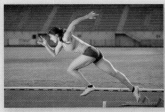
100% ATP-CP

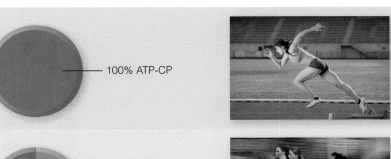

100-M DASH (10–12 seconds)
ATP and CP provide energy for about 10 seconds of quick, intense activity, after which energy is provided as ATP from the breakdown of carbohydrates.

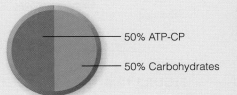
50% ATP-CP
50% Carbohydrates

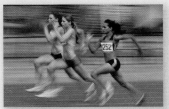

1500-M RACE (4–6 minutes)
Energy derived from ATP and CP is small and would be exhausted after about 10 seconds of the race. At this point, most of the energy is derived from aerobic metabolism of primarily carbohydrates.

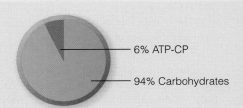
6% ATP-CP
94% Carbohydrates

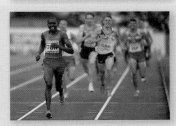

10-KM RACE (30–40 minutes)
During moderately intense activities such as a 10-kilometer race, ATP is provided by fat and carbohydrate metabolism. As the intensity increases, so does the utilization of carbohydrates for energy.

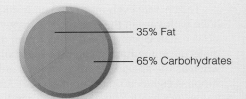
35% Fat
65% Carbohydrates

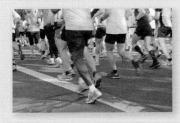

MARATHON (2.5–3 hours)
During endurance events such as marathons, ATP is primarily derived from carbohydrates, and to a lesser extent, fat. A very small amount of energy is provided by the breakdown of amino acids to form glucose.

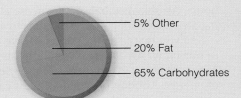
5% Other
20% Fat
65% Carbohydrates

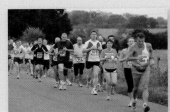

DAY-LONG HIKE (5.5–7 hours)
The primary energy source for events lasting several hours at low intensity is fat (free fatty acids in the bloodstream) which derive from triglycerides stored in fat cells. Carbohydrates contribute a relatively smaller percentage of energy needs.

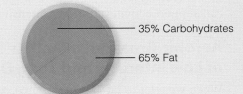
35% Carbohydrates
65% Fat

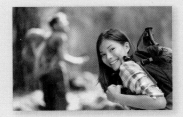

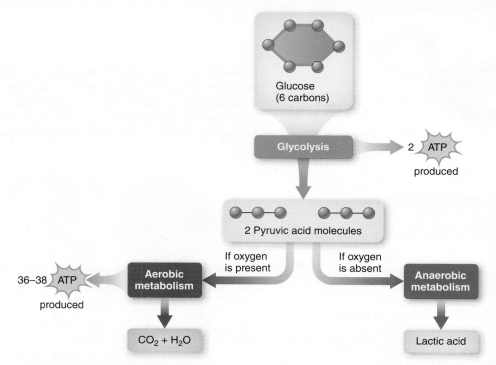

FIGURE 12.8 The breakdown of one molecule of glucose, or the process of glycolysis, yields two molecules of pyruvic acid and two ATP molecules. The further metabolism of pyruvic acid in the presence of insufficient oxygen (anaerobic process) results in the production of lactic acid. The metabolism of pyruvic acid in the presence of adequate oxygen (aerobic process) yields 36 to 38 molecules of ATP.

The major advantage of glycolysis is that it is the fastest way that we can regenerate ATP for exercise, other than the ATP-CP system. However, this high rate of ATP production can be sustained only briefly, generally less than 3 minutes. To perform exercise that lasts longer than 3 minutes, we must rely on the aerobic energy system to provide adequate ATP.

To generate even more ATP molecules, pyruvic acid can go through additional metabolic pathways in the presence of oxygen (see Figure 12.8). Although this process is slower than glycolysis occurring under anaerobic conditions, the breakdown of 1 glucose molecule going through aerobic metabolism yields 36 to 38 ATP molecules for energy, whereas the anaerobic process yields only 2 ATP molecules. Thus, this aerobic process supplies eighteen times more energy! Another advantage of the aerobic process is that it does not result in the significant production of acids and other compounds that contribute to muscle fatigue, which means that a low-intensity activity can be performed for hours. Aerobic metabolism of glucose is the primary source of fuel for our muscles during activities lasting from 3 minutes to 4 hours (see Figure 12.7).

As you learned (in Chapter 4), we can store only a limited amount of glycogen in our body. An average, well-nourished man who weighs about 154 pounds (70 kg) can store about 200 to 500 g of muscle glycogen, which is equal to 800 to 2,000 kcal of energy. Although trained athletes can store more muscle glycogen than the average person, even their bodies do not have enough stored glycogen to provide an unlimited energy supply for long-term activities. Thus, we also need a fuel source that is very abundant and can be broken down under aerobic conditions, so that it can support activities of lower intensity and longer duration. This fuel source is fat.

Aerobic Breakdown of Fats Supports Exercise of Low Intensity and Long Duration

When we refer to fat as a fuel source, we mean stored triglycerides, which is the primary storage form of fat in our cells. As you learned (in Chapter 5), a triglyceride

nutrition myth or fact?

Does Lactic Acid Cause Muscle Fatigue and Soreness?

Theo and his teammates won their basketball game last night, but just barely. With two of the players sick, Theo got more court time than usual, and when he got back to the dorm, he could hardly get his legs to carry him up the stairs. This morning, Theo's muscles ache all over, and he wonders if a build-up of lactic acid is to blame.

Lactic acid is a by-product of glycolysis. For many years, scientists and athletes believed that lactic acid caused muscle fatigue and soreness. Does recent scientific evidence support this belief?

The exact causes of muscle fatigue are not known, and there appear to be many contributing factors. Recent evidence suggests that fatigue may be due not only to the accumulation of many acids and other metabolic by-products, such as inorganic phosphate,[12] but also to the depletion of creatine phosphate and changes in calcium in the cells that affect muscle contraction. Depletion of muscle glycogen, liver glycogen, and blood glucose, as well as psychological factors, can all contribute to fatigue.[13] Thus, it appears that lactic acid only contributes to fatigue but does not cause fatigue independently.

So what causes muscle soreness? As with fatigue, there are probably many factors. It is hypothesized that soreness usually results from microscopic tears in the muscle fibers as a result of strenuous exercise. This damage triggers an inflammatory reaction, which causes an influx of fluid and various chemicals to the damaged area. These substances work to

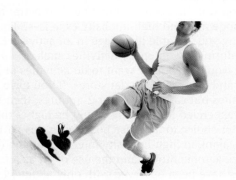

remove damaged tissue and initiate tissue repair, but they may also stimulate pain. However, it appears highly unlikely that lactic acid is an independent cause of muscle soreness.

Recent studies indicate that lactic acid is produced even under aerobic conditions! This means it is produced at rest as well as during exercise at any intensity. The reasons for this constant production of lactic acid are still being studied. What we do know is that lactic acid is an important fuel for resting tissues, for working cardiac and skeletal muscles, and even for the brain both at rest and during exercise[14,15] That's right—skeletal muscles not only *produce* lactic acid but also *use* it for energy, both directly and after it is converted into glucose and glycogen in the liver. We also know that endurance training improves the muscles' ability to use lactic acid for energy. Thus, contrary to being a waste product of glucose metabolism, lactic acid is actually an important energy source for muscle cells during rest and exercise.

CRITICAL THINKING QUESTIONS

1. What factors likely contributed to Theo's muscle soreness after the game?
2. Based on what you've learned about developing a sound fitness plan, what strategies could Theo undertake to reduce the level of muscle soreness he experienced?

molecule is composed of a glycerol backbone attached to three fatty acid molecules (see Figure 5.1 in Chapter 5). It is these fatty acid molecules that provide much of the energy we need to support long-term activity. Fatty acids are classified by their length—that is, by the number of carbons they contain. The longer the fatty acid, the more ATP that can be generated from its breakdown. For instance, palmitic acid is a fatty acid with 16 carbons. If palmitic acid is broken down completely, it yields 129 ATP molecules! Obviously, far more energy is produced from this one fatty acid molecule than from the aerobic breakdown of a glucose molecule.

There are two major advantages of using fat as a fuel. First, fat is an abundant energy source, even in lean people. For example, a man who weighs 154 pounds (70 kg) who has a body fat level of 10% has approximately 15 pounds of body fat, which is equivalent to more than 50,000 kcal of energy! This is significantly more energy than can be provided by his stored muscle glycogen (800 to 2,000 kcal). Second, fat provides 9 kcal of energy per gram, more than twice as much energy per gram as carbohydrate. The primary disadvantage of using fat as a fuel is that the breakdown process is relatively slow; thus, fat is used predominantly as a fuel source during activities of lower intensity and longer duration. Fat is also our primary energy source during rest, sitting, and standing in place.

What specific activities are primarily fueled by fat? Walking long distances uses fat stores, as do hiking, long-distance cycling, and other low- to moderate-intensity forms of exercise. Fat is also an important fuel source during endurance events such as marathons (26.2 miles) and ultra-marathon races (49.9 miles). Endurance exercise training improves our ability to use fat for energy, which may be one reason that people who exercise regularly tend to have lower body fat levels than people who do not exercise.

It is important to remember that we are almost always using some combination of carbohydrate and fat for energy. At rest, we use very little carbohydrate, relying mostly on fat. During maximal exercise (100% effort), we are using mostly carbohydrate and very little fat. However, most activities we do each day involve some use of both fuels (**FIGURE 12.9**).

If you want to decrease body fat, is it better to do low-intensity exercise, or perform moderate- and high-intensity exercises? The answer to this question depends on how long you are able to engage in an activity. Even though fat is the primary fuel source during low-intensity activities such as sitting and standing, to decrease body fat you would obviously want to do activities of higher intensity to expend additional energy and decrease body fat stores. If you have a low fitness level and can walk for 20 minutes but can only jog for 2 minutes, then the overall amount of fat utilized and energy expended for walking would be higher than for jogging, and walking would be the better choice to decrease body fat in this particular case. Recent evidence suggests that engaging in high-intensity interval training (or HIT) is a time-efficient strategy to optimize aerobic fitness and the use of fat as a fuel to support exercise.[16] Beneficial changes have been observed with only about 15 minutes of very intense exercise; however, the potential of applying this type of training to people who are highly unfit or with disease is not known.

When it comes to eating properly to support regular physical activity or exercise training, the nutrient to focus on is carbohydrate. This is because most people store more than enough fat to support exercise, whereas our storage of carbohydrate is limited. It is especially important that we maintain adequate stores of glycogen for moderate to intense exercise. Dietary recommendations for fat, carbohydrate, and protein are reviewed later in this chapter.

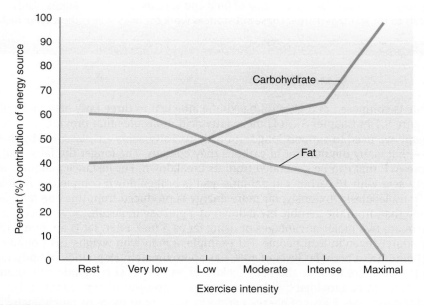

FIGURE 12.9 For most daily activities, including exercise, we use a mixture of carbohydrate and fat for energy. At lower exercise intensities, we rely more on fat as a fuel source. As exercise intensity increases, we rely more on carbohydrate for energy.

Data adapted from: Brooks, G. A., and J. Mercier. 1994. Balance of carbohydrate and lipid utilization during exercise: the "crossover" concept. *J. Appl. Physiol.* 76(6):2253–2261.

Amino Acids Are Not Major Sources of Fuel During Exercise

Proteins, or more specifically amino acids, are not major energy sources during exercise. As previously discussed (in Chapter 6), amino acids can be used directly for energy if necessary, but they are more often used to make glucose to maintain our blood glucose levels during exercise. Amino acids also help build and repair tissues after exercise. Depending on the intensity and duration of the activity, amino acids may contribute about 1–6% of the energy needed.[17]

Given this, why is it that so many people are concerned about their protein intakes? As you learned (in Chapter 6), our muscles are stimulated to grow only by appropriate physical training, not by eating extra dietary protein. Thus, although adequate dietary protein is needed to support activity and recovery, consuming very high amounts does not provide an added benefit. Although the protein needs of athletes are somewhat higher than the needs of non-athletes, most of us eat more than enough protein to support even the highest requirements for competitive athletes! Thus, there is generally no need for recreationally active people or even competitive athletes to consume protein or amino acid supplements.

recap The amount of ATP stored in a muscle cell is limited and can keep a muscle active for only about 1 to 3 seconds. For intense activities lasting about 3 to 15 seconds, creatine phosphate can be broken down to provide energy and support the regeneration of ATP. To support activities that last from 30 seconds to 2 minutes, energy is produced from glycolysis. Fatty acids can be broken down aerobically to support activities of low intensity and longer duration. The two major advantages of using fat as a fuel are that it is an abundant energy source and it provides more than twice the energy per gram as compared with carbohydrate. Amino acids may contribute from 3% to 6% of the energy needed during exercise, depending on the intensity and duration of the activity. Amino acids help build and repair tissues after exercise.

What kind of diet supports physical activity?

Lots of people wonder, "Do my nutrient needs change if I become more physically active?" The answer to this question depends on the type, intensity, frequency, and duration of the activity in which you participate. It is not necessarily true that our requirement for every nutrient is greater if we are physically active.

People who are performing moderate-intensity daily activities for health can follow the dietary guidelines put forth in the USDA Food Patterns. For smaller or less active people, the lower end of the range of recommendations for each food group may be appropriate. For larger or more active people, the higher end of the range is suggested. Modifications may be necessary for people who exercise vigorously every day, particularly for athletes training for competition. **TABLE 12.2** provides an overview of the nutrients that can be affected by regular, vigorous exercise training. Each of these nutrients is described in more detail in the following section.

Vigorous Exercise Increases Energy Needs

Athletes generally have higher energy needs than moderately physically active or sedentary people. The amount of extra energy needed to support regular training is determined by the type, intensity, and duration of the activity. In addition, the energy needs of male athletes are higher than those of female athletes because male athletes typically weigh more, have more muscle mass, and expend more energy during activity. This is relative, of course: a large woman who trains 3 to 5 hours each day will probably need

Small snacks can be helpful to meet daily energy demands.

TABLE 12.2   Suggested Intakes of Nutrients to Support Vigorous Exercise

Nutrient	Functions	Suggested Intake
Energy	Supports exercise, activities of daily living, and basic body functions	Depends on body size and the type, intensity, and duration of activity For many female athletes: 1,800 to 3,500 kcal/day For many male athletes: 2,500 to 7,500 kcal/day
Carbohydrate	Provides energy, maintains adequate muscle glycogen and blood glucose; high complex carbohydrate foods provide vitamins and minerals	45–65% of total energy intake Depending on sport and gender, should consume 6–10 g of carbohydrate per kg body weight per day
Fat	Provides energy, fat-soluble vitamins, and essential fatty acids; supports production of hormones and transport of nutrients	20–35% of total energy intake
Protein	Helps build and maintain muscle; provides building material for glucose; energy source during endurance exercise; aids recovery from exercise	10–35% of total energy intake Endurance athletes: 1.2–1.5 g per kg body weight Strength athletes: 1.3–1.8 g per kg body weight
Water	Maintains temperature regulation (adequate cooling); maintains blood volume and blood pressure; supports all cell functions	Consume fluid before, during, and after exercise Consume enough to maintain body weight Consume at least 8 cups (64 fl. oz) of water daily to maintain regular health and activity Athletes may need up to 10 liters (170 fl. oz) every day; more is required if exercising in a hot environment
B-vitamins	Critical for energy production from carbohydrate, fat, and protein	May need slightly more (one to two times the RDA) for thiamin, riboflavin, and vitamin B$_6$
Calcium	Builds and maintains bone mass; assists with nervous system function, muscle contraction, hormone function, and transport of nutrients across cell membrane	Meet the current RDA: 14–18 years: 1,300 mg/day 19–50 years: 1,000 mg/day 51–70 years: 1,000 mg/day (men); 1,200 mg/day (women) 71 and older: 1,200 mg/day
Iron	Primarily responsible for the transport of oxygen in blood to cells; assists with energy production	Consume at least the RDA: Males: 14–18 years: 11 mg/day 19 and older: 8 mg/day Females: 14–18 years: 15 mg/day 19–50 years: 18 mg/day 51 and older: 8 mg/day

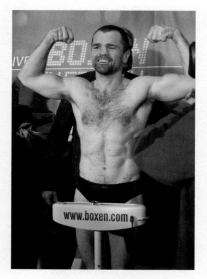

◄ Some athletes diet to meet a predefined weight category.

grazing Consistently eating small meals throughout the day; done by many athletes to meet their high energy demands.

more energy than a small man who trains 1 hour each day. The energy needs of athletes can range from only 1,500 to 1,800 kcal/day for a small female gymnast to more than 7,500 kcal/day for a male cyclist competing in the Tour de France cross-country cycling race.

FIGURE 12.10 shows a sample of 1-day's meals and snacks, totaling about 1,800 kcal and 4,000 kcal, with the carbohydrate content of these foods meeting more than 60% of total energy intake. As you can see, athletes who require more than 4,000 kcal per day need to consume very large quantities of food. However, the heavy demands of daily physical training, work, school, and family responsibilities often leave these athletes with little time to eat adequately. Thus, many athletes meet their energy demands by planning regular meals and snacks and **grazing** (eating small meals throughout the day) consistently. They may also take advantage of the energy-dense snack foods and meal replacements specifically designed for athletes participating in vigorous training. These steps help athletes maintain their blood glucose and energy stores.

If an athlete is losing body weight, then his or her energy intake is inadequate. Conversely, weight gain may indicate that energy intake is too high. Weight maintenance is generally recommended to maximize performance. If weight loss is warranted, food intake should be lowered no more than 200 to 500 kcal per day, and athletes should try to lose weight prior to the competitive season, if at all possible. Weight gain may be necessary for some athletes and can usually be accomplished by consuming 500 to 700 kcal/day more than needed for weight maintenance. The extra energy should come from a healthy balance of carbohydrate (45–65% of total energy intake), fat (20–35% of total energy intake), and protein (10–35% of total energy intake).

Eating for Athletes: Meeting High Energy Demands

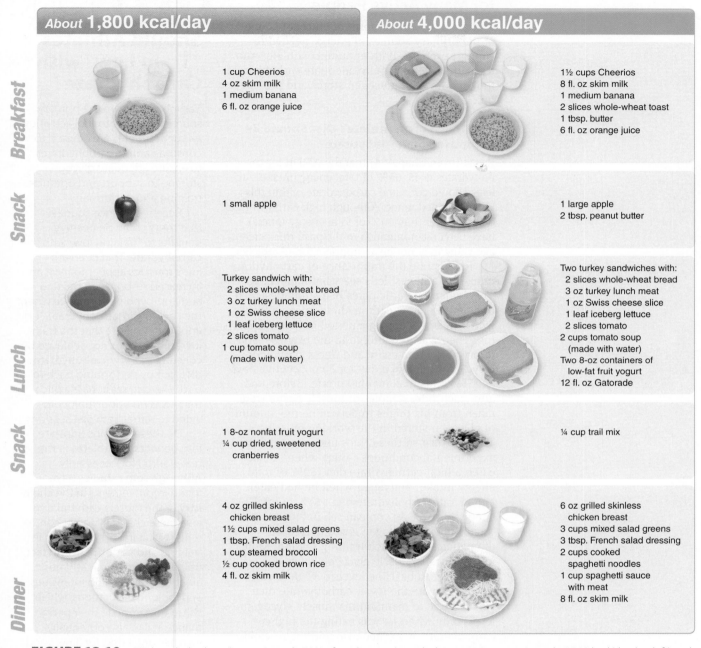

About **1,800 kcal/day**	About **4,000 kcal/day**

Breakfast

1 cup Cheerios
4 oz skim milk
1 medium banana
6 fl. oz orange juice

1½ cups Cheerios
8 fl. oz skim milk
1 medium banana
2 slices whole-wheat toast
1 tbsp. butter
6 fl. oz orange juice

Snack

1 small apple

1 large apple
2 tbsp. peanut butter

Lunch

Turkey sandwich with:
 2 slices whole-wheat bread
 3 oz turkey lunch meat
 1 oz Swiss cheese slice
 1 leaf iceberg lettuce
 2 slices tomato
 1 cup tomato soup
  (made with water)

Two turkey sandwiches with:
 2 slices whole-wheat bread
 3 oz turkey lunch meat
 1 oz Swiss cheese slice
 1 leaf iceberg lettuce
 2 slices tomato
 2 cups tomato soup
  (made with water)
Two 8-oz containers of
 low-fat fruit yogurt
12 fl. oz Gatorade

Snack

1 8-oz nonfat fruit yogurt
¼ cup dried, sweetened
 cranberries

¼ cup trail mix

Dinner

4 oz grilled skinless
 chicken breast
1½ cups mixed salad greens
1 tbsp. French salad dressing
1 cup steamed broccoli
½ cup cooked brown rice
4 fl. oz skim milk

6 oz grilled skinless
 chicken breast
3 cups mixed salad greens
3 tbsp. French salad dressing
2 cups cooked
 spaghetti noodles
1 cup spaghetti sauce
 with meat
8 fl. oz skim milk

FIGURE 12.10 High-carbohydrate (approximately 60% of total energy) meals that contain approximately 1,800 kcal/day (on left) and 4,000 kcal/day (on right). Athletes, particularly those with very high energy needs, must plan their meals carefully to meet energy demands.

Many athletes are concerned about their weight. Jockeys, boxers, wrestlers, judo athletes, and others are required to "make weight"—to meet a predefined weight category. Others, such as distance runners, gymnasts, figure skaters, and dancers, are required to maintain a very lean figure for performance and aesthetic reasons. These athletes tend to eat less energy than they need to support vigorous training, which puts them at risk for inadequate intakes of all nutrients. These athletes are also at a higher risk of suffering from health consequences resulting from poor energy and nutrient intake, including eating disorders, osteoporosis, menstrual disturbances (in women), dehydration, heat and physical injuries, and even death. It is also important to understand that athletes should not adopt low-carbohydrate diets in an attempt to lose weight. As we discuss next, carbohydrates are a critical energy source for maintaining exercise performance.

Carbohydrate Needs Increase for Many Active People

Carbohydrate (in the form of glucose) is one of the primary sources of energy needed to support exercise. Both endurance athletes and strength athletes require adequate carbohydrate to maintain their glycogen stores and provide quick energy.

How Much of an Athlete's Diet Should Be Composed of Carbohydrate?

Recall (from Chapter 4) that the AMDR for carbohydrates is 45–65% of total energy intake. Athletes should consume carbohydrate within this recommended range. Although high-carbohydrate diets (greater than 60% of total energy intake) have been recommended in the past, this percentage value may not be appropriate for all athletes.

To illustrate the importance of carbohydrate intake for athletes, let's see what happens to Theo when he participates in a study designed to determine how carbohydrate intake affects glycogen stores during a period of heavy training. Theo was asked to go to the exercise laboratory at the university and ride a stationary bicycle for 2 hours a day for 3 consecutive days at 75% of his maximal heart rate. Before and after each ride, samples of muscle tissue were taken from his thighs to determine the amount of glycogen stored in the working muscles. Theo performed these rides under two different experimental conditions—once when he had eaten a high-carbohydrate diet (80% of total energy intake) and again when he had eaten a moderate-carbohydrate diet (40% of total energy intake). As you can see in **FIGURE 12.11**, Theo's muscle glycogen levels decreased dramatically after each training session. More important, his muscle glycogen levels did not recover to baseline levels over the 3 days when Theo ate the lower-carbohydrate diet. He was able to maintain his muscle glycogen levels only when he was eating the higher-carbohydrate diet. Theo also told the researchers that completing the 2-hour rides was much more difficult when he had eaten the moderate-carbohydrate diet as compared to when he ate the diet that was higher in carbohydrate.

When Should Carbohydrates Be Consumed?

It is important for athletes not only to consume enough carbohydrate to maintain glycogen stores but also to time their intake optimally. Our body stores glycogen very rapidly during the first 24 hours of recovery from exercise, with the highest storage rates occurring during the first few hours.[18] Higher carbohydrate intakes during the first 24 hours of recovery from exercise are associated with higher amounts of glucose being stored as muscle glycogen. It is recommended that athletes consume a daily carbohydrate

HOT TOPIC

Should Athletes "Train Low" with Carbohydrate?

Carbohydrates are the primary source of energy to fuel activities. As such, athletes are advised to consume ample carbohydrates to ensure adequate glycogen storage to support and optimize training and performance.

Recent evidence suggests that there could be positive benefits to "training low" with carbohydrate. That is, an athlete's muscles appear to have an increased response to training and improved performance when they are low in carbohydrate. It is important to note that the train-low stimulus was not achieved by consuming a low-carbohydrate diet, but by performing back-to-back exercise sessions in which there was no opportunity provided to refuel between sessions.

Do these findings translate into benefits for athletes in the real world? Not necessarily. Although some studies have found improvements in the chemistry of the muscle with training low, these changes do not consistently result in improvements in training and performance. In fact, training low can limit athletes' ability to train at high intensities and for longer durations, which will in turn impede their performance. It can also potentially increase one's risks for illness and injury. As a relatively new area of research, more studies are needed to determine if periods of training low can be combined with traditional high carbohydrate approaches to optimize exercise training and performance.

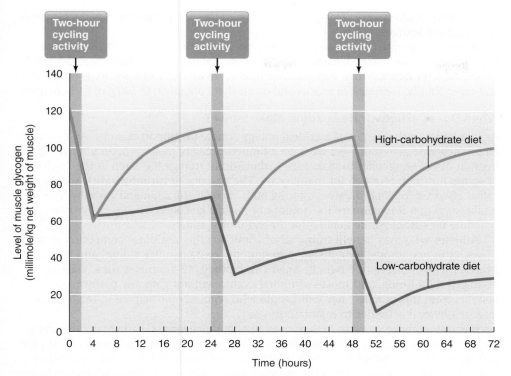

FIGURE 12.11 The effects of a low-carbohydrate diet on muscle glycogen stores. When a low-carbohydrate diet is consumed, glycogen stores cannot be restored during a period of regular vigorous training.
Data from: Costill, D. L., and J. M. Miller. 1980. Nutrition for endurance sport: CHO and fluid balance. *Int. J. Sports Med.* 1:2–14. Copyright © 1980 Georg Thieme Verlag. Used with permission.

intake of approximately 6 to 10 g of carbohydrate per kg body weight to optimize muscle glycogen stores.

If an athlete has to perform or participate in training bouts that are scheduled less than 8 hours apart, then he or she should try to consume enough carbohydrate in the few hours following training to allow for ample glycogen storage. However, with a longer recovery time (generally 12 hours or more), the athlete can eat when he or she chooses, and glycogen levels should be restored as long as the total carbohydrate eaten is sufficient.

Interestingly, studies have shown that muscle glycogen can be restored to adequate levels whether the food is eaten in small, multiple snacks or in larger meals,[18] although some studies show enhanced muscle glycogen storage during the first 4 to 6 hours of recovery when athletes are fed large amounts of carbohydrate every 15 to 30 minutes.[19,20] There is also evidence that consuming high glycemic index foods during the immediate postrecovery period results in higher glycogen storage than is achieved as a result of eating low glycemic index foods. This may be due to a greater malabsorption of the carbohydrate in low glycemic index foods, because these foods contain more indigestible forms of carbohydrate.[18]

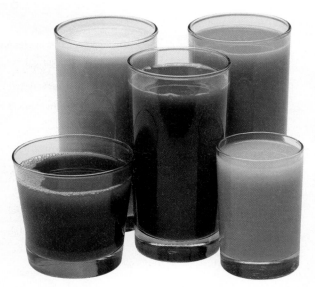

Fruit and vegetable juices can be a good source of carbohydrates.

What Food Sources of Carbohydrates Are Good for Athletes?

What are good carbohydrate sources to support vigorous training? In general, fiber-rich, less processed carbohydrate foods, such as whole grains and cereals, fruits, vegetables, and juices, are excellent sources that also supply fiber, vitamins, and minerals. Guidelines recommend that intake of simple sugars be less than 10% of total energy intake, but some athletes who require very large energy intakes to support training may need to consume more. In addition, as previously mentioned, glycogen storage can be enhanced by consuming foods with a high glycemic index

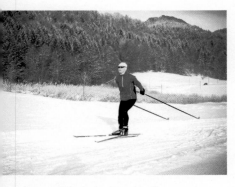

↖ Carbohydrate loading may benefit endurance athletes, such as cross-country skiers.

immediately postrecovery. Thus, there are advantages to consuming a wide variety of carbohydrate sources.

As a result of time constraints, many athletes have difficulties consuming enough food to meet carbohydrate demands. Sports drinks and energy bars have been designed to help athletes increase their carbohydrate intake. TABLE 12.3 identifies some energy bars and other simple, inexpensive snacks and meals that contain 50 to 100 g of carbohydrate.

When Does Carbohydrate Loading Make Sense?

As you know, carbohydrate is a critical energy source to support exercise—particularly endurance-type activities—yet we have a limited capacity to store it. So it's not surprising that discovering ways to maximize carbohydrate storage has been at the forefront of sports nutrition research for many years. The practice of **carbohydrate loading**, also called *glycogen loading,* involves altering both exercise duration and carbohydrate intake such that it maximizes the amount of muscle glycogen. TABLE 12.4 reviews a schedule for carbohydrate loading for an endurance athlete.

Athletes who may benefit from carbohydrate loading are those competing in marathons, ultra-marathons, long-distance swimming, cross-country skiing, and triathlons. Athletes who compete in baseball, American football, 10-kilometer runs, walking, hiking, weight lifting, and most swimming events will not gain any performance benefits from this practice, nor will people who regularly participate in moderately intense physical activities to maintain fitness.

It is important to emphasize that, even in endurance events, carbohydrate loading does not always improve performance. There are many adverse side effects of this practice, including extreme gastrointestinal distress, particularly diarrhea. We store water along with the extra glycogen in the muscles, which leaves many athletes feeling heavy and sluggish. Athletes who want to try carbohydrate loading should experiment prior to competition to determine whether it is an acceptable and beneficial approach for them.

carbohydrate loading Also known as glycogen loading. A process that involves altering training and carbohydrate intake, so that muscle glycogen storage is maximized.

TABLE 12.3 Carbohydrate and Total Energy in Various Foods

Food	Amount	Carbohydrate (g)	Energy from Carbohydrate (%)	Total Energy (kcal)
Sweetened applesauce	1 cup	50	97	207
Large apple with	1 each	50	82	248
saltine crackers	8 each			
Whole-wheat bread	1-oz slice	50	71	282
with jelly	4 tsp.			
and skim milk	12 fl. oz			
Spaghetti (cooked)	1 cup	50	75	268
with tomato sauce	1/4 cup			
Brown rice (cooked)	1 cup	100	88	450
with mixed vegetables	1/2 cup			
and apple juice	12 fl. oz			
Grape-Nuts cereal	1/2 cup	100	84	473
with raisins	3/8 cup			
and skim milk	8 fl. oz			
Clif Bar (chocolate chip)	2.4 oz	43	75	230
Meta-Rx (fudge brownie)	100 g	41	41	400
Power Bar (chocolate)	1 bar	45	75	240
PR Bar Ironman	50 g	22	44	200

Data adapted from: Manore, M. M., N. L. Meyer, and J. L. Thompson. 2009. *Sport Nutrition for Health and Performance,* 2nd edn. Champaign, IL: Human Kinetics.

TABLE 12.4 **Recommended Carbohydrate Loading Guidelines for Endurance Athletes**

Days Prior to Event	Exercise Duration (in minutes)	Carbohydrate Content of Diet (g per kg body weight)
6	90 (at 70% max effort)	5 (moderate)
5	40 (at 70% max effort)	5 (moderate)
4	40 (at 70% max effort)	5 (moderate)
3	20 (light training)	10 (high)
2	20 (light training)	10 (high)
1	Rest	10 (high)
Day of race	Competition	Precompetition food and fluid

Data adapted from: Current Trends in Performance Nutrition, by Marie Dunford. Copyright © 2005 by Human Kinetics, Champaign, IL. Reprinted with permission.

Moderate Fat Consumption Is Enough to Support Most Activities

Fat is an important energy source for both moderate physical activity and vigorous endurance training. When athletes reach a physically trained state, they are able to use more fat for energy; in other words, they become better "fat burners." This can also occur in people who are not athletes but who regularly participate in aerobic-type fitness activities. This training effect occurs for a number of reasons, including an increase in the number and activity of various enzymes involved in fat metabolism, improved ability of the muscle to store fat, and improved ability to extract fat from the blood for use during exercise. By using fat as a fuel, athletes can spare carbohydrate, so that they can use it during prolonged, intense training or competition.

Many athletes concerned with body weight and physical appearance believe they should eat less than 15% of their total energy intake as fat, but this is inadequate for vigorous activity. Instead, a fat intake of 20–35% of total energy intake is generally recommended for most athletes, with less than 10% of total energy intake as saturated fat. The same recommendations are put forth for non-athletes. Fat provides not only energy but also fat-soluble vitamins and essential fatty acids that are critical to maintaining general health. If fat consumption is too low, inadequate levels of these nutrients can eventually prove detrimental to training and performance. Athletes who have chronic disease risk factors, such as high blood lipids, high blood pressure, or unhealthful blood glucose levels, should work with their physician to adjust their intake of fat and carbohydrate according to their health risks.

Many Athletes Have Increased Protein Needs

The protein intakes suggested for active people range from 1.0 to 1.8 grams per kg body weight. At the lower end of this range are people who exercise four to five times a week for 30 minutes or less. At the upper end are athletes who train five to seven times a week for more than an hour a day. Protein intakes as high as 1.8 to 2.0 grams per kg per day may help to prevent the loss of lean body mass during periods when an athlete may be restricting energy to promote fat loss.[21]

Most inactive people and many athletes in the United States consume more than enough protein to support their needs.[22] However, some athletes do not consume enough protein, including those with very low energy intakes, vegetarians or vegans who do not consume high-protein food sources, and young athletes who are growing and are not aware of their higher protein needs.

In 1995, Dr. Barry Sears published *The Zone: A Dietary Road Map*, a book that claims numerous benefits of a high-protein, low-carbohydrate diet for athletes.[23] Since that time, Sears has published more than a dozen spin-offs, all of which recommend the consumption of a 40–30–30 diet, or one composed

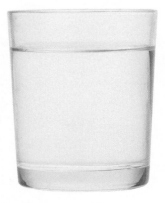

Water is essential for maintaining fluid balance and preventing dehydration.

of 40% carbohydrate, 30% fat, and 30% protein. Dr. Sears claims that high-carbohydrate diets impair athletic performance because of the unhealthful effects of insulin. These claims have not been supported by research, and, in fact, many of Dr. Sears' claims are not consistent with human physiology. The primary problem with the Zone Diet for athletes is that it is too low in both energy and carbohydrate to support training and performance.

High-quality protein sources include lean meats, poultry, fish, eggs, low-fat dairy products, legumes, and soy products. By following their personalized MyPlate food patterns, people of all fitness levels can consume more than enough protein without the use of supplements or specially formulated foods. Many athletes use protein shakes and other products in an attempt to build muscle mass and strength; some even use ergogenic aids to try to enhance performance. To learn more about whether ergogenic aids are effective and safe, refer to the *In Depth* following this chapter.

recap The type, intensity, and duration of activities a person participates in determine his or her nutrient needs. Carbohydrate needs may increase for some active people. In general, athletes should consume 45–65% of their total energy as carbohydrate. Carbohydrate loading involves altering physical training and the diet such that the storage of muscle glycogen is maximized. Active people use more fat than carbohydrates for energy because they experience an increase in the number and activity of the enzymes involved in fat metabolism and they have an improved ability to store fat and extract it from the blood for use during exercise. A dietary fat intake of 20–35% is recommended for athletes, with less than 10% of total energy intake as saturated fat. Although protein needs can be higher for athletes, most people in the United States already consume more than twice their daily needs for protein.

Regular Exercise Increases Our Need for Fluids

In this chapter, we will focus on the role of water during exercise. (A detailed discussion of fluid and electrolyte balance is provided in Chapter 7.)

Cooling Mechanisms

Heat production can increase fifteen to twenty times during heavy exercise! The primary way in which we dissipate this heat is through sweating, which is also called **evaporative cooling**. When body temperature rises, more blood (which contains water) flows to the surface of the skin. Heat is carried in this way from the core of our body to the surface of our skin. By sweating, the water (and body heat) leaves our body and the air around us picks up the evaporating water from our skin, cooling our body.

Dehydration and Heat-Related Illnesses

Heat illnesses occur because, when we exercise in the heat, our muscles and skin constantly compete for blood flow. When there is no longer enough blood flow to simultaneously provide adequate blood to both our muscles and our skin, muscle blood flow takes priority and evaporative cooling is inhibited. Exercising in heat plus humidity is especially dangerous; whereas the heat dramatically raises body temperature, the high humidity inhibits evaporative cooling—that is, the environmental air is already so saturated with water that it is unable to absorb the water in sweat. Body temperature becomes dangerously high, and heat illness is likely.

Dehydration significantly increases our risk for heat illnesses. **FIGURE 12.12** identifies the symptoms of dehydration during heavy exercise.

Heat illnesses include heat syncope, heat cramps, heat exhaustion, and heatstroke:

- *Heat syncope* is dizziness that occurs when people stand for too long in the heat and the blood pools in their lower extremities. It can also occur when people stop suddenly after a race or stand suddenly from a lying position.
- *Heat cramps* are muscle spasms that occur during exercise or several hours after strenuous exercise or manual labor in the heat. They are most commonly felt in the legs, arms, or abdomen after a person cools down.

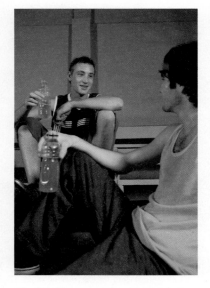

Drinking sports beverages during training and competition lasting more than 1 hour replaces fluid, carbohydrates, and electrolytes.

evaporative cooling Another term for sweating, which is the primary way in which we dissipate heat.

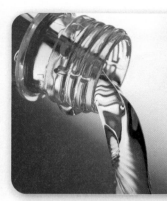

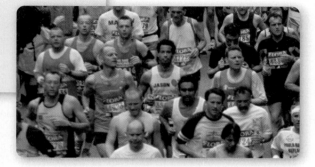

Symptoms of Dehydration During Heavy Exercise:
- Decreased exercise performance
- Increased level in perceived exertion
- Dark yellow or brown urine color
- Increased heart rate at a given exercise intensity
- Decreased appetite
- Decreased ability to concentrate
- Decreased urine output
- Fatigue and weakness
- Headache and dizziness

- *Heat exhaustion* and *heatstroke* occur on a continuum, with unchecked heat exhaustion leading to heatstroke. Early signs of heat exhaustion include excessive sweating, cold and clammy skin, rapid but weak pulse, weakness, nausea, dizziness, headache, and difficulty concentrating. Signs that a person is progressing to heatstroke are hot, dry skin; rapid and strong pulse; vomiting; diarrhea; a body temperature greater than or equal to 104°F; hallucinations; and coma. Prompt medical care is essential to save the person's life. (For more information about heat illnesses, see Chapter 7.)

Guidelines for Proper Fluid Replacement

How can we prevent dehydration and heat illnesses? Obviously, adequate fluid intake is critical before, during, and after exercise. Unfortunately, our thirst mechanism cannot be relied on to signal when we need to drink. If we rely only on our feelings of thirst, we will not consume enough fluid to support exercise.

General fluid replacement recommendations are based on maintaining body weight. Athletes who are training and competing in hot environments should weigh themselves before and after the training session or event and should regain the weight lost over the subsequent 24-hour period. They should avoid losing more than 2–3% of body weight during exercise because performance can be impaired with fluid losses as small as 1% of body weight.

TABLE 12.5 reviews the guidelines for proper fluid replacement. For activities lasting less than 1 hour, plain water is generally adequate to replace fluid losses. However, for training and competition lasting longer than 1 hour in any weather, sports beverages containing carbohydrates and electrolytes are recommended. These beverages are also recommended for people who will not drink enough water because they don't like the taste. If drinking these beverages will guarantee adequate hydration, they are appropriate to use. (For more specific information about sports beverages, refer to Chapter 7, page 261.)

Inadequate Micronutrient Intake Can Diminish Health and Performance

When people train vigorously for athletic events, their requirements for certain vitamins and minerals may be altered. Many highly active people do not eat enough food or a variety of foods that allows them to consume enough of these nutrients, yet it is imperative that active people do their very best to eat an adequate, varied, and balanced diet to try to meet the increased needs associated with vigorous training.

TABLE 12.5 Guidelines for Fluid Replacement

Activity Level	Environment	Fluid Requirements (liters per day)
Sedentary	Cool	2–3
Active	Cool	3–6
Sedentary	Warm	3–5
Active	Warm	5–10

Before Exercise or Competition:
- Drink adequate fluids during the 24 hours before event; should be able to maintain body weight.
- Slowly drink about 0.17 to 0.24 fl. oz per kg body weight of water or a sports drink at least 4 hours prior to exercise or event to allow time for excretion of excess fluid prior to event.
- Slowly drink another 0.10 to 0.17 fl. oz per kg body weight about 2 hours before event.
- Consuming beverages with sodium and/or small amounts of salted snacks at a meal will help stimulate thirst and retain fluids consumed.

During Exercise or Competition:
- Drink early and regularly throughout event to sufficiently replace all water lost through sweating.
- Amount and rate of fluid replacement depend on individual sweating rate, exercise duration, weather conditions, and opportunities to drink.
- Fluids should be cooler than the environmental temperature and flavored to enhance taste and promote fluid replacement.

During Exercise or Competition That Lasts More Than 1 Hour:
- Fluid replacement beverage should contain 5–10% carbohydrate to maintain blood glucose levels; sodium and other electrolytes should be included in the beverage in amounts of 0.5–0.7 g of sodium per liter of water to replace the sodium lost by sweating.

Following Exercise or Competition:
- Consume about 3 cups of fluid for each pound of body weight lost.
- Fluids after exercise should contain water to restore hydration status, carbohydrates to replenish glycogen stores, and electrolytes (for example, sodium and potassium) to speed rehydration.
- Consume enough fluid to permit regular urination and to ensure the urine color is very light or light yellow in color; drinking about 125–150% of fluid loss is usually sufficient to ensure complete rehydration.

In General:
- Products that contain fructose should be limited, as these may cause gastrointestinal distress.
- Caffeine and alcohol should be avoided, as these products increase urine output and reduce fluid retention.
- Carbonated beverages should be avoided, as they reduce the desire for fluid intake due to stomach fullness.

Data adapted from: Murray, R. 1997. Drink more! Advice from a world class expert. *ACSM's Health and Fitness Journal* 1:19–23; American College of Sports Medicine Position Stand. 2007. Exercise and fluid replacement. *Med. Sci. Sports Exerc.* 39(2):377–390; and Casa, D. J., L. E. Armstrong, S. K. Hillman, S. J. Montain, R. V. Reiff, B. S. E. Rich, W. O. Roberts, and J. A. Stone. 2000. National Athletic Trainers' Association position statement: fluid replacement for athletes. *J. Athl. Train.* 35:212–224.

B-Vitamins

The B-vitamins are directly involved in energy metabolism (see Chapter 10). There is reliable evidence that—as a population—active people may require slightly more thiamin, riboflavin, and vitamin B_6 than the current RDA due to increased production of energy in active people and inadequate dietary intake in some individuals.[22] However, these increased needs are easily met by consuming adequate energy and plenty of fiber-rich carbohydrates. Active people at risk for poor B-vitamin status are those who consume inadequate energy or who consume mostly refined carbohydrate foods, such as soda pop and sugary snacks. Vegan athletes and active individuals may be at risk for inadequate intake of vitamin B_{12}; food sources enriched with this nutrient include soy and cereal products.

Calcium

Calcium supports proper muscle contraction and ensures bone health. Calcium intakes are inadequate for most women in the United States, including both sedentary and active women. This is most likely due to a failure to consume foods that are high in calcium, particularly dairy products. Although vigorous training does not appear to directly increase our need for calcium, we need to consume enough calcium to support bone health. If we do not, stress fractures and severe loss of bone can result.

Some female athletes suffer from a syndrome known as the *female athlete triad* (see the **In Depth** on Disordered Eating, pages 429–439). In the female athlete triad, nutritional inadequacies cause irregularities in the menstrual cycle and hormonal disturbances that lead to a significant loss of bone mass. Thus, for female athletes, consuming the recommended amounts of calcium is critical. For female athletes who are physically small and have lower energy intakes, calcium supplementation may be needed to meet current recommendations.

Iron

Iron is a part of the hemoglobin molecule and is critical for the transport of oxygen in our blood to our cells and working muscles. Iron also is involved in energy production. Active individuals lose more iron in the sweat, feces, and urine than do inactive people, and endurance runners lose iron when their red blood cells break down in their feet as a consequence of the high impact of running. Female athletes and non-athletes lose more iron than male athletes because of menstrual blood losses, and females in general tend to eat less iron in their diet. Vegetarian athletes and active people may also consume less iron. Thus, many athletes and active people are at higher risk for iron deficiency. Depending on its severity, poor iron status can impair athletic performance and our ability to maintain regular physical activity.

A phenomenon known as *sports anemia* was identified in the 1960s. Sports anemia is not true anemia, but rather a transient decrease in iron stores that occurs at the start of an exercise program for some people, and it is seen in athletes who increase their training intensity. Exercise training increases the amount of water in our blood (called *plasma volume*); however, the amount of hemoglobin does not increase until later into the training period. Thus, the iron content in the blood appears to be low but instead is falsely depressed due to increases in plasma volume. Sports anemia, because it is not true anemia, does not affect performance.

In general, it appears that physically active females are at relatively high risk of suffering from the first stage of iron depletion, in which iron stores are low.[24] Because of this, it is suggested that blood tests of iron stores and monitoring of dietary iron intake be done routinely for active people.[24] In some cases, iron needs cannot be met through the diet, and supplementation is necessary. Iron supplementation should be done with a physician's approval and proper medical supervision.

recap   Regular exercise increases fluid needs. Fluid is critical to cool our internal body temperature and prevent heat illnesses. Dehydration is a serious threat during exercise in extreme heat and high humidity. Heat illnesses include heat syncope, heat cramps, heat exhaustion, and heat stroke. Active people may need more thiamin, riboflavin, and vitamin B_6 than inactive people. Exercise itself does not increase our calcium needs, but most women, including active women, do not consume enough calcium. Many active individuals require more iron, particularly female athletes and vegetarian athletes.

*behavior change... getting started!

Now that you've read this chapter, try making these changes:

For yourself:

- Complete the President's Fitness Challenge with a friend, and use this information to determine your level of fitness.
- Set two specific, realistic goals for the coming week that will help you work toward increasing your physical activity levels and reduce the time you spend sitting.

For your community:

- Start a walking group in your local neighborhood or at your school: for tips on how to start, to go www.mayoclinic.com, and search under "health walking."
- Volunteer with the Disabled Athlete Sports Association to become an activity buddy with an individual with a permanent physical or visual disability or hearing impairment. To learn more go to www.dasasports.org.

How Much Physical Activity Is Enough?

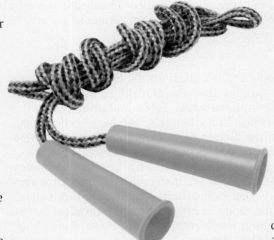

Your aerobics instructor tells you to work out at your target heart rate for 20 minutes a day, whereas your doctor tells you to walk for half an hour three or four times a week. A magazine article exhorts you to work out to the point of exhaustion, while a new weight-loss book claims that you can be perfectly healthy without ever breaking a sweat. As if these mixed messages about what constitutes "regular physical activity" weren't enough, a report from the Institute of Medicine (IOM) published in 2002 inadvertently added to the confusion. This report recommended that Americans be active 60 minutes per day to optimize health.[8] This message appears contradictory to the Surgeon General's report published in 1996, which recommended that Americans accumulate 30 minutes of physical activity on most, if not all, days of the week to optimize health.[1]

So how much activity is really enough? To try to answer this question, let's take a closer look at how the two reports differ. The IOM recommendation was derived from metabolic studies specifically examining the energy expenditure associated with maintaining a healthful body weight (defined as a body mass index [BMI] of 18.5 to 25 kg/m²). After reviewing a large number of studies that assessed energy expenditure and BMI, the IOM concluded that participating in about 60 minutes of moderately intense physical activity per day will move people to an active lifestyle and will allow them to maintain a healthful body weight.

The Surgeon General's report considers a combination of what we have learned from two types of studies not used by the IOM: exercise training studies and population-based epidemiological studies. *Exercise training studies* involve putting individuals through a clearly defined training program and assessing fitness and health outcomes. These studies consistently show that less fit and older individuals can significantly improve their cardiorespiratory fitness and reduce their risk for chronic diseases by participating in moderate levels of physical activity. In contrast, *population-based epidemiological studies* compare self-reports of physical activity and/or fitness to rates of illness and mortality. In other words, these studies do not assess the direct effect of exercise training; instead, they assess only the relationship between level of physical activity/fitness and rates of disease and premature death. These studies show that unfit, sedentary people suffer from the highest rates of disease and premature mortality and that increased physical activity significantly correlates to decreased risks for chronic diseases and premature mortality.

The IOM recommendation was not based on evidence supporting the wider range of health benefits that result when a person moves from doing no physical activity to at least some level of physical activity. The growing body of evidence regarding the health benefits of physical activity clearly indicates that doing at least some physical activity is better than doing none, and doing more physical activity is better than doing less.

Although the IOM recommendation appears to be very different from that of the Surgeon General's report, and may seem unrealistic, the IOM emphasizes that it includes all activities a person does above resting levels, including gardening, dog walking, housekeeping, and shopping.

In 2008, the United States Department of Health and Human Services released the Physical Activity Guidelines for Americans.[7] These include guidelines for children and adolescents, adults, and older adults, with additional information for women who are pregnant; people with disabilities, type 2 diabetes, or osteoarthritis; and people who are cancer survivors. These guidelines build upon the Surgeon General's recommendation of 30 minutes per day on most, if not all, days of the week. They incorporate the range of available evidence and promote a *minimum* of 150 minutes per week of moderate-intensity aerobic physical activity, with additional encouragement to increase both the intensity and duration of activity throughout the week to gain even more health benefits. Thus, these latest guidelines illustrate that the IOM and Surgeon General's recommendations are not really that different after all.

CRITICAL THINKING QUESTIONS

1. How might an overweight person gain substantial health benefits by shifting from doing no physical activity to meeting the minimum recommendation of 30 minutes per day on most days of the week?
2. Would there be health benefits even if those changes did not result in weight loss? If so, what would they be?

chapter **review**

test yourself | answers

1. **True.** Almost 50% of Americans do not get enough physical activity. Moreover, about half of these people—25% of the population—report doing no leisure-time physical activity at all.

2. **False.** Our muscles are not stimulated to grow when we eat extra protein, whether as food or supplements. Weight-bearing exercise appropriately stresses the body and produces increased muscle mass and strength.

3. **False.** Unfortunately, our thirst mechanism cannot be relied upon to signal when we need to drink. If we rely solely on our feelings of thirst, we will not consume enough fluid to support exercise.

MasteringNutrition™

Check out these additional resources in the MasteringNutrition Study Area at www.masteringhealthandnutrition.pearson.com:

- Read It: Chapter Summary and RSS Feeds
- See It: ABC News videos and nutrition animations
- Hear It: MP3s
- Study It: Get Ready for Nutrition Math and Chemistry review
- Do It: NutriTools and "Find the Quack" feature
- Review It: Quizzes, flashcards, and glossary

review questions

1. Exercise is
   a. a subcategory of leisure-time physical activity.
   b. activity that is purposeful, planned, and structured.
   c. not related to a person's occupation.
   d. all of the above.

2. The four components of physical fitness are
   a. cardiorespiratory fitness, musculoskeletal fitness, flexibility, and body composition.
   b. cardiorespiratory fitness, strength, stamina, and flexibility.
   c. aerobic capacity, muscular strength, chronic disease resistance, and maintenance of a healthful body weight.
   d. cardiorespiratory efficiency, musculoskeletal strength, optimal immunity, and weight management.

3. Which of the following is a benefit of regular physical activity?
   a. reduces body cells' uptake of glucose from the blood
   b. reduces the risk of nearly all forms of cancer
   c. reduces anxiety and mental stress
   d. all of the above

4. For achieving and maintaining cardiorespiratory fitness, the intensity range typically recommended is
   a. 25–50% of your estimated maximal heart rate.
   b. 35–75% of your estimated maximal heart rate.
   c. 50–70% of your estimated maximal heart rate.
   d. 75–95% of your estimated maximal heart rate.

5. The amount of ATP stored in a muscle cell can keep a muscle active for about
   a. 1 to 3 seconds.
   b. 10 to 30 seconds.
   c. 1 to 3 minutes.
   d. 1 to 3 hours.

6. To support a long afternoon of gardening, the body predominantly uses which nutrient for energy?
   a. carbohydrate
   b. fat
   c. amino acids
   d. lactic acid

7. Athletes participating in an intense athletic competition lasting more than 1 hour should
   a. drink caffeinated beverages to improve their performance while maintaining their hydration.
   b. drink plain warm water copiously both before and during the event in response to fluid losses from sweating and the desire to drink.
   c. drink plain ice water both before and during the event in response to thirst.
   d. drink a beverage containing carbohydrate and electrolytes both before and during the event in amounts that balance hydration with energy, carbohydrate, and electrolyte needs.

8. Which of the following statements about carbohydrate loading is true?
   a. Carbohydrate loading involves altering the duration and intensity of exercise and intake of carbohydrate such that the storage of fat is minimized.
   b. Carbohydrate loading results in increased storage of glycogen in muscles and the liver.
   c. Carbohydrate loading is beneficial for most athletes prior to most competitive events.
   d. All of the above are true.

9. **True or false?** A sound fitness program overloads the body.

10. **True or false?** Sports anemia is a chronic decrease in iron stores that occurs in some athletes who have been training intensely for several months to years.

math review

11. Liz is a dance major. She participates in two 90-minute dance classes each day 5 days a week, plus does a 60-minute strength training workout during her lunch break twice a week. She is a vegetarian, and her current energy intake is 1,800 kcal per day. She weighs 105 lb. After referring to Table 6.2 (page 209) she estimates that her protein intake should be 1.5 grams per kilogram of body weight, and she wants to keep her fat intake relatively low at 20% of her total daily energy intake. Based on this information, calculate how many grams of protein, fat, and carbohydrate Liz needs to consume daily to support this activity program. Does Liz's carbohydrate intake fall within the AMDR, which is 45–65% of total energy intake?

Answers to Review Questions and Math Review are located at the back of this text and in the MasteringNutrition Study Area.

web resources

www.heart.org
American Heart Association

The "Getting Healthy" section of this site has sections on health tools, exercise and fitness, healthy diet, managing your lifestyle, and more.

www.acsm.org
American College of Sports Medicine

Click on "Access Public Information" under the "Brochures and Fact Sheets" section for guidelines on healthy aerobic activity and calculating your exercise heart rate range, and under the "Newsletters" section to access the ACSM's Fit Society Page newsletter.

www.choosemyplate.gov
USDA ChooseMyPlate.gov

Visit this site to learn more about physical activity and how to find ways to incorporate more physical activity into your daily life.

www.webmd.com
WebMD

Visit this site to learn about a variety of lifestyle topics, including fitness and exercise.

www.hhs.gov
U.S. Department of Health and Human Services

Review this site for multiple statistics on health, exercise, and weight as well as information on supplements, wellness, and more.

www.win.niddk.nih.gov
Weight-Control Information Network

To find out more about healthy fitness programs log onto this site and search under "Publications" and "Weight Control."

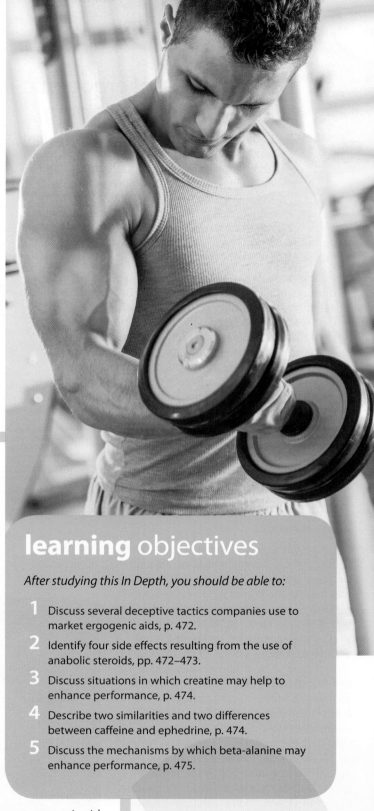

in depth 12.5

Do Active People Need Ergogenic Aids?

Many competitive athletes and even some recreationally active people continually search for that something extra that will enhance their performance. That search often leads them to **ergogenic aids**, substances used to improve exercise and athletic performance. For example, nutrition supplements can be classified as ergogenic aids, as can anabolic steroids and other pharmaceuticals. Interestingly, people report using ergogenic aids not only to enhance athletic performance but also to improve their physical appearance, prevent or treat injuries and diseases, and help them cope with stress. Some people even report using them because of peer pressure!

As you've learned (in Chapter 12), adequate nutrition is critical to athletic performance and to regular physical activity, and products such as sports bars and beverages can help athletes maintain their competitive edge. However, as we will explore shortly, many ergogenic aids are not effective, some are dangerous, and most are very expensive. For the average consumer, it's virtually impossible to track the latest research findings for these products. In addition, many have not been adequately studied, and unsubstantiated claims surrounding them are rampant. How can you become a more educated consumer about ergogenic aids?

learning objectives

After studying this In Depth, you should be able to:

1 Discuss several deceptive tactics companies use to market ergogenic aids, p. 472.

2 Identify four side effects resulting from the use of anabolic steroids, pp. 472–473.

3 Discuss situations in which creatine may help to enhance performance, p. 474.

4 Describe two similarities and two differences between caffeine and ephedrine, p. 474.

5 Discuss the mechanisms by which beta-alanine may enhance performance, p. 475.

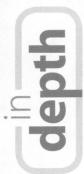

Marketing of ergogenic aids can be misleading

Early in the text (in Chapter 1) we explained how to determine if a website is reliable, and how to evaluate research and claims made by companies promoting their products. The sale of ergogenic aids is a multi-billion-dollar industry, and some companies resort to misleading claims to boost their share of the market. Beware of the following deceptive tactics used to market ergogenic aids:

- Taking published research out of context, applying the findings in an unproven manner, or having inappropriate control over study results. Some companies claim that research has been done or is currently being done but fail to provide specific information.
- Paying celebrities to endorse products—remember that testimonials can be faked, bought, and exaggerated.
- Stating that the product is patented and that this proves its effectiveness. Patents are granted to indicate differences among products; they do not indicate effectiveness.
- Advertising through infomercials and mass-media marketing videos. Although the Federal Trade Commission (FTC) regulates false claims in advertising, products are generally investigated only if they pose significant public danger.
- Offering mail-order fitness evaluations or anabolic measurements. Most of these evaluations are inappropriate and inaccurate.

A recent review of the evidence underpinning sports performance products, which includes drinks, supplements, clothing, and footwear, found that there was inadequate information available to perform a critical appraisal of approximately half of the products.[1] In addition, when studies were conducted to assess a product's effectiveness, only 2.7% of the studies were judged to be of high quality and at low risk of bias. Thus, the authors of this review concluded that the currently available evidence is not of sufficient quality to inform the public about the benefits and risks of these products.

New ergogenic aids are available virtually every month. It is therefore not possible to discuss every available product in this *In Depth*. **TABLE 1** details a list of commonly used erogenic aids, and below we provide additional details on a number of currently popular ergogenic aids.

---

ergogenic aids Substances used to improve exercise and athletic performance.

anabolic The term applied to a substance that builds muscle and increases strength.

Anabolic products are said to enhance muscle and strength

Many ergogenic aids are said to be **anabolic**, meaning that they build muscle and increase strength. Although some are effective, many are associated with harmful side effects.

Anabolic Steroids

Anabolic steroids are testosterone-based drugs. Testosterone is a reproductive system hormone that is associated with male sex characteristics and increased muscle size and strength. Because anabolic steroids are known to be effective in increasing muscle size, strength, power, and speed, they have been used by strength and power athletes worldwide; however, these products are illegal in the United States, and their use is banned by all major collegiate and professional sports organizations, in addition to both the U.S. and the International Olympic Committees.

Proven long-term and irreversible harmful effects of anabolic steroid use include:

- Infertility
- Early closure of the plates of the long bones, resulting in permanent shortened stature
- Shriveled testicles, enlarged breast tissue (that can be removed only surgically), and other signs of "feminization" in men
- Enlarged clitoris, facial hair growth, and other signs of "masculinization" in women
- Increased risk for certain forms of cancer
- Liver damage
- Unhealthful changes in blood lipids
- Hypertension
- Severe acne
- Hair thinning or baldness
- Disorders such as depression, delusions, sleep disturbances, and extreme anger (so-called *roid rage*)

Androstenedione and Dehydroepiandrosterone

Androstenedione ("andro") and dehydroepiandrosterone (DHEA) are precursors of testosterone. Manufacturers of these products claim that taking them will increase testosterone levels and muscle strength. Androstenedione became very popular after baseball player Mark McGwire claimed he used it during the time he was breaking home run records. A national survey found that, in 2002, about one of every forty high school seniors had used it in the past year.[2] Contrary to popular claims, studies have found that neither androstenedione nor DHEA increases testosterone levels, and androstenedione has been shown to increase the risk for heart disease in men

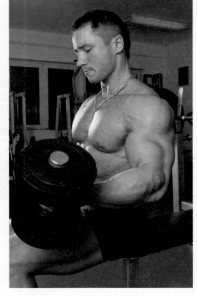

Anabolic substances are often marketed to people wishing to increase muscle size, but many cause harmful side effects.

TABLE 1 An Overview of Commonly Used Ergogenic Aids

Ergogenic Aid	Claimed Mechanism of Action	Does Evidence Support or Refute Claims?	Side Effects
Anabolic Steroids	Increases muscle size, strength, power, and speed	Yes	Infertility; early closure of the plates of the long bones, resulting in permanently shortened stature; shriveled testicles, enlarged breast tissue, and other signs of "feminization" in men; enlarged clitoris, facial hair growth, and other signs of "masculinization" in women; increased risk of cancer; liver damage; unhealthful changes in blood lipids; hypertension; severe acne; hair thinning or baldness; and depression, delusions, sleep disturbances, and "roid rage"
Androstenedione and Dehydroepiandrosterone	Increase testosterone levels and muscle strength	No	Increased risk of heart disease (in middle-aged men)
Gamma-hydroxybutyric Acid	Builds muscle mass	No	Dizziness, tremors, vomiting, seizures, respiratory depression, sedation, coma, death
Creatine	Enhances availability of creatine phosphate, which increases the replenishment of ATP, thus prolonging one's ability to train and perform in short-term, explosive activities, such as weight lifting and sprinting	Yes—has been shown to increase the work performed and the amount of strength gained during resistance exercise and to enhance sprint performance in swimming, running, and cycling	Dehydration, muscle cramps, and gastrointestinal disturbances
Caffeine	Increases alertness and energy, and decreases feelings of fatigue during exercise; also may increase the use of fat as a fuel during endurance exercise, which spares muscle glycogen and improves performance	Yes—has been shown to enhance training and performance	Dehydration, increased blood pressure, increased heart rate, dizziness, insomnia, headache, and gastrointestinal distress
Ephedrine	Promotes weight loss and enhances energy for performance	No—ephedra alone does not enhance performance energy, but supplements containing both caffeine and ephedra have been shown to prolong exercise time to exhaustion; effect on weight loss in athletes is unknown	Headaches, nausea, nervousness, anxiety, irregular heart rate, high blood pressure, and death
Carnitine	Restores carnitine levels after exercise, thereby improving the ability to use fat as a fuel source	No	Nausea, diarrhea, cramps, vomiting
Chromium	Enhances uptake of amino acids into muscle cells, which may increase muscle growth and strength; also marketed as a fat burner because it is speculated that its effect on insulin stimulates the brain to decrease food intake	No	Irregular heartbeat, sleep disturbances, headaches, mood disturbances, allergic reactions, increased risk for liver or kidney damage in those with liver or kidney disease
Ribose	Improves athletic performance by increasing production of ATP, subsequently increasing work output and promoting a faster recovery time from vigorous training	No	Diarrhea, gastrointestinal discomfort, nausea, headache, low blood sugar (when combined with diabetes drugs)
Beta-alanine	Increases the production of carnosine, which plays a key role in the regulation of pH in the muscle, and is said to buffer acids produced during exercise, enhancing ability to perform short-term, high-intensity activities	Yes	Flushing and tingling at high doses

aged 35 to 65.[3] There are no studies that support claims that these products improve strength or increase muscle mass.

Gamma-Hydroxybutyric Acid

Gamma-hydroxybutyric acid, or GHB, is a central nervous system depressant. It was once promoted as an alternative to anabolic steroids for building muscle. The production and sale of GHB were never approved in the United States; however, it was illegally produced and sold on the black market as a dietary supplement. For many users, GHB caused only dizziness, tremors, or vomiting, but others experienced severe side effects, including seizures, respiratory depression, sedation, and coma. Many people were hospitalized, and some died.

In 2001, the federal government placed GHB on the controlled substances list, making its manufacture, sale, and possession illegal. A form of GHB is available by prescription for the treatment of narcolepsy, a rare sleep disorder, but extra paperwork is required by the prescribing physician, and prescriptions are closely monitored. After the ban, a similar product (gamma-butyrolactone, or GBL) was marketed in its place. This product was also found to be dangerous and was removed from the market. Recently, another replacement product called BD (also known as 1,4-butanediol) was banned by the Food and Drug Administration (FDA) because it has caused at least seventy-one deaths, with forty more under investigation. BD is an industrial solvent and is listed on ingredient labels as tetramethylene glycol, butylene glycol, or sucol-B. Side effects include wild, aggressive behavior; nausea; incontinence; and sudden loss of consciousness.

Creatine

Creatine supplements have become wildly popular with strength and power athletes. Creatine, or creatine phosphate, is found in meat and fish and stored in our muscles. As described earlier (in Chapter 12), we use creatine phosphate (CP) to regenerate ATP. It is hypothesized that creatine supplements make more CP available to replenish ATP, which prolongs a person's ability to train and perform in short-term, explosive activities, such as weight lifting and sprinting. Between 1994 and 2013, more than 1,700 research articles related to creatine and exercise in humans were published. This research indicates that creatine does not enhance performance in aerobic-type events but does increase the work performed and the amount of strength gained during resistance exercise and enhance sprint performance in swimming, running, and cycling.[4]

In 2001, claims surfaced that creatine use could lead to cancer.[5] These claims were found to be false, as no studies in humans suggest an increased risk for cancer with creatine use. In fact, numerous studies show an anticancer effect.[6,7] Although side effects such as dehydration, muscle cramps, and gastrointestinal disturbances have been reported with creatine use, there is very little information on how the long-term use of creatine impacts health. Further research is needed to determine its effectiveness and safety over prolonged periods.

Protein and Amino Acid Supplements

Protein and amino acid supplements have long been popular and are widely available in health food stores and on the Internet. Examples of these products include various protein powders and individual amino acids, such as glutamine and arginine. Although manufacturers claim that these products build muscle mass and enhance strength, research indicates that they do not.[8–10]

Some products are said to improve fuel use or pH during exercise

Certain ergogenic aids are touted as increasing energy levels and improving athletic performance by optimizing our use of fat, carbohydrate, and protein. Other products have been identified that may enhance our capacity to buffer acids during exercise, resulting in delayed onset of fatigue. The products reviewed here are caffeine, ephedrine, carnitine, chromium, ribose, and beta-alanine.

Caffeine

Caffeine is a stimulant that makes us feel more alert and energetic, decreasing feelings of fatigue during exercise. In addition, caffeine has been shown to increase the use of fat as a fuel during endurance exercise, which spares muscle glycogen and improves performance.[11,12] Energy drinks that contain high amounts of caffeine, such as Red Bull, have become popular with athletes and many college students. These drinks should be avoided during exercise because severe dehydration can result due to the combination of fluid loss from exercise and caffeine consumption. Research also indicates that energy drinks are associated with serious side effects in children, adolescents, and young adults with conditions such as seizures, diabetes, and mood behavior disorders.[13] It should be recognized that caffeine is a controlled or restricted drug in the athletic world, and athletes can be banned from Olympic competition if urine caffeine levels are too high. However, the amount of caffeine that is banned is quite high, and athletes would need to consume caffeine in pill form to reach this level. Side effects of caffeine use include increased blood pressure, increased heart rate, dizziness, insomnia, headache, and gastrointestinal distress.

Ephedrine

Ephedrine, also known as ephedra, Chinese ephedra, or *ma huang,* is a strong stimulant marketed as a weight-loss supplement and energy enhancer. Many products sold as "all natural" Chinese ephedra (or herbal ephedra) contain ephedrine synthesized in a laboratory, as well as other stimulants, such as caffeine. The use of ephedra does not appear to enhance performance, but supplements containing both caffeine and ephedra have been shown to prolong the amount of exercise that can be done until exhaustion is reached.[14] Ephedra is known to reduce body weight and body fat in sedentary women, but its impact on weight loss and body fat levels in athletes is unknown.

The risks of ephedra use are considerable. Side effects include headaches, nausea, nervousness, anxiety, irregular heart rate, and high blood pressure; moreover, at least seventeen deaths have been attributed to its use. It is currently illegal to sell ephedra-containing supplements in the United States.

Carnitine

Our bodies synthesize carnitine from the amino acids lysine and methionine. In our cells, carnitine is found in the membranes of mitochondria, where it helps shuttle fatty acids into the mitochondria interior so that they can be used for energy. It has been

Ephedrine is made from the herb *Ephedra sinica* (Chinese ephedra).

proposed that exercise training depletes our cells of carnitine and that supplementation should restore carnitine levels, thereby enabling us to be able to improve our use of fat as a fuel source. Thus, carnitine is marketed not only as a performance-enhancing substance but also as a "fat burner." Research studies of carnitine supplementation do not support these claims because neither the transport of fatty acids nor their oxidation appears to be enhanced with supplementation.[15] The use of carnitine supplements has not been associated with significant side effects.

Chromium

Chromium is a trace mineral that enhances insulin's action of increasing the transport of amino acids into the cell. It is found in whole-grain foods, cheese, nuts, mushrooms, and asparagus. It is theorized that many people are chromium deficient and that supplementation will enhance the uptake of amino acids into muscle cells, which will increase muscle growth and strength. Like carnitine, chromium is marketed as a fat burner due to speculation that its effect on insulin stimulates the brain to decrease food intake. Chromium supplements are available as chromium picolinate and chromium nicotinate. Early studies of chromium supplementation showed promise, but more recent, better-designed studies do not support any benefit of chromium supplementation on muscle mass, muscle strength, body fat, or exercise performance.[16]

Ribose

Ribose is a five-carbon sugar that is critical to the production of ATP. Ribose supplementation is claimed to improve athletic performance by increasing work output and promoting a faster recovery time from vigorous training. Although ribose has been shown to improve exercise tolerance in patients with heart disease, several studies have reported that ribose supplementation has no impact on athletic performance.[17–20]

Beta-Alanine

Beta-alanine is a nonessential amino acid that has been identified as the limiting factor in the production of carnosine, a dipeptide composed of beta-alanine and L-histidine and synthesized in skeletal muscle. Carnosine plays a key role in the regulation of pH in the muscle and is thought to buffer acids produced during exercise, thereby enhancing a person's ability to perform short-term, high-intensity activities.[21,22] Recent evidence suggests that beta-alanine supplementation can increase muscle carnosine levels and delay the onset of muscle fatigue. Additionally, beta-alanine supplementation results in improved exercise performance during single or repeated high-intensity exercise bouts or maximal muscle contractions.[21,22] It appears that several weeks of supplementation is needed to increase muscle carnosine levels and positively affect performance.[22]

As this review indicates, many ergogenic aids fail to live up to their claims of enhancing athletic performance, strength, or body composition. And many have uncomfortable or even dangerous side effects. Be a savvy consumer. Before purchasing these products, do some homework to make sure you wouldn't be wasting your money or putting your health at risk by using them.

nutri-case | THEO

"All season long I've been watching my diet, but lately I feel really wiped out after games. I'm eating about 500 grams of carbs a day, but only 150 grams of protein, so maybe I'm not getting enough protein. I'm planning to try a protein powder they sell at my gym. I guess I just feel like, when I'm competing, I need some extra insurance."

Theo's weight averages about 190 pounds during basketball season. Given what you've learned about the role of the energy nutrients in vigorous physical activity, what do you think might be causing Theo to feel "wiped out" after games? Do you think his plan to boost his protein intake with a protein powder makes sense? What other strategies might be helpful for him to consider?

MasteringNutrition™

Check out these additional resources in the MasteringNutrition Study Area:

- Read It: Chapter Summary and RSS Feeds
- See It: ABC News videos and nutrition animations
- Hear It: MP3s
- Study It: Get Ready for Nutrition Math and Chemistry review
- Do It: NutriTools and "Find the Quack" feature
- Review It: Quizzes, flashcards, and glossary

web resources

www.ods.od.nih.gov
NIH Office of Dietary Supplements

Look on this National Institutes of Health site to learn more about the health effects of specific nutritional supplements.

www.nal.usda.gov
Food and Nutrition Information Center

Visit this site, searching on "fnic," for links to detailed information about ergogenic aids and sports nutrition.

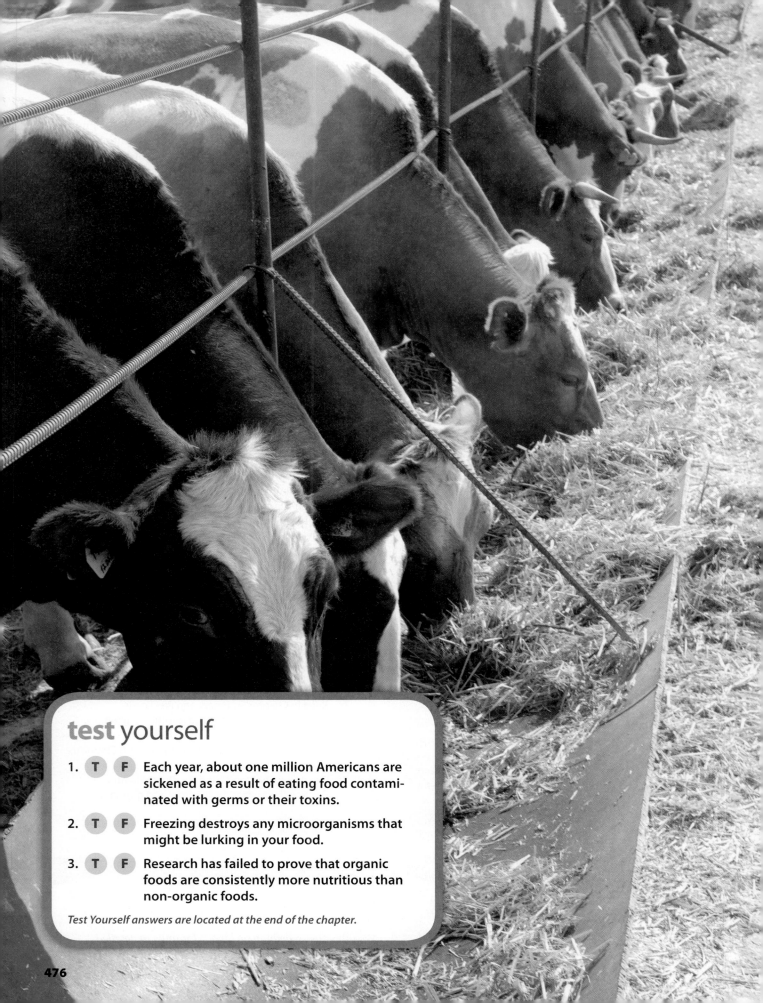

test yourself

1. **T** **F** Each year, about one million Americans are sickened as a result of eating food contaminated with germs or their toxins.

2. **T** **F** Freezing destroys any microorganisms that might be lurking in your food.

3. **T** **F** Research has failed to prove that organic foods are consistently more nutritious than non-organic foods.

Test Yourself answers are located at the end of the chapter.

Food Safety and Technology
Impact on consumers

13

A cruise: The epitome of luxury. The ads promised panoramic views of romantic landscapes, indulgent comfort, family fun, and delicious food. . . So why did passengers on numerous cruise lines sailing during the winter of 2012–2013 describe the experience as like being on "a plague ship"?

The answer was, in a word, *norovirus*. Infection with this highly contagious virus typically causes 1–3 days of forceful vomiting and diarrhea, but it can be more severe and even fatal. In any given year, over 90% of diarrheal disease outbreaks on cruise ships are caused by norovirus, but a new, more potent strain arose in Australia early in 2012 and quickly made its way around the world.[1] It hit not just cruise lines, but hospitals and nursing homes, schools and colleges, restaurants, and workplaces.

Norovirus is spread by direct person-to-person contact as well as in food or water. Food can become contaminated while it is being grown, shipped, handled, or prepared, most commonly when workers with virus particles on their hands touch the food. Although a variety of foods have been associated with outbreaks, foods that are eaten raw, such as leafy vegetables, fruit, and shellfish, are most commonly involved.[2]

But norovirus is not the only microbe contaminating our food supply. *Salmonella* bacteria are routinely found in raw poultry and eggs, and in 2012 it also showed up in mangoes, cantaloupes, and peanut butter.[3] And *E. coli* is a common resident of raw and undercooked meats: in recent years, *E. coli*–contaminated beef has caused several outbreaks of severe illness, including kidney failure and death.[4] What's worse, *Salmonella* and *E. coli* are just two of several bacteria that cause foodborne illness.

Continued next page

learning objectives

After studying this chapter you should be able to:

1 Summarize the two main reasons that foodborne illness is a critical concern in the United States, pp. 478–479.

2 Identify the types of microorganisms most commonly involved in foodborne illness, pp. 479–485.

3 Describe strategies for preventing foodborne illness at home, while eating out, and when traveling to other countries, pp. 486–491.

4 Compare and contrast the different methods manufacturers use to preserve foods, pp. 491–492.

5 Debate the safety of food additives, including the role of the GRAS list, pp. 492–493.

6 Describe the process of genetic modification and discuss the potential risks and benefits associated with genetically modified organisms, pp. 495–496.

7 Describe the processes by which residues, persistant organic pollutants, and pesticides affect foods and the food supply, pp. 496–499.

8 Discuss the regulation, labeling, benefits, and limitations of organic foods, pp. 499–500.

MasteringNutrition™

Go online for chapter quizzes, pre-tests, Interactive Activities, and more!

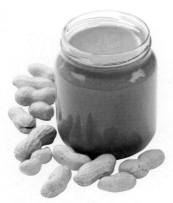

Nationwide food recalls as a result of *Salmonella* contamination in recent years included hundreds of products made from peanuts.

Continued—How do disease-causing agents enter our food and water supplies, and how can we protect ourselves from them? What makes food spoil, and what keeps it fresh? Which aspects of industrial food production help consumers, and which put us at risk? We explore these and other questions in this chapter.

Why is foodborne illness a critical concern?

Foodborne illness is a term used to encompass any symptom or disorder that arises from ingesting food or water contaminated with disease-causing (*pathogenic*) microscopic organisms (called *microorganisms*), their toxic secretions, or chemicals (such as mercury or pesticides). You probably refer to foodborne illness as *food poisoning*.

Foodborne Illness Affects Millions of Americans Annually

According to the Centers for Disease Control and Prevention (CDC), approximately 48 million Americans—1 out of every 6—report experiencing foodborne illness each year. Of these, 128,000 are hospitalized and 3,000 die.[5] The people most at risk for serious foodborne illness include:

- Developing fetuses, infants, and young children because their immune system is immature
- People who are very old or have a chronic illness because their immune system may be compromised
- People with acquired immunodeficiency syndrome (AIDS)
- People who are receiving immune system–suppressing drugs, such as transplant recipients and cancer patients

Although the statistics may seem frightening, most experts consider our food supply safe. That's partly because not all cases of food contamination make all people sick; in fact, even virulent strains cause illness in only a small percentage of people who consume the tainted food. Moreover, modern technology has given us an array of techniques to preserve foods. We discuss these later in this chapter.

Moreover, food safety in the United States is monitored by several government agencies. In addition to the CDC, mentioned earlier, the United States Department of Agriculture (USDA), Food and Drug Administration (FDA), and Environmental Protection Agency (EPA) monitor and regulate food safety, production, and preservation. Information about these agencies and how to access them appear in **TABLE 13.1**.

Food Production Is Increasingly Complex

foodborne illness An illness transmitted by food or water contaminated by a pathogenic microorganism, its toxic secretions, or a toxic chemical.

Despite safeguards, foodborne illness has emerged as a major public health threat in recent years. One reason is that more foods are mass-produced than ever before, with a combination of ingredients from a much greater number of sources, including

TABLE 13.1 Government Agencies That Regulate Food Safety

Name of Agency	Year Established	Role in Food Regulations	Website
U.S. Department of Agriculture (USDA)	1785	Oversees safety of meat, poultry, and eggs sold across state lines; also regulates which drugs can be used to treat sick cattle and poultry	www.usda.gov
U.S. Food and Drug Administration (FDA)	1862	Regulates food standards of food products (except meat, poultry, and eggs) and bottled water; regulates food labeling and enforces pesticide use as established by the EPA	www.fda.gov
Centers for Disease Control and Prevention (CDC)	1946	Works with public health officials to promote and educate the public about health and safety; able to track information needed in identifying foodborne illness outbreaks	www.cdc.gov
Environmental Protection Agency (EPA)	1970	Regulates use of pesticides and which crops they can be applied to; establishes standards for water quality	www.epa.gov

fields, feedlots, and a variety of processing facilities all over the world. These various sources can remain hidden not only to consumers but even to food companies using the ingredients. Contamination can occur at any point from farm to table (**FIGURE 13.1** on page 480), and when it does, it can be difficult to trace.

Moreover, oversight of food safety, according to the government's own descriptions, is both fragmented and underfunded.[6] Over the last few decades, for example, government inspection of food-production facilities has declined just as the number of facilities, both here and overseas, has skyrocketed. Farms and production facilities are often inspected by private auditors who have a financial interest in completing the job quickly and perfunctorily: In September 2011, for example, a farm that just a few weeks earlier had passed its inspection with a score of 96 out of 100 was found to be the source of an outbreak of *Listeria monocytogenes* infections—spread via contaminated cantaloupe—that sickened over 140 people and caused a miscarriage and thirty deaths.[7]

New food safety legislation, the FDA Food Safety Modernization Act (FSMA), which was signed into law in January 2011, is beginning to strengthen our food safety system.[6] Among its provisions are the following:

- New requirements for food processors to prevent contamination
- New requirements for food importers to verify the safety of food from their suppliers
- New FDA enforcement tools, including mandatory recall authority
- A new, more rigorous inspection schedule

It is too soon to judge the effectiveness of these provisions; however, in 2013, the CDC published data showing that the overall rate of foodborne infections with six key pathogens was significantly lower in 2011 compared with 1996–1998.[8] Moreover, in January of 2013, the FDA proposed two new rulings requiring farmers and food processors, whether foreign or domestic, to develop a formal plan for preventing contamination and for correcting any problems that arise. Additional rules are expected to follow.[9]

recap Foodborne illness affects 48 million Americans a year. Contamination can occur at any point from farm to table. The Centers for Disease Control and Prevention, the Food and Drug Administration, the United States Department of Agriculture, and the Environmental Protection Agency monitor and regulate food production and preservation. The Food Safety Modernization Act of 2011 increased the oversight of food production by federal agencies and authorized the FDA to swiftly recall contaminated foods from the market; in addition, new rules are under development.

> To get information and access numerous resources on food safety topics, go to www.cdc.gov, and enter "food safety spotlight" into the search bar.

What causes most foodborne illness?

A *pathogen* is any agent capable of generating disease. The consumption of food containing pathogenic microorganisms results in *food infections*. *Food intoxications* result from consuming food tainted with harmful substances called *toxins*. Chemical residues in foods, such as pesticides and pollutants, can also cause illness. Residues are discussed later in this chapter.

Several Types of Microorganisms Contaminate Foods

The two types of microorganisms that most commonly cause food infections are viruses and bacteria.

Viruses Involved in Foodborne Illness

Viruses are non-cellular agents that can survive only by infecting living cells. Norovirus, the species introduced at the beginning of this chapter, causes more than 21 million infections annually in the United States, and more than 5 million of

viruses A group of infectious agents that are usually much smaller than bacteria, lack independent metabolism, and are incapable of growth or reproduction outside of living cells.

FIGURE 13.1 Food is at risk for contamination at any of the five stages from farm to table, but following food safety guidelines can reduce the risks.

Farms

Animals raised for meat can harbor harmful microorganisms, and crops can be contaminated with pollutants from irrigation, runoff from streams, microorganisms or toxins in soil, or pesticides. Contamination can also occur during animal slaughter or from harvesting, sorting, washing, packing, and/or storage of crops.

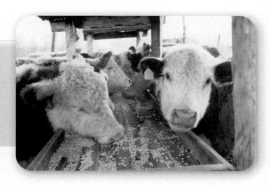

Processing

Some foods, such as produce, may go from the farm directly to the market, but most foods are processed. Processed foods may go through several steps at different facilities. At each site, people, equipment, or environments may contaminate foods. Federal safeguards, such as cleaning protocols, testing, and training, can help prevent contamination.

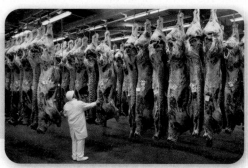

Transportation

Foods must be transported in clean, refrigerated vehicles and containers to prevent multiplication of microorganisms and microbial toxins.

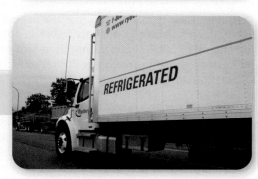

Retail

Employees of food markets and restaurants may contaminate food during storage, preparation, or service. Conditions such as inadequate refrigeration or heating may promote multiplication of microorganisms or microbial toxins. Establishments must follow FDA guidelines for food safety and pass local health inspections.

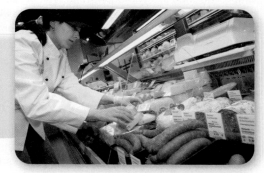

Table

Consumers may contaminate foods with unclean hands, utensils, or surfaces. They can allow the multiplication of microorganisms and microbial toxins by failing to follow the food-safety guidelines for storing, preparing, cooking, and serving foods discussed in this chapter.

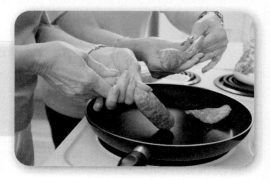

these are foodborne.[5] In fact, norovirus causes more foodborne illness than the other thirty known pathogens put together (**FIGURE 13.2**).[5]

Norovirus is so common and contagious that many people refer to it simply as "the stomach flu"; however, it is not a strain of influenza. Symptoms of infection typically come on suddenly as *gastroenteritis*, inflammation of the lining of the stomach and intestines. This causes stomach cramps as well as both vomiting and diarrhea. Because the vomiting begins abruptly, the person is likely to be in a social setting. Because it is forceful, anyone nearby is likely to become contaminated. Another characteristic that makes norovirus so contagious is that, whereas most viruses perish quickly in a dry environment, norovirus is able to survive on dry surfaces and objects, from countertops to utensils, for days or even weeks. Also, ingestion of even a few "particles" of norovirus can result in full-blown illness.[10]

College campuses commonly report outbreaks. In 2013, for instance, several campuses in the Northeast experienced norovirus outbreaks, sending hundreds of students to their campus health center or to the hospital. The best way to prevent the spread of norovirus is to wash your hands, kitchen surfaces, and utensils with warm, soapy water. Alcohol-based hand sanitizers may be used in addition to hand washing but not as a substitute.[10] If you experience vomiting or diarrhea, immediately clean and disinfect all nearby surfaces and remove and wash laundry thoroughly.

Whereas norovirus is estimated to infect about 21 million Americans annually, hepatitis A virus (HAV) causes about 21,000 infections.[11] Like norovirus, HAV can be transmitted person-to-person or via contaminated foods and water supplies. The term *hepatitis* means inflammation of the liver. This causes jaundice (a yellowish skin tone), the most common sign of HAV infection.[11] Typically, the symptoms of HAV infection include a mild fever, abdominal pain, and nausea and vomiting that lasts a few weeks. Rarely, in elderly patients and those with preexisting liver disease, HAV infection can lead to liver failure and even death.

Bacteria Involved in Foodborne Illness

In contrast to viruses, **bacteria** are cellular microorganisms; however, they lack the true cell nucleus common to plant and animals cells, and they reproduce either by dividing in two or by forming reproductive spores. Many thrive in the intestines of birds and mammals, including humans; as we've discussed earlier in this text, our bodies contain more bacterial cells than human cells, and many of these bacteria contribute to our health and functioning.

In contrast, pathogenic bacteria are capable of causing mild to severe disease. Foodborne bacterial illness commonly occurs when we ingest pathogenic bacteria living in or on undercooked or raw foods or fluids. These bacteria, which often come from human or animal feces, can damage our cells and tissues either directly or by secreting a destructive toxin. Of the eight pathogens causing the greatest number of foodborne illnesses, hospitalizations, and deaths among Americans, six are species of bacteria.[5] These are identified in **TABLE 13.2**. Of these, the most deadly is *Salmonella* (**FIGURE 13.3**).

Other Microorganisms Involved in Foodborne Illness

Parasites are microorganisms that simultaneously derive benefit from and harm their host. They are responsible for only about 2% of foodborne illnesses. The following are the most common culprits:

- **Helminths** are multicellular worms, such as tapeworms (**FIGURE 13.4**, page 483), flukes, and roundworms. They reproduce by releasing their eggs into vegetation or water. Animals, including fish, then consume the contaminated matter. The eggs hatch inside their host, and larvae develop in the host's tissue. The larvae can survive in the flesh long after the host is killed for food. Thoroughly cooking beef, pork, or fish destroys the larvae. In contrast, people who eat contaminated foods either raw or undercooked consume living larvae, which then mature into adult worms in their small intestine. Some worms cause mild symptoms, such as nausea and diarrhea, but others can grow large enough to cause intestinal obstruction or even death.
- **Protozoa** are single-celled parasites implicated in food- and waterborne illness. One of these, *Toxoplasma gondii*, is the last of our top eight culprits in foodborne illness and is second only to *Salmonella* as a cause of death.[5] Another common

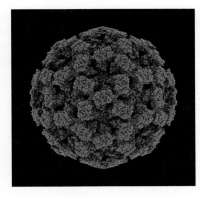

FIGURE 13.2   Norovirus is the leading cause of foodborne infection in the United States. It is responsible for more foodborne illness from known agents than all other viruses, bacteria, and parasites combined.

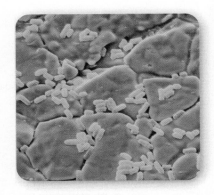

FIGURE 13.3   *Salmonella* is the leading cause of bacterial foodborne illness. Infection can cause fever, diarrhea, and abdominal cramps, and cells of some strains of *Salmonella* can perforate the intestines and invade the blood, causing systemic infection and death.

bacteria Microorganisms that lack a true nucleus and reproduce by division or by forming spores.

parasite A microorganism that simultaneously derives benefit from and harms its host.

helminth A multicellular microscopic worm.

protozoa Single-celled, mobile microorganisms.

TABLE 13.2 Six Most Common Bacterial Causes of Foodborne Illness

Bacteria	Incubation Period	Duration	Symptoms	Foods Most Commonly Affected	Usual Sources of Contamination	Steps for Prevention
Salmonella (more than 2,300 types)	12–24 hours	4–7 days	Diarrhea Abdominal pain Chills Fever Vomiting Dehydration	Raw or undercooked eggs, poultry, and meat Raw milk and dairy products Seafood Fruits and vegetables	Intestinal tract and feces of poultry *Salmonella enteritidis* in raw eggs	Cook foods thoroughly. Avoid cross-contamination. Use sanitary practices.
Clostridium perfringens	6–24 hours	1 day	Abdominal cramps Diarrhea	Beef Poultry Gravies Dried foods Cooked foods prepared in large quantities Leftovers	Widely found in environment and in intestinal tracts of animals and humans Can survive in little or no oxygen	Cook foods thoroughly. Serve hot. Refrigerate leftovers promptly. Reheat leftovers thoroughly before serving.
Campylobacter (several species)	1–7 days	7–10 days	Fever Headache and muscle pain followed by diarrhea (sometimes bloody) Nausea Abdominal cramps	Raw and undercooked meat, poultry, or shellfish Raw eggs Cake icing Untreated water Unpasteurized milk	Intestinal tracts of animals and birds Raw milk Untreated water and sewage sludge	Only drink pasteurized milk. Cook foods properly. Avoid cross-contamination.
Staphylococcus aureus	1–6 hours	2–3 days	Severe nausea and vomiting Abdominal cramps Diarrhea	Custard- or cream-filled baked goods Ham Poultry Dressings, sauces, and gravies Eggs Mayonnaise-based salads	Human skin Infected cuts Pimples Noses and throats	Refrigerate foods. Use sanitary practices.
Escherichia coli (O157:H7 and other strains that can cause human illness)	2–4 days	5–10 days	Diarrhea (may be bloody) Abdominal cramps Nausea Can lead to kidney and blood complications	Contaminated water Raw milk Raw or rare ground beef, sausages Unpasteurized apple juice or cider Uncooked fruits and vegetables	Intestinal tracts of cattle Raw milk Unchlorinated water	Thoroughly cook meat. Avoid cross-contamination.
Listeria monocytogenes	2 days–3 weeks	None reported	Fever Muscle aches Nausea Diarrhea Headache, stiff neck, confusion, loss of balance, or convulsions if infection spreads to nervous system Infections during pregnancy can lead to miscarriage or stillbirth	Uncooked meats and vegetables Soft cheeses Lunch meats and hot dogs Unpasteurized milk	Intestinal tract and feces of animals Soil and manure used as fertilizer Raw milk	Thoroughly cook all meats. Heat hot dogs until they are steaming hot. Wash produce before eating. Avoid cross-contamination. Wash hands after handling hot dogs, lunch meats, and other meats. Avoid unpasteurized milk and foods made with unpasteurized milk. People at high risk should avoid eating refrigerated smoked seafood unless it is cooked.

Data from: Iowa State University Extension, Food Safety and Quality Project. 2000. Safe Food: It's Your Job Too!; U.S. Food and Drug Administration (FDA). How Can I Prevent Foodborne Illness?; and Centers for Disease Control and Prevention (CDC). 2012. 2011 Estimates of Foodborne Illness in the United States.

agent is *Giardia*, various species of which cause a diarrheal illness called *giardiasis*. Both *T. gondii* and *Giardia* live in the intestines of infected animals and humans and are passed into food and water from stools. People typically ingest these parasites by swallowing contaminated water or by eating undercooked or raw contaminated food. Many people infected with these parasites never develop symptoms, or experience only a mild, flulike illness; however, in vulnerable populations, *T. gondii* can lead to organ damage, and infection during pregnancy can cause a miscarriage, stillbirth, or eye or brain damage in the newborn.[12, 13]

- **Fungi** are plantlike, spore-forming organisms that can grow as either single cells or multicellular colonies. Three common types are yeasts, which are globular; molds, which are long and thin; and the familiar mushrooms. Foodborne illnesses are rarely caused by microscopic fungi, in part because very few species are capable of causing serious disease in people with healthy immune systems, and these few are not typically foodborne. The CDC lists only one foodborne fungus, *Cryptococcus*, which almost exclusively affects patients with compromised immunity.[14] In addition, unlike bacterial growth, which is invisible and often tasteless, fungal growth typically makes food look and taste so unappealing that we immediately discard it (**FIGURE 13.5**).

A foodborne illness in beef cattle that has had front-page exposure in recent years is mad cow disease, or *bovine spongiform encephalopathy* (*BSE*). This neurological disorder is caused by a **prion**, a proteinaceous infectious particle that is self-replicating. Prions are normal proteins of animal tissues that can misfold and become infectious. When they do, they can transform other normal proteins into abnormally shaped prions until they eventually cause illness.

The human form of BSE can develop in people who consume contaminated meat or tissue. If you eat beef, are you at risk? See the **Nutrition Myth or Fact?** feature and find out.

Some Foodborne Illness Is Due to Toxins

Some species of bacteria and fungi secrete chemicals, called **toxins**, that are responsible for serious and even life-threatening illnesses. These toxins bind to body cells and can cause a variety of symptoms, such as diarrhea, vomiting, organ damage, convulsions, and paralysis. Toxins can be categorized depending on the type of cell they bind to; the two primary types of toxins associated with foodborne illness are neurotoxins, which damage the nervous system and can cause paralysis, and enterotoxins, which target the gastrointestinal system and generally cause severe diarrhea and vomiting.

Bacterial Toxins

One of the most common and deadly neurotoxins is produced by the bacterium *Clostridium botulinum*. The botulism toxin blocks nerve transmission to muscle cells and causes paralysis, including of the muscles required for breathing. A common source of contamination is food in a damaged (split, pierced, or bulging) can. If you spot damaged canned goods while shopping, notify the store manager. If you inadvertently purchase food in a damaged can, or find that the container spurts liquid when you open it, throw it out immediately. *Never* taste the food because even a microscopic amount of botulism toxin can be deadly.[15] Other common sources of *C. botulinum* are foods improperly canned at home and raw honey.

Some strains of *E. coli* are particularly dangerous because they produce a toxin called *Shiga toxin*. These types are referred to as Shiga toxin–producing *E. coli*, or STEC. The most common STEC is *E. coli* O157. In vulnerable populations, infection with one of the STECs can result in kidney failure and, in some cases, death.

Eating spoiled fish, commonly tuna or mackerel, is unwise because bacteria responsible for the spoilage release toxins into the fish. The result is *scombrotoxic fish poisoning*, which causes headache, vomiting, a rash, sweating, and flushing within a few minutes to 2 hours after consumption. Symptoms are usually mild and resolve within a few hours in healthy people.[16]

Fungal Toxins

Some fungi produce poisonous chemicals called *mycotoxins*. (The prefix *myco-* means "fungus.") These toxins are typically found in grains stored in moist environments. In some instances, moist conditions in the field encourage fungi to reproduce and release their toxins on the surface of growing crops. Long-term consumption of mycotoxins can cause organ damage or cancer.

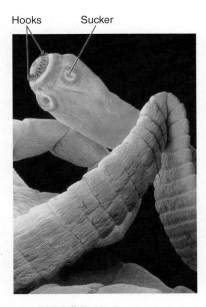

Hooks   Sucker

FIGURE 13.4 Tapeworms have long, wormlike bodies and hooks and suckers, which help them attach to human tissues.

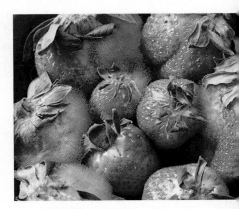

FIGURE 13.5 Molds rarely cause foodborne illness, in part because they look so unappealing that we throw the food away.

fungi Plantlike, spore-forming organisms that can grow as either single cells or multicellular colonies.

prion A protein that misfolds and becomes infectious; prions are not living cellular organisms or viruses.

toxin Any harmful substance; in microbiology, a chemical produced by a microorganism that harms tissues or causes harmful immune responses.

nutrition myth or fact?

Mad Cow Disease: Is It Safe to Eat Beef?

Mad cow disease is a fatal neurological disorder in cattle caused by a *prion*, which is an abnormally folded, infectious protein. Prions influence other proteins to take on their abnormal shape, and these abnormal proteins damage nerve tissue, notably in the brain and spinal cord. The disease can occur in sheep and other animals as well as cows.

Mad cow disease is technically known as *bovine spongiform* (sponge-like) *encephalopathy (BSE)* because the disease eats away at a cow's brain, leaving it full of holes. Eventually, the brain can no longer control vital functions and the cow literally "goes mad" and dies. Unfortunately, people who eat contaminated meat from infected cattle will also be infected. Symptoms may take years to appear, but eventually the person may develop the human form of mad cow disease, called *variant Creutzfeldt-Jakob disease (vCJD)*. As of June 2012, this disease had killed 176 people in Great Britain as well as 25 people in France and several in other nations.[17]

Scientists are not certain how the prions are introduced to cattle. They think that cattle become infected by eating feed containing tissue from the brains and spinal cords of other infected cattle. Decades ago in Great Britain and Europe, it was common practice to feed livestock with meal made from other animals. This practice has ceased, and the number of deaths attributed to vCJD has declined from its peak of twenty-eight in the year 2000 to just five in 2011.[17]

For many years, experts in North America believed BSE to be a problem limited to Europe. But then, eight cases of BSE were found in cows in Canada from 2003 to 2006. And in December 2003, the first case of mad cow disease was reported in the United States. Since then, three additional cases have been confirmed, the most recent in April 2012.[18] So if you eat beef, are you at risk?

To date, only one case of vCJD has been confirmed in Canada and one in the United States, and these individuals are thought to have acquired the disease while in the United Kingdom. The low incidence of vCJD in North America may reflect longstanding preventive practices. For instance, the United States has a system of three interlocking safeguards against BSE. The first and most important of these is the practice of removing, prior to slaughter, the parts of an animal that would contain BSE should an animal have the disease. The second is rigorous control of the quality of animal feed. The third safeguard—which led to the April 2012 detection in a cow culled for lameness—is an ongoing BSE surveillance program in which carcasses are routinely sampled for BSE.[18]

So is it safe for Americans to eat beef? The USDA is working together with other government agencies and the U.S. beef industry to eliminate the use of unapproved animal feed and to improve technologies and procedures to detect BSE before an animal is approved for consumption. The beef industry is highly motivated to maintain food safety because reduced beef consumption would translate into millions of dollars in lost income. Although it may not be possible to guarantee the safety of U.S. beef, adherence to strict safety standards minimizes the risk of an outbreak of vCJD.

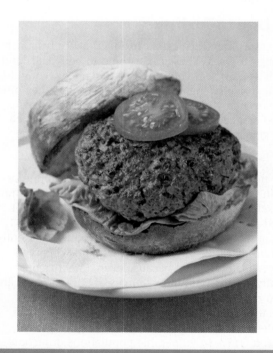

CRITICAL THINKING QUESTIONS

1. How is vCJD related to "mad cow disease"?
2. When the cases of vCJD began to spike in Europe a decade ago, consumers were often advised to avoid salami, sausages, burgers, and other processed, ground meats and to choose lean meats cut "further from the bone." Why do you think this is?

A highly visible fungus that causes food intoxication is the poisonous mushroom. Most mushrooms are not toxic, but a few, such as the deathcap mushroom (*Amanita phalloides*), can be fatal. Some poisonous mushrooms are quite colorful (**FIGURE 13.6**), a fact that helps explain why the victims of mushroom poisoning are often children.[19]

Toxic Algae

In April 2012, scientists predicted that a "red tide" could cause the closure of shellfish beds along as much as 250 miles of the northern New England coastline. Shellfish beds are closed to protect the public from a foodborne illness called *paralytic shellfish poisoning* (*PSP*) in anyone consuming mussels or clams harvested during a red tide.[20]

Red tides are caused by an excessive production of certain species of toxic algae whose bloom turns ocean waters purple, pink, or red. The blooms commonly occur along the Gulf of Maine and on the Gulf Coast of Florida. Humans don't consume these marine toxins directly; rather, mussels, clams, and other seafood consume the toxic algae. When humans consume the seafood, which typically looks, smells, and tastes normal, PSP results.[20]

Finfish can also be contaminated with toxic algae. Ciguatoxins are marine toxins commonly found in fresh fish caught off the coasts of Hawaii, Puerto Rico, the Virgin Islands, and other tropical regions. They are produced by algae called *dinoflagellates*, which are consumed by small fish. The toxins become progressively more concentrated as larger fish eat these small fish, and high concentrations can be present in grouper, sea bass, snapper, and a number of other large fish from tropical regions. Symptoms of ciguatoxin poisoning include nausea, vomiting, diarrhea, headache, itching, a "pins-and-needles" feeling, and even nightmares or hallucinations, but the illness is rarely fatal and typically resolves within a few weeks.[18]

Plant Toxins

A variety of plants contain toxins that, if consumed, can cause illness. As humans evolved, we learned to avoid such plants. However, one plant toxin is still commonly found in kitchens. Potatoes that have turned green contain the toxin solanine, which forms during the greening process. The green color is actually due to chlorophyll, a harmless pigment that forms when the potatoes are exposed to light. Although the production of solanine occurs simultaneously with the production of chlorophyll, the two processes are separate and unrelated. The toxin also occurs in the sprouts that form on stored potatoes, whether or not they have turned green.

Solanine is very toxic even in small amounts. Potatoes that appear green beneath the skin should be thrown away, and any sprouts forming on a stored potato should be removed. Toxicity causes vomiting, diarrhea, fever, headache, and other symptoms, and can progress to shock. Very rarely, the poisoning can be fatal.[21] You can avoid the greening and sprouting of potatoes by storing them for only short periods in a dark cupboard or brown paper bag in a cool area.

The Body Responds to Contaminants with Acute Illness

Many contaminants are killed in the mouth by antimicrobial enzymes in saliva or in the stomach by hydrochloric acid. Any that survive these chemical assaults usually trigger vomiting and/or diarrhea as the gastrointestinal tract attempts to expel them. Simultaneously, the white blood cells of the immune system are activated, and a generalized inflammatory response causes the person to experience nausea, fatigue, fever, and muscle aches. Depending on the state of one's health, the precise microorganism or toxin involved, and the "dose" ingested, the symptoms can range from mild to severe.

To diagnose a foodborne illness, a specimen—usually blood or stool—must be analyzed. Treatment usually involves keeping the person hydrated and comfortable because most foodborne illness tends to be self-limiting; the person's vomiting and/or diarrhea, though unpleasant, rid the body of the offending agent. In more severe cases, hospitalization may be necessary.

In the United States, all confirmed cases of foodborne illness must be reported to the state health department, which in turn reports these illnesses to the CDC in Atlanta, Georgia. The CDC monitors its reports for indications of epidemics of foodborne illness and assists local and state agencies in controlling such outbreaks.

Certain Conditions Help Microorganisms Multiply in Foods

Given the correct environmental conditions, microorganisms can thrive in many types of food. Four factors affect the survival and reproduction of food microorganisms:

- **Temperature.** Many microorganisms capable of causing human illness thrive at moderately cool to warm temperatures, from about 40°F to 140°F (4°C to 60°C). You can think of this range of temperatures as the **danger zone** (**FIGURE 13.7**, page 486). These microorganisms can be destroyed by thoroughly heating or cooking foods,

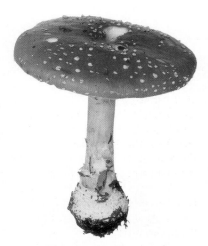

FIGURE 13.6 Some mushrooms, such as this fly agaric, contain toxins that can cause illness or even death.

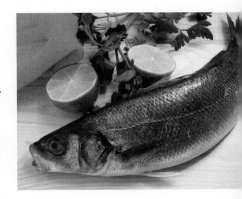

Sea bass may look appealing, but like several other large predatory tropical fish, it can be contaminated with a high concentration of marine toxins.

danger zone Range of temperature (about 40°F to 140°F, or 4°C to 60°C) at which many microorganisms capable of causing human disease thrive.

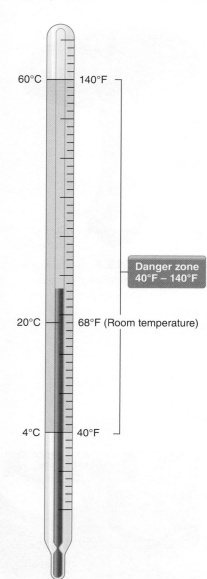

FIGURE 13.7 The danger zone is a range of temperature at which many pathogenic microorganisms thrive. Notice that "room temperature" (about 68°F) is within the danger zone!

and their reproduction can be slowed by refrigeration and freezing. We identify safe cooking and food-storage temperatures later in this chapter.

- **Humidity.** Many microorganisms require a high level of moisture; thus, foods such as boxed dried pasta do not make suitable microbial homes, although cooked pasta left at room temperature would prove hospitable.
- **Acidity.** Most microorganisms have a preferred pH range in which they thrive. For instance, *Clostridium botulinum* loves alkaline environments. It cannot grow or produce its toxin in acidic environments, so the risk for botulism is decreased in citrus fruits, pickles, and tomato-based foods. In contrast, alkaline foods, such as fish and most vegetables, are a magnet for *C. botulinum*.
- **Oxygen content.** Many microorganisms require oxygen to function; thus, food-preservation techniques that remove oxygen, such as industrial canning and bottling, keep foods safe for consumption. In contrast, *C. botulinum* thrives in an oxygen-free environment. For this reason, the canning process heats foods to an extremely high temperature to destroy this organism. It is not uncommon for food producers to voluntarily recall canned goods because of concerns that the food had not been heated high enough to destroy *C. botulinum*.

In addition, microorganisms need an entryway into a food. Just as our skin protects our body from microbial invasion, the peels, rinds, and shells of many foods seal off access to the nutrients within. Eggshells are a good example of a natural food barrier. Once such a barrier is removed, however, the food loses its primary defense against contamination.

recap Food infections result from the consumption of food containing living microorganisms, such as bacteria, whereas food intoxications result from consuming food containing toxins. The body has several defense mechanisms that help rid us of offending microorganisms or their toxins. In order to reproduce in foods, microorganisms require a precise range of temperature, humidity, acidity, and oxygen content.

How can you prevent foodborne illness?

The United States Department of Agriculture's Fight BAC! logo identifies four basic rules for food safety **(FIGURE 13.8)**.

Clean: Wash Your Hands and Kitchen Surfaces Often

One of the easiest and most effective ways to prevent foodborne illness is to wash your hands before and after handling food. Remove any rings or bracelets before you begin, because jewelry can harbor bacteria. Scrub for at least 20 seconds with a mild soap, being sure to wash underneath your fingernails and between your fingers. Rinse under warm, running water. Although you should wash dishes in hot water, it's too harsh for hand washing: it causes the surface layer of the skin to break down, increasing the risk that microorganisms will be able to penetrate your skin. Dry your hands on a clean towel or fresh paper towel.

Thoroughly wash utensils, containers, cutting boards, and countertops with soap and hot water. Rinse. You may sanitize them with a solution of 1 tablespoon (or more) of chlorine bleach to 1 gallon of water. Flood the surface with the bleach solution and allow it to air dry. Wash fruits and vegetables thoroughly under running water just before eating, cutting, or cooking them. Washing fruits and vegetables with soap or detergent or using commercial produce washes is not recommended.[22]

Separate: Don't Cross-Contaminate

cross-contamination Contamination of one food by another via the unintended transfer of microorganisms through physical contact.

Cross-contamination is the spread of microorganisms from one food to another. This commonly occurs when raw foods, such as chicken and vegetables, are cut using the same knife, prepared on the same cutting board, or stored on the same plate. Keep raw meat, poultry, eggs, and seafood and their juices away from ready-to-eat

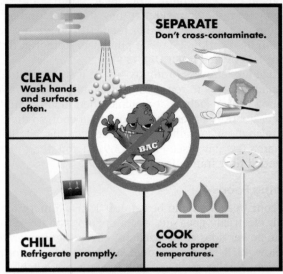

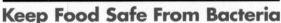

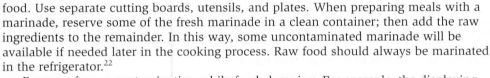

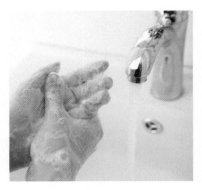

One of the most effective strategies for preventing foodborne illness is simply to wash your hands thoroughly.

➤ **FIGURE 13.8** Fight BAC! is the food-safety logo of the U.S. Department of Agriculture.

food. Use separate cutting boards, utensils, and plates. When preparing meals with a marinade, reserve some of the fresh marinade in a clean container; then add the raw ingredients to the remainder. In this way, some uncontaminated marinade will be available if needed later in the cooking process. Raw food should always be marinated in the refrigerator.[22]

Beware of cross-contamination while food shopping. For example, the displaying of food products such as cooked shrimp on the same bed of ice as raw seafood is not safe, nor is slicing cold cuts with the same knife used to trim raw meat. Report such practices to your local health authorities.

Chill: Store Foods in the Refrigerator or Freezer

The third rule for keeping food safe from bacteria is to promptly refrigerate or freeze it. Remember the danger zone: microorganisms that cause foodborne illness can reproduce rapidly in foods left at room temperature. Refrigeration (at or below 40°F) and freezing (at or below 0°F)[23] do not kill all microorganisms, but cold temperatures diminish their ability to reproduce in quantities large enough to cause illness. Also, many naturally occurring enzymes that cause food spoilage are deactivated at cold temperatures.

Shopping for Perishable Foods

When shopping for food, purchase refrigerated and frozen foods last. Put packaged meat, poultry, or fish into a plastic bag before placing it in your shopping cart. This prevents drippings from those foods from coming into contact with others in your cart.

When choosing perishable foods, check the "sell by" or "best used by" date on the label. The "sell by" date indicates the last day a product can be sold and still maintain its quality during normal home storage and consumption. The "best used by" date tells you how long a product will maintain optimum quality before eating.[24] If the stamped date has passed, don't purchase the item and notify the store manager. These foods should be promptly removed from the shelves.

After you purchase perishable foods, get them home and into the refrigerator or freezer within 1 hour. If your trip home will be longer than an hour, take along a cooler to transport them in.

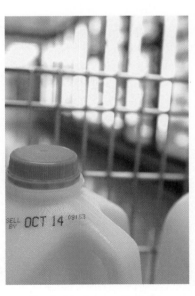

The "sell by" date tells the store how long to display the product for sale.

Refrigerating Foods at Home

As soon as you get home from shopping, put meats, eggs, cheeses, milk, and any other perishable foods in the refrigerator. Store meat, poultry, and seafood in the back of the refrigerator away from the door, so that they stay cold, and on the lowest shelf, so that their juices do not drip onto any other foods. If you are not going to use raw poultry, fish, or ground beef within 2 days of purchase, store it in the freezer. A guide for refrigerating foods is provided in **FIGURE 13.9**.

After a meal, refrigerate leftovers promptly—even if still hot—to discourage microbial growth. The standard rule is to refrigerate leftovers within *2 hours* of serving.[23] If the temperature is above 90°F, such as at a picnic, then foods should be refrigerated within 1 hour. A larger quantity of food takes longer to cool, so divide and conquer: separate leftovers into shallow containers for quicker cooling.[23] Finally, avoid keeping leftovers for more than a few days (see Figure 13.9). If you don't plan to finish a dish within the recommended time frame, freeze it.

Freezing and Thawing Foods

The temperature in your freezer should be set at 0°F. Use a thermometer and check it periodically. If your electricity goes out, avoid opening the freezer until the power is restored. When the power does come back on, check the temperature on the top shelf. If it is at or below 40°F, the food should still be safe to eat, or refreeze.

As with refrigeration, smaller packages will freeze more quickly. So rather than attempting to freeze an entire casserole, divide the food into multiple small portions in freezer-safe containers; then freeze.

Sufficient thawing will ensure adequate cooking throughout, which is essential to preventing foodborne illness. Thaw poultry on the bottom shelf of the refrigerator in a large bowl to catch its juices. Never thaw frozen meat, poultry, or seafood on a kitchen counter or in a basin of warm water. Room temperatures allow growth of bacteria on the surface of food. You can also thaw foods in your microwave, following the manufacturer's instructions.

Dealing with Molds in Refrigerated Foods

Some molds like cool temperatures. Mold spores are common in the atmosphere, and they randomly land on food in open containers. If the temperature and acidity of the food are hospitable, they will grow.

> For more information about thawing foods safely, check out www.fsis.usda.gov. Click through on "Topics," then "Fact Sheets," then "Safe Food Handling," and finally click on "The Big Thaw."

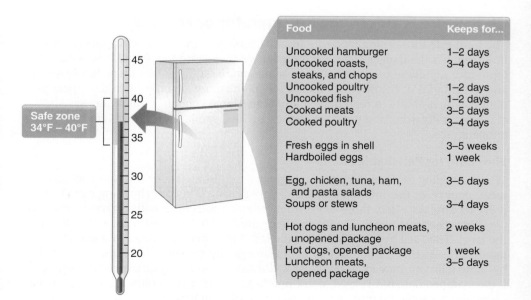

Food	Keeps for...
Uncooked hamburger	1–2 days
Uncooked roasts, steaks, and chops	3–4 days
Uncooked poultry	1–2 days
Uncooked fish	1–2 days
Cooked meats	3–5 days
Cooked poultry	3–4 days
Fresh eggs in shell	3–5 weeks
Hardboiled eggs	1 week
Egg, chicken, tuna, ham, and pasta salads	3–5 days
Soups or stews	3–4 days
Hot dogs and luncheon meats, unopened package	2 weeks
Hot dogs, opened package	1 week
Luncheon meats, opened package	3–5 days

Safe zone 34°F – 40°F

FIGURE 13.9 Although it's important to keep a well-stocked refrigerator, it's also important to know how long foods will keep.

Data from: U.S. Department of Agriculture, Food Safety and Inspection Service. May 11, 2010. Fact Sheets. Safe Food Handling. Refrigeration and Food Safety.

If the surface of a small portion of a solid food, such as hard cheese, becomes moldy, it is generally safe to cut off that section down to about an inch and eat the unspoiled portion. However, if soft cheese, sour cream, tomato sauce, or another soft or fluid product becomes moldy, discard it.

Cook: Heat Foods Thoroughly

Thoroughly cooking food is a sure way to kill the intestinal worms discussed earlier and many other microorganisms. Color and texture are unreliable indicators of safety. Use a food thermometer to ensure that you have cooked food to a safe minimum internal temperature to destroy any harmful bacteria. Place the thermometer in the thickest part of the food, away from bone, fat, or gristle.[22] See the **Quick Tips** box for advice on grilling and barbequing foods.

Microwave cooking is convenient, but you need to be sure your food is thoroughly and evenly cooked and that there are no cold spots in the food where bacteria can thrive. For best results, cover food, stir often, and rotate for even cooking. Raw and semi-raw (such as marinated or partly cooked) fish delicacies, including sushi and sashimi, may be tempting, but their safety cannot be guaranteed. Always cook fish thoroughly. When done, fish should be opaque and flake easily with a fork. If you're wondering how sushi restaurants can guarantee the safety of their food, the short answer is they can't. All fish to be used for sushi must be flash frozen in a process that effectively kills any parasites that are in the fish, but does not necessarily kill bacteria or viruses. In April 2012, 316 people in 26 states experienced foodborne illness after consuming sushi made with tuna contaminated with *Salmonella* bacteria.[26] Thus, eating raw seafood remains risky. For this reason pregnant women and others at increased risk for foodborne illness are advised to avoid it.[27]

> The safe minimum cooking temperatures for the doneness of meat, poultry, seafood, eggs, and leftovers are identified in a table at www.foodsafety.gov. Go to the pull-down menu for "Keep Food Safe" and scroll down to "Charts: Food Safety at a Glance."

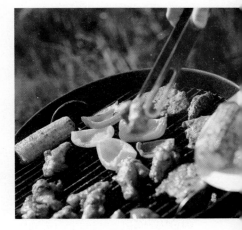

At a barbecue, it's essential to heat foods to the proper temperature.

QuickTips

Staying Food-Safe at Your Next Barbecue

It's the end of the term and you and your friends are planning a lakeside barbecue to celebrate! Here are some tips from the U.S. Food and Drug Administration for preventing foodborne illness at any outdoor gathering.[25]

✓ **Wash your hands, utensils, and food-preparation surfaces.** Even in outdoor settings, food safety begins with hand washing. Take along a water jug, some soap, and paper towels or a box of moist disposable towelettes. Keep all utensils and platters clean when preparing foods.

✓ **Keep foods cold during transport.** Use coolers with ice or frozen gel packs to keep food at or below 40°F. It's easier to maintain a cold temperature in small coolers. Consider packing three: put beverages in one cooler, washed fruits and vegetables and containers of potato salad in another, and wrapped, frozen meat, poultry, and seafood in another. Keep coolers in the air-conditioned passenger compartment of your car, rather than in a hot trunk.

✓ **Grill foods thoroughly.** Use a food thermometer to be sure the food has reached an adequate internal temperature before serving.

✓ **Avoid cross-contamination.** When taking food from the grill to the table, never use the same platter or utensils that previously held raw meat or seafood!

✓ **Keep hot foods hot.** Keep grilled food hot until it is served by moving it to the side of the grill, just away from the coals, so that it stays at or above 140°F. If grilled food isn't going to be eaten right away, wrap it well and place it in an insulated container.

✓ **Keep cold foods cold.** Cold foods, such as chicken salad, should be kept in a bowl of ice during your barbecue. Drain off water as the ice melts and replace the ice frequently. Don't let any perishable food sit out longer than 2 hours. In temperatures above 90°F, don't let food sit out for more than 1 hour.

You may have memories of licking cake batter off a spoon when you were a kid, but such practices are no longer considered safe. That's because most cake batter contains raw eggs, one of the most common sources of *Salmonella*. The USDA recommends that you cook eggs until firm.

Protect Yourself from Toxins in Foods

Killing microorganisms with heat is an important step in keeping food safe, but it won't protect you against their toxins. That's because many toxins are unaffected by heat and are capable of causing severe illness even when the microorganisms that produced them have been destroyed. For example, let's say you prepare a casserole for a team picnic. Too bad you forget to wash your hands before serving it to your teammates because you contaminate the casserole with the bacterium *Staphylococcus aureus*, which is commonly found on skin. You and your friends go off and play soccer, leaving the food in the sun, and a few hours later you take the rest of the casserole home. At supper, you heat the leftovers thoroughly, thinking that this will kill any bacteria that multiplied while it was left out. That night you experience nausea, severe vomiting, and abdominal pain. What happened? While your food was left out, *Staphylococcus* multiplied in the casserole and produced a toxin (**FIGURE 13.10**). When

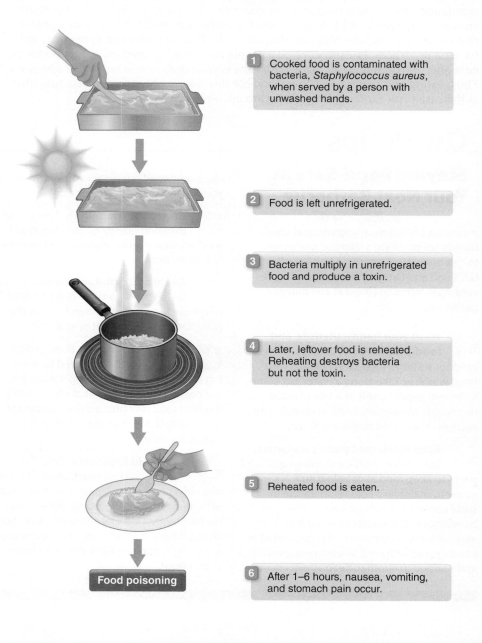

1. Cooked food is contaminated with bacteria, *Staphylococcus aureus*, when served by a person with unwashed hands.

2. Food is left unrefrigerated.

3. Bacteria multiply in unrefrigerated food and produce a toxin.

4. Later, leftover food is reheated. Reheating destroys bacteria but not the toxin.

5. Reheated food is eaten.

Food poisoning

6. After 1–6 hours, nausea, vomiting, and stomach pain occur.

▶ **FIGURE 13.10** Food contamination can occur long after the microorganism itself has been destroyed.

you reheated the food, you killed the microorganisms, but their toxin was unaffected by the heat. When you then ate the food, the toxin made you sick.

Be Choosy When Eating Out—Close to Home or Far Away

When choosing a place to eat out, avoid restaurants that don't look clean. Grimy tabletops and dirty restrooms indicate indifference to hygiene. On the other hand, cleanliness of areas used by the public doesn't guarantee that the kitchen is clean. That is why health inspections are important. Public health inspectors randomly visit and inspect the food-preparation areas of all businesses that serve food, whether eaten in or taken out. When in doubt, check the inspection results posted in the restaurant.

Another way to protect yourself when dining out is by ordering foods to be cooked thoroughly. If you order a hamburger and it arrives pink in the middle, or scrambled eggs and they arrive runny, send the food back to be cooked thoroughly.

When planning a trip, tell your physician your travel plans and ask about vaccinations needed or any medications that you should take along in case you get sick. Pack a waterless antibacterial hand cleanser and use it frequently. When dining, select foods and beverages carefully (see Chapter 3). All raw food has the potential for contamination.

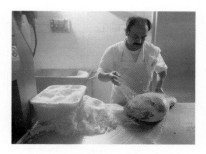

◆ A worker salting a Parma ham.

recap Foodborne illness can be prevented at home by following four tips: Clean: wash your hands and kitchen surfaces often. Separate: isolate foods to prevent cross-contamination. Chill: store foods in the refrigerator or freezer. Cook: heat foods long enough and at the correct temperatures to ensure proper cooking. When eating out, avoid restaurants that don't look clean, and ask that all food be cooked thoroughly.

How is food spoilage prevented?

Any food that has been harvested and that people aren't ready to eat must be preserved in some way or, before long, it will degrade enzymatically and become home to a variety of microorganisms. Even **processed foods** have the potential to spoil.

The most ancient methods of preserving foods include salting, sugaring, drying, and smoking, all of which draw the water out of the plant or animal cells. By dehydrating the food, these methods make it inhospitable to microorganisms and dramatically slow the action of enzymes that would otherwise degrade the food. Natural methods of cooling also have been used for centuries, including storing foods in underground cellars, caves, running streams, and even "cold pantries"—north-facing rooms of the house that were kept dark and unheated and often were stocked with ice.

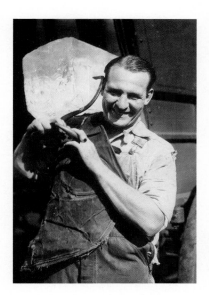

◆ Before the modern refrigerator, an iceman would deliver ice to homes and businesses.

nutri-case | THEO

"I got really sick yesterday after eating lunch in the cafeteria. I had a turkey sandwich, potato salad, and a cola. A few hours later, in the middle of basketball practice, I started to shake and sweat. I felt really nauseated and barely made it to the bathroom before vomiting. Then I went back to my dorm room and crawled into bed. This morning I still feel a little sick to my stomach, and sort of weak. I asked a couple of my friends who ate in the cafeteria yesterday if they got sick, and neither of them did, but I still think it was the food. I'm going off-campus for lunch from now on!"

Do you think that Theo's illness was foodborne? If so, what food(s) do you most suspect? What do you think of his plan to go off-campus for lunch from now on?

processed foods Foods that are manipulated mechanically or chemically.

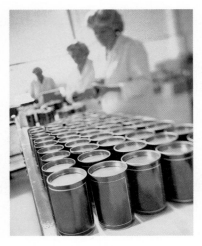

⬆ Canning food involves several steps to ensure all microorganisms in the food are killed.

More recently, technological advances have helped food producers preserve the integrity of their products for months and even years between harvesting and consumption:

- **Canning.** Developed in the late 1700s, canning involves washing and blanching the food, placing it in cans, siphoning out the air, sealing the cans, and then heating them to a very high temperature. Canned food has an average shelf life of at least 2 years from the date of purchase.

- **Pasteurization.** The technique called **pasteurization** exposes a beverage or other food to heat high enough to destroy microorganisms but for a short enough period that the taste and quality of the food are not affected. For example, in *flash pasteurization*, milk or other liquids are heated to 162°F (72°C) for 15 seconds. Although some people claim that unpasteurized juices and ciders taste better, drinking these products puts you at risk for foodborne illness.

- **Irradiation.** In **irradiation**—a process that exposes foods to gamma rays from radioactive metals—energy from the rays penetrates food and its packaging, killing or disabling microorganisms in the food. The process does not cause foods to become radioactive! A few nutrients, including thiamin and vitamins A, E, and K, are lost, but these losses are also incurred in conventional processing and preparation. Although irradiated food has been shown to be safe, the FDA requires that all irradiated foods be labeled with a "radura" symbol and a caution against irradiating the food again (**FIGURE 13.11**).

- **Aseptic packaging.** You probably know aseptic packaging best as "juice boxes." Food and beverages are first heated, then cooled, then placed in sterile containers. The process uses less energy and materials than traditional canning, and the average shelf life is about 6 months.

- **Modified atmosphere packaging.** In this process, the oxygen in a package of food is replaced with an inert gas, such as nitrogen or carbon dioxide. This prevents a number of chemical reactions that spoil food, and it slows the growth of bacteria that require oxygen. The process can be used with a variety of foods, including meats, fish, vegetables, and fruits.

- **High-pressure processing** is a technique in which the food to be preserved is subjected to an extremely high pressure. This inactivates most bacteria while retaining the food's quality and freshness.

⬆ **FIGURE 13.11** The U.S. Food and Drug Administration requires the Radura—the international symbol of irradiated food—to be displayed on all irradiated food sold in the United States.

recap Salting, sugaring, drying, smoking, and cooling have been used for centuries to preserve food. Canning, pasteurization, irradiation, and several packaging techniques are used to preserve a variety of foods during shipping as well as on grocer and consumer shelves.

What are food additives, and are they safe?

Have you ever picked up a loaf of bread and started reading its ingredients? You'd expect to see flour, yeast, water, and some sugar, but what are all those other items? They are collectively called *food additives,* and they are in almost every processed food. **Food additives** are chemicals that don't occur naturally in the food but are added to enhance the food in some way. More than 3,000 different food additives are currently used in the United States. **TABLE 13.3** identifies only a few of the most common.

Food Additives Include Nutrients and Preservatives

Vitamins and minerals are added to foods as nutrients and as preservatives. Vitamin E is usually added to fat-based products to keep them from going rancid, and vitamin C is used as an antioxidant in many foods. Iodine is added to table salt to help decrease the incidence of goiter, a condition that causes the thyroid gland to enlarge. Vitamin D is added to milk, and calcium is added to soy milk, rice milk, almond milk, and some juices to promote bone health. Folate is added to cereals, breads, and other foods to help prevent certain types of birth defects.

pasteurization A form of sterilization using high temperatures for short periods.

irradiation A sterilization process in which food is exposed to gamma rays or high-energy electron beams to kill microorganisms. Irradiation does not impart any radiation to the food being treated.

food additive A substance or mixture of substances intentionally put into food to enhance its appearance, safety, palatability, and quality.

Polluted Packaging?

In December 2009, *Consumer Reports* magazine reported that it had found a chemical called bisphenol A, or BPA, in nearly all of the canned foods it had tested, from soups to infant formula. BPA is a synthetic hormone, which some research has linked to genital abnormalities, breast and prostate cancer, miscarriage, and other disorders. In addition to cans, BPA is found in plastic bottles, cups, dinnerware, toys, and many other products.

Weeks after the report, the FDA began conducting research into the effects of BPA. In 2012, the agency published its conclusions. Reviews of hundreds of studies did not suggest that the very low levels of human exposure to BPA through the diet were unsafe.[28] Nonetheless, later that year, the FDA banned the use of BPA in baby bottles and sippy cups.[29]

Here is information from the FDA for consumers who want to limit their exposure to BPA:[28, 29]

- Reduce your consumption of canned foods.

- Plastic containers have recycle codes on the bottom. Some plastics marked with codes 3 or 7 may be made with BPA. Do not put hot or boiling beverages or foods (coffee, soups, and others) in these containers, and do not microwave foods in these containers. BPA levels in beverages and foods rise when the containers become heated.

- Discard all plastic containers with scratches because these may harbor bacteria and, if they contain BPA, may lead to greater release.

- Whenever possible, opt for glass, porcelain, or stainless steel containers for beverages and foods.

The following two preservatives have raised health concerns:

- **Sulfites.** A small segment of the population is sensitive to sulfites, preservatives used in many beers and wines and some other processed foods. These people can experience asthma, headaches, or other symptoms after eating food containing the offending preservatives.
- **Nitrites.** Commonly used to preserve processed meats, nitrites can be converted to *nitrosamines* during the cooking process. Nitrosamines have been found to be carcinogenic in animals, so the FDA has required all foods with nitrites to contain additional antioxidants to decrease the formation of nitrosamines.

Other Food Additives Include Flavorings, Colorings, and Other Agents

Flavoring agents are used to replace the natural flavors lost during food processing. In contrast, *flavor enhancers* have little or no flavor of their own but accentuate the natural flavor of foods. One of the most common flavor enhancers used is monosodium glutamate (MSG). In some people, MSG causes symptoms such as headaches, difficulty breathing, and heart palpitations.

Common food *colorings* include beet juice, which imparts a red color; beta-carotene, which gives a yellow color; and caramel, which adds brown color. The coloring tartrazine (FD&C Yellow #5) causes an allergic reaction in some people, and its use must be indicated on the product packaging.

Texturizers are added to foods to improve their texture. *Emulsifiers* help keep fats evenly dispersed within foods. *Stabilizers* give foods "body" and help them maintain a desired texture or color. *Humectants* keep foods such as marshmallows, chewing gum, and shredded coconut moist and stretchy. *Desiccants* prevent moisture absorption from the air; for example, they are used to prevent table salt from forming clumps.[30]

Are Food Additives Safe?

Federal legislation was passed in 1958 to regulate food additives. The Delaney Clause, also enacted in 1958, states, "No additive may be permitted in any amount if tests show it produces cancer when fed to man or animals or by other appropriate tests." Before a new additive can be used in food, the producer of the additive must submit data

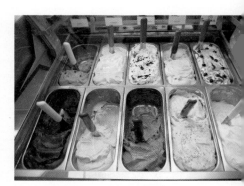

Many foods, such as ice cream, contain colorings.

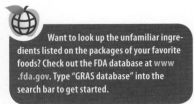

Want to look up the unfamiliar ingredients listed on the packages of your favorite foods? Check out the FDA database at www.fda.gov. Type "GRAS database" into the search bar to get started.

TABLE 13.3   Examples of Common Food Additives

Food Additive	Foods Found In
Coloring Agents	
Beet extract	Beverages, candies, ice cream
Beta-carotene	Beverages, sauces, soups, baked goods, candies, macaroni and cheese mixes
Caramel	Beverages, sauces, soups, baked goods
Tartrazine	Beverages, cakes and cookies, ice cream
Preservatives	
Alpha-tocopherol (vitamin E)	Vegetable oils
Ascorbic acid (vitamin C)	Breakfast cereals, cured meats, fruit drinks
BHA	Breakfast cereals, chewing gum, oils, potato chips
BHT	Breakfast cereals, chewing gum, oils, potato chips
Calcium proprionate/sodium proprionate	Bread, cakes, pies, rolls
EDTA	Beverages, canned shellfish, margarine, mayonnaise, processed fruits and vegetables, sandwich spreads
Propyl gallate	Mayonnaise, chewing gum, chicken soup base, vegetable oils, meat products, potato products, fruits, ice cream
Sodium benzoate	Carbonated beverages, fruit juice, pickles, preserves
Sodium chloride (salt)	Most processed foods
Sodium nitrate/sodium nitrite	Bacon, corned beef, lunch meats, smoked fish
Sorbic acid/potassium sorbate	Cakes, cheese, dried fruits, jellies, syrups, wine
Sulfites (sodium bisulfite, sulfur dioxide)	Dried fruits, processed potatoes, wine
Texturizers, Emulsifiers, and Stabilizers	
Calcium chloride	Canned fruits and vegetables
Carageenan/pectin	Ice cream, chocolate milk, soy milk, frostings, jams, jellies, cheese, salad dressings, sour cream, puddings, syrups
Cellulose gum/guar gum/gum arabic/locust gum/xanthan gum	Soups and sauces, gravies, sour cream, ricotta cheese, ice cream, syrups
Gelatin	Desserts, canned meats
Lecithin	Mayonnaise, ice cream
Humectants	
Glycerin	Chewing gum, marshmallows, shredded coconut
Propylene glycol	Chewing gum, gummy candies

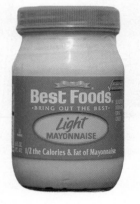

Mayonnaise contains emulsifiers to prevent separation of fats.

Generally Recognized as Safe (GRAS) List established by Congress to identify substances used in foods that are generally recognized as safe based on a history of long-term use or on the consensus of qualified research experts.

demonstrating its safety to the FDA, which then determines the additive's safety based on these data.

Also in 1958, the U.S. Congress recognized that many substances added to foods would not require this type of formal review by the FDA prior to marketing and use because their safety had already been established through long-term use or because their safety had been recognized by qualified experts through scientific studies. These substances are exempt from the more stringent testing criteria for new food additives and are referred to as substances that are **Generally Recognized as Safe (GRAS)**.

In 1985, the FDA established the Adverse Reaction Monitoring System (ARMS). Under this system, the FDA investigates complaints from consumers, physicians, and food companies about food additives.

recap Food additives are chemicals intentionally added to foods to enhance their color, flavor, texture, nutrient density, moisture level, or shelf life. Although there is continuing controversy over food additives in the United States, the FDA regulates additives used in our food supply and considers safe those it approves. The GRAS list identifies substances that have either been tested and determined by the FDA to be safe and approved for use in the food industry or are deemed safe as a result of consensus among experts qualified by scientific training and experience

How is genetic modification used in food production?

In **genetic modification**, also referred to as *genetic engineering,* the genetic material, or DNA, of an organism is altered to bring about specific changes in its seeds or offspring. Selective breeding is one example of genetic modification; for example, Brahman cattle, which have poor-quality meat but high resistance to heat and humidity, are bred with English shorthorn cattle, which have good meat but low resistance to heat and humidity. The outcome of this selective breeding process is Santa Gertrudis cattle, which have the desired characteristics of higher-quality meat and resistance to heat and humidity. Although selective breeding is effective and has helped increase crop yields and improve the quality and quantity of our food supply, it is a relatively slow and imprecise process because a great deal of trial and error typically occurs before the desired characteristics are achieved.

Recently, advances in biotechnology have moved genetic modification beyond selective breeding. These advances include the manipulation of the DNA of living cells of one organism to produce the desired characteristics of a different organism. Called **recombinant DNA technology**, the process commonly begins when scientists isolate from an animal, a plant, or a microbial cell a particular segment of DNA—one or more genes—that codes for a protein conferring a desirable trait, such as salt tolerance in tomato plants **(FIGURE 13.12)**. Scientists then splice the DNA into a "host cell," usually a microorganism. The cell is cultured to produce many copies—a *gene library*—of the beneficial gene. Then, many scientists can readily obtain the gene to modify other organisms that lack the desired trait—for example, traditional tomato plants. The modified DNA causes the plant's cells to build the protein of interest, and the plant expresses the desired trait. The term *genetically modified organism* (GMO) refers to any organism in which the DNA has been altered using recombinant DNA technology.

Cultivation of GMO food crops began in 1996. Typically, they have been used to induce resistance to pesticides. This means that genetically modified crops can be sprayed more liberally with chemicals that kill weeds and insects—in theory, without harming the crops or the surrounding ecology. Genetic modification can also increase a plant's resistance to disease or make crops more tolerant of environmental

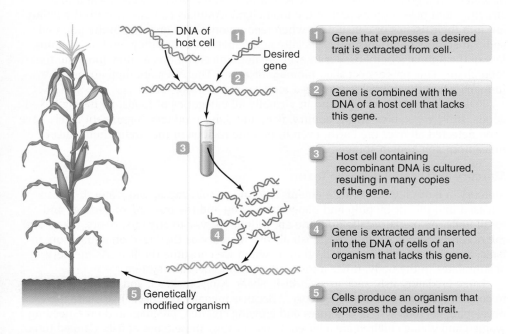

1 Gene that expresses a desired trait is extracted from cell.

2 Gene is combined with the DNA of a host cell that lacks this gene.

3 Host cell containing recombinant DNA is cultured, resulting in many copies of the gene.

4 Gene is extracted and inserted into the DNA of cells of an organism that lacks this gene.

5 Cells produce an organism that expresses the desired trait.

◆ **FIGURE 13.12** Recombinant DNA technology involves producing plants and other organisms that contain modified DNA, which enables them to express desirable traits that are not present in the original organism.

genetic modification The process of changing an organism by manipulating its genetic material.

recombinant DNA technology A type of genetic modification in which scientists combine DNA from different sources to produce a transgenic organism that expresses a desired trait.

conditions, such as drought or poor soil. Another use is to increase the nutritional value of a crop. Researchers have modified soybeans and canola, for instance, to increase their content of monounsaturated fatty acids.

Since 1996, an increasing number and quantity of food crops have been genetically modified. The most common are corn and soybeans. The USDA reports that, in 2012, 88% of all corn crops and 93% of all soybean crops grown in the United States were genetically engineered varieties.[31] As the use of genetic modification increases, however, critics are pointing to research indicating that their risks may outweigh their benefits, not only to the environment but also to human health. For more information on this controversy, see the **Nutrition Debate** at the end of this chapter.

recap In genetic modification, the genetic material, or DNA, of an organism is altered to enhance certain qualities. In agriculture, genetic modification is often used to improve crop protection or to increase nutrients in the resulting food. Genetic modification is also used in animals and microorganisms.

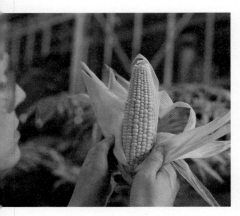

⬆ Corn is one of the most widely cultivated genetically modified crops.

How do residues harm our food supply?

Food **residues** are chemicals that remain in foods despite cleaning and processing. Three types of residues of global concern are persistent organic pollutants, pesticides, and the hormones and antibiotics used in animals. The health concerns related to residues include skin rashes, nerve damage, cancer, and the development of antibiotic-resistant pathogenic bacteria.

Persistent Organic Pollutants Can Cause Illness

Some chemicals released into the atmosphere as a result of industry, agriculture, automobile emissions, and improper waste disposal can persist in soil or water for years or even decades. These chemicals, collectively referred to as **persistent organic pollutants (POPs)**, can travel thousands of miles in gases or as airborne particles in rain, snow, rivers, and oceans, eventually entering the food supply through the soil or water.[32] If a pollutant gets into the soil, a plant can absorb the chemical into its structure and pass it on as part of the food chain. Animals can also absorb the pollutant into their tissues or consume it when feeding on plants growing in the polluted soil. Fat-soluble pollutants are especially problematic because they tend to accumulate in the animal's body tissues in ever greater concentrations as they move up the food chain. This process is called **biomagnification**. The POPs are then absorbed by humans when the animal is used as a food source **(FIGURE 13.13)**.

POP residues have been found in virtually all categories of foods, including baked goods, fruit, vegetables, meat, poultry, fish, and dairy products. Significant levels have been detected all over the Earth, even in pristine regions of the Arctic thousands of miles from any known source.[32]

Mercury and Lead Are Nerve Toxins

Mercury, a naturally occurring element, is found in soil, rocks, and water. It is also released into the air by pulp and paper processing and the burning of garbage and fossil fuels. As mercury falls from the air, it finds its way to streams, rivers, lakes, and the ocean, where it accumulates. Fish absorb mercury as they feed on aquatic organisms, and this mercury is passed on to us when we consume the fish. As mercury accumulates in the body, it has a toxic effect on the nervous system.

Large predatory fish, such as swordfish, shark, King mackerel, and tilefish, tend to contain the highest levels of mercury.[33] Because mercury is especially toxic to the developing nervous system of fetuses and growing children, pregnant and breastfeeding women and young children are advised to avoid eating these types of fish. Canned tuna, salmon, cod, pollock, sole, shrimp, mussels, and scallops do not contain high levels of mercury and are safe to consume; however, the FDA recommends that pregnant women and young children eat no more than two servings (12 oz) per week of any type of fish.[33]

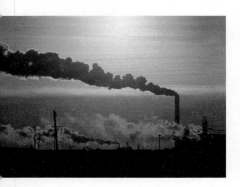

⬆ One of the ways mercury is released into the environment is by burning fossil fuels.

residues Chemicals that remain in the foods we eat despite cleaning and processing.

persistent organic pollutants (POPs) Chemicals released into the environment as a result of industry, agriculture, or improper waste disposal; automobile emissions also are considered POPs.

biomagnification Process by which persistent organic pollutants become more concentrated in animal tissues as they move from one creature to another through the food chain.

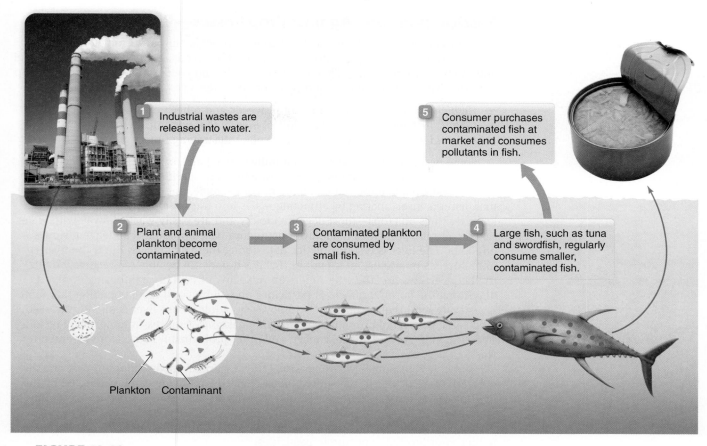

1 Industrial wastes are released into water.

2 Plant and animal plankton become contaminated.

3 Contaminated plankton are consumed by small fish.

4 Large fish, such as tuna and swordfish, regularly consume smaller, contaminated fish.

5 Consumer purchases contaminated fish at market and consumes pollutants in fish.

Plankton   Contaminant

FIGURE 13.13   Biomagnification of persistent organic pollutants in the food supply.

Lead is another POP of concern. It can be found naturally in the soil, water, and air but also occurs as industrial waste from leaded gasoline, lead-based paints, and lead-soldered cans, now outlawed but decomposing in landfills. Older homes may have high levels of lead paint dust, or the lead paint may be peeling in chips, which young children may put it their mouths. Some ceramic mugs and other dishes are fired with lead-based glaze, allowing residues to build up in foods. Excessive lead exposure can cause serious learning and behavioral disorders in children and cardio-vascular and kidney disease in adults.

Dioxins Are Carcinogens

Dioxins are industrial pollutants typically formed as a result of combustion processes, such as waste incineration or the burning of wood, coal, or oil. Dioxins enter the soil and can persist in the environment for many years. Thus, even though dioxin levels have been declining for the last 30 years, largely as a result of increased regulation, some of the dioxins emitted decades ago will still be in the environment years from now.

There is concern that long-term exposure to dioxins can result in an increased risk for cancer and other disorders.[34] Because dioxins easily accumulate in the fatty tissues of animals, most dioxin exposure in humans occurs through dietary intake of animal fats.[35] Whereas the EPA has been working to reduce dioxin emissions into the environment, the USDA and the FDA have been collaborating on efforts to monitor the dioxin levels in the U.S. food supply and to reduce levels of all types of dioxins. If a particular food is shown to have high dioxin levels and the source can be determined, the agencies work to eliminate that source. To reduce your personal exposure to dioxins, eat meat less frequently, trim the fat from the meats you consume, and avoid fatty meats. Choose non-fat milk and yogurt and low-fat cheeses, and replace butter with plant oils.

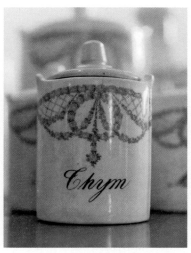

Antique porcelain is often coated with lead-based glaze.

Pesticides Protect Against Crop Losses—But at a Cost

Pesticides are a family of chemicals used in both fields and farm storage areas to decrease the destruction and crop losses caused by weeds, animals, insects, and fungi and other microorganisms. They increase overall crop yield and allow for greater crop diversity. The three most common types of pesticides used in food production are:

- *Herbicides,* which are used to control weeds and other unwanted plant growth
- *Insecticides,* which are used to control insects that can infest crops
- *Fungicides,* which are used to control plant-destroying fungal growth

Some pesticides used today are naturally derived and/or have a low impact on the environment. These include **biopesticides**, which are species-specific and work to suppress a pest's population, not eliminate it. For example, pheromones are a biopesticide that disrupts insect mating by attracting males into traps. Biopesticides also do not leave residues on crops—most degrade rapidly and are easily washed away with water.

In contrast, pesticides made from petroleum-based products can leave residues on foods. The liver is responsible for detoxifying these chemicals. But if the liver is immature, as in a fetus, an infant, or a child, it may not be able to effectively detoxify the pesticides. In 2012, the American Academy of Pediatrics published a report describing the harmful effects of pesticides on children and recommending that families strictly limit their exposure.[36] Moreover, an adult whose liver is already stressed by disease or alcohol abuse may suffer physical consequences from pesticide residues. These include nerve damage, cancer, and other problems. It is therefore essential to wash all produce carefully.

The EPA is responsible for regulating the labeling, sale, distribution, use, and disposal of all pesticides in the United States. Before a pesticide can be accepted by the EPA for use, it must be determined that it performs its intended function with minimal impact to the environment. Once the EPA has certified a pesticide, states can set their own regulations for its use. The nearby **Quick Tips** from the EPA can help you reduce your level of exposure to pesticides.

Growth Hormones and Antibiotics Are Used in Animals

Introduced in the U.S. food supply in 1994, **recombinant bovine growth hormone (rBGH)** is a genetically engineered growth hormone. It is used in beef herds to induce animals to grow more muscle tissue and less fat. It is also injected into a third of U.S. dairy cows to increase milk output.

Quick Tips

Reducing Your Exposure to Pesticides

The EPA offers the following strategies for reducing your level of exposure to pesticides.[37]

✓ Wash and scrub all fresh fruits and vegetables thoroughly under running water.

✓ Peel fruits and vegetables whenever possible, and discard the outer leaves of leafy vegetables, such as cabbage and lettuce. Trim the excess fat from meat and remove the skin from poultry and fish because some pesticide residues collect in the fat.

✓ Eat a variety of foods from various sources because this can reduce the risk of exposure to a single pesticide.

✓ Consume more organically grown foods.

✓ If you garden, avoid using fertilizers and pesticides to keep these chemicals out of your groundwater as well as your foods.

✓ Filter your tap water, whether it comes from a municipal water system or a well, to reduce your exposure to pesticides, fertilizers, and other contaminants.

pesticides Chemicals used either in the field or in storage to decrease destruction by predators or disease.

biopesticides Primarily insecticides, these chemicals use natural methods to reduce damage to crops.

recombinant bovine growth hormone (rBGH) A genetically engineered hormone injected into dairy cows to enhance their milk output.

Although the FDA has allowed the use of rBGH in the United States, both Canada and the European Union have banned its use for two reasons:

- The available evidence shows an increased risk for mastitis (inflamed udders) in dairy cows injected with rBGH.[38] Farmers treat mastitis with antibiotics, promoting the development of strains of pathogenic bacteria that are resistant to antibiotics.
- The milk of cows receiving rBGH has higher levels of a hormone called insulin-like growth factor (IGF-1). This hormone can pass into the bloodstream of humans who drink milk from cows that receive rBGH, and some studies have shown that an elevated level of IGF-1 in humans may increase the risk for certain cancers. However, the evidence from these studies is inconclusive.[38]

The American Cancer Society suggests that more research is needed to help better appraise these health risks. In the meantime, consumer concerns about rBGH have caused a significant decline in sales of milk from cows treated with rBGH.[38]

Antibiotics are also routinely given to animals raised for food. For example, they are added to the feed of swine to reduce the number of disease outbreaks in over-crowded pork-production facilities. Many researchers are concerned that cows, pigs, and other animals treated with antibiotics are becoming significant reservoirs for the development of virulent antibiotic-resistant strains of bacteria—so-called "superbugs." In 2011, the National Antimicrobial Resistance Monitoring System, a program of the CDC, FDA, and USDA, conducted tests on supermarket meats. It found that 39% of chicken products, 55% of ground beef, 69% of pork, and 81% of ground turkey harbored significant amounts of superbug bacteria.[39] Another study found a particularly dangerous superbug, methicillin-resistant *Staphylococcus aureus* (MRSA), in 100% of swine 9 to 12 weeks old on hog farms in Illinois and Iowa.[40] This subtype of *Staphylococcus aureus* cannot be effectively treated with methicillin or other beta-lactam antibiotics, including penicillin and amoxicillin. Infection with MRSA can cause symptoms ranging from a mild skin rash to widespread invasion of tissues, including the bloodstream. MRSA blood infections are often fatal.[41]

You can reduce your exposure to growth hormones and antibiotics by choosing organic eggs, milk, yogurt, and cheeses and by eating free-range meat from animals raised without the use of these chemicals. You can also reduce your risk by eating vegetarian and vegan meals more often.

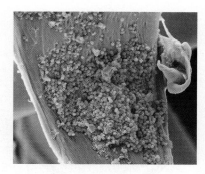

The resistant strain of bacteria responsible for methicillin-resistant *Staphylococcus aureus* (MRSA).

Organic Agriculture Reduces Residues

In the population boom that followed the end of World War II, the demand for food increased dramatically. The American chemical industry helped increase agricultural production by providing a variety of new fertilizers and pesticides, including an insecticide called DDT, which began poisoning not just insects, but fish and birds, from the time it was first released for agricultural use in 1945. Then, in 1962, marine biologist Rachel Carson published *Silent Spring,* a book in which she described the harmful effects of DDT and other synthetic pesticides. The book's title, for example, referred to the effect of pesticides on songbirds, whose extinction would someday lead to a "silent spring." Scientists found Carson's research convincing and readers flocked to her cause, creating a small but ever-growing demand for organic food.

The term **organic** describes foods that are grown without the use of synthetic fertilizers, toxic and persistent pesticides, genetic engineering, or irradiation. A recent national survey indicates that more than 4% of all food products sold in the United States are now organic. Between 1990 and 2011, sales of organic products in the United States skyrocketed from $1 billion to over $31 billion.[42]

To Be Labeled Organic, Foods Must Meet Federal Standards

In 2002, the National Organic Program (NOP) of the USDA established organic standards that provide uniform definitions for all organic products. Any product claiming to be organic must comply with the following definitions:[43]

- *100% organic:* products containing only organically produced ingredients, excluding water and salt

organic Produced without the use of synthetic fertilizers, toxic and persistent pesticides, genetic engineering, or irradiation.

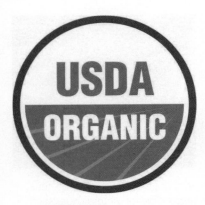

FIGURE 13.14 The USDA organic seal identifies foods that are at least 95% organic.

■ *Organic:* products containing 95% organically produced ingredients by weight, excluding water and salt, with the remaining ingredients consisting of those products not commercially available in organic form

■ *Made with organic ingredients:* a product containing more than 70% organic ingredients

If a processed product contains less than 70% organically produced ingredients, then those products cannot use the term *organic* in the principal display panel, but ingredients that are organically produced can be specified on the ingredients statement on the information panel. Products that are "100% organic" and "organic" may display the USDA organic seal **(FIGURE 13.14)**.

Farms certified as organic must pass an inspection by a government-approved certifier who verifies that the farmer is following all USDA organic standards.[43] Organic farming methods are strict and require farmers to find natural alternatives to many common problems, such as weeds and insects. Contrary to common belief, organic farmers can use pesticides as a final option for pest control when all other methods have proven insufficient, but they are restricted to a limited number that have been approved for use in organic production.[43] Also, to be certified organic, farmers must employ practices that conserve resources, including soil and water, and promote ecological balance and biodiversity.

Organic meat, poultry, eggs, and dairy products come from animals fed only organic feed, and if the animals become ill, they are removed from the others until well again. None of these animals are given growth hormones to increase their size or ability to produce milk.

Research on Nutritional Advantages of Organic Foods Is Inconclusive

Over the past few decades, some studies have found organically grown fruits and vegetables, from strawberries to corn, to be somewhat higher in a limited number of vitamins, minerals, and antioxidant phytochemicals than their non-organic counterparts.[44, 45] However, three recent review studies have not found conclusive evidence of a significant nutritional superiority of organically produced animal and plant foods over the same foods conventionally produced.[46-48] Still, many people choose organic foods because of concerns about their exposure to residues, and, indeed, a 2012 study found that organically produced foods were about 30% less likely to be contaminated with detectable pesticide residues or antibiotic-resistant bacteria.[48]

Earlier we noted that the EPA does advise Americans to reduce their total exposure to pesticides by consuming more organically grown foods. Unfortunately, these tend to cost more than foods conventionally grown. So it makes sense to spend more for organic when the alternative—the conventionally grown version—is likely to retain a high pesticide residue. **TABLE 13.4** identifies twelve foods that the Environmental Working Group advises should be your priority organic purchases. If your food budget is limited, spend your money on the organically grown versions of these foods. The table also identifies the fifteen foods that tend to be lowest in pesticide residues. You can feel confident purchasing conventional versions of these.

recap Persistent organic pollutants (POPs) of concern include mercury, lead, and dioxins. Pesticides are used to prevent or reduce food crop losses but are potential toxins; therefore, it is essential to wash all produce carefully. Use of recombinant bovine growth hormone (rBGH) and antibiotics raises concerns about bovine and human health. The USDA organic seal identifies foods that are at least 95% organic; that is, they have been produced without the use of synthetic fertilizers, toxic and persistent pesticides, genetic engineering, or irradiation.

TABLE 13.4   Shopper's Guide to Pesticides in Produce

The "Dirty Dozen": Buy These Organic	The "Clean Fifteen": Lowest in Pesticides
1. Apples	1. Onions
2. Celery	2. Sweet corn
3. Bell peppers	3. Pineapples
4. Peaches	4. Avocados
5. Strawberries	5. Cabbage
6. Nectarines—imported	6. Sweet peas
7. Grapes	7. Asparagus
8. Spinach	8. Mangoes
9. Lettuce	9. Eggplant
10. Cucumbers	10. Kiwi
11. Blueberries	11. Cantaloupe—domestic
12. Potatoes	12. Sweet potatoes
	13. Grapefruit
	14. Watermelon
	15. Mushrooms

Data from: Environmental Working Group. 2012. EWG's 2012 Shopper's Guide to Pesticides in Produce.

*behavior change . . . getting started!

Now that you've read this chapter, try making these changes:

For yourself:

- Wash your hands before you begin to prepare food or eat!
- Buy a thermometer for your refrigerator and freezer. If you eat meat, buy a meat thermometer. Then start to use them!
- Next time you buy an apple, pay the extra cash for organic. Apples top the list of high-pesticide foods.

For your community:

- Choose an issue covered in this chapter that you'd like to raise awareness of among your friends. Research organizations covering this issue, such as the Worldwatch Institute, the Environmental Working Group, or the Cornucopia Institute. Choose one and "Like it" on your Facebook page.

Genetically Modified Organisms: A Blessing or a Curse?

Genetically modified organisms (GMOs) represent arguably one of the most controversial topics in food science. GMOs are created through *genetic engineering*, a process in which foreign genes are spliced into a nonrelated species, creating an entirely new (*transgenic*) organism. Many GMOs are, of course, animal and plant foods. The terms for these foods—biotech foods, gene foods, and "frankenfoods"—suggest divergent views of their potential benefits and risks to the environment and to human health.

Supporters envision an ever-expanding role for genetic engineering in food production. They identify numerous potential benefits resulting from the application of this technology. These benefits include:

- Enhanced taste and nutritional quality of food
- Crops that grow faster, have higher yields, can be grown in inhospitable soils, and have increased resistance to pests, diseases, herbicides, and spoilage
- Increased production of high-quality meat, eggs, and milk
- Improved animal health due to increased disease resistance and overall hardiness
- Environmentally responsible outcomes such as a reduction in use of an insecticide called Bt; use of less harmful pesticides; conservation of water due largely to the development of drought-tolerant species of corn; reduced use of energy and emmission of greenhouse gases because of reduced need for ploughing and pesticide spraying; and conservation of soil due to higher productivity[49]
- Increased food security for countries struggling with food insecurity and starvation by increasing the income of small farmers, improving crop yields, and producing food crops with greater resistance to drought[49]

Despite these claims, there is significant opposition to genetic engineering. Detractors cite a wide range of concerns related to environmental hazards, human health risks, and economic instability. These include the following:

- Genes have been transferred to nontarget species through cross-pollination, resulting in the spread of undesirable plants, including superweeds that are tolerant to conventional herbicides.[50] Indeed, from 1996 to 2011, despite the decline in the use of the insecticide Bt, the rapid spread of herbicide-resistant superweeds in the United States led to an overall 7% increase in pesticide use.[51] In short, the magnitude of the increase in the use of herbicides on these superweeds has dwarfed the more modest reductions in insecticide use, and the problem is estimated to increase dramatically in the future.[51]
- Genes have been transferred from non-food crops to crops intended for food, tainting them with non–food-grade ingredients. This was demonstrated when traces of a type

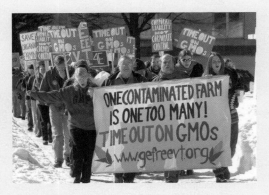

▲ Many people oppose the genetic engineering of foods for environmental, health, or economic reasons.

of maize that was approved for use only in animal feed appeared in food products in the United States.[50]

- Undesirable genes could be transferred from genetically modified foods to cells of the body or to the gastrointestinal flora, adversely affecting human health. For example, if antibiotic-resistant genes were transferred, susceptibility to infectious disease could increase.[50]
- There is a potential for significant loss of biodiversity. Not only could GMOs, superweeds, and increased use of herbicides decimate populations of beneficial insects, microorganisms, and native plants and animals, but also the diversity of food crops in cultivation could be reduced.[50]
- Monopolization and privatization of farming has reduced economic opportunity. For example, the seed industry has become increasingly controlled by just three large bioengineering firms that have bought up small, local seed companies, then increased prices to farmers for their genetically engineered seed. At the same time, the firms require farmers to sign contracts promising that they will not save the seeds from their future crops.[52] Critics say that monopoly control of genetically modified, nonrenewable seed has had tragic consequences. By one estimate, a quarter million farmers have taken their lives because of debt induced by the high cost of nonrenewable genetically engineered seed.[53]

Other concerns commonly cited include the potential for the creation of new biological weapons and an increased risk for bioterrorism as well as the development of new diseases that can attack plants, animals, and humans.[50] Many argue that, at the very least, all genetically modified foods should be labeled so that consumers know what they're purchasing. As of 2012, the U.S. Food and Drug Administration did not require that all genetically engineered foods be identified as such; however, nationwide polls over the past several years have continually shown that more than 90% of Americans support labeling of GMO foods.[54]

Because GMOs and genetically modified foods have been available only since 1996, we do not as yet have any long-term human health or environmental impact studies of genetically engineered foods or crops. It may thus be many years before we can begin to understand their impact on the world.

CRITICAL THINKING QUESTIONS

1. Based on your knowledge of GMOs and genetically modified foods, do you support their production within the United States and around the world? Why or why not?
2. Do you think genetically modified foods should be clearly identified for consumers? What are the arguments, pro and con, for labeling genetically modified foods?

chapter **review**

test yourself | answers

1. **False.** Foodborne illness actually sickens about 48 million Americans each year, and about 3,000 die.

2. **False.** Freezing destroys some microorganisms but only inhibits the ability of other microorganisms to reproduce. When the food is thawed, these cold-tolerant microorganisms resume reproduction.

3. **True.** Although some studies have found higher levels of certain vitamins and phytochemicals in organic foods, there is insufficient research evidence to support a claim that organic foods are consistently more nutritious than conventionally grown foods. Still, organic foods do have lower levels of pesticides.

MasteringNutrition™

Check out these additional resources in the MasteringNutrition Study Area at www.masteringhealthandnutrition.pearson.com:

- Read It: Chapter Summary and RSS Feeds
- See It: ABC News videos and nutrition animations
- Hear It: MP3s
- Study It: Get Ready for Nutrition Math and Chemistry review
- Do It: NutriTools and "Find the Quack" feature
- Review It: Quizzes, flashcards, and glossary

review questions

1. Which of the following statements about food safety is true?
   a. Federal inspections of food production facilities have decreased over the last few decades.
   b. The United States Department of Agriculture oversees the safety of all foods produced in or imported into the United States.
   c. Foodborne illness causes 3 million hospitalizations in the United States each year.
   d. Both a and b are true.

2. The two non-bacterial microorganisms most commonly involved in foodborne illnesses, hospitalizations, and deaths are
   a. norovirus and prions.
   b. norovirus and *Toxoplasma gondii*.
   c. hepatitis A virus and *Giardia*.
   d. helminths and *Cryptococcus*.

3. The temperature in your refrigerator should be at or below
   a. 0°F.
   b. 20°F.
   c. 40°F.
   d. 60°F.

4. A food preservation technique in which the oxygen in a food is replaced with an inert gas is
   a. pasteurization.
   b. irradiation.
   c. modified atmosphere packaging.
   d. high-pressure processing.

5. Food additives that have raised health concerns include
   a. sodium chloride and potassium sorbate.
   b. sulfites and nitrites.
   c. lecithin and glycerin.
   d. all of the above.

6. The process in which a gene conferring a beneficial trait is spliced into another organism is technically known as
   a. biodiversification.
   b. genetic breeding.
   c. gene therapy.
   d. recombinant DNA technology.

7. Which of the following best describes how biomagnification occurs?
   a. Conventional fertilizers and pesticides are sprayed onto food crops.
   b. Industrial pollutants initiate DNA mutations that lead to cancer.
   c. Animal wastes contaminate soils where food crops are grown.
   d. Industrial contaminants become more concentrated in animal tissues as they move up the food chain.

8. Foods that are labeled *100% organic*
   a. contain only organically produced ingredients, excluding water and salt.
   b. may display the EPA's organic seal.
   c. can include genetically modified organisms.
   d. contain foods from plant sources only.

9. **True or False?** You prepare a potato, egg, and red onion salad with mayonnaise at 10:00 AM for a 2:00 PM barbecue. It is safe to leave the salad at room temperature until the barbecue.

10. **True or False?** In the United States, farms certified as organic are allowed to use pesticides under certain conditions.

math review

11. What percentage of Americans who contract foodborne illness each year die as a result? Propose an explanation for your finding.

Answers to Review Questions and Math Review are located at the back of this text and in the MasteringNutrition Study Area.

web resources

www.foodsafety.gov
Use this website as a gateway to food safety information from recalls to updates, food safety tips, and more.

www.cdc.gov
CDC Food Safety Homepage

Enter "Food Safety" into the search bar on the home page. This is the CDC's site for information about foodborne illness outbreaks, food safety tips, and more.

www.fightbac.org
Partnership for Food Safety Education

This is the official website for the USDA's Fight BAC! Initiative.

www.epa.gov
U.S. Environmental Protection Agency

Enter "Pesticides" into the search bar on the home page. This site provides information on safe pesticide use in your home or garden, how to reduce pesticide residues in foods, and regulation of pesticides.

www.ota.com
Organic Trade Association

This website provides lots of information about the production and marketing of organic food.

in depth 13.5

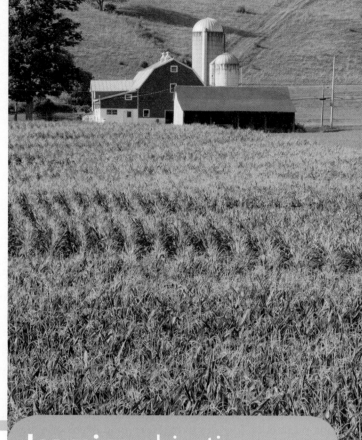

Food Ethics: Sustainability, Equity, and the New Food Movement

In 1993, four children in Washington State died after eating fast-food hamburgers contaminated with *E. coli.* Although certainly not the first food-safety incident to capture public attention, it marked a turning point, after which Americans increasingly questioned the assumption that all of our food is always entirely safe to eat. A national debate about food safety and food politics began; a series of investigative news articles, books, and films explored not only the health risks but also the environmental and social costs of contemporary methods of food production. Advocates for public health, animal welfare, farmland preservation, the rights of farmworkers, and environmental quality all came together in a common cause. The food movement was born. Although a comprehensive discussion of the food movement isn't undertaken here, let's take an **In Depth** look at two of its broadest concerns: sustainability and food equity.

learning objectives

After studying this In Depth, you should be able to:

1 Explain how sustainable agricultural practices help to preserve environmental resources and maintain food diversity, pp. 506–507.

2 Identify several initiatives embraced by the food movement to protect the environment and promote food diversity, pp. 507–508.

3 Summarize the problem of food insecurity globally and in the United States, pp. 509–510.

4 Identify the goals of partnerships committed to fair trade, p. 510.

5 Discuss how your own personal choices can help protect the environment, promote food diversity, combat poverty, and support fair trade, pp. 510–511.

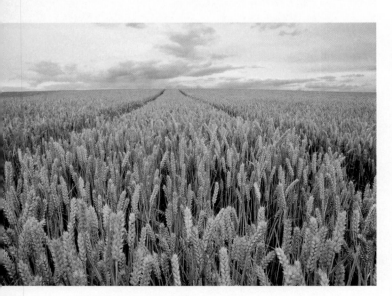

Sustainability preserves the environment and food diversity

The U.S. Environmental Protection Agency (EPA) defines **sustainability** as the ability to satisfy basic economic, social, and security needs now and in the future without undermining the natural resource base and environmental quality on which life depends.[1] Whereas some people view sustainability as a lofty but impractical ideal, others point out that it's a necessary condition of human survival. That's because sustainable practices can reduce pollution of our soil and water and help reverse America's declining food diversity. To achieve both of these goals, experts argue that we must reduce our dependence on corporate farming. To understand the impact of corporate farming, let's review some history.

Environmental Impact of Corporate Farming

Throughout history, wars have prompted innovation. World War II was no different, leading to advances in industrial technology, engineering, and chemistry. After the war ended, these innovations were directed toward agriculture, specifically toward increasing worldwide food production in order to meet the food needs of a dramatically increasing post-war population. Together, the new technologies and procedures became known as the **green revolution**, a massive program that led to improved seed quality, fertilizers, and pesticides, as well as new techniques for farming and irrigation, which doubled crop yields throughout the world.[2] As part of the green revolution, for example, new **high-yield varieties** of grain were produced by cross-breeding plants and selecting for the most desirable traits. It's estimated that these new varieties of rice, corn, and wheat have saved millions of people from starvation since the 1960s. In addition, they have reduced the need to cut forests for new agricultural land, a factor in global warming.[3]

Although it has achieved higher yields at lower costs, the green revolution has also created new problems. Because it requires the use of expensive chemical fertilizers, pesticides, irrigation, and mechanical harvesters to reduce labor costs, it has mostly benefited larger, wealthier landowners rather than small, family farms. Moreover, environmental costs associated with the green revolution have included:

- Loss of topsoil due to erosion from heavy tilling, from extensive planting of row crops such as corn and soybeans, and from run-off due to irrigation
- Diminished biodiversity as traditional, resistant local species have been replaced with high-yield varieties that are more fragile
- Development of insecticide-resistant species of insects and herbicide-resistant varieties of weeds as use of agrochemical products has intensified
- Depletion and pollution of water supplies from irrigation techniques requiring heavy water consumption and from agrochemical run-off
- Depletion of fossil fuels and increased release of greenhouse gases[2]

In response to these drawbacks of the green revolution, a new global movement toward **sustainable agriculture** has evolved. The goal of the sustainable agriculture movement is to develop local, site-specific farming methods that improve soil conservation, crop yields, and food security in a sustainable manner, minimizing the adverse environmental impact. For example, soil erosion can be controlled by **crop rotation**, by terracing sloped land for

---

sustainability The ability to meet or satisfy basic economic, social, and security needs now and in the future without undermining the natural resource base and environmental quality on which life depends.

green revolution The period of significant increase in global productivity between 1944 and 2000 as a result of selective cross-breeding or hybridization that produced high-yield grains and industrial farming techniques.

high-yield varieties Semi-dwarf varieties of plants that are unlikely to fall over in wind and heavy rains and thus can carry larger amounts of seeds, greatly increasing the yield per acre.

sustainable agriculture Techniques of food production that preserve the environment indefinitely.

crop rotation The practice of alternating crops in a particular field to prevent nutrient depletion and erosion of the soil and to help with control of crop-specific pests.

New varieties of crops such as wheat, rice, and corn are produced by cross-breeding plants and selecting for the most desirable traits.

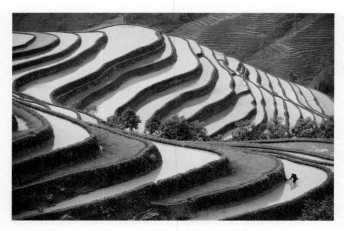

FIGURE 1 Terracing sloped land to avoid soil erosion is one practice of sustainable agriculture.

the cultivation of crops (**FIGURE 1**), and by tillage that minimizes disturbance to the topsoil. Organic farming is one method of sustainable agriculture because to be certified organic, farms must commit to sustainable agricultural practices, including avoiding the use of synthetic fertilizers and toxic and persistent pesticides.

Meat production is a particularly controversial issue within the sustainable agriculture movement. Research data points to the inefficiency of eating meat from grain-fed cattle instead of eating the grains themselves, both in terms of the resources required and the level of methane and other emissions generated (see the Chapter 6 Nutrition Debate, page 221). Livestock production also leads to deforestation, further contributing to global warming. Sustainable meat production minimizes the use of antibiotics and synthetic hormones, allows for the use of otherwise unusable plants for high-quality animal feed, recycles animal wastes for fertilizers and fuel, and practices humane treatment of animals.

Impact of Corporate Farming on Food Diversity

How have corporate farms reduced food diversity? Beginning in the 1960s, revisions of the federal Agricultural Adjustment Act, commonly called the farm bill, provided financial incentives for America's farmers to "get big or get out."[4] The number of small farms dwindled, and the remaining industrial operations focused on increasing their production of the few subsidized crops such as corn. To do so, industrial farming relied on the techniques of the green revolution, including pesticides, fertilizers, and the use of antibiotics on feedlots, practices that prompted a sharp increase in soil and water pollution. In the Salinas and lower San Joaquin Valleys of California, for example, pollution from chemical fertilizers and manure has contaminated the groundwater, making it undrinkable for at least the next 30 years.[4]

When the farm bill began to subsidize target crops, those crops—especially corn—began to monopolize the food supply. As a result, the average American diet lost its variety,

which is a key component of a healthful diet. As food expert Michael Pollan writes, if you are what you eat, most Americans are "corn": meat and poultry are corn-fed, french fries are cooked in corn oil, soft drinks are sweetened with high-fructose corn syrup, and fillers, binders, and dozens of other additives in processed foods are derived from corn.[5] Since no subsidies were paid for production of fresh fruits and vegetables, their availability and variety plummeted, and they became more expensive. Americans soon discovered that they could enjoy an entire meal of corn-based foods for less than the cost of a pint of fresh raspberries.

Food Movement Initiatives to Promote Sustainability

Recently, the **food movement** has embraced a variety of initiatives to protect the environment and challenge the monopolization of our food supply. The following are a few examples of the many ways that individuals, communities, and corporations are promoting sustainability and food diversity:

- *Family farms.* For the first time in decades, the number of farms in the United States has been increasing. The U.S. Department of Agriculture's (USDA's) most recent Census of Agriculture showed a 4% increase in the number of farms between 2002 and 2007—a net increase of more than 75,000 farms.[6] And many of the new farmers are young adults taking advantage of programs offering land, financial support, and mentoring. Moreover, many are dedicated to organic farming, crop diversity, and other practices of sustainable agriculture.
- *Community supported agriculture (CSA).* In CSA programs, a farmer sells a certain number of "shares" to the public. Shares typically consist of a box of produce from the farm on a regular basis, such as once weekly throughout the growing season. Farmers get cash early on as well as guaranteed buyers. Consumers get fresh, locally grown food. Together, farmers and consumers develop ongoing relationships as they share the bounty in a good year as well as the losses when extreme weather or blight reduces yield. Although there is no national database on CSA programs, the organization LocalHarvest lists over 4,000.[7]
- *Farmers' markets.* There are now more than 7,000 farmers' markets in the United States, more than four times the number when the USDA began compiling these data in 1994.[8] Along with CSAs, farmers' markets represent a growing trend toward the consumption of "local food"— that is, food grown within a few hundred miles of the consumer. Supporters claim that consuming local food limits energy use and greenhouse gas emissions from transportation (so-called food miles) and that these foods are fresher and nutritionally superior. Although researchers agree that the lowest environmental impact is associated with

---

food movement A group of local, regional, and national initiatives aimed at promoting sustainable agriculture, food diversity, and food equity, including affordability and fair trade.

consuming foods harvested in-season from a local farm, this is not possible year-round in the many regions of the world with short growing seasons. In such cases, the resource costs of both greenhouse cultivation and long-term storage of foods may exceed the energy costs of transported foods.[9]

- *Urban agriculture.* Urban agriculture is on the rise. From Pittsburgh to San Francisco, city governments are changing zoning codes to encourage the cultivation of vegetable gardens on rooftops, in abandoned parking lots, and even as part of the landscaping on municipal properties.[10]

- *School gardens.* The School Garden Association of America was founded in 1910, and in 1914 the federal government created the Office of School and Home Gardening within the U.S. Bureau of Education.[11] During World Wars I and II, school gardening became part of the war effort; however, in the post-war decades, school gardens dwindled. Recently, growing concerns about childhood obesity, the poor quality of children's diets, and their reduced opportunities for physical activity has renewed interest in school gardens. In partnership with the AmeriCorps Service Network, a new effort called FoodCorps was launched in 2009 to increase school garden programs across the United States. In addition to promoting student acceptance of fruits and vegetables, school garden programs teach valuable lessons in nutrition, agriculture, and even cooking. In many schools, cafeterias incorporate the foods into the school lunch menu. In the 2011–2012 school year, FoodCorps served nearly 50,000 children.[12]

- *Entrepreneurship.* A number of prominent venture capital (VC) firms in Silicon Valley are now investing in food start-ups dedicated to preserving human health and the environment. In 2012 alone, VCs poured about $350 million into organic foods, vegan versions of cheese, eggs, burgers, and other animal foods, and services that bring fresh produce from local farms directly to consumers' doors.[13]

- *Corporate involvement.* Whereas many smaller natural-food companies have long made sustainable agriculture

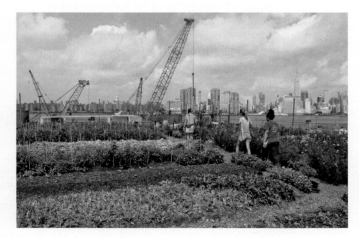

Eagle Street Rooftop Farm is a 6,000 square foot organic vegetable garden located on top of a warehouse in Brooklyn, New York.

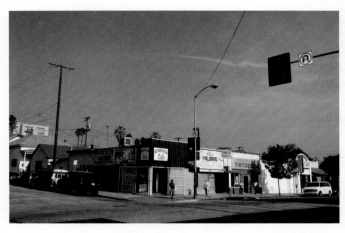

"Food deserts" are geographic areas where people lack access to affordable, nutritious food, often characterized by an absence of grocery stores.

part of their company identity, only recently has the food movement moved into corporate America. In 2010, Walmart, the world's largest retailer, unveiled a set of global sustainable agriculture goals the company intends to reach by the year 2015. Those goals include selling $1 billion in foods from small and mid-size local farms and providing training in sustainable farming practices to 1 million farmers.[14] Since the Walmart announcement, Kellogg, McDonald's, and several other corporations have announced their own commitments to sustainable agriculture.

Public health experts point out that these efforts to promote sustainability also have the potential to reduce the number of so-called **food deserts**—geographic areas where people lack access to affordable, nutritious food. There are no reliable statistics on how many Americans live in food deserts because there is no standard definition; however, the CDC reports that the problem does affect a small percentage of Americans, mostly those who live far from a large grocery store and do not have access to transportation.[15] Not only isolated rural regions, but also inner-city neighborhoods can be food deserts. For example, Philadelphia, which has the highest obesity rate and the greatest percentage of people in poverty of any large American city, has many neighborhoods that qualify as food deserts. As part of a new national initiative called Healthy Corner Stores, Philadelphia in 2012 invested $900,000 into 600 of the city's corner stores to increase city residents' access to healthy foods such as fresh produce.[16]

Find a farmers' market near you! Go to the USDA's Farmers' Market Search page at http://apps.ams.usda.gov. Enter "Farmers Markets" into the search bar.

food desert An area or community in which residents lack reliable access to affordable fresh produce and other healthful foods.

Food Equity promotes a fair sharing of resources

You might think of the food movement as affluent Americans shopping at a farmer's market. However, the second broad issue in the food movement is food equity: sharing the world's food and other resources fairly.

Food Insecurity

Despite the dramatic advances in food production brought about by the green revolution, 925 million people worldwide were hungry in 2010.[17] The World Hunger Education Service estimates that one in seven people in the world is chronically undernourished and that 98% of these people live in developing nations.[17]

Any situation that results in inadequate food for an individual or community will prompt undernutrition. Natural disasters, wars, overpopulation, poor farming practices, disease, inequities in resource distribution, and other factors can result in a food supply that is inadequate to support the needs of all of the people in a particular place. However, the major cause of undernutrition in the world is unequal distribution of food because of poverty. In the developing world, more than three-fourths of malnourished children live in countries with food surpluses.[18] The most at-risk populations

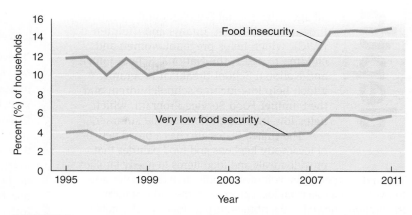

FIGURE 2 Prevalence of food insecurity and very low food security in U.S. households, 1995–2011.
Data from: "Food Security in the U.S.: Key Statistics and Graphics."

are the rural poor. Lacking sufficient land to grow their own foods, the rural poor must work for others to earn money to buy food, but because they live in rural areas, employment opportunities are limited.

Unequal distribution also occurs in the United States, again largely because of poverty. As shown in **FIGURE 2**, the USDA estimates that 14.9% of U.S. households (about 17.9 million households) experienced **food insecurity** in 2011.[19] This means that the people living in these homes were unable to obtain enough food to meet their physical needs every day. About one-third of these households—about 6.8 million—had *very low food security*, meaning that normal eating patterns of one or more members of the household were disrupted and food intake was reduced at times during the year because they had insufficient money or other resources for food.

Those at higher risk for food insecurity are households with income ranging from below the official U.S. poverty threshold (which was $23,550 for a family of four in 2013) to as much as 185% of the poverty threshold. Also at increased risk are families consisting of single mothers or single fathers and their children, African American households, and Hispanic households.[19] Other vulnerable groups are the homeless, the unemployed, elderly people living on a fixed income, migrant laborers, and other workers in minimum-wage jobs.

Sometimes illness or disability contributes to food insecurity among Americans. For instance, people may lose work hours due to illness, have to accept lower-wage jobs, or have medical expenses that limit money for food. Depression, substance abuse, and other psychological disorders can similarly limit productivity and reduce income.

In the United States, several government programs help low-income citizens acquire food over extended periods. Among these programs are the Supplemental Nutrition Assistance Program (SNAP, previously called the Food Stamp Program), which helps low-income individuals of

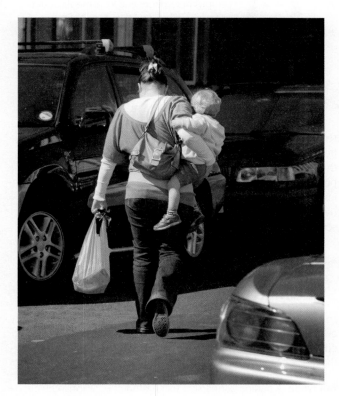

Single parents face unique economic challenges that can leave them and their children vulnerable to food insecurity.

food insecurity A condition in which an individual is unable to regularly obtain enough food to provide sufficient energy and nutrients to meet physical needs.

all ages; the Special Supplemental Nutrition Program for Women, Infants and Children (WIC), which helps pregnant women and children to age 5; the National School Lunch and National School Breakfast Programs, which help low-income schoolchildren; and the Summer Food Service Program, which helps low-income children in the summer.

The United States also has a broad network of local soup kitchens and food pantries that provide meals and food items to needy families. They are supported by volunteers, individual donations, and food contributions from local grocery stores and restaurants. In addition, the USDA distributes surplus foods to charitable agencies for distribution to needy families.

In the less developed nations, many international organizations help improve the nutrient status of the poor by enabling them to produce their own foods. For example, both USAID and the Peace Corps have agricultural education programs, the World Bank provides loans to fund small business ventures, and many nonprofit and nongovernmental organizations (NGOs) support community and family farms.

Fair Trade

The introduction of corporate farming has displaced small-scale farmers and reduced food diversity in developing as well as developed nations. Currently, for example, just four companies control 75% of the international grain trade.[20] But corporate farming has also monopolized agricultural labor, forcing farmworkers to accept poverty-level wages and substandard and even dangerous living conditions. In the past decade, for example, the owners of seven Florida farms have been convicted of beating, chaining, and stealing from laborers in conditions that a Florida District Attorney described as "slavery." While performing backbreaking labor, America's 6 million farmworkers are continually exposed to ultraviolet (UV) radiation, pesticides, and crop dusts and pests, and often lack basic sanitation as well as access to healthcare.[4] Not surprisingly, the life expectancy of U.S. farmworkers is just 49 years.[20]

The **fair trade** movement was born in response to the exploitation of farm laborers around the world. It began decades ago in North America and Europe, but is now a global effort that depends on support from consumers worldwide to purchase fruits, vegetables, coffee, tea, cocoa, wine, and many other products that display the Fair Trade Certified logo (**FIGURE 3**). Fair trade empowers farm laborers to demand living wages and humane treatment. It also

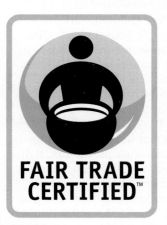

FIGURE 3 The Fair Trade Certified logo guarantees that the product has been produced equitably without exploitation of workers or the environment. (Fair Trade Logo)

nutri-case | JUDY

"I never seem to be able to make ends meet. I keep hoping next month will be different, but rent and utilities eat up most of my paycheck, so when something unexpected happens, I'm short. Last week, my car broke down and I'm way behind on my credit card payments. Today, a collections guy called and said that if I didn't pay at least $100 right away, they'd take me to court! When I got off the phone, I started to cry, and Hannah asked me what was wrong. When I told her how bad the money situation is, she thought we might qualify for food stamps. I have a full-time job, so I don't think we'll qualify, but even if we do, I wonder if it'll help much."

In 2012, the federal minimum wage was $7.25 an hour. As a nurse's aide, Judy earns $9 an hour, or $1,560 a month. She is eligible for the Supplemental Nutrition Assistance Program (food stamps). Are you surprised that someone making almost 25% more than the minimum wage, and working full-time, qualifies for food assistance?

Before you're too certain that Judy's eligibility will solve her problems, consider that the average food stamp allotment in 2012 was $4.30 per person per day, or about $30 per week for one person.* If you had just $30 to keep yourself fed for a week, what would you buy?

Take this challenge one step further and follow the example of some U.S. college students to raise local awareness of food insecurity: For 1 week, restrict yourself to just $30 for all your food purchases. Let your campus newspaper and local media outlets know what you're doing, and ask readers to make donations to local food banks.

*Congressional Budget Office. 2012. An Overview of the Supplemental Nutrition Assistance Program.

reduces child labor and increases access of children to education because parents earning higher wages are able to allow their children to leave the fields and attend school. Fair trade purchases also support the building of schools and health clinics, provide funds to help farmers adopt sustainable agricultural practices, and provide financial assistance for women to set up in small businesses.[21]

What can you do to increase sustainability and food equity?

In a climate in which power over food is ever more tightly controlled, the food movement is providing ordinary citizens a means to promote change. Across national

fair trade A trading partnership that promotes equity in international trading relationships, and contributes to sustainable development by securing the rights of marginalized producers and workers.

boundaries, people like you are making simple choices—such as to support local farms or to purchase only fair trade goods—that are making a difference. Let's explore a few ways that you can join the food movement.

The choices you make when you shop can contribute to sustainability and food equity because your purchases influence local and global markets. If you choose vegetables, fruits, nuts, whole grains, and beans and other legumes, then you will influence greater production of these healthful foods. If you buy organic foods, you encourage reduction in the use of chemical pesticides and herbicides. If you buy produce from a local farmer's market, you encourage greater local availability of fresh foods. This reduces the costs and resources devoted to distribution, transportation, and storage of foods. And if you purchase Fair Trade foods, you support equitable production worldwide.

The amount of meat you eat also affects the environment and the global food supply. Because the production of plant-based foods requires a lower expenditure of natural resources and releases fewer greenhouse gases than the production of animal-based foods, adopting a plant-based diet preserves land, water, and global energy, and reduces global warming. However, animal-based foods do contribute high-quality nutrients, such as iron, zinc, and vitamin B_{12}, and can be consumed in modest amounts without harm to the environment. To promote reduced meat consumption on campus, talk with your food services manager about sponsoring "Meatless Mondays." See the Web Resources for a link to the Meatless Monday website, where you can download a Meatless Monday Goes to College toolkit.

You know that physical activity is important in maintaining health, but walking, biking, and taking public transportation also limits your consumption of nonrenewable fossil fuels. When it's time to purchase a car, research your options and choose the one with the best fuel economy.

To fight food insecurity in the United States, consider joining the National Student Campaign Against Hunger and Homelessness. The campaign is committed to ending hunger and homelessness in America by training students to meet individuals' immediate needs while advocating for long-term, systemic solutions. It holds "Hunger Cleanups," staffs relief agencies, solicits donations of food and money, and promotes community activism. Alternatively, you can gather foods for local food banks, volunteer to work in a soup kitchen, help distribute food to homebound elderly, or start a community or school garden. You can also hold fund-raisers and donate cash directly.

Get the word out! If you find an organization whose goals you share, recommend them on your social networking page. Or send a short article about the organization's work to your campus news site with suggestions about how other students can support its work.

As Francis Moore Lappe, author of the groundbreaking book *Diet for a Small Planet*, explains, the food movement encourages us to think with an "eco-mind," refusing to accept scarcity and oppression for some in the name of production for many. By promoting the values of fairness, connection, and abundance, involvement in the food movement encourages us to make choices that can create positive changes in our world.[20]

MasteringNutrition™

Check out these additional resources in the MasteringNutrition Study Area:

- Read It: Chapter Summary and RSS Feeds
- See It: ABC News videos and nutrition animations
- Hear It: MP3s
- Study It: Get Ready for Nutrition Math and Chemistry review
- Do It: NutriTools and "Find the Quack" feature
- Review It: Quizzes, flashcards, and glossary

web resources

www.slowfoodusa.org
Slow Food USA

Slow Food links the pleasure of growing, preparing, and consuming food with commitment to our communities and environment. Visit this site to learn more about the slow food movement and get involved.

www.fairtradeusa.org
Fair Trade USA

Visit this website to find out why "Every Purchase Matters!"

www.meatlessmonday.com
Meatless Monday

This website offers information on the environmental and health benefits of going meatless one day a week, as well as recipes for vegetarian meals and a toolkit to promote Meatless Mondays on your campus.

www.epa.gov
Environmental Protection Agency's Sustainability Tips

This site offers a wide variety of tips and tools to help you reduce your environmental footprint. Enter "green living" into the search box, then click on the top-most link.

www.studentsagainsthunger.org
National Student Campaign Against Hunger and Homelessness

Visit their site to find out what they're up to and how to get involved.

www.bread.org
Bread for the World

Find out about this faith-based effort to advocate local and global policies that help the poor obtain food.

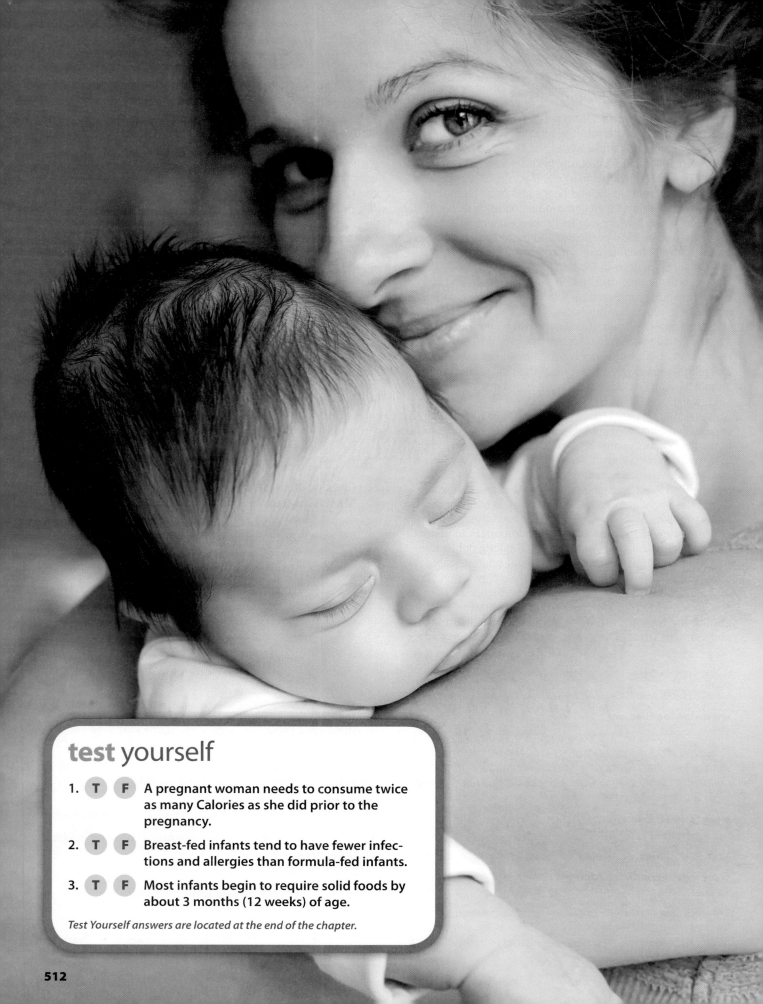

test yourself

1. **T** **F** A pregnant woman needs to consume twice as many Calories as she did prior to the pregnancy.

2. **T** **F** Breast-fed infants tend to have fewer infections and allergies than formula-fed infants.

3. **T** **F** Most infants begin to require solid foods by about 3 months (12 weeks) of age.

Test Yourself answers are located at the end of the chapter.

Nutrition Through the Life Cycle
Pregnancy and the first year of life

14

The birth of baby Tomas brought new joy to his parents and family. However, little Tomas weighed just over 3 lb 5 oz at birth—about half of what an average full-term newborn weighs. Although the United States has an extensive and expensive healthcare system, the prevalence of low-, very-low-, and extremely low-birth-weight infants, such as Tomas, remains around 8%.[1] Moreover, our infant mortality rate—the number of deaths of infants before their first birthday—is higher than the rate in 47 other countries: in 2012, the United States recorded 5.98 infant deaths for every 1,000 live births, as compared to just 2.74 for Sweden and 2.21 for Japan, the best-ranked large nation.[2]

What contributes to these troubling statistics? On a broader scale, what role does prenatal diet play in determining the future health and well-being of the child? In this chapter, we'll discuss how adequate nutrition supports fetal development, maintains a pregnant woman's health, and contributes to lactation. We'll then explore the nutrient needs of breastfeeding and formula-feeding infants.

learning objectives

After studying this chapter you should be able to:

1 Describe the relationship among increased nutrient requirements, fetal development, and physiologic changes in the mother during the course of a pregnancy, pp. 514–518.

2 Identify the range of optimal weight gain for a pregnant woman in the first, second, and third trimesters, pp. 518–519.

3 Discuss recommendations for addressing some common nutrition-related concerns during pregnancy as well as for engaging in exercise, pp. 519–529.

4 Describe the physiologic events involved in lactation, pp. 530–531.

5 Detail the nutrient requirements of lactating women, pp. 531–533.

6 Identify the advantages and challenges of breast-feeding, pp. 533–537.

7 Relate the growth and activity patterns of infants to their nutrient needs, pp. 538–542.

8 Discuss some common nutrition-related concerns for infants, pp. 542–544.

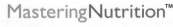

MasteringNutrition™

Go online for chapter quizzes, pre-tests, Interactive Activities, and more!

Starting out right: healthful nutrition in pregnancy

From conception through the end of the first year of life, adequate nutrition is essential for tissue formation, neurologic development, and bone growth, modeling, and remodeling. The ability to reach peak physical and intellectual potential in adult life is in part determined by the nutrition received during the earliest stages of development.

Is Nutrition Important Before Conception?

Several factors make adequate nutrition important even before **conception**, the point at which a woman's ovum (egg) is fertilized with a man's sperm. First, some deficiency-related problems develop extremely early in the pregnancy, typically before the mother even realizes she is pregnant. An adequate and varied preconception diet reduces the risk for such early-onset problems. For example, inadequate levels of folate during the first few weeks following conception can result in brain and spinal cord defects. This problem is discussed in more detail shortly. To reduce the incidence of such defects, federal guidelines advise all women capable of becoming pregnant to consume 400 µg of folic acid daily, whether or not they plan to become pregnant.

Second, adopting a healthful diet prior to conception includes the avoidance of alcohol, illegal drugs, and other known **teratogens** (substances that cause birth defects). Women should also consult their healthcare provider about their consumption of caffeine, medications, herbs, and supplements, and if they smoke they should attempt to quit.

Third, a healthful diet and an appropriate level of physical activity can help women achieve and maintain an optimal body weight prior to pregnancy. Women with a prepregnancy body mass index (BMI) between 19.8 and 26.0 kg/m² have the best chance of a successful pregnancy. As we will discuss shortly, women with a BMI above or below this range are at greater risk for pregnancy-related complications.

Finally, maintaining a balanced and nourishing diet before conception reduces a woman's risk of developing a nutrition-related disorder during her pregnancy. These disorders, which we discuss later in the chapter, include gestational diabetes and hypertensive disorders. Although genetic and metabolic abnormalities are beyond the woman's control, following a healthful diet prior to conception is something a woman can do to help her fetus develop into a healthy baby.

The man's nutrition prior to pregnancy is important as well because malnutrition contributes to abnormalities in sperm.[3,4] Both sperm number and motility (ability to move) are reduced by alcohol consumption as well as by the use of certain prescription and illegal drugs. Zinc, calcium, vitamin D, folic acid, and dietary antioxidants such as vitamin C have also been linked to improved sperm health and male fertility. In contrast, high saturated fat diets, obesity, and diabetes have been linked to impaired male fertility.

Why Is Nutrition Important During Pregnancy?

A balanced, nourishing diet is important throughout pregnancy to provide the nutrients needed to support fetal development without depriving the mother of the nutrients she needs to maintain her own health. It also minimizes the risk of excess energy intake. A full-term pregnancy lasts 38 to 42 weeks and is divided into three **trimesters**, with each trimester lasting about 13 to 14 weeks.

The First Trimester

About once each month, a nonpregnant woman of childbearing age experiences **ovulation**, the release of an ovum from an ovary. The ovum is then drawn into the uterine tube. The first trimester of pregnancy begins when the ovum and sperm unite to form a single, fertilized cell called a **zygote**. As the zygote travels through the uterine tube, it divides into a ball of 12 to 16 cells, which, at about day 4, arrives in the uterus (**FIGURE 14.1**). By day 10, the inner portion of the zygote, called the *blastocyst*, has implanted into the uterine lining. The outer portion becomes part of the placenta, which is discussed shortly.

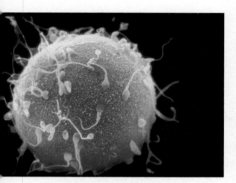

⬆ During conception, a sperm fertilizes an egg, creating a zygote.

conception The uniting of an ovum (egg) and sperm to create a fertilized egg, or zygote. Also called *fertilization*.

teratogen Any substance that can cause a birth defect.

trimester Any one of three stages of pregnancy, each lasting 13 to 14 weeks.

ovulation The release of an ovum (egg) from a woman's ovary.

zygote A fertilized ovum (egg) consisting of a single cell.

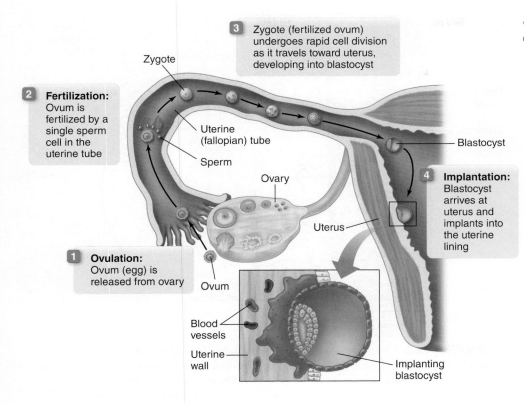

▲ **FIGURE 14.1** Ovulation, conception, and implantation.

1 Ovulation: Ovum (egg) is released from ovary

2 Fertilization: Ovum is fertilized by a single sperm cell in the uterine tube

3 Zygote (fertilized ovum) undergoes rapid cell division as it travels toward uterus, developing into blastocyst

4 Implantation: Blastocyst arrives at uterus and implants into the uterine lining

Zygote

Uterine (fallopian) tube

Sperm

Ovary

Uterus

Blastocyst

Ovum

Blood vessels

Uterine wall

Implanting blastocyst

Further cell growth, multiplication, and differentiation occur, resulting in the formation of an **embryo**. Over the next 6 weeks, embryonic tissues continue to differentiate and fold into a primitive, tubelike structure with limb buds, organs, and facial features (**FIGURE 14.2**). It isn't surprising, then, that the embryo is most vulnerable to teratogens during this time. Not only alcohol and illegal drugs, but also some prescription and over-the-counter medications, megadoses of certain supplements, several herbs, some viruses, cigarette smoking, and radiation can interfere with embryonic development and cause birth defects. In some cases, the damage is so severe that the pregnancy ends in a **spontaneous abortion** (*miscarriage*), most of which occur in the first trimester.

During the first weeks of pregnancy, the embryo obtains its nutrients from cells lining the uterus. But by the fourth week, a primitive **placenta** has formed in the uterus from both embryonic and maternal tissue. Within a few more weeks, the placenta will be a fully functioning organ through which the mother will provide nutrients and remove fetal wastes (**FIGURE 14.3** on page 516).

embryo The human growth and developmental stage lasting from the third week to the end of the eighth week after fertilization.

spontaneous abortion The natural termination of a pregnancy and expulsion of pregnancy tissues because of a genetic, developmental, or physiologic abnormality that is so severe that the pregnancy cannot be maintained. Also called *miscarriage*.

placenta A pregnancy-specific organ formed from both maternal and embryonic tissues. It is responsible for oxygen, nutrient, and waste exchange between mother and fetus.

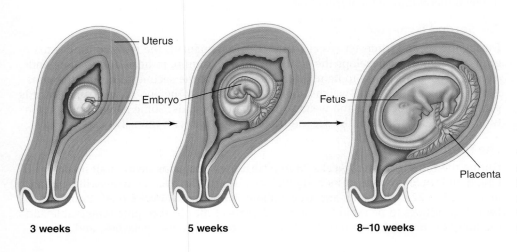

Uterus

Embryo

Fetus

Placenta

3 weeks   **5 weeks**   **8–10 weeks**

▲ **FIGURE 14.2** Human embryonic development during the first 10 weeks. Organ systems are most vulnerable to teratogens during this time, when cells are dividing and differentiating.

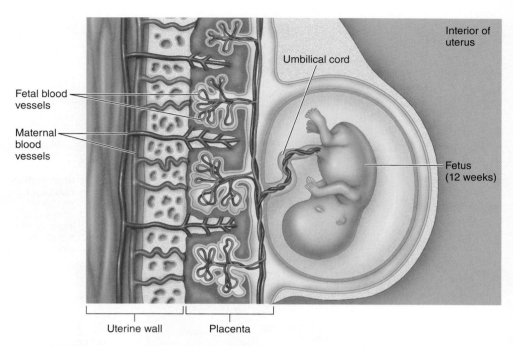

FIGURE 14.3 Placental development. The placenta is formed from both embryonic and maternal tissues. When the placenta is fully functional, fetal blood vessels and maternal blood vessels are intimately intertwined, allowing the exchange of nutrients and wastes between the two. The mother transfers nutrients and oxygen to the fetus, and the fetus transfers wastes to the mother for disposal.

By the end of the embryonic stage, about 8 weeks postconception, the embryo's tissues and organs have differentiated dramatically. A primitive skeleton, including fingers and toes, has formed. Muscles have begun to develop in the trunk and limbs, and some movement is possible. A primitive heart has begun to beat, and the digestive organs are becoming distinct. The brain has differentiated, and the head has a mouth, eyespots with eyelids, and primitive ears.

The third month of pregnancy marks the transition from embryo to **fetus**. To support its dramatic growth, the fetus requires abundant nutrients from the placenta. It is connected to the fetal circulatory system via the **umbilical cord**, an extension of fetal blood vessels emerging from the fetus's navel (called the *umbilicus*). Blood rich in oxygen and nutrients flows through the placenta and into the umbilical vein (see Figure 14.3). Wastes are excreted in blood returning from the fetus to the placenta via the umbilical arteries. Although many people think there is a mixing of blood from the fetus and the mother, the two blood supplies remain separate. Nutrients move from the maternal blood into the fetal blood and waste products are transferred out of the fetal blood into the maternal blood.

The Second Trimester

During the second trimester (weeks 14 to 27 of pregnancy), the fetus continues to grow and mature. It develops the ability to suck its thumb, to hear, and to open and close its eyes in response to light. At the beginning of the second trimester, the fetus is about 3 inches long and weighs about 1.5 pounds. By the end of this trimester, it is generally over a foot long and weighs more than 2 pounds. Some babies born prematurely in the last weeks of the second trimester survive with intensive care.

The Third Trimester

During the third trimester (weeks 28 to birth), the fetus gains nearly half its body length and three-quarters of its body weight! At birth, an average baby will be approximately 18 to 22 inches long and weigh about 7.5 pounds **(FIGURE 14.4)**. Brain growth (which continues to be rapid for the first 2 years of life) is also quite remarkable and the lungs become fully mature. The fetus acquires eyebrows, eyelashes, and hair on

fetus The human growth and developmental stage lasting from the beginning of the ninth week after conception to birth.

umbilical cord The cord containing the arteries and veins that connect the baby (from the navel) to the mother via the placenta.

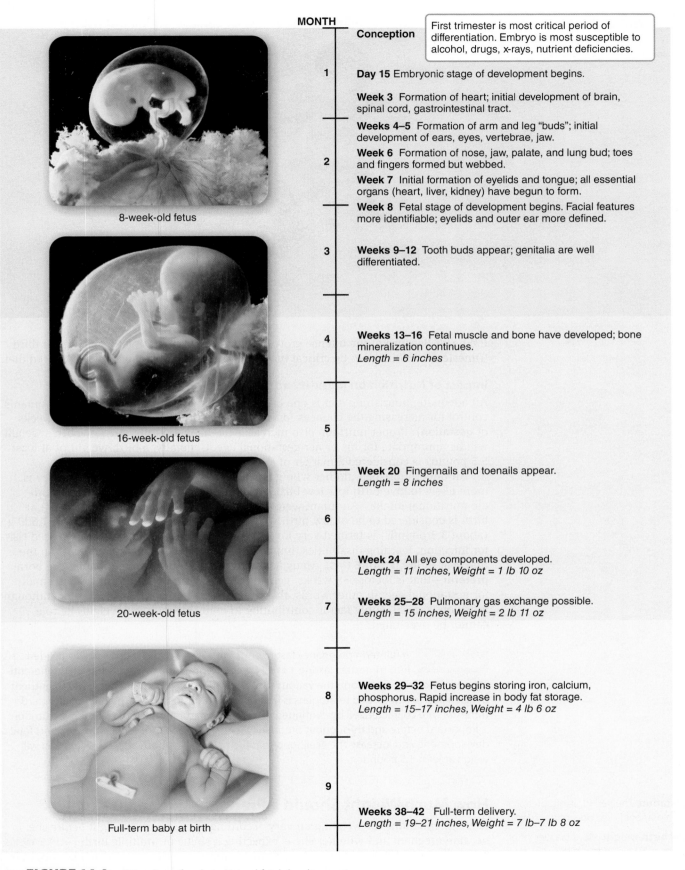

MONTH

Conception

First trimester is most critical period of differentiation. Embryo is most susceptible to alcohol, drugs, x-rays, nutrient deficiencies.

1

Day 15 Embryonic stage of development begins.

Week 3 Formation of heart; initial development of brain, spinal cord, gastrointestinal tract.

Weeks 4–5 Formation of arm and leg "buds"; initial development of ears, eyes, vertebrae, jaw.

2

Week 6 Formation of nose, jaw, palate, and lung bud; toes and fingers formed but webbed.

Week 7 Initial formation of eyelids and tongue; all essential organs (heart, liver, kidney) have begun to form.

Week 8 Fetal stage of development begins. Facial features more identifiable; eyelids and outer ear more defined.

3

Weeks 9–12 Tooth buds appear; genitalia are well differentiated.

8-week-old fetus

4

Weeks 13–16 Fetal muscle and bone have developed; bone mineralization continues.
Length = 6 inches

5

16-week-old fetus

Week 20 Fingernails and toenails appear.
Length = 8 inches

6

Week 24 All eye components developed.
Length = 11 inches, Weight = 1 lb 10 oz

7

Weeks 25–28 Pulmonary gas exchange possible.
Length = 15 inches, Weight = 2 lb 11 oz

20-week-old fetus

8

Weeks 29–32 Fetus begins storing iron, calcium, phosphorus. Rapid increase in body fat storage.
Length = 15–17 inches, Weight = 4 lb 6 oz

9

Full-term baby at birth

Weeks 38–42 Full-term delivery.
Length = 19–21 inches, Weight = 7 lb–7 lb 8 oz

FIGURE 14.4 A timeline of embryonic and fetal development.

▶ **FIGURE 14.5** A healthy 2-day-old infant (right) compared to two low-birth-weight infants.

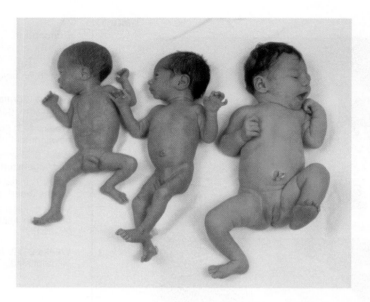

the head. Because of the intense growth and maturation of the fetus during the third trimester, it continues to be critical that the mother eat an adequate and balanced diet.

Impact of Nutrition on Maturity and Birth Weight

An adequate, nourishing diet is one of the most important variables under a woman's control for increasing the chances for birth of a mature newborn (at 38 to 42 weeks of **gestation**). Proper nutrition also increases the likelihood that the newborn's weight will be appropriate for his or her gestational age. Generally, a birth weight of at least 5.5 pounds is considered a marker of a successful pregnancy.

An undernourished mother who gains too little weight during her pregnancy is more likely to give birth to a **low-birth-weight** baby than a woman with appropriate nutritional intake.[3] An infant weighing less than 2,500 g (about 5.5 pounds) at birth is considered to be of low birth weight and an infant weighing less than 1,500 g (about 3.3 pounds) is termed very low birth weight. Both groups are at increased risk for infection, learning disabilities, impaired physical development, and death in the first year of life **(FIGURE 14.5)**. Many low- and very-low-birth-weight babies are born **preterm**—that is, before 38 weeks' gestation. Others are born at term but are small for gestational age; in other words, they weigh less than would be expected. Although nutrition is not the only factor contributing to maturity and birth weight, its role cannot be overstated.

recap A full-term pregnancy lasts from 38 to 42 weeks and is traditionally divided into trimesters lasting 13 to 14 weeks. During the first trimester, cells differentiate and divide rapidly to form the various tissues of the human body. Vulnerability to nutrient deficiencies, toxicities, and teratogens is highest during this trimester. The second and third trimesters are characterized by continued growth and maturation of organ systems. Nutrition is important before and throughout pregnancy to maintain the mother's health, support fetal development, and increase the likelihood that the baby will be born after 37 weeks and will weigh at least 5.5 pounds.

gestation The period of intrauterine development from conception to birth.

low birth weight Having a weight of less than 5.5 pounds at birth.

preterm The birth of a baby prior to 38 weeks' gestation.

How Much Weight Should a Pregnant Woman Gain?

Recommendations for weight gain vary according to a woman's weight *before* she became pregnant and whether she is expecting a single or multiple birth **(TABLE 14.1)**. The average recommended weight gain for women of normal prepregnancy weight is 25 to 35 pounds; underweight women should gain a little more than this amount, and overweight and obese women should gain less. Adolescents should follow the same

TABLE 14.1   Recommended Weight Gain for Women During Pregnancy

Prepregnancy Weight Status	Body Mass Index (kg/m^2)	Recommended Weight Gain (lb)
Normal	18.5–24.9	25–35
Underweight	<18.5	28–40
Overweight	25.0–29.9	15–25

Data adapted from: Rasmussen, K. M., and A. L. Yaktine, eds. 2009. *Weight Gain During Pregnancy: Reexamining the Guidelines.* Institute of Medicine; National Research Council. Washington, DC: National Academies Press.

recommendations as those for adult women.[5] Women of normal prepregnancy weight who are pregnant with twins are advised to gain 37 to 54 pounds.[5]

Women who have a low prepregnancy BMI (<18.5 kg/m^2) or gain too little weight during their pregnancy increase their risk of having a preterm or low-birth-weight baby; the pregnancy may also dangerously deplete their own nutrient reserves.

Gaining *too* much weight or being overweight (BMI ≥25 kg/m^2) or obese (BMI ≥30 kg/m^2) prior to conception is also risky and much more common. Excessive prepregnancy weight or prenatal weight gain increases the risk that the fetus will be large for gestational age, increasing the likelihood of trauma during vaginal delivery and of cesarean birth. Also, children born to overweight or obese mothers have higher rates of childhood obesity and insulin resistance.[6] In addition, the more weight a woman gains during pregnancy, the more difficult it will be for her to return to prepregnancy weight and the more likely it is that her weight gain will be permanent.

In addition to amount of weight, the *pattern* of weight gain is important. During the first trimester, a woman of normal weight should gain no more than 3 to 5 pounds. During the second and third trimesters, about 1 pound a week is considered healthful. Overweight women should gain only 0.6 lb/week and, for obese women, a gain of 0.5 lb/week is appropriate.[5] If weight gain is excessive in a single week, month, or trimester, the woman should not attempt to lose weight. Instead, the woman should merely attempt to slow the rate of weight gain. In short, weight gain throughout pregnancy should be slow and steady.

In a society obsessed with thinness, it is easy for pregnant women to worry about weight gain. Focusing on the quality of food consumed, rather than the quantity, can help women feel more in control. In addition, following a physician-approved exercise program helps women maintain a positive body image and prevent excessive weight gain. The 2010 Dietary Guidelines for Americans advises pregnant women to aim for and achieve an appropriate weight gain as defined by the Institute of Medicine (see Table 14.1).[7]

A pregnant woman may also feel less anxious about her weight gain if she understands how that weight is distributed. Of the total weight gained in pregnancy, 10 to 12 pounds are accounted for by the fetus itself, the amniotic fluid, and the placenta (**FIGURE 14.6** on page 520). In addition, the woman's blood volume increases 40–50%, accounting for another 3 to 4 pounds. A woman can expect to be about 10 to 12 pounds lighter immediately after the birth and, within about 2 weeks, another 5 to 8 pounds lighter because of fluid loss. After that, losing the remainder of pregnancy weight depends on more energy being expended than is taken in. Although the production of breast milk requires significant energy, the effect of breastfeeding on postpartum weight loss varies. Moderate weight loss while breastfeeding is safe and will not interfere with the weight gain of the nursing infant. (Breastfeeding is discussed later in this chapter on pages 530–537.)

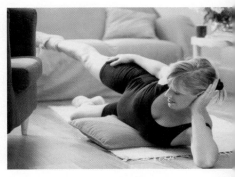

Following a physician-approved exercise program helps pregnant women maintain a positive body image and prevent excess weight gain.

What Are a Pregnant Woman's Nutrient Needs?

The requirement for nearly all nutrients increases during pregnancy to accommodate the growth and development of the fetus without depriving the mother of the nutrients she needs to maintain her own health. With the exception of iron, most of these increased needs can be met by carefully selecting foods high in nutrient density. The Choose MyPlate.gov website provides useful information that emphasizes the need for

For a useful video on recommended weight gain during pregnancy, visit www.youtube.com. Enter "weight gain during pregnancy 461737986," then click on the first link.

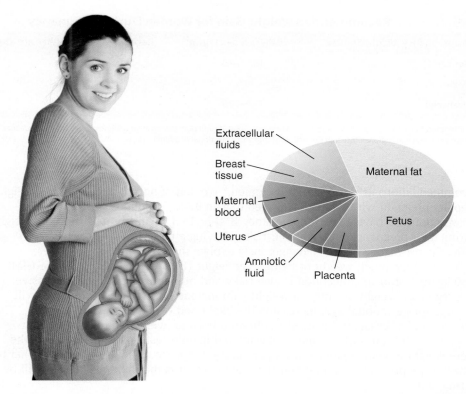

Extracellular fluids

Breast tissue

Maternal blood

Uterus

Amniotic fluid

Maternal fat

Fetus

Placenta

⬆ **FIGURE 14.6** The weight gained during pregnancy is distributed between the mother's own tissues and the pregnancy-specific tissues.

dietary adequacy, balance, and variety in food choices; it also suggests food patterns for pregnant women (see Web Resources at the end of this chapter).

Macronutrient Needs of Pregnant Women

During pregnancy, macronutrients provide necessary energy for building tissue. They are also the building blocks for the physical form and structure of the fetus as well as for other pregnancy-associated tissues.

Energy Energy requirements increase only modestly during pregnancy.[8] In fact, during the first trimester, a woman should consume approximately the same number of Calories daily as during her nonpregnant days. Instead of eating more, she should attempt to maximize the nutrient density of what she eats. For example, drinking low-fat milk is preferable to drinking soft drinks. Low-fat milk provides valuable protein, vitamins, and minerals to feed the fetus's rapidly dividing cells, whereas soft drinks provide nutritionally empty Calories.

During the last two trimesters of pregnancy, caloric needs increase by about 350 to 450 kcal/day. For a woman consuming 2,000 kcal/day, an extra 400 kcal represents only a 20% increase in Calorie intake. For example, 1 cup of low-fat yogurt and a graham cracker with jam is about 400 kcal. At the same time, some vitamin and mineral needs increase by as much as 50%, so again, the key for getting adequate micronutrients while not consuming too many extra Calories is choosing nutrient-dense foods.

Protein and Carbohydrate During pregnancy, protein needs increase to 1.1 g/day/kg body weight (an additional 25 g or so of protein per day).[8] Many women already eat this much protein each day. Dairy products, meats, eggs, and soy products are all rich sources of protein, as are legumes, nuts, and seeds.

Carbohydrate intake should be at least 175 g/day.[8] The majority of carbohydrate intake should come from whole-grain breads and cereals, brown rice, fruits, vegetables, and legumes. Not only are these carbohydrate-rich foods good sources of the

B-vitamins and other nutrients, but they also contain a lot of fiber. Fiber-rich foods contribute to one's sense of fullness, helping to avoid excess weight gain, and may lower risk of constipation.

Fat   The guideline for the percentage of daily Calories that come from fat does not change during pregnancy.[8] Pregnant women should be aware that, because new tissues and cells are being built, some fat in the diet is essential.

Moderation in the amount of dietary fat and consumption of the right kinds of fats is important. Like anyone else, pregnant women should limit their intakes of saturated and *trans* fats because of their negative impact on cardiovascular health (see Chapter 5 for more detail on fats). The omega-3 polyunsaturated fatty acid *docosahexaenoic acid (DHA)* and the omega-6 arachidonic acid *(ARA)* have been linked in some, but not all, studies to both enhanced brain growth and eye development. Because the fetal brain grows dramatically during the third trimester, DHA is especially important in the maternal diet. Good sources of DHA are oily fish, such as salmon, sardines, anchovies, and mackerel. It is also found in smaller amounts in tuna, chicken, and eggs (some eggs are DHA enhanced by feeding hens a DHA-rich diet). ARA is found in most types of meat, fish, and poultry.

Pregnant women who eat fish should be aware of the potential for mercury contamination because even a limited intake of mercury during pregnancy can impair a fetus's developing nervous system. Although pregnant women should avoid large fish, such as swordfish, shark, tile fish, and king mackerel, they can safely consume up to 12 oz of most other types of fish per week, as long as it is properly cooked. Albacore tuna, however, should be limited to 6 oz per week because it is higher in mercury than other types of tuna.[7]

Micronutrient Needs of Pregnant Women

During pregnancy, expansion of the mother's blood supply and growth of the uterus, placenta, breasts, body fat levels, and the fetus itself all contribute to an increased need for micronutrients. In addition, the increased need for energy during pregnancy correlates with an increased need for the micronutrients involved in energy metabolism. Discussions of the micronutrients that are most critical during pregnancy follow. See **TABLE 14.2** for an overview of the changes in micronutrient needs with pregnancy.

Folate   Because folate is necessary for cell division, it follows that, during a time when both maternal and fetal cells are dividing rapidly, the requirement for this vitamin increases. Adequate folate is especially critical during the first 28 days after conception, when it is required for the formation and closure of the **neural tube**, an embryonic structure that eventually becomes the brain and spinal cord. Folate deficiency is associated with neural tube defects, such as **anencephaly**, a fatal defect

TABLE 14.2   Changes in Nutrient Recommendations with Pregnancy for Adult Women

Micronutrient	Prepregnancy	Pregnancy	% Increase
Folate	400 µg/day	600 µg/day	50
Vitamin B$_{12}$	2.4 µg/day	2.6 µg/day	8
Vitamin C	75 mg/day	85 mg/day	13
Vitamin A	700 µg/day	770 µg/day	10
Vitamin D	600 IU/day	600 IU/day	0
Calcium	1,000 mg/day	1,000 mg/day	0
Iron	18 mg/day	27 mg/day	50
Zinc	8 mg/day	11 mg/day	38
Sodium	1,500 mg/day	1,500 mg/day	0
Iodine	150 µg/day	220 µg/day	47

neural tube Embryonic tissue that forms a tube, which eventually becomes the brain and spinal cord.

anencephaly A fatal neural tube defect in which there is partial absence of brain tissue, most likely caused by failure of the neural tube to close.

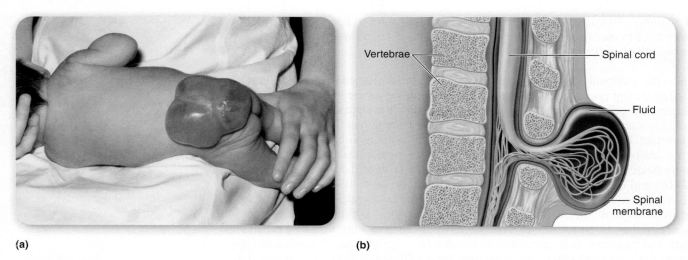

(a)   (b)

⬤ **FIGURE 14.7** Spina bifida, a common neural tube defect. **(a)** An external view of an infant with spina bifida. **(b)** An internal view of the protruding spinal membrane and fluid-filled sac.

in which brain tissue is partially or fully absent, and **spina bifida**, in which a portion of the spinal cord protrudes through the spinal vertebrae, causing varying degrees of paralysis **(FIGURE 14.7)**. Adequate folate intake does not guarantee normal neural tube development because the precise cause of neural tube defects is unknown, and there is a genetic component in some cases. Still, it is estimated that 70% of all neural tube defects could be prevented if all women of childbearing age consumed enough folate or folic acid.[9]

To reduce the risk for a neural tube defect, all women capable of becoming pregnant are encouraged to consume 400 µg of folate per day. Of course, folate remains very important even after the neural tube has closed. The RDA for folate for pregnant women is therefore 600 µg/day, a full 50% increase over the RDA for a nonpregnant female.[10] A deficiency of folate during pregnancy can result in macrocytic anemia (a condition in which blood cells do not mature properly) and has been associated with low birth weight, preterm delivery, and failure of the fetus to grow properly. Sources of folate include fortified cereals and grains, spinach, and lentils.

Vitamin B$_{12}$ Vitamin B$_{12}$ (cobalamin) is vital during pregnancy because it regenerates the active form of folate. Not surprisingly, deficiencies of vitamin B$_{12}$ can also result in macrocytic anemia. Yet the RDA for vitamin B$_{12}$ for pregnant women is only 2.6 µg/day, a mere 8% increase over the RDA of 2.4 µg/day for nonpregnant women.[10] How can this be? One reason is that, during pregnancy, absorption of vitamin B$_{12}$ is more efficient. The required amount of vitamin B$_{12}$ can easily be obtained from animal food sources. However, deficiencies have been observed in women who follow a vegan diet. Fortified foods or supplementation provides these women with the needed B$_{12}$.

Vitamin C   Vitamin C is necessary for the synthesis of collagen, a component of connective tissue (including skin, blood vessels, and tendons) and part of the organic matrix of bones. The RDA for vitamin C during pregnancy is increased by a little more than 10% over the RDA for nonpregnant women (from 75 to 85 mg/day).[11] A deficiency of vitamin C during pregnancy increases the risk for preterm birth and other complications. Abundant amounts of vitamin C are found in many food sources, such as citrus fruits and juices and numerous other fruits and vegetables.

Vitamin A   Vitamin A needs increase during pregnancy by about 10%, to 770 µg/day.[12] However, excess preformed vitamin A can cause fetal abnormalities, particularly heart defects and facial malformations. A well-balanced diet supplies sufficient vitamin A, so supplementation during pregnancy is not recommended. Beta-carotene (which is converted to vitamin A in the body) has not been associated with birth defects.

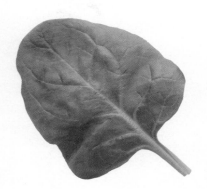

⬤ Spinach is an excellent source of folate.

spina bifida The embryotic neural tube defect that occurs when the spinal vertebrae fail to completely enclose the spinal cord, allowing it to protrude.

Vitamin D   Despite the role of vitamin D in calcium absorption, the RDA for this nutrient does not increase during pregnancy.[13] Pregnant women who receive adequate exposure to sunlight do not need vitamin D supplements. However, pregnant women with darkly pigmented skin and/or limited sun exposure who do not regularly drink milk (which is fortified with vitamin D) will benefit from vitamin D supplementation. Most prenatal vitamin supplements contain 10 µg/day of vitamin D, which is considered safe and acceptable.[10] Pregnant women should be cautious and avoid consuming excessive vitamin D from supplements because toxicity can cause developmental disability in the newborn.

Calcium   Growth of the fetal skeleton requires a significant amount of calcium. However, the RDA for adult pregnant women is the same as that for nonpregnant women, 1,000 mg/day, for two reasons.[13] First, pregnant women absorb calcium from the diet more efficiently than do nonpregnant women. Second, the extra demand for calcium has not been found to cause demineralization of the mother's bones or to increase fracture risk; thus, there is no justification for higher intakes. Sources of calcium include milk, yogurt, and cheese; nondairy foods, such as kale, collard greens, and broccoli; and calcium-fortified soy milk, juices, and cereals.

Iron   Recall (from Chapter 10) the importance of iron in the formation of red blood cells, which transport oxygen throughout the body. During pregnancy, the demand for red blood cells increases to accommodate the needs of the mother's expanded blood volume, the growing uterus, the placenta, and the fetus itself. Thus, more iron is needed. Fetal demand for iron increases even further during the last trimester, when the fetus stores iron in the liver for use during the first few months of life.

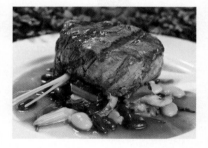

Meats provide protein, vitamin B_{12}, heme iron, and zinc.

Severely inadequate iron intake has the potential to harm the fetus, resulting in an increased risk for low birth weight, preterm birth, and death of the newborn in the first weeks after birth. However, in most cases, the fetus builds adequate stores by "robbing" maternal iron, prompting iron-deficiency anemia in the mother. During pregnancy, maternal iron deficiency causes paleness and exhaustion, but at birth it endangers her life: anemic women are more likely to die during or shortly following childbirth because they are less able to tolerate blood loss and fight infection.

The RDA for iron for pregnant women is 27 mg/day, compared to 18 mg/day for nonpregnant women.[12] This represents a 50% increase, despite the fact that iron loss is minimized during pregnancy because menstruation ceases. Typically, women of childbearing age have poor iron stores, and the demands of pregnancy are likely to produce a deficiency. To ensure adequate iron stores during pregnancy, an iron supplement (as part of, or distinct from, a total prenatal supplement) is routinely prescribed during the last two trimesters. Vitamin C enhances iron absorption, as do dietary sources of heme iron, whereas substances in coffee, tea, milk, bran, and oxalates decrease iron absorption. Therefore, many healthcare providers recommend taking iron supplements with foods high in vitamin C and/or heme iron. Sources of iron include clams, fortified cereals, legumes, spinach, and meats.

Zinc   The RDA for zinc for adult pregnant women increases by about 38% over the RDA for nonpregnant women, from 8 mg/day to 11 mg/day.[12] Zinc is critical in DNA, RNA, and protein synthesis, and inadequate intake can lead to malformations in the fetus, premature labor, and extended labor. It should be noted that the absorption of zinc is inhibited by high intakes of non-heme iron, such as high-potency iron supplements, when these two minerals are taken with water.[11] However, when food sources of iron and zinc are consumed together in a meal, absorption of zinc is not affected. In addition, the heme form of iron does not appear to inhibit zinc absorption.

Sodium and Iodine   During pregnancy, the AI for sodium is the same as for a nonpregnant adult woman, or 1,500 mg (1.5 g) per day.[14] Although too much sodium is associated with fluid retention, bloating, and high blood pressure, an increase in body fluids is a normal and necessary part of pregnancy, so some sodium is necessary to maintain fluid balance.

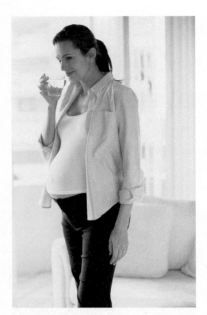

⬆ It's important for pregnant women to drink about 10 cups of fluid a day.

Iodine needs increase significantly during pregnancy, but the RDA of 220 µg/day is easy to achieve by using a modest amount of iodized salt (sodium chloride) during cooking.

Do Pregnant Women Need Supplements?

Prenatal multivitamin and mineral supplements are not strictly necessary during pregnancy, but most healthcare providers recommend them. Meeting all the nutrient needs would otherwise take careful and somewhat complex dietary planning. Prenatal supplements are especially good insurance for special populations, such as vegans, adolescents, and others whose diet might normally be low in one or more micronutrients. It is important that pregnant women understand, however, that supplements are to be taken *in addition to,* not as a substitute for, a nutrient-rich diet.

Fluid Needs of Pregnant Women

Fluid allows for the necessary increase in the mother's blood volume, aids in regulating body temperature, and helps maintain the **amniotic fluid** that surrounds, cushions, and protects the fetus in the uterus. The AI for total fluid intake, which includes drinking water, beverages, and food, is 3 liters/day (or about 12.7 cups). This recommendation includes approximately 2.3 liters (10 cups) of fluid as total beverages, including drinking water.[14]

Drinking adequate fluid also helps combat two common discomforts of pregnancy: fluid retention and, possibly, constipation. Drinking lots of fluids may also lower the risk for **urinary tract infections**, which are common in pregnancy. Fluids also combat dehydration, which can develop if a woman has frequent bouts of vomiting. For these women, fluids such as soups, juices, and sports beverages are usually well tolerated.

recap Sufficient Calories should be consumed, so that a pregnant woman gains an appropriate amount of weight, typically 25 to 35 pounds, to ensure adequate growth of the fetus. The Calories consumed during pregnancy should be nutrient-dense. Protein, carbohydrates, and fats provide the building blocks for fetal growth. Folate deficiency has been associated with neural tube defects. Most healthcare providers recommend prenatal supplements for pregnant women. Fluid provides for increased maternal blood volume and amniotic fluid.

Nutrition-Related Concerns for Pregnant Women

Pregnancy-related conditions involving a particular nutrient, such as iron-deficiency anemia, have already been discussed. The following sections describe some of the most common discomforts and disorders of pregnant women that are related to their general nutrition.

Morning Sickness

Morning sickness, or *nausea and vomiting of pregnancy (NVP),* is a potentially serious medical condition.[15] The symptoms vary in severity, from occasional mild queasiness to constant nausea with bouts of vomiting. In truth, "morning sickness" is not an appropriate name because the nausea and vomiting can begin at any time of the day and may last all day. NVP usually peaks between weeks 8 and 12, then resolves by weeks 12 to 16, but some women experience it throughout the pregnancy. Usually, the mother and fetus do not suffer lasting harm. However, some women experience such frequent vomiting that they are unable to nourish or hydrate themselves or their fetus adequately and may require hospitalization or in-home intravenous (IV) therapy.

There is no cure for morning sickness. However, some women find the following strategies helpful for reducing its severity:

- Eating small, frequent meals and snacks throughout the day. An empty stomach can trigger nausea.
- Consuming the majority of fluids between meals. Frozen ice pops, watermelon, gelatin desserts, and mild broths are some well-tolerated sources of fluid.

amniotic fluid The watery fluid contained within the innermost membrane of the sac containing the fetus. It cushions and protects the growing fetus.

urinary tract infection A bacterial infection of the urethra, the tube leading from the bladder to the body exterior.

morning sickness Varying degrees of nausea and vomiting associated with pregnancy, most commonly in the first trimester.

- Keeping snacks such as dry cereal or crackers at the bedside to ease nighttime queasiness or to eat before rising.
- Taking prenatal supplements at a time of day when vomiting is least likely.
- Avoiding sights, sounds, smells, and tastes that bring on or worsen queasiness. Cold or room-temperature foods are often easier to tolerate than hot foods.

For some women, alternative therapies, such as acupuncture, acupressure wrist bands, biofeedback, meditation, and hypnosis, help. Women should always check with their healthcare provider that the therapy they are using is safe and does not interact with other treatments, medications, or supplements.

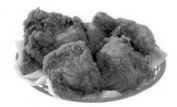

Deep-fried foods are often unappealing to pregnant women.

Cravings and Aversions

It seems like nothing is more stereotypical about pregnancy than the image of a frazzled husband getting up in the middle of the night to run to the convenience store to get his pregnant wife some pickles and ice cream. This image, although humorous, is far from reality for most women. Although some women have specific cravings, most crave a general type of food ("something sweet" or "something salty") rather than a particular food.

Why do pregnant women crave certain tastes? Does a desire for salty foods mean that the woman is experiencing a sodium deficit? Although some people believe that we crave what we need, scientific evidence is lacking. It is more likely that cravings during pregnancy are due to hormonal fluctuations or physiologic changes or have familial or cultural roots. Most cravings are, of course, for edible substances. But a surprising number of pregnant women crave nonfoods, such as laundry starch and clay. This craving, called **pica**, can result in nutritional or health problems for the mother and fetus.[16]

Food aversions are also common during pregnancy and may originate from social, cultural, or religious beliefs. In some cultures, for example, pregnant women avoid shellfish ("causes allergies") or citrus fruits ("may increase risk for a miscarriage"). These types of aversions may not be scientifically valid, but they are often strongly woven into the family's belief system.

Gastroesophageal Reflux

Gastroesophageal reflux (GER) is common during pregnancy because pregnancy-related hormones relax the smooth muscle of the lower esophagus. During the last two trimesters, the enlarging uterus pushes up on the stomach, worsening the problem. (GER is discussed in detail in Chapter 3.) Practical tips for minimizing GER during pregnancy include the following:

- Avoid excessive weight gain, tight clothing, overeating, and foods that seem to trigger the problem.
- Chew food slowly.
- Wait for at least 1 hour after eating before lying down.
- Sleep with the head of the bed elevated.

In addition, the woman's healthcare provider may be able to suggest an antacid that is safe for use during pregnancy.

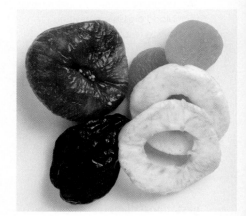

Foods high in fiber, such as dried fruits, reduce the chances of constipation.

Constipation

Hormone production during pregnancy causes the smooth muscles to relax, including the muscles of the large intestine, slowing colonic movement of food residue. In addition, pressure exerted by the growing uterus on the colon can slow movement even further, making elimination difficult. Practical hints that may help a pregnant woman avoid constipation include the following:

- Eat 25 to 35 g of fiber each day, concentrating on fresh fruits and vegetables, legumes, and whole grains.
- Keep fluid intake high as fiber intake increases. Drink plenty of water and eat water-rich fruits and vegetables, such as melons, citrus, and lettuce.
- Keep physically active because exercise is one of many factors that help increase motility of the large intestine.

pica An abnormal craving to eat nonfood substances such as clay, paint, or chalk.

Gestational Diabetes

Gestational diabetes, diagnosed in as many as 10% of U.S. pregnancies, is generally a temporary condition in which a pregnant woman is unable to produce sufficient insulin or becomes insulin resistant, resulting in elevated levels of blood glucose. Screening for gestational diabetes is a routine aspect of prenatal care because the symptoms, which include frequent urination, fatigue, and an increase in thirst and appetite, appear to be the same as normal pregnancy symptoms.

Fortunately, gestational diabetes has no ill effects on either the mother or the fetus if blood glucose levels are strictly controlled through diet, exercise, and/or medication. If not controlled, gestational diabetes can result in a baby who is too large as a result of receiving too much glucose across the placenta during fetal life. Inappropriately large infants are at risk for early delivery and trauma during vaginal birth, and they may need to be born by cesarean section. There is also evidence that exposing a fetus to maternal diabetes significantly increases the risk for overweight and metabolic disorders later in life.[17,18]

Women who are obese, women who are age 35 years or older, and women of Native American, African American, or Hispanic origin have a greater risk of developing gestational diabetes. Any woman who develops gestational diabetes has a 40–60% risk of developing type 2 diabetes within the next 5 to 10 years—particularly if she is obese to begin with or fails to maintain normal body weight after pregnancy. As with any form of diabetes, attention to diet, weight control, and physical activity reduces the risk for gestational diabetes.

Hypertensive Disorders of Pregnancy

About 7% to 8% of U.S. pregnancies are complicated by some form of hypertension, and it accounts for almost 16% of pregnancy-related deaths in developed nations such as the United States.[19] The term *hypertensive disorders of pregnancy* encompasses several different conditions. A woman who develops high blood pressure, with no other symptoms, during her pregnancy is said to have *gestational hypertension*. **Preeclampsia** is characterized by a sudden increase in maternal blood pressure with swelling, excessive and rapid weight gain unrelated to food intake, and protein in the urine. If left untreated, it can progress to *eclampsia*, a very serious condition characterized by seizures, kidney failure, and, potentially, fetal and/or maternal death.

No one knows exactly what causes the various hypertensive disorders of pregnancy, but deficiencies in dietary protein, vitamin C, vitamin E, calcium, and magnesium seem to increase the risk. Other risk factors include first pregnancy, age under 20 or over 35, African American race, diabetes, and a family history of eclampsia. Management focuses mainly on blood pressure control. Typical treatments include medication and close monitoring, with hospitalization if necessary. Ultimately, the only thing that will cure the condition is childbirth. Today, with good prenatal care, gestational hypertension is nearly always detected early and can be appropriately managed, and outcomes for both mother and fetus are usually very good. In nearly all women without prior chronic high blood pressure, maternal blood pressure returns to normal within about a day after the birth.

Adolescent Pregnancy

The adolescent birth rate in the United States is currently 34.3 births for every 1,000 women aged 15 to 19 years. Although this is the lowest rate in the past 60 years, it is still one of the highest among all industrialized nations.[20]

Throughout the adolescent years, a woman's body continues to change and grow. Peak bone mass has not yet been reached. Full physical stature may not have been attained, and teens are more likely to be underweight than are young adult women. Thus, pregnant adolescents have higher needs for Calories and bone-related nutrients, such as calcium. Teens also commonly begin pregnancy in an iron-deficient state and so have an increased iron need. In addition, many adolescents have not established healthful nutritional patterns. At the same time, higher rates of alcohol use, smoking, and drug use contribute to a greater frequency of nutritional deficiencies.

With regular prenatal care and close attention to proper nutrition and other healthful behaviors, the likelihood of a positive outcome for both the adolescent mother and the infant is similar to that for older mothers and their infants.[21]

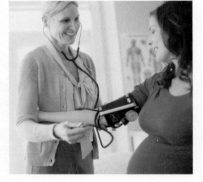

⬆ Pregnant women should have their blood pressure measured regularly to test for gestational hypertension.

gestational diabetes A condition of insufficient insulin production or insulin resistance that results in consistently high blood glucose levels, specifically during pregnancy; the condition typically resolves after birth occurs.

preeclampsia High blood pressure that is pregnancy specific and accompanied by protein in the urine, edema, and unexpected weight gain.

Vegetarianism

With the possible exception of iron and zinc, vegetarian women who consume dairy products and/or eggs (lacto-ovo-vegetarians) have no nutritional concerns beyond those encountered by every pregnant woman. In contrast, women who are totally vegetarian (vegan) need to be more vigilant than usual about their intake of nutrients that are derived primarily or wholly from animal products. These include vitamin D (unless fair skinned and regularly exposed to adequate sunlight throughout pregnancy), vitamin B_6, vitamin B_{12}, calcium, iron, and zinc. Supplements containing these nutrients are usually necessary. A regular prenatal supplement will fully meet the vitamin and iron needs of a vegan woman but does not fulfill calcium needs, so a separate calcium supplement, or consumption of calcium-fortified soy milk or orange juice, is usually required.

Exercise

Physical activity during pregnancy is recommended for all women experiencing normal pregnancies. Women who rarely, if ever, exercised before becoming pregnant and overweight or obese women can benefit greatly from increased activity but should begin slowly and progress gradually under the guidance of their healthcare provider. Women should avoid exercising outdoors when it is hot and humid and should always maintain appropriate fluid intake. Exercise during pregnancy benefits both mother and fetus in the following ways:

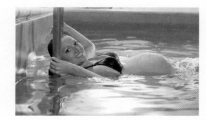

◆ During pregnancy, women should adjust their physical activity toward comfortable low-impact exercises.

- Reduces risk of gestational diabetes and preeclampsia
- Helps prevent excessive prenatal weight and body fat gain
- Improves mood, energy level, sleep patterns
- Enhances posture and balance
- Improves muscle tone, strength, and endurance
- Reduces lower back pain and shortens the duration of active labor
- Reduces the risk of preterm birth and large-for-gestational age infants

Recent guidelines suggest exercises that engage large muscle groups in a continuous manner, including a combination of moderate intensity aerobic activity (brisk walking, leisurely swimming, dancing), vigorous intensity aerobic activity (very brisk walking, swimming at a moderate-to-hard pace, cycling on a stationary bike, indoor rowing), and muscle strengthening activities.[21] The terms "moderate" and "vigorous" are relative because each woman enters and moves through her pregnancy at an individual level of fitness. Moderate activity is often described as one during which it is still possible to carry on a normal conversation; vigorous activity produces sweating, noticeable increases in breathing rate and depth, and an inability to converse normally. The more vigorous the activity, the less total time is needed to reap its benefits: 6.5 hours/week of brisk walking versus fewer than 3 hours/week of stationary cycling.

Recommendations for muscle strengthening exercise during pregnancy are straightforward:[22]

- Choose lighter weights and more repetitions.
- Opt for resistance bands over free weights, which might accidently hit or fall on the abdomen.
- Don't lift weights while lying on your back because this might compress a major blood vessel and restrict blood flow to the fetus.
- Avoid moves that require sudden movements or might place you off balance, such as lunges or twists.
- Pay attention to your body's signals!

What about yoga and pilates? Both offer classes tailored to pregnant women, adapting certain exercises to accommodate the body's changing center of gravity and increased joint flexibility. Activities that strengthen body core, abdominals, and pelvic floor or Kegel muscles make for an easier pregnancy and birth. See **TABLE 14.3** for a sample program of physical activity for a pregnant woman.

Pregnant women should avoid activities such as horseback riding, scuba diving, water or snow skiing, hockey, gymnastics, and soccer. They need to stay hydrated, especially in hot and humid weather, and dress comfortably. If symptoms of stress,

TABLE 14.3 Exercise Plan for Pregnant Women*

Day of the Week	Warm-Up	Aerobic Activity	Muscle Strengthening	Cool-Down
Monday	5–10 min	30–45 min moderate intensity (leisurely lap swimming)		5 min
Tuesday	5–10 min		30 min light weights, high repetitions; upper and lower body	5 min
Wednesday	5–10 min	30 min vigorous activity (indoor cycling or rowing)		5 min
Thursday	5–10 min		45 min yoga, Pilates, or other core exercises	5 min
Friday	5–10 min	30–45 min moderate intensity (outdoor hike, flat or gentle slope)		5 min
Saturday	5–10 min		30 min light weights, high repetitions; upper and lower body	5 min

Note: *Women with established prepregnancy exercise routines should aim for the higher duration; women who rarely/never exercised before pregnancy should start with short durations of low-intensity activity and gradually build endurance.

Want more details on maintaining fitness while pregnant? Watch this slideshow on exercise during and after pregnancy: www.webmd.com. Enter "pregnancy fitness moves slideshow" into the search bar, then click on the first link.

such as dizziness, shortness of breath, chest pain, vaginal bleeding or leakage, or uterine contractions occur, all physical activity should stop and a healthcare provider contacted immediately.[22]

Caffeine Consumption

Caffeine is a stimulant found in several foods, including coffee, tea, soft drinks, and chocolate. Caffeine crosses the placenta and thus reaches the fetus. Current thinking holds that women who consume less than about 200–300 mg per day (the equivalent of one to two cups of coffee) are very likely doing no harm to the fetus.[23] Evidence suggests that consuming higher daily doses of caffeine (the higher the dose, the more compelling the evidence) may slightly increase the risk for miscarriage and stillbirth and impair fetal growth. In addition, maternal intakes as low as 200–300 mg/day have been associated with decreased birth weight.[24] Finally, coffee and colas have no nutritional value and, if sweetened, provide considerable Calories. A low- or nonfat decaf latte, known to Latinas as *café con leche*, offers a more healthful nutrient profile than just coffee alone.

Alcohol Consumption

Frequent drinking (more than seven drinks per week) or occasional binge drinking (more than four to five drinks on one occasion) during pregnancy increases the risk for miscarriage, complications during delivery, preterm birth, and sudden infant death syndrome. In addition, alcohol is a known teratogen, and its consumption during pregnancy increases the risk that the baby will be born with any of a variety of birth defects. (See the **In Depth** on Alcohol following Chapter 7.)

The more a mother drinks, the greater the potential harm to the fetus. Heavy drinking (more than three to four drinks per day) throughout pregnancy can result in a condition called fetal alcohol syndrome (FAS).[25] Babies born with FAS have characteristic malformations, particularly of the face, limbs, heart, and nervous system. They have a high mortality rate, and those who survive typically have emotional, behavioral, social, learning, and developmental problems throughout life. Other birth defects associated with maternal alcohol consumption include heart, skeletal, kidney, ear, and eye malformations as well as a range of lifelong developmental, behavioral, and mental problems (for example, hyperactivity and attention deficit disorder).

Although some women do have the occasional alcoholic drink with no apparent ill effects, there is no amount of alcohol that is known to be safe. The best advice regarding alcohol during pregnancy is to abstain, if not from before conception then as soon as pregnancy is suspected.

Smoking

Although the dangers of smoking are well known, currently more than 13% of pregnant women smoke during pregnancy, and the rate is even higher among pregnant adolescents.[26,27] Maternal smoking exposes the fetus to toxins such as lead, cadmium, cyanide, nicotine, and carbon monoxide. Fetal blood flow is reduced, which limits the delivery of oxygen and nutrients, resulting in impaired fetal growth and development. Maternal smoking greatly increases the risk for miscarriage, stillbirth, placental abnormalities, preterm delivery, and low birth weight. Rates of sudden infant death syndrome, respiratory illness, and allergies are higher in the infants and children of smokers compared to those of nonsmokers.

Illegal Drug Use

Despite the fact that the use of illegal drugs is unquestionably harmful to the fetus, nearly 5% of pregnant women in the United States report having used illicit drugs, with rates highest among pregnant adolescents between 15 and 18 years of age.[28] Most drugs pass through the placenta into fetal blood, where they accumulate in fetal tissues and organs, including the liver and brain. Prenatal use of illegal drugs also impairs placental blood flow (thereby reducing the transfer of nutrients to the fetus) and increases the risk for low birth weight, premature delivery, miscarriage, and placental defects. Newborns suffer signs of withdrawal, including tremors, excessive crying, sleeplessness, and poor feeding. Even after several years, children are at greater risk for developmental delays, impaired learning, and behavioral problems. All women are strongly advised to stop taking drugs before becoming pregnant. There is no safe level of use for illegal drugs during pregnancy.

Food Safety

The U.S. Department of Health and Human Services recommends that pregnant women avoid unpasteurized milk, raw or partially cooked eggs, raw or undercooked meat/fish/poultry, unpasteurized juices, and raw sprouts.[29] Women who are or could become pregnant, as well as breastfeeding mothers, are advised to avoid eating large fish, such as shark, swordfish, and king mackerel, and to limit their intake of canned albacore tuna because of their high mercury content. Pregnant women should consult their state or county health department for information on the safety of locally caught fish.

Fish, shellfish, and a variety of meats may be contaminated with dioxins, persistent organic pollutants associated with a variety of health problems. The effect of dioxins may be most significant on the developing fetal organs, including the nervous system.[30] As with mercury, state and county health departments can provide information about dioxin levels in the local food supply.

Soft cheeses, such as Brie, feta, Camembert, and Mexican-style cheeses—also called *queso blanco* or *queso fresco*—should be avoided unless the label specifically states the product is made with pasteurized milk. Unpasteurized milk and cheeses may be contaminated with the bacterium *Listeria monocytogenes*, which triggers miscarriage, premature birth, or fetal infection when consumed during pregnancy. (Safe food-handling practices are discussed in Chapter 13.)

recap   About half of all pregnant women experience morning sickness. Heartburn and constipation in pregnancy are related to hormonal relaxation of smooth muscle. Gestational diabetes and hypertensive disorders can seriously affect maternal and fetal well-being. The nutrient needs of pregnant adolescents are so high that adequate nourishment becomes difficult. Women who follow a vegan diet usually need to consume supplements during pregnancy. Exercise (provided the mother has no contraindications) can enhance the health of a pregnant woman. Caffeine intake should be limited and the use of alcohol, cigarettes, and illegal drugs should be completely avoided during pregnancy. Safe food choices and handling practices are especially important during pregnancy.

nutri-case | JUDY

"Back when I was pregnant with Hannah, the doctor told me I had gestational diabetes but said I shouldn't worry about it. He said I didn't need any medication, and I don't remember changing my diet. In fact, I just kept eating whatever I wanted, and by the time Hannah was born, I had gained almost 60 pounds! I never did lose all that extra weight."

Review what you learned about diabetes in the **In Depth** following Chapter 4 (pages 139–145). What information would have been important for Judy to learn while she was pregnant? Is it common for women with gestational diabetes to develop type 2 diabetes later? What are some things Judy could have done to lower her risk for type 2 diabetes?

Lactation: Nutrition for breastfeeding mothers

Throughout most of human history, infants have thrived on only one food: breast milk. But during the first half of the 20th century, commercially prepared infant formulas slowly began to replace breast milk as the mother's preferred feeding method. Aggressive marketing campaigns convinced many families, even in developing nations, to switch. Soon formula-feeding had become a status symbol, proof of the family's wealth and modern thinking. In the 1970s, this trend began to reverse with a renewed appreciation for the natural simplicity of breastfeeding. At the same time, several international organizations, including the World Health Organization, UNICEF, and La Leche League, began to promote the nutritional, immunologic, financial, and emotional advantages of breastfeeding and developed programs to encourage and support breastfeeding worldwide. These efforts have paid off: in 2012, almost 77% of new mothers initiated breastfeeding in the hospital and over 47% of mothers were still breastfeeding their babies at 6 months of age.[31] Worldwide, more than half of all women breastfeed *exclusively* for at least 6 months; however, only 16% of U.S. infants are exclusively breastfed at 6 months of age.

How, exactly, does breastfeeding occur? What nutrients are important for breastfeeding mothers? And what exactly are the advantages that everyone is talking about? The answers to these questions are presented in the following sections.

How Does Lactation Occur?

Lactation, the production of breast milk, is a process that is set in motion during pregnancy in response to several hormones. Once established, lactation can be sustained as long as the mammary glands continue to receive the proper stimuli.

The Body Prepares During Pregnancy

Throughout pregnancy, the placenta produces estrogen and progesterone. In addition to performing various functions to maintain the pregnancy, these hormones prepare the breasts physically for lactation. The breasts increase in size, and milk-producing glands (alveoli) and milk ducts are formed **(FIGURE 14.8)**. Toward the end of pregnancy, the hormone *prolactin* increases. Prolactin is released by the anterior pituitary gland and is responsible for milk

lactation The production of breast milk.

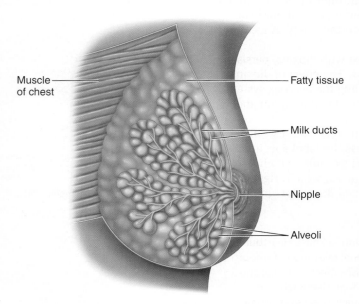

Muscle of chest

Fatty tissue

Milk ducts

Nipple

Alveoli

FIGURE 14.8 Anatomy of the breast. During pregnancy, estrogen and progesterone secreted by the placenta foster the preparation of breast tissue for lactation. This process includes breast enlargement and development of the milk-producing glands, or alveoli.

HOT TOPIC

Can a Mother Breastfeed Her Adopted Baby?

It might sound impossible, but it's not! Some women who wish to breastfeed their adopted baby have induced lactation by stimulating production of the hormones that naturally cause milk production and letdown. How? The most common method is to pump both breasts using a hospital-grade breast pump three times a day, beginning about 2 months before the expected adoption date. The woman's physician can also prescribe pharmaceutical estrogen, progesterone, or other medications that mimic the effects of pregnancy. If used, these are discontinued before breastfeeding begins, at which point the infant's suckling should stimulate and maintain milk production. Additional information can be found by going to the Mayo Clinic website (www.mayoclinic.org) and searching on the terms "health" and "induced lactation."

synthesis. However, estrogen and progesterone suppress the effects of prolactin during pregnancy.

What Happens After Childbirth

By the time a pregnancy has come to full term, the level of prolactin is about ten times higher than it was at the beginning of pregnancy. At birth, the suppressive effect of estrogen and progesterone ends, and prolactin is free to stimulate milk production. The first substance released is **colostrum**, sometimes called pre-milk or first milk. It is thick, yellowish in color, and rich in protein and micronutrients, and it includes antibodies that help protect the newborn from infection. Colostrum also contains a factor that fosters the growth of a particular species of "friendly" bacteria in the infant gastrointestinal tract. These bacteria in turn prevent the growth of other, potentially harmful bacteria. Finally, colostrum has a laxative effect in infants, helping the infant expel *meconium*, the sticky "first stool."

Within 4 to 6 days in most women, colostrum is fully replaced by mature milk. Mature breast milk contains protein, fat, and carbohydrate (in the form of the sugar lactose). Much of the protein and fat is synthesized in the breast, while the rest enters the milk from the mother's bloodstream.

Mother–Infant Interaction Maintains Milk Production

Continued, sustained breast milk production depends entirely on infant suckling (or a similar stimulus, such as a mechanical breast pump). Infant suckling stimulates the continued production of prolactin, which in turn stimulates more milk production. The longer and more vigorous the feeding, the more milk will be produced. Thus, even multiples (twins, triplets) can be successfully breastfed.

Prolactin allows for milk to be produced, but that milk has to move through the milk ducts to the nipple in order to reach the baby's mouth. The hormone responsible for this "let down" of milk is *oxytocin*. Like prolactin, oxytocin is produced by the pituitary gland, and its production is dependent on the suckling stimulus at the beginning of a feeding (**FIGURE 14.9** on page 532). This response usually occurs within 10 to 30 seconds but can be significantly inhibited by stress. Finding a relaxed environment in which to breastfeed is therefore important.

What Are a Breastfeeding Woman's Nutrient Needs?

You might be surprised to learn that breastfeeding requires even more energy than pregnancy! This is because breast milk has to supply an adequate amount of all the nutrients an infant needs to grow and develop.

Nutrient Recommendations for Breastfeeding Women

It is estimated that milk production requires about 700 to 800 kcal/day. It is generally recommended that lactating women 19 and older consume 330 kcal/day above their prepregnancy energy needs during the first 6 months of lactation and 400 additional kcal/day during the second 6 months.[8] This additional energy is sufficient to support

colostrum The first fluid made and secreted by the breasts from late in pregnancy to about a week after birth. It is rich in immune factors and protein.

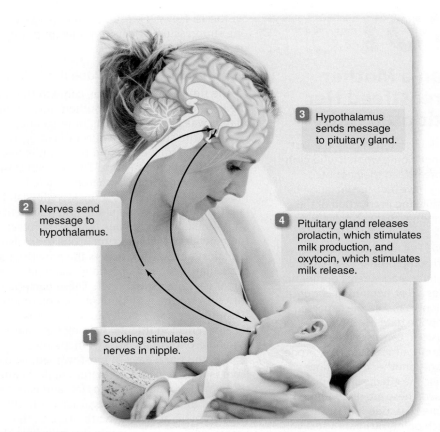

3 Hypothalamus sends message to pituitary gland.

2 Nerves send message to hypothalamus.

4 Pituitary gland releases prolactin, which stimulates milk production, and oxytocin, which stimulates milk release.

1 Suckling stimulates nerves in nipple.

FIGURE 14.9 Sustained milk production depends on the mother–child interaction during breastfeeding, specifically the suckling of the infant. Suckling stimulates the continued production of prolactin, which is responsible for milk production, and oxytocin, which is responsible for the let-down response.

adequate milk production. The remaining energy deficit will assist in the gradual loss of excess fat and body weight gained during pregnancy. It is critical that lactating women avoid severe energy restriction because this practice can result in decreased milk production.

The weight loss that occurs during breastfeeding should be gradual, approximately 1 to 4 pounds per month. Both breastfeeding and participation in regular physical activity can assist with weight loss. The 2010 Dietary Guidelines for Americans confirm that neither occasional nor regular exercise negatively affects a woman's ability to breastfeed successfully.[7] Some active women, however, may lose too much weight during breastfeeding and must either increase their energy intake or reduce their activity level to maintain health.

Of the macronutrients, protein and carbohydrate needs are different from pregnancy requirements. Increases of 15 to 20 g of protein per day and 80 g of carbohydrate per day above prepregnancy requirements are recommended during lactation.[8] Women who breastfeed also need good dietary sources of the essential fatty acids.

The needs for several vitamins and minerals increase over the requirements of pregnancy. These include vitamins A, C, and E, riboflavin, vitamin B_{12}, biotin, and choline, as well as the minerals copper, chromium, manganese, iodine, selenium, and zinc. The requirement for folate during lactation is 500 µg/day, which is decreased from the 600 µg/day required during pregnancy, but it is still higher than prepregnancy needs (400 µg/day).[10]

Requirements for iron decrease significantly during lactation to a mere 9 mg/day.[12] This is because iron is not a significant component of breast milk, and breastfeeding usually suppresses menstruation for at least a few months, minimizing iron losses.

Calcium is a significant component of breast milk; however, as in pregnancy, calcium absorption is enhanced during lactation, and urinary loss of calcium is decreased. In addition, some calcium appears to come from the demineralization of the mother's bones, and increased dietary calcium does not prevent this. Thus, the recommended intake for calcium for a lactating woman is unchanged from pregnancy and nonpregnant guidelines—that is, 1,000 mg/day (for mothers over age 18).[13] Because of their own continuing growth, however, teen mothers who are breastfeeding should continue to consume 1,300 mg/day.[13] Typically, if calcium intake is adequate, a woman's bone density returns to normal shortly after lactation ends.

ChooseMyPlate.gov provides a Daily Food Plan for Moms with specific, individualized dietary advice for women who are pregnant, or who are exclusively or partially breastfeeding their infants (see Web Resources at the end of this chapter).

Do Breastfeeding Women Need Supplements?

If a breastfeeding woman appropriately increases her energy intake, and does so with nutrient-dense foods, her nutrient needs can usually be met without supplements. However, there is nothing wrong with taking a basic multivitamin for insurance, as long as it is not considered a substitute for proper nutrition. Lactating women should consume either fish or fish oil supplements to increase the levels of DHA in their breast milk in order to support the infant's developing nervous system. Women who don't consume dairy products should monitor their calcium intake carefully.

Fluid Recommendations for Breastfeeding Women

Because extra fluid is expended with every feeding, lactating women need to consume about an extra quart (about 1 liter) of fluid per day.[14] This extra fluid facilitates milk production and reduces risk for dehydration. Many women report that, within a minute or two of beginning to nurse their baby, they become intensely thirsty. To prevent this thirst and achieve the recommended fluid intake, women are encouraged to drink a nutritious beverage, such as water, juice, or milk, each time they nurse their baby. However, it is not good practice to drink hot beverages while nursing because accidental spills could burn the infant.

recap Lactation is the result of the coordinated effort of several hormones, including estrogen, progesterone, prolactin, and oxytocin. Breasts are prepared for lactation during pregnancy, and infant suckling provides the stimulus that sustains the production of the prolactin and oxytocin needed to maintain the milk supply. It is recommended that lactating women consume an extra 300–400 kcal/day above prepregnancy energy intake, including increased protein, DHA, certain vitamins and minerals, and fluids. The requirements for folate and iron decrease from pregnancy levels, whereas the requirement for calcium remains the same.

Getting Real About Breastfeeding: Advantages and Challenges

Breastfeeding is the perfect way to nourish a baby for the first 6 months of life. However, the technique does require patience and practice, and teaching by an experienced mother or a certified lactation consultant is important. La Leche League International (see Web Resources at the end of this chapter) and "Baby Friendly" hospitals can provide ongoing support and advice. For some women, illness, medication use, or other factors may make breastfeeding a difficult choice. The decision to breastfeed or use formula must be made by each family after careful consideration of all the factors that apply to their situation.

Advantages of Breastfeeding

As adept as formula manufacturers have been at simulating the components of breast milk, an exact replica has never been produced. In addition, there are benefits that mother and baby can access only through breastfeeding.

Nutritional Quality of Breast Milk The amount and types of protein in breast milk are ideally suited to the human infant. The main protein in breast milk, lactalbumin,

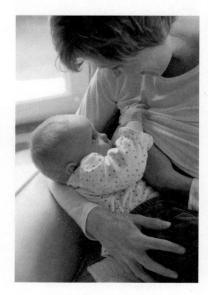

Breastfeeding has benefits for both the mother and her infant.

is easily digested in infants' immature gastrointestinal tracts, reducing the risk for gastric distress. Other proteins in breast milk bind iron and prevent the growth of harmful bacteria that require iron. Antibodies from the mother are additional proteins that help prevent infection while the infant's immune system is still immature. Certain proteins in human milk improve the absorption of iron; this is important because breast milk is low in iron. Cow's milk contains too much protein for infants, and the types of protein in cow's milk are harder for the infant to digest.

The primary carbohydrate in milk is lactose, a disaccharide composed of glucose and galactose. The galactose component is important in nervous system development. Lactose provides energy and prevents ketosis in the infant, promotes the growth of beneficial bacteria, and increases the absorption of calcium. Breast milk has more lactose than cow's milk.

The amounts and types of fats in breast milk are ideally suited to the human infant. DHA and ARA have been shown in many studies to be essential for growth and development of the infant's nervous system and for development of the retina (neural tissue) of the eyes. Interestingly, the concentration of DHA in breast milk varies considerably, reflecting the amount of DHA in the mother's diet, and is highest in women who regularly consume fish.

The fat content of breast milk, which is higher than that of whole cow's milk, changes according to the gestational age of the infant and during the course of every feeding: The milk that is initially released (called *foremilk*) is watery and low in fat, somewhat like skim milk. This milk is thought to satisfy the infant's initial thirst. As the feeding progresses, the milk acquires more fat and becomes more like whole milk. Finally, the very last 5% or so of the milk produced during a feeding (called the *hind-milk*) is very high in fat, similar to cream. This milk is thought to satiate the infant. It is important to let infants suckle for at least 20 minutes at each feeding, so that they get this hindmilk. Breast milk is also relatively high in cholesterol, which supports the rapid growth and development of the brain.

Another important aspect of breastfeeding (or any type of feeding) is the fluid it provides the infant. Because of their small size, infants are at risk for dehydration, which is one reason feedings must be consistent and frequent. This topic is discussed at greater length in the section on infant nutrition.

In terms of micronutrients, breast milk is a good source of readily absorbed calcium and magnesium. It is low in iron, but the iron it does contain is easily absorbed. Because healthy full-term infants store iron in preparation for the first few months of life, most experts agree that their iron needs can be met by breast milk alone for the first 6 months, after which iron-rich foods are needed. Although breast milk has some vitamin D, the American Academy of Pediatrics and other professional groups recommend that all infants, including those who are breastfed, be provided a vitamin D supplement, particularly those infants with highly pigmented skin.[32]

Breast milk composition continues to change as the infant grows and develops. Because of this ability to change as the baby matures, breast milk alone is entirely sufficient to sustain infant growth for the first 6 months of life. In addition, exclusively breast-fed infants maintain total control over their food intake, allowing them to self-regulate energy intake during a critical period of growth and development. Some researchers believe this self-regulation accounts for the finding that breast-fed babies grow in length and weight at a slower rate than formula-fed infants. The relationship between breastfeeding and lifelong patterns of weight gain are explored in more detail in the Nutrition Debate at the end of this chapter.

Throughout the next 6 months of infancy, as solid foods are gradually introduced, breast milk remains the baby's primary source of superior-quality nutrition. The American Academy of Pediatrics recommends exclusive breastfeeding for the first 6 months of life, continuing breastfeeding for at least the first year of life, and, if acceptable within the family, into the second year of life.[33]

Protection from Infections, Allergies, and Residues Immune factors from the mother, including antibodies and immune cells, are passed directly from the mother to the newborn through breast milk. These factors provide important disease protection for the infant while its immune system is still immature. It has been shown that

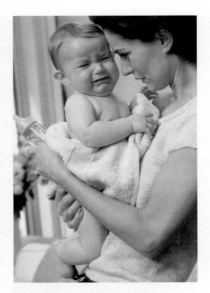

Although there are many benefits to breastfeeding, some breast-fed babies may resist taking a bottle.

breast-fed infants have a lower incidence of respiratory tract, gastrointestinal tract, and ear infections than formula-fed infants.[33] Even a few weeks of breastfeeding is beneficial, but the longer a child is breastfed, the greater the level of passive immunity from the mother. In the United States, exclusive breastfeeding for 6 months has the potential to lower healthcare costs by as much as $13 billion per year, in large part due to a reduction in infant mortality rates related to **sudden infant death syndrome (SIDS)** and necrotizing enterocolitis (a disorder that causes tissue death in the intestine) in breast-fed infants.[34]

In addition, breast milk is nonallergenic, and breastfeeding is associated with a reduced risk for allergies during childhood and adulthood. Breast-fed babies also have a decreased risk of developing diabetes, overweight and obesity, and chronic digestive disorders.[34]

Breast-fed infants are known to have a different profile of gastrointestinal (GI) flora compared to formula-fed infants. Specifically, breast-fed infants have greater numbers of health-promoting *Bifidobacteria* and lower counts of infection-producing bacteria. These differences in the infant GI microbiome are due not only to the bacteria found in breast milk, but also to the presence of oligosaccharides and other prebiotics within breast milk. Moreover, it is thought that the microbiome of breast-fed infants reduces future risk of obesity, allergies, inflammatory disorders, and metabolic diseases.[35]

Exclusively breast-fed infants are also protected from exposure to known and unknown contaminants and residues that may be found in baby bottles and cans of infant formulas. Recent concerns have centered on bisphenol A (BPA), a toxic chemical that has been found in some brands of reusable bottles and formula cans. As of 2009, the major U.S. manufacturers of baby bottles and infant feeding cups, which account for 90% of U.S. sales, had discontinued the sale of products using BPA for the U.S. market[36] (see the Hot Topic box in Chapter 13, page 493).

Physiologic Benefits for Mother Breastfeeding causes uterine contractions, which quicken the return of the uterus to prepregnancy size and reduce bleeding. Many women also find that breastfeeding helps them lose the weight they gained during pregnancy, particularly if it continues for more than 6 months. In addition, breastfeeding appears to be associated with a decreased risk for breast cancer.[37] The relationship between breastfeeding and osteoporosis is still unclear, and more research on this topic is needed.

Breastfeeding also suppresses ovulation, lengthening the time between pregnancies and giving a mother's body the chance to recover before she conceives again. This benefit can be lifesaving for malnourished women living in countries that discourage or outlaw the use of contraceptives. Ovulation may not cease completely, however, so it is still possible to become pregnant while breastfeeding. Healthcare providers typically recommend the use of additional birth control methods while breastfeeding to avoid another conception occurring too soon to allow a mother's body to recover from the earlier pregnancy.

Mother–Infant Bonding Breastfeeding is among the most intimate of human interactions. Ideally, it is a quiet time away from distractions when mother and baby begin to develop an enduring bond of affection known as *attachment*. Breastfeeding enhances attachment by providing the opportunity for frequent, direct skin-to-skin contact, which stimulates the baby's sense of touch and is a primary means of communication. Most hospitals now permit round-the-clock rooming-in of breast-fed infants in order to encourage breastfeeding. The cuddling and intense watching that occur during breastfeeding begin to teach the mother and baby about the other's behavioral cues. Breastfeeding also reassures the mother that she is providing the best possible nutrition for her baby.

Undoubtedly, bottle-feeding does not preclude parent–infant attachment! As long as attention is paid to closeness, cuddling, and skin and eye contact, bottle-feeding can foster bonding as well.

Convenience and Cost Breast milk is always ready, clean, at the right temperature, and available on demand, whenever and wherever it's needed. In the middle of the

sudden infant death syndrome (SIDS) The sudden death of a previously healthy infant; the most common cause of death in infants over 1 month of age.

night, when the baby wakes up hungry, a breastfeeding mother can respond almost instantaneously, and both are soon back to sleep. In contrast, formula-feeding is a time-consuming process: parents have to continually wash and sterilize bottles, and each batch of formula must be mixed and heated to the proper temperature.

In addition, breastfeeding costs nothing other than the price of a modest amount of additional food for the mother. In contrast, formula can be relatively expensive, and there are the additional costs of bottles and other supplies as well as the cost of energy used for washing and sterilization. A hidden cost of formula-feeding is its effect on the environment: the energy used and waste produced during formula manufacturing, marketing, shipping and distribution, preparation, and disposal of used packaging. In contrast, breastfeeding is environmentally responsible, using no external energy and producing no external wastes.

Challenges Associated with Breastfeeding

For some women and infants, breastfeeding is easy from the very first day. Others experience some initial difficulty, but with support from an experienced nurse, lactation consultant, or volunteer mother from La Leche League, the experience becomes successful and pleasurable. In contrast, some families encounter difficulties that make formula-feeding their best choice. This section discusses some challenges that may impede the success of breastfeeding.

Effects of Drugs and Other Substances on Breast Milk   Many substances, including illegal, prescription, and over-the-counter drugs, pass into breast milk. Breastfeeding mothers should inform their physician that they are breastfeeding. If a safe and effective form of a necessary medication cannot be found, the mother will have to avoid breastfeeding while she is taking the drug. During this time, she can pump and discard her breast milk, so that her milk supply will be adequate when she resumes breastfeeding.

Caffeine, alcohol, nicotine, and illicit drugs also enter breast milk. Caffeine, nicotine, and other stimulant drugs can make the baby agitated and fussy and disturb infant sleep patterns. Breastfeeding women should reduce their caffeine intake to no more than two or three cups of coffee per day (or the equivalent of other caffeine containing beverages and foods) and avoid caffeine intake within 2 hours prior to nursing their infant. They should also quit smoking and avoid the use of illicit drugs. Alcohol can make the baby sleepy, depress the central nervous system, and slow motor development, in addition to inhibiting the mother's milk supply. Breastfeeding women should abstain from alcohol in the early stages of lactation because it easily passes into the breast milk and infants 0 to 3 months of age metabolize alcohol at a rate half that of adults. It takes about 2 to 3 hours for the alcohol from a single serving of beer or wine to be eliminated from the body, so it is possible but challenging for breastfeeding women to coordinate moderate alcohol intake with their breastfeeding schedule.

Environmental contaminants, including pesticides, industrial solvents, dioxins, and heavy metals (such as lead and mercury), can pass into breast milk when breastfeeding mothers are exposed to these chemicals. Mothers can limit their infants' exposure to these harmful substances by controlling their own environments. Fresh fruits and vegetables should be thoroughly washed and peeled to minimize exposure to pesticides and fertilizer residues. Exposure to paint fumes, gasoline, solvents, and similar products should be greatly limited. Even with some exposure to these environmental contaminants, U.S. and international health agencies all agree that the benefits of breastfeeding almost always outweigh potential concerns.

Food components that pass into the breast milk may seem innocuous; however, some substances, such as those found in garlic, onions, peppers, broccoli, and cabbage, are distasteful enough to the infant to prevent proper feeding. Some babies have allergic reactions to foods the mother has eaten, such as wheat, cow's milk, eggs, or citrus, and suffer gastrointestinal upset, diaper rash, or another reaction. The offending foods must then be identified and avoided.

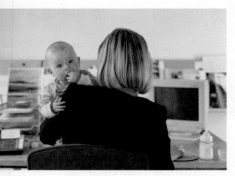

Working moms can be discouraged from—or supported in—breastfeeding in a variety of ways.

Maternal HIV Infection   HIV, which causes AIDS, can be transmitted from mother to baby through breast milk. Thus, HIV-positive women in the United States and Canada are encouraged to feed their infants formula. This recommendation does not apply to all women worldwide, however, because the low cost and sanitary nature of breast milk, as compared to the potential for waterborne diseases with formula-feeding, often make breastfeeding the best choice for women in developing countries.[38]

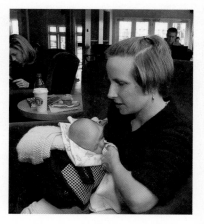

Although a much more common practice today than in the past, breast-feeding in public can still meet with disapproval.

Conflict Between Breastfeeding and the Mother's Employment   Breast milk is absorbed more readily than formula, making more frequent feedings necessary. Newborns commonly require breastfeedings every 1 to 3 hours versus every 2 to 4 hours for formula-feedings. Mothers who are exclusively breastfeeding and return to work within the first 6 months after the baby's birth must leave several bottles of pumped breast milk for others to feed the baby in their absence each day. This means that working women have to pump their breasts to express the breast milk during the workday. This can be a challenge in companies that do not provide the time, space, and privacy required.

Work-related travel is also a concern: if the mother needs to be away from home for longer than 24 to 48 hours, she can typically pump and freeze enough breast milk for others to give the baby in her absence. When longer business trips are required, some mothers take the baby with them and arrange for childcare at their destination. Others resort to pumping, freezing, and shipping breast milk home via overnight mail. Understandably, many women cite returning to work as the reason they switch to formula-feeding.

Some working women successfully combine breastfeeding with commercial formula-feeding. For example, a woman might breastfeed in the morning before she leaves for work, as soon as she returns home, and once again before retiring at night. The remainder of the feedings is formula given by the infant's father or a child-care provider. Women who choose supplemental formula-feedings usually find that their bodies adapt quickly to the change and produce ample milk for the remaining breastfeedings.

Social Concerns   In North America, women have been conditioned to keep their breasts covered in public, even when feeding an infant. Over the past decade, however, both social customs and state laws have become more accommodating and supportive of nursing mothers. Some states have even passed legislation preserving a woman's right to breastfeed in public. With both legal and cultural support, women feel free to nurse their infants upon demand, whether they are at home or out in public.

What About Bonding for Fathers and Siblings?

With all the attention given to attachment between a breastfeeding mother and her infant, it is easy for fathers and siblings to feel left out. One option that allows other family members to participate in infant feeding is to supplement breastfeed-ings with bottle-feedings of stored breast milk or formula. If a family decides to share infant feeding in this manner, bottle-feedings can begin as soon as breastfeed-ing has become well established. That way, the infant will not become confused by the artificial nipple. Fathers and other family members can also bond with the infant when bathing and/or clothing the infant as well as through everyday cud-dling and play.

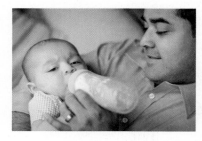

Fathers and siblings can bond with infants through bottle-feeding and other forms of close contact.

recap   Breastfeeding provides many benefits to both mother and newborn, including superior nutrition, heightened immunity, mother–infant bonding, convenience, and cost. However, breastfeeding may not be the best option for every family. The mother may need to use a medication that enters the breast milk and makes it unsafe for consumption. A mother's job may interfere with the baby's requirement for frequent feedings. The infant's father and siblings can participate in feedings using a bottle filled with either pumped breast milk or formula.

Infant nutrition: from birth to 1 year

Most first-time parents are amazed at how rapidly their infant grows. Optimal nutrition is extremely important during the first year, as the baby's organs and nervous system continue to develop and the baby grows physically. In fact, physicians use length and weight measurements as the main tools for assessing an infant's nutritional status. These measurements are plotted on growth charts (there are separate charts for boys and girls), which track an infant's growth over time (**FIGURE 14.10**). Although every infant is unique, in general, physicians look for a correlation between length and weight. In other words, an infant who is in the 60th percentile for length is usually in about the 50th to 70th percentile for weight. An infant who is in the 90th percentile for weight but is in the 20th percentile for length might be overfed.

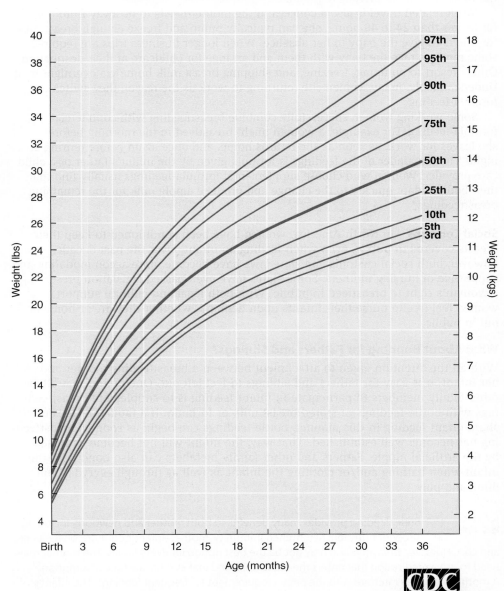

Weight-for-age percentiles: Girls, birth to 36 months

★ FIGURE 14.10 This weight-for-age growth chart is a much smaller version of charts used by healthcare practitioners to monitor and assess the growth of an infant/toddler from birth to 36 months. This example shows the growth curves of girls over time, each at different percentiles.
Data adapted from: "Clinical Growth Charts: Infants, birth to 36 months." Centers for Disease Control and Prevention.

Consistency over time is also a consideration: for example, an infant who suddenly drops well below her established profile for weight might be underfed or ill.

Typical Infant Growth and Activity Patterns

Babies' basal metabolic rates are high, in part because their body surface area is large compared to their body size. Still, their limited physical activity keeps total energy expenditure relatively low. For the first few months of life, an infant's activities consist mainly of eating and sleeping. As the first year progresses, the repertoire of activity gradually expands to include rolling over, sitting up, crawling, standing, and finally taking the first few wobbly steps. Nevertheless, relatively few Calories are expended in movement, and the primary use of energy is to support growth.

In the first year of life, an infant generally grows about 10 inches in length and triples in weight—a growth rate more rapid than will ever occur again. Not surprisingly, energy needs per unit body weight are also the highest they will ever be in order to support this phenomenal growth and metabolism.

The infant's growth surge includes the brain. To accommodate such a large increase in brain size, the bones of the skull do not fuse until the second year of life. An infant's head is typically quite large in proportion to the rest of the body. Pediatricians use head circumference as an additional tool for the assessment of growth and nutritional status. After around 18 months of age, the rate of brain growth slows, and gradually the body "catches up" to head size.

An infant's physical activity will progress beyond crawling before the first year of life is over.

Nutrient Needs for Infants

Three characteristics of infants combine to make their nutritional needs unique: 1) their high energy needs per unit body weight to support rapid growth, 2) their immature digestive tract and kidneys, and 3) their small size.

Macronutrient Needs of Infants

An infant needs to consume about 40–50 kcal/lb of body weight per day.[8] This amounts to about 600–650 kcal/day at around 6 months of age. Given the immature digestive tract and kidneys of infants, as well as their high fluid needs, providing this much energy may seem difficult. Fortunately, breast milk and commercial formulas are energy dense, contributing about 650 kcal/liter of fluid. When complementary (solid) foods are introduced after about 4 to 6 months of age, they provide even more energy in addition to the breast milk or formula.

Infants are not merely small versions of adults. The proportions of macronutrients they require differ from adult proportions, as do the types of food they can tolerate. It is generally agreed that about 40–50% of an infant's energy should come from fat during the first year of life and that fat intake below this level can be harmful before the age of 2. Given the high energy needs of infants, it makes sense to take advantage of the energy density of fat (9 kcal/g) to help meet these requirements. Breast milk and commercial formulas are both high in fat (about 50% of total energy). As noted earlier, breast milk is an excellent source of the fatty acids ARA and DHA, although DHA levels vary considerably with the mother's diet. Many formula manufacturers now add ARA and DHA to their products.

Infants 0 to 6 months of age need approximately 9 g of protein/day, whereas infants 7 to 12 months need almost 10 g/day.[8] These amounts accommodate an infant's rapid growth. Infants have immature kidneys, which are not able to process and excrete the excess nitrogen groups from higher-protein diets; thus, no more than 20% of an infant's daily energy requirement should come from protein. Breast milk and commercial formulas both provide adequate total protein and appropriate essential amino acids to support growth and development.

The recommended intake for carbohydrate is set at 60 g/day for infants 0 to 6 months of age and 95 g/day for infants 7 to 12 months old.[8] These levels reflect the lactose content of human milk, which is used as the reference point for most infant nutrient guidelines.

Micronutrient Needs of Infants

Infants need micronutrients to accommodate their rapid growth and development. The micronutrients of particular concern are iron, vitamin D, zinc, fluoride, and iodine. Fortunately, breast milk and commercial formulas provide most of the micronutrients needed for infant growth and development, with some special considerations, discussed shortly.

In addition, all infants are routinely given an injection of vitamin K shortly after birth. This provides vitamin K until the infant's intestine can develop its own healthful bacteria, which then contribute to the infant's supply of vitamin K.

Do Infants Need Supplements?

Breast milk and commercial formulas provide most of the vitamins and minerals infants need. However, several micronutrients may warrant supplementation.

For breast-fed infants, a supplement containing vitamin D is commonly prescribed from birth to around 6 months of age, even in sunny climates, because exposure of a young infant's skin to adequate direct sunlight for vitamin D synthesis is not advised. Vitamin D deficiency is actually quite common among U.S. infants with dark skin and those with limited sunlight exposure.[32]

Iron is extremely important for cognitive development and prevention of iron-deficiency anemia. Breast-fed infants require additional iron beginning no later than 6 months of age because the infant's iron stores become depleted and breast milk is a poor source of iron. At 4 to 6 months of age, breast-fed infants should be started on complementary (solid) foods that are high in iron, such as pureed meats or iron-fortified infant rice cereal.

If the mother is a vegan, her breast milk may be low in vitamin B_{12}, and a supplement of this vitamin should be given to the baby. Fluoride is important for strong tooth development, but fluoride supplementation is not recommended during the first 6 months of life.

For formula-fed infants, supplementation depends on the formula composition and the water supply used to make the formula. Many formulas are already fortified with iron, for example, and some municipal water supplies contain fluoride. If this is the case, and the baby is getting adequate vitamin D through the intake of at least 1 liter of formula per day, then an extra supplement may not be necessary.

Consultation with the infant's pediatrician is essential before giving a supplement. The supplement should be formulated specifically for infants, and the daily dose should not be exceeded. High doses of micronutrients can be dangerous. Too much iron can be fatal, too much fluoride can cause discoloration and pitting of the teeth, and too much vitamin D can lead to calcification of soft tissue, such as the kidneys.

Fluid Recommendations for Infants

Fluid is critical for everyone, but for infants the balance is more delicate for two reasons. First, because infants are so small, they proportionally lose more water through evaporation than adults. Second, their kidneys are immature and unable to concentrate urine. Hence, they are at even greater risk for dehydration. An infant needs about 2 oz of fluid per pound of body weight, and either breast milk or formula is almost always enough to provide this amount. Experts recently confirmed that "infants exclusively fed human milk do not require supplemental water."[14]

Certain conditions, such as diarrhea, vomiting, fever, or hot weather, can greatly increase fluid loss. In these instances, supplemental fluid, ideally as water, may be necessary. Because too much fluid can be particularly dangerous for an infant, supplemental fluids (whether water or an infant electrolyte formula) should be given only under the advice of a physician. Generally, it is advised that supplemental fluids not exceed 4 oz per day, and parents should avoid giving sugar water, fruit juices, or any sweetened beverage in a bottle. Parents can be sure that their infant's fluid intake is appropriate if the infant produces six to eight wet diapers per day.

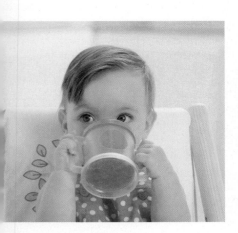

⬆ Infants are at high risk for dehydration, but breast milk and formula are almost always adequate to meet their fluid needs.

What Types of Formula Are Available?

We discussed the advantages of breastfeeding earlier in this chapter, and indeed both national and international healthcare organizations consider breastfeeding the best choice for infant nutrition, when possible. However, if breastfeeding is not feasible, several types of commercial formulas provide nutritious alternatives. By law, formula manufacturers must meet standards for 29 different nutrients.

Most formulas are based on cow's milk proteins, casein and whey, that have been modified to make them more appropriate for human infants. The sugars lactose and

nutrition label activity

Reading Infant Food Labels

Imagine that you are a new parent shopping for infant formula. **FIGURE 14.11** shows the label from a typical can of formula. As you can see, the ingredients list is long and has many technical terms. Even well-informed parents would probably be stumped by many of them. Fortunately, with the information you learned in previous chapters, you can probably answer the following questions.

■ The first ingredient listed is a modified form of *whey protein*. What common food is the source of whey?

■ The fourth ingredient listed is *lactose*. Is lactose a form of protein, fat, or carbohydrate? Why is it important for infants?

■ The front label states that the formula has a blend of *docosahexaenoic acid (DHA)* and *arachidonic acid (ARA)*. Are DHA and ARA forms of protein, fat, or carbohydrate? Why are these two nutrients thought to be important for infants?

The label also claims that this formula is "Our Closest Formula to Breast Milk." Can you think of some differences between breast milk and this formula that still exist?

Look at the list of nutrients on the label. You'll notice that there is no "% Daily Value" column, which you see on most food labels. The next time you are at the grocery store, look at other baby food items, such as baby cereal or pureed fruits. Do their labels simply list the nutrient content or is the "% Daily Value" column used? Why do you think infant formula has a different label format?

Let's say you are feeding a 6-month-old infant who needs about 500 kcal/day. Using the information from the nutrition section of the label, you can calculate the number of fluid ounces of formula the baby needs (this assumes that no cereal or other foods are eaten):

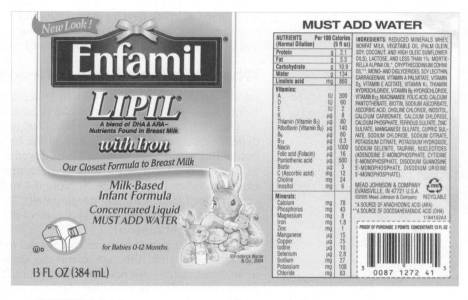

▲ **FIGURE 14.11** An infant formula label. Notice that there is a long list of ingredients and no % Daily Value.

There are 100 kcal (Calories) per 5 fl. oz.

100 kcal ÷ 5 fl. oz = 20 kcal/fl. oz

500 kcal ÷ 20 kcal/fl. oz = 25 fl. oz of formula per day to meet the baby's energy needs

A 6-month-old infant needs about 210 mg calcium per day. Based on an intake of 25 fl. oz of formula per day, as just calculated, you can use the label nutrition information to calculate the amount of calcium that is provided:

There are 78 mg calcium per 5 fl. oz serving of formula.

78 mg ÷ 5 fl. oz = 15.6 mg calcium per fl. oz

15.6 mg calcium per fl. oz × 25 fl. oz = 390 mg of calcium per day

You can see that the infant's need for calcium is easily met by the formula alone.

sucrose, alone or in combination, provide carbohydrates, and vegetable oils and/or synthetic fatty acids provide the fat component. Recently, some manufacturers have added other nutrients, such as taurine, carnitine, and the fatty acids ARA and DHA, to more closely mimic the nutrient profile of human milk. The **Nutrition Label Activity** feature (this page) provides on opportunity to review some of these ingredients.

Soy-based formulas are a viable alternative for infants who are lactose intolerant (although this is rare provides an infants) or cannot tolerate the proteins in cow's milk–based formulas. Soy formulas may also satisfy the requirements of families who are strict vegans. However, soy-based formulas are not without controversy. Because soy contains isoflavones, or plant forms of estrogens, there is some concern over the effects these compounds may have on growing infants, and that they may promote early onset of menstruation.[39] Babies can also have allergic reactions to soy-based formulas. Soy-based formulas are not the same as soy milk, which is not suitable for infant feeding.

There are specialized formula preparations for specific medical conditions. Some contain proteins that have been predigested, for example, or have compositions designed to accommodate certain diseases. Some have been specially formulated for preterm infants, older infants, and toddlers. The final choice of formula should depend on infant tolerance, stage of infant development, cost, and the advice of the infant's pediatrician. It is important to note that the use of cow's milk (fresh, dried, evaporated, or condensed) is inappropriate for infants under the age of 1 year, as is the use of goat's milk.

When Do Infants Begin to Need Solid Foods?

Infants begin to need solid, or complementary, foods at around 6 months of age. Before this age, several factors make most infants unable to consume solid food.

One factor is the *extrusion reflex*. During infant feeding, the suckling response depends on a particular movement of the tongue that draws liquid out of the breast or bottle. But when solid foods are introduced with a spoon, this tongue movement (the extrusion reflex) causes the baby to push most of the food back out of the mouth. The extrusion reflex begins to lessen around 4 to 5 months of age.

Another factor is muscle development. To minimize the risk for choking, the infant must have gained muscular control of the head and neck and be able to sit up (with or without support).

Still another part of being ready for solid foods is sufficient maturity of the digestive and kidney systems. Although infants can digest and absorb lactose from birth, the ability to digest starch does not fully develop until the age of 3 to 4 months. Feeding cereal, for example, before an infant can digest the starch may cause diarrhea and discomfort. In addition, early introduction of solid foods can lead to improper absorption of intact, undigested proteins, setting the stage for allergies. Finally, the kidneys must have matured so that they are better able to process nitrogen wastes from proteins and concentrate urine.

The need for solid foods is also related to nutrient needs. At about 6 months of age, infant iron stores become depleted; thus, iron-fortified infant cereals are often the first foods introduced. Iron-fortified rice cereal, a source of non-heme iron, rarely provokes an allergic response and is easy to digest. Pureed meats and poultry also provide well-absorbed heme iron. Once a child reaches 6 months of age, other single-grain cereals, strained vegetables, fruits, and protein sources can gradually be incorporated into the diet.

Infant foods should be introduced one at a time, with no other new foods for about 1 week, so that parents can watch for signs of allergies, such as a rash, gastrointestinal problems, a runny nose, or wheezing. Gradually, a variety of foods should be introduced by the end of the first year. Commercial baby foods are convenient, nutritious, and typically made without added salt or sugar; however, home-prepared baby foods are usually cheaper and reflect the cultural food patterns of the family. Throughout the first year, solid foods should only be a supplement to, not a substitute for, breast milk or iron-fortified formula. Infants still need the nutrient density and energy that breast milk and formula provide.

What *Not* to Feed an Infant

The following foods should never be offered to an infant:

- **Foods that can cause choking.** Infants cannot adequately chew foods such as grapes, hot dogs, nuts, popcorn, raw carrots, raisins, and hard candies. These can cause choking.
- **Corn syrup and honey.** These may contain spores of the bacterium *Clostridium botulinum*. These spores can germinate and grow into viable bacteria in the immature digestive tract of infants, whereupon they produce a potent toxin, which can be fatal. Children older than 1 year can safely consume these substances because their digestive tract is mature enough to kill any *C. botulinum* bacteria.
- **Goat's milk.** Goat's milk is notoriously low in many nutrients that infants need, such as folate, vitamin C, vitamin D, and iron. Moreover, it is too high in protein.
- **Cow's milk.** For children under 1 year, cow's milk is too concentrated in minerals and protein and contains too few carbohydrates to meet infant energy needs. Infants

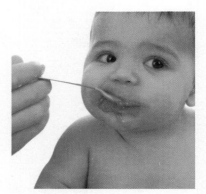

The extrusion reflex will push solid food out of an infant's mouth.

For a list of foods associated with choking, visit http://www.nal.usda.gov. Enter "infant choking risks" into the search box to get underway.

can begin to consume whole cow's milk after the age of 1 year. Infants and toddlers should not be given reduced-fat cow's milk before the age of 2 because it does not contain enough fat and is too high in mineral content for the kidneys to handle effectively. Infants should not be given evaporated milk or sweetened condensed milk.

- **Too much salt and sugar.** Infant foods should not be seasoned with salt or other seasonings. Naturally occurring sugars, such as those found in fruits, are acceptable, but cookies and other processed desserts should be avoided.

- **Too much breast milk or formula.** As nutritious as breast milk and formula are, once infants reach the age of 6 months, solid foods should be introduced gradually. Over-reliance on breast milk or formula can limit the infant's intake of iron-rich foods, resulting in a condition known as *milk anemia*. In addition, infants are physically and psychologically ready to eat solid foods at this time, and solid foods can help appease their increasing appetites. Between 6 months and the time of weaning (from breast or bottle), solid foods should gradually make up an increasing proportion of the infant's diet.

Nutrition-Related Concerns for Infants

Nutrition is one of the biggest concerns of new parents. Infants cannot speak, and their cries are sometimes indecipherable. Feeding time can be very frustrating for parents, especially if the child is not eating, is not growing appropriately, or has problems such as diarrhea, vomiting, or persistent skin rashes. The following are some nutrition-related concerns for infants.

Allergies

Many foods have the potential to stimulate an allergic reaction. Breastfeeding helps deter allergy development, as does delaying the introduction of solid foods until the age of 6 months. One of the most common allergies in infants is to the proteins in cow's milk–based formulas. Egg white, peanut, and wheat are other common triggers of food allergies. Symptoms vary but may include gastrointestinal distress, such as diarrhea, constipation, bloating, blood in the stool, and vomiting. As stated earlier, every food should be introduced in isolation, so that any allergic reaction can be identified and the offending food avoided.

Dehydration

Whether the cause is diarrhea, vomiting, or inadequate fluid intake, dehydration is extremely dangerous to infants and, if left untreated, can quickly result in death. (The factors behind infants' increased risk for dehydration were detailed on page 540.) Treatment includes providing fluids, a task that is difficult if vomiting is occurring. In some cases, the physician may recommend that a pediatric electrolyte solution be administered on a temporary basis. In more severe cases, hospitalization may be necessary. If possible, breastfeeding should continue throughout an illness. A physician should be consulted concerning formula-feeding and solid foods.

Colic

Perhaps nothing is more frustrating to new parents than the relentless crying spells of some infants, typically referred to as **colic**. In this condition, newborns and young infants who appear happy, healthy, and well nourished suddenly begin to cry or even shriek, continuing for several minutes to 3 hours or more, no matter what their caregiver does to console them. The spells tend to occur at the same time of day, typically late in the afternoon or early in the evening, and often occur daily for a period of several weeks. Overstimulation of the nervous system, feeding too rapidly, swallowing of air, and intestinal gas pain are considered possible culprits, but the precise cause is unknown.

As with allergies, if a colicky infant is breastfed, breastfeeding should be continued, but the mother should try to determine whether eating certain foods seems to prompt crying and, if so, eliminate the offending food(s) from her diet. Formula-fed infants may benefit from a change in type of formula. In the worst cases of colic, a physician may prescribe medication. Fortunately, most cases disappear spontaneously, possibly because of the maturity of the gastrointestinal tract, around 3 months of age.

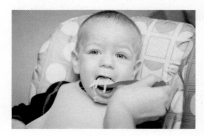

◀ Early introduction of solid foods may play a role in the development of food allergies, especially if infants are introduced to highly allergenic foods early on.

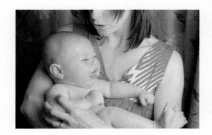

◀ Colicky babies will begin crying for no apparent reason, even if they otherwise appear well nourished and happy.

colic A condition of inconsolable infant crying that lasts for hours at a time.

Anemia

As stated earlier, full-term infants are born with sufficient iron stores to last for approximately the first 6 months of life. In older infants and toddlers, however, iron is the mineral most likely to be deficient. Iron-deficiency anemia causes pallor, lethargy, and impaired growth. Iron-fortified formula is a good source for formula-fed infants. Some pediatricians prescribe a supplement containing iron especially formulated for infants. Iron for older infants is typically supplied by iron-fortified rice cereal.

Nursing Bottle Syndrome

Infants should not be left alone with a bottle, whether lying down or sitting up. As infants manipulate the nipple of the bottle in their mouth, the high-carbohydrate fluid (whether breast milk, formula, or fruit juice) drips out, coming into prolonged contact with the developing teeth. This high-carbohydrate fluid provides an optimal food source for the bacteria that are the underlying cause of **dental caries** (cavities). Severe tooth decay can result (**FIGURE 14.12**). Encouraging the use of a cup around the age of 8 months helps prevent nursing bottle syndrome, along with weaning the baby from a bottle entirely by the age of 15 to 18 months.

FIGURE 14.12 Leaving a baby alone with a bottle can result in the tooth decay of nursing bottle syndrome.

Lead Poisoning

Lead is especially toxic to infants and children because their brain and central nervous system are still developing. Lead poisoning can result in decreased mental capacity, behavioral problems, impaired growth, impaired hearing, and other problems. Unfortunately, leaded pipes and lead paint can still be found in older homes and buildings. The following measures can reduce lead exposure:

- Allowing tap water to run for a minute or so before use to clear the pipes of any lead-contaminated water
- Using only cold tap water for drinking and cooking because hot tap water is more likely to leach lead
- Professionally removing lead-based paint or painting over it with latex paint

recap Infancy is characterized by the most rapid growth a human being will ever experience, and appropriate growth is the most reliable long-term indicator of adequate infant nutrition. Infants need large amounts of energy per unit body weight to keep up with growth. Breast milk or iron-fortified formula provides all necessary nutrients for the first 6 months of life. After that, solid foods can gradually be introduced into an infant's diet. Micronutrient supplements should be given only if prescribed. Infants must be monitored for allergies, dehydration, and other signs of distress.

✳behavior change . . . getting started!

Now that you've read this chapter, try making these changes:

For yourself:

- Whether you're single or married with children, start taking better care of your own health. Eat a moderate and nutritious diet, and get regular physical activity. If you smoke or abuse illegal substances, stop. If you drink alcohol, keep it moderate, and, if female, avoid drinking entirely if you're pregnant or think you might be.
- If you're a female of childbearing age, make sure your diet is providing at least 400 μg of folic acid daily, whether or not you intend to become pregnant.

For your community:

- Many colleges and universities offer lactation rooms, on-campus childcare, and other services to help student-moms to breastfeed on campus. Men and women should show support for these efforts, and if your campus doesn't offer them, contact the office of family services and lobby for them. Mention the benefits: improved infant health and well-being, reduced student absenteeism to care for an infant who is ill, increased student productivity, and enhanced student recruitment and retention.

dental caries Dental erosion and decay caused by acid-secreting bacteria in the mouth and on the teeth. The acid produced is a by-product of bacterial metabolism of carbohydrates deposited on the teeth.

Should Breastfeeding Throughout Infancy Be Mandatory?

The year is 2021. Obesity rates have remained unacceptably high, especially among children, many of whom are experiencing high blood glucose, high blood pressure, and other signs of metabolic syndrome. In this climate, Marcy goes shopping for infant formula. Although her daughter has been exclusively breastfed since her birth 4 months ago, Marcy needs to go back to work full-time and has decided to switch to formula. At the check-out, Marcy is horrified at the price of the can of powdered formula she has selected. "It's not our fault," the clerk replies. "There's a new state surcharge to discourage families from using formula!"

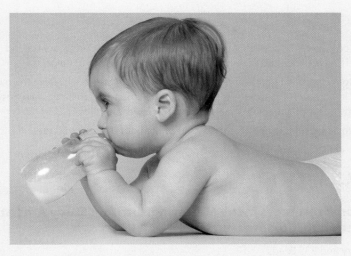

Formula-feeding has been associated with an increased risk for obesity in childhood and adulthood.

If this scenario sounds preposterous, you might be interested to learn that some healthcare providers are actually proposing that states implement a system of rewards for breastfeeding and penalties for formula-feeding—and a surcharge like the one just described is among the various proposals. What's behind these recommendations? Let's have a look.

As obesity rates have climbed, more researchers have posed the question, "Do adults and children who were breastfed as infants have lower rates of obesity and metabolic disorder than adults and children who were formula-fed?"[40–42] The theory of *metabolic programming* states that infant-feeding practices and other factors in early postnatal life can influence an infant's physiology and subsequent risk for obesity and chronic diseases. Supporting this theory is the established fact that breast-fed infants grow in length and weight at a slower rate than formula-fed infants. But does this lower weight persist into childhood and adulthood?

Although some studies show no protective effect, most have concluded that breastfeeding for longer than 3 to 6 months does, in fact, lower rates of child and adult overweight and obesity. Exclusive breastfeeding appears to provide greater protection than partial breastfeeding, and the longer breastfeeding persists, the greater the protection against obesity.[40–42]

The obesity risk reduction may stem from the lower protein and energy intakes of breast-fed infants, alterations in insulin secretion, and/or differences in metabolism. In contrast, rapid weight gain during infancy, which is more common among formula-fed infants, is associated with a higher risk for obesity later in life. Some scientists have suggested that differences in feeding patterns also play a role: formula-fed infants suck at a faster and more powerful rate, consume a larger volume at each feeding, and have fewer feedings per day with longer intervals between feedings compared to breast-fed infants. It is possible that these differences translate into different eating habits as the infant transitions to child and adult diets.

Do these research data suggest that our society should do more to encourage or even require prolonged breastfeeding? Before you answer, consider the costs of obesity. A well-established risk factor for heart disease, stroke, type 2 diabetes, and some forms of cancer, obesity costs the United States an estimated \$147 to \$210 billion in healthcare expenditures annually, with additional costs due to lost productivity, reduced longevity, and impaired quality of life.[43,44]

Much of this financial burden is borne by the public in the form of higher healthcare costs and insurance premiums, reduced tax revenues (from lost productivity), and increased disability payments. Does the public have the right to legislate actions that could reduce this burden? After all, we have laws restricting and taxing sales of alcohol and tobacco. Although some would argue that such laws take away our "personal freedoms," others point out that they help us make choices that improve our own health and the health of our children.

CRITICAL THINKING QUESTIONS

1. If breastfeeding were conclusively shown to lower obesity rates (along with its other established benefits for infants) should it be required by law? Or should the decision to breast- or formula-feed an infant rest only with the mother or family? Why or why not?

2. If legislation to discourage formula-feeding were in effect, how would such laws affect women as compared to men? Would this type of regulation be a form of gender discrimination?

3. Would you support a tax credit to families or mothers who breastfeed their children for 6 months or more? Why or why not?

chapter **review**

test yourself | answers

1. **False.** Pregnant women need only 350–450 additional Calories per day, and only during the second and third trimesters of pregnancy. This is an increase of only 20% or less, not a doubling of Calories.

2. **True.** Breast milk contains various immune factors (antibodies and immune system cells) from the mother that protect the infant against infection. The nutrients in breast milk are structured to be easily digested by an infant, resulting in fewer symptoms of gastrointestinal distress and fewer allergies.

3. **False.** Most infants do not have a physiologic need for solid food until about 6 months of age.

MasteringNutrition™

review questions

1. Folate deficiency in the first weeks after conception has been linked with which of the following problems in the newborn?
   a. anemia
   b. neural tube defects
   c. low birth weight
   d. preterm delivery

2. A pregnancy weight gain of 28 to 40 pounds is recommended for
   a. all women.
   b. women who begin their pregnancy underweight.
   c. women who begin their pregnancy overweight.
   d. women who begin their pregnancy at a normal weight.

3. Which of the following is a valid recommendation for reducing symptoms of morning sickness?
   a. Eat as much as possible at each meal, as a full stomach can reduce nausea.
   b. Consume fluids only at mealtimes because fluids on an empty stomach can increase nausea.
   c. Nibble on dry cereal or crackers before bedtime to ease nighttime nausea and before rising to prevent morning nausea.
   d. Drink colas and other caffeinated, carbonated beverages because these reduce nausea.

4. Which of the following hormones is responsible for the letdown response?
   a. progesterone
   b. estrogen
   c. oxytocin
   d. prolactin

5. Which of the following statements about maternal nutrition is true?
   a. Lactating women need more Calories than pregnant women.
   b. Pregnant women need more iron than lactating women.
   c. Pregnant women need more folate than lactating women.
   d. All of the above are true.

6. Which of the following statements about breast milk is true?
   a. Certain proteins in breast milk improve the absorption of iron.
   b. The fat content of breast milk is lower than that of cow's milk.
   c. Breast milk is cholesterol-free.
   d. All of the above are true.

7. Which of the following nutrients should be added to the diet of breast-fed infants when they are around 6 months of age?

   a. fiber

   b. fat

   c. iron

   d. vitamin A

8. After 6 months of age, it is safe and healthful to give infants

   a. cow's milk.

   b. goat's milk.

   c. soy milk.

   d. none of the above.

9. **True or false?** Major developmental errors and birth defects are most likely to occur in the third trimester of pregnancy.

10. **True or false?** If gestational diabetes is uncontrolled, the fetus may not receive enough glucose and may be born small for gestational age.

math review

11. Mature breast milk averages about 700 kcal per liter, with 35 g of fat and 9 g of protein. Calculate the % of kcal from fat and protein. How do these values compare to those recommended for a healthy young adult? Why are the nutrient proportions of breast milk appropriate for infants?

Answers to Review Questions and Math Review are located at the back of this text and in the MasteringNutrition Study Area.

web resources

www.drspock.com
Dr. Spock.com

Check out this website for a quiz testing your readiness for parenthood.

www.aap.org
American Academy of Pediatrics

Visit this website for information on infants' and children's health. Searches can be performed for topics such as "neural tube defects" and "infant formulas."

www.emedicine.com
eMedicine: Pediatrics

Enter "Pediatrics" into the search bar, then select "toxicology," and then "iron toxicity" to learn about accidental iron poisoning in children and infants.

www.marchofdimes.com
March of Dimes

Click on "During Your Pregnancy" to find links on nutrition during pregnancy, exercise, and things to avoid.

www.diabetes.org
American Diabetes Association

Search for "gestational diabetes" to find information about diabetes that develops during pregnancy.

www.choosemyplate.gov
USDA ChooseMyPlate

Search on the term "Daily Food Plan for Moms" and enter your information to get specific, individualized dietary advice for pregnant, or exclusively or partially breastfeeding, women via the Supertracker feature.

www.lalecheleague.org
La Leche League

Search this site to find multiple articles on the health effects of breastfeeding for mother and infant.

www.obgyn.net
OBGYN.net

Visit this site to learn about pregnancy health and nutrition as well as breastfeeding and infant nutrition.

www.nofas.org
National Organization on Fetal Alcohol Syndrome

This site provides news and information relating to fetal alcohol syndrome.

www.helppregnantsmokersquit.org
The National Partnership for Smoke-Free Families

This site was created for healthcare providers and smokers with the purpose of educating about the dangers of smoking while pregnant and providing tools to help pregnant smokers quit.

in depth
14.5

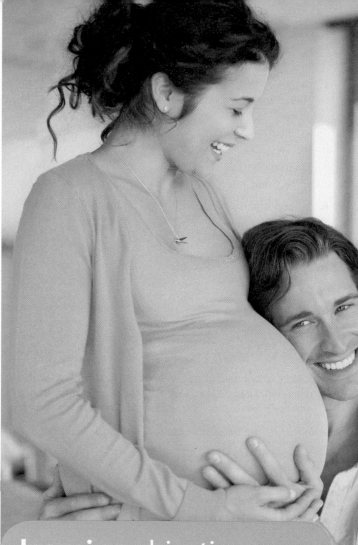

The Fetal Environment: A Lasting Impression

Would you be surprised to learn that your risk of developing obesity and certain chronic diseases as an adult can be influenced by what happened before your birth? Over the last several decades, a growing body of evidence has revealed that the fetal environment, including the mother's nutritional status, influences the risks for obesity and chronic diseases later in life. This relationship is described as the "fetal origins theory" or the theory of "developmental origins of adult health and disease." This **In Depth** explores this relationship and describes the lifelong effects of a variety of factors in the fetal environment.

learning objectives

After studying this In Depth, you should be able to:

1 Identify three health problems seen in adults whose mothers were exposed to famine during their first trimester of pregnancy, pp. 549–550.

2 Identify the effects seen later in life among children born to mothers with calcium, folate, and zinc deficiencies, p. 550.

3 List three infant/child health risks associated with maternal obesity or gestational diabetes, p. 550.

4 Describe the long-term health consequences suffered by the offspring of women who smoke during pregnancy, pp. 550–551.

Exposure to famine

Some of the earliest research into the *fetal origins theory* investigated the health of adults born during or shortly after a famine in the Netherlands from 1944 to 1945. During World War II, the Dutch population had been relatively well nourished until October 1944, when the Germans placed an embargo on all food transport into the western Netherlands. At the same time, an unusually early and harsh winter set in. As a result, a severe

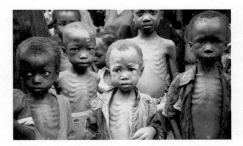

We are still learning about the long-term effects of low birth weight and fetal nutrient privation.

famine hit the western Netherlands. For the next several months, food intake was limited and energy intakes were as low as 500 kcal/day. In May 1945, with the liberation of the country, food supplies were once again plentiful and dietary intake rapidly normalized. Luckily for scientists, the Dutch maintained an excellent system of healthcare records, providing important information not only about pregnancy outcomes but also the health of the offspring over the next 60 years. Not surprisingly, maternal weight gain and infant birth weight were much lower than normal. What was surprising, however, was the long-term impact of the famine as these "embargo babies" progressed through adulthood.[1,2]

Exposure to famine during the first trimester of pregnancy resulted in a much higher risk among the offspring for obesity, abdominal obesity, coronary heart disease, abnormal serum lipid profile, and metabolic syndrome during adulthood. Exposure during mid-gestation increased risk of renal disorders. There is also evidence that prenatal exposure to famine affected the health not only of the individuals deprived *in utero*, but also of their children.[1]

Why, you might wonder, would low pregnancy weight gain and low birth weight lead to an increased risk of obesity and other diseases some 50 years later? Although there are many theories, most relate to a process known as **fetal adaptation**.[3,4] A fetus exposed to a stressful environment, such as maternal starvation or malnutrition, goes into survival mode. The body's production of hormones shifts in favor of those that promote energy storage, the activity of certain enzymes may change, and the size and functioning of body organs such as the liver, kidney, and pancreas are affected. There may even be changes in the activation—and thus the expression—of certain genes. Although these adaptations are beneficial to the fetus, allowing it to survive the harmful prenatal environment, these same hormonal, enzymatic, organ, and genetic changes may contribute to the development of chronic diseases over the life span.

The results of other "natural experiments" suggest that the effects of the prenatal environment on adult health depend quite heavily on the precise circumstances in each situation. For example, Leningrad (now St. Petersburg) was under siege by the Germans during World War II for over 2-1/2 years, and as a result the population experienced starvation—over a million people died. And yet, adults who were born during this period did not have the same increased disease risks as found in those exposed, *in utero*, to the Dutch famine.[5,6] How could this be, since the Leningrad babies were exposed to conditions far worse than those experienced by the Dutch babies? Researchers theorize that the impact of fetal exposure to malnutrition is actually worsened if followed by high nutrient intakes shortly after birth.[6] This was a key difference between the Netherlands and Leningrad famines: once the Dutch embargo was lifted, the population returned to a nourishing, adequate diet. This allowed the underweight infants to experience rapid weight gain and catch-up growth during their first year of life (**FIGURE 1**, page 550). In contrast, the Leningrad infants who survived into adulthood may have continued to suffer from malnutrition throughout infancy and even into toddlerhood, remaining underweight and underfed. Catch-up growth in the post-natal period is associated with a more severe increase in blood pressure and other chronic diseases during adulthood.

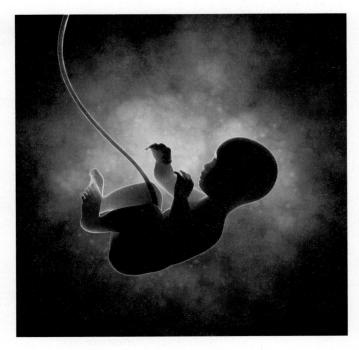

Exposure to prenatal famine can lead to lifelong health consequences for the infant.

---

fetal adaptation The process by which fetal metabolism, hormone production, and other physiologic processes shift in response to factors, such as inadequate energy intake, in the maternal environment.

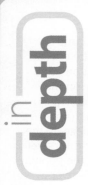
More recently, people born during weather- and war-related famines in Africa and other parts of the world have provided researchers with additional information on the impact of the fetal environment on adult health/disease outcomes. For instance, some recent studies confirm the association between low birth weight and high blood pressure and other forms of cardiovascular disease.[7]

Exposure to specific nutrient deficiencies

By definition, a famine is a widespread lack or severe reduction in all food. Thus, research on the long-term health effects of famines cannot identify or describe the impact of *in utero* deficiencies of specific nutrients. Other studies, however, have been able to look at the impact of specific food patterns or nutrient deficiencies. For example, evidence suggests that poor maternal intake of calcium increases risk of hypertension in adult offspring. Moreover, poor maternal folate status has been linked not only to neural tube defects in the newborn but also to early signs of atherosclerosis in adult offspring. Prenatal deficiencies of zinc have also been linked to later-life disorders such as diabetes and atherosclerosis.[8] Thus, fetal stressors that influence adult health include not only starvation and inadequate energy but also specific micronutrient deficiencies.

Exposure to dietary excesses

Strong evidence also links maternal dietary excesses to health problems in adult offspring. Maternal obesity has been linked not only to an increased risk of childhood[9] and adult[10] obesity, but also to changes in the "programming" of the fetal brain, resulting in altered feeding behaviors.[11] It is also linked to a higher risk of birth defects, including neural tube defects, many of which have lifelong implications for health.[12] Population studies have also reported an association between high birth weight, common in infants born to obese women, and an increased risk of breast cancer in adulthood.

Maternal diabetes and its high-glucose environment has been shown to greatly increase the risk of type 2 diabetes, overweight, excess adiposity, and metabolic syndrome in adult offspring.[13,14] The children of diabetic women are up to eight times more likely to develop type 2 diabetes or prediabetes as adults compared to the general population.[14] High blood levels of triglycerides, increased waist circumference, and increased blood pressure are other measures of adult-onset diseases associated with maternal diabetes.

Prenatal exposure to excessive levels of individual nutrients also has lifelong implications. A high maternal intake of vitamin A as retinol (but not as its precursor beta-carotene) is associated with an increased risk of congenital heart defects,[15] skull abnormalities, and other defects.[16] Scientists continue to investigate the possible lifelong effects of other nutrient excesses, including the impact of high maternal intake of sodium on risk of hypertension in their adult offspring and the effect of high maternal saturated fat intake on risk for congenital defects.

In short, research suggests that there are lifelong consequences to any type of nutrient imbalance during pregnancy, whether the imbalance is a total energy deficit, a single nutrient deficiency, or an energy or nutrient excess.

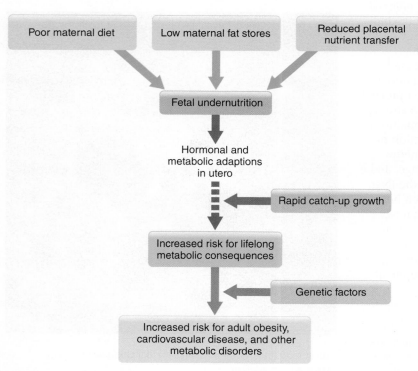

FIGURE 1 Fetal adaptation to undernutrition can lead to a variety of diseases in childhood and throughout adulthood.

Exposure to alcohol, tobacco, and other toxic agents

You've already learned of the lifelong impact of fetal alcohol syndrome, resulting from exposure to alcohol *in utero*. In addition, maternal smoking has been shown to have long-term harmful effects on offspring. Not only are the children of women who smoked during pregnancy at high risk for preterm birth and low birth weight, they are also at higher risk for childhood allergies and respiratory diseases, adult-onset high blood pressure, childhood behavioral problems, and cleft lip and palate.[16] New evidence also confirms a link between maternal smoking and increased risk for

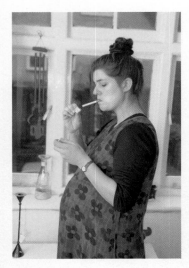

Maternal smoking is extremely harmful to the fetus and increases its risk for many health problems in childhood and adulthood.

adult-onset diabetes among offspring as well as a lifelong higher risk for obesity.[17]

Not surprisingly, maternal exposure to persistent organic pollutants also has lifelong effects on offspring. For example, *in utero* exposure to lead increases the risk of developmental delays, behavioral and learning problems, hearing loss, and elevated blood pressure.[18] Maternal exposure to even low levels of mercury can result in irreversible damage to the baby's nervous system and subsequent learning disabilities.[19]

Implications for your health

If your mother experienced some type of nutritional, metabolic, or environmental stress during pregnancy, you certainly are not doomed to suffer from one or more of the health problems mentioned previously. That's because the research described previously reported on large groups of people, not individuals. Moreover, it calculated increases in risk of—or susceptibility to—certain conditions, but it did not and cannot condemn anyone to any particular disease.

Any type of fetal programming or genetic influence that develops as a result of the fetal environment is just one factor in your wellness. A much more significant influence is your own lifestyle, especially your personal food choices, dietary patterns, activity habits, alcohol intake, and smoking. In fact, the Centers for Disease Control and Prevention cite these as the primary factors influencing your risk of actually experiencing any of the most common chronic diseases.[20] In short, you have the power to optimize your health by making smart lifestyle choices every day.

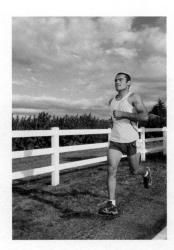

Regular physical activity is one of the most significant factors in maintaining wellness.

nutri-case | HANNAH

"In my nutrition class, I learned that having a mother with diabetes increases the risk that you'll develop diabetes in childhood or adulthood. That helps me understand why my blood sugar test showed I have pre-diabetes, but it doesn't help me understand what to do about it."

Is Hannah destined to develop type 2 diabetes? Why or why not? Identify the factors that increase her risk, as well as the steps she can take to reduce her blood glucose levels and avoid the disease. (Review the **In Depth** on diabetes on pages 139–145.)

MasteringNutrition™

Check out these additional resources in the MasteringNutrition Study Area:

- Read It: Chapter Summary and RSS Feeds
- See It: ABC News videos and nutrition animations
- Hear It: MP3s
- Study It: Get Ready for Nutrition Math and Chemistry review
- Do It: NutriTools and "Find the Quack" feature
- Review It: Quizzes, flashcards, and glossary

web resources

www.marchofdimes.com
March of Dimes

This website provides information on the potential risks of maternal dietary imbalances and exposure to environmental pollutants.

www.epa.gov
Environmental Protection Agency

The latest information on health effects of mercury can be found in this resource. Enter "mercury exposure" into the home page search bar.

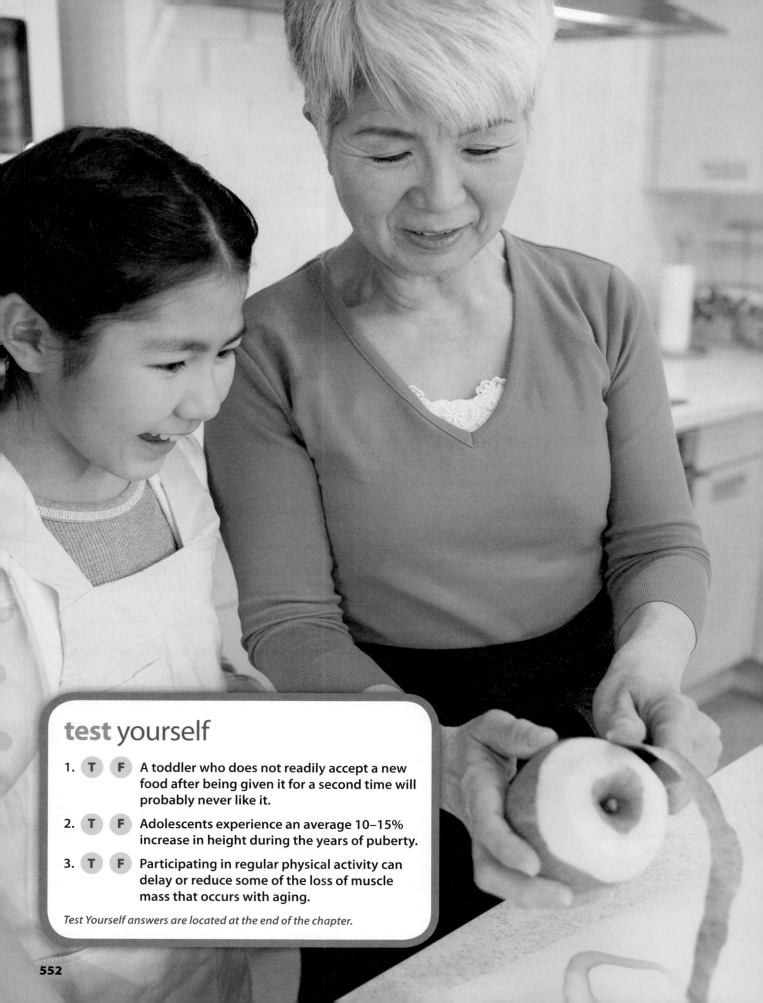

test yourself

1. **T** **F** A toddler who does not readily accept a new food after being given it for a second time will probably never like it.

2. **T** **F** Adolescents experience an average 10–15% increase in height during the years of puberty.

3. **T** **F** Participating in regular physical activity can delay or reduce some of the loss of muscle mass that occurs with aging.

Test Yourself answers are located at the end of the chapter.

Nutrition Through the Life Cycle
Childhood to late adulthood

15

On Sunday afternoons, the Hsiao family gathers for dinner at the Long Beach apartment of their 88-year-old matriarch, Leng. Leng is petite and slender, as are her 70-year-old daughter and 67-year-old son. But when her granddaughters, who are cooking the family meal, send everyone to the table, a change becomes evident. Many of Leng's grandchildren and their spouses are overweight, as are some of her great-grandchildren. Leng worries about everyone's weight. Back home in China, overweight was still relatively rare, but here in America, it seems to bring illness. One of her grandsons has had a heart attack, and some in her family have been diagnosed with type 2 diabetes. Leng's family isn't alone in their weight problems: in the United States, although the prevalence of obesity has recently stabilized, rates remain unacceptably high.[1] Currently, about 12% of preschoolers and 18% of youth age 6 to 19 are classified as obese, leading to both short- and long-term health problems.

Why are the rates of obesity and its associated chronic diseases so high, and what can be done to promote weight management across the life span? How do our nutrient needs change as we grow and age, and what other nutrition-related concerns develop in each life stage? This chapter will help you answer these questions.

learning objectives

After studying this chapter you should be able to:

1. Discuss nutrient recommendations and appropriate serving sizes for toddlers, pp. 554–557.

2. Describe the nutrition-related concerns for toddlers and very young children being fed a vegetarian or vegan diet, pp. 558–560.

3. Discuss the nutrient needs of school-age children and the role of school attendance in children's nutrition, pp. 559, 561–565.

4. Define *puberty* and describe how it influences changes in the body, pp. 566–567.

5. Describe the nutrient needs and nutrition-related concerns of adolescents, p. 567–571.

6. Discuss the problem of pediatric obesity, including risk factors and preventive measures, pp. 572–573.

7. Discuss the growth of the U.S. elderly population, and explain the effect of at least three normal age-related physiologic changes on the nutrient needs of older adults, pp. 574–576.

8. Discuss the nutritional needs and nutrition-related health concerns of older adults, pp. 576–583.

MasteringNutrition™

Go online for chapter quizzes, pre-tests, Interactive Activities, and more!

Nutrition for toddlers

As babies begin to walk and explore, they transition out of infancy and into the active world of toddlers. From their first to their third birthday, a toddler will grow a total of about 5.5 to 7.5 inches and gain an average of 9 to 11 pounds. Toddlers need to consume a lot of energy to fuel their increasing levels of activity as they explore their ever-expanding world and develop new skills. But feeding a toddler raises new challenges for parents and caregivers.

What Are a Toddler's Nutrient Needs?

Nutrient needs increase as a child progresses from infancy to toddlerhood. Although toddlers' rate of growth has slowed, their increased nutrient needs reflect their larger body size and increased activity. Refer to **TABLE 15.1** for a review of specific nutrient recommendations.

Energy and Macronutrient Recommendations for Toddlers

Although the energy requirement per kilogram of body weight for toddlers is slightly less than for infants, *total* energy requirements are higher because toddlers are larger and much more active than infants. The estimated energy requirements (EERs) vary according to the toddler's age, body weight, and level of activity.[2] In general, toddlers should consume a diet that provides enough energy to sustain a healthy and appropriate rate of growth.

Healthy toddlers of appropriate body weight should consume 30–40% of their total daily energy intake as fat.[2] We know that fat provides a concentrated source of energy in a relatively small amount of food, and this is important for toddlers, especially those who are fussy eaters or have little appetite. Fat is also necessary to support the toddler's continuously developing nervous system.

Toddlers' protein needs increase modestly because they weigh more than infants and are still growing rapidly. The RDA for protein for toddlers is 1.10 g/kg body weight per day, or approximately 13 g of protein daily.[2] Remember that 2 cups of milk alone provide 16 g of protein; thus, most toddlers have little trouble meeting their protein needs.

The RDA for carbohydrate for toddlers is 130 g/day, and carbohydrate intake should be about 45–65% of total energy intake.[2] As is the case for older children and

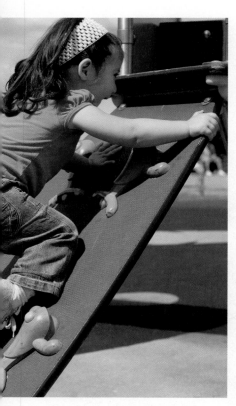

⬆ Toddlers expend significant amounts of energy exploring their world.

TABLE 15.1   Nutrient Recommendations for Children and Adolescents

Nutrient	Toddlers (1–3 Years)	Children (4–8 Years)	Children (9–13 Years)	Adolescents (14–18 Years)
Fat	No RDA	No RDA	No RDA	No RDA
Protein	1.10 g/kg body weight per day	0.95 g/kg body weight per day	0.95 g/kg body weight per day	0.85 g/kg body weight per day
Carbohydrate	130 g/day	130 g/day	130 g/day	130 g/day
Vitamin A	300 µg/day	400 µg/day	600 µg/day	Boys: 900 µg/day Girls: 700 µg/day
Vitamin C	15 mg/day	25 mg/day	45 mg/day	Boys: 75 mg/day Girls: 65 mg/day
Vitamin E	6 mg/day	7 mg/day	11 mg/day	15 mg/day
Calcium	700 mg/day	1,000 mg/day	1,300 mg/day	1,300 mg/day
Iron	7 mg/day	10 mg/day	8 mg/day	Boys: 11 mg/day Girls: 15 mg/day
Zinc	3 mg/day	5 mg/day	8 mg/day	Boys: 11 mg/day Girls: 9 mg/day
Fluid	1.3 liters/day	1.7 liters/day	Boys: 2.4 liters/day Girls: 2.1 liters/day	Boys: 3.3 liters/day Girls: 2.3 liters/day

adults, most of the carbohydrates eaten should be complex, and refined carbohydrates from high-fat/high-sugar items, such as desserts and snack foods, should be kept to a minimum. Fruits and fruit juices are nutritious sources of simple carbohydrates; however, too much fruit juice can displace other foods, including milk and whole fruits, and can cause diarrhea. The American Academy of Pediatrics recommends that the intake of fruit juice be limited to 4–6 fl. oz/day for children 1 to 6 years of age.[3]

Adequate fiber is important for toddlers to maintain bowel regularity. The AI is 14 g of fiber per 1,000 kcal of energy, or, on average, 19 g/day.[2] Whole-grain breads and cereals and fresh fruits and vegetables are healthful choices for toddlers. Too much fiber, however, can inhibit the absorption of iron, zinc, and other essential nutrients; can harm the toddler's small digestive tract; and cause satiation before the toddler has consumed adequate nutrients.

Determining the macronutrient requirements of toddlers can be challenging. See the **You Do the Math** box for an analysis of the macronutrient levels in one toddler's daily diet.

Micronutrient Recommendations for Toddlers

As toddlers grow, their micronutrient needs increase (see Table 15.1). Of particular concern with toddlers is an adequate intake of the minerals calcium and iron.

Calcium is necessary for children to promote optimal bone mass, which continues to accumulate until early adulthood. For toddlers, the RDA for calcium is 700 mg/day.[4] Dairy products are excellent sources of calcium. When a child reaches the age of 1 year, whole cow's milk can be given; however, reduced-fat milk (2% or less) should *not* be given until age 2 due to the relatively high need for total energy in young children. If consumption of dairy products is not feasible, calcium-fortified orange juice or soy milk can supply calcium, or children's calcium supplements can be given. Toddlers generally cannot consume enough dark-green vegetables and similar plant foods to depend on them for adequate calcium.

Iron-deficiency anemia is the most common nutrient deficiency in young children in the United States and around the world. Iron-deficiency anemia can affect a child's energy level, attention span, and mood. The RDA for iron for toddlers is 7 mg/day.[5] Good sources of well-absorbed heme iron include lean meats, fish, and poultry; non-heme iron is provided by eggs, legumes, greens, and fortified foods, such as breakfast cereals. When toddlers consume non-heme sources of iron, eating vitamin C at the same meal will enhance the absorption of iron from these sources.

Given toddlers' typically erratic eating habits, pediatricians often recommend a multivitamin and mineral supplement as a precaution against deficiencies. The toddler's physician or dentist may also prescribe a fluoride supplement if the community water supply is not fluoridated. Any supplement given should be formulated especially for toddlers, and the recommended dose should not be exceeded. A supplement should not contain more than 100% of the Daily Value of any nutrient per dose. Toddlers are at particularly high risk of overdosing on iron supplements, so parents must be careful to keep such products out of reach of their children.

Fluid Recommendations for Toddlers

Toddlers lose less fluid from evaporation than infants, and their more mature kidneys are able to concentrate urine, thereby sparing fluid. However, as toddlers become active, they start to lose significant fluid through sweat, especially in hot weather. Parents need to make sure an active toddler is drinking adequately. The recommended fluid intake for toddlers—about 4 cups as beverages, including drinking water—is listed in Table 15.1.[6] Suggested beverages are plain water, milk and soy milk, diluted fruit juice, and foods high in water content, such as vegetables and fruits.

recap Growth during toddlerhood is slower than during infancy; however, toddlers are highly active, and total energy, fat, and protein requirements are higher for toddlers than for infants. Although all forms of milk can be used to meet calcium requirements, until age 2, toddlers should drink whole milk. Iron deficiency can be avoided by feeding toddlers lean meats/fish/poultry, eggs, and iron-fortified foods. Toddlers need to drink about 4 cups of water or other beverages per day.

you do the math

Is This Menu Good for a Toddler?

A dedicated mother and father want to provide the best nutrition for their son, Ethan, who is now 1-½ years old and has just been completely weaned from breast milk. Ethan weighs about 26 pounds (11.8 kg). In the accompanying table is a typical day's menu for Ethan. Grams of protein, fat, and carbohydrate are given for each food. The day's total energy intake is 1,168 kcal. Calculate the percentage of Ethan's Calories that come from protein, fat, and carbohydrate (the numbers may not add up to exactly 100% because of rounding). In what areas are Ethan's parents doing well, and where can they improve?

Note: This activity focuses on the macronutrients. It does not ask you to consider Ethan's intake of micronutrients or fluids.

Calculations:

There is a total of 47.5 g protein in Ethan's menu.

$$47.5 \text{ g} \times 4 \text{ kcal/g} = 190 \text{ kcal}$$
$$190 \text{ kcal protein}/1{,}168 \text{ total kcal} \times 100 = 16\% \text{ protein}$$

There is a total of 25.75 g fat in Ethan's menu.

$$25.75 \text{ g} \times 9 \text{ kcal/g} = 232 \text{ kcal}$$
$$232 \text{ kcal fat}/1{,}168 \text{ total kcal} \times 100 = 20\% \text{ fat}$$

There is a total of 186.5 g carbohydrate in Ethan's menu.

$$186.5 \text{ g} \times 4 \text{ kcal/g} = 746 \text{ kcal}$$
$$746 \text{ kcal carbohydrate}/1{,}168 \text{ total kcal} \times 100$$
$$= 64\% \text{ carbohydrate}$$

Analysis:

Ethan's parents are doing very well at offering a wide variety of foods from various food groups; they are especially doing well with fruits and vegetables. Also, according to his estimated energy requirement, Ethan requires about 970 kcal/day, and he is consuming 1,168 kcal/day, thus meeting his energy needs.

Ethan's total carbohydrate intake for the day is 186.5 g, which is higher than the RDA of 130 g/day; however, this value falls within the recommended 45–65% of total energy intake that should come from carbohydrates. Thus, high carbohydrate intake is adequate to meet his energy needs.

However, Ethan is being offered far more than enough protein. The DRI for protein for toddlers is about 13 g/day, and Ethan is eating more than three times that much!

It is also readily apparent that Ethan is being offered too little fat for his age. Toddlers need at least 30–40% of their total energy intake from fat, and Ethan is consuming only about 20% of his Calories from fat. He should be drinking whole milk, not 1% milk. He should occasionally be offered higher-fat foods,

Meal	Foods	Protein (g)	Fat (g)	Carbo-hydrate (g)
Breakfast	Oatmeal (½ cup, cooked)	2.5	1.5	13.5
	Brown sugar (1 tsp.)	0	0	4
	Milk (1%, 4 fl. oz)	4	1.25	5.5
	Grape juice (4 fl. oz)	0	0	20
Mid-morning snack	Banana slices (1 small banana)	0	0	16
	Yogurt (nonfat, fruit-flavored 1.3 fl. oz)	5.5	0	15.5
	Orange juice (4 fl. oz)	1	0	13
Lunch	Whole-wheat bread (1 slice)	1.5	0.5	10
	Peanut butter (1 tbsp.)	4	8	3.5
	Strawberry jam (1 tbsp.)	0	0	13
	Carrots (cooked, ⅛ cup)	0	0	2
	Applesauce (sweetened, ¼ cup)	0	0	12
	Milk (1%, 4 fl. oz)	4	1.25	5.5
Afternoon snack	Bagel (½)	3	1	20
	American cheese product (1 slice)	3	5	1
	Water	0	0	0
Dinner	Scrambled egg (1)	11	5	1
	Baby food spinach (3 oz)	2	0.5	5.5
	Whole-wheat toast (1 slice)	1.5	0.5	10
	Mandarin orange slices (¼ cup)	0.5	0	10
	Milk (1%, 4 fl. oz)	4	1.25	5.5

such as cheese for his snacks or macaroni and cheese for a meal. Yogurt is fine, but it shouldn't be nonfat at Ethan's age. In conclusion, Ethan's parents should continue to offer a variety of nutritious foods but should shift some of the energy Ethan currently consumes as protein and carbohydrate to fat.

Encouraging Nutritious Food Choices with Toddlers

Parents and pediatricians have long known that toddlers tend to be choosy about what they eat. Some avoid entire food groups, such as all meats or vegetables. Others will refuse all but one or two favorite foods (such as peanut butter on crackers) for several days or longer. Still others eat extremely small amounts, seemingly satisfied by a single slice of apple or two bites of toast. These behaviors frustrate and worry many parents, but in fact, as long as a variety of healthful food is available, most toddlers have the ability to match their intake with their needs. A toddler will most likely make up for one day's deficiency later on in the week. Parents who offer only nutritious foods can usually feel confident that their children are being well fed, even if a child's choices seem odd or erratic on any particular day. Food should never be "forced" on a child because doing so sets the stage for eating and control issues later in life.

It is also important to recognize that toddlers' stomachs are still very small, and they cannot consume all of the Calories they need in three meals. Toddlers need small meals, alternated with nutritious snacks, every 2 to 3 hours. A successful technique is to create a snack tray filled with small portions of nutritious food choices, such as one-third of a banana, a few cubes of tofu, and two whole-grain crackers, and leave it within reach of the child's play area. The child can then "graze" on these healthful foods while he or she plays. A snack tray plus a spill-proof cup of milk or water is particularly useful on car trips.

Foods prepared for toddlers should be developmentally appropriate. Nuts, carrots, grapes, raisins, cherry tomatoes, and firm cheese are difficult for a toddler to chew and pose a choking hazard. Foods should be soft and sliced into thin strips or wedges that are easy for children to grasp. As the child develops more teeth and becomes more coordinated, the range of food can expand.

Foods prepared for toddlers can also be fun **(FIGURE 15.1)**. Parents can use cookie cutters to turn a peanut butter sandwich into a pumpkin face, or arrange cooked peas or carrot slices to look like a smiling face on top of mashed potatoes. Juice and yogurt can be frozen into "popsicles" or blended into "milkshakes."

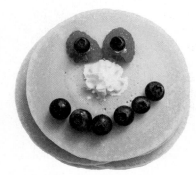

◀ **FIGURE 15.1** Most toddlers are delighted by food prepared in a fun way.

Even at mealtime, portion sizes should be small. One tablespoon of a food for each year of age constitutes a serving throughout the toddler and preschool years **(FIGURE 15.2)**. Realistic portion sizes can give toddlers a sense of accomplishment when they "eat it all up" and minimize parents' fears that their child is not eating enough.

New foods should be introduced gradually. Most toddlers are leery of new foods, spicy foods, hot (temperature) foods, mixed foods (such as casseroles), and foods with strange textures. A helpful rule is to encourage the child to eat at least one bite of a new food: if the child does not want the rest, nothing negative should be said and the child should be praised just for the willingness to try. The food should be reintroduced a few weeks later. Toddlers may need as many as 15 exposures to a new food before accepting it.[7] Parents should never bribe with food—for example, promising dessert if the child finishes her squash. Bribing teaches children that food can be used to reward and manipulate. Instead, parents can try to positively reinforce good behaviors—for example, "Wow! You ate every bite of your squash! That's going to help you grow big and strong!"

Role modeling is important because toddlers mimic older children and adults: if they see their parents eating a variety of healthful foods, they are likely to do so as well. Providing limited healthful alternatives will also help toddlers make nutritious food choices. For example, parents might say, "It's snack time! Would you like apples and cottage cheese or bananas and yogurt?" Finally, toddlers are more likely to eat food they help prepare: encourage them to assist in the preparation of simple foods, such as helping pour a bowl of cereal or arrange vegetables on a plate.

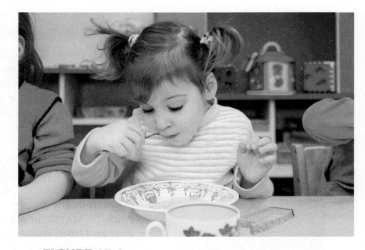

◀ **FIGURE 15.2** Portion sizes for preschoolers are much smaller than those for older children. Use the following guideline: 1 tbsp. of the food for each year of age equals 1 serving. For example, 2 tbsp. of rice, 2 tbsp. of black beans, and 2 tbsp. of chopped tomatoes is appropriate for a 2-year-old.

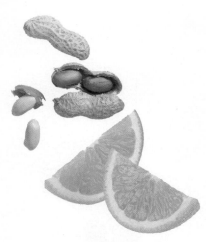

Foods that may cause allergies, such as peanuts and citrus fruits, should be introduced to toddlers one at a time.

Nutrition-Related Concerns for Toddlers

Just as toddlers have their own specific nutrient needs, they also have toddler-specific nutrition concerns, while others continue from infancy.

Continued Allergy Watch

As during infancy, new foods should be presented one at a time, and the toddler should be monitored for allergic reactions for a week before additional new foods are introduced. To prevent the development of food allergies, even foods that are established in the diet should be rotated, rather than served every day.

Overweight: A Concern Now?

Believe it or not, the signs of a tendency toward overweight can occur as early as the toddler years. Toddlers should *not* be denied nutritious food; however, they should not be forced or encouraged to eat when they are full.

Parents and other caregivers can use growth charts to help identify children at risk for overweight or obesity. The Centers for Disease Control and Prevention (CDC) publish a series of growth charts for boys and girls ages 2 through 19 years of age that document stature-for-age, weight-for-age, and BMI-for-age, as well as length-for-age and head circumference for infants (see Appendix E). These charts are also available at the CDC website listed in the Web Resources. Children, including toddlers over the age of 2, who are at or above the 95th percentile for their gender-specific BMI-for-age are defined as obese, whereas those at or above the 85th percentile but below the 95th percentile on BMI-for-age charts are defined as overweight. Parents and health-care providers can easily track a child's growth over time and observe the pattern that develops from year to year. Children who begin to track toward higher and higher BMI-for-age percentiles should be encouraged and supported in increasing their physical activity, and, as for all children, their intake of foods with low nutritional value should be limited. A comprehensive discussion of obesity in children is provided later in this chapter.

Vegetarian Families

For toddlers, a lacto-ovo-vegetarian diet, in which dairy foods and eggs are included, can be as wholesome as a diet that includes meats and fish. However, because red meat is an important source of zinc and heme iron, families who do not serve red meat must be careful to include enough zinc and iron from other sources in their child's diet.

In contrast, a vegan diet, in which no foods of animal origin are consumed, poses several potential nutritional risks for toddlers:

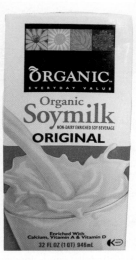

Enriched foods, such as fortified soy milk, should be given to toddlers consuming vegan diets to ensure they get key nutrients.

- **Protein.** Vegan diets can be too low in total protein or protein quality for toddlers, who need adequate amounts of high-quality protein for growth and increasing activity. Few toddlers can consume enough legumes and whole grains to provide sufficient protein. The high fiber content of legumes and whole grains results in a rapid sense of fullness for toddlers, decreasing their total food intake. Soy milk, tofu, and other soy-based products are excellent sources of complete dietary protein.
- **Calcium.** Children who consume no milk, yogurt, or cheese are at risk for calcium deficiency. As with protein, few children can consume enough calcium from plant sources to meet their daily requirement. Although some brands of soy milk and other milk alternatives, and certain fruit juices and cereals, are now fortified with calcium, supplementation is advised.
- **Zinc and Iron.** These minerals, which are abundant in meat, poultry, and seafood, are commonly low in vegan diets. Although both zinc and iron are found in legumes, young children simply cannot eat enough legumes to meet their needs, and supplementation is advised.
- **Vitamins D and B$_{12}$.** Children consuming strict vegan diets are at risk for deficiencies of both of these vitamins. Some cereals and soy milks are fortified with vitamin D; however, many toddlers may still need a vitamin D–containing

supplement. Vitamin B$_{12}$ is not available in any amount from plant foods and must be obtained from fortified foods or supplements.

- **Fiber.** Vegan diets often contain a higher amount of fiber than is recommended for toddlers, resulting in lowered absorption of iron and zinc, as well as the early onset of fullness or satiety.

Although adults who follow a vegan diet have the ability to choose alternative foods and/or supplements to meet the demands for these nutrients, toddlers depend on their parents to make appropriate food choices for them. If parents are determined to maintain a vegan diet for their toddler, choosing to include fortified juices, soy milk, and other soy products, along with an appropriate pediatric supplement and ongoing consultation with a pediatrician or pediatric dietitian, can ensure adequate nutrition in the toddler's diet.

The practice of feeding a vegan diet to infants and young children is highly controversial. See the **Nutrition Myth or Fact?** box (page 560) for more information about this controversy.

> Children who follow a vegetarian diet can meet their protein needs by following the guidelines illustrated by the Power Plate graphic, which can be found at http://pcrm.org. Select the pull-down menus for "health and nutrition," then "vegetarian and vegan diets," and then click on "The Power Plate" near the page bottom.

recap Toddlers require small, frequent, nutritious meals and snacks, and food should be soft and cut in small pieces, so that it is easy to handle, mash, and swallow. Because toddlers are becoming more independent and can self-feed, parents need to be alert for choking and should watch for allergies and monitor weight gain. Role modeling by parents and access to ample healthful foods can help toddlers make nutritious choices. Feeding vegan diets to toddlers poses the potential for deficiencies in protein, calcium, zinc, iron, vitamin D, and vitamin B$_{12}$.

Nutrition for preschool and school-age children

During the preschool and school-age years, children become even more active, but their growth rate slows. Children grow an average of 2 to 4 inches per year at a slow and steady pace, the "calm before the storm" of adolescence, when growth rates again become very rapid.

What Are a Child's Nutrient Needs?

Until the age of 8 or 9 years, the nutrient needs of young boys and girls do not differ; because of this, the DRI values for the macronutrients, fiber, and micronutrients are grouped together for children age 4 to 8 years. The beginning of sexual maturation, however, has a dramatic impact on the nutrient needs of children. Boys' and girls' bodies develop differently in response to gender-specific hormones. These changes in sexual maturation can begin subtly between the ages of 8 and 9 years; thus, the DRI

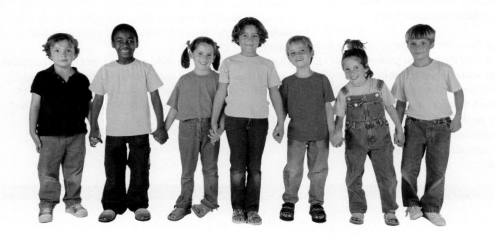

◀ School-age children grow an average of 2 to 4 inches per year.

nutrition myth or fact?

Are Vegan Diets Appropriate for Young Children?

Feeding a vegan diet to young children is a controversial issue. Some supporters of vegan diets assert that feeding animal products to children is forcing them into a life of obesity and chronic diseases. Some note that the consumption of animal products wastes natural resources and contributes to climate change and is therefore unethical. In contrast, some who oppose a vegan diet for young children assert that it deprives developing children of certain essential nutrients that can be found only or primarily in animal products. Some people even suggest that veganism for young children is, in essence, a form of child abuse.

As with many controversies, there is some truth on both sides. For example, there have been documented cases of children failing to thrive, and even dying, on extreme vegan diets. Cases of protein deficiency as well as micronutrient deficiencies have also been cited. These deficiencies can have serious and lifelong consequences. For example, not all of the neurologic impairments caused by vitamin B_{12} deficiency can be reversed by timely B_{12} supplement intervention. In addition, inadequate zinc, calcium, vitamin D, and omega-3 fatty acids can result in impaired bone growth and strength, failure to reach peak bone mass, and impaired development.

However, cases of nutrition-related illness in vegan children are typically due to lack of education, fanaticism, and/or extremism. Informed parents following a responsible vegan diet, in conjunction with pediatric monitoring, are rarely involved. This points to the vital importance of education when administering this diet to young children. Specifically, parents need to know *which nutrients are not available in plant products and therefore must be supplemented*. They also need to understand that typical vegan diets are high in fiber and low in fat, a combination that can be dangerous for very young children. Moreover, certain staples of the vegan diet, such as wheat, soy, and nuts, commonly provoke allergic reactions in children; when this happens, finding a plant-based substitute that contains adequate nutrients can be challenging.

Both the Academy of Nutrition and Dietetics and the American Academy of Pediatrics have stated that a well-planned vegan diet can promote normal growth and development in childhood, although vegetarian children tend to be slightly smaller and leaner. It has also been shown that well-planned vegan diets have no negative effect on final adult height or weight. Parents should ensure that adequate supplements and/or fortified foods are consumed to account for the nutrients that are normally found in animal products.

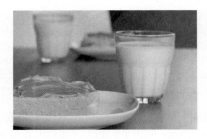

⬆ Most nutrition experts recommend a more balanced diet—including protein sources such as fish, dairy products, and eggs—rather than a strictly vegan diet for developing young children. This snack of a peanut butter sandwich and milk is a healthful choice.

Many health organizations, however, continue to advocate a more moderate approach during the early childhood years. There are several reasons for this level of caution:

- Some vegan parents are not adequately educated on the planning of meals, the balancing of foods, and the inclusion of supplements to ensure adequate intake of all nutrients.
- Most young children are picky eaters and are hesitant to eat certain food groups, particularly vegetables, a staple in the vegan diet.
- The high-fiber content of vegan diets may not be appropriate for very young children.
- Young children have small stomachs, and they may not be able to consume enough plant-based foods to ensure adequate intakes of all nutrients and energy.

Because of these concerns, these organizations advise parents to take a more moderate dietary approach, one that emphasizes plant foods but also includes some animal-based foods, such as fish, dairy, and/or eggs.

Once children reach school age, the abundant fiber, antioxidants, and many micronutrients in a vegan diet, coupled with its lower-fat profile, will promote their health as they progress into adulthood. However, those who consume animal products can derive similar benefits from choosing low-fat, nutrient-dense foods, such as lean meats, nonfat dairy products, whole grains, and fruits and vegetables. When a varied diet is consumed, there are fewer worries about consuming adequate amounts of all nutrients.

CRITICAL THINKING QUESTIONS

1. Some parents have been charged with child endangerment or neglect when their child is found to be very underweight due to vegan or other extreme diets. The same is rarely true for parents of very obese children. Why do you think that is the case?
2. At what age do you think a child is mature and knowledgeable enough to make his or her own decision to follow a vegan diet? If you were the parent of a 14-year-old who wanted to adopt a vegan diet, would you support your child's decision?

values are separately defined for boys and girls age 9 to 13 years.[2] Table 15.1 (page 554) identifies the nutrient needs of children and adolescents.

Energy and Macronutrient Recommendations for Children

Total energy requirements continue to increase throughout childhood because of increasing body size and, for some children, higher levels of physical activity.[2] The estimated energy requirement (EER) varies according to the child's age, body weight, and level of activity. Parents should provide diets that allow for normal growth and support physical activity while minimizing the risk for excess weight gain.

The U.S. Department of Agriculture (USDA) has produced a Daily Food Plan for preschoolers, helping parents to lead their child on the path to healthy eating (**FIGURE 15.3** on page 562). This Plan meets the nutrient requirements for preschoolers as discussed in this section.

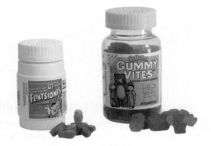

◄ Children's multivitamins often appear in shapes or bright colors.

Fat   Although dietary fat remains a key macronutrient in the preschool years, total fat intake should gradually be reduced to a level closer to that of an adult, 25–35% of total energy.[2] One easy way to start reducing dietary fat is to gradually introduce lower-fat dairy products, such as 2% or 1% milk, and to minimize the intake of fried foods. A diet providing less than 25% of Calories from fat is not recommended for children because they are still growing, developing, and maturing. Foods such as meats and dairy products should not be withheld solely because of their fat content, since they have important nutrient value. In fact, parents should avoid putting too much emphasis on fat at this age. Impressionable and peer-influenced children can easily be led to categorize foods as "good" or "bad," leading to skewed views of food and inappropriate eating habits.

Carbohydrate   The RDA for carbohydrate for children is 130 g/day, which is about 45–65% of total daily energy intake.[2] Complex carbohydrates from whole grains, fruits, vegetables, and legumes should be emphasized. Simple sugars should come from fruits and fruit juices, with foods high in refined sugars, such as cakes, cookies, and candies, saved for occasional indulgences. The AI for fiber for children is 14 g/1,000 kcal of energy consumed.[2] As is the case with toddlers, too much fiber can be harmful because it can make a child feel prematurely full and interfere with adequate food intake and nutrient absorption.

Protein   As seen in Table 15.1, the protein recommendation for boys and girls is 0.95 g/kg body weight per day.[2] Although the recommended protein intake per kilogram of body weight for children ages 4 to 13 years is lower than that of toddlers, the total protein intake of school-age children is higher due to their higher body weight. Lean meats/fish/poultry, lower-fat dairy products, soy-based foods, and legumes are nutritious sources of protein that can be provided to children of all ages.

Micronutrient Recommendations for Children

The need for most micronutrients increases slightly for children up to age 8 because of their increasing size. A sharper increase in micronutrient needs occurs during the transition into full adolescence; this increase is due to the beginning of sexual maturation and in preparation for the impending adolescent growth spurt. Children who fail to consume the USDA-recommended 4 cups of fruits and vegetables each day may become deficient in vitamins A, C, and E. Minerals of concern continue to be calcium, iron, and zinc, which come primarily from animal-based foods.[4,5] Notice that the RDA for iron is based on the assumption that most girls do not begin menstruation until after age 13.[5] Refer again to Table 15.1 for a review of the nutrient needs of children.

If there is any concern that a child's nutrient needs are not being met for any reason (for instance, breakfasts are skipped, lunches are traded, or parents lack money for nourishing food), a pediatric vitamin/mineral supplement that provides no more than 100% of the Daily Value for the micronutrients may help correct any existing deficit.

Fluid Recommendations for Children

The fluid recommendations for children are about 5 to 8 cups of beverages, including drinking water (see Table 15.1).[6] The exact amount of fluid needed varies according to

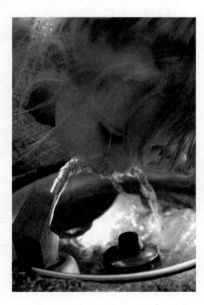

◄ Fluid intake is important for children, who may become so involved in their play that they ignore the sensation of thirst.

Healthy Eating *for* Preschoolers Daily Food Plan

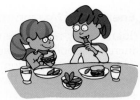

Use this Plan as a general guide.

- These food plans are based on average needs. Do not be concerned if your child does not eat the exact amounts suggested. Your child may need more or less than average. For example, food needs increase during growth spurts.

- Children's appetites vary from day to day. Some days they may eat less than these amounts; other days they may want more. Offer these amounts and let your child decide how much to eat.

Food group	2 year olds	3 year olds	4 and 5 year olds	What counts as:
Fruits	1 cup	1 - 1½ cups	1 - 1½ cups	½ cup of fruit? ½ cup mashed, sliced, or chopped fruit ½ cup 100% fruit juice ½ medium banana 4-5 large strawberries
Vegetables	1 cup	1½ cups	1½ - 2 cups	½ cup of veggies? ½ cup mashed, sliced, or chopped vegetables 1 cup raw leafy greens ½ cup vegetable juice 1 small ear of corn
Grains Make half your grains whole	3 ounces	4 - 5 ounces	4 - 5 ounces	1 ounce of grains? 1 slice bread 1 cup ready-to-eat cereal flakes ½ cup cooked rice or pasta 1 tortilla (6" across)
Protein Foods	2 ounces	3 - 4 ounces	3 - 5 ounces	1 ounce of protein foods? 1 ounce cooked meat, poultry, or seafood 1 egg 1 Tablespoon peanut butter ¼ cup cooked beans or peas (kidney, pinto, lentils)
Dairy Choose low-fat or fat-free	2 cups	2 cups	2½ cups	½ cup of dairy? ½ cup milk 4 ounces yogurt ¾ ounce cheese 1 string cheese

 Some foods are easy for your child to choke on while eating. Skip hard, small, whole foods, such as popcorn, nuts, seeds, and hard candy. Cut up foods such as hot dogs, grapes, and raw carrots into pieces smaller than the size of your child's throat—about the size of a nickel.

There are many ways to divide the Daily Food Plan into meals and snacks. View the "Meal and Snack Patterns and Ideas" to see how these amounts might look on your preschooler's plate at www.choosemyplate.gov/preschoolers.html.

▲ **FIGURE 15.3** MyPlate Healthy Eating for Preschoolers: Daily Food Plan.
Data adapted from: *My Plate, Healthy Eating for Preschoolers: Daily Food Plan*. USDA Food and Nutrition Service.

a child's level of physical activity and the weather conditions. At this point in life, children are mostly in control of their own fluid intake. However, as they engage in physical activity at school and in sports and play, young children in particular may need reminders to drink in order to stay properly hydrated, especially if the weather is hot.

recap Total protein and energy needs are higher for children due to their larger size and higher activity levels. Dietary fat should be gradually reduced to the level of 25–35% of total energy. Calcium, iron, and zinc requirements are higher for children than toddlers. Children need to drink from 5 to 8 cups of water and other beverages throughout the day.

Encouraging Nutritious Food Choices with Children

Peer pressure can be extremely difficult for both parents and their children to deal with during this life stage. Most children want to feel as if they "belong," and they admire and like to mimic children they believe to be popular. If the popular children at school are eating chips and drinking sugared soft drinks, it may be hard for a child to consume a peanut butter on whole-wheat sandwich, an apple, and a low-fat milk without embarrassment.

One strategy for combating peer pressure is to introduce kids to "cool" role models, such as star athletes and popular entertainers who follow nutritious diets. Involving children in growing their own food, shopping, and preparing meals is also a good idea. If they have input into what is going into their bodies, children may be more likely to take an active role in their health. In addition, adults should consistently model healthful eating and physical activity patterns. Families should also choose restaurants where "children's meals" reflect the standards of the National Restaurant Association's *Kids LiveWell* program, which defines goals for total Calories, fat, and sodium, or help their children select healthful menu choices.

What Is the Effect of School Attendance on Nutrition?

Children's school attendance can affect their nutrition in several ways. First, in the hectic time between waking and getting out the door, many children minimize or skip breakfast completely. Many nutrition and education experts believe that children who skip breakfast are at increased risk for behavioral and learning problems associated with hunger in the classroom. Many schools offer a free "in-class breakfast" to all students, helping them optimize their nutrient intake and avoid these problems, but not all children take advantage of them. You've probably heard people say that breakfast is the most important meal of the day. Is that so? Read the **Nutrition Myth or Fact?** box to find out.

Another consequence of attending school is that, with little or no supervision of what they eat, children do not always consume appropriate types or amounts of food. If they purchase a school lunch, they might not like all the foods being served, or their friends might influence them to skip certain foods with comments such as "This broccoli's nasty!" Even homemade lunches that contain nutritious foods may be left uneaten or traded for less nutritious fare.

Finally, schools continue to sell foods with low nutrient value at bake sales and other fund-raisers. Also, despite recent legislation and industry-sponsored initiatives, some schools still have vending machines offering snacks that are high in empty Calories.

Do School Lunches Improve Child Health and Nutrition?

The impact of the National School Lunch Program (NSLP) on children's diets is enormous: 99% of public schools participate, serving nearly 32 million children.[8] On the surface, it would appear that school lunches would be expected to improve children's diets, because they must meet the nutritional standards of the newly implemented Healthy, Hunger-Free Kids Act:

- Students must be offered both fruits and vegetables every day.
- Milk must be fat-free or low fat.

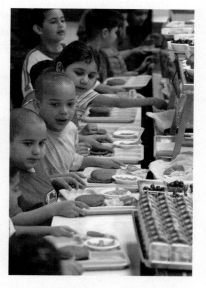

School-age children may receive a standard school lunch, but many choose less healthful foods when given the chance.

Download a free, 112-page cookbook chock full of healthy, kid-friendly recipes from the National Heart, Lung, and Blood Institute. Go to www.nhlbi.nih.gov, enter "family cookbook" into the search box, then click on the top-most link to "NHLBI Deliciously Healthy Eating Recipies."

nutrition myth or fact?

Is Breakfast the Most Important Meal of the Day?

What did you eat for breakfast this morning? Whole-grain cereal with low-fat milk? A strawberry Pop-Tart? Nothing at all? What does it matter, anyway? Sure, you've heard that breakfast is the most important meal of the day, but that's just a myth—right? As long as you eat a nutritious lunch and dinner, why should breakfast matter?

Over the past 20 years, dozens of published research studies have confirmed the importance of a healthful breakfast. Many of these studies highlight the ability of breakfast to support our physical and mental functioning. Let's examine the evidence for this claim.

The word *breakfast* was first used as a verb meaning "to break the fast"—that is, to end the hours of fasting that naturally occur while we sleep. When we fast, our body breaks down stored nutrients to provide fuel for the resting body. First, cells break down glycogen stores in the liver and muscle tissues, using the newly released glucose for energy. These stores last about 12 hours. But people who skip breakfast typically go without food for much longer than that: if they finish dinner about 7:00 PM and don't eat again until noon the next day, they are fasting (going without fuel) for 17 hours! Long before that point, essentially all stored glycogen is used up, and the body has turned to fatty acids and amino acids as fuel sources.

If you're like most people, when your blood glucose is low, you are not only hungry but also weak, shaky, and irritable, and you have poor concentration. So it's not surprising that children and teens who skip breakfast don't function as well as their breakfast-eating peers: their physical, academic, and behavioral performances are all negatively affected.[9,10] Recent research confirms the following:

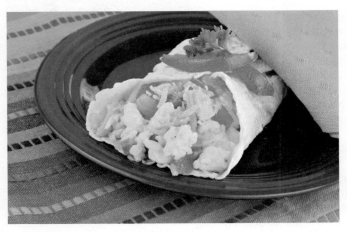

⬆ Breakfast doesn't have to be boring! A breakfast burrito with scrambled eggs, low-fat cheese, and vegetables wrapped in a whole-grain tortilla provides energy and nutrients to start your day off right.

- Missing breakfast and experiencing hunger impair students' ability to learn. Exam scores are lower, their attention span is reduced, and they have more behavioral problems than students who arrive at school in a well-nourished state.

- Eating breakfast at school helps students perform better on demanding mental tasks and improves attention and memory. Children who eat a complete breakfast make fewer mistakes and work faster in math and vocabulary.

- Breakfast improves students' behavior, decreases their tardiness, and improves their school attendance.

What do you think? Is breakfast the most important meal of the day? And what—if anything—will you be having for breakfast tomorrow?

- Offerings of whole grain-rich foods must be substantially increased and, by July 2014, all grains must be whole-grain rich.
- Calories, averaged over a week, and portion sizes must be appropriate for the age of the children being served.
- Sodium, saturated fats, and *trans* fats must be reduced to specified levels.[11]

These same guidelines will apply to the School Breakfast Program. In addition, vending machines and other sources of food on school campuses must meet specific nutrient guidelines.

As a result of such standards, schools nationwide are paying more attention to the quality of food they offer to their students. Some, for example, have installed salad bars, baked potato bars, and soup stations to entice students into more healthful choices. Many schools now cultivate a garden on school grounds or even on the school rooftop where children help to grow the vegetables that will be used in their lunches. Many have implemented programs from the USDA that encourage children to adopt healthy lifestyles, for example, by providing children with less common fruits and vegetables they might not otherwise have had the chance to try. Schools that succeed in improving their meals get additional federal funding.

Although these new regulations represent the first major enhancement of nutritional standards in over 15 years, some caution remains. The actual amount of nutrients a student *gets* depends on what the student actually *eats*. So, a child might eat the slice of whole-wheat veggie pizza and the low-fat milk but skip the carrot sticks and apple. Also keep in mind that children can still bring high-fat and high-sugar snacks and beverages from home or trade with classmates who bring them.

recap Peer pressure has a strong influence on children's nutritional choices. Involving children in growing, purchasing, and preparing foods can help them make more healthful food choices. Skipping breakfast can impair a child's school performance. School lunches are nutritious as planned and must meet new strict federal guidelines, but the foods that children choose to eat at school can still be higher in fat, sugar, and energy and lower in complex carbohydrates and micronutrients than desired. Recent efforts, including state, federal, and industry guidelines, represent a shift toward improved nutrition at school.

Nutrition-Related Concerns for Children

In addition to the potential nutrient deficiencies that have already been discussed, new concerns arise during childhood. Foremost among these are overweight and obesity, a topic we discuss in detail ahead.

Dental Caries

Dental caries, or cavities, occur when bacteria in the mouth feed on carbohydrates deposited on teeth. As a result of metabolizing the carbohydrates, the bacteria then secrete acid, which begins to erode tooth enamel, leading to tooth decay. The development of dental caries can be minimized by limiting sugary sweets, especially those that stick to teeth, such as jelly beans. Frequent brushing helps eliminate the sugars on teeth as well as the bacteria that feed on them.

Fluoride, through a municipal water supply, through fluoridated toothpaste or mouthwash, or through supplements, also helps deter the development of dental caries. Even though the teeth of a young child will be replaced by permanent teeth in several years, it is critical to keep them healthy and strong. This is because they make room for and guide the permanent teeth into position. Children should start having regular dental visits at the age of 3.

Inadequate Calcium Intake

Another nutrition-related concern for children is an inadequate intake of calcium. Adequate calcium is necessary to achieve peak bone mass as well as for numerous other critical body and cell functions. Peak bone mass is achieved by the late teens or early twenties, and childhood and adolescence are critical times to ensure an adequate deposition of bone tissue. Inadequate calcium intake during childhood and adolescence can set the stage for osteoporosis in later years.

Dairy products are the most common source of calcium for children in the United States.[4] During the infant, toddler, and preschool years, milk consumption can largely be monitored by parents and other caregivers. However, older children often choose soft drinks, sports beverages, fruit punch, and other high-sugar, low-nutrient beverages in place of milk. This "milk displacement" is associated with lower intakes of protein, calcium, phosphorus, magnesium, potassium, and vitamin A, increasing subsequent risk for poor bone health.[12]

Body Image Concerns

As children, particularly girls, approach puberty, concerns about their appearance play increasingly important roles in their food choices. These concerns are not necessarily detrimental to health, particularly if they prompt children to make more healthful food choices, such as eating more whole grains, fruits, and vegetables. However, it is important for children to understand that being thin does not guarantee health, popularity, or happiness and that we can be physically fit and healthy at a variety of weights, shapes, and sizes. Children who are physically active may be more confident

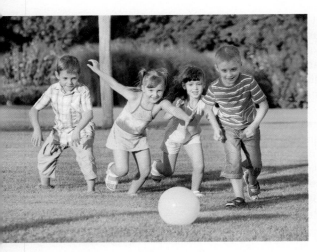

▲ Engaging in physical play with friends is a good way for children to maintain self-confidence and a positive body image.

and accepting of their body image; thus, it is important to encourage daily participation in organized sports or active play and games. Excessive concern with thinness can lead children to experiment with fad diets, food restriction, and other behaviors that can result in undernutrition and perhaps even trigger a clinical eating disorder. (Disordered eating is discussed **In Depth** following Chapter 11.)

Childhood Food Insecurity

Although most children in the United States grow up with an abundant and healthful supply of food, millions of American children are faced with *food insecurity*, a term used to describe a household's inability to ensure a consistent, dependable supply of safe and nutritious food.[13]

Approximately 21% of U.S. households with children can be classified as food insecure, and the rate is much higher among low-income households with children (47%).[13] These statistics are definitely at odds with America's image as "the land of plenty."

The effects of food insecurity can be very harmful to children.[13] Without an adequate breakfast, they will not be able to concentrate or pay attention to their parents and teachers. Impaired nutrient status can blunt children's immune responses, making them more susceptible to common childhood illnesses. Increased rates of hospitalizations have been linked to food insecurity. Children's rates of anxiety and suicide are also increased with food insecurity. Finally, maternal depression is more common within food-insecure households, creating an environment that often leads to poor mental health outcomes in the child.

Options for families facing food insecurity include a number of government and privately funded programs, including school breakfast and lunch programs and the Supplemental Nutrition Assistance Program (SNAP; previously known as the Food Stamp program). Families who face economic difficulties should be referred to public health or social service agencies and encouraged to apply for available nutrition benefits. Private and faith-based food pantries and kitchens can provide a narrow range of foods for a limited period but cannot be relied on to meet the nutritional needs of children and their families over a prolonged time.

recap Parents can communicate effectively with children to encourage healthful eating and can act as role models in regard to food choices and level of physical activity. To prevent dental caries, children should brush their teeth regularly, limit sweets, and visit the dentist regularly beginning at age 3. Consuming adequate calcium to support the development of peak bone mass is also a primary concern for school-age children. Body image is increasingly important to children as they grow older, and disordered eating behaviors can result. Food insecurity is a growing threat to the health and well-being of American children.

Nutrition for adolescents

Although there is no consensus on the exact age range corresponding to the term *adolescence*, this life stage begins with the onset of **puberty**, the period in life in which secondary sexual characteristics develop and we become capable of reproducing, and continues through age 18. This is a physically and emotionally tumultuous time for adolescents and their families. The nutritional needs of adolescents are influenced by their rapid growth in height, increased weight, changes in body composition, and individual levels of physical activity.

Adolescent Growth and Activity Patterns

puberty The period of life in which secondary sexual characteristics develop and people become biologically capable of reproducing.

Growth during adolescence is driven primarily by hormonal changes, including increased levels of testosterone for boys and estrogen for girls. Both boys and girls experience growth spurts, or periods of accelerated increase in height, during later childhood and adolescence. The timing and length of these growth spurts vary by race, gender, nutritional status, and other factors. Growth spurts for girls can begin as early as 9 to 10 years of age, whereas growth spurts for boys can begin as early as 10 or 11 years.

Skeletal growth ceases once closure of the **epiphyseal plates** occurs (**FIGURE 15.4**). These are plates of cartilage located toward the end of the long bones that provide for their growth in length. Although most girls reach their full adult height by about age 18, some continue to increase in height past age 19, although the rate of growth slows considerably. Most boys continue to grow up to the age of 21, although their rate of growth also slows over time.

In some circumstances, the epiphyseal plates close early and the adolescent fails to reach full stature. The most common causes of this failure are malnutrition, such as may occur with an eating disorder, and the use of anabolic steroids during this critical growth period.

About half of peak bone mass is deposited during the adolescent years. Weight and body composition also change dramatically. Weight gain is extremely variable and reflects the adolescent's energy intake, physical activity level, and genetics. The average weight gained by girls and boys during this time is 39 and 52 pounds, respectively. The weight gained by girls and boys is considerably different in terms of its composition. Girls tend to gain significantly more body fat than boys, with this fat accumulating around the buttocks, hips, breasts, thighs, and upper arms. Although many girls are uncomfortable or embarrassed by these changes, they are a natural result of maturation. Boys gain significantly more muscle mass than girls, and they experience an increase in muscle definition.

The physical activity levels of adolescents are highly variable. Many are physically active in sports or other organized physical activities, whereas others become less interested in sports and more interested in intellectual or artistic pursuits. This variability in activity levels results in highly individual energy needs. Although the rapid growth and maturation that occur during puberty require a significant amount of energy, adolescence is often a time in which overweight begins.

What Are an Adolescent's Nutrient Needs?

The nutrient needs of adolescents are influenced by rapid growth, weight gain, and sexual maturation, in addition to the demands of physical activity (see Table 15.1).

Energy and Macronutrient Recommendations for Adolescents

Adequate energy intake is necessary to maintain adolescents' health, support their dramatic growth and maturation, and fuel their physical activity. Because of these competing demands, the energy needs of adolescents can be quite high. Although it is possible to calculate estimated energy requirements of an adolescent by using a published equation, it is more practical to monitor the growth pattern of the adolescent to ensure that weight remains in proportion to height.[2]

Fat   Adolescents are at risk for the same chronic diseases as adults, including type 2 diabetes, obesity, cardiovascular disease, and various cancers. Thus, it is prudent for adolescents to consume no more than 25–35% of total energy from fat and no more than 10% of total energy from saturated fat sources.[2]

Carbohydrate   The RDA for carbohydrate for adolescents is 130 g/day.[2] As with adults, this amount of carbohydrate covers what is needed to supply adequate glucose to the brain, but it does not cover the amount of carbohydrate needed to support daily activities. Thus, it is recommended that adolescents consume more than the RDA, or about 45–65% of their total energy as carbohydrate, and most should come from fiber-rich carbohydrates. The AI for fiber for adolescents is 26 g/day, which is similar to adult values.

Protein   The RDA for protein for adolescents is similar to that of adults, 0.85 g of protein per kilogram of body weight per day.[2] This value was selected because data are not available to determine protein maintenance requirements for this age group,

Want an overview of the typical adolescent growth spurt? Watch this short video for a summary of this process. www .howcast.com. Enter "puberty growth spurts" into the search box, then click on the video by Dr. Jennifer Wider called "What Are Growth Spurts?"

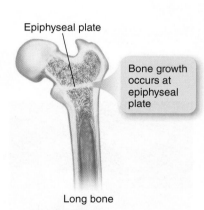

Epiphyseal plate

Bone growth occurs at epiphyseal plate

Long bone

FIGURE 15.4   Skeletal growth ceases once closure of the epiphyseal plates occurs.

epiphyseal plates   Plates of cartilage located toward the end of long bones that provide for growth in the length of long bones.

and the amount of nitrogen needed to maintain protein balance in children is similar to that of adults.[3] This amount is assumed to be sufficient to support health and to cover the additional needs of growth and development during the adolescent stage.

Micronutrient Recommendations for Adolescents

The micronutrients of particular concern for adolescents are calcium, iron, and vitamins A and D.

Calcium and Vitamin D Adequate calcium and vitamin D intakes are critical to achieve peak bone density. The RDA for calcium from age 9 through adolescence is 1,300 mg/day.[4] This amount of calcium can be difficult for many adolescents to consume because the quality of the foods they select is often less than optimal to meet their nutrient needs. However, this level of calcium intake is easily achieved by eating at least 4 servings of dairy foods or calcium-fortified products daily.

The RDA for vitamin D for adolescents is 600 IU/day.[4] Most foods are naturally low in vitamin D; thus, fortified foods, such as milk and cereals, are important sources of this vitamin. If an adolescent is not consuming adequate milk and does not get enough sunlight year round, he or she may need to take a supplement providing both calcium and vitamin D.

Iron The iron requirements of adolescents are relatively high; this is because iron is needed to replace the blood lost during menstruation in girls and to support the growth of muscle mass in boys. Between the ages of 14 and 18 years, the RDA for iron for boys is 11 mg/day, whereas the RDA for girls is 15 mg/day.[5] If energy intake is adequate and adolescents consume food sources of heme iron, such as lean meat/fish/poultry, each day, they should be able to meet the RDA for iron. However, many young people adopt a vegetarian lifestyle during this life stage, or they consume foods that have limited amounts of iron. Both of these situations can prevent adolescents from meeting the RDA for iron and, particularly in females, can increase their risk for iron-deficiency anemia.

Vitamin A Vitamin A is critical to support the rapid growth and development that occur during adolescence. The RDA for vitamin A is 900 μg/day for boys and 700 μg/day for girls ages 14 to 18 years.[5] The RDA can be met by consuming at least 5 servings of dark-green, yellow, and orange fruits and vegetables each day. As with iron and calcium, meeting the RDA for vitamin A can be a challenging goal if the adolescent fails to make healthful food choices. In such cases, a multivitamin and mineral supplement that provides no more than 100% of the Daily Value for the micronutrients can be beneficial as a safety net. As with younger children and adults, a supplement should not be considered a substitute for a balanced, healthful diet.

Fluid Recommendations for Adolescents

The fluid needs of adolescents are higher than those of children because of their higher physical activity levels and the extensive growth and development that occur during this phase of life. The AI for total fluid for adolescent girls and boys is listed in Table 15.1; it includes about 8 and 11 cups, respectively, as beverages, including drinking water.[7] Boys require a higher fluid intake because they are often more active than girls and have more lean tissue. Highly active adolescents of either gender who are exercising in the heat may have higher fluid needs than the AI, and these individuals should be encouraged to drink often to quench their thirst and avoid dehydration.

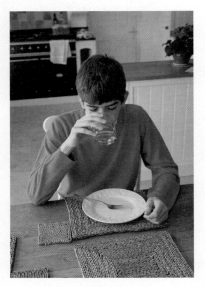

⬅ Adolescents have higher fluid needs than younger children.

recap Puberty is the period in life in which secondary sexual characteristics develop and the ability to reproduce begins. Adolescents experience rapid increases in height, weight, and lean body mass and fat mass. Energy needs can be very high. Fat intake should be 25–35% of total energy, and carbohydrate intake should be 45–65%. Calcium is needed to optimize bone growth and to achieve peak bone density, and iron needs are increased due to increased muscle mass in boys and to menstruation in girls. Adolescents need to drink about 8 cups (girls) and 11 cups (boys) of water or other beverages daily.

Encouraging Nutritious Food Choices with Adolescents

At this point in their lives, adolescents are making most of their own food choices, and many are buying and preparing a significant amount of the foods they consume. Although parents can still be effective role models, adolescents are generally strongly influenced by their peers, their personal food preferences, and their own developing sense of which foods constitute a healthful and adequate diet. Adolescents are anxious to develop their own identity and establish a more self-reliant lifestyle. The decision to adopt a vegetarian diet, for example, may represent an adolescent's effort to establish some distance from the family unit.

One area of concern in most adolescents' diets is a lack of vegetables, fruits, and whole grains. Many teens eat on the run, skip meals, and select fast foods and convenience foods because they are inexpensive, are accessible, and taste good. High school students are often allowed to leave campus for lunch, increasing their opportunities to eat high-fat, low-nutrient fast foods. Parents and school food service personnel can capitalize on adolescents' preferences for pizza, burgers, spaghetti, and sandwiches by providing more healthful meat and cheese alternatives, whole-grain breads, and plenty of appealing vegetable-based sides or additions to these foods. In addition, keeping healthful snacks accessible, such as fruits and vegetables that are cleaned and prepared in easy-to-eat pieces, may encourage adolescents to choose more of these foods as between-meal snacks. Teens should also be encouraged to consume adequate milk and other calcium-enriched beverages, while minimizing sodas, sports drinks, and other high-sugar beverages.

As adolescents leave the nest for college or their own apartments, it is important that they set the foundation for healthful eating. One question teens often have is how to stock their first kitchen. What basic foods—or staples—should they always have on hand, so that they can quickly and easily assemble healthful meals and snacks? The **Quick Tips** checklist (page 570) includes the foods that many Americans consider to be staples. It can be modified to include items that are staples in non-Western cultures and to address vegetarian, vegan, low-fat, low-sodium, or other diets. By stocking healthful foods such as those listed here, they'll be much more likely to make healthful food choices every day!

Nutrition-Related Concerns for Adolescents

Nutrition-related concerns for adolescents include bone density, body image issues, acne, cigarette smoking, and the use of alcohol and illegal drugs.

Bone Density Watch

Early adolescence, 13 to 15 years of age, is a crucial time for ensuring adequate calcium and vitamin D levels to maximize bone calcium uptake and bone mineral density over the next several years.[4] Achieving and maintaining optimal bone density during adolescence and into young adulthood is critical for delaying or preventing the onset of osteoporosis.

As previously noted, meeting the adolescent DRIs for calcium (1,300 mg/day) and vitamin D (600 IU/day) can be challenging. Milk is one of the most reliable sources of both nutrients, yet average milk intake has decreased by nearly one-half over the past 3 decades.[14] By age 18, average milk consumption has fallen by more than 25% compared to intake at age 8 years, whereas soda intake has tripled. A national "Milk Matters" campaign, coordinated by the National Institutes of Health, distributes teen-friendly materials to encourage greater intakes of milk and other dairy foods (FIGURE 15.5). (See the Web Resources at the end of this chapter.)

Body Image and Eating Disorders

An initially healthful concern about body image and weight can turn into a dangerous obsession during this emotionally challenging life stage. Eating disorders frequently begin during adolescence and can occur in boys as well as girls. Parents, teachers, and friends should be aware of the warning signs, which include rapid and excessive weight loss, a preoccupation with weight and body image, regular trips to the bathroom after meals, and signs of frequent vomiting or laxative use. (For more information, see the **In Depth** following Chapter 11, pages 429–439.)

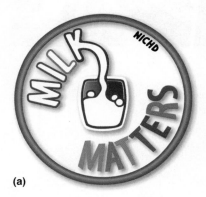

(a)

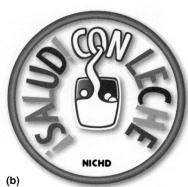

(b)

◆ **FIGURE 15.5** Milk Matters/Salud con Leche. These logos are part of a new government program to encourage milk consumption by children and adolescents. They are provided **(a)** in English and **(b)** in Spanish.
Source: National Institute of Child Health and Development.

QuickTips

Stocking Your First Kitchen

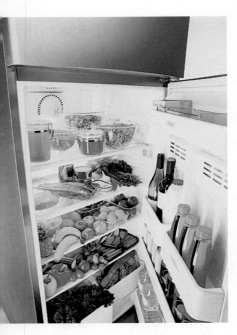

Keep your refrigerator stocked with:

✓ Low-fat or skim milk or soy milk

✓ Calcium-enriched orange juice

✓ Hard cheeses

✓ Eggs

✓ Lean deli meats or soy meat alternatives

✓ Lower-fat hummus, peanut butter, and other perishable spreads

✓ A 2- to 3-day supply of dark-green lettuce and other salad fixings, or ready-to-eat salads

✓ A 2- to 3-day supply of other fresh veggies

✓ A 2- to 3-day supply of fresh fruits

✓ Low-fat salad dressings, mustards, and salsas

✓ Whole-grain breads, rolls, bagels, pizza crusts, and tortillas

Stock your freezer with:

✓ Individual servings of chicken breast, extra-lean ground beef, pork loin chops, fish fillets, or soy meat alternatives

✓ Lower-fat frozen entrées ("boost" with salad, whole-grain roll, and extra veggies)

✓ Frozen veggies (no sauce)

✓ Frozen cheese or veggie pizza ("boost" with added mushrooms, green peppers, and other veggie toppings)

✓ Low-fat ice cream, sherbet, or sorbet

Stock your pantry with:

✓ Staples such as potatoes, sweet potatoes, onions, and garlic

✓ Canned or vacuum-packed tuna, salmon, and crab (in water, not oil)

✓ Canned legumes, such as black beans, refried beans, pinto/kidney beans, and garbanzo beans

✓ Low-sodium, low-fat, high-fiber canned soups (read the label!)

✓ Dried beans and/or lentils

✓ Whole-grain pasta and rice

✓ Tomato-based pasta sauces

✓ Canned fruit in juice with no added sugar

✓ Dried fruits, such as golden raisins, cranberries, and apricots

✓ Nuts, such as peanuts, almonds, and walnuts

✓ Whole-grain ready-to-eat cereals or oatmeal

✓ Whole-grain, low-fat crackers

✓ Low-salt pretzels, low-fat tortilla/corn chips, and low-fat or nonfat microwave popcorn

✓ Salt, pepper, balsamic vinegar, low-sodium soy sauce, and similar condiments and spices

✓ Olive and canola oils

Adolescent Acne

The hormonal changes that occur during puberty are largely responsible for the acne flare-ups that plague many adolescents. Emotional stress, genetic factors, and personal hygiene are secondary contributors. But what about foods? For years, chocolate, fried foods, and fatty foods were linked to acne. In the 1960s, however, these theories were discounted and researchers came to agree that diet had virtually no role in its development. Currently, however, evidence is growing that dietary choices may indeed influence the risk or severity of acne.[15] Whereas some studies have found an association between a high glycemic-load diet and increased acne (see Chapter 4), others have found a reduced risk for acne among people following a Mediterranean dietary pattern (see Chapter 2).[9] These studies are not conclusive; however, the Mediterranean diet is rich in fruits, vegetables, whole grains, olive oil, and fish—foods that provide vitamin A, vitamin C, zinc, and other nutrients that help to maintain skin health and immune function.

Prescription medications, including the vitamin A derivative 13-*cis*-retinoic acid (Accutane), effectively control severe forms of acne. Prescription topical creams, applied directly to the skin, may also be used under the guidance of a physician. Neither Accutane nor any other prescription vitamin A derivative should be used by women who are pregnant, are planning a pregnancy, or may become pregnant. Accutane is a known teratogen, causing severe fetal malformations. Adolescent females who treat their acne with vitamin A–derivative prescription drugs must protect themselves against pregnancy and immediately contact their physician if they discover or believe they are pregnant. Incidentally, vitamin A taken in supplement form is not effective in acne treatment and, due to its own risk for toxicity, should not be used in amounts that exceed 100% of the Daily Value.

Use of Tobacco, Alcohol, and Illegal Drugs

Adolescents are naturally curious and many are open to experimenting with tobacco, alcohol, and illegal drugs. Cigarette smoking diminishes appetite and can interfere with nutrient metabolism. In fact, it is often used by adolescent girls to achieve or maintain a lower body weight.[10] Other effects of smoking on young people include the following:

- Addiction to nicotine
- Reduced rate of lung growth
- Impaired athletic performance and endurance
- Shortness of breath
- Early signs of heart disease and stroke
- Increased risk for lung cancer and other smoking-related cancers

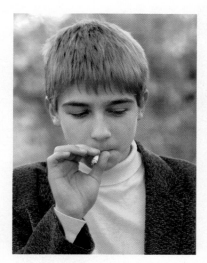

Cigarette smoking can interfere with nutrient metabolism, in addition to having other harmful effects.

Among adolescents, smoking is also associated with an increased incidence of participation in other risky behaviors, such as abusing alcohol and other drugs, fighting, and engaging in unprotected sex. There is also a link between adolescent smoking and early onset of depression and anxiety disorders.[16]

Alcohol and illegal drug use can start at early ages, even in school-age children. Motor vehicle accidents are the leading cause of death among adolescents; the risk of being involved in an accident is greatly increased by using alcohol and illegal drugs. Alcohol can also interfere with proper nutrient absorption and metabolism, and it can take the place of foods in an adolescent's diet; these adverse effects of alcohol put adolescents at risk for various nutrient deficiencies. Alcohol consumption and the use of certain illegal drugs are also associated with "the munchies," a feeling of food craving that usually results in the intake of large quantities of high-fat, high-sugar, nutrient-poor foods. This behavior can result in overweight or obesity, and it increases the risk for nutrient imbalance. Teens who use illegal drugs and alcohol are typically in poor physical condition, are either underweight or overweight, have poor appetites, and perform poorly in school.

recap Adolescents' food choices are influenced by peer pressure, personal preferences, and their own developing sense of what foods are healthful. Adolescents are at risk of skipping meals and selecting fast foods and snack foods in place of whole grains, fruits, and vegetables. Milk is commonly replaced with sugared soft drinks, reducing the calcium available for building bone density. Disordered eating behaviors, eating disorders, acne, cigarette smoking, and use of alcohol and illegal drugs are also concerns for this age group.

nutri-case | LIZ

"High school was really hard for me. Because dance took up such a big part of my life, I just didn't make a lot of friends. When I looked at the popular girls, I always noticed how slender they all were. So I started skipping lunch and eating less at dinner. This went on until I went to an audition for a production of *The Nutcracker*. I wanted so badly to dance in it, but I was feeling so spaced out—I guess from hunger—that before I knew what had happened, I was on the floor! I sprained my ankle and didn't get to dance at all that year! So that's why, while I've been preparing for my audition with the City Ballet, I made sure I'm getting at least 1,000 Calories a day. The audition's tomorrow, and I'm not going to end up on the floor this time!"

Do you—or does someone you know—equate body weight with popularity and desirability? Why are adolescents or young adults particularly prone to this type of thinking? If Liz succeeds in getting into the City Ballet—given what you've learned throughout this text—what health risks do you think she is likely to face in the future? How could she reduce these risks?

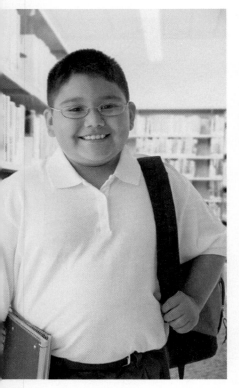

The rates of obesity among U.S. children remain unacceptably high.

Pediatric obesity watch: A concern for children and adolescents

Although the prevalence of obesity has stabilized for U.S children and adolescents since 2007, rates remain unacceptably high.[17] Currently, about 12% of preschoolers and 18% of youth age 6 to 19 are classified as obese. The CDC classifies children as obese if their body mass index (BMI) is at or above the 95th percentile; that is, their BMI is higher than that of 95% of U.S. children of the same age and gender who made up the reference group at the time these charts were developed.[18]

We may feel shocked at the sight of an obese preschooler or school-age child, but children's health experts point out that we should be more concerned by what we don't see. Even in early childhood, obesity can worsen asthma, cause sleep apnea, impair the child's mobility, reduce academic performance, and lead to intense teasing, low self-esteem, depression, and social isolation. Fatty liver is diagnosed in one-third of obese children, and increasing numbers of obese children are experiencing abnormal blood lipids, high blood pressure, high blood glucose, metabolic syndrome, skeletal disorders, and other medical problems.[18] Also, it has been estimated that about 70% of children who are obese maintain their higher weight as adults.[19]

Parents should not be offended if the child's pediatrician or other healthcare provider expresses concern over the child's weight status; early intervention is often the most effective measure against lifelong obesity. The best approach to preventing pediatric obesity combines constructive support for healthful, balanced eating and increased physical activity.

Prevention Through a Healthful Diet

The introduction and retention of healthful eating habits within the family unit are among the most effective strategies in the fight against pediatric obesity. Rather than singling out overweight children and placing them on restrictive diets, experts encourage family-wide improvements in food choices and mealtime habits. Parents should strive to consistently provide nutritious food choices, encourage children to eat a healthful breakfast every morning, and sit down to a shared family meal each evening or as often as possible. The television should be off throughout mealtimes to encourage attentive eating and true enjoyment of the food.

Parents should retain control over the purchase and preparation of foods until older children and teens are responsible and knowledgeable enough to make healthful decisions. For children "on the run," parents can keep a supply of nonperishable snacks—such as granola bars, dried fruits and nuts, and kid-friendly fruits, including apples,

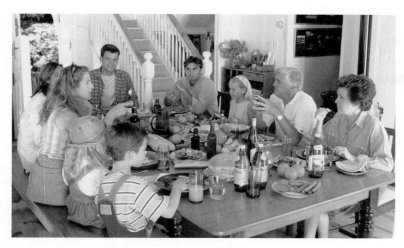

Families should try to have shared meals whenever possible.

bananas, and oranges—to grab as everyone dashes out the door. Mealtimes should offer a colorful variety of vegetables, and children should drink milk or water, not soda.

Whenever possible, parents should minimize the number of meals eaten in restaurants, especially fast-food franchises. When families do eat out, large portion sizes can be shared; moreover, the family can order grilled, broiled, or baked foods instead of fried foods.

As discussed earlier, schools play a role in shaping eating behaviors. Parents can work with local school boards to eliminate or restrict the sale of soda, candy, chips, and pastries. Schools can set aside land or construct raised beds for vegetable gardens, and food service providers can use the produce in lunch menus. Consistent and repeated school-based messages on good nutrition can reinforce the efforts of parents and healthcare providers.

Prevention Through an Active Lifestyle

Television, computer use, and electronic games often tempt children into a sedentary lifestyle, but increased energy expenditure through increased physical activity is essential for successful weight management. The Institute of Medicine recommends that children participate in daily physical activity and exercise for at least an hour each day.[2] For younger children, this can be divided into two or three shorter sessions, allowing them to regroup, recoup, and refocus between activity sessions. Overweight children are more likely to engage in physical activities that are noncompetitive, fun, and structured in a way that allows them to proceed at their own pace. All children can be encouraged to have fun using their muscles in various ways that suit their interests (TABLE 15.2, page 574). Activity-based interactive DVD games are ideal for children who must remain indoors for extended periods.

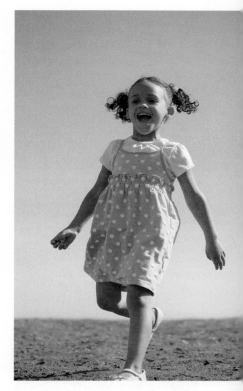

Active, healthy-weight children are less likely to become overweight adults.

recap Obesity is an important concern for children of all ages, their families, and their communities. Parents should model healthy eating and activity behaviors. Schools play an important role in providing nutritious breakfasts and lunches and varied opportunities for daily physical activity.

Nutrition for older adults

The U.S. population is getting older each year. Consider the following statistics:

- In 2010, average life expectancy at birth was projected at 78.3 years.[20]
- It is estimated that, by the year 2030, the elderly (those 65 years and above) will account for about 20% of Americans.[21,22]

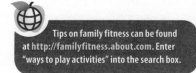

Tips on family fitness can be found at http://familyfitness.about.com. Enter "ways to play activities" into the search box.

TABLE 15.2 Examples of Physical Activities for Children and Adolescents*

Type of Physical Activity	Age Group: Children	Age Group: Adolescents
Moderate-intensity aerobic	• Active recreation, such as hiking, skateboarding, rollerblading • Bicycle riding • Brisk walking	• Active recreation, such as canoeing, hiking, skateboarding, rollerblading • Brisk walking • Bicycle riding (stationary or road bike) • Housework and yard work, such as sweeping or pushing a lawn mower • Games that require catching and throwing, such as baseball and softball
Vigorous-intensity aerobic	• Active games involving running and chasing, such as tag • Bicycle riding • Jumping rope • Martial arts, such as karate • Running • Sports such as soccer, ice or field hockey, basketball, swimming, tennis • Cross-country skiing	• Active games involving running and chasing, such as flag football • Bicycle riding • Jumping rope • Martial arts, such as karate • Running • Sports such as soccer, ice or field hockey, basketball, swimming, tennis • Vigorous dancing • Cross-country skiing
Muscle-strengthening	• Games such as tug-of-war • Modified push-ups (with knees on the floor) • Resistance exercises using body weight or resistance bands • Rope or tree climbing • Sit-ups (curl-ups or crunches) • Swinging on playground equipment/bars	• Games such as tug-of-war • Push-ups and pull-ups • Resistance exercises with exercise bands, weight machines, hand-held weights • Climbing wall • Sit-ups (curl-ups or crunches)
Bone-strengthening	• Games such as hopscotch • Hopping, skipping, jumping • Jumping rope • Running • Sports such as gymnastics, basketball, volleyball, tennis	• Hopping, skipping, jumping • Jumping rope • Running • Sports such as gymnastics, basketball, volleyball, tennis

Note: *Some activities, such as bicycling, can be moderate or vigorous intensity, depending upon level of effort.

Data from: *2008 Physical Activity Guidelines for Americans*, U.S. Department of Health and Human Services.

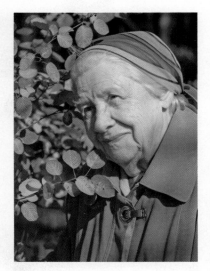

Centenarians represent the future of U.S. elderly.

• People 85 years of age and older currently represent the fastest-growing U.S. population subgroup, projected to increase from 5.5 million in 2010 to nearly 20 million by the year 2050.[22] These so-called very elderly or oldest old account for the majority of healthcare expenditures and nursing home admissions in the United States.

• The number of *centenarians*, persons over the age of 100 years, and *super centenarians*, over 110 years, continues to grow as well.[23] Between 1980 and 2010, the number of centenarians grew by 66%, and there are now over 50,000 centenarians in the United States.

These statistics have important nutrition-related implications even for younger adults because a nutritious diet and regular physical activity throughout life can help prevent or delay the onset of chronic diseases and keep adults happy and productive in their later years. Throughout this book, our exploration of nutrition and physical activity has focused mainly on young and middle-age adults. In the following section, we discuss the unique nutritional needs and concerns of older adults, and we identify ways in which diet and lifestyle affect the aging process.

What Physiologic Changes Accompany Aging?

Older adulthood is a time in which body systems begin to slow and degenerate. If the following discussion of this degeneration seems disturbing or depressing, remember that the changes described are at least partly within an individual's control. For instance, some of the decrease in muscle mass, bone mass, and muscle strength is due to low physical activity levels. In addition, there are intriguing lines of research actively searching for a modern-day "Fountain of Youth," some of which are discussed in the **In Depth** following this chapter.

Age-Related Changes in Sensory Perception

For most individuals, eating is a social and pleasurable process; the sights, sounds, odors, and textures associated with food stimulate and enhance one's appetite. However, odor, taste, touch, and vision all decline with age and negatively affect the food intake and nutritional status of older adults.

It has been estimated that over half of older adults experience a significant impairment in their sense of smell. The nerve receptors for taste and smell are complementary; thus, enjoyment of food relies heavily on the sense of smell. Older adults who cannot adequately appreciate the appealing aromas of food may be unable to fully enjoy the foods offered in a meal. Although often a simple consequence of aging, loss of odor perception can also be caused by a zinc deficiency or a medication. If this is the case, a zinc supplement or change of medication may be a simple solution.

Because the sense of smell contributes significantly to the sense of taste, *dysgeusia*, or an impaired sense of taste, is also common. Most often diminished are the abilities to detect salt and bitter tastes. The perception of sweetness and sourness also declines, but to a lesser extent.

Loss of visual acuity has unexpected consequences for the nutritional health of older adults. Many have difficulty reading food labels, including nutrient information and "pull dates" for perishable foods. Driving skills decline, limiting the ability of some older Americans to get to a market offering healthful, affordable foods. Older adults with vision loss may not be able to see the temperature knobs on stoves or the controls on microwave ovens and may therefore choose cold meals, such as sandwiches, rather than meals that require heating. Also, the visual appeal of a colorful, attractively arranged plate of food is lost to visually impaired elderly people, further reducing their desire to eat healthful meals.

Age-Related Changes in Gastrointestinal Function

Significant changes in the mouth, stomach, intestinal tract, and related organs occur with aging. Some of these changes can increase the risk for nutrient deficiency.

With increasing age, salivary production declines. A dry mouth reduces taste perception, increases tooth decay, and makes chewing and swallowing more difficult. Thus, a diet rich in moist foods, including fruits and vegetables; sauces or gravies on meats; and high-fluid desserts, such as puddings, is advised. Difficulty swallowing, clinically known as *dysphagia*, can also result from a stroke or a condition such as Parkinsonism. Smooth, thick foods, such as cream soups, applesauce, milkshakes, fruit nectars, yogurt, and puddings, are usually well tolerated.

Older adults are also at risk for a reduced secretion of hydrochloric acid, which limits the absorption of minerals such as calcium, iron, and zinc and food sources of folic acid and vitamin B_{12}. A decline in intrinsic factor greatly reduces the absorption of vitamin B_{12} (see Chapter 10). Thus, vitamin B_{12} supplements and/or B_{12} injections are advised.

Age-Related Changes in Body Composition

With aging, body fat increases and muscle mass declines, leading to impaired physical functioning in the elderly.[24] It has been estimated that women and men lose 20–25% of their lean body mass, respectively, as they age from 35 to 70 years. The decreased production of certain hormones, including testosterone and growth hormone, and chronic diseases contribute to this loss of muscle, as do poor diet and an increasingly sedentary lifestyle. Along with adequate dietary intake, regular physical activity,

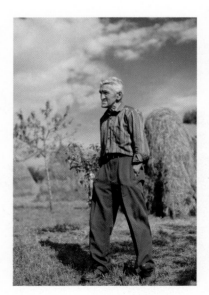

▲ A variety of gastrointestinal and other physiologic changes can lead to weight loss in older adults.

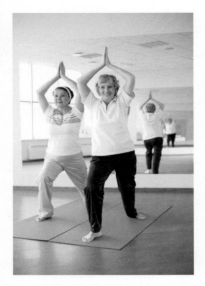

◀ Regular physical activity slows the progression of age-related loss of muscle mass.

including strength or resistance training, can help older adults maintain their muscle mass and strength.

Body fat increases from young adulthood through middle age, peaking at approximately 55 to 65 years of age, then declining in persons over the age of 70. With aging, body fat shifts from subcutaneous stores, just below the skin, to internal, or visceral, fat stores. Older men and women tend to deposit more fat in their abdominal region compared to younger adults. Among women, this shift in body fat stores is most dramatic after the onset of menopause and coincides with an increased risk for heart disease, diabetes, and metabolic syndrome.

Bone mineral density declines with age and may eventually drop to the critical fracture zone. Among older women, the onset of menopause leads to a sudden and dramatic loss of bone due to the lack of estrogen. Although it is less dramatic, elderly men also experience this loss of bone, due in part to decreasing levels of testosterone. In addition to the well-known benefits of calcium and vitamin D, intakes of vitamins A, C, and K; phosphorus; magnesium; fluoride; and protein are now recognized as influencing bone density. As noted in the **Nutrition Debate** on physical activity in the elderly (page 584), bone health can be promoted through regular weight-bearing activity in adults well into their nineties and beyond.

recap   The physiologic changes that can occur with aging include sensory declines; an impaired ability to chew, swallow, and absorb and metabolize various nutrients; a loss of muscle mass and lean tissue; increased fat mass; and decreased bone density. These age-related changes influence the nutritional needs of older adults and their ability to consume a healthful diet.

What Are an Older Adult's Nutrient Needs?

The requirements for many nutrients are the same for older adults as for young and middle-aged adults. A few nutrient requirements increase, and a few are actually lower. **TABLE 15.3** identifies the nutrient recommendations that change as well as the physiologic reasons behind these changes.

Energy and Macronutrient Recommendations for Older Adults

The energy needs of older adults are lower than those of younger adults. This decrease is due to a loss of muscle mass and lean tissue, a reduction in thyroid hormones, and an increasingly sedentary lifestyle. It is estimated that total daily energy expenditure decreases approximately 10 kcal each year for men and 7 kcal each year

TABLE 15.3   Nutrient Recommendations That Change with Increased Age

Changes in Nutrient Recommendations	Rationale for Changes
Vitamin D	Decreased bone density
Increased need for vitamin D from 600 IU/day for adults age 18–70 years to 800 IU/day for adults over age 70 years	Decreased ability to synthesize vitamin D in the skin
Calcium	Decreased bone density
Increased need for calcium from 1,000 mg/day for adults 19–50 years to 1,200 mg/day for women 51 years of age and older, and men 71 years and older	Decreased absorption of dietary calcium
Fiber	Decreased energy intake
Decreased need for fiber from 38 g/day for young men to 30 g/day for men 51 years and older; decreases for women from 25 g/day for young women to 21 g/day for women 51 years and older	
B-Vitamins	Lower levels of gastric juice
Increased need for vitamin B$_6$ and need for vitamin B$_{12}$ as a supplement or from fortified foods	Decreased absorption of food B$_{12}$ from gastrointestinal tract
	Increased need to reduce homocysteine levels and to optimize immune function

for women ages 19 and older.[2] This adds up over time; for example, a woman who needs 2,000 kcal at age 20 needs just 1,650 at age 70. Some of this decrease in energy expenditure is an inevitable response to aging, but some of the decrease can be delayed or minimized by staying physically active. To avoid weight gain, older adults need to consume a diet high in nutrient-dense foods but not too high in energy. The Human Nutrition Research Center at Tufts University has released a MyPlate for Older Adults to help guide food choices (**FIGURE 15.6**). See the **In Depth** following this chapter to learn more about the theory and practice of Caloric restriction, which proposes that low-energy diets may significantly prolong life.

Fat   To reduce their risk for heart disease and other chronic diseases, it is recommended that older adults maintain a total fat intake within 20–35% of total daily energy intake, with no more than 10% of total energy intake coming from saturated fat.

Carbohydrate   The RDA for carbohydrate for older adults is 130 g/day.[2] Complex carbohydrates should be emphasized over simple sugars: it is recommended that older individuals consume a diet that contains no more than 30% of total energy intake as sugars.[2] The fiber recommendations are slightly lower for older adults than for younger adults because older adults eat less energy. After age 50, 30 g of fiber per day for men and 21 g for women is assumed sufficient to reduce the risks for constipation and diverticular disease, maintain healthful blood levels of glucose and lipids, and provide good sources of nutrient-dense, low-energy foods.

Protein   The DRI for protein is the same for adults of all ages: 0.80 g protein/kg body weight per day.[2] Some researchers have argued for a protein allowance of 1.0 to 1.2 g protein/kg body weight for older adults in order to optimize their protein status; however, the issue remains unresolved.[25] Protein is important to help minimize

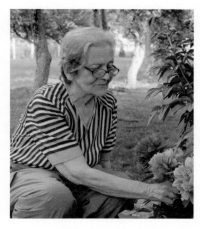

Older adults have lower total energy requirements as a result of several factors, including a less physically active lifestyle.

MyPlate for Older Adults

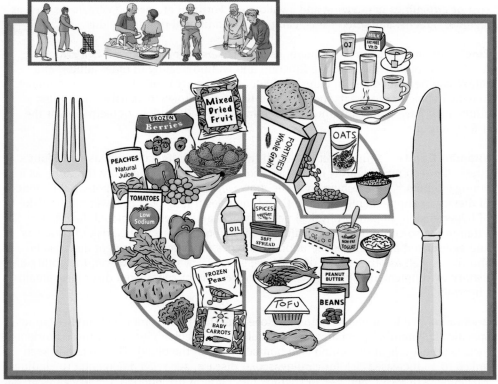

FIGURE 15.6   The Tufts University MyPlate for Older Adults illustrates healthful food and fluid choices appropriate for older adults.
Source: Tufts University School of Nutrition.

the loss of muscle and lean tissue, optimize healing after injury or disease, maintain immunity, and help prevent excessive bone loss. Many protein-rich foods are also important sources of the vitamins and minerals that are typically low in the diets of older adults; thus, protein is an important nutrient for this age group.

Micronutrient Recommendations for Older Adults

The vitamins and minerals of particular concern for older adults are identified in Table 15.3.

Calcium and Vitamin D   Preventing or minimizing the consequences of osteoporosis is a top priority for older adults. The RDA for calcium is higher for all adults over the age of 70 years and for women aged 51 to 70 years compared to younger adults.[4] The calcium requirement increases at an earlier age for women compared to men due to the earlier onset of bone loss, typically at the onset of menopause, in women compared to men.

Older adults living in long-term care facilities are at risk for vitamin D deficiency because they may not be exposed to amounts of sunlight adequate for vitamin D synthesis in the skin. Even among older adults leading active lives, the use of sunscreen may block the sunlight needed for vitamin D synthesis. It is critical, therefore, that older adults consume foods that are high in calcium and vitamin D and, when needed, use supplements in appropriate amounts and under the guidance of a healthcare provider. Recent research suggests that the elderly experience a reduced risk for fracture only when the intake of vitamin D falls between 800 and 1,000 IU/day.[26]

Iron   Iron needs decrease with aging. This decrease is primarily due to reduced muscle and lean tissue in both men and women and the cessation of menstruation in women. The decreased need for iron in older men is not significant enough to change the recommendations for iron intake in this group; thus, the RDA for iron is the same for older and younger men, 8 mg/day. However, the RDA for iron for older women is 8 mg/day, which is 10 mg/day lower than the RDA for younger women.[5] Heme iron from meat, fish, and poultry represents the most available source of dietary iron; however, some older adults reduce their intake of these foods because of cost or difficulties in chewing and swallowing. Fortified grains and cereals, as well as legumes, greens, and dried fruits, can provide additional iron in the diet.

Zinc   Although zinc recommendations are the same for all adults, it is a critical nutrient for optimizing immune function and wound healing in older adults. Zinc intake can be inadequate in older adults for the same reasons that heme iron intake may be deficient: red meats, poultry, and fish are relatively expensive, and older adults may have a difficult time chewing meats because of loss of teeth and/or the use of dentures.

Vitamins C and E   Although it is thought that older adults have increased oxidative stress, the recommendations for the antioxidant vitamins C and E are the same as for younger adults.[27] Researchers continue, however, to investigate the potential benefits of dietary or supplemental vitamin C and the roles it may play in lowering the risk of hypertension, impaired physical performance, and other age-related disorders.[28,29] Vitamin E also continues to be evaluated for its potential to reduce risk of cataracts and age-related macular degeneration, two types of vision impairment discussed shortly, as well as other forms of oxidative stress.[30,31] Overall, however, the ability of dietary or supplemental vitamin C or E to lower risk of age-related disorders remains uncertain.[32]

B-vitamins   Older adults need to pay close attention to their intake of the B-vitamins—specifically, vitamin B_{12}, vitamin B_6, and folate.[33] Inadequate intakes of these nutrients increase the levels of the amino acid homocysteine in the blood. This state has been linked to an increased risk for cardiovascular disease, age-related dementia (including Alzheimer's disease), and loss of cognitive function in the elderly.[34]

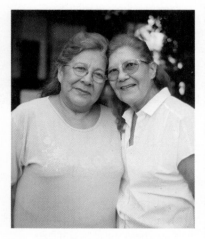

Older adults have unique nutritional needs.

HOT TOPIC

Senior Supplements: A Marketing Ploy?

Are the so-called silver supplements really better for seniors than ordinary formulations? Only minor differences exist between most standard and silver products. Let's take a look.

Iron is omitted from the silver supplement, reducing a senior's increased risk for iron overload. Vitamin K is reduced because many seniors take prescription anti-clotting medications. Less vitamin K therefore reduces the risk for a negative drug–nutrient interaction.

Silver supplements provide 40 mg more calcium than standard versions, which helps supply a little more of the additional 200 mg of calcium that older adults need. Vitamins E and B_6 are also increased. The DRI for vitamin E does not change with age; however, increased oxidative stress and age-associated eye disorders explain the modest increase in the silver version. The increase in vitamin B_6 may help lower serum homocysteine.

The silver supplement also provides four times more vitamin B_{12}. Why? Many adults over age 50 malabsorb vitamin B_{12} from foods so it is better absorbed in a supplement.

Seniors should evaluate the potential benefits of silver supplements. The bottom line is, their differences can be small but appropriate.

The RDA for both folate and vitamin B_{12} is the same for younger and older adults, but up to 30% of older adults cannot absorb enough vitamin B_{12} from foods because of reduced production of gastric juice. It is recommended that older adults consume supplements or foods that are fortified with vitamin B_{12} because the vitamin B_{12} in these products is absorbed more readily. Vitamin B_{12} is also available via injection. Vitamin B_6 recommendations are slightly higher for adults age 51 and older because these higher levels appear necessary to reduce homocysteine levels and optimize cognitive function in this population.[35]

Vitamin A   Vitamin A requirements are the same for adults of all ages; however, older adults should be careful not to consume more than the RDA because the absorption of vitamin A is actually greater in older adults. Thus, this group is at greater risk for vitamin A toxicity, which can cause liver damage and neurologic problems. In addition, high intakes of vitamin A by older adults have been linked increased risk for hip fractures.[5] Although older adults should avoid high dietary vitamin A and high-potency vitamin A supplements, consuming fruits and vegetables high in beta-carotene or other carotenoids is safe and does not lead to vitamin A toxicity.

Supplementation   A variety of factors may limit an older adult's ability to eat healthfully. These include limited financial resources, reduced appetite, social isolation, an inability to prepare foods, and illnesses and physiologic changes that limit the absorption and metabolism of many nutrients. Thus, some older adults may benefit from taking a multivitamin and mineral supplement that contains no more than the RDA for all the nutrients contained in the supplement. Additional supplementation may be necessary for nutrients such as calcium, vitamin D, and vitamin B_{12}. However, supplementation with individual nutrients should be done only under the supervision of the individual's primary healthcare provider because the risk of nutrient toxicity is high in this population. For a closer look at supplements marketed specifically for seniors, see the nearby Hot Topic.

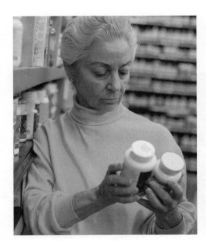

Many supplements are targeted at the elderly.

Fluid Recommendations for Older Adults

The AI for fluid is the same for older and younger adults.[6] Men should consume 3.7 liters of total water per day, which includes 3.0 liters (about 13 cups) as beverages, including drinking water. Women should consume 2.7 liters of total water per day, which includes 2.2 liters (about 9 cups) as beverages. Kidney function changes with age, and the thirst mechanism of older people can be impaired. These changes can result in chronic dehydration and hypernatremia (elevated blood sodium levels)

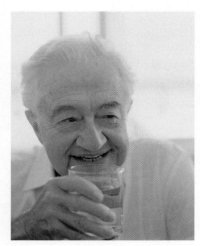

Older adults need the same amount of fluids as other adults.

in this population. Some older adults intentionally limit their beverage intake because they have urinary incontinence or don't want to be awakened for nighttime urination. This practice can endanger their health, so it is important for them to seek treatment for the incontinence and continue to drink plenty of fluids.

recap Older adults have lower energy needs as a result of their loss of lean tissue and lower physical activity levels. They should consume 20–35% of total energy as fat and 45–65% of their energy as carbohydrate. Protein recommendations are the same as for younger adults. The micronutrients of concern are calcium, vitamin D, iron, zinc, vitamin B_{12}, vitamin B_6, and folate. Supplementation may be necessary. Older adults are at risk for chronic dehydration. Men need to drink about 13 cups of water and other beverages per day, and women need about 9 cups.

Nutrition-Related Concerns for Older Adults

Older adults have a number of unique nutritional concerns. In addition to overweight and underweight, they commonly face dental problems, eye disorders, and potential interactions between nutrients and medications. Also, some older adults face financial difficulties that affect their nutritional choices. Each of these concerns is discussed briefly in the following sections.

Obesity and Underweight

In the United States, nearly 41% of adults between the ages of 65 and 74 are obese, while the incidence drops to just below 28% for those 75 years and older.[22] The elderly population as a whole has a high risk for heart disease, hypertension, type 2 diabetes, and cancer, and these diseases are more prevalent in older adults who are obese. Obesity also increases the severity and consequences of osteoarthritis, limits mobility, and is associated with functional declines in daily activities.

Underweight is also risky for older adults; mortality rates are actually higher in the underweight elderly than in the overweight elderly.[36] Significantly underweight older adults have fewer protein reserves to call upon during periods of catabolic stress, such as post-surgery or trauma, and are more susceptible to infection. Inappropriate weight loss suggests inadequate energy intake, which also implies inadequate nutrient intake. Chronic deficiencies of protein, vitamins, and minerals leave older adults at risk for poor wound healing and a depressed immune response.

Gerontologists have identified "nine Ds" that account for most cases of geriatric weight loss (**FIGURE 15.7**). Several of these factors promote weight loss by reducing energy intake, others by increasing energy expenditure or loss of nutrients. A condition known as *geriatric failure-to-thrive*—also called "the dwindles"—illustrates the complexity of inappropriate age-related weight loss and related health issues.

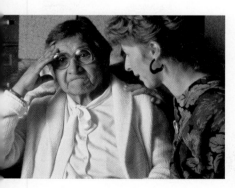

Dementia in older adults is one factor that can affect weight loss and overall nutritional status.

Dental Health Issues

Diet plays an important role in the maintenance of dental health in the elderly.[37] Deficiencies of the B-vitamins can lead to irritation, inflammation, and cracking of the lips and tongue, whereas vitamin C deficiency increases the risk for periodontal (gum) disease. A lack of adequate calcium, vitamin D, and protein contributes to bone loss in the oral cavity, which increases risk for tooth loss. Saliva helps neutralize the decay-promoting acids produced by oral bacteria; however, with aging, saliva production decreases.

Despite great advances in dental health, older adults remain at high risk of losing some or all of their teeth, suffering from gum disease, or having poorly fitting dentures, which cause considerable mouth pain and make chewing difficult. Adults with poorly fitted dentures or chewing problems tend to avoid meats and firm fruits and vegetables, leading to nutrient deficiencies. Older adults can compensate for a loss of chewing ability by selecting soft, protein-rich foods, such as eggs, peanut butter, cheese, yogurt, ground meat, fish, and well-cooked legumes. Red meats and poultry can be stewed or cooked in liquid for a long period. Oatmeal and other whole-grain cooked cereals can provide needed fiber, as do mashed berries and bananas, ripened melons, and canned vegetables. Shredded and minced raw vegetables can be

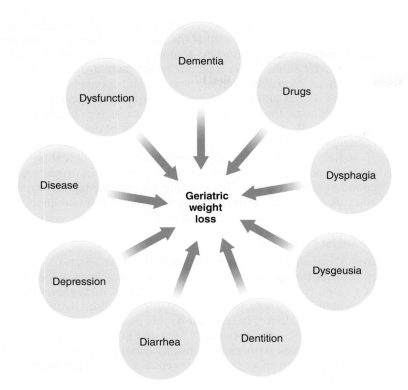

◀ **FIGURE 15.7** The nine Ds of geriatric weight loss. These are among the most significant factors contributing to inappropriate weight loss in the elderly.

added to dishes. With planning, older adults with oral health problems can maintain a varied, healthful diet.

Age-Related Eye Diseases

Two age-related eye disorders are responsible for vision impairment and blindness in older adults. *Macular degeneration* is damage to the macula, a portion of the retina of the eye (**FIGURE 15.8A**). Impacting more than 1.75 million U.S. adults, it is the leading cause of blindness in the elderly. A *cataract* is a cloudiness in the lens of the eye (Figure 15.8b). This condition affects 20% of adults in their sixties and almost 70% of those in their eighties. Although these are different conditions, sunlight exposure and smoking are lifestyle practices that increase the risk for both.

Recent research suggests, but does not prove, that dietary choices may slow the progress of these two degenerative eye diseases, saving millions of dollars and preventing or delaying the functional losses associated with impaired vision. Several studies have shown the beneficial effects of antioxidants, including vitamins C and E, on cataract formation, whereas others have reported no significant benefit.[32] Two phytochemicals, lutein and zeaxanthin, have also been identified as protective by some, but not all, studies.[38] These four antioxidants, as well as zinc, may also provide protection against macular degeneration. Although the research is not yet conclusive, older adults can benefit by consuming foods rich in these nutrients, primarily colorful fruits and vegetables, nuts, and whole grains. Vision-enhancing nutrient supplements remain an unproved therapy.

Interactions Between Medications and Nutrition

Although persons 65 years of age and above account for only 13% of the U.S. population, they are prescribed about 35% of all medications, and they experience almost 40% of all adverse drug effects, in part because of **polypharmacy**, or the use of five or more prescription drugs at any given time.[39] A small but significant number of older adults use ten or more medications, a practice known as *excessive polypharmacy*.[40] The more medications older adults take, the more likely they are to experience adverse effects from the medications' interactions, including toxicity. It should come as no surprise then that older adults make more than 175,000 emergency department

polypharmacy The use of five or more prescription drugs at any one time.

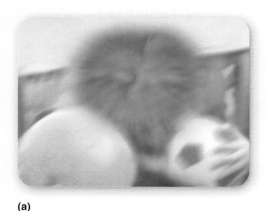

(a)

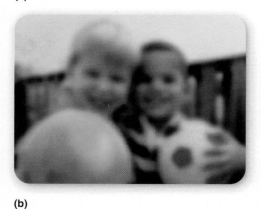

(b)

⬥ **FIGURE 15.8** These photos simulate two forms of vision loss common in older adults. **(a)** Macular degeneration results in a loss of central vision. **(b)** Cataracts impair vision across the visual field.

visits annually for medication-related problems.[39] Medications can interact not only with each other but also with herbs and other dietary supplements. A survey from the National Institutes of Health found that 75% of older adults use at least one prescription drug plus one dietary supplement. Moreover, both medications and supplements can alter food intake as well as nutrient digestion, absorption, or excretion—for example, by reducing the metabolism of nutrients such as vitamin D, folate, and vitamin B_6. **TABLE 15.4** summarizes some of the more common drug–nutrient interactions.

Individual foods such as grapefruit juice, spinach, and aged cheese are also known to react negatively with a number of drugs.[41] A compound in grapefruit juice, for example, inhibits the breakdown of as many as 85 different drugs, leading to as much as a tenfold increase in blood drug levels and potential overdose.[42]

Financial Problems

Over 8% of elderly men and women in the United States, or 4 million adults over the age of 60 years, experience some form of food insecurity. At greatest risk are African American, Hispanic, and other minorities; those living in the southern United States; and those living with one or more grandchildren.[43] In response to this problem, the federal government has developed a network of food and nutrition services for older Americans. These services are typically coordinated with state and local governments as well as nonprofit or community organizations. They include the following:

- **Supplemental Nutrition Assistance Program (SNAP):** Previously known as the Food Stamp program, this USDA program provides food assistance for low-income households. It is designed to meet the basic nutritional needs of eligible people of all ages. Participants are provided with a monthly allotment, typically in the form of a prepaid debit card or food coupons. Food insecure seniors participating in SNAP are less likely to suffer from depression compared to nonparticipants. Unfortunately, older Americans who are eligible for SNAP are far less likely to participate compared to younger groups.[44]

- **Child and Adult Care Program:** This program provides healthy meals and snacks to 120,000 older and functionally impaired adults in qualified adult day-care settings.

TABLE 15.4 **Examples of Common Drug–Nutrient Interactions**

Category of Drug	Interactions
Antacids	May decrease the absorption of iron, calcium, folate, vitamin B_{12}
Antibiotics	May reduce the absorption of calcium, fat-soluble vitamins; reduces the production of vitamin K by gut bacteria
Anticonvulsants	Interfere with activation of vitamin D
Anticoagulants ("blood thinners")	Reduce the activity of vitamin K
Antidepressants	May cause weight gain as a result of increased appetite
Antiretroviral agents (used in treatment of HIV/AIDS)	Reduce absorption of most nutrients
Aspirin	Lowers blood folate levels; increases iron loss due to gastrointestinal bleeding
Diuretics	May increase urinary excretion of potassium, sodium, calcium, magnesium; may cause retention of potassium, other electrolytes
Laxatives	Increase fecal excretion of dietary fat, fat-soluble vitamins, calcium, and other minerals

- **Commodity Supplemental Food Program:** This program targets low-income pregnant women, infants and young children, and adults 60 years and older. Nearly 600,000 elderly participate in this program. Income guidelines must be met. Specific commodity foods are distributed, including cereals, peanut butter, dry beans, rice or pasta, and canned juice, fruits, vegetables, meat, poultry, and tuna. This program is not intended to provide a complete array of foods but distributes specific foods rich in nutrients typically lacking in the diets of targeted populations.
- **Senior Farmers' Market Nutrition Program:** This program, sponsored by the USDA, provides coupons to 865,000 low-income seniors, so that they can buy eligible foods at farmers' markets and roadside stands. Seniors enjoy the nutritional benefits of fresh local produce and the opportunity to increase the variety of their meals.
- **Nutrition Services Incentive Program:** The Department of Health and Human Services provides funds and USDA commodity foods to state agencies for meals for senior citizens. There are no income criteria; any person 60 years or older (plus his or her spouse, even if younger) can take part. Meals, designed to provide one-third of the RDA for key nutrients, are served at senior centers and similar locations in the community and can be delivered to qualified homebound elders. Although the meals are free, participants are encouraged to contribute what they can to cover the cost of each meal. Participation in the Nutrition Services Incentive Program improves the nutrient intakes of older adults; however, the program may have a long waiting list and be unable to meet the current demand in the community.

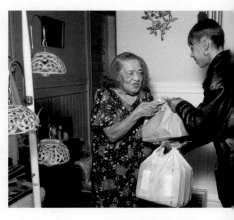

For many homebound, disabled, and older adults, community programs that supply food and other assistance are lifelines that provide nourishing meals as well as vital social contact.

recap Overweight and obesity are important concerns for older adults because they increase the risk for chronic diseases. Underweight is also a concern because it can lead to increased illness and injury. Older adults may lose their sense of smell and taste, and dental and vision problems can limit their intake of meats, fruits, and vegetables, leading to nutrient deficiencies. Medications and certain nutrients can have adverse interactions. Several government and community programs are available for older adults in need of food assistance.

*behavior change ... getting started!

Now that you've read this chapter, try making these changes:

For yourself:

- The changes in body composition and function associated with aging are at least partly within your control. For instance, some of the decrease in muscle and bone mass and strength are due to lack of physical activity. So to age well, eat a nutritious diet and get plenty of regular physical activity throughout life—starting right now!
- If you smoke, get the help you need to stop. Smoking directly causes cancer and contributes to many other diseases. Plus it reduces life expectancy by more than a dozen years.

For your community:

- Host a fundraising party and donate the proceeds to a food bank or your local chapter of Meals on Wheels.
- Volunteer to help kids, teens or older adults get the physical activity they need to maintain fitness and a healthy weight. Depending on your area of expertise, you might offer to coach an after-school cross-country team, or offer a free dance class at the local senior center.

Physical Activity in Older Adulthood: Should Seniors "Go for the Gold"?

Participation in vigorous physical activity is uncommon among older adults. Fewer than 14% of the "young elderly" (65–74 years) and only 7% of the "older elderly" (75 years and above) report participating in a regular program of vigorous exercise.[45]

We know that physically active elders live longer and enjoy better health. A regular program of physical activity lowers the risk for heart disease, hypertension, type 2 diabetes, obesity, depression, and cognitive decline or dementia. The complications of arthritis can also be reduced with appropriate exercise, as can the risk for falls and bone fractures. The need for healthcare visits, diagnostic tests, medication, and other treatments to control blood glucose, serum cholesterol, blood pressure, and other factors in chronic illness can be reduced or eliminated with regular exercise.[46]

How much physical activity do older adults need in order to achieve these health benefits—and does moderate activity count, or should seniors "go for the gold"? Here are the most recent CDC guidelines:[47]

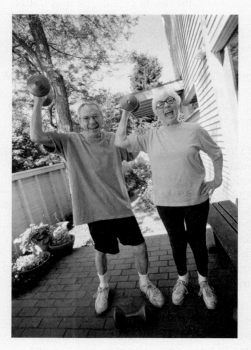

- Aerobic activity: Seniors should engage in a minimum of 150 minutes of moderate-intensity aerobic activity (brisk walking, bicycling, swimming) or 75 minutes of vigorous aerobic activity (running or jogging) every week.
- Muscle strengthening: Seniors should engage in muscle-strengthening activities, such as resistance or strength training, on 2 or more days a week. These activities should work all the major muscle groups. Free weights, weight machines, resistance bands, push-ups, and heavy physical work (digging, shoveling) all contribute to muscle strengthening. Older adults can gain even greater health benefits by increasing their aerobic exercise to either 300 minutes of moderate-intensity or 150 minutes of vigorous activity each week.
- Flexibility and balance: Seniors should do a few minutes of flexibility and balance exercises, such as stretches, tai chi, Pilates, or yoga, most days of the week. Daily balance exercises are also important to reduce the risk for falls as we age. In addition to tai chi, toe raises, side leg raises, and rear leg swings are examples of effective balance activities.

Are older adults more susceptible to injury or harm from vigorous exercise? A review of exercise-related sudden cardiac death in adults concluded that vigorous activity can, in fact, increase the risk for heart attack and/or sudden cardiac death in susceptible persons.[48] But who qualifies as susceptible? At greatest risk are people who perform activities at an intensity or a duration they are not used to. Think of the "weekend warrior": a person who is very sedentary most days of the week but goes "all out" on a Saturday afternoon. This person is at high risk for a heart attack or sudden cardiac death during or shortly after vigorous activity. A second vulnerable group includes older adults with diagnosed or undiagnosed heart disease. Seniors may also be more vulnerable to dehydration, heat stress, fractures, falls, knee pain, and muscle soreness or stiffness with intense exercise.[48]

To minimize the risk for exercise-related cardiac events and other complications of vigorous exercise, older adults should follow these guidelines:

- Work with a qualified healthcare provider to determine the optimal types, intensities, and duration of physical activities appropriate for them.
- Become familiar with the signs of cardiac impairment: shortness of breath, chest pain, neck pain, dizziness or palpitations, and unusual fatigue. Recognize the need to modify activity patterns under conditions of stress, such as very cold temperatures, high heat or humidity, or during recovery from an illness.
- Exercise in rooms with appropriate temperature, ventilation, and lighting; wear appropriate clothing and comfortable shoes; and have water readily available.
- Engage in supervised warm-up and cool-down activities.

For most older adults, the potential risks of vigorous physical activity are almost always outweighed by the benefits—better health, more independence, less disability, and a longer, happier life!

CRITICAL THINKING QUESTIONS

1. What approaches might you use to encourage an older adult to start a regular program of physical activity after a lifetime of mostly sedentary behavior? What incentives or advantages could you offer him or her?
2. If you were the manager of a fitness center popular with young adults, what modifications to the facility might you propose to make it more attractive to older adults? Do you think one fitness center can effectively serve both young and older adults? Why or why not?
3. What barriers to physical activity do older adults face as compared to younger adults? How might communities increase exercise opportunities for the elderly?

chapter **review**

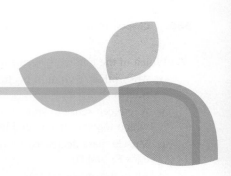

test yourself | answers

1. **False.** Toddlers may need ten or more exposures to a specific food before accepting it.
2. **False.** Adolescents experience an average 20–25% increase in height during puberty.
3. **True.** Although a reduction in muscle mass and lean tissue is inevitable with aging, some of this loss can be attenuated with regular physical activity.

MasteringNutrition™

Check out these additional resources in the MasteringNutrition Study Area at www.masteringhealthandnutrition.pearson.com:

- Read It: Chapter Summary and RSS Feeds
- See It: ABC News videos and nutrition animations
- Hear It: MP3s
- Study It: Get Ready for Nutrition Math and Chemistry review
- Do It: NutriTools and "Find the Quack" feature
- Review It: Quizzes, flashcards, and glossary

review questions

1. Which of the following breakfasts would be most appropriate to serve a 20-month-old child?

   a. 1/2 cup of iron-fortified cooked oat cereal, 2 tbsp. of mashed pineapple, and 1 cup of whole milk

   b. 2 tbsp. of nonfat yogurt, 2 tbsp. of applesauce, one slice of melba toast spread with strawberry preserves, and 1 cup of calcium-fortified orange juice

   c. 1/2 cup of iron-fortified cooked oat cereal, 1/4 cup of cubed pineapple, and 1 cup of low-fat milk

   d. two small link sausages cut in 1-inch pieces, 2 tbsp. of scrambled egg, one slice of whole-wheat toast, four cherry tomatoes, 2 tbsp. of applesauce, and 1 cup of whole milk

2. Which of the following is most likely to be deficient in the diet of a vegetarian toddler?

   a. carbohydrate and fat
   b. vitamin C
   c. iron and zinc
   d. fiber

3. Carbohydrate should make up what percentage of total energy for school-age children?

   a. 25–40%
   b. 35–50%
   c. 45–65%
   d. 65–85%

4. An adolescent continues to grow in height until

   a. production of testosterone and estrogen ceases.
   b. the epiphyseal plates close.
   c. peak bone density is reached.
   d. approximately age 13 in girls and age 16 in boys.

5. The RDA for calcium increases to 1,300 mg for which of the following age groups?

   a. both boys and girls, beginning at age 4
   b. girls only, beginning at age 9
   c. both boys and girls, beginning at age 9
   d. girls only, beginning at age 14

6. Which of the following statements about pediatric obesity is true?

   a. The prevalence of obesity among U.S children and adolescents increased by nearly 5% between 2007 and 2012.
   b. To control energy intake, parents should encourage obese children to skip breakfast.
   c. Among adolescents, cigarette smoking increases the risk for obesity.
   d. None of the above is true.

7. Which of the following events occurs with normal aging?

    a. Absorption of vitamin B_{12} from the gastrointestinal tract is reduced.

    b. A reduced sense of smell contributes to dysphagia, which together make food less appealing.

    c. Muscle mass decreases an average of 5–10% between ages 35 and 70.

    d. All of the above are true.

8. Among older adults

    a. cataracts are the most common cause of blindness.

    b. northerners living alone have the highest rate of food insecurity.

    c. 75% use five or more prescription drugs at any given time.

    d. the prevalence of obesity declines after age 75.

9. True or false? The food choice patterns of children are heavily influenced by circumstances at school.

10. True or false? Mortality rates are higher in the underweight elderly than in the overweight elderly.

math review

11. While helping her 72-year-old grandmother put away groceries, Kristina notices three new supplement bottles. One is a single-nutrient vitamin A supplement, which provides 3,333 µg/dose. The second is a "Healthy Skin Formula" providing 1,500 µg vitamin A/dose. The third is a multivitamin-mineral supplement that provides 2,200 µg vitamin A/dose. When Kristina asks her grandmother about these new products, her grandmother explains that she read online that vitamin A makes your skin look younger, so she was taking the three supplements every day to make her wrinkles go away faster! If Kristina's grandmother takes one dose of each of the three supplements per day, what percentage of the RDA does she consume? Of the UL? Do you see any potential problems with this level of vitamin A intake?

Answers to Review Questions and Math Review are located at the back of this text and in the MasteringNutrition Study Area.

web resources

www.cdc.gov
The Centers for Disease Control and Prevention

Click on Life Stages & Populations. Next, select topics such as Children, where you'll find milestones and growth charts; Adolescents & Teens, where you'll find a link to the BAM! Body and Mind site; or Older Adults & Seniors, which provides information and services on healthy aging.

www.kidsnutrition.org
USDA/ARS Children's Nutrition Research Center

This site provides information about current research projects, nutrition web links, and consumer and nutrition news.

www.keepkidshealthy.com
Keep Kids Healthy.com

Find information about nutrition and health for toddlers, children, and adolescents on this website.

www.vrg.org
The Vegetarian Resource Group

Learn more about vegetarianism for all ages. Included on the site are sections for teens and kids as well as recipes and eating guides.

www.nichd.nih.gov
Milk Matters

This website provides practical tips and menus for children and adolescents. Enter "milk matters" into the home page search bar.

www.nutrition.wsu.edu
Eat Better, Eat Together

This website offers educational materials for strengthening family meal time. Suggestions for community events, media interviews, and educational materials are available. Enter "eat better" into the search bar to get underway.

www.fns.usda.gov
USDA Food & Nutrition Service

Read about government programs to provide food to people of all ages, including school meals programs, the Child and Adult Care Food program, and the WIC program.

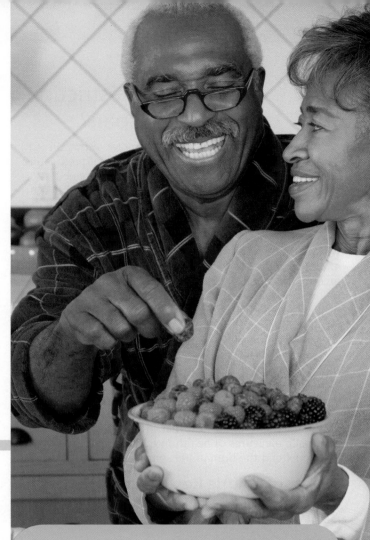

in depth 15.5

Searching for the Fountain of Youth

How old do you want to live to be—80 years, 90, 100? Worldwide, throughout human history, legends have told of a "fountain of youth" that reverses decades of aging in anyone who drinks its waters. Of course no one believes such tales any longer, but pick up a fashion or fitness magazine and you're likely to find modern equivalents: anti-aging diets, supplements, cosmetics, spa treatments, and other therapies. For instance, if you were to read that you could live to celebrate your 100th birthday in good health by eating about a quarter less than the average energy intake for your gender and height, would you do it? Or would you assume that this is just a fairy tale, too? Believe it or not, a growing number of people are drastically cutting their Calorie intake in an effort to extend both their youthfulness and their longevity. Is this effective? What other actions can you take right now to live longer in good health? Let's find out.

learning objectives

After studying this In Depth, you should be able to:

1 Discuss the evidence linking Calorie restriction to life span, pp. 588–589.

2 Refute the claim that single-nutrient, herbal, and other dietary supplements increase longevity, pp. 589–590.

3 Evaluate the potential of your current health-related behaviors to increase or reduce the likelihood of your living a long and healthy life, p. 590.

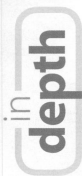
Does calorie restriction increase life span?

A practice known as *Calorie restriction* (CR) has been getting a great deal of press lately. Although researchers haven't defined a precise number of Calories, or level of nutrients, that qualify as a Calorie-restricted diet, the practice typically involves eating fewer Calories than your body needs to maintain your normal weight while still getting enough vitamins and other nutrients to keep your body functioning in good health. In general—allowing for differences in how many Calories people are consuming prior to CR, as well as their gender, age, body composition, level of activity, and so forth—CR may call for a person to consume 20–30% fewer Calories than usual.[1]

Research has shown that CR can significantly extend the life span of rats, mice, fish, flies, and yeast cells as well as non-human primates such as monkeys.[2] But only in the past few years have researchers begun to design and conduct studies of CR in humans. The results of these preliminary studies suggest that CR can also improve metabolic measures of health in humans and thus may be able to extend the human life span.[3]

Effects of Calorie Restriction

How might CR prolong life span? The answer to this question is not fully understood, but it is thought that

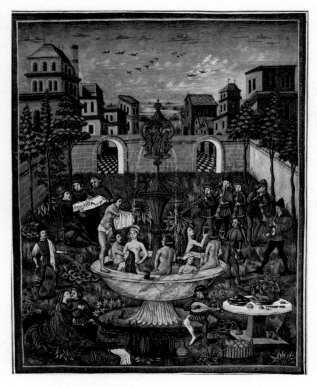

We may no longer believe in an actual "fountain of youth," but our search for health and longevity continues today.

the reduction in metabolic rate that occurs with restricting energy intake results in a much lower production of free radicals, which in turn reduces oxidative damage to DNA, cell membranes, and other cell structures, possibly lowering chronic disease risk and prolonging life. Calorie restriction also improves cells' sensitivity to insulin and prompts other hormonal changes that can lower the risk of chronic diseases such as heart disease, stroke, and diabetes. There is also evidence that CR can alter gene expression in ways that reduce the effects of aging and lower the risk of cancer and other diseases. Some of the metabolic effects of CR reported in several, but not all, human studies include:[1,3,4,5]

- Decreased fat mass and lean body mass
- Decreased blood glucose levels
- Decreased serum low-density lipoprotein (LDL) and total cholesterol; increased serum high-density lipoprotein (HDL) cholesterol
- Decreased core body temperature and blood pressure
- Decreased energy expenditure beyond that expected for the weight loss that occurred, which suggests a generalized slowing of metabolic rate
- Decreased oxidative stress
- Reduced levels of DNA damage
- Lower levels of chronic inflammation
- Protective changes in various hormone levels

It is important to emphasize that, in laboratory studies, species found to live longer with CR are fed highly nutritious diets. Situations such as starvation, anorexia nervosa, and extreme fad dieting, in which both energy and nutrient intakes are severely restricted, do not result in prolonged life but are associated with an increased risk for premature death. It's also essential to understand that the benefits of CR are thought to correlate to the age at which the program begins. The later in life the CR protocol is started, the lower the expected benefit. For example, if a person did not start CR until the age of 55 years, he or she would be expected to gain only 4 months of extended life![3]

Challenges of Calorie Restriction

Although the benefits listed previously appear promising, the research data supporting these benefits in humans are only preliminary. Research that can precisely study CR in humans might never be conducted because of logistical and ethical concerns. For instance, most people find it challenging to follow a Calorie-restricted diet for just a few months; compliance with this type of diet for a decades-long study could be almost impossible. There are also ethical concerns about the potential malnutrition that could occur.

In the absence of high-quality human studies, several CR groups, including the "CRONies" (Caloric Restriction with Optimal Nutrition), have provided researchers with some data. Most of the CRONies are males in their late thirties to mid-fifties. One report indicated that most CRONies had followed the CR diet for about 10 years and reduced their caloric intake by about 30%. Overall, members report improved blood lipids and the other health benefits listed earlier. Still, researchers lack specific data on how well free-living adults actually follow the rigid and extensive demands of CR protocols.

You may be wondering how much less energy *you* would have to consume to meet the definition of Calorie restriction—and when you'd have to begin. It has been estimated that humans would need to restrict their typical energy intake by at least 20% for 40 years or more in order to gain an additional 4 to 5 years of healthy living. If you normally eat about 2,000 kcal/day, a 20% reduction would result in an energy intake of about 1,600 kcal per day. Although this might not seem excessive, it would be very difficult to maintain it every day for 40 years.

Also keep in mind the requirement that your diet must be of very high nutritional quality. This presents a huge number of challenges, including meticulous planning of meals, limited options for eating meals outside of your home, and the challenge of working the demands of your special diet around the eating behaviors of family members and friends.

Also, those who follow the CR program report several side effects. The top three complaints are constant hunger, frequently feeling cold, and a loss of libido (sex drive).[3] Moreover, the long-term effects of the diet are not known. There is concern that, if initiated in early adulthood, CR might reduce bone density or lead to inappropriate loss of muscle mass. And because the production of female reproductive hormones is linked to a certain level of body fat, CR could impair a woman's fertility. Interestingly, as noted earlier, most of the members of the CRONies are males. Finally, it is well known that being significantly underweight is associated with increased mortality, especially among older adults.

Alternatives to Calorie Restriction

An interesting alternative to caloric restriction is the practice of *intermittent fasting* (*IF*), also known as every-other-day-feeding (EODF) or alternate-day fasting (ADF).[6,7,8] This approach, which does *not* reduce average energy intake but simply alters the pattern of food intake, has also been shown, in animals, to prolong life span and improve a range of metabolic measures of health. Although not as well studied as CR, IF has produced beneficial changes in insulin and glucose status, blood lipid levels, and blood pressure in humans in at least some studies.

Additionally, some researchers have proposed that limiting total protein, which is much easier to implement than extreme caloric restriction, may limit the onset of cancer and aging. Surveys indicate that Americans eat 15–17% of their total daily energy intake as protein, so limiting total protein might mean consuming a diet with 10% of energy

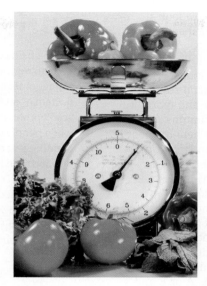

On a Calorie-restricted diet, all food must be highly nutritious, and both nutrients and energy must be calculated precisely.

intake from protein, which is still within the AMDR for protein intake.

Finally, other research suggests that exercise-induced leanness may slow the aging process without the need for caloric restriction.[9] That is, it may not be the energy intake per se that extends life span but the overall energy balance a person maintains. A person would not have to strictly limit energy intake as long as his or her energy expenditure was high enough to maintain a lean body profile.

Can supplements slow aging?

Recently, some researchers have speculated that consuming the optimum level of nutrients could extend a person's healthy life span. Could micronutrient supplements take the place of whole foods in providing this "optimum level of nutrients"? And could other ingredients, besides vitamins and minerals, also slow aging?

The anti-aging market accounts for nearly $100 billion in sales, with individuals spending as much as $20,000 a year on various treatments. Among the most popular are "anti-aging" or "age-management" supplements. Some of these supplements provide specific vitamins and minerals, whereas others provide exotic "metabolites," "glandular extracts," or "food concentrates." Many of these products are heavily marketed and, as just noted, can be very expensive. Are they

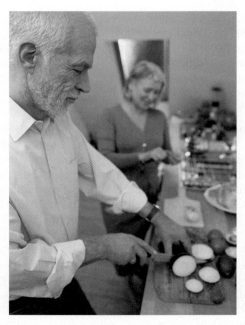

Maintaining an energy-restricted diet that is also highly nutritious requires significant meal planning and preparation.

worth the investment? Let's take a look at some of the research into supplements promoted for longevity.

Many well-designed, carefully conducted research studies have looked at the effects of vitamin and/or mineral supplements on chronic disease risk and mortality rates. Antioxidants such as vitamins A, E, and C and the phytochemical beta-carotene have gotten the most attention.[10,11,12] Unfortunately, not even one trial of these nutrients (alone or in combination) has shown them to lower rates of death from heart disease or other causes. In fact, some of the studies actually reported a *higher* risk of death with high doses of vitamins A or E and beta-carotene supplements.[13] However, a quick search on your computer will open up a world of promises, all guaranteeing better health and longer life spans if you use the advertised supplements!

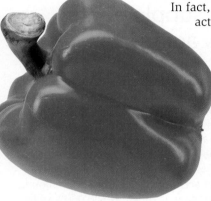

Anyone can benefit from the antioxidant nutrients in fresh fruits and vegetables.

Other supplements that claim to enhance longevity include products containing

- food extracts, such as resveratrol from red wines and other foods
- herbs, including Siberian ginseng, ginkgo biloba, and various combinations of botanicals from Asia
- animal extracts, such as royal jelly and dried glandulars
- hormone-based preparations, such as DHEA (dehydroepiandrosterone), HGH (human growth hormone), and melatonin
- metabolites, such as alpha lipoic acid

Manufacturers promote these products with claims such as "revered in the Far East for centuries" and "nature's own therapeutic powers." However, no well-designed research studies support the claims of life-extending effectiveness for any of these products in humans. Moreover, researchers have been unable to identify any plausible scientific explanation for why or how these supplements might increase longevity.

More disturbingly, like antioxidant supplements, many of these non-nutrient supplements have serious side effects. For example, ginkgo biloba can cause gastrointestinal upset, nausea, diarrhea, headache, dizziness, or an allergic reaction, and recent studies have found an increased risk of cancer in laboratory animals administered ginkgo.[14]

nutri-case | GUSTAVO

"I don't believe in taking pills. If you eat good food, you get everything you need and it's the way nature intended it. My daughter kept nagging my wife and me to start taking B vitamins and some kind of Chinese herb with a name I can't pronounce. She said we need this stuff because when people get to be our age they have problems with their nerves and circulation. I didn't fall for it, but my wife did, and then her doctor told her she needs calcium pills and vitamin D, too. The kitchen counter is starting to look like a medicine cabinet! Our ancestors never took pills their whole lives! So how come we need them? I think the whole thing is a hoax to get you to empty your wallet."

Would you support Gustavo's decision to avoid taking supplements? Given what you have learned in previous Nutri-Cases about Gustavo's wife, would you support or oppose her taking ginkgo biloba, B-vitamins, calcium, or vitamin D? Explain your choices.

HGH can contribute to high cholesterol levels, increase the risk of diabetes, and cause joint pain, muscle pain, and other symptoms.[15] DHEA may decrease HDL-cholesterol and increase risk for certain types of cancer. However, despite these concerns, sales of such supplements continue to grow.

QuickTips

Promoting Your Longevity

✓ Engage in at least 30 minutes of moderate physical activity most days of the week.

✓ Eat a diet based on the USDA Food Guide.

✓ Use only the nutrient supplements that have been recommended to you by your healthcare provider and within the recommended amounts.

✓ Maintain a healthful weight and body composition. Both underweight and overweight are associated with increased mortality.

✓ If you smoke or use any other form of tobacco, stop. If you don't smoke, don't start. On average, smokers die 13 to 14 years earlier than nonsmokers.

✓ If you drink alcohol, do so only in moderation, meaning no more than two drinks per day for men and one drink per day for women.

How Long Are You Likely to Live?

First, let's get one thing straight: no "longevity calculator," game, or quiz, no matter how complex or high-tech, can predict how long you'll live. That's not only because death from traumatic injury is unpredictable, but also because chronic diseases, as we've discussed throughout this text, are multifactorial, and we have a long way to go before we understand fully how all the factors interact to produce or prevent disease. That said, studies of large populations have demonstrably linked certain behaviors with an increased life span. These include regular physical activity, a nourishing diet, no tobacco use, and no excessive alcohol consumption. These factors are included in *all* longevity tools. In addition, most tools ask about other factors, such as drug abuse, stress, sleep quality and duration, seat belt use, and social support.

Want to learn more? If so, you'll find longevity games and quizzes on many websites. Here are two popular options:

The Longevity Game
www.northwesternmutual.com
Enter "longevity game" into the home page search box. This game was developed using the company's actuarial statistics tracking longevity for more than 150 years.

Living to 100
www.livingto100.com
This quiz, developed by Dr. Thomas Perls, has forty questions related to your family and health. It provides some brief feedback and a list of suggested lifestyle changes to improve your health.

Are your actions today promoting a longer, healthier life?

If none of these options interest you, is there anything else you can do to increase your chances of living a long and healthful life? The CDC reminds us that chronic disease is responsible for seven out of every ten deaths of Americans. Moreover, just four behaviors within your control are responsible for chronic disease:

- Lack of physical activity
- Poor nutrition
- Tobacco use
- Excessive consumption of alcohol

So if you want to live a longer, healthier life, the CDC advises that you adopt the health habits identified in the nearby **Quick Tips** box.

Maybe you're already engaging in these healthful behaviors but still wonder how long you're likely to live. If so, check out the **What About You?** feature for some fun longevity quizzes: your results might make you laugh, or put you on track to more healthful choices starting today!

MasteringNutrition™

Check out these additional resources in the MasteringNutrition Study Area:

- Read It: Chapter Summary and RSS Feeds
- See It: ABC News videos and nutrition animations
- Hear It: MP3s
- Study It: Get Ready for Nutrition Math and Chemistry review
- Do It: NutriTools and "Find the Quack" feature
- Review It: Quizzes, flashcards, and glossary

web resources

www.nia.nih.gov
The National Institute on Aging

The National Institute on Aging provides information about how older adults can benefit from physical activity and a good diet.

www.nihseniorhealth.gov
National Institutes of Health, Senior Health

This website, written in large print, offers up-to-date information on popular health topics for older Americans.

www.agingblueprint.org
American College of Sports Medicine, Active Aging Partnership

Get information for health professionals and the general public on The National Blueprint: Increasing Physical Activity Among Adults Age 50 and Older. Enter "partnership" into the home page search box.

www.aarp.org
The American Association of Retired Persons

Visit this gateway site for a wide range of articles on promoting physical activity in older adults. Enter "health fitness" into the search box to get started.

Appendices

appendix A

2010 Dietary Guidelines, Upper Intake Levels, and Dietary Reference Intakes

Dietary Guidelines for Americans, 2010

Key Recommendations for Each Area of the Guidelines:

Adequate Nutrients Within Calorie Needs

a. Consume a variety of nutrient-dense foods and beverages within and among the basic food groups while choosing foods that limit the intake of saturated and *trans* fats, cholesterol, added sugars, salt, and alcohol.

b. Meet recommended intakes by adopting a balanced eating pattern, such as the USDA Food Patterns or the DASH Eating Plan.

Weight Management

a. To maintain body weight in a healthy range, balance Calories from foods and beverages with Calories expended.

b. To prevent gradual weight gain over time, make small decreases in food and beverage Calories and increase physical activity.

Physical Activity

a. Engage in regular physical activity and reduce sedentary activities to promote health, psychological well-being, and a healthy body weight.

b. Achieve physical fitness by including cardiovascular conditioning, stretching exercises for flexibility, and resistance exercises or calisthenics for muscle strength and endurance.

Food Groups to Encourage

a. Consume a sufficient amount of fruits and vegetables while staying within energy needs. Two cups of fruit and 2-½ cups of vegetables per day are recommended for a reference 2,000-Calorie intake, with higher or lower amounts depending on the Calorie level.

b. Choose a variety of fruits and vegetables each day. In particular, select from all five vegetable subgroups (dark green, orange, legumes, starchy vegetables, and other vegetables) several times a week.

c. Consume 3 or more ounce-equivalents of whole-grain products per day, with the rest of the recommended grains coming from enriched or whole-grain products.

d. Consume 3 cups per day of fat-free or low-fat milk or equivalent milk products.

Fats

a. Consume less than 10% of Calories from saturated fatty acids and less than 300 mg/day of cholesterol, and keep *trans* fatty acid consumption as low as possible.

b. Keep total fat intake between 20% and 35% of Calories, with most fats coming from sources of polyunsaturated and monounsaturated fatty acids, such as fish, nuts, and vegetable oils.

c. Choose foods that are lean, low-fat, or fat-free, and limit intake of fats and oils high in saturated and/or *trans* fatty acids.

Carbohydrates

a. Choose fiber-rich fruits, vegetables, and whole grains often.

b. Choose and prepare foods and beverages with little added sugars or caloric sweeteners, such as amounts suggested by the USDA Food Patterns and the DASH Eating Plan.

c. Reduce the incidence of dental caries by practicing good oral hygiene and consuming sugar- and starch-containing foods and beverages less frequently.

Sodium and Potassium

a. Consume less than 2,300 mg (approximately 1 tsp. of salt) of sodium per day.

b. Consume potassium-rich foods, such as fruits and vegetables.

Alcoholic Beverages

a. Those who choose to drink alcoholic beverages should do so sensibly and in moderation—defined as the consumption of up to one drink per day for women and up to two drinks per day for men.

b. Alcoholic beverages should not be consumed by some individuals, including those who cannot restrict their alcohol intake, women of childbearing age who may become pregnant, pregnant and lactating women, children and adolescents, individuals taking medications that can interact with alcohol, and those with specific medical conditions.

c. Alcoholic beverages should be avoided by individuals engaging in activities that require attention, skill, or coordination, such as driving or operating machinery.

Food Safety

a. To avoid microbial foodborne illness, clean hands, food contact surfaces, and fruits and vegetables; separate raw, cooked, and ready-to-eat foods; cook foods to a safe temperature; and refrigerate perishable food promptly and defrost foods properly. Meat and poultry should not be washed or rinsed.

b. Avoid unpasteurized milk or products made from unpasteurized milk or juices, or raw or partially cooked eggs, meat, or poultry.

There are additional key recommendations for specific population groups. You can access all the Guidelines on the web at: www.health.gov.

Data from: U.S. Department of Agriculture and U.S. Department of Health and Human Services. 2010. Dietary Guidelines for Americans, 2010. 7th edn.

Tolerable Upper Intake Levels (UL[a])

Vitamins

Life-Stage Group	Vitamin A (µg/d)[b]	Vitamin C (mg/d)	Vitamin D (IU/d)	Vitamin E (mg/d)[c,d]	Niacin (mg/d)[d]	Vitamin B₆ (mg/d)	Folate (µg/d)[d]	Choline (g/d)
Infants								
0–6 mo	600	ND[e]	1,000	ND	ND	ND	ND	ND
7–12 mo	600	ND	1,500	ND	ND	ND	ND	ND
Children								
1–3 y	600	400	2,500	200	10	30	300	1.0
4–8 y	900	650	3,000	300	15	40	400	1.0
Males, Females								
9–13 y	1,700	1,200	4,000	600	20	60	600	2.0
14–18 y	2,800	1,800	4,000	800	30	80	800	3.0
19–70 y	3,000	2,000	4,000	1,000	35	100	1,000	3.5
≥70 y	3,000	2,000	4,000	1,000	35	100	1,000	3.5
Pregnancy								
≤18 y	2,800	1,800	4,000	800	30	80	800	3.0
19–50 y	3,000	2,000	4,000	1,000	35	100	1,000	3.5
Lactation								
≤18 y	2,800	1,800	4,000	800	30	80	800	3.0
19–50 y	3,000	2,000	4,000	1,000	35	100	1,000	3.5

Elements

Life-Stage Group	Boron (mg/d)	Calcium (mg/d)	Copper (µg/d)	Fluoride (mg/d)	Iodine (µg/d)	Iron (mg/d)	Magnesium (mg/d)[f]	Manganese (mg/d)	Molybdenum (µg/d)	Nickel (mg/d)	Phosphorus (g/d)	Selenium (µg/d)	Vanadium (mg/d)[g]	Zinc (mg/d)
Infants														
0–6 mo	ND	1,000	ND	0.7	ND	40	ND	ND	ND	ND	ND	45	ND	4
7–12 mo	ND	1,500	ND	0.9	ND	40	ND	ND	ND	ND	ND	60	ND	5
Children														
1–3 y	3	2,500	1,000	1.3	200	40	65	2	300	0.2	3	90	ND	7
4–8 y	6	2,500	3,000	2.2	300	40	110	3	600	0.3	3	150	ND	12
Males, Females														
9–13 y	11	3,000	5,000	10	600	40	350	6	1,100	0.6	4	280	ND	23
14–18 y	17	3,000	8,000	10	900	45	350	9	1,700	1.0	4	400	ND	34
19–50 y	20	2,500	10,000	10	1,100	45	350	11	2,000	1.0	4	400	1.8	40
51–70 y	20	2,000	10,000	10	1,100	45	350	11	2,000	1.0	4	400	1.8	40
≥70 y	20	2,000	10,000	10	1,100	45	350	11	2,000	1.0	3	400	1.8	40
Pregnancy														
≤18 y	17	3,000	8,000	10	900	45	350	9	1,700	1.0	3.5	400	ND	34
19–50 y	20	2,500	10,000	10	1,100	45	350	11	2,000	1.0	3.5	400	ND	40
Lactation														
≤18 y	17	3,000	8,000	10	900	45	350	9	1,700	1.0	4	400	ND	34
19–50 y	20	2,500	10,000	10	1,100	45	350	11	2,000	1.0	4	400	ND	40

[a] UL = The maximum level of daily nutrient intake that is likely to pose no risk of adverse effects. Unless otherwise specified, the UL represents total intake from food, water, and supplements. Due to lack of suitable data, ULs could not be established for vitamin K, thiamin, riboflavin, vitamin B₁₂, pantothenic acid, biotin, or carotenoids. In the absence of ULs, extra caution may be warranted in consuming levels above recommended intakes.

[b] As preformed vitamin A only.

[c] As α-tocopherol; applies to any form of supplemental α-tocopherol.

[d] The ULs for vitamin E, niacin, and folate apply to synthetic forms obtained from supplements, fortified foods, or a combination of the two.

[e] ND = Not determinable due to lack of data of adverse effects in this age group and concern with regard to lack of ability to handle excess amounts. Source of intake should be from food only to prevent high levels of intake.

[f] The ULs for magnesium represent intake from a pharmacological agent only and do not include intake from food and water.

[g] Although vanadium in food has not been shown to cause adverse effects in humans, there is no justification for adding vanadium to food, and vanadium supplements should be used with caution. The UL is based on adverse effects in laboratory animals, and this data could be used to set a UL for adults but not children and adolescents.

Data from the Dietary Reference Intakes series, National Academies Press. Copyright 1997, 1998, 2000, 2001, and 2010, by the National Academy of Sciences. Courtesy of the National Academies Press, Washington, DC. Reprinted with permission.

Dietary Reference Intakes: RDA, AI*, (AMDR)

Macronutrients

Life-Stage Group	Carbohydrate—Total Digestible (g/d)	Total Fiber (g/d)	Total Fat (g/d)	n-6 polyunsaturated fatty acids (linoleic acid) (g/d)	n-3 polyunsaturated fatty acids (?-linoleic acid) (g/d)	Protein and Amino Acids (g/d)[a]
Infants						
0–6 mo	60* (ND[b])[c]	ND	31*	4.4* (ND)	0.5* (ND)	9.1* (ND)
7–12 mo	95* (ND)	ND	30*	4.6* (ND)	0.5* (ND)	13.5 (ND)
Children						
1–3 y	130 (45–65)	19*	(30–40)	7* (5–10)	0.7* (0.6–1.2)	13 (5–20)
4–8 y	130 (45–65)	25*	(25–35)	10* (5–10)	0.9* (0.6–1.2)	19 (10–30)
Males						
9–13 y	130 (45–65)	31*	(25–35)	12* (5–10)	1.2* (0.6–1.2)	34 (10–30)
14–18 y	130 (45–65)	38*	(25–35)	16* (5–10)	1.6* (0.6–1.2)	52 (10–30)
19–30 y	130 (45–65)	38*	(20–35)	17* (5–10)	1.6* (0.6–1.2)	56 (10–35)
31–50 y	130 (45–65)	38*	(20–35)	17* (5–10)	1.6* (0.6–1.2)	56 (10–35)
51–70 y	130 (45–65)	30*	(20–35)	14* (5–10)	1.6* (0.6–1.2)	56 (10–35)
≥70 y	130 (45–65)	30*	(20–35)	14* (5–10)	1.6* (0.6–1.2)	56 (10–35)
Females						
9–13 y	130 (45–65)	26*	(25–35)	10* (5–10)	1.0* (0.6–1.2)	34 (10–30)
14–18 y	130 (45–65)	26*	(25–35)	11* (5–10)	1.1* (0.6–1.2)	46 (10–30)
19–30 y	130 (45–65)	25*	(20–35)	12* (5–10)	1.1* (0.6–1.2)	46 (10–35)
31–50 y	130 (45–65)	25*	(20–35)	12* (5–10)	1.1* (0.6–1.2)	46 (10–35)
51–70 y	130 (45–65)	21*	(20–35)	11* (5–10)	1.1* (0.6–1.2)	46 (10–35)
≥70 y	130 (45–65)	21*	(20–35)	11* (5–10)	1.1* (0.6–1.2)	46 (10–35)
Pregnancy						
≤18 y	175 (45–65)	28*	(20–35)	13* (5–10)	1.4* (0.6–1.2)	71 (10–35)
19–30 y	175 (45–65)	28*	(20–35)	13* (5–10)	1.4* (0.6–1.2)	71 (10–35)
31–50 y	175 (45–65)	28*	(20–35)	13* (5–10)	1.4* (0.6–1.2)	71 (10–35)
Lactation						
≤18 y	210 (45–65)	29*	(20–35)	13* (5–10)	1.3* (0.6–1.2)	71 (10–35)
19–30 y	210 (45–65)	29*	(20–35)	13* (5–10)	1.3* (0.6–1.2)	71 (10–35)
31–50 y	210 (45–65)	29*	(20–35)	13* (5–10)	1.3* (0.6–1.2)	71 (10–35)

Note: This table is adapted from the DRI reports, see www.nap.edu. It lists Recommended Dietary Allowances (RDAs), with Adequate Intakes (AIs) indicated by an asterisk (*), and Acceptable Macronutrient Distribution Range (AMDR) data provided in parentheses. RDAs and AIs may both be used as goals for individual intake. RDAs are set to meet the needs of almost all (97% to 98%) individuals in a group. For healthy breastfed infants, the AI is the mean intake. The AI for other life stage and gender groups is believed to cover the needs of all individuals in the group, but lack of data prevent being able to specify with confidence the percentage of individuals covered by this intake.

[a] Based on 1.5 g/kg/day for infants, 1.1 g/kg/day for 1–3 y, 0.95 g/kg/day for 4–13 y, 0.85 g/kg/day for 14–18 y, 0.8 g/kg/day for adults, and 1.1 g/kg/day for pregnant (using pre-pregnancy weight) and lactating women.

[b] ND = Not determinable due to lack of data of adverse effects in this age group and concern with regard to lack of ability to handle excess amounts. Source of intake should be from food only to prevent high levels of intake.

[c] Data in parentheses are Acceptable Macronutrient Distribution Range (AMDR). This is the range of intake for a particular energy source that is associated with reduced risk of chronic disease while providing intakes of essential nutrients. If an individual consumes in excess of the AMDR, there is a potential of increasing the risk of chronic diseases and/or insufficient intakes of essential nutrients.

Data from "Dietary Reference Intakes for Energy, Carbohydrates, Fiber, Fat, Fatty Acids, Cholesterol, Protein, and Amino Acids (Macronutrients)," © 2002 by the National Academy of Sciences, courtesy of the National Academies Press, Washington, DC. Reprinted with permission.

Dietary Reference Intakes: RDA, AI*

Vitamins

Life-Stage Group	Vitamin A (µg/d)[a]	Vitamin D (IU/d)[b]	Vitamin E (mg/d)[c]	Vitamin K (µg/d)	Thiamin (mg/d)	Riboflavin (mg/d)	Niacin (mg/d)[d]	Pantothenic Acid (mg/d)	Biotin (µg/d)	Vitamin B_6 (mg/d)	Folate (µg/d)[e]	Vitamin B_{12} (µg/d)	Vitamin C (mg/d)	Choline (mg/d)
Infants														
0–6 mo	400*	400*	4*	2.0*	0.2*	0.3*	2*	1.7*	5*	0.1*	65*	0.4*	40*	125*
7–12 mo	500*	400*	5*	2.5*	0.3*	0.4*	4*	1.8*	6*	0.3*	80*	0.5*	50*	150*
Children														
1–3 y	300	600	6	30*	0.5	0.5	6	2*	8*	0.5	150	0.9	15	200*
4–8 y	400	600	7	55*	0.6	0.6	8	3*	12*	0.6	200	1.2	25	250*
Males														
9–13 y	600	600	11	60*	0.9	0.9	12	4*	20*	1.0	300	1.8	45	375*
14–18 y	900	600	15	75*	1.2	1.3	16	5*	25*	1.3	400	2.4	75	550*
19–30 y	900	600	15	120*	1.2	1.3	16	5*	30*	1.3	400	2.4	90	550*
31–50 y	900	600	15	120*	1.2	1.3	16	5*	30*	1.3	400	2.4	90	550*
51–70 y	900	600	15	120*	1.2	1.3	16	5*	30*	1.7	400	2.4	90	550*
≥70 y	900	800	15	120*	1.2	1.3	16	5*	30*	1.7	400	2.4	90	550*
Females														
9–13 y	600	600	11	60*	0.9	0.9	12	4*	20*	1.0	300	1.8	45	375*
14–18 y	700	600	15	75*	1.0	1.0	14	5*	25*	1.2	400	2.4	65	400*
19–30 y	700	600	15	90*	1.1	1.1	14	5*	30*	1.3	400	2.4	75	425*
31–50 y	700	600	15	90*	1.1	1.1	14	5*	30*	1.3	400	2.4	75	425*
51–70 y	700	600	15	90*	1.1	1.1	14	5*	30*	1.5	400	2.4	75	425*
≥70 y	700	800	15	90*	1.1	1.1	14	5*	30*	1.5	400	2.4	75	425*
Pregnancy														
≤18 y	750	600	15	75*	1.4	1.4	18	6*	30*	1.9	600	2.6	80	450*
19–30 y	770	600	15	90*	1.4	1.4	18	6*	30*	1.9	600	2.6	85	450*
31–50 y	770	600	15	90*	1.4	1.4	18	6*	30*	1.9	600	2.6	85	450*
Lactation														
≤18 y	1,200	600	19	75*	1.4	1.4	17	7*	35*	2.0	500	2.8	115	550*
19–30 y	1,300	600	19	90*	1.4	1.4	17	7*	35*	2.0	500	2.8	120	550*
31–50 y	1,300	600	19	90*	1.4	1.4	17	7*	35*	2.0	500	2.8	120	550*

Note: This table is adapted from the DRI reports; see www.nap.edu. It lists Recommended Dietary Allowances (RDAs), with Adequate Intakes (AIs) indicated by an asterisk (*). RDAs and AIs may both be used as goals for individual intake. RDAs are set to meet the needs of almost all (97% to 98%) individuals in a group. For healthy breastfed infants, the AI is the mean intake. The AI for other life stage and gender groups is believed to cover the needs of all individuals in the group, but lack of data prevent being able to specify with confidence the percentage of individuals covered by this intake.
[a] Given as retinal activity equivalents (RAE).
[b] Also known as calciferol. The DRI values are based on the absence of adequate exposure to sunlight.
[c] Also known as α-tocopherol.
[d] Given as niacin equivalents (NE), except for infants 0–6 months, which are expressed as preformed niacin.
[e] Given as dietary folate equivalents (DFE).
Data from the Dietary Reference Intakes series, National Academies Press. Copyright 1997, 1998, 2000, 2001, and 2010, by the National Academy of Sciences. Courtesy of the National Academies Press, Washington, DC. Reprinted with permission.

Dietary Reference Intakes: RDA, AI*

Elements

Life-Stage Group	Calcium (mg/d)	Phosphorus (mg/d)	Magnesium (mg/d)	Iron (mg/d)	Zinc (mg/d)	Selenium (µg/d)	Iodine (µg/d)	Copper (µg/d)	Manganese (mg/d)	Fluoride (mg/d)	Chromium (µg/d)	Molybdenum (µg/d)
Infants												
0–6 mo	200*	100*	30*	0.27*	2*	15*	110*	200*	0.003*	0.01*	0.2*	2*
7–12 mo	260*	275*	75*	11	3	20*	130*	220*	0.6*	0.5*	5.5*	3*
Children												
1–3 y	700	460	80	7	3	20	90	340	1.2*	0.7*	11*	17
4–8 y	1,000	500	130	10	5	30	90	440	1.5*	1*	15*	22
Males												
9–13 y	1,300	1,250	240	8	8	40	120	700	1.9*	2*	25*	34
14–18 y	1,300	1,250	410	11	11	55	150	890	2.2*	3*	35*	43
19–30 y	1,000	700	400	8	11	55	150	900	2.3*	4*	35*	45
31–50 y	1,000	700	420	8	11	55	150	900	2.3*	4*	35*	45
51–70 y	1,000	700	420	8	11	55	150	900	2.3*	4*	30*	45
≥70 y	1,200	700	420	8	11	55	150	900	2.3*	4*	30*	45
Females												
9–13 y	1,300	1,250	240	8	8	40	120	700	1.6*	2*	21*	34
14–18 y	1,300	1,250	360	15	9	55	150	890	1.6*	3*	24*	43
19–30 y	1,000	700	310	18	8	55	150	900	1.8*	3*	25*	45
31–50 y	1,000	700	320	18	8	55	150	900	1.8*	3*	25*	45
51–70 y	1,200	700	320	8	8	55	150	900	1.8*	3*	20*	45
≥70 y	1,200	700	320	8	8	55	150	900	1.8*	3*	20*	45
Pregnancy												
≤18 y	1,300	1,250	400	27	12	60	220	1,000	2.0*	3*	29*	50
19–30 y	1,000	700	350	27	11	60	220	1,000	2.0*	3*	30*	50
31–50 y	1,000	700	360	27	11	60	220	1000	2.0*	3*	30*	50
Lactation												
≤18 y	1,300	1,250	360	10	13	70	290	1,300	2.6*	3*	44*	50
19–30 y	1,000	700	310	9	12	70	290	1,300	2.6*	3*	45*	50
31–50 y	1,000	700	320	9	12	70	290	1,300	2.6*	3*	45*	50

Note: This table is adapted from the DRI reports; see www.nap.edu. It lists Recommended Dietary Allowances (RDAs), with Adequate Intakes (AIs) indicated by an asterisk (*). RDAs and AIs may both be used as goals for individual intake. RDAs are set to meet the needs of almost all (97% to 98%) individuals in a group. For healthy breastfed infants, the AI is the mean intake. The AI for other life stage and gender groups is believed to cover the needs of all individuals in the group, but lack of data prevent being able to specify with confidence the percentage of individuals covered by this intake.

Data from the Dietary Reference Intakes series, National Academies Press. Copyright 1997, 1998, 2000, 2001, and 2010, by the National Academy of Sciences. Courtesy of the National Academies Press, Washington, DC. Reprinted with permission.

appendix B

Calculations and Conversions

Calculation and Conversion Aids

Commonly Used Metric Units

millimeter (mm): one-thousandth of a meter (0.001)
centimeter (cm): one-hundredth of a meter (0.01)
kilometer (km): one-thousand times a meter (1000)
kilogram (kg): one-thousand times a gram (1000)
milligram (mg): one-thousandth of a gram (0.001)
microgram (μg): one-millionth of a gram (0.000001)
milliliter (ml): one-thousandth of a liter (0.001)

International Units

Some vitamin supplements may report vitamin content as International Units (IU).

To convert IU to:

- Micrograms of vitamin D (cholecalciferol), divide the IU value by 40 or multiply by 0.025.
- Milligrams of vitamin E (alpha-tocopherol), divide the IU value by 1.5 if vitamin E is from natural sources. Divide the IU value by 2.22 if vitamin E is from synthetic sources.
- Vitamin A: 1 IU = 0.3 μg retinol or 3.6 μg beta-carotene.

Retinol Activity Equivalents

Retinol Activity Equivalents (RAE) are a standardized unit of measure for vitamin A. RAE account for the various differences in bioavailability from sources of vitamin A. Many supplements will report vitamin A content in IU, as just shown, or Retinol Equivalents (RE).

1 RAE = 1 μg retinol
12 μg beta-carotene
24 μg other vitamin A carotenoids

To calculate RAE from the RE value of vitamin carotenoids in foods, divide RE by 2.

For vitamin A supplements and foods fortified with vitamin A, 1 RE = 1 RAE.

Folate

Folate is measured as Dietary Folate Equivalents (DFE). DFE account for the different factors affecting bioavailability of folate sources.

1 DFE =   1 μg food folate
0.6 μg folate from fortified foods
0.5 μg folate supplement taken on an
empty stomach
0.6 μg folate as a supplement consumed
with a meal

To convert micrograms of synthetic folate, such as that found in supplements or fortified foods, to DFE:

μg synthetic × folate 1.7 = μg DFE

For naturally occurring food folate, such as spinach, each microgram of folate equals 1 microgram DFE:

μg folate = μg DFE

Conversion Factors

Use the following table to convert U.S. measurements to metric equivalents:

Original Unit	Multiply by	To Get
ounces avdp	28.3495	grams
ounces	0.0625	pounds
pounds	0.4536	kilograms
pounds	16	ounces
grams	0.0353	ounces
grams	0.002205	pounds
kilograms	2.2046	pounds
liters	1.8162	pints (dry)
liters	2.1134	pints (liquid)
liters	0.9081	quarts (dry)
liters	1.0567	quarts (liquid)
liters	0.2642	gallons (U.S.)
pints (dry)	0.5506	liters
pints (liquid)	0.4732	liters
quarts (dry)	1.1012	liters
quarts (liquid)	0.9463	liters
gallons (U.S.)	3.7853	liters
millimeters	0.0394	inches
centimeters	0.3937	inches
centimeters	0.03281	feet
inches	25.4000	millimeters
inches	2.5400	centimeters
inches	0.0254	meters
feet	0.3048	meters
meters	3.2808	feet
meters	1.0936	yards
cubic feet	0.0283	cubic meters
cubic meters	35.3145	cubic feet
cubic meters	1.3079	cubic yards
cubic yards	0.7646	cubic meters

Length: U.S. and Metric Equivalents

¼ inch = 0.6 centimeter
1 inch = 2.5 centimeters
1 foot = 0.3048 meter
30.48 centimeters
1 yard = 0.91144 meter
1 millimeter = 0.03937 inch
1 centimeter = 0.3937 inch
1 decimeter = 3.937 inches
1 meter = 39.37 inches
1.094 yards
1 micrometer = 0.00003937 inch

Weights and Measures

Food Measurement Equivalencies from U.S. to Metric

Capacity

1/5 teaspoon	=	1 milliliter
1/4 teaspoon	=	1.25 milliliters
1/2 teaspoon	=	2.5 milliliters
1 teaspoon	=	5 milliliters
1 tablespoon	=	15 milliliters
1 fluid ounce	=	28.4 milliliters
1/4 cup	=	60 milliliters
1/3 cup	=	80 milliliters
1/2 cup	=	120 milliliters
1 cup	=	225 milliliters
1 pint (2 cups)	=	473 milliliters
1 quart (4 cups)	=	0.95 liter
1 liter (1.06 quarts)	=	1,000 milliliters
1 gallon (4 quarts)	=	3.84 liters

Weight

0.035 ounce	=	1 gram
1 ounce	=	28 grams
1/4 pound (4 ounces)	=	114 grams
1 pound (16 ounces)	=	454 grams
2.2 pounds (35 ounces)	=	1 kilogram

U.S. Food Measurement Equivalents

3 teaspoons	=	1 tablespoon
1/2 tablespoon	=	1-1/2 teaspoons
2 tablespoons	=	1/8 cup
4 tablespoons	=	1/4 cup
5 tablespoons + 1 teaspoon	=	1/3 cup
8 tablespoons	=	1/2 cup
10 tablespoons + 2 teaspoons	=	2/3 cup
12 tablespoons	=	3/4 cup
16 tablespoons	=	1 cup
2 cups	=	1 pint
4 cups	=	1 quart
2 pints	=	1 quart
4 quarts	=	1 gallon

Volumes and Capacities

1 cup	=	8 fluid ounces
		1/2 liquid pint
1 milliliter	=	0.061 cubic inch
1 liter	=	1.057 liquid quarts
		0.908 dry quart
		61.024 cubic inches
1 U.S. gallon	=	231 cubic inches
		3.785 liters
		0.833 British gallon
		128 U.S. fluid ounces

1 British Imperial gallon	=	277.42 cubic inches
		1.201 U.S. gallons
		4.546 liters
		160 British fluid ounces
1 U.S. ounce, liquid or fluid	=	1.805 cubic inches
		29.574 milliliters
		1.041 British fluid ounces
1 pint, dry	=	33.600 cubic inches
		0.551 liter
1 pint, liquid	=	28.875 cubic inches
		0.473 liter
1 U.S. quart, dry	=	67.201 cubic inches
		1.101 liters
1 U.S. quart, liquid	=	57.75 cubic inches
		0.946 liter
1 British quart	=	69.354 cubic inches
		1.032 U.S. quarts, dry
		1.201 U.S. quarts, liquid

Energy Units

1 kilocalorie (kcal)	=	4.2 kilojoules
1 millijoule (MJ)	=	240 kilocalories
1 kilojoule (kJ)	=	0.24 kcal
1 gram carbohydrate	=	4 kcal
1 gram fat	=	9 kcal
1 gram protein	=	4 kcal

Temperature Standards

	°Fahrenheit	°Celsius
Body temperature	98.6°	37°
Comfortable room temperature	65–75°	18–24°
Boiling point of water	212°	100°
Freezing point of water	32°	0°

Temperature Scales

To Convert Fahrenheit to Celsius:

$[(°F - 32) 5]/9$

1. Subtract 32 from °F.
2. Multiply (°F – 32) by 5, then divide by 9.

To Convert Celsius to Fahrenheit:

$[(°C \times 9)/5] + 32$

1. Multiply °C by 9, then divide by 5.
2. Add 32 to (°C × 9/5).

appendix C

Foods Containing Caffeine | Data from: USDA Nutrient Database for Standard Reference, Release 23.

Beverages

Food Name	Serving	Caffeine/Serving (mg)
Beverage mix, chocolate flavor, dry mix, prepared w/milk	1 cup (8 fl. oz)	7.98
Beverage mix, chocolate malt powder, fortified, prepared w/milk	1 cup (8 fl. oz)	5.3
Beverage mix, chocolate malted milk powder, no added nutrients, prepared w/milk	1 cup (8 fl. oz)	7.95
Beverage, chocolate syrup w/o added nutrients, prepared w/milk	1 cup (8 fl. oz)	5.64
Beverage, chocolate syrup, fortified, mixed w/milk	1 cup milk and 1 tbsp syrup	2.63
Cocoa mix w/aspartame and calcium and phosphorus, no sodium or vitamin A, low kcal, dry, prepared	6 fl. oz water and 0.53-oz packet	5
Cocoa mix w/aspartame, dry, low kcal, prepared w/water	1 packet dry mix with 6 fl. oz water	1.92
Cocoa mix, dry mix	1 serving (3 heaping tsp. or 1 envelope)	5.04
Cocoa mix, dry, w/o added nutrients, prepared w/water	1-oz packet with 6 fl. oz water	4.12
Cocoa mix, fortified, dry, prepared w/water	6 fl. oz H_2O and 1 packet	6.27
Cocoa, dry powder, high-fat or breakfast, plain	1 piece	6.895
Cocoa, hot, homemade w/whole milk	1 cup	5
Coffee liqueur, 53 proof	1 fl. oz	9.048
Coffee liqueur, 63 proof	1 fl. oz	9.05
Coffee w/cream liqueur, 34 proof	1 fl. oz	2.488
Coffee mix w/sugar (cappuccino), dry, prepared w/water	6 fl. oz H_2O and 2 rounded tsp. mix	74.88
Coffee mix w/sugar (French), dry, prepared w/water	6 fl. oz H_2O and 2 rounded tsp. mix	51.03
Coffee mix w/sugar (mocha), dry, prepared w/water	6 fl. oz and 2 round tsp. mix	33.84
Coffee, brewed	1 cup (8 fl. oz)	94.8
Coffee, brewed, prepared with tap water, decaffeinated	1 cup (8 fl. oz)	2.37
Coffee, instant, prepared	1 cup (8 fl. oz)	61.98
Coffee, instant, regular, powder, half the caffeine	1 cup (8 fl. oz)	30.99
Coffee, instant, decaffeinated	1 cup (8 fl. oz)	1.79
Coffee and cocoa (mocha) powder, with whitener and low-Calorie sweetener	1 cup	405.48
Coffee, brewed, espresso, restaurant-prepared	1 cup (8 fl. oz)	502.44
Coffee, brewed, espresso, restaurant-prepared, decaffeinated	1 cup (8 fl. oz)	2.37
Energy drink, with caffeine, niacin, pantothenic acid, vitamin B_6	1 fl. oz	9.517
Milk beverage mix, dairy drink w/aspartame, low kcal, dry, prep	6 fl. oz	4.08
Milk, low-fat, 1% fat, chocolate	1 cup	5
Milk, whole, chocolate	1 cup	5
Soft drink, cola w/caffeine	1 fl. oz	2
Soft drink, cola, w/higher caffeine	1 fl. oz	8.33
Soft drink, cola or pepper type, low kcal w/saccharin and caffeine	1 fl. oz	3.256
Soft drink, cola, low kcal w/saccharin and aspartame, w/caffeine	1 fl. oz	4.144
Soft drink, lemon-lime soda, w/caffeine	1 fl. oz	4.605
Soft drink, low kcal, not cola or pepper, with aspartame and caffeine	1 fl. oz	4.44
Soft drink, pepper type, w/caffeine	1 fl. oz	3.07
Tea mix, instant w/lemon flavor, w/saccharin, dry, prepared	1 cup (8 fl. oz)	16.59
Tea mix, instant w/lemon, unsweetened, dry, prepared	1 cup (8 fl. oz)	26.18
Tea mix, instant w/sugar and lemon, dry, no added vitamin C, prepared	1 cup (8 fl. oz)	28.49
Tea mix, instant, unsweetened, dry, prepared	1 cup (8 fl. oz)	30.81
Tea, brewed	1 cup (8 fl. oz)	47.36
Tea, brewed, prepared with tap water, decaffeinated	1 cup (8 fl. oz)	2.37
Tea, instant, unsweetened, powder, decaffeinated	1 tsp.	1.183
Tea, instant, w/o sugar, lemon-flavored, w/added vitamin C, dry prepared	1 cup (8 fl. oz)	26.05
Tea, instant, with sugar, lemon-flavored, decaffeinated, no added vitamin	1 cup	9.1

Cake, Cookies, and Desserts

Food Name	Serving	Caffeine/serving (mg)
Brownie, square, large (2-¾″ × ⅞″)	1 piece	1.12
Cake, chocolate pudding, dry mix	1 oz	1.701
Cake, chocolate, dry mix, regular	1 oz	3.118
Cake, German chocolate pudding, dry mix	1 oz	1.985
Cake, marble pudding, dry mix	1 oz	1.985
Candies, chocolate-covered, caramel with nuts	1 cup	35.34
Candies, chocolate-covered, dietetic or low-Calorie	1 cup	16.74
Candy, milk chocolate w/almonds	1 bar (1.45 oz)	9.02
Candy, milk chocolate w/rice cereal	1 bar (1.4 oz)	9.2
Candy, raisins, milk-chocolate-coated	1 cup	45
Chocolate chips, semisweet, mini	1 cup chips (6-oz package)	107.12
Chocolate, baking, unsweetened, square	1 piece	22.72
Chocolate, baking, Mexican, square	1 piece	2.8
Chocolate, sweet	1 oz	18.711
Cookie Cake, Snackwell Fat Free Devil's Food, Nabisco	1 serving	1.28
Cookie, Snackwell Caramel Delights, Nabisco	1 serving	1.44
Cookie, chocolate chip, enriched, commercially prepared	1 oz	3.118
Cookie, chocolate chip, homemade w/margarine	1 oz	4.536
Cookie, chocolate chip, lower-fat, commercially prepared	3 pieces	2.1
Cookie, chocolate chip, refrigerated dough	1 portion, dough spooned from roll	2.61
Cookie, chocolate chip, soft, commercially prepared	1 oz	1.985
Cookie, chocolate wafers	1 cup, crumbs	7.84
Cookie, graham crackers, chocolate-coated	1 oz	13.041
Cookie, sandwich, chocolate, cream-filled	3 pieces	3.9
Cookie, sandwich, chocolate, cream-filled, special dietary	1 oz	0.85
Cupcake, chocolate w/frosting, low-fat	1 oz	0.86
Donut, cake, chocolate w/sugar or glaze	1 oz	0.284
Donut, cake, plain w/chocolate icing, large (3-1/2″)	1 each	1.14
Fast food, ice cream sundae, hot fudge	1 sundae	1.58
Fast food, milk beverage, chocolate shake	1 cup (8 fl. oz)	1.66
Frosting, chocolate, creamy, ready-to-eat	2 tbsp creamy	0.82
Frozen yogurt, chocolate	1 cup	5.58
Fudge, chocolate w/nuts, homemade	1 oz	1.984
Granola bar, soft, milk-chocolate-coated, peanut butter	1 oz	0.85
Granola bar, with coconut, chocolate-coated	1 cup	5.58
Ice cream, chocolate	1 individual (3.5 fl. oz)	1.74
Ice cream, chocolate, light	1 oz	0.85
Ice cream, chocolate, rich	1 cup	5.92
M&M's Peanut Chocolate	1 cup	18.7
M&M's Plain Chocolate	1 cup	22.88
Milk chocolate	1 cup chips	33.6
Milk-chocolate-coated coffee beans	1 NLEA serving	48
Milk dessert, frozen, fat-free milk, chocolate	1 oz	0.85
Milk shake, thick, chocolate	1 fl. oz	0.568
Pastry, eclair/cream puff, homemade, custard-filled w/chocolate	1 oz	0.567
Pie crust, chocolate-wafer-cookie-type, chilled	1 crust, single 9″	11.15
Pie, chocolate mousse, no bake mix	1 oz	0.284
Pudding, chocolate, instant dry mix prepared w/reduced-fat (2%) milk	1 oz	0.283
Pudding, chocolate, regular dry mix prepared w/reduced-fat (2%) milk	1 oz	0.567
Pudding, chocolate, ready-to-eat, fat-free	4 oz can	2.27
Syrups, chocolate, genuine chocolate flavor, light, Hershey	2 tbsp.	1.05
Topping, chocolate-flavored hazelnut spread	1 oz	1.984
Yogurt, chocolate, nonfat milk	1 oz	0.567
Yogurt, frozen, chocolate, soft serve	0.5 cup (4 fl. oz)	2.16

appendix D

U.S. Exchange Lists for Meal Planning

Adapted from: Choose Your Foods: Exchange Lists For Diabetes. © 2008 by the American Diabetes Association and the Academy of Nutrition and Dietetics. Used by permission of the Academy of Nutrition and Dietetics.

Starch List

1 starch choice = 15 g carbohydrate, 0–3 g protein, 0–1 g fat, and 80 cal

Icon Key

☺ = More than 3 g of dietary fiber per serving.

! = Extra fat, or prepared with added fat. (Count as 1 starch + 1 fat.)

▮ = 480 mg or more of sodium per serving.

Food	Serving Size	Food	Serving Size
Bread		☺ Bulgur (cooked)	½ c
Bagel, 4 oz	¼ (1 oz)	Cereals	½ c
! Biscuit, 2½" across	1	☺ bran	½ c
Bread		cooked (oats, oatmeal)	½ c
☺ reduced-calorie	2 slices (1½ oz)	puffed	1½ c
white, whole-grain, pumpernickel, rye,		shredded wheat, plain	½ c
unfrosted raisin	1 slice (1 oz)	sugar-coated	½ c
Chapatti, small, 6" across	1	unsweetened, ready-to-eat	¾ c
! Cornbread, 1¾" cube	1 (1½ oz)	Couscous	⅓ c
English muffin	½	Granola	
Hot dog bun or hamburger bun	½ (1 oz)	low-fat	¼ c
Naan, 8" by 2"	¼	! regular	¼ c
Pancake, 4" across, ¼" thick	1	Grits, cooked	½ c
Pita, 6" across	½	Kasha	½ c
Roll, plain small	1 (1 oz)	Millet, cooked	⅓ c
! Stuffing, bread	⅓ cup	Muesli	¼ c
! Taco shell, 5" across	2	Pasta, cooked	⅓ c
Tortilla		Polenta, cooked	⅓ c
Corn, 6" across	1	Quinoa, cooked	⅓ c
Flour, 6" across	1	Rice, white or brown, cooked	⅓ c
Flour, 10" across	⅓ tortilla	Tabbouleh (tabouli), prepared	½ c
! Waffle, 4"-square or 4" across	1	Wheat germ, dry	3 tbs
		Wild rice, cooked	½ c
Cereals and Grains		**Starchy Vegetables**	
Barley, cooked	⅓ cup	Cassava	⅓ c
Bran, dry		Corn	½ c
☺ oat	¼ c	on cob, large	½ cob (5 oz)
☺ wheat	½ c		

Food	Serving Size	Food	Serving Size
☺ Hominy, canned	¾ c	Graham crackers, 2½" square	3
☺ Mixed vegetables with corn, peas, or pasta	1 c	Matzoh	¾ oz
☺ Parsnips	½ c	Melba toast, about 2" by 4" piece	4 pieces
☺ Peas, green	½ c	Oyster crackers	20
Plantain, ripe	⅓ c	Popcorn	3 c
Potato		! ☺ with butter	3 c
baked with skin	¼ large (3 oz)	☺ no fat added	3 c
boiled, all kinds	½ c or ½ medium (3 oz)	☺ lower fat	3 c
! mashed, with milk and fat	½ c	Pretzels	¾ oz
French fried (oven-baked)	1 cup (2 oz)	Rice cakes, 4" across	2
☺ Pumpkin, canned, no sugar added	1 c	Snack chips	
Spaghetti/pasta sauce	½ c	fat-free or baked (tortilla, potato),	
☺ Squash, winter (acorn, butternut)	1 c	baked pita chips	15–20 (¾ oz)
☺ Succotash	½ c	! regular (tortilla, potato)	9–13 (¾ oz)
Yam, sweet potato, plain	½ c		

Crackers and Snacks

Food	Serving Size
Animal crackers	8
Crackers	
! round-butter type	6
saltine-type	6
! sandwich-style, cheese or peanut butter filling	3
! whole-wheat regular	2–5 (¾ oz)
! whole-wheat lower fat or crispbreads	2–5 (¾ oz)

Beans, Peas, and Lentils

(Count as 1 starch + 1 lean meat)

Food	Serving Size
☺ Baked beans	⅓ c
☺ Beans, cooked (black, garbanzo, kidney, lima, navy, pinto, white)	½ c
☺ Lentils, cooked (brown, green, yellow)	½ c
☺ Peas, cooked (black-eyed, split)	½ c
▮ ☺ Refried beans, canned	½ c

Fruit List

1 fruit choice = 15 g carbohydrate, 0 g protein, 0 g fat, and 60 cal
Weight includes skin, core, seeds, and rind.

Icon Key

☺ = More than 3 g of dietary fiber per serving.

! = Extra fat, or prepared with added fat.

▮ = 480 mg or more of sodium per serving.

Food	Serving Size	Food	Serving Size
Apples		Dried fruits (blueberries, cherries, cranberries, mixed fruit, raisins)	2 tbs
unpeeled, small	1 (4 oz)	Figs	
dried	4 rings	dried	1½
Applesauce, unsweetened	½ c	☺ fresh	1½ large or 2 medium (3½ oz)
Apricots		Fruit cocktail	½ c
canned	½ c	Grapefruit	
dried	8 halves	large	½ (11 oz)
▮ fresh	4 whole (5½ oz)	sections, canned	¾ c
Banana, extra small	1 (4 oz)	Grapes, small	17 (3 oz)
Blackberries	¾ c	Honeydew melon	1 slice or 1 c cubed (10 oz)
▮ Blueberries	¾ c	☺ Kiwi	1 (3½ oz)
Cantaloupe, small	⅓ melon or 1 c cubed (11 oz)	Mandarin oranges, canned	¾ c
Cherries		Mango, small	½ fruit (5½ oz) or ½ c
sweet, canned	½ c	Nectarine, small	1 (5 oz)
sweet, fresh	12 (3 oz)	☺ Orange, small	1 (6½ oz)
Dates	3		

Food	Serving Size	Food	Serving Size
Papaya	½ fruit or 1 c cubed (8 oz)	☺ Raspberries	1 c
Peaches		☺ Strawberries	1¼ c whole berries
canned	½ c	☺ Tangerines, small	2 (8 oz)
fresh, medium	1 (6 oz)	Watermelon	1 slice or 1¼ c cubes (13½ oz)
Pears			
canned	½ c		
fresh, large	½ (4 oz)	**Fruit Juice**	
Pineapple		Apple juice/cider	½ c
canned	½ c	Fruit juice blends, 100% juice	⅓ c
fresh	¾ c	Grape juice	⅓ c
Plums		Grapefruit juice	½ c
canned	½ c	Orange juice	½ c
dried (prunes)	3	Pineapple juice	½ c
small	2 (5 oz)	Prune juice	⅓ c

Milk and Yogurts

1 milk choice = 12 g carbohydrate and 8 g protein

Food	Serving Size	Count As
Fat-Free or Low-Fat (1%)		
(0–3 g fat per serving, 100 calories per serving)		
Milk, buttermilk, acidophilus milk, Lactaid	1 c	1 fat-free milk
Evaporated milk	½ c	1 fat-free milk
Yogurt, plain or flavored with an artificial sweetener	⅔ c (6 oz)	1 fat-free milk
Reduced-Fat (2%)		
(5 g fat per serving, 120 calories per serving)		
Milk, acidophilus milk, kefir, Lactaid	1 c	1 reduced-fat milk
Yogurt, plain	⅔ c (6 oz)	1 reduced-fat milk
Whole		
(8 g fat per serving, 160 calories per serving)		
Milk, buttermilk, goat's milk	1 c	1 whole milk
Evaporated milk	½ c	1 whole milk
Yogurt, plain	8 oz	1 whole milk
Dairy-Like Foods		
Chocolate milk		
fat-free	1 c	1 fat-free milk + 1 carbohydrate
whole	1 c	1 whole milk + 1 carbohydrate
Eggnog, whole milk	½ c	1 carbohydrate + 2 fats
Rice drink		
flavored, low-fat	1 c	2 carbohydrates
plain, fat-free	1 c	1 carbohydrate
Smoothies, flavored, regular	10 oz	1 fat-free milk + 2½ carbohydrates
Soy milk		
light	1 c	1 carbohydrate + ½ fat
regular, plain	1 c	1 carbohydrate + 1 fat
Yogurt		
and juice blends	1 c	1 fat-free milk + 1 carbohydrate
low carbohydrate (less than 6 g carbohydrate per choice)	⅔ c (6 oz)	½ fat-free milk
with fruit, low-fat	⅔ c (6 oz)	1 fat-free milk + 1 carbohydrate

Sweets, Desserts, and Other Carbohydrates List

1 other carbohydrate choice = 15 g carbohydrate and variable protein, fat, and calories.

Icon Key

▮ = 480 mg or more of sodium per serving.

Food	Serving Size	Count As
Beverages, Soda, and Energy/Sports Drinks		
Cranberry juice cocktail	½ c	1 carbohydrate
Energy drink	1 can (8.3 oz)	2 carbohydrates
Fruit drink or lemonade	1 c (8 oz)	2 carbohydrates
Hot chocolate		
regular	1 envelope added to 8 oz water	1 carbohydrate + 1 fat
sugar-free or light	1 envelope added to 8 oz water	1 carbohydrate
Soft drink (soda), regular	1 can (12 oz)	2½ carbohydrates
Sports drink	1 cup (8 oz)	1 carbohydrate
Brownies, Cake, Cookies, Gelatin, Pie, and Pudding		
Brownie, small, unfrosted	1¼" square, ⅞", high (about 1 oz)	1 carbohydrate + 1 fat
Cake		
angel food, unfrosted	1½ of cake (about 2 oz)	2 carbohydrates
frosted	2" square (about 2 oz)	2 carbohydrates + 1 fat
unfrosted	2" square (about 2 oz)	1 carbohydrate + 1 fat
Cookies		
chocolate chip	2 cookies (2¼" across)	1 carbohydrate + 2 fats
gingersnap	3 cookies	1 carbohydrate
sandwich, with creme filling	2 small (about ⅔ oz)	1 carbohydrate + 1 fat
sugar-free	3 small or 1 large (¾ oz–1 oz)	1 carbohydrate + 1–2 fats
vanilla wafer	5 cookies	1 carbohydrate + 1 fat
Cupcake, frosted	1 small (about 1¾ oz)	2 carbohydrates + 1–1½ fats
Fruit cobbler	½ c (3½ oz)	3 carbohydrates + 1 fat
Gelatin, regular	½ c	1 carbohydrate
Pie		
commercially prepared fruit, 2 crusts	⅙ of 8" pie	3 carbohydrates + 2 fats
pumpkin or custard	⅙ of 8" pie	1½ carbohydrates + 1½ fats
Pudding		
regular (made with reduced-fat milk)	½ c	2 carbohydrates
sugar-free, or sugar-free and fat-free (made with fat-free milk)	½ c	1 carbohydrate
Candy, Spreads, Sweets, Sweeteners, Syrups, and Toppings		
Candy bar, chocolate/peanut	2 "fun size" bars (1 oz)	1½ carbohydrates + 1½ fats
Candy, hard	3 pieces	1 carbohydrate
Chocolate "kisses"	5 pieces	1 carbohydrate + 1 fat
Coffee creamer		
dry, flavored	4 tsp	½ carbohydrate + ½ fat
liquid, flavored	2 tbs	1 carbohydrate
Fruit snacks, chewy (pureed fruit concentrate)	1 roll (¾ oz)	1 carbohydrate
Fruit spreads, 100% fruit	1½ tbs	1 carbohydrate
Honey	1 tbs	1 carbohydrate

Food	Serving Size	Count As
Jam or jelly, regular	1 tbs	1 carbohydrate
Sugar	1 tbs	1 carbohydrate
Syrup		
chocolate	2 tbs	2 carbohydrates
light (pancake type)	2 tbs	1 carbohydrate
regular (pancake type)	1 tbs	1 carbohydrate
Condiments and Sauces		
Barbeque sauce	3 tbs	1 carbohydrate
Cranberry sauce, jellied	¼ c	1½ carbohydrates
Gravy, canned or bottled	½ c	½ carbohydrate + ½ fat
Salad dressing, fat-free, low-fat, cream-based	3 tbs	1 carbohydrate
Sweet and sour sauce	3 tbs	1 carbohydrate
Doughnuts, Muffins, Pastries, and Sweet Breads		
Banana nut bread	1" slice (1 oz)	2 carbohydrates + 1 fat
Doughnut		
cake, plain	1 medium, (1½ oz)	1½ carbohydrates + 2 fats
yeast type, glazed	3¾" across (2 oz)	2 carbohydrates + 2 fats
Muffin (4 oz)	¼ muffin (1 oz)	1 carbohydrate + ½ fat
Sweet roll or Danish	1 (2½ oz)	2½ carbohydrates + 2 fats
Frozen Bars, Frozen Dessert, Frozen Yogurt, and Ice Cream		
Frozen pops	1	½ carbohydrate
Fruit juice bars, frozen, 100% juice	1 bar (3 oz)	1 carbohydrate
Ice cream		
fat-free	½ c	1½ carbohydrates
light	½ c	1 carbohydrate + 1 fat
no sugar added	½ c	1 carbohydrate + 1 fat
regular	½ c	1 carbohydrate + 2 fats
Sherbet, sorbet	½ c	2 carbohydrates
Yogurt, frozen		
fat-free	⅓ c	1 carbohydrate
regular	½ c	1 carbohydrate + 0–1 fat
Granola Bars, Meal Replacement Bars/Shakes, and Trail Mix		
Granola or snack bar, regular or low-fat	1 bar (1 oz)	1½ carbohydrates
Meal replacement bar	1 bar (1⅓ oz)	1½ carbohydrates + 0–1 fat
Meal replacement bar	1 bar (2 oz)	2 carbohydrates + 1 fat
Meal replacement shake, reduced-calorie	1 can (10–11 oz)	1½ carbohydrates + 0–1 fat
Trail mix		
candy/nut-based	1 oz	1 carbohydrates + 2 fats
dried-fruit-based	1 oz	1 carbohydrate + 1 fat

Nonstarchy Vegetable List

1 vegetable choice = 5 g carbohydrate, 2 g protein, 0 g fat, 25 cal

Icon Key

☺ = More than 3 g of dietary fiber per serving.

❙ = 480 mg or more of sodium per serving.

Amaranth or Chinese spinach	Kohlrabi
Artichoke	Leeks
Artichoke hearts	Mixed vegetables (without corn, peas, or pasta)
Asparagus	Mung bean sprouts
Baby corn	Mushrooms, all kinds, fresh
Bamboo shoots	Okra
Beans (green, wax, Italian)	Onions
Bean sprouts	Oriental radish or daikon
Beets	Pea pods
❙ Borscht	☺ Peppers (all varieties)
Broccoli	Radishes
☺ Brussels sprouts	Rutabaga
Cabbage (green, bok choy, Chinese)	❙ Sauerkraut
Carrots	Soybean sprouts
Cauliflower	Spinach
Celery	Squash (summer, crookneck, zucchini)
☺ Chayote	Sugar pea snaps
Coleslaw, packaged, no dressing	❙ Swiss chard
Cucumber	Tomato
Eggplant	Tomatoes, canned
Gourds (bitter, bottle, luffa, bitter melon)	❙ Tomato sauce
Green onions or scallions	❙ Tomato/vegetable juice
Greens (collard, kale, mustard, turnip)	Turnips
Hearts of palm	Water chestnuts
Jicama	Yard-long beans

Meat and Meat Substitutes List

Icon Key

❗ = Extra fat, or prepared with added fat. (Add an additional fat choice to this food.)

❙ = 480 mg or more of sodium per serving (based on the sodium content of a typical 3 oz serving of meat, unless 1 or 2 is the normal serving size).

Food	Amount	Food	Amount
Lean Meats and Meat Substitutes		*Fish, fresh or frozen, plain:* catfish, cod, flounder,	
(1 lean meat choice = 7 g protein, 0–3 g fat,		haddock, halibut, orange roughy, salmon,	
45 calories)		tilapia, trout, tuna	1 oz
Beef: Select or Choice grades trimmed of fat:		❙ *Fish, smoked:* herring or salmon (lox)	1 oz
ground round, roast (chuck, rib, rump),		*Game:* buffalo, ostrich, rabbit, venison	1 oz
round, sirloin, steak (cubed, flank,		❙ Hot dog with 3 g of fat or less per oz (8 dogs	
porterhouse, T-bone), tenderloin	1 oz	per 14 oz package) (*Note: May be high in*	
❙ Beef jerky	1 oz	*carbohydrate.*)	1
Cheeses with 3 g of fat or less per oz	1 oz	*Lamb:* chop, leg, or roast	1 oz
Cottage cheese	¼ cup	*Organ meats:* heart, kidney, liver (*Note: May*	
Egg substitutes, plain	¼ cup	*be high in cholesterol*)	1 oz
Egg whites	2		

Food	Amount	Food	Amount

Oysters, fresh or frozen. . . . . .6 medium

Pork, lean

ı Canadian bacon . . . . .1 oz

rib or loin chop/roast, ham, tenderloin . . . . . .1 oz

Poultry without skin: Cornish hen, chicken,
domestic duck or goose (well drained
of fat), turkey . . . . .1 oz

*Processed sandwich meats with 3 g of
fat or less per oz:* chipped beef, deli
thin-sliced meats, turkey ham, turkey
kielbasa, turkey pastrami . . . . .1 oz

Salmon, canned . . . . .1 oz

Sardines, canned . . . . .2 medium

ı Sausage with 3 g or less fat per oz . . . . .1 oz

Shellfish: clams, crab, imitation shellfish,
lobster, scallops, shrimp. . . . . .1 oz

Tuna, canned in water or oil, drained . . . . .1 oz

Veal: Lean chop, roast . . . . .1 oz

Medium-Fat Meat and Meat Substitutes

(1 medium-fat meat choice = 7 g protein, 4–7 g fat, and 75 calories)

Beef: corned beef, ground beef, meatloaf,
Prime grades trimmed of fat (prime rib),
short ribs, tongue . . . . .1 oz

Cheeses with 4–7 g of fat per oz: feta,
mozzarella, pasteurized processed
cheese spread, reduced-fat
cheeses, string . . . . .1 oz

Egg (*Note: High in cholesterol, limit
to 3 per week.*) 1

Fish, any fried product . . . . .1 oz

Lamb: ground, rib roast . . . . .1 oz

Pork: cutlet, shoulder roast .1 oz

Poultry: chicken with skin; dove, pheasant,
wild duck, or goose; fried chicken;
ground turkey . . . . .1 oz

Ricotta cheese. . . . . .2 oz or ¼ c

ı Sausage with 4–7 g fat per oz . . . . .1 oz

Veal: Cutlet (no breading) .1 oz

High-Fat Meat and Meat Substitutes[a]

(1 high-fat meat choice = 7 g protein, 8 + g fat, 100 calories)

Bacon

ı pork . . . . .2 slices (16 slices
per lb or 1 oz
each, before
cooking)

ı turkey. . . . . .3 slices (½ oz
each before
cooking)

Cheese, regular: American, bleu, brie, cheddar,
hard goat, Monterey Jack, queso, Swiss . . . .1 oz

ı! *Hot dog:* beef, pork, or combination
(10 per lb-sized package) 1

ı *Hot dog:* turkey or chicken (10 per lb-sized
package) 1

Pork: ground, sausage, spareribs . . . . .1 oz

*Processed sandwich meats with 8 g of fat or
more per oz:* bologna, pastrami,
hard salami . . . . .1 oz

ı *Sausage with 8 g of fat or more per oz:*
bratwurst, chorizo, Italian, knockwurst,
Polish, smoked, summer . . . . .1 oz

[a]These foods are high in saturated fat, cholesterol, and calories and may raise blood cholesterol levels if eaten on a regular basis. Try to eat 3 or fewer servings from this group per week.

Plant-Based Proteins

Because carbohydrate and fat content varies among plant-based proteins, you should read the food label.

Icon Key

☺ =More than 3 g of dietary fiber per serving; 7 g protein; calories vary.

ı = 480 mg or more of sodium per serving (based on the sodium content of a typical 3-oz serving of meat, unless 1 or 2 oz is the normal serving size).

	Food	Amount	Count As
	"Bacon" strips, soy-based	3 strips	1 medium-fat meat
☺	Baked beans	⅓ c	1 starch + 1 lean meat
☺	*Beans, cooked:* black, garbanzo, kidney, lima, navy, pinto, white	½ c	1 starch + 1 lean meat
☺	"Beef" or "sausage" crumbles, soy-based	2 oz	½ carbohydrate + 1 lean meat
	"Chicken" nuggets, soy-based	2 nuggets (1½ oz)	½ carbohydrate + 1 medium-fat meat
☺	Edamame	½ c	½ carbohydrate + 1 lean meat
	Falafel (spiced chickpea and wheat patties)	3 patties (about 2 inches across)	1 carbohydrate + 1 high-fat meat
	Hot dog, soy-based	1 (1½ oz)	½ carbohydrate + 1 lean meat

Food	Amount	Count As
☺ Hummus	⅓ c	1 carbohydrate + 1 high-fat meat
☺ Lentils, brown, green, or yellow	½ c	1 carbohydrate + 1 lean meat
☺ Meatless burger, soy-based	3 oz	½ carbohydrate + 2 lean meats
☺ Meatless burger, vegetable- and starch-based	1 patty (about 2½ oz)	1 carbohydrate + 2 lean meats
Nut spreads: almond butter, cashew butter, peanut butter, soy nut butter	1 tbs	1 high-fat meat
☺ *Peas, cooked:* black-eyed and split peas	½ c	1 starch + 1 lean meat
▯☺ Refried beans, canned	½ c	1 starch + 1 lean meat
"Sausage" patties, soy-based	1 (1½ oz)	1 medium-fat meat
Soy nuts, unsalted	¾ oz	½ carbohydrate + 1 medium-fat meat
Tempeh	¼ cup	1 medium-fat meat
Tofu, 4 oz (½ cup)		1 medium-fat meat
Tofu, light	4 oz (½ cup)	1 lean meat

Fat List

1 fat choice = 5 g fat, 45 cal

Icon Key

▯ = 480 mg or more of sodium per serving.

Food	Serving Size
Unsaturated Fats—	
Monounsaturated Fats	
Avocado, medium	2 tbs (1 oz)
Nut butters (trans fat-free): almond butter, cashew butter, peanut butter (smooth or crunchy)	1½ tsp
Nuts	
almonds	6 nuts
Brazil	2 nuts
cashews	6 nuts
filberts (hazelnuts)	5 nuts
macadamia	3 nuts
mixed (50% peanuts)	6 nuts
peanuts	10 nuts
pecans	4 halves
pistachios	16 nuts
Oil: canola, olive, peanut	1 tsp
Olives	
black (ripe)	8 large
green, stuffed	10 large
Polyunsaturated Fats	
Margarine: lower-fat spread (30% to 50% vegetable oil, *trans* fat-free)	1 tbs
Margarine: stick, tub (*trans* fat-free), or squeeze (*trans* fat-free)	1 tsp
Mayonnaise	
reduced-fat	1 tbs
regular	1 tsp

Food	Serving Size
Mayonnaise-style salad dressing	
reduced-fat	1 tbs
regular	2 tsp
Nuts	
Pignolia (pine nuts)	1 tbs
walnuts, English	4 halves
Oil: corn, cottonseed, flaxseed, grape seed, safflower, soybean, sunflower	1 tsp
Oil: made from soybean and canola oil—Enova	1 tsp
Plant stanol esters	
light	1 tbs
regular	2 tsp
Salad dressing	
▯ reduced-fat (*Note: May be high in carbohydrate.*)	2 tbs
▯ regular	1 tbs
Seeds	1 tbs
flaxseed, whole	1 tbs
pumpkin, sunflower	1 tbs
sesame seeds	1 tbs
Tahini or sesame paste	2 tsp
Saturated Fats	
Bacon, cooked, regular or turkey	1 slice
Butter	
reduced-fat	1 tbs
stick	1 tsp
whipped	2 tsp

Food	Serving Size	Food	Serving Size
Butter blends made with oil		whipped	2 tbs
reduced-fat or light	1 tbs	whipped, pressurized	¼ c
regular	1½ tsp	Cream cheese	
Chitterlings, boiled	2 tbs (½ oz)	reduced-fat	1½ tbs (¾ oz)
Coconut, sweetened, shredded	2 tbs	regular	1 tbs (½ oz)
Coconut milk		Lard	1 tsp
light	¼ c	*Oil:* coconut, palm, palm kernel	1 tsp
regular	1½ tbs	Salt pork	¼ oz
Cream		Shortening, solid	1 tsp
half and half	2 tbs	Sour cream	
heavy	1 tbs	reduced-fat or light	3 tbs
light	1½ tbs	regular	2 tbs

Free Foods List

A *free food* is any food or drink that has less than 20 calories and 5 g or less of carbohydrate per serving. Foods with a serving size listed should be limited to three servings per day. Foods listed without a serving size can be eaten as often as you like.

Icon Key

▮ = 480 mg or more of sodium per serving.

Food	Serving Size	Food	Serving Size
Low Carbohydrate Foods		Salad dressing	
Cabbage, raw	½ c	fat-free or low-fat	1 tbs
Candy, hard (regular or sugar-free)	1 piece	fat-free, Italian	2 tbs
Carrots, cauliflower, or green beans, cooked	¼ c	Sour cream, fat-free, reduced-fat	1 tbs
Cranberries, sweetened with sugar substitute	½ c	Whipped topping	
Cucumber, sliced	½ c	light or fat-free	2 tbs
Gelatin		regular	1 tbs
dessert, sugar-free			
unflavored		**Condiments**	
Gum		Barbecue sauce	2 tsp
Jam or jelly, light or no sugar added	2 tsp	Catsup (ketchup)	1 tbs
Rhubarb, sweetened with sugar substitute	½ c	Honey mustard	1 tbs
Salad greens		Horseradish	
Sugar substitutes (artificial sweeteners)		Lemon juice	
Syrup, sugar-free	2 tbs	Miso	1½ tsp
		Mustard	
Modified Fat Foods with Carbohydrate		Parmesan cheese, freshly grated	1 tbs
Cream cheese, fat-free	1 tbs (½ oz)	Pickle relish	1 tbs
Creamers		Pickles	
nondairy, liquid	1 tbs	▮ dill	1½ medium
nondairy, powdered	2 tsp	sweet, bread and butter	2 slices
Margarine spread		sweet, gherkin	¾ oz
fat-free	1 tbs	Salsa	¼ c
reduced-fat	1 tsp	▮ Soy sauce, regular or light	1 tbs
Mayonnaise		Sweet and sour sauce	2 tsp
fat-free	1 tbs	Sweet chili sauce	2 tsp
reduced-fat	1 tsp	Taco sauce	1 tbs
Mayonnaise-style salad dressing		Vinegar	
fat-free	1 tbs	Yogurt, any type	2 tbs
reduced-fat	1 tsp		

Drinks/Mixes

Any food on this list—without serving size listed—can be consumed in any moderate amount.

Icon Key

▮ = 480 mg or more of sodium per serving.

▮ Bouillon, broth, consommé

Bouillon or broth, low sodium

Carbonated or mineral water

Club soda

Cocoa powder, unsweetened (1 tbs)

Coffee, unsweetened or with sugar substitute

Diet soft drinks, sugar-free

Drink mixes, sugar-free

Tea, unsweetened or with sugar substitute

Tonic water, diet

Water

Water, flavored, carbohydrate free

Seasonings

Any food on this list can be consumed in any moderate amount.

Flavoring extracts (for example, vanilla, almond, peppermint)

Garlic

Herbs, fresh or dried

Nonstick cooking spray

Pimento

Spices

Hot pepper sauce

Wine, used in cooking

Worcestershire sauce

Combination Foods List

Icon Key

☺ = More than 3 g of dietary fiber per serving.

▮ = 600 mg or more of sodium per serving (for combination food main dishes/meals).

Food	Serving Size	Count As
Entrées		
▮ Casserole type (tuna noodle, lasagna, spaghetti with meatballs, chili with beans, macaroni and cheese)	1 c (8 oz)	2 carbohydrates + 2 medium-fat meats
▮ Stews (beef/other meats and vegetables)	1 c (8 oz)	1 carbohydrate + 1 medium-fat meat + 0–3 fats
Tuna salad or chicken salad	½ c (3½ oz)	½ carbohydrate + 2 lean meats + 1 fat
Frozen Meals/Entrées		
▮☺ Burrito (beef and bean)	1 (5 oz)	3 carbohydrates + 1 lean meat + 2 fats
▮ Dinner-type meal	generally 14–17 oz	3 carbohydrates + 3 medium-fat meats + 3 fats
▮ Entrée or meal with less than 340 calories	about 8–11 oz	2–3 carbohydrates + 1–2 lean meats
Pizza		
▮ cheese/vegetarian thin crust	¼ of 12" (4½ to 5 oz)	2 carbohydrates + 2 medium-fat meats
▮ meat topping, thin crust	¼ of 12" (5 oz)	2 carbohydrates + 2 medium-fat meats, + 1½ fats
▮ Pocket sandwich	1 (4½ oz)	3 carbohydrates + 1 lean meat + 1–2 fats
▮ Pot pie	1 (7 oz)	2½ carbohydrates + 1 medium-fat meat + 3 fats
Salads (Deli-Style)		
Coleslaw	½ c	1 carbohydrate + 1½ fats
Macaroni/pasta salad	½ c	2 carbohydrates + 3 fats
▮ Potato salad	½ c	1½ carbohydrates + 1–2 fats
Soups		
▮ Bean, lentil, or split pea	1 cup	1 carbohydrate + 1 lean meat

Food	Serving Size	Count As
▮Chowder (made with milk)	1 c (8 oz)	1 carbohydrate + 1 lean meat + 1½ fats
▮Cream (made with water)	1 c (8 oz)	1 carbohydrate + 1 fat
▮Instant	6 oz prepared	1 carbohydrate
▮ with beans or lentils	8 oz prepared	2½ carbohydrates + 1 lean meat
▮Miso soup	1 c	½ carbohydrate + 1 fat
▮Oriental noodle	1 c	2 carbohydrates + 2 fats
Rice (congee)	1 c	1 carbohydrate
▮Tomato (made with water)	1 c (8 oz)	1 carbohydrate
▮Vegetable beef, chicken noodle, or other broth-type	1 c (8 oz)	1 carbohydrate

Fast Foods List[a]

Icon Key

☺ = More than 3 g of dietary fiber per serving.

! = Extra fat, or prepared with added fat.

▮ = 600 mg or more sodium per serving (for fast food main dishes/meals).

Food	Serving Size	Exchanges per Serving
Breakfast Sandwiches		
▮ Egg, cheese, meat, English muffin	1 sandwich	2 carbohydrates + 2 medium-fat meats
▮ Sausage biscuit sandwich	1 sandwich	2 carbohydrates + 2 high-fat meats + 3½ fats
Main Dishes/Entrées		
▮☺Burrito (beef and beans)	1 (about 8 oz)	3 carbohydrates + 3 medium-fat meats + 3 fats
▮ Chicken breast, breaded and fried	1 (about 5 oz)	1 carbohydrate + 4 medium-fat meats
Chicken drumstick, breaded and fried	1 (about 2 oz)	2 medium-fat meats
▮ Chicken nuggets	6 (about 3½ oz)	1 carbohydrate + 2 medium-fat meats + 1 fat
▮ Chicken thigh, breaded and fried	1 (about 4 oz)	½ carbohydrate + 3 medium-fat meats + 1½ fats
▮ Chicken wings, hot	6 (5 oz)	5 medium-fat meats + 1½ fats
Oriental		
▮ Beef/chicken/shrimp with vegetables in sauce	1 c (about 5 oz)	1 carbohydrate + 1 lean meat + 1 fat
▮ Egg roll, meat	1 (about 3 oz)	1 carbohydrate + 1 lean meat + 1 fat
Fried rice, meatless	½ c	1½ carbohydrates + 1½ fats
▮ Meat and sweet sauce (orange chicken)	1 c	3 carbohydrates + 3 medium-fat meats + 2 fats
▮☺Noodles and vegetables in sauce (chow mein, lo mein)	1 c	2 carbohydrates + 1 fat
Pizza		
▮ Cheese, pepperoni, regular crust	⅛ of 14" (about 4 oz)	2½ carbohydrates + 1 medium-fat meat + 1½ fats
▮ Cheese/vegetarian, thin crust	¼ of 12" (about 6 oz)	2½ carbohydrates + 2 medium-fat meats + 1½ fats
Sandwiches		
▮ Chicken sandwich, grilled	1	3 carbohydrates + 4 lean meats
▮ Chicken sandwich, crispy	1	3½ carbohydrates + 3 medium-fat meats + 1 fat
Fish sandwich with tartar sauce	1	2½ carbohydrates + 2 medium-fat meats + 2 fats
Hamburger		
▮ large with cheese	1	2½ carbohydrates + 4 medium-fat meats + 1 fat
regular	1	2 carbohydrates + 1 medium-fat meat + 1 fat
▮ Hot dog with bun	1	1 carbohydrate + 1 high-fat meat + 1 fat
Submarine sandwich		
▮ less than 6 grams fat	6" sub	3 carbohydrates + 2 lean meats
▮ regular	6" sub	3½ carbohydrates + 2 medium-fat meats + 1 fat

[a]The choices in the Fast Foods list are not specific fast food meals or items, but are estimates based on popular foods. You can get specific nutrition information for almost every fast food or restaurant chain. Ask the restaurant or check its website for nutrition information about your favorite fast foods.

Food	Serving Size	Exchanges per Serving
Taco, hard or soft shell (meat and cheese)	1 small	1 carbohydrate + 1 medium-fat meat + 1½ fats

Salads

☺ Salad, main dish (grilled chicken type, no dressing or croutons)	Salad	1 carbohydrate + 4 lean meats
Salad, side, no dressing or cheese	Small (about 5 oz)	1 vegetable

Sides/Appetizers

French fries, restaurant style	Small	3 carbohydrates + 3 fats
Medium		4 carbohydrates + 4 fats
Large		5 carbohydrates + 6 fats
Nachos with cheese	Small (about 4½ oz)	2½ carbohydrates + 4 fats
Onion rings	1 serving (about 3 oz)	2½ carbohydrates + 3 fats

Desserts

Milkshake, any flavor	12 oz	6 carbohydrates + 2 fats
Soft-serve ice cream cone	1 small	2½ carbohydrates + 1 fat

Alcohol List

In general, 1 alcohol choice (½ oz absolute alcohol) has about 100 calories.

Alcoholic Beverage	Serving Size	Count As
Beer		
light (4.2%)	12 fl. oz.	1 alcohol equivalent + ½ carbohydrate
regular (4.9%)	12 fl. oz.	1 alcohol equivalent + 1 carbohydrate
Distilled spirits: vodka, rum, gin, whiskey, 80 or 86 proof	1½ fl. oz.	1 alcohol equivalent
Liqueur, coffee (53 proof)	1 fl. oz.	1 alcohol equivalent + 1 carbohydrate
Sake	1 fl. oz.	½ alcohol equivalent
Wine		
dessert (sherry)	3½ fl. oz.	1 alcohol equivalent + 1 carbohydrate
dry, red or white (10%)	5 fl. oz.	1 alcohol equivalent

appendix E

Stature-for-Age Charts

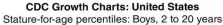

CDC Growth Charts: United States
Stature-for-age percentiles: Boys, 2 to 20 years

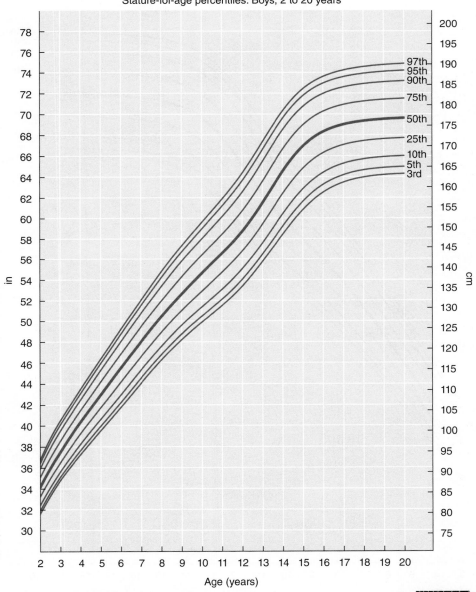

Age (years)

Source: "CDC Growth Charts, United States" Developed by the National Center for Health Statistics in collaboration with the National Center for Chronic Disease Prevention and Health Promotion,from the Centers For Disease Control and Prevention website, 2000.

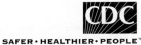

SAFER • HEALTHIER • PEOPLE™

CDC Growth Charts: United States
Stature-for-age percentiles: Girls, 2 to 20 years

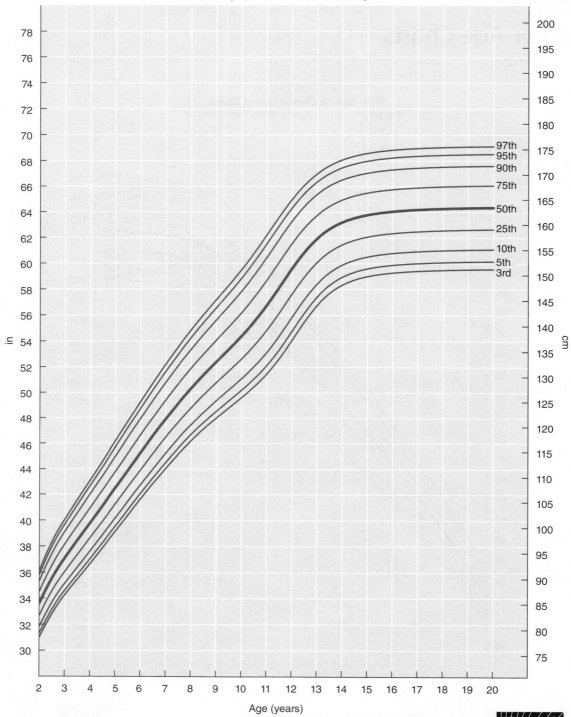

Age (years)

Source: "CDC Growth Charts, United States" Developed by the National Center for Health Statistics in collaboration with the National Center for Chronic Disease Prevention and Health Promotion,from the Centers For Disease Control and Prevention website, 2000.

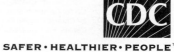

SAFER • HEALTHIER • PEOPLE™

appendix F

Organizations and Resources

Academic Journals

International Journal of Sport Nutrition and Exercise Metabolism
Human Kinetics
P.O. Box 5076
Champaign, IL 61825-5076
(800) 747-4457
www.humankinetics.com

Journal of Nutrition
Department of Nutrition
Pennsylvania State University
126-S Henderson Building
University Park, PA 16802-6504
(814) 865-4721
www.nutrition.org

Nutrition Research
Elsevier: Journals Customer Service
6277 Sea Harbor Drive
Orlando, FL 32887
(877) 839-7126
www.journals.elsevierhealth.com

Nutrition
Elsevier: Journals Customer Service
6277 Sea Harbor Drive
Orlando, FL 32887
(877) 839-7126
www.journals.elsevierhealth.com

Nutrition Reviews
International Life Sciences Institute
Subscription Office
P.O. Box 830430
Birmingham, AL 35283
(800) 633-4931
www.ingentaconnect.com

Obesity Research
North American Association for the Study of Obesity (NAASO)
8630 Fenton Street, Suite 918
Silver Spring, MD 20910
(301) 563-6526

International Journal of Obesity
Journal of the International Association
for the Study of Obesity
Nature Publishing Group
The Macmillan Building
4 Crinan Street
London N1 9XW
United Kingdom

Journal of the American Medical Association
American Medical Association
P.O. Box 10946
Chicago, IL 60610-0946
(800) 262-2350
www.jama.ama-assn.org

New England Journal of Medicine
10 Shattuck Street
Boston, MA 02115-6094
(617) 734-9800
www.content.nejm.org

American Journal of Clinical Nutrition
The American Journal of Clinical Nutrition
9650 Rockville Pike
Bethesda, MD 20814-3998
(301) 634-7038
www.ajcn.org

Journal of the Academy of Nutrition and Dietetics
Elsevier, Health Sciences Division
Subscription Customer Service
6277 Sea Harbor Drive
Orlando, FL 32887
(800) 654-2452
www.eatright.org

Aging

Administration on Aging
U.S. Health & Human Services
200 Independence Avenue, SW
Washington, DC 20201
(877) 696-6775
www.aoa.gov

American Association of Retired Persons (AARP)
601 E. Street, NW
Washington, DC 20049
(888) 687-2277
www.aarp.org

Health and Age
Sponsored by the Novartis Foundation for Gerontology &
The Web-Based Health Education Foundation
Robert Griffith, MD
Executive Director
573 Vista de la Ciudad
Santa Fe, NM 87501
www.healthandage.com

National Council on the Aging
300 D Street, SW, Suite 801
Washington, DC 20024
(202) 479-1200
www.ncoa.org

International Osteoporosis Foundation
5 Rue Perdtemps
1260 Nyon
Switzerland
41 22 994 01 00
www.osteofound.org

National Institute on Aging
Building 31, Room 5C27
31 Center Drive, MSC 2292
Bethesda, MD 20892
(301) 496-1752
www.nia.nih.gov

Osteoporosis and Related Bone Diseases National Resource Center
2 AMS Circle
Bethesda, MD 20892-3676
(800) 624-BONE
www.osteo.org

American Geriatrics Society
The Empire State Building
350 Fifth Avenue, Suite 801
New York, NY 10118
(212) 308-1414
www.americangeriatrics.org

National Osteoporosis Foundation
1232 22nd Street, NW
Washington, DC 20037-1292
(202) 223-2226
www.nof.org

Alcohol and Drug Abuse

National Institute on Drug Abuse
6001 Executive Boulevard, Room 5213
Bethesda, MD 20892-9561
(301) 443-1124
www.nida.nih.gov

National Institute on Alcohol Abuse and Alcoholism
5635 Fishers Lane, MSC 9304
Bethesda, MD 20892-9304
www.niaaa.nih.gov

Alcoholics Anonymous
Grand Central Station
P.O. Box 459
New York, NY 10163
www.alcoholics-anonymous.org

Narcotics Anonymous
P.O. Box 9999
Van Nuys, California 91409
(818) 773-9999
www.na.org

National Council on Alcoholism and Drug Dependence
20 Exchange Place, Suite 2902
New York, NY 10005
(212) 269-7797
www.ncadd.org

National Clearinghouse for Alcohol and Drug Information
11420 Rockville Pike
Rockville, MD 20852
(800) 729-6686
www.health.org

Canadian Government

Health Canada
A.L. 0900C2
Ottawa, ON
K1A 0K9
(613) 957-2991
www.hc-sc.gc.ca

National Institute of Nutrition
408 Queen Street, 3rd Floor
Ottawa, ON K1R 5A7
(613) 235-3355
www.nin.ca/public_html

Agricultural and Agri-Food Canada
Public Information Request Service
Sir John Carling Building
930 Carling Avenue
Ottawa, ON K1A 0C5
(613) 759-1000
www.arg.gc.ca

Bureau of Nutritional Sciences
Sir Frederick G. Banting Research Centre
Tunney's Pasture (2203A)
Ottawa, ON K1A 0L2
(613) 957-0352
www.hc-sc.gc.ca

Canadian Food Inspection Agency
59 Camelot Drive
Ottawa, ON K1A 0Y9
(613) 225-2342
www.inspection.gc.ca

Canadian Institute for Health Information
CIHI Ottawa
377 Dalhousie Street, Suite 200
Ottawa, ON K1N 9N8
(613) 241-7860
www.cihi.ca

Canadian Public Health Association
1565 Carling Avenue, Suite 400
Ottawa, ON K1Z 8R1
(613) 725-3769
www.cpha.ca

Canadian Nutrition and Professional Organizations

Dietitians of Canada
480 University Avenue, Suite 604
Toronto, ON M5G 1V2
(416) 596-0857
www.dietitians.ca

Canadian Diabetes Association
National Life Building
1400-522 University Avenue
Toronto, ON M5G 2R5
(800) 226-8464
www.diabetes.ca

National Eating Disorder Information Centre
CW 1-211, 200 Elizabeth Street
Toronto, ON M5G 2C4
(866) NEDIC-20
www.nedic.ca

Canadian Pediatric Society
100-2204 Walkley Road
Ottawa, ON K1G 4G8
(613) 526-9397
www.cps.ca

Canadian Dietetic Association
480 University Avenue, Suite 604
Toronto, ON M5G 1V2
(416) 596-0857
www.dietitians.ca

Disordered Eating

American Psychiatric Association
1000 Wilson Boulevard, Suite 1825
Arlington, VA 22209
(703) 907-7300
www.psych.org

Harvard Eating Disorders Center
WACC 725
15 Parkman Street
Boston, MA 02114
(617) 236-7766
www.hedc.org

National Institute of Mental Health
Office of Communications
6001 Executive Boulevard, Room 8184, MSC 9663
Bethesda, MD 20892
(866) 615-6464
www.nimh.nih.gov

National Association of Anorexia Nervosa and Associated Disorders (ANAD)
Box 7
Highland Park, IL 60035
(847) 831-3438
www.anad.org

National Eating Disorders Association
603 Stewart Street, Suite 803
Seattle, WA 98101
(206) 382-3587
www.nationaleatingdisorders.org

Eating Disorder Referral and Information Center
2923 Sandy Pointe, Suite 6
Del Mar, CA 92014
(858) 792-7463
www.edreferral.com

Anorexia Nervosa and Related Eating Disorders, Inc. (ANRED)
E-mail: jarinor@rio.com
www.anred.com

Overeaters Anonymous
P.O. Box 44020
Rio Rancho, NM 87174
(505) 891-2664
www.oa.org

Exercise, Physical Activity, and Sports

American College of Sports Medicine (ACSM)
P.O. Box 1440
Indianapolis, IN 46206-1440
(317) 637-9200
www.acsm.org

American Physical Therapy Association (ASNA)
1111 North Fairfax Street
Alexandria, VA 22314
(800) 999-APTA
www.apta.org

Gatorade Sports Science Institute (GSSI)
617 West Main Street
Barrington, IL 60010
(800) 616-GSSI
www.gssiweb.com

National Coalition for Promoting Physical Activity (NCPPA)
1010 Massachusetts Avenue, Suite 350
Washington, DC 20001
(202) 454-7518
www.ncppa.org

Sports, Wellness, Eating Disorder and Cardiovascular Nutritionists (SCAN)
P.O. Box 60820
Colorado Springs, CO 80960
(719) 635-6005
www.scandpg.org

President's Council on Physical Fitness and Sports
Department W
200 Independence Avenue, SW
Room 738-H
Washington, DC 20201-0004
(202) 690-9000
www.fitness.gov

American Council on Exercise
4851 Paramount Drive
San Diego, CA 92123
(858) 279-8227
www.acefitness.org

The International Association for Fitness Professionals (IDEA)
10455 Pacific Center Court
San Diego, CA 92121
(800) 999-4332, ext. 7
www.ideafit.com

Food Safety

Food Marketing Institute
655 15th Street, NW
Washington, DC 20005
(202) 452-8444
www.fmi.org

Agency for Toxic Substances and Disease Registry (ATSDR)
ORO Washington Office
Ariel Rios Building
1200 Pennsylvania Avenue, NW
M/C 5204G
Washington, DC 20460
(888) 422-8737
www.atsdr.cdc.gov

Food Allergy and Anaphylaxis Network
11781 Lee Jackson Highway, Suite 160
Fairfax, VA 22033-3309
(800) 929-4040
www.foodallergy.org

Foodsafety.gov
www.foodsafety.gov

The USDA Food Safety and Inspection Service
Food Safety and Inspection Service
United States Department of Agriculture
Washington, DC 20250
www.fsis.usda.gov

Consumer Reports
Web Site Customer Relations Department
101 Truman Avenue
Yonkers, NY 10703
www.consumerreports.org

Center for Science in the Public Interest: Food Safety
1875 Connecticut Avenue, NW
Washington, DC 20009
(202) 332-9110
www.cspinet.org

Center for Food Safety and Applied Nutrition
5100 Paint Branch Parkway
College Park, MD 20740
(888) SAFEFOOD
www.cfsan.fda.gov

Food Safety Project
Dan Henroid, MS, RD, CFSP
HRIM Extension Specialist and Website Coordinator
Hotel, Restaurant and Institution Management
9e MacKay Hall
Iowa State University
Ames, IA 50011
(515) 294-3527
www.extension.iastate.edu

Organic Consumers Association
6101 Cliff Estate Road
Little Marais, MN 55614
(218) 226-4164
www.organicconsumers.org

Infancy and Childhood

Administration for Children and Families
370 L'Enfant Promenade, SW
Washington, DC 20447
www.acf.dhhs.gov

The American Academy of Pediatrics
141 Northwest Point Boulevard
Elk Grove Village, IL 60007
(847) 434-4000
www.aap.orgKidnetic.com
www.kidnetic.com

Kidshealth: The Nemours Foundation
12735 West Gran Bay Parkway
Jacksonville, FL 32258
(866) 390-3610
www.kidshealth.org

National Center for Education in Maternal and Child Health
Georgetown University
Box 571272
Washington, DC 20057
(202) 784-9770
www.ncemch.org

Birth Defects Research for Children, Inc.
930 Woodcock Road, Suite 225
Orlando, FL 32803
(407) 895-0802
www.birthdefects.org

USDA/ARS Children's Nutrition Research Center at Baylor College of Medicine
1100 Bates Street
Houston, TX 77030
www.kidsnutrition.org

Keep Kids Healthy.com
www.keepkidshealthy.com

International Agencies

UNICEF
3 United Nations Plaza
New York, NY 10017
(212) 326-7000
www.unicef.org

World Health Organization
Avenue Appia 20
1211 Geneva 27
Switzerland
41 22 791 21 11
www.who.int

The Stockholm Convention on Persistent Organic Pollutants
11–13 Chemin des Anémones
1219 Châtelaine
Geneva, Switzerland
41 22 917 8191
www.pops.int

Food and Agricultural Organization of the United Nations
Viale delle Terme di Caracalla
00100 Rome, Italy
39 06 57051
www.fao.org

International Food Information Council Foundation
1100 Connecticut Avenue, NW
Suite 430
Washington, DC 20036
(202) 296-6540

Pregnancy and Lactation

San Diego County Breastfeeding Coalition
c/o Children's Hospital and Health Center
3020 Children's Way, MC 5073
San Diego, CA 92123
(800) 371-MILK
www.breastfeeding.org

National Alliance for Breastfeeding Advocacy
Barbara Heiser, Executive Director
9684 Oak Hill Drive
Ellicott City, MD 21042-6321
OR
Marsha Walker, Executive Director
254 Conant Road
Weston, MA 02493-1756
www.naba-breastfeeding.org

American College of Obstetricians and Gynecologists
409 12th Street, SW, P.O. Box 96920
Washington, DC 20090
www.acog.org

La Leche League
1400 N. Meacham Road
Schaumburg, IL 60173
(847) 519-7730
www.lalecheleague.org

National Organization on Fetal Alcohol Syndrome
900 17th Street, NW
Suite 910
Washington, DC 20006
(800) 66 NOFAS
www.nofas.org

March of Dimes Birth Defects Foundation
1275 Mamaroneck Avenue
White Plains, NY 10605
(888) 663-4637
www.modimes.org

Professional Nutrition Organizations

Association of Departments and Programs of Nutrition (ANDP)
Dr. Marilynn Schnepf, ANDP Chair
316 Ruth Leverton Hall
Nutrition and Health Sciences
University of Nebraska-Lincoln
Lincoln, NE 68583-0806
www.andpnet.org

North American Association for the Study of Obesity (NAASO)
8630 Fenton Street, Suite 918
Silver Spring, MD 20910
(301) 563-6526
www.naaso.org

American Dental Association
211 East Chicago Avenue
Chicago, IL 60611-2678
(312) 440-2500
www.ada.org

American Heart Association
National Center
7272 Greenville Avenue
Dallas, TX 75231
(800) 242-8721
www.americanheart.org

Academy of Nutrition and Dietetics
120 South Riverside Plaza, Suite 2000
Chicago, IL 60606-6995
(800) 877-1600
www.eatright.org

The American Society for Nutrition (ASN)
9650 Rockville Pike, Suite L-4500
Bethesda, MD 20814-3998
(301) 634-7050
www.nutrition.org

The Society for Nutrition Education
7150 Winton Drive, Suite 300
Indianapolis, IN 46268
(800) 235-6690
www.sne.org

American College of Nutrition
300 S. Duncan Avenue, Suite 225
Clearwater, FL 33755
(727) 446-6086
www.amcollnutr.org

American Obesity Association
1250 24th Street, NW, Suite 300
Washington, DC 20037
(800) 98-OBESE

American Council on Health and Science
1995 Broadway
Second Floor
New York, NY 10023
(212) 362-7044
www.acsh.org

American Diabetes Association
ATTN: National Call Center
1701 North Beauregard Street
Alexandria, VA 22311
(800) 342-2383
www.diabetes.org

Institute of Food Technologies
525 W. Van Buren, Suite 1000
Chicago, IL 60607
(312) 782-8424
www.ift.org

ILSI Human Nutrition Institute
One Thomas Circle, Ninth Floor
Washington, DC 20005
(202) 659-0524
www.hni.ilsi.org

Trade Organizations

American Meat Institute
1700 North Moore Street
Suite 1600
Arlington, VA 22209
(703) 841-2400
www.meatami.com

National Dairy Council
10255 W. Higgins Road, Suite 900
Rosemont, IL 60018
(312) 240-2880
www.nationaldairycouncil.org

United Fresh Fruit and Vegetable Association
1901 Pennsylvania Ave. NW, Suite 1100
Washington, DC 20006
(202) 303-3400
www.uffva.org

U.S.A. Rice Federation
Washington, DC
4301 North Fairfax Drive, Suite 425
Arlington, VA 22203
(703) 236-2300
www.usarice.com

U.S. Government

The USDA National Organic Program
Agricultural Marketing Service
USDA-AMS-TMP-NOP
Room 4008-South Building
1400 Independence Avenue, SW
Washington, DC 20250-0020
(202) 720-3252
www.ams.usda.gov

U.S. Department of Health and Human Services
200 Independence Avenue, SW
Washington, DC 20201
(877) 696-6775
www.os.dhhs.gov

Food and Drug Administration (FDA)
5600 Fishers Lane
Rockville, MD 20857
(888) 463-6332
www.fda.gov

Environmental Protection Agency
Ariel Rios Building
1200 Pennsylvania Avenue, NW
Washington, DC 20460
(202) 272-0167
www.epa.gov

Federal Trade Commission
600 Pennsylvania Avenue, NW
Washington, DC 20580
(202) 326-2222
www.ftc.gov

Partnership for Healthy Weight Management
www.consumer.gov

Office of Dietary Supplements
National Institutes of Health
6100 Executive Boulevard, Room 3B01, MSC 7517
Bethesda, MD 20892
(301) 435-2920
www.dietary-supplements.info.nih.gov

Nutrient Data Laboratory Homepage
Beltsville Human Nutrition Center
10300 Baltimore Avenue
Building 307-C, Room 117
BARC-East
Beltsville, MD 20705
(301) 504-8157
www.nal.usda.gov

National Digestive Disease Clearinghouse
2 Information Way
Bethesda, MD 20892-3570
(800) 891-5389
www.digestive.niddk.nih.gov

The National Cancer Institute
NCI Public Inquiries Office
Suite 3036A
6116 Executive Boulevard, MSC 8322
Bethesda, MD 20892-8322
(800) 4-CANCER
www.cancer.gov

The National Eye Institute
31 Center Drive, MSC 2510
Bethesda, MD 20892-2510
(301) 496-5248
www.nei.nih.gov

The National Heart, Lung, and Blood Institute
Building 31, Room 5A52
31 Center Drive, MSC 2486
Bethesda, MD 20892
(301) 592-8573
www.nhlbi.nih.gov

Institute of Diabetes and Digestive and Kidney Diseases
Office of Communications and Public Liaison
NIDDK, NIH, Building 31, Room 9A04
Center Drive, MSC 2560
Bethesda, MD 20892
(301) 496-4000
www.niddk.nih.gov

National Center for Complementary and Alternative Medicine
NCCAM Clearinghouse
P.O. Box 7923
Gaithersburg, MD 20898
(888) 644-6226
www.nccam.nih.gov

U.S. Department of Agriculture (USDA)
14th Street, SW
Washington, DC 20250
(202) 720-2791
www.usda.gov

Centers for Disease Control and Prevention (CDC)
1600 Clifton Rd
Atlanta, GA 30333
(404) 639-3311 / Public Inquiries: (800) 311-3435
www.cdc.gov

National Institutes of Health (NIH)
9000 Rockville Pike
Bethesda, MD 20892
(301) 496-4000
www.nih.gov

Food and Nutrition Information Center
Agricultural Research Service, USDA
National Agricultural Library, Room 105
10301 Baltimore Avenue
Beltsville, MD 20705-2351
(301) 504-5719
www.nal.usda.gov

National Institute of Allergy and Infectious Diseases
NIAID Office of Communications and Public Liaison
6610 Rockledge Drive, MSC 6612
Bethesda, MD 20892
(301) 496-5717
www.niaid.nih.gov

Weight and Health Management

The Vegetarian Resource Group
P.O. Box 1463, Dept. IN
Baltimore, MD 21203
(410) 366-VEGE
www.vrg.org

American Obesity Association
1250 24th Street, NW
Suite 300
Washington, DC 20037
(202) 776-7711

Anemia Lifeline
(888) 722-4407
www.anemia.com

The Arc
(301) 565-3842
E-mail: info@thearc.org
www.thearc.org

Bottled Water Web
P.O. Box 5658
Santa Barbara, CA 93150
(805) 879-1564
www.bottledwaterweb.com

The Food and Nutrition Board
Institute of Medicine
500 Fifth Street, NW
Washington, DC 20001
(202) 334-2352
www.iom.edu

The Calorie Control Council
www.caloriecontrol.org

TOPS (Take Off Pounds Sensibly)
4575 South Fifth Street
P.O. Box 07360
Milwaukee, WI 53207
(800) 932-8677
www.tops.org

Shape Up America!
15009 Native Dancer Road
N. Potomac, MD 20878
(240) 631-6533
www.shapeup.org

World Hunger

Center on Hunger, Poverty, and Nutrition Policy
Tufts University
Medford, MA 02155
(617) 627-3020
www.tufts.edu

Freedom from Hunger
1644 DaVinci Court
Davis, CA 95616
(800) 708-2555
www.freefromhunger.org

Oxfam International
1112 16th Street, NW, Suite 600
Washington, DC 20036
(202) 496-1170
www.oxfam.org

WorldWatch Institute
1776 Massachusetts Avenue, NW
Washington, DC 20036
(202) 452-1999
www.worldwatch.org

Food First
398 60th Street
Oakland, CA 94618
(510) 654-4400
www.foodfirst.org

The Hunger Project
15 East 26th Street
New York, NY 10010
(212) 251-9100
www.thp.org

U.S. Agency for International Development
Information Center
Ronald Reagan Building
Washington, DC 20523
(202) 712-0000
www.usaid.gov

appendix G

The USDA Food Guide Evolution

Early History of Food Guides

Did you know that in the United States food guides in one form or another have been around for over 125 years?

That's right. Back in 1885 a college chemistry professor named Wilber Olin Atwater helped bring the fledgling science of nutrition to a broader audience by introducing dietary standards that became the basis for the first U.S. food guide. Those early standards focused on defining the daily needs of an "average man" for proteins and Calories. They soon expanded into food composition tables with three sweeping categories: protein, fat, and carbohydrate; mineral matter; and "fuel values." As early as 1902, Atwater advocated for three foundational nutritional principles that we still support today: variety, proportionality, and moderation in food choices and eating.

These ideas were adapted a few years later by a nutritionist named Caroline Hunt, who developed a food "buying" guide divided into five categories: meats and proteins; cereals and starches; vegetables and fruits; fatty foods; and sugar.

From the 1930s to the early 1970s, these guidelines kept changing—from twelve food groups to seven to four, and from there to a "Hassle-Free" guide that briefly increased the number of groups back up to five. Although critics identified many drawbacks of these approaches, they were necessary attempts to provide Americans with reliable guidelines based on the best scientific data and practices available at the time.

Contemporary Food Guides: From Pyramid to Plate

By the early 1980s, public health experts began to recognize that, to be effective, a national food guide had to reflect key philosophical values. These core values included the following:

- it must encompass a broad focus on *overall health*;
- it should emphasize the use of *current research*;
- it should be an approach that includes the *total diet*, rather than parts or pieces;
- it should be *useful*;
- it should be *realistic*;
- it should be *flexible*;
- it should be *practical*;
- and it must be *evolutionary*, able to adapt as new information comes to light.

These values guided the development of the USDA Food Guide Pyramid, released in 1992, which also was the first guide to include a graphic representation of the Dietary Guidelines

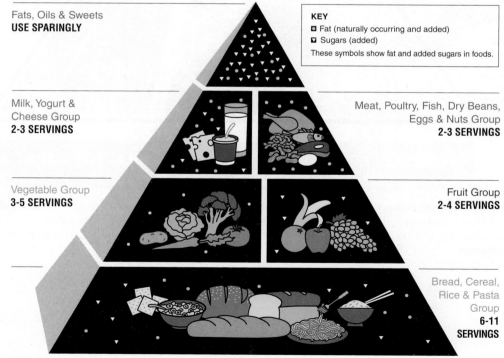

Fats, Oils & Sweets
USE SPARINGLY

KEY
◻ Fat (naturally occurring and added)
▽ Sugars (added)
These symbols show fat and added sugars in foods.

Milk, Yogurt & Cheese Group
2-3 SERVINGS

Meat, Poultry, Fish, Dry Beans, Eggs & Nuts Group
2-3 SERVINGS

Vegetable Group
3-5 SERVINGS

Fruit Group
2-4 SERVINGS

Bread, Cereal, Rice & Pasta Group
6-11 SERVINGS

Source: U.S. Department of Agriculture/U.S. Department of Health and Human Services

The 1992 Food Guide Pyramid. This representation of the USDA guidelines took several years to develop and attempted to convey in a single image all the key aspects of a nutritional guide.
Data from: The 1992 Food Guide Pyramid.

for Americans—in the shape of a pyramid. The 1992 Guide included the following components:

- Nutritional Goals
- Food Groups
- Serving Sizes
- Nutrient Profiles
- Numbers of Servings

The 1992 Guide did not have an enthusiastic reception. Instead, critics quickly began pointing out flaws in the design, recommendations, and ease of use. Many nutritionists trying to use the Guide to teach different population groups basic nutrition messages found that it was out of touch with people's day-to-day lives. Back to the drawing board!

The USDA addressed these complaints by revising—and then radically reinventing—the 1992 Guide. Let's take a look at this evolution of the USDA Food Guide over the past two decades by examining the following graphics.

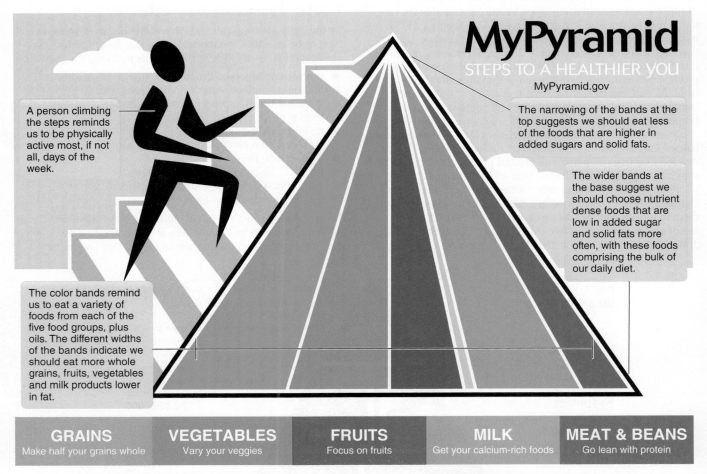

The USDA revised the Guide in 2005 to address concerns regarding the recommendations and ease of use for a general audience. The result was the MyPyramid Food Guidance System, which retained the "pyramid" graphic, but in a simpler presentation that included an emphasis on daily physical activity, and introduced an interactive MyPyramid website where consumers could enter personal data and print out a personalized guide.

Data from: USDA ChooseMyPlate. www.choosemyplate.org

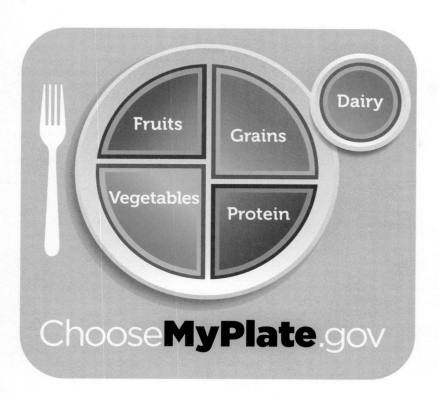

In May 2011 the USDA again changed the food guide—this time dramatically. Dropping the pyramid concept, as well as the previous attempts to teach detailed lessons about foods and physical activity, the new MyPlate guide uses simple icons to directly convey a few key pointers for maintaining a healthy diet. The accompanying website, www.choosemyplate.gov, includes more detailed information as well as interactive tools and multimedia for professionals and consumers.

Data from: www.nal.usda.gov and www.choosemyplate.gov.

references

Chapter 1

1. Kraut, A., Dr. Joseph Goldberger, and the War on Pellagra. National Institutes of Health, Office of NIH History; and H. Markel. 2003. The New Yorker who changed the diet of the South. *New York Times*, August 12, 2003, D5.
2. U.S. Department of Health and Human Services. 2012. HealthyPeople.gov.
3. Institute of Medicine, Food and Nutrition Board. 2003. *Dietary Reference Intakes: Applications in Dietary Planning.* Washington, DC: National Academies Press.
4. Institute of Medicine, Food and Nutrition Board. 2002. *Dietary Reference Intakes for Energy, Carbohydrates, Fiber, Fat, Protein and Amino Acids (Macronutrients).* Washington, DC: National Academies Press.
5. Rising, K., P. Bacchetti, and L. Bero. 2008. Reporting bias in drug trials submitted to the Food and Drug Administration: review of publication and presentation. *PLoS Med.* 5(11):e217. doi:10.1371/journal.pmed.0050217
6. Schott, G., H. Pachl, U. Limbach, U. Gundert-Remy, W. Ludwig, and K. Lieb. 2010. The financing of drug trials by pharmaceutical companies and its consequences: part 1. A qualitative systematic review of the literature on possible influences on the findings, protocols, and quality of drug trials. *Dtsch. Arztebl. Int.* 107(16):279–285.
7. Fogel, J., and S. B. S. Shlivko. 2010. Weight problems and spam e-mail for weight loss products. *South. Med. J.* 103(1):31–36.
8. Winterfeldt, E. A., M. L. Bogle, and L. L. Ebro. 2005. *Dietetics. Practice and Future Trends*, 2nd edn. Sudbury, MA: Jones and Bartlett.
9. Danaei, G., E. L. Ding, D. Mozaffarian, B. Taylor, J. Rehm, C. J. L. Murray, and M. Ezzati. 2009. The preventable causes of death in the United States: Comparative risk assessment of dietary, lifestyle, and metabolic risk factors. *PLoS Med.* 6(4):e1000058. doi:10.1371/journal.pmed.1000058
10. Academy of Nutrition and Dietetics. 2013. Position of the Academy of Nutrition and Dietetics. Total diet approach to healthy eating. *J. Acad. Nutr. Diet.* 113:307–317.
11. Nestle, M., and L. B. Dixon. 2004. *Taking Sides: Clashing Views on Controversial Issues in Food and Nutrition.* New York: McGraw-Hill/Dushkin. pp. 24–39.
12. QSR. 2013. The QSR 50.
13. Elbel, B., J. Gyamfi, and R. Kersh. 2011. Child and adolescent fast food choice and the influence of calorie labelling: a natural experiment. *Int. J. Obes. (Lond)* 35(4):493–500.

InDepth: New Frontiers in Nutrition and Health

1. Waterland, R. A., and R. L. Jirtle. 2003. Transposable elements: targets for early nutritional effects on epigenetic gene regulation. *Mol. Cell. Biol.* 23(15):5293–5300.
2. Corella, D., and J. M. Ordovas. 2009. Nutrigenomics in cardiovascular medicine. *Circ. Cardiovasc. Genet.* 2:637–651.
3. Young-Joon, S. 2008. NF-kB and Nrf2 as potential chemopreventive targets of some anti-inflammatory and antioxidative phytonutrients with anti-inflammatory and antioxidative activities. *Asia Pac. J. Clin. Nutr.* 17(S1):269–272.
4. Zeisel, S. H. 2010. A grand challenge for nutrigenomics. *Front Genet.* 1(2). doi: 10.3389/fgene.2010.00002.
5. Janssens, A. C. J. W., M. Gwinn, L. A. Bradley, B. A. Oostra, C. M. van Duijn, and M. J. Khoury. 2008. A critical appraisal of the scientific basis of commercial genomic profiles used to assess health risks and personalize health interventions. *Am. J. Hum. Genet.* 82(3):593–599.
6. Sterling, R. 2008. The on-line promotion and sale of nutrigenomic services. *Genet. Med.* 10(11):784–796.
7. Tsai, F., and W. J. Coyle. 2009. The microbiome and obesity: is obesity linked to our gut flora? *Curr. Gastroenterol. Rep.* 11(4):307–313.
8. National Institutes of Health. 2012. NIH Human Microbiome Project defines normal bacterial makeup of the body. *NIH News.* June 13, 2012.
9. Hemarajata, P., and J. Versalovic. 2013. Effects of probiotics on gut microbiota: mechanisms of intestinal immunomodulation and neuromodulation. *Therap. Adv. Gastroenterol.* 6(1):39–51.
10. Stanghellini, V., et al. 2010. Gut microbiota and related diseases: clinical features. *Intern. Emerg. Med.* 5(suppl. 1):S57–S63.
11. Draganov, P. V. 2009. Recent advances and remaining gaps in our knowledge of associations between gut microbiota and human health. *World J. Gastroenterol.* 15(1):81–85.
12. Krajmalnik-Brown, R., Z. E. Ilhan, D. W. Kang, and J. K. DiBaise. 2012. Effects of gut microbes on nutrient absorption and energy regulation. *Nutr. Clin. Pract.* 27(2):201–214.
13. United States Food and Drug Administration. 2012, April 6. Regulatory Information: Complementary and Alternative Medicine Products and their Regulation by the Food and Drug Administration.
14. Russo, M., C. Spagnuolo, I. Tedesco, and G. L. Russo. 2010. Phytochemicals in cancer prevention and therapy: truth or dare? *Toxins.* 2(4):517–551.
15. Bellik, Y., S. M. Hammoudi, F. Abdellah, M. Iguer-Ouada, and L. Boukraa. 2012. Phytochemicals to prevent inflammation and allergy. *Recent Pat. Inflamm. Allergy Drug Discov.* 6(2):147–158.
16. Huang, W. Y., Y. A. Cal, and Y. Zhang. 2010. Natural phenolic compounds from medicinal herbs and dietary plants: potential use for cancer prevention. *Nutr. Cancer* 62(1):1–20.
17. Gibbons, S. 2008. Phytochemicals for bacterial resistance: strengths, weaknesses, and opportunities. *Planta Med.* 74(6):594–602.
18. Vasanthi, H. R., N. Shrishrimal, and D. K. Das. 2012. Phytochemicals from plants to combat cardiovascular disease. *Curr. Med. Chem.* 19(14):2242–2251.
19. Ban, J. O., D. H. Lee, E. J. Kim, J. W. Kang, M. S. Kim, et al. 2012. Antiobesity effects of a sulfur compound thiacremonone mediated via down-regulation of serum triglyceride and glucose levels and lipid accumulation in the liver of db/db mice. *Phytother. Res.* doi: 10.1002/ptr.3729[e-pub ahead of print]
20. Huang, B., H. D. Yuan, Y. Kim do, H. Y. Quan, and S. H. Chung. 2011. Cinnamaldehyde prevents adipocyte differentiation and adipogenesis via regulation of peroxisome proliferators-activated receptor-Y (PPARγ) and AMP-activated protein kinase (AMPK) pathways. *J. Agric. Food Chem.* 59(8):3666–3673.
21. Wenwen, X., J. J. Huang, and P. C. K. Cheung. 2012. Extract of *Pleurotus pulmonarius* suppresses liver cancer development and progression through inhibition of VEGF-induced P13K/AKT signaling pathway. *PLoS One* 7(3):e34406.
22. Meyskens, F. L., and E. Szabo. 2005. Diet and cancer: the disconnect between epidemiology and randomized clinical trials. *Cancer Epidemiol. Biomarkers Prev.* 14(6):1366–1369.
23. The Alpha-Tocopherol, Beta-Carotene Cancer Prevention Study Group. 1994. The effect of vitamin E and beta carotene on the incidence of lung cancer and other cancers in male smokers. *N. Engl. J. Med.* 330(15):1029–1035.
24. Omenn, G. S., et al. 1996. Risk factors for lung cancer and for intervention effects in CARET, the Beta-Carotene and Retinol Efficacy Trial. *J. Natl. Cancer Inst.* 88(21):1550–1559.
25. U.S. Preventive Services Task Force. 2006. Multivitamin/Mineral Supplements and Prevention of Chronic Disease: Evidence Report and Technology Assessment Number 139. AHRQ Publication No. 06-E012.

Chapter 2

1. Ogden, C. L., M. D. Carroll, B. K. Kit, and K. M. Flegal. 2012. Prevalence of obesity in the United States, 2009–2010. *NCHS Data Brief Number 82*, January.
2. The Associated Press. 2011. New food nutrition labels from FDA coming [television broadcast]. CBSNews. September 3, 2011.
3. U.S. Department of Agriculture and U.S. Department of Health and Human Services. 2010. *Dietary Guidelines for Americans, 2010*, 7th edn. Washington, DC: U.S. Government Printing Office.
4. Nielsen, S. J., and B. M. Popkin. 2003. Patterns and trends in food portion sizes, 1977–1998. *JAMA* 289(4):450–453.
5. Young, L. R., and M. Nestle. 2002. The contribution of expanding portion sizes to the US obesity epidemic. *Am. J. Pub. Health.* 92(2):246–249.
6. Steward, H., N. Blisard, and D. Joliffe. 2006. Let's eat out. Americans weight taste, convenience and nutrition. *U.S. Department of Agriculture. Economic Research Service. Economic Information Bulletin Number 19.*
7. Chou, S.-Y., M. Grossman, and H. Saffer. 2004. An economic analysis of adult obesity: results from the Behavior Risk Factor Surveillance System. *J. Health Econ.* 23:565–587.
8. Robert Wood Johnson Foundation. 2013. Healthy eating research. Building evidence to prevent childhood obesity. Research results. Menu labeling.
9. Willett, W. C., and D. S. Ludwig. 2011. The 2010 Dietary Guidelines—the best recipe for health? *New Engl. J. Med.* 365(17):1563–1565.
10. World Cancer Research Fund. 2007. *Food, nutrition, physical activity, and the prevention of cancer: A global perspective.* Washington, DC: American Institute for Cancer Research.

InDepth: Eating Wisely

1. Yeomans, M. R. 2006. Olfactory influences on appetite and satiety in humans. *Physiol. Behav.* 87(4):800–804.
2. Brown, K. W., and R. M. Ryan. 2003. The benefits of being present: Mindfulness and its role in psychological well-being. *J. Pers. Soc. Psychol.* 84:822–848.
3. Davidson, R. J., J. Kabat-Zinn, J. Schumacher, M. Rosenkranz, D. Muller, S. F. Santorelli, F. Urbanowski, A. Harrington, K. Bonus, and J. F. Sheridan. 2003. Alterations in brain and immune function produced by mindfulness meditation. *Psychosom. Med.* 65:564–570.
4. Framson, C., A. R. Kristal, J. M. Schenk, A. J. Littman, S. Zeliat, and D. Benitez. 2009. Development and validation of the Mindful Eating Questionnaire. *J. Am. Diet. Assoc.* 109:1439–1444.
5. Timmerman, G. M., and A. Brown. 2012. The effect of a *Mindful Restaurant Eating* intervention on weight management in women. *J. Nutr. Educ. Behav.* 44:22–28.
6. Dalen, J., B. W. Smith, B. M. Shelley, A. L. Sloan, L. Leahigh, and D. Begay. 2010. Pilot study: Mindful Eating and Living (MEAL): Weight, eating behaviour, and psychological outcomes associated with a mindfulness-based intervention for people with obesity. *Complement. Ther. Med.* 18:260–264.
7. Miller, C. K., J. L. Kristeller, A. Headings, H. Nagaraja, and W. F. Miser. 2012. Comparative effectiveness of a mindful eating intervention to a diabetes self-management intervention among adults with type 2 diabetes: a pilot study. *J. Acad. Nutr. Diet.* 112:1835–1842.

Chapter 3

1. Fundukian, L. J., ed. 2011. *Gale Encyclopedia of Medicine*, 4th edn. Farmington Hills, MI: The Gale Group.
2. Yu, J. H., and M-S. Kim. 2012. Molecular mechanisms of appetite regulation. *Diabetes Metab J.* 2012 Dec; 36(6):391–398.
3. Abou-Samra, R., et al. 2011. Effect of different protein sources on satiation and short-term satiety when consumed as a starter. *Nutrition Journal 2011*, December 23(10):139.
4. Marieb, E., and K. Hoehn. 2013. *Human Anatomy and Physiology*, 9th edn. San Francisco: Benjamin Cummings, p. 569.

5. Saulnier, D. M., Kolida, S., and Gibson, G. R. 2009. Microbiology of the human intestinal tract and approaches for its dietary modulation. *Curr Pharm Des.* 2009;15(13):1403–14.
6. National Digestive Diseases Information Clearinghouse (NDDIC). April 30, 2012. Heartburn, gastroesophageal reflux (GER), and gastroesophageal reflux disease (GERD). NIH Publication No. 07–0882.
7. National Digestive Diseases Information Clearinghouse (NDDIC). April 30, 2012. NSAIDs and peptic ulcers. NIH Publication No. 10–4644.
8. National Digestive Diseases Information Clearinghouse (NDDIC). April 23, 2012. Cyclic vomiting syndrome. NIH Publication No. 09-4548.
9. National Digestive Diseases Information Clearinghouse (NDDIC). September 24, 2012. Diarrhea. NIH Publication No. 11–2749.
10. National Digestive Diseases Information Clearinghouse (NDDIC). July 2, 2012. Irritable bowel syndrome. NIH Publication No. 12–693.
11. American Cancer Society. 2012. *Cancer Facts and Figures 2012.*
12. Bernstein, C., Holubec, H., Bhattacharyya, A. K., Nguyen, H., Payne, C. M., Zaitlin, B., and Bernstein, H. 2011. Carcinogenicity of deoxycholate, a secondary bile acid. *Arch Toxicol.* 2011 August;85(8):863–867.
13. Murphy, K. October 31, 2011. In some cases, even bad bacteria may be good. *The New York Times.*
14. Specter, M. October 22, 2012. Germs are us. *The New Yorker.*
15. Chen, Y. and M. J. Blaser. April 15, 2012. Association between gastric *Helicobacter pylori* colonization and glycated hemoglobin levels. *J. Infect. Dis.* 2012 Apr 15;205(8):1195–1202.
16. Arnold, I. C., et al. 2011. *Helicobacter pylori* infection prevents allergic asthma in mouse models through the induction of regulatory T cells. *J Clin Invest.* 2011;121(8):3088–3093.
17. Brazowski, J., A. Nowak, and A. Szaflarska-Poplawska. 2006. Prevalence of *Helicobacter pylori* infection among children and youth with gastroesophageal reflux. *Przegl Lek* 2006;63(3):128–130; Peek, R. M. 2004. *Helicobacter pylori* and gastroesophageal reflux disease. *Current Treatment Options in Gastroenterology* 2004;7(1):59–70; and Richter, J. E. 2001. *H. pylori:* The bug is not all bad. *Gut* 2001;49:319–320.
18. Wu, J. C. 2011. Does *Helicobacter pylori* infection protect against esophageal diseases in Asia? *Indian J Gastroenterol.* 2011 Jul;30(4):149–153.
19. Trasande, L., et al. 2013. Infant antibiotic exposures and early-life body mass. *International Journal of Obesity* 2013;37(1):16–23.

InDepth: Disorders Related to Specific Foods

1. National Digestive Diseases Information Clearinghouse (NDDIC). April 23, 2012. Lactose intolerance. NIH Publication No. 09-2751.
2. U.S. Food and Drug Administration (FDA). May 14, 2012. Food allergies: What you need to know.
3. National Institutes of Health (NIH). June 17, 2012. Allergy testing. *MedlinePlus.*
4. National Digestive Diseases Information Clearinghouse (NDDIC). January 27, 2012. Celiac disease. NIH Publication No. 12-4269.
5. National Institutes of Health (NIH). March 1, 2012. Celiac disease awareness campaign: Frequently asked questions about the campaign.
6. National Institutes of Health. 2011. NIH-funded scientists discover gluten-degrading enzymes in the mouth. *Celiac Disease News.* Summer 2011.

Chapter 4

1. Sears, B. 1995. *The Zone. A Dietary Road Map.* New York: HarperCollins.
2. Steward, H. L., M. C. Bethea, S. S. Andrews, and L. A. Balart. 1995. *Sugar Busters! Cut Sugar to Trim Fat.* New York: Ballantine Books.
3. Atkins, R. C. 1992. *Dr. Atkins' New Diet Revolution.* New York: M. Evans & Company, Inc.
4. Scharlau, D., A. Borowicki, N. Habermann, T. Hofmann, S. Klenow, C. Miene, U. Munjal, K. Stein, and M. Glei. 2009. Mechanisms of primary prevention by butyrate and other products formed during gut flora-mediated fermentation of dietary fibre. *Mutat. Res.* 682(1):39–53.
5. Institute of Medicine, Food and Nutrition Board. 2002. *Dietary Reference Intakes for Energy, Carbohydrates, Fiber, Fat, Protein and*

Amino Acids (Macronutrients). Washington, DC: The National Academy of Sciences.

6. U.S. Department of Agriculture and U.S. Department of Health and Human Services. 2010. *Dietary Guidelines for Americans, 2010*, 7th edn. Washington, DC: U.S. Government Printing Office.

7. Foster-Powell, K., S. H. A. Holt, and J. C. Brand-Miller. 2002. International table of glycemic index and glycemic load values: 2002. *Am. J. Clin. Nutr.* 76:5–56.

8. Levitan, E. B., N. R. Cook, M. J. Stampfer, P. M. Ridker, K. M. Rexrode, J. E. Buring, J. E. Manson, and S. Liu. 2008. Dietary glycemic index, dietary glycemic load, blood lipids, and C-reactive protein. *Metab.* 57(3):437–443.

9. Denova-Gutiérrez, E., G. Huitrón-Bravo, J. O. Talavera, S. Castañon, K. Gallegos-Carrillo, Y. Flores, and J. Salmerón. 2010. Dietary glycemic index, dietary glycemic load, blood lipids, and coronary heart disease. *J. Nutr. Metab.* doi:10.1155/2010/170680

10. Augustin, L. S. A., C. Galeone, L. Dal Maso, C. Pelucchi, V. Ramazzotti, D. J. A. Jenkins, M. Montella, R. Talamini, E. Negri, S. Franceschi, and C. La Vecchia. 2004. Glycemic index, glycemic load and risk of prostate cancer. *Int. J. Cancer* 112:446–450.

11. Welsh, J. A., A. Sharma, J. L. Abramson, V. Vaccarino, C. Gillespie, and M. B. Vos. 2010. Caloric sweetener consumption and dyslipidemia among US adults. *JAMA* 303:1490–1497.

12. Fung, T. T., V. Malik, K. M. Rexrode, J. E. Manson, W. C. Willett, and F. B. Hu. 2009. Sweetened beverage consumption and risk of coronary heart disease in women. *Am. J. Clin. Nutr.* 89:1037–1042.

13. De Koning, L., V. S. Malik, M. D. Kellogg, E. B. Rimm, W. C. Willett, and F. B. Hu. 2012. Sweetened beverage consumption, incident coronary heart disease, and biomarkers of risk in men. *Circulation* 125:1735–1741.

14. Johnson, R. K., L. J. Appel, M. Brands, B. V. Howard, M. Lefevre, R. H. Lustig, F. Sacks, L. M. Steffen, and J. Wylie-Rosett. 2009. Dietary sugars intake and cardiovascular health: a scientific statement from the American Heart Association. *Circulation* 120:1011–1020.

15. Schultze, M. B., J. E. Manson, D. S. Ludwig, G. A. Colditz, M. J. Stampfer, W. C. Willett, and F. B. Hu. 2004. Sugar-sweetened beverages, weight gain, and incidence of type 2 diabetes in young and middle-aged women. *JAMA*. 292:927–934.

16. Bazzano, L. A., T. Y. Li, K. J. Joshipura, and F. B. Hu. 2008. Intake of fruit, vegetables, and fruit juices and risk of diabetes in women. *Diabetes Care* 31:1311–1317.

17. Basu, S., P. Yoffee, N. Hills, and R. H. Lustig. 2013. The relationship of sugar to population-level diabetes prevalence: an econometric analysis of repeated cross-sectional data. *PLoS ONE* 8(2):e57873. doi:10.1371/journal.pone.0057873

18. Malik, V. S., B. M. Popkin, G. A. Gray, J.-P. Deprés, and F. B. Hu. 2010. Sugar-sweetened beverages, obesity, type 2 diabetes mellitus, and cardiovascular disease risk. *Circulation* 121:1356–1364.

19. Te Moranga, L., S. Mallard, and J. Mann. 2013. Dietary sugars and body weight: systematic review and meta-analyses of randomised controlled trials and cohort studies. *BMJ* 346:e7492.

20. International Food Information Council Foundation. 2012. Facts about low-calorie sweeteners.

21. International Food Information Council Foundation. 2012. Everything you need to know about aspartame.

22. Bray, G. A., S. J. Nielsen, and B. M. Popkin. 2004. Consumption of high-fructose corn syrup in beverages may play a role in the epidemic of obesity. *Am. J. Clin. Nutr.* 79:537–543.

23. Jacobson, M. F. 2004. Letter to the editor. High-fructose corn syrup and the obesity epidemic. *Am. J. Clin. Nutr.* 80:1081–1090.

InDepth: Diabetes

1. Kleinfield, N. R. 2006. Diabetes and its awful toll quietly emerge as a crisis. *The New York Times*, January 9, 2006.

2. National Diabetes Information Clearinghouse (NDIC). 2011. National diabetes statistics, 2011. National Institutes of Health Publication No. 11–3892.

3. Gebel, E. 2010, February. High blood glucose and diabetes complications. *Diabetes Forecast*: American Diabetes Association.

4. Hoyert, D. L., and J. Xu. 2012. *National Vital Statistics Reports*, 61(6): October 10, 2012.

5. American Diabetes Association. 2013. Diabetes basics. Genetics of Diabetes.

6. Savage, D. B., K. F. Petersen, and G. I. Shulman. 2005. Mechanisms of insulin resistance in humans and possible links with inflammation. *Hypertension* 45:828–833.

7. Dalleck, L. C., and E. M. Kjelland. 2012. The prevalence of metabolic syndrome and metabolic syndrome risk factors in college-aged students. *Am. J. Health Promot.* 270(1):37–42.

8. American College Health Association (ACHA) National College Health Assessment (NCHA). 2012. ACHA NCHA II. Reference Group Executive Summary Spring 2012.

9. American College of Sports Medicine and the American Diabetes Association. 2010. Exercise and type 2 diabetes: American College of Sports Medicine and American Diabetes Association joint position statement. *Med. Sci. Sports Exerc.* 42(12):2282–2303.

10. Academy of Nutrition and Dietetics. 2012. Diabetes and diet.

11. TODAY Study Group. 2012. A clinical trial to maintain glycemic control in youth with type 2 diabetes. *N. Engl. J. Med.* 366:2247–2256.

Chapter 5

1. Harvey, R. A., and D. R. Ferrier. 2013. *Lippincott's Illustrated Reviews: Biochemistry*, 5th edn. Philadelphia: Lippincott Williams & Wilkins.

2. Pan, A., M. Chen, R. Chowdhury, J. H. Wu, Q. Sun, H. Campos, et al. 2012. α-Linolenic acid and risk of cardiovascular disease: a systematic review and meta-analysis. *Am. J. Clin. Nutr.* 96(6):1262–1273.

3. Gropper, S. S., and J. L. Smith. 2013. *Advanced Nutrition and Human Metabolism*, 6th edn. Belmont, CA: Wadsworth, Cengage Learning.

4. Mozaffarian, D., and J. H. Wu. 2011. Omega-3 fatty acids and cardiovascular disease: effects on risk factors, molecular pathways, and clinical events. *J. Am. Coll. Cardiol.* 58(20):2047–2067.

5. Jump, D. B., C. M. Depner, and S. Tripathy. 2012. Omega-3 fatty acid supplementation and cardiovascular disease. *J. Lipid Res.* 53:2525–2545.

6. Manore, M. M., N. L. Meyer, and J. Thompson. 2009. *Sport Nutrition for Health and Performance*, 2nd edn. Champaign, IL: Human Kinetics.

7. Institute of Medicine (IOM), Food and Nutrition Board. 2005. *Dietary Reference Intakes for Energy, Carbohydrate, Fiber, Fat, Fatty Acids, Cholesterol, Protein, and Amino Acids (Macronutrients)*. Washington, DC: National Academies Press.

8. Cialdella-Kam, L. C., and M. M. Manore. 2009. Macronutrient requirements of active individuals: an update. *Nutrition Today* 44(3):104–111.

9. Rodriguez, N. R., N. M. DiMarco, and S. Langley. 2009. Position of the American Dietetic Association, Dietitians of Canada, and the American College of Sports Medicine: nutrition and athletic performance. *J. Am. Diet. Assoc.* 109:509–527.

10. Lichtenstein, A. H., and L. Van Horn. 1998. Very low fat diets. *Circulation* 98:935–939.

11. Baum, S. J., P. M. Kris-Etherton, W. C. Willett, A. H. Lichtenstein, L. L. Rudel, K. C. Maki, et al. 2012. Fatty acids in cardiovascular health and disease: a comprehensive update. *J. Clin. Lipidol.* 6(3):216–234.

12. Expert Panel on Detection, Evaluation, and Treatment of High Blood Cholesterol in Adults, National Institutes of Health. 2001. Executive summary of the Third Report of the National Cholesterol Education Program (NCEP) Expert Panel on Detection, Evaluation, and Treatment of High Blood Cholesterol in Adults (Adult Treatment Panel III). *JAMA* 285(19):2486–2509.

13. USDA, Weighing in on Fats. Agricultural Research Service (ARS). 2008.

14. Ratnayake, W. M. N., M. R. L. L'Abee, S. Farnworth, L. Dumais, C. Gagnon, B. Lampi, V. Casey, D. Mohottalage, I. Rondeau, and L. Underhill. 2009. Trans fatty acids: current contents in Canadian food and estimated intake levels for the Canadian population. *J AOAC Int.* 92(5):1258–1276.

15. Teegala, S. M., W. C. Willett, and D. Mazaffarian. 2009. Consumption and health effects of trans fatty acids: a review. *J AOAC Int.* 92(5):1250–1257.

16. Mozaffarian, D., M. B. Katan, A. Ascherio, M. J. Stampher, and W. C. Willet. 2006. Trans fatty acids and cardiovascular disease. *N. Engl. J. Med.* 354(15):1601–1613.

17. Othman, R. A., M. H. Moghadasian, and P. J. Jones. 2011. Cholesterol-lowering effects of oat β-glucan. *Nutr. Rev.* 69(6):299–309.

18. Lichtenstein, A. H., and P. J. H. Jones. 2012. Lipids: absorption and transport. In: Erdman, J. W., I. A. Macdonald, and S. H. Zeisel, eds. *Present Knowledge in Nutrition*, 10th edn. Oxford, UK: Wiley-Blackwell.

19. Flock, M. R., P. M. Kris-Etherton. 2011. Dietary Guidelines for Americans 2010: Implications for Cardiovascular Disease. *Current Atherosclerosis Reports* 13(6):449–507.

20. Grundy, S. M. 2006. Nutrition in the management of disorders of serum lipids and lipoproteins. In: Shils, M. E., M. Shike, A. C. Ross, B. Caballero, and R. J. Cousins, eds. *Modern Nutrition in Health and Disease*, 10th edn. Philadelphia: Lippincott Williams & Wilkins.

21. Sabastian, R., C. Enns, J. Goldman, and A. Moshfegh. 2008. Effect of fast food consumption on dietary intake and likelihood of meeting MyPyramid recommendations in adults: results from What We Eat in America, NHANES 2003–04. *FASEB Journal* 22:868.7.

22. Jones, P. J. H., and A. A. Papamandjaris. 2012. Lipids: Cellular metabolism. In: Erdman, J. W., I. A. Macdonald, and S. H. Zeisel, eds. *Present Knowledge in Nutrition*, 10th edn. Oxford, UK: Wiley-Blackwell.

23. Prentice, R. L., C. Bette, R. Chlebowski, et al. 2006. Low-fat dietary patterns and risk of invasive breast cancer. The Women's Health Initiative Randomized Controlled Dietary Modification Trial. *JAMA* 295:629–642.

24. Ormrod, D. J., C. C. Holmes, and T. E. Miller. 1998. Dietary chitosan inhibits hypercholesterolaemia and atherogenesis in the apolipoprotein E-deficient mouse model of atherosclerosis. *Atherosclerosis* 138(2):329–334.

25. Mhurchu, C. N., C. Dunshea-Mooij, D. Bennet, and A. Rodgers. 2005a. Effect of chitosan on weight loss in overweight and obese individuals: a systemic review of randomized control trials. *Obesity Rev* 6:35–42.

26. Mhurchu, C. N., C. A. Dunshea-Mooij, D. Bennett, and A. Rodgers. 2005b. Chitosan for overweight or obesity. *Cochrane Database Syst. Rev.* (Online) 3:CD003892. 2005b.

27. Jull, A. B., C. Ni Mhurchu, D. A. Bennett, C. A. Dunshea-Mooij, and A. Rodgers. 2008. Chitosan for overweight or obesity. *Cochrane Database Syst. Rev.* (Online) 3:CD003892. 2008;3.

28. Kaats, G. R., J. E. Michalek, and H. G. Preuss. 2006. Evaluating efficacy of a chitosan product using a double-blinded, placebo-controlled protocol. *J. Am. Coll. Nutr.* 25(5):389–394.

29. Gades, M. D., and J. S. Stern. 2005. Chitosan supplementation and fat absorption in men and women. *J. Am. Diet. Assoc.* 105:72–77.

InDepth: Cardiovascular Disease

1. Mizuno, Y., R. F. Jacob, and R. P. Mason. 2011. Inflammation and the development of atherosclerosis. *J. Atheros. Thromb.* 18(5):351–358.

2. Ostchega, Y., S. S. Yoon, J. Hughes, and T. Louise. 2008. *Hypertension Awareness, Treatment and Control—Continued Disparities in Adults: United States, 2005–2006*. National Center for Health Statistics (NCHS) data brief no. Hyattsville, MD: NCHS.

3. Lloyd-Jones, D., R. J. Adams, T. M. Brown, M. Carnethon, S. Dai, G. DeSimone, et al. 2010. Heart disease and stroke statistics 2010 update. A report from the American Heart Association. *Circulation* 121:e1–e170.

4. National Center for Chronic Disease Prevention and Health Promotion (NCCDPHP). 2008. *Division for Heart Disease and Stroke Prevention addressing the nation's leading killers. At a glance 2008*.

5. Miller, M., N. J. Stone, C. Ballantyne, V. Bittner, M. H. Criqui, H. N. Ginsberg, et al. 2011. Triglycerides and cardiovascular disease: a scientific statement from the American Heart Association. *Circulation*. 123(20):2292–2333.

6. Rippe, J. M., T. J. Angelopoulos, and L. Zukley. 2007. The rationale for intervention to reduce the risk of coronary heart disease. *Am. J. Lifestyle Med.* 1(1):10–19.

7. Marwick, T. H., M. D. Hordern, T. Miller, D. A. Chyun, A. G. Bertoni, R. S. Blumenthal, G. Philippides, and A. Rocchini. 2009. Exercise training for type 2 diabetes mellitus: impact on cardiovascular risk: a scientific statement from the American Heart Association. *Circulation* 119:3244–3262.

8. Department of Health and Human Services (DHHS). 2008. *Physical Activity Guidelines Advisory Committee, Physical Activity Guidelines Advisory Committee Report, 2008*. Washington, DC: Author.

9. Department of Health and Human Services (DHHS). 2010. *How Tobacco Smoke Causes Disease: The Biology and Behavioral Basis for Smoking-Attributable Disease: A Report of the Surgeon General*. Atlanta, GA: U.S. Department of Health and Human Services (DHHS), Centers for Disease Control and Prevention, National Center for Chronic Disease Prevention and Health Promotion, Office on Smoking and Health.

10. Hohensinner, P. J., A. Niessner, K. Huber, C. M. Weyand, and J. Wojta. 2011. Inflammation and cardiac outcome. *Curr. Opin. Infect. Dis.* 24(3):259–264.

11. Chowdhury, R., S. Stevens, D. Gorman, A. Pan, S. Warnakula, S. Chowdhury, et al. 2012. Association between fish consumption, long chain omega 3 fatty acids, and risk of cerebrovascular disease: systematic review and meta-analysis. *Br. J. Med.* 345:e6698.

12. Mozaffarian, D., and J. H. Wu. 2011. Omega-3 fatty acids and cardiovascular disease: effects on risk factors, molecular pathways, and clinical events. *J. Am. Coll. Cardiol.* 58(20):2047–2067.

13. Zoeller, R. F. 2007. Physical activity and fitness in the prevention of coronary heart disease and associated risk factors. *Am. J. Lifestyle Med.* 1(1):29–33.

14. Flock, M. R., P. M. Kris-Etherton. 2011. Dietary Guidelines for Americans 2010: Implications for Cardiovascular Disease. *Current Atherosclerosis Reports* 13(6):449–507.

15. Center for Disease Control and Prevention (CDC). 2012. *Stroke Facts*.

16. National Institutes of Health (NIH), Expert Panel on Detection, Evaluation, and Treatment of High Blood Cholesterol in Adults. 2002. Third Report of the National Cholesterol Education Program (NCEP) Expert Panel on Detection, Evaluation, and Treatment of High Blood Cholesterol in Adults (Adult Treatment Panel III) final report. *Circulation* 106:3143–3421.

17. Institute of Medicine (IOM), Food and Nutrition Board. 2005. *Dietary Reference Intakes for Energy, Carbohydrate, Fiber, Fat, Fatty Acids, Cholesterol, Protein, and Amino Acids (Macronutrients)*. Washington, DC: National Academies Press.

18. Kris-Etherton, P. M., W. S. Harris, L. J. Appel, and the Nutrition Committee of the American Heart Association. 2002. Fish consumption, fish oil, omega-3 fatty acids and cardiovascular disease. *Circulation* 106:2747–2757.

19. Lichtenstein, A. H., L. J. Appel, M. Brands, M. Carnethon, S. Daniels, H. A. Franch, B. Franklin, P. Kris-Ethergon, W. S. Harris, B. Howard, N. Karanja, M. Lefevre, L. Rudel, F. Sancks, L. Van Horn, M. Winston, and J. Wylie-Rosett. 2006. Diet and lifestyle recommendations revision 2006: a scientific statement from the American Heart Association Nutrition Committee. *Circulation* 114:82–96.

20. Gidding, S. S., A. H. Lichtenstein, M. S. Faith, A. Karpyn, J. A. Mennella, B. Popkin, J. Rowe, L. Van Horn, and L. Whitsel. 2009. Implementing American Heart Association Pediatric and Adult Nutrition Guidelines. *Circulation* 119:1161–1175.

21. Othman, R. A., M. H. Moghadasian, and P. J. Jones. 2011. Cholesterol-lowering effects of oat β-glucan. *Nutr. Rev.* 69(6):299–309.

22. Despres, J. P., and I. Lemieux. 2006. Abdominal obesity and metabolic syndrome. *Nature* 444(14):881–887.

23. Appel, L. J., T. J. Moare, E. Obarzanek, W. M. Vollmer, L. P. Svetkey, F. M. Sacks, G. A. Bray, T. M. Vogt, J. A. Cutler, M. M. Windhauser, P. H. Lin, and N. Karanja. 1997. A clinical trial of the

effects of dietary patterns on blood pressure. *New Engl. J. Med.* 336:1117–1124.

24. Libby, P., P. M. Ridker, and A. Maseri. 2002. Inflammation and atherosclerosis. *Circulation* 105:1135–1143.

25. Sacks, F. M., L. P. Svetkey, W. M. Vollmer, L. J. Appel, G. A. Bray, D. Harsha, E. Obarzanek, P. R. Conlin, E. R. Miller III, D. G. Simons-Morton, N. Karanja, and P. H. Lin. 2001. Effects of blood pressure on reduced dietary sodium and the Dietary Approaches to Stop Hypertension (DASH) diet. *New Engl. J. Med.* 244:3–10.

26. Department of Health and Human Services (DHS). 2008. Physical Activity Guidelines Advisory Committee Report, 2008. Washington DC.

27. Freedman, M. R., J. King, and E. Kennedy. 2001. Popular Diets: a scientific overview. *Obes. Res.* (suppl. 1):1S–40S.

Chapter 6

1. *Huffington Post*. 2011. Vegetarian Celebrities Highlighted on World Vegetarian Day.

2. The Vegetarian Resource Group. 2012, May 18. How often do Americans eat vegetarian meals? and how many adults in the U.S. are vegetarian?

3. American College of Sports Medicine, American Dietetic Association, and Dietitians of Canada. 2009. Joint position statement. Nutrition and athletic performance. *Med. Sci. Sports Exerc.* 41(3):709–731.

4. Phillips, S. M., and L. J. C. van Loon. 2011. Dietary protein for athletes: from requirements to optimum adaptation. *J. Sports Sci.* 29(suppl. 1):S29–S38.

5. Fulgoni, V. L. 2008. Current protein intake in America: analysis of the National Health and Nutrition Examination Survey, 2003–2004. *Am. J. Clin. Nutr.* 87(suppl.):1554S–1557S.

6. Manore, M. M., N. L. Meyer, and J. Thompson. 2009. *Sport Nutrition for Health and Performance.* 2nd edn. Champaign, IL: Human Kinetics.

7. Halton, T. L., and F. B. Hu. 2004. The effects of high protein diets on thermogenesis, satiety and weight loss: a critical review. *J. Am. Coll. Nutr.* 23(5):373–385.

8. Leitzmann, C. 2005. Vegetarian diets: what are the advantages? *Forum Nutr.* 57:147–156.

9. Szeto, Y. T., T. C. Y. Kwok, and I. F. F. Benzie. 2004. Effects of a long-term vegetarian diet on biomarkers of antioxidant status and cardiovascular disease risk. *Nutrition* 20:863–866.

10. Calvez, J., N. Poupin, C. Chesneau, C. Lassale, and D. Tomé. 2012. Protein intake, calcium balance and health consequences. *Eur. J. Clin. Nutr.* 66:281–295.

11. American Diabetes Association (ADA). 2003. Evidence-based nutrition principles and recommendations for the treatment and prevention of diabetes and related complications. *Diabet. Care* 26:S51–S61.

12. Martin, W. F., L. E. Armstrong, and N. R. Rodriguez. 2005. Dietary protein intake and renal function. *Nutr. Metabol.* 2:25.

13. Sabaté, J. M., and Y. Ang. 2009. Nuts and health outcomes: new epidemiological evidence. *Am. J. Clin. Nutr.* 89(suppl.):1643S–1648S.

14. Li, T. Y., A. M. Brennan, N. M. Wedick, C. Mantzoros, N. Rifai, and F. B. Hu. 2009. Regular consumption of nuts is associated with a lower risk of cardiovascular disease in women with type 2 diabetes. *J. Nutr.* 139(7):1333–1338.

15. Pan, A., Q. Sun, J. E. Manson, W. C. Willett, and F. B. Hu. 2013. Walnut consumption is associated with lower risk of type 2 diabetes in women. *J. Nutr.* 143:512–518.

16. American Dietetic Association. 2009. Position of the American Dietetic Association: vegetarian diets. *J. Am. Diet. Assoc.* 109:1266–1282.

17. World Cancer Research Fund and the American Institute for Cancer Research. 2012. Continuous update project. Colorectal cancer. latest evidence.

18. Barr, S. I., and C. A. Rideout. 2004. Nutrition considerations for vegetarian athletes. *Nutrition* 20:696–703.

19. Institute of Medicine, Food and Nutrition Board. 2005. *Dietary Reference Intakes for Energy, Carbohydrate, Fiber, Fat, Fatty Acids, Cholesterol, Protein, and Amino Acids (Macronutrients).* Washington, DC: National Academies Press.

20. Smith, M. I., T. Yatsunenko, M. J. Manary, I. Trehan, R. Mkakosya, J. Cheng, A. L. Kau, S. S. Rich, P. Concannon, J. C. Mychaleckyj, J. Liu, E. Houpt, J. V. Li, E. Holmes, J. Nicholson, D. Knights, L. K. Ursell, R. Knight, and J. I. Gordon. 2013. Gut microbiomes of Malawian twin pairs discordant for kwashiorkor. *Science* 339:548–554.

21. Food and Agriculture Organization of the United Nations. 2006. Livestock's long shadow: environmental issues and options.

22. Jowit, J. 2008. UN says eat less meat to curb global warming. *The Observer.*

23. Water Footprint Network. 2012. Direct and indirect water use.

24. Cattlemen's Beef Board and National Cattlemen's Beef Association. 2010. Explore beef.

25. Hamerschlag, K. 2011, July. Meat-eater's guide to climate change and health. Environmental Working Group.

InDepth: Vitamins and Minerals: Micronutrients with Macro Powers

1. Institute of Medicine, Food and Nutrition Board. 2001. *Dietary Reference Intakes for Vitamin A, Vitamin K, Arsenic, Boron, Chromium, Copper, Iodine, Iron, Manganese, Molybdenum, Nickel, Silicon, Vanadium, and Zinc.* Washington, DC: National Academy Press.

2. Mursu, J., K. Robien, L. J. Harnack, K. Park, and D. R. Jacobs Jr. 2011. Less is more: Dietary supplements and mortality rate in older women: The Iowa Women's Health Study. *Arch. Intern. Med.* 171:1625–1633.

3. Caire-Juvera, G., C. Ritenbaugh, J. Wactawski-Wende, L. G. Snetselaar, and Z. Chen. 2009. Vitamin A and retinol intakes and the risk of fractures among participants of the Women's Health Initiative Observational Study. *Am. J. Clin. Nutr.* 89:323–330.

4. Pollan, M. 2007. The age of nutritionism. *The New York Times Magazine*, January 28.

5. Pollan, M. 2008. *In Defense of Foods*. New York: Penguin Press.

6. Solis, C., K. Veenema, A. A. Ivanov, S. Tran, R. Li, W. Wang, D. J. Moriarty, C. V. Maletz, and M. A. Caudill. 2008. Folate intake at RDA levels is inadequate for Mexican American men with the methylenetetrahydrofolate reductase 677TT genotype. *J. Nutr.* 138:67–72.

Chapter 7

1. Ruxton, C. H., and V. A. Hart. 2011. Black tea is not significantly different from water in the maintenance of normal hydration in human subjects: results from a randomized controlled trial. *Brit. J. Nutr.* 106:588–595.

2. Institute of Medicine. 2004. *Dietary Reference Intakes for Water, Potassium, Sodium, Chloride, and Sulfate.* Washington, DC: The National Academies Press.

3. Godek, S. F., C. Peduzzi, R. Burkholder, S. Condon, G. Dorshimer, and A. R. Bartolozzi. 2010. Sweat rates, sweat sodium concentrations, and sodium losses in 3 groups of professional football players. *J. Athletic Training* 45:364–371.

4. Fishman, C. 2012. U.S. bottled water sales are booming (again) despite opposition. *News Watch.*

5. International Bottled Water Association. 2011. U.S. bottled water volume grew 3.5% in 2010 as economic conditions begin to improve.

6. Zhang, Y., E. T. Lee, L. D. Cowan, R. R. Fabsitz, and B. V. Howard. 2011. Coffee consumption and the incidence of type 2 diabetes in men and women with normal glucose tolerance: the Strong Heart Study. *Nutr., Metab., Cardiovasc. Dis.* 21:418–423.

7. Larsson, S. C., J. Virtamo, and A. Wolk. 2011. Coffee consumption and risk of stroke in women. *Stroke* 42:908–912.

8. da Silva Pinto, M. 2013. Tea: a new perspective on health benefits. *Food Res. Int.*

9. Laine, M. L., and W. Crielaard. 2012. Functional foods/ingredients and periodontal diseases. *Eur. J. Nutr.* 51(suppl 2):S27–S30.

10. Zomer, E., A. Owen, J. Magliano, D. Liew, and C. M. Reid. 2012. The effectiveness and cost effectiveness of dark chocolate consumption as prevention therapy in people at risk of cardiovascular disease: best case scenario analysis using a Markov model. *BMJ* 344:e3657. doi:10.1136/bmj.e3657

11. Seifert, S. M., J. L. Schaechter, E. R. Hershorin, and S. E. Lipshultz. 2011. Health effects of energy drinks on children, adolescents, and young adults. *Pediatrics* 127:511–528.

12. Committee on Nutrition and the Council on Sports Medicine and Fitness. 2011. Clinical report—sports drinks and energy drinks for children and adolescents: are they appropriate? *Pediatrics* 127:1182–1189.

13. U.S. Department of Agriculture and U.S. Department of Health and Human Services. 2010. *Dietary Guidelines for Americans, 2010.* 7th edn. Washington, DC: U.S. Government Printing Office.

14. Kipps, C., S. Sharma, and D. T. Pedoe. 2011. The incidence of exercise-associated hyponatremia in the London marathon. *Brit. J. Sports Med.* 45:14–19.

15. Drewnowski, A., M. Maillot, and C. Rehm. 2012. Reducing the sodium-potassium ratio in the US diet: a challenge for public health. *Am. J. Clin. Nutr.* 96:439–444.

16. Roan, S. 2011. Scientists study surge in heat-related football deaths. *Los Angeles Times*, August 8, 2011.

17. Kreider, R. B., C. D. Wilborn, L. Taylor, B. Campbell, A. L. Almada, R. Collins, M. Cooke, C. P. Earnest, M. Greenwood, D. K. Kalman, C. M. Kerksick, S. M. Kleiner, B. Leutholtz, H. Lopez, L. M. Lowery, R. Mendel, A. Smith, M. Spano, R. Wildman, D. S. Willoughby, T. N. Ziegenfuss, and J. Antonio. 2010. ISSN exercise & sport nutrition review: research & recommendations. *J. Intern. Soc. Sports Nutr.* 7:7–51.

18. American College of Sports Medicine, American Dietetic Association and Dietitians of Canada. 2009. Joint position statement: nutrition and athletic performance. *Med. Sci. Sports Exerc* 41:709–731.

19. Committee on Nutrition and the Council on Sports Medicine and Fitness. 2011. Clinical report—sports drinks and energy drinks for children and adolescents: are they appropriate? *Pediatrics* 127:1182–1189.

20. Institute of Medicine. 2007. *Nutrition Standards for Foods in Schools: Leading the Way Toward Healthier Youth.* Washington, DC: National Academies Press.

InDepth: Alcohol

1. Yeomans, M. R. 2010. Alcohol, appetite and energy balance: is alcohol intake a risk factor for obesity? *Physiol. Behav.* 100:82–89.

2. Rajpathak, S. N., M. S. Freiber, C. Wang, J. Wylie-Rosett, R. P. Wildman, T. E. Rohan, J. G. Robinson, S. Liu, and S. Wassertheil-Smoller. 2010. Alcohol consumption and the risk of coronary heart disease in postmenopausal women with diabetes: Women's Health Initiative Observational Study. *Eur. J. Nutr.* 49:211–218.

3. National Institutes of Health. 2012. NIH study uncovers probable mechanism underlying resveratrol activity. *NIH News* February 2, 2012.

4. Wakabayaski, I., and Y. Araki. 2010. Influences of gender and age on relationships between alcohol drinking and atherosclerotic risk factors. *Alcohol Clin. Exp. Res.* 34(suppl 1):S54–60.

5. Jimenez, M., S. E. Chiuve, R. J. Glynn, M. J. Stampfer, C. A. Camargo, W. C. Willett, J. E. Manson, and K. M. Rexrode. 2012. Alcohol consumption and risk of stroke in women. *Stroke* 43:939–945.

6. Lourenço, S., A. Oliveira, and C. Lopes. 2012. The effect of current and lifetime alcohol consumption on overall and central obesity. *Eur. J. Clin. Nutr.* 1–6.

7. NIAAA. 2012. *Alcohol Use Disorders*.

8. Xiao-Jun, W., D. Kanny, W. W. Thompson, C. A. Okoro, M. Town, and L. S. Balluz. 2012. Binge drinking intensity and health-related quality of life among US adult binge drinkers. *Prev. Chronic Dis.* 9:110204.

9. Centers for Disease Control and Prevention. 2013. Vital signs: binge drinking among women and high school girls—United States, 2011. *MMWR Morb. Mortal. Wkly. Rep.* 62:913.

10. Parada, M., M. Corral, N. Mota, A. Crego, S. Rodríquez Holguín, and F. Cadaveira. 2012. Executive functioning and alcohol binge drinking in university students. *Addictive Behaviors* 37:167–172.

11. de Wit, H., and T. J. Phillips. 2012. Do initial responses to drugs predict future use or abuse? *Neurosci. Biobehav. Rev.* 36:1565–1576.

12. Maurel, D. B., N. Boisseau, C. L. Benhamou, and C. Jaffre. 2012. Alcohol and bone: review of dose effects and mechanisms. *Osteoporosis* 23:1–16.

13. Chen, W. Y., B. Rosner, S. E. Hankinson, et al. 2011. Moderate alcohol consumption during adult life, drinking pattern, and breast cancer risk. *JAMA* 306: 1884–1890.

14. Tramacere, I., E. Negri, C. Pelucchi, V. Bagnardi, M. Rota, L. Scotti, F. Islami, G. Corrao, C. La Vecchia, and P. Boffetta. 2012. A meta-analysis on alcohol drinking and gastric cancer risk. *Ann. Oncol.* 23:28–36.

15. Dalye, J. I., M. A. Stahre, F. J. Chaloupka, and T. S. Naimi. 2012. The impact of a 25-cent-per-drink alcohol tax increase. *Am. J. Prev. Med.* 42:382–389.

16. Centers for Disease Control and Prevention. 2012. Alcohol use and binge drinking among women of childbearing age—United States, 2006–2010. *MMWR Morb. Mortal. Wkly. Rep.* 61:534–538.

Chapter 8

1. Institute of Medicine. Food and Nutrition Board. 2000. *Dietary Reference Intakes for Vitamin C, Vitamin E, Selenium and Carotenoids.* Washington, DC: National Academy Press.

2. The HOPE and HOPE-TOO Trial Investigators. 2005. Effects of long-term vitamin E supplementation on cardiovascular events and cancer. A randomized controlled trial. *JAMA* 293:1338–1347.

3. Miller, E. R. 3rd, R. Pastor-Barriuso, D. Dalal, R. A. Riemersma, L. J. Appel, and E. Guallar. 2005. Meta-analysis: high-dosage vitamin E supplementation may increase all-cause mortality. *Ann. Intern. Med.* 142:37–46.

4. Bjelakovic, G., D. Nikolova, L. L. Gluud, R. G. Simonetti, and C. Gluud. 2007. Mortality in randomized trials of antioxidant supplements for primary and secondary prevention: systematic review and meta-analysis. *JAMA* 297:842–857.

5. Klein, E. A., I. M. Thompson Jr., C. M. Tangen, J. J. Crowley, M. S. Lucia, P. J. Goodman, L. M. Minasian, L. G. Ford, H. L. Parnes, J. M. Gaziano, D. D. Karp, M. M. Lieber, P. J. Walther, L. Klotz, J. K. Parsons, J. L. Chin, A. K. Darke, S. M. Lippman, G. E. Goodman, F. L. Myeskens, Jr., and L. H. Baker. 2011. Vitamin E and the risk of prostate cancer: the Selenium and Vitamin E Cancer Prevention Trial (SELECT). *JAMA* 306:1549–1556.

6. Sesso, H. D., J. E. Buring, W. G. Christen, T. Kurth, C. Belanger, J.MacFadyn, V. Bubes, J. E. Manson, R. J. Glynn, and J. M. Gaziano. 2008. Vitamins E and C in the prevention of cardiovascular disease in men: the Physicians' Health Study II randomized controlled trial. *JAMA* 300(18):2123–2133.

7. Gao, X., P. E. Wilde, A. H. Lichtenstein, O. I. Bermudez, and K. L. Tucker. 2006. The maximal amount of dietary α-tocopherol intake in U.S. adults (NHANES 2001–2002). *J. Nutr.* 136:1021–1026.

8. Maras, J. E., O. I. Bermudez, N. Qiao, P. J. Bakun, E. L. Boody-Alter, and K. L. Tucker. 2004. Intake of alpha-tocopherol is limited among US adults. *J. Am. Diet. Assoc.* 104(4):567–575.

9. Hemilä, H., E. Chalker, B. Treacy, and B. Douglas. 2007. Vitamin C for preventing and treating the common cold. *Cochrane Database Syst. Rev.* 3:CD000980. doi: 10.1002/14651858.CD000980.pub3

10. U.S. National Library of Medicine. National Institutes of Health. 2011. Medline Plus. Beta-carotene.

11. U.S. Department of Agriculture (USDA), Agricultural Research Service. 2012. USDA National Nutrient Database for Standard Reference, Release 25.

12. El-akawi, Z., N. Abdel-Latif, and K. Abdul-Razzak. 2006. Does the plasma level of vitamins A and E affect acne condition? *Clin. Experimen. Dermatol.* 31:430–434.

13. Institute of Medicine. Food and Nutrition Board. 2001. *Dietary Reference Intakes for Vitamin A, Vitamin K, Arsenic, Boron, Chromium, Copper, Iodine, Iron, Manganese, Molybdenum, Nickel,*

Silicon, Vanadium, and Zinc. Washington, DC: National Academy Press.

14. World Health Organization (WHO). 2013. Micronutrient deficiencies. Vitamin A deficiency.

15. Albanes, D., O. P. Heinonen, J. K. Huttunen, P. R. Taylor, J. Virtamo, B. K. Edwards, J. Haapakoski, M. Rautalahti, A. M. Hartman, J. Palmgren, and P. Greenwald. 1995. Effects of alpha-tocopherol and beta-carotene supplements on cancer incidence in the Alpha-Tocopherol Beta-Carotene Cancer Prevention Study. *Am. J. Clin. Nutr.* 62(suppl.):1427S–1430S.

16. Omenn, G. S., G. E. Goodman, M. D. Thornquist, J. Balmes, M. R. Cullen, A. Glass, J. P. Keogh, F. L. Meyskens, B. Valanis, J. H. Williams, S. Barnhart, and S. Hammar. 1996. Effects of a combination of beta carotene and vitamin A on lung cancer and cardiovascular disease. *New Engl. J. Med.* 334:1150–1155.

17. Druesne-Pecollo, N., P. Latino-Martel, T. Norat, E. Barrandon, S. Bertrais, P. Galan, and S. Hercberg. 2010. Beta-carotene supplementation and cancer risk: a systematic review and meta-analysis of randomized controlled trials. *Int. J. Cancer* 127(1):172–184.

18. Joshipura, K. J., F. B. Hu, J. E. Manson, M. J. Stampfer, E. B. Rimm, F. E. Speizer, G. Colditz, A. Ascherio, B. Rosner, D. Spiegelman, and W. C. Willett. 2001. The effect of fruit and vegetable intake on risk for coronary heart disease. *Ann. Intern. Med.* 134:1106–1114.

19. Liu, S., I.-M. Lee, U. Ajani, S. R. Cole, J. E. Buring, and J. E. Manson. 2001. Intake of vegetables rich in carotenoids and risk of coronary heart disease in men: The Physicians' Health Study. *Int. J. Epidemiol.* 30:130–135.

20. The Alpha-Tocopherol, Beta-Carotene Cancer Prevention Study Group (The ATBC Study Group). 1994. The effect of vitamin E and beta carotene on the incidence of lung cancer and other cancers in male smokers. *N. Engl. J. Med.* 330:1029–1035.

21. Lee, I. M., N. R. Cook, J. M. Gaziano, D. Gordon, P. M. Ridker, J. E. Manson, C. H. Hennekens, and J. E. Buring. 2005. Vitamin E in the primary prevention of cardiovascular disease and cancer: The Women's Health Study: A randomized controlled trial. *JAMA* 294(1):56–65.

22. Geleijnse, J. M., L. J. Launer, D. A. M. van der Kuip, A. Hofman, and J. C. M. Witteman. 2002. Inverse association of tea and flavonoid intakes with incident myocardial infarction: The Rotterdam Study. *Am. J. Clin. Nutr.* 75:880–886.

InDepth: Cancer

1. American Cancer Society. 2013. Cancer Facts & Figures 2013.

2. Kimball, J. W. 2013, April 19. Cancers become more common as one gets older. *Kimball's Biology Pages*.

3. Copstead, L., and J. Banasik. 2013. *Pathophysiology*, 5th edn. St. Louis, MO: Elsevier. p. 128.

4. American Cancer Society. 2013. ACS Guide to Quitting Smoking.

5. U.S. Department of Health and Human Services (USDHHS). 2004. *The Health Consequences of Smoking: A Report of the Surgeon General*. Washington, DC: U.S. Department of Health and Human Services, Centers for Disease Control and Prevention, National Center for Chronic Disease Prevention and Health Promotion, Office on Smoking and Health.

6. American Cancer Society. 2011. *Global Cancer Facts & Figures*, 2nd edn. Atlanta, GA: American Cancer Society.

7. World Cancer Research Fund/American Institute for Cancer Research (AICR). 2007. *Food, Nutrition, Physical Activity and the Prevention of Cancer: A Global Perspective*. Washington, DC: AICR.

8. Pfahlberg, A., K. F. Kolmel, and O. Gefeller. 2002. Adult vs. childhood susceptibility to melanoma. Is there a difference? *Arch. Dermatol.* 138:1234–1235.

9. National Cancer Institute. 2010. Tanning bed study shows best evidence yet of increased melanoma risk. *NCI Cancer Bulletin.* 7(11).

10. American Cancer Society. 2012. Signs and symptoms of cancer.

11. American Cancer Society. 2013. Stay healthy.

12. American Cancer Society. 2012. Stay healthy. Fitting in Fitness.

13. American Cancer Society. 2012. ACS Guidelines on Nutrition and Physical Activity for Cancer Prevention.

14. Shukla, S., and S. Gupta. 2010. Apigenin: a promising molecule for cancer prevention. *Pharm. Res.* 27(6):962–978.

15. Ohio State University. 2013, May 20. Compound in Mediterranean diet makes cancer cells 'mortal'. *ScienceDaily*.

16. Abdull Razis, A. F., and N. M. Noor. 2013. Cruciferous vegetables: dietary phytochemicals for cancer prevention. *Asian Pac. J. Cancer Prev.* 14(3):1565–1570.

Chapter 9

1. Zmuda, N. 2011. Bottoms up! A look at America's drinking habits. *AdvertisingAge*.

2. NIH Osteoporosis and Related Bone Diseases National Resource Center. 2012. Osteoporosis: peak bone mass in women.

3. Ho, A. Y. Y., and A. W. C. Kung. 2005. Determinants of peak bone mineral density and bone area in young women. *J. Bone Miner. Metab.* 23:470–475.

4. Chevalley, T., R. Rizzoli, D. Hans, S. Ferrari, and J. P. Bonjour. 2005. Interaction between calcium intake and menarcheal age on bone mass gain: an eight-year follow-up study from prepuberty to postmenarche. *J. Clin. Endocrinol. Metab.* 90:44–51.

5. Kindblom, J. M., M. Lorentzon, E. Norjavaara, A. Hellqvist, S. Nilsson, D. Mellström, and C. Ohlsson. 2006. Pubertal timing predicts previous fractures and BMD in young adult men: the GOOD study. *J. Bone Miner. Res.* 21:790–795.

6. Institute of Medicine, Food and Nutrition Board. 1997. *Dietary Reference Intakes for Calcium, Phosphorus, Magnesium, Vitamin D, and Fluoride*. Washington, DC: National Academies Press.

7. U.S. Department of Agriculture, Economic Research Service. 2008. Dietary assessment of major trends in U.S. food consumption, 1970–2005. *Economic Information Bulletin* No. EIB-33, 1–27.

8. U.S. Department of Health and Human Services, National Kidney and Urologic Diseases Information Clearinghouse. 2013. Diet for kidney stone formation. NIH Publication No. 13-6425.

9. Zemel, M. B., W. Thompson, A. Milstead, K. Morris, and P. Campbell. 2004. Calcium and dairy acceleration of weight and fat loss during energy restriction in obese adults. *Obes. Res.* 12:582–590.

10. Wagner, G., S. Kindrick, S. M. Hertzler, and R. A. DiSilvesto. 2007. Effects of various forms of calcium on body weight and bone turnover markers in women participating in a weight loss program. *J. Am. Coll. Nutr.* 26:456–461.

11. Major, G. C., F. Alarie, J. Dore, S. Phouttama, and A. Tremblay. 2007. Supplementation with calcium + vitamin D enhances the beneficial effect of weight loss on plasma lipid and lipoprotein concentrations. *Am. J. Clin. Nutr.* 85:54–59.

12. Witbracht, M. G., M. Van Loan, S. H. Adams, N. L. Keim, and K. D. Laugero. 2013. Dairy food consumption and meal-induced cortisol response interacted to influence weight loss in overweight women undergoing a 12-week, meal-controlled, weight loss intervention. *J. Nutr.* 143(1):46–52.

13. Institute of Medicine, Food and Nutrition Board. 2010. *Dietary Reference Intakes for Calcium and Vitamin D*. Washington, DC: National Academies Press.

14. Florez, H., R. Martinez, W. Chacra, N. Strickman-Stein, and S. Levis. 2007. Outdoor exercise reduces the risk of hypovitaminosis D in the obese. *J. Steroid Biochem. Mol. Biol.* 103:679–681.

15. Holick, M. F. 2005. The vitamin D epidemic and its health consequences. *J. Nutr.* 135:2739S–2748S.

16. Holick, M. F. 2007. Vitamin D deficiency. *N. Engl. J. Med.* 357:266–281.

17. Heaney, R. P. 2007. The case for improving vitamin D status. *J. Steroid Biochem. Mol. Biol.* 103:635–641.

18. Office of Dietary Supplements, National Institutes of Health. 2011. Dietary Supplement Fact Sheet: Vitamin D; and, Holick, M. F. 2006. Resurrection of vitamin D deficiency and rickets. *J. Clin. Invest.* 116:2062–2072.

19. Weisberg, P., K. S. Scanlon, R. Li, and M. E. Cogswell. 2004. Nutritional rickets among children in the United States: review of cases reported between 1986 and 2003. *Am. J. Clin. Nutr.* 80(suppl.):1697S–1705S.

20. Institute of Medicine, Food and Nutrition Board. 2002. *Dietary Reference Intakes for Vitamin A, Vitamin K, Arsenic, Boron, Chromium, Copper, Iodine, Iron, Manganese, Molybdenum, Nickel, Silicon, Vanadium, and Zinc.* Washington, DC: National Academies Press.

21. Fang, Y., C. Hu, X. Tao, Y. Wan, and F. Tao. 2012. Effect of vitamin K on bone mineral density: a meta-analysis of randomized controlled trials. *J. Bone Miner. Metab.* 30(1):60–68.

22. Briefel, R. R., and C. L. Johnson. 2004. Secular trends in dietary intake in the United States. *Ann. Rev. Nutr.* 24:401–431.

23. Wyshak, G., R. E. Frisch, T. E. Albright, N. L. Albright, I. Schiff, and J. Witschi. 1989. Nonalcoholic carbonated beverage consumption and bone fractures among women former college athletes. *J. Orthop. Res.* 7:91–99.

24. Wyshak, G., and R. E. Frisch. 1994. Carbonated beverages, dietary calcium, the dietary calcium/phosphorus ratio, and bone fractures in girls and boys. *J. Adolesc. Health* 15:210–215.

25. Wyshak, G. 2000. Teenaged girls, carbonated beverage consumption, and bone fractures. *Arch. Pediatr. Adolesc. Med.* 154:610–613.

26. Tucker, K. L., K. Morita, N. Qiao, M. T. Hannan, L. A. Cupples, and D. P. Kiel. 2006. Colas, but not other carbonated beverages, are associated with low bone mineral density in older women: The Framingham Osteoporosis Study. *Am. J. Clin. Nutr.* 84(4):936–942.

27. Fitzpatrick, L., and R. P. Heaney. 2003. Got soda? *J. Bone Miner. Res.* 18:1570–1572.

28. Rodríquez-Morán, M., and F. Guerrero-Romero. 2003. Oral magnesium supplementation improves insulin sensitivity and metabolic control in type 2 diabetic subjects. *Diab. Care* 26(4):1147–1152.

29. Larsson, S. C., L. Bergkvist, and A. Wolk. 2005. Magnesium intake in relation to risk of colorectal cancer in women. *JAMA* 293:86–89.

30. American Dietetic Association. 2005. Position of the American Dietetic Association: the impact of fluoride on health. *J. Am. Diet. Assoc.* 105:1620–1628.

31. U.S. Department of Health and Human Services. Public Health Service. 1991. Review of fluoride: benefits and risks. Report of the Ad Hoc Subcommittee on Fluoride of the Committee to Coordinate Environmental Health and Related Programs.

32. National Cancer Institute, National Institutes of Health. 2012. National Cancer Institute FactSheet. Fluoridated Water.

33. Centers for Disease Control and Prevention. 2012. Community water fluoridation: questions and answers.

34. Ginde, A. A., M. C. Liu, and C. A. Camargo, Jr. 2009. Demographic differences and trends of vitamin D insufficiency in the U.S. population, 1988-2004. *Arch. Intern. Med.* 169:626–632.

35. Weaver, C. M., and J. C. Fleet. 2004. Vitamin D requirements: current and future. *Am. J. Clin. Nutr.* 80(suppl):1735S–1739S.

36. Adams, J. S., and M. Hewison. 2010. Update on vitamin D. *J. Clin. Endocrinol. Metab.* 95:471–478.

37. Holick, M. F., N. C. Binkley, H. A. Bischoff-Ferrari, C. M. Gordon, D. A. Hanley, R. P. Heaney, M. Hassan Murad, and C. M. Weaver. 2011. Evaluation, treatment, and prevention of vitamin D deficiency: an Endocrine Society Clinical Practice Guideline. *J. Clin. Endocrinol. Metab.* 96:1911–1930.

38. Yetley, E. A., et al. 2009. Dietary Reference Intakes for Vitamin D: Justification for a review of the 1997 values. *Am. J. Clin. Nut.* 89:719–727.

39. Looker, A. C., C. M. Pfeiffer, D. A. Lacher, R. L. Schleicher, M. F. Picciano, and E. A. Yetley. 2008. Serum 25-hydroxyvitamin D status of the U.S. population: 1988–1994 compared with 2000–2004. *Am. J. Clin. Nutr.* 88:1519–1527.

40. Wolpowitz, D., and B. A. Gilchrest. 2006. The vitamin D questions: how much do we need and how should we get it? *J. Am. Acad. Dermatol.* 54(2):301–317.

41. Lucas, R. M., and A. L. Ponsonby. 2006. Considering the potential benefits as well as adverse effects of sun exposure: can all the potential benefits be provided by oral vitamin D supplementation? *Prog. Biophys. Mol. Biol.* 92:140–149.

42. Reichrath, J. 2006. The challenge resulting from positive and negative effects of sunlight: how much solar UV exposure is appropriate to balance between risks of vitamin D deficiency and skin cancer? *Prog. Biophys. Mol. Biol.* 92:9–16.

InDepth: Osteoporosis

1. National Osteoporosis Foundation. 2013. What is osteoporosis?

2. National Osteoporosis Foundation. 2013. Just for men.

3. Berg, K. M., H. V. Kunins, J. L. Jackson, S. Nahvi, A. Chaudhry, K. A. Harris Jr., R. Malik, and J. H. Arnsten. 2008. Association between alcohol consumption and bone osteoporotic fracture and bone density. *Am. J. Med.* 121(5):406–418.

4. Massey, L. K. 2001. Is caffeine a risk factor for bone loss in the elderly? *Am. J. Clin. Nutr.* 74:569–570.

5. Rapuri, P. B., J. C. Gallagher, H. K. Kinyamu, and K. L. Ryschon. 2001. Caffeine intake increases the rate of bone loss in elderly women and interacts with vitamin D receptor genotypes. *Am. J. Clin. Nutr.* 74:694–700.

6. New, S. A. 2004. Intake of fruit and vegetables: implications for bone health. *Proc. Nutr. Soc.* 62(4):889–899.

7. Prynne, C. J., G. D. Mishra, M. A. O'Connell, G. Muniz, M. A. Laskey, L. Yan, A. Prentice, and F. Ginty. 2006. Fruit and vegetable intakes and bone mineral status: a cross-sectional study in 5 age and sex cohorts. *Am. J. Clin. Nutr.* 83(6):1420–1428.

8. Dawson-Hughes, B., and S. S. Harris. 2002. Calcium intake influences the association of protein intake with rates of bone loss in elderly men and women. *Am. J. Clin. Nutr.* 75:773–779.

9. Moyer, V. A., on behalf of the U.S. Preventive Services Task Force. 2013. Vitamin D and calcium supplementation to prevent fractures in older adults: U.S. Preventive Services Task Force Recommendation Statement. *Ann. Intern. Med.* 158(9):691–696.

10. Langsetmo, L., C. Berger, N. Kreiger, C. S. Kovacs, D. A. Hanley, S. A. Jamal, S. J. Whiting, J. Genest, S. N. Morin, A. Hodsman, J. C. Prior, B. Lentle, M. S. Patel, J. P. Brown, T. Anastasiades, T. Towheed, R. G. Josse, A. Papaioannou, J. D. Adachi, W. D. Leslie, K. S. Davison, D. Goltzman; the CaMos Group. 2013. Calcium and vitamin D intake and mortality: results from the Canadian Multicentre Osteoporosis Study (CaMos). *J. Clin. Endocrinol. Metab.* doi: 10.1210/jc.2013-1516. [Epub ahead of print, May 23, 2013]

11. Nuti, R. 2012. Calcium supplementation and risk for cardiovascular disease. *Clin. Cases Miner. Bone Metab.* 9(3):133–134.

12. Reid, I. R. 2013. Osteoporosis treatment: focus on safety. *Eur. J. Intern. Med.* pii: S0953-6205(13)00096-4. doi: 10.1016/j.ejim.2013.03.012. [Epub ahead of print, April 19].

13. Teucher, B., J. R. Dainty, C. A. Spinks, G. Majsak-Newman, D. J. Berry, J. A. Hoogewerff, R. J. Foxall, J. Jakobsen, K. D. Cashman, A. Flynn, and S. J. Fairweather-Tait. 2008. Sodium and bone health: impact of moderately high and low salt intakes on calcium metabolism in postmenopausal women. *J. Bone Miner. Res.* 23(9):1477–1485.

14. Institute of Medicine, Food and Nutrition Board. 1997. *Dietary Reference Intakes for Calcium, Phosphorus, Magnesium, Vitamin D, and Fluoride.* Washington, DC: National Academies Press.

15. National Institute of Arthritis and Musculoskeletal and Skin Diseases. NIH Osteoporosis and Related Bone Diseases National Resource Center. 2012. Exercise for Your Bone Health.

16. Black, D. M., M. P. Kelly, H. K. Genant, L. Palermo, R. Eastell, C. Bucci-Rechweg, J. Cauley, P. C. Leung, S. Boonen, A. Santora, A. de Papp, and D. C. Bauer for the Fracture Intervention Trial and HORIZON Pivotal Fracture Trial Steering Committees. 2010. Bisphosphonates and fractures of the subtrochanteric or diaphyseal femur. *N. Engl. J. Med.* 362:1761–1777.

17. Schilcher, J., K. Michaëlsson, and P. Aspenberg. 2011. Bisphosphonate use and atypical fractures of the femoral shaft. *N. Engl. J. Med.* 364:1728–1737.

18. Writing Group for the Women's Health Initiative Investigators. 2002. Risks and benefits of estrogen plus progestin in healthy postmenopausal women. Principal results from the Women's Health Initiative randomized control trial. *JAMA* 288:321–332.

19. U.S. Preventive Services Task Force. 2012. Understanding task force recommendations. Menopausal hormone therapy for the primary prevention of chronic conditions.

20. Bischoff-Ferrari, H. A., W. C. Willett, J. B. Wong, A. E. Stuck, H. B. Staehelin, E. J. Orav, A. Thoma, D. P. Kiel, and J. Henschkowski. 2009. Prevention of nonvertabral fractures with oral vitamin D and dose dependency: a meta-analysis of randomized controlled trials. *Arch. Intern. Med.* 169:551–561.

21. National Institutes of Health, Office of Dietary Supplements. 2009. Dietary supplement fact sheet: vitamin D.

Chapter 10

1. Bernstein, L. 2000. Dementia without a cause: Lack of vitamin B_{12} can cause dementia. *Discover Magazine,* February 2000.

2. Bates, C. J. 2005. Thiamin. In: Bowman, B. A., and R. M. Russell, eds. *Present Knowledge in Nutrition,* 9th edn., pp. 242–249. Washington, DC: ILSI Press.

3. Bettendorff, L. 2012. Thiamin. In: Erdman, J. W., I. A. Macdonald, and S. H. Zeisel, eds. *Present Knowledge in Nutrition,* 10th edn., pp. 261–279. Washington, DC: ILSI Press.

4. McCollum, E. V. 1957. *A History of Nutrition.* Boston: Houghton Mifflin Co.

5. Institute of Medicine, Food and Nutrition Board. 1998. *Dietary Reference Intakes for Thiamin, Riboflavin, Niacin, Vitamin B_6, Folate, Vitamin B_{12}, Pantothenic Acid, Biotin, and Choline.* Washington, DC: National Academies Press.

6. McCormick, D. B. 2006. Riboflavin. Niacin, riboflavin, and thiamin. In: M. H. Stipanuk, ed. *Biological and Physiological Aspects of Human Nutrition,* 2nd edn. Philadelphia: W. B. Saunders.

7. McCormick, D. B. 2012. Riboflavin. In: Erdman, J. W., I. A. Macdonald, and S. H. Zeisel, eds. *Present Knowledge in Nutrition,* 10th edn., pp. 280–292. Washington, DC: ILSI Press.

8. Jacques, P. F., A. Taylor, S. Moeller, et al. 2005. Long-term nutrient intake and 5-year change in nuclear lens opacities. *Arch. Ophthalmol.* 123:517–526.

9. Rivlin, R. S. 2006. Riboflavin. In: Bowman, B. A., and R. M. Russel, eds. *Present Knowledge in Nutrition,* 9th edn., pp. 250–259. Washington, DC: ILSI Press.

10. Penberthy, W. T., and J. B. Kirkland. 2012. Niacin. In: Erdman, J. W., I. A. Macdonald, and S. H. Zeisel, eds. *Present Knowledge in Nutrition,* 10th edn., pp. 293–306. Washington, DC: ILSI Press.

11. Jacob, R. A. 2006. Niacin. In: Bowman, B. A., and R. M. Russel, eds. *Present Knowledge in Nutrition,* 9th edn., pp. 260–268. Washington, DC: ILSI Press.

12. Da Silva, V. R., K. A. Russel, and J. F. Gregory. 2012. Vitamin B_6. In: Erdman, J. W., I. A. Macdonald, and S. H. Zeisel, eds. *Present Knowledge in Nutrition,* 10th edn., pp. 307–320. Washington, DC: ILSI Press.

13. Mackey, A. D., S. R. Davis, and J. F. Gregory III. 2006. Vitamin B_6. In: Shils, M. E., M. Shike, A. C. Ross, B. Caballero, and R. Cousins, eds. *Modern Nutrition in Health and Disease,* 10th edn., pp. 452–261. Philadelphia: Lippincott Williams & Wilkins.

14. Joubert, L. M., and M.M. Manore. 2006. Exercise, nutrition and homocysteine. *Int. J. Sport Nutr. Exer. Metab.* 16:341–361.

15. Carmel, R. 2006. Folic acid. In: Shils, M. E., M. Shike, A. C. Ross, B. Caballero, and R. Cousins, eds. *Modern Nutrition in Health and Disease,* 10th edn., pp. 470–481. Philadelphia: Lippincott Williams & Wilkins.

16. Kim, Y. 2006. Does a high folate intake increase the risk of breast cancer? *Nutr. Rev.* 64(10):468–475.

17. Shane, B. 2006. Folic acid, vitamin B_{12} and vitamin B_6. In: Stipanuk, M. H., ed. *Biochemical, Physiological and Molecular Aspects of Human Nutrition,* pp 693–732. Philadelphia: W. B. Saunders.

18. Arbor Clinical Nutrition Updates. 2010, December. Can folate supplements be dangerous? Part 2. 327:1–5.

19. Connolly, M. 2001. Premenstrual syndrome: an update on definitions, diagnosis and management. *Advances in Psychiatric Treatment.* 7:469–477.

20. Kashanian, M., R. Mazinani, and S. Jalalmanesh. 2007. Pyridoxine (vitamin B_6) therapy for premenstrual syndrome. *Int. J. Gynaecol. Obstet.* 96(1):43–44.

21. Sánchez-Moreno, C., A. Jiménez-Escrig, and A. Martín. 2009. Stroke: roles of B vitamins, homocysteine and antioxidants. *Nutr. Res. Rev.* 2009;22(1):49–67.

22. Holligan, S. D., C. E. Berryman, L. Wang, M. R. Flock, K. A. Harris, and P. M. Kris-Etherton. 2012. Atherosclerotic cardiovascular disease. In: Erdman, J. W., I. A. Macdonald, and S. H. Zeisel, eds. *Present Knowledge in Nutrition,* 10th edn., pp. 745–805. Washington, DC: ILSI Press.

23. Huang, T. Y. Chen, B. Yang, J. Yang, M. L. Wahlqvist, and D. Li. 2012. Meta-analysis of B vitamin supplementation on plasma homocysteine, cardiovascular and all-cause mortality. *Clin. Nutr.* 31(4):448–454.

24. Stabler, S. P. 2012. Vitamin B_{12}. In: Erdman, J. W., I. A. Macdonald, and S. H. Zeisel, eds. *Present Knowledge in Nutrition,* 10th edn., pp. 343–358. Washington, DC: ILSI Press.

25. Carmel, R. 2006. Cobalamin (vitamin B_{12}). In: Shils, M. E., M. Shike, A. C. Ross, B. Caballero, and R. Cousins, eds. *Modern Nutrition in Health and Disease,* 10th edn., pp. 482–497. Philadelphia: Lippincott Williams & Wilkins.

26. Miller, J. W., and R. B. Rucker. 2013. Pantothenic acid. 2013. In: Erdman, J. W., I. A. Macdonald, and S. H. Zeisel, eds. *Present Knowledge in Nutrition,* 10th edn., pp. 375–390. Washington, DC: ILSI Press.

27. Kolata, Gina. April 24, 2013. Eggs, too, may provoke bacteria to raise heart risk. New York Times.

28. Tang, W. H. Wilson, Z. Wang, B. S. Levison, R. A. Koeth, E. B. Britt, X. Fu, Y. Wu, and S. L. Hazen. 2013. Intestinal microbial metabolism of phosphatidylcholine and cardiovascular risk. *New Eng. J. Med.* 368: 1575–1584.

29. Freake, H. C. 2006. Iodine. In: Stipanuk, M. H., ed. *Biochemical and Physiological Aspects of Human Nutrition,* 2nd edn., pp. 1068–1090. Philadelphia: W. B. Saunders.

30. World Health Organization. 2004. Nutrition. Micronutrient deficiencies. International Council of Control of Iodine Deficiency Disorders.

31. Institute of Medicine, Food and Nutrition Board. 2001. *Dietary Reference Intakes for Vitamin A, Vitamin K, Arsenic, Boron, Chromium, Copper, Iodine, Iron, Manganese, Molybdenum, Nickel, Silicon, Vanadium, and Zinc.* Washington, DC: National Academy Press.

32. Evans, G. W. 1989. The effect of chromium picolinate on insulin controlled parameters in humans. *Int. J. Biosoc. Med. Res.* 11:163–180.

33. Hasten, D. L., E. P. Rome, D. B. Franks, and M. Hegsted. 1992. Effects of chromium picolinate on beginning weight training students. *Int. J. Sports Nutr.* 2:343–350.

34. Lukaski, H. C., W. W. Bolonchuk, W. A. Siders, and D. B. Milne. 1996. Chromium supplementation and resistance training: effects on body composition, strength, and trace element status of men. *Am. J. Clin. Nutr.* 63:954–965.

35. Hallmark, M. A., T. H. Reynolds, C. A. DeSouza, C. O. Dotson, R. A. Anderson, and M. A. Rogers. 1996. Effects of chromium and resistive training on muscle strength and body composition. *Med. Sci. Sports Exerc.* 28:139–144.

36. Pasman, W. J., M. S. Westerterp-Plantenga, and W. H. Saris. 1997. The effectiveness of long-term supplementation of carbohydrate, chromium, fibre and caffeine on weight maintenance. *Int. J. Obes. Relat. Metab. Disord.* 21:1143–1151.

37. Walker, L. S., M. G. Bemben, D. A. Bemben, and A. W. Knehans. 1998. Chromium picolinate effects on body composition and muscular performance in wrestlers. *Med. Sci. Sports Exerc.* 30:1730–1737.

38. Campbell, W. W., L. J. Joseph, S. L. Davey, D. Cyr-Campbell, R. A. Anderson, and W. J. Evans. 1999. Effects of resistance training and chromium picolinate on body composition and skeletal muscle in older men. *J. Appl. Physiol.* 86:29–39.

39. Volpe, S. L., H. W. Huang, K. Larpadisorn, and I. I. Lesser. 2001. Effect of chromium supplementation and exercise on body composition, resting metabolic rate and selected biochemical parameters in moderately obese women following an exercise program. *J. Am. Coll. Nutr.* 20:293–306.

40. Campbell, W. W., L. J. O. Joseph, R. A. Anderson, S. L. Davey, J. Hinton, and W. J. Evans. 2002. Effects of resistive training and chromium picolinate on body composition and skeletal muscle size in older women. *Int. J. Sports Nutr. Exerc. Metab.* 12:125–135.

41. Lukaski H. C., W. A. Siders, and J. G. Penland. 2007. Chromium picolinate supplementation in women: effects on body weight, composition and iron status. *Nutrition* 23:187–195.

42. Diaz, M. L., B. A. Watkins, Y. Li, R. A. Anderson, and W. W. Campbell. 2008. Chromium picolinate and conjugated linoleic acid do not synergistically influence diet- and exercise-induced changes in body composition and health indexes in overweight women. *J. Nutr. Biochem.* 19:61–68.

43. Arbor Nutrition Clinical Nutrition Updates. 2007. October. Chromium, body building and weight loss. 284:1–3.

44. Ferland, G. 2012. Vitamin K. In: Erdman, J. W., I A. Macdonald, and S. H. Zeisel, eds. *Present Knowledge in Nutrition*, 10th edn., pp. 230–247. Washington, DC: ILSI Press.

45. World Health Organization. 2012. Nutrition. Micronutrient deficiencies: iron deficiency anemia.

46. Aggett, P. J. 2012. Iron. In: Erdman, J. W., I. A. Macdonald, and S. H. Zeisel, eds. *Present Knowledge in Nutrition*, 10th edn., pp. 506–520. Washington, DC: ILSI Press.

47. Sharp, P. A. 2010. Intestinal iron absorption: regulation by dietary and systemic factors. *Int. J. Vitam. Nutr. Res.* 80(4–5):231–242.

48. Spanierman, C. S. 2011. Iron toxicity in emergency medicine. Medscape Reference. Drugs, Disease and Procedures.

49. Duchini, A. 2011. Hemochromatosis. Medscape Reference. Drugs, Disease and Procedures.

50. Milman, N. 2012. Postpartum anemia II: prevention and treatment. *Ann. Hematol.* 91(2):143–154. PubMed PMID: PMID: 22160256. English.

51. Center for Disease Control and Prevention (CDC). 2013. Common colds: protect yourself and others.

52. National Institute of Allergy and Infectious Diseases, National Institutes of Health. 2012. The common cold.

53. Singh, M., and R. R. Das. 2011a. Zinc for the common cold. Cochrane Database Syst. Rev. Issue 2. Art. No. Cd001364, DOI:10.1002/14651858.

54. Prasad, A. 1996. Zinc: the biology and therapeutics of an ion. *Ann. Intern. Med.* 125:142–143.

55. Jackson, J. L., E. Lesho, and C. Peterson. 2000. Zinc and the common cold: A meta-analysis revisited. *J. Nutr.* 130:1512S–1515S.

56. Singh, M., and R. R. Das. 2011b. Clinic potential of zinc in prophylaxis of the common cold. *Expert Rev. Respir. Med.* 5(3):301–303.

57. Hemila, H. 2011. Zinc lozenges may shorten the duration of colds: a systemic review. *Open Respir. Med. J.* 5:51–58.

InDepth: Dietary Supplements: Necessity or Waste?

1. *Nutrition Business Journal.* 2012. Considering a post-DSHEA world. 17:1–9.

2. Bailey, R. L., J. J. Gahche, C. V. Lentino, J. T. Dwyer, J. S. Engel, P. R. Thomas, et al. 2011. Dietary supplement use in the United States, 2003-2006. *J. Nutr.* 141(2):261–266.

3. Bailey, R. L., J. J. Gahche, P. E. Miller, P. R. Thomas, and J. T. Dwyer. 2013. Why US adults use dietary supplements. *JAMA* 173(5):355–361.

4. U.S. Food and Drug Administration (FDA). Center for Food Safety and Applied Nutrition. 2008. FDA 101: dietary supplements.

5. U.S. Food and Drug Administration (FDA). Center for Food Safety and Applied Nutrition. 2013. 6 tip-offs to rip-offs: don't fall for health fraud scams.

6. National Center for Complementary and Alternative Medicine (NCCAM). 2010. Using dietary supplements wisely.

7. U.S. Government Accountability Office. 2010. Herbal dietary supplements: examples of deceptive or questionable marketing practices and potentially dangerous advice. May 26, 2010. GAO-10_662T.

8. National Institutes of Health. 2012. Important information to know when you are taking Coumadine and Vitamin K.

9. Marra, M. V., and A. P. Boyar. 2009. Position of the American Dietetic Association: nutrient supplementation. *J. Am. Diet. Assoc.* 109(12):2073–2085.

Chapter 11

1. 60 Minutes Overtime Staff. 2012, February 12. Adele talks about her body image and weight. *CBS News.*

2. Manore, M. M., N. L. Meyer, and J. L. Thompson. 2009. *Sport Nutrition for Health and Performance*, 2nd edn. Champaign, IL: Human Kinetics.

3. Flegal, K. M., B. K. Kit, H. Orpana, and B. I. Graubard. 2013. Association of all-cause mortality with overweight and obesity using standard body mass index categories. A systematic review and meta-analysis. *JAMA* 309(1):71–82.

4. Willett, W. C., F. B. Hu, and M. Thun. 2013. Letters. Overweight, obesity and all-cause mortality. *JAMA* 309(16):1681–1682.

5. Hughes, V. 2013. The big fat truth. *Nature* 497:428–430.

6. Wang, Y. 2004. Epidemiology of childhood obesity—methodological aspects and guidelines: What is new? *Int. J. Obes.* 23:S21–S28.

7. Shai, I., R. Jiang, J. E. Manson, M. J. Stampfer, W. C. Willett, G. A. Colditz, and F. B. Hu. 2006. Ethnicity, obesity, and risk of type 2 diabetes in women. *Diab. Care* 29:1585–1590.

8. Galgani, J., and E. Ravussin. 2008. Energy metabolism, fuel selection and body weight regulation. *Int. J. Obes.* 32:S109–S119.

9. Stunkard, A. J., T. I. A. Sørensen, C. Hanis, T. W. Teasdale, R. Chakraborty, W. J. Schull, and F. Schulsinger. 1986. An adoption study of human obesity. *N. Engl. J. Med.* 314:193–198.

10. Bouchard, C. 2010. Defining the genetic architecture of the predisposition to obesity: a challenging but not insurmountable task. *Am. J. Clin. Nutr.* 91:5–6.

11. Bloss, C. S., N. J. Stork, and E. J. Topol. 2011. Effect of direct-to-consumer genomewide profiling to assess disease risk. *N. Engl. J. Med.* 364(6):524–534.

12. Razquin, C., A. Marti, and J. A. Martinez. 2011. Evidences on three relevant obesogenes: MC4R, FTO, and PPARY. *Mol. Nutr. Food Res.* 55(1):136–149.

13. Kilpeläinen, T. O., L. Qi, S. Brage, S. J. Sharp, E. Sonestedt, E. Demerath, . . . R. J. Loos. 2011. Physical activity attenuates the influence of FTO variants on obesity risk: a meta-analysis of 218,166 adults and 19,268 children. *PLoS Med.* 8(11):e1001116. [Epub November 1, 2011]

14. Bouchard, C., A. Tremblay, J. P. Després, A. Nadeau, P. J. Lupien, G. Thériault, . . . G. Fournier. 1990. The response to long-term overfeeding in identical twins. *N. Engl. J. Med.* 322:1477–1482.

15. Sumithran, P., L. A. Prendergast, E. Delbridge, K. Purcell, A. Shulkes, A. Kriketos, and J. Proietto. 2011. Long-term persistence of hormonal adaptations to weight loss. *N. Engl. J. Med.* 365:1597–1604.

16. Druce, M. R., A. M. Wren, A. J. Park, J. E. Milton, M. Patterson, G. Frost, M. A. Ghatei, C. Small, and S. R. Bloom. 2005. Ghrelin increases food intake in obese as well as lean subjects. *Int. J. Obes.* 29:1130–1136.

17. Suzuki, K., C. N. Jayasena, and S. R. Bloom. 2011. The gut hormones in appetite regulation. *J. Obes.* doi: 10.1155/2011/528401.

18. Virtanen, K. A., M. E. Lidell, J. Orava, M. Heglind, R. Westergren, T. Niemi, M. Taittonen, J. Laine, N-J. Savito, S. Enerbäck, and P. Nuutila. 2009. Functional brown adipose tissue in healthy adults. *N. Engl. J. Med.* 360(15):1518–1525.

19. Cypess, A. M., S. Lehman, G. Williams, I. Tal, D. Rodman, A. B. Goldfine, F. C. Kuo, E. L. Palmer, Y-H. Tseng, A. Doria, G. M. Kolodny, and C. R. Kahn. 2009. Identification and importance of brown adipose tissue in adult humans. *N. Engl. J. Med.* 360(15):1509–1517.

20. Eyler, A. E., D. Matson-Koffman, D. Rohm-Young, S. Wilcox, J. Wilbur, J. L. Thompson, B. Sanderson, and K. R. Evenson. 2003. Quantitative study of correlates of physical activity in women from

diverse racial/ethnic groups: The Women's Cardiovascular Health Network Project. *Am. J. Prev. Med.* 25(3Si):93–103.

21. Eyler, A. E., D. Matson-Koffman, J. R. Vest, K. R. Evenson, B. Sanderson, J. L. Thompson, J. Wilbur, S. Wilcox, and D. Rohm-Young. 2002. Environmental, policy, and cultural factors related to physical activity in a diverse sample of women: The Women's Cardiovascular Health Network Project—Summary and Discussion. *Women and Health* 36:123–134.

22. Black, J. L., and J. Macinko. (2008). Neighborhoods and obesity. *Nutr. Rev.* 66 (1), 2–20.

23. Ding, D., T. Sugiyama, and N. Owen. 2012. Habitual active transport, TV viewing and weight gain: a four-year follow-up study. *Prev. Med.* 54:201–204.

24. Lumeng, J. C., P. Forrest, D. P. Appugliese, N. Kaciroti, R. F. Corwyn, and R. H. Bradley. 2010. Weight status as a predictor of being bullied in third through sixth grades. *Pediatrics* 125(6):1301–1307.

25. Academy of Nutrition and Dietetics. 2012. Tip of the day. say no to the dangers of fad diets.

26. Prentice, R. L., B. Caan, R. T. Chlebowski, R. Patterson, L. H. Kuller, J. K. Ockene, . . . M. Henderson. 2006. Low-fat dietary pattern and risk of invasive breast cancer: the Women's Health Initiative Randomized Controlled Dietary Modification Trial. *JAMA* 295:629–642.

27. Beresford, S. A., K. C. Johnson, C. Ritenbaugh, N. L. Lasser, L. G. Snetselaar, H. R. Black, . . . E. Whitlock. 2006. Low-fat dietary pattern and risk of colorectal cancer: the Women's Health Initiative Randomized Controlled Dietary Modification Trial. *JAMA* 295:643–654.

28. Howard, B. V., L. Van Horn, J. Hsia, J. E. Manson, M. L. Stefanick, S. Wassertheil-Smoller, J. M. Kotchen. 2006. Low-fat dietary pattern and risk of cardiovascular disease: the Women's Health Initiative Randomized Controlled Dietary Modification Trial. *JAMA* 295:655–666.

29. Howard, B. V., J. E. Manson, M. L. Stefanick, S. A. Beresford, G. Frank, B. Jones, R. Prentice. 2006. Low-fat dietary pattern and weight change over 7 years: the Women's Health Initiative Dietary Modification Trial. *JAMA* 295:39–49.

30. Hession, M., C. Rolland, U. Kulkarni, A. Wise, and J. Broom. 2009. Systematic review of randomized controlled trials of low-carbohydrate vs. low-fat/low-calorie diets in the management of obesity and its co-morbidities. *Obes. Rev.* 10(1):36–50.

31. Ello-Martin, J. A., J. H. Ledikwe, and B. J. Rolls. 2005. The influence of food portion size and energy density on energy intake: implications for weight management. *Am. J. Clin. Nutr.* 82(suppl.):236S–241S.

32. Flood, J. E., L. S. Roe, and B. J. Rolls. 2006. The effect of increased beverage portion size on energy intake at a meal. *J. Am. Diet. Assoc.* 106:1984–1990.

33. Ello-Martin, J. A., L. S. Roe, J. H. Ledikwe, A. M. Beach, and B. J. Rolls. 2007. Dietary energy density in the treatment of obesity: a year-long trial comparing 2 weight-loss diets. *Am. J. Clin. Nutr.* 85(6):1465–1477.

34. Rolls, B. J., L. S. Roe, and J. S. Meengs. 2006. Reductions in portion size and energy density of foods are additive and lead to sustained decreases in energy intake. *Am. J. Clin. Nutr.* 83(1):11–17.

35. Wing, R. R., and S. Phelan. 2005. Long-term weight loss maintenance. *Am. J. Clin. Nutr.* 82(suppl):222S–225S.

36. American College of Sports Medicine, American Dietetic Association, and Dietitians of Canada. 2009. Nutrition and athletic performance. Joint Position Stand. *Med. Sci. Sports Exerc.* 41(3):709–731.

37. Ogden, C. L., M. D. Carroll, B. K. Kitt, and K. M. Flegal. 2012. Prevalence of obesity in the United States, 2009-10. NCHS Data Brief No. 82.

38. Grundy, S. M., B. Hansen, S. C. Smith, J. I. Cleeman, and R. A. Kahn. 2004. Clinical management of metabolic syndrome: Report of the American Heart Association/National Heart, Lung, and Blood Institute/American Diabetes Association Conference on Scientific Issues Related to Management. *Circulation* 109:551–556.

39. MyHealthyWaist.org. 2011. The Concept of CMR.

40. Agency for Healthcare Research and Quality, National Guideline Clearinghouse. 2011. Cardiometabolic risk management in primary care.

41. Ervin, R. B. 2009. Prevalence of metabolic syndrome among adults 20 years of age and over, by sex, age, race and ethnicity, and body mass index: United States, 2003-2006. *Nat. Health Stat. Rep.* 13:1–4.

42. National Institute of Diabetes and Digestive and Kidney Diseases. Weight-control Information Network. 2012. Understanding adult obesity. NIH Publication No. 06-3680.

43. Bibbins-Domingo, K., P. Coxson, M. J. Pletcher, J. Lightwood, and L. Goldman. 2007. Adolescent overweight and future adult coronary heart disease. *N. Engl. J. Med.* 357:2371–2379.

44. Christakis, N. A., and J. H. Fowler. 2007. The spread of obesity in a large social network over 32 years. *N. Engl. J. Med.* 357(4):370–379.

45. Institute of Medicine, Food and Nutrition Board. 2002. *Dietary Reference Intakes for Energy, Carbohydrate, Fiber, Fat, Fatty Acids, Cholesterol, Protein, and Amino Acids (Macronutrients).* Washington, DC: The National Academies Press.

46. Mayo Clinic. 2013. Weight loss. Prescription drugs: can they help you?

47. Saper, R. B., D. M. Eisenberg, and R. S. Phillips. 2004. Common dietary supplements for weight loss. *Am. Fam. Phys.* 70(9):1731–1738.

48. Blanck, H. M., M. K. Serdula, C. Gillespie, D. A. Galuska, P. A. Sharpe, J. M. Conway, L. K. Khan, and B. E. Ainsworth. 2007. Use of nonprescription dietary supplements for weight loss is common among Americans. *J. Am. Diet. Assoc.* 107(3):441–447.

49. Padwal, R., S. Klarenbach, N. Wiebe, D. Birch, S. Karmali, B. Manns, M. Hazel, A. M. Sharma, and M. Tonelli. 2011. Bariatric surgery: a systematic review and network meta-analysis of randomized trials. *Obes. Rev.* 12:602–621.

50. Buchwald, H., R. Estok, K. Fahrbach, D. Banel, M. D. Jensen, W. J. Pories, J. P. Bantle, and I. Sledge. Weight and type 2 diabetes after bariatric surgery: systematic review and meta-analysis. *Am. J. Med.* 122(3):248–256.

51. Sjöström, L., A-K. Lindroos, M. Peltonen, J. Torgerson, C. Bouchard, B. Carlsson, S. Dahlgren, B. Larsson, K. Narbro, C. D. Sjöström, M. Sullivan, and H. Wedel. 2004. Lifestyle, diabetes, and cardiovascular risk factors 10 years after bariatric surgery. *N. Engl. J. Med.* 351(26):2683–2693.

52. Howard, B. V., L. Van Horn, J. Hsia, J. E. Manson, M. L. Stefanick, S. Wassertheil-Smoller, . . . J. M. Kotchen. 2006. Low-fat dietary pattern and risk of cardiovascular disease. The Women's Health Initiative Randomized Controlled Dietary Modification Trial. *JAMA* 295(6):655–666.

53. Prentice, R. L., B. Caan, R. T. Chlebowski, R. Patterson, L. H. Kuller, J. K. Ockene, M. M. Henderson. 2006. Low-fat dietary pattern and risk of invasive breast cancer. The Women's Health Initiative Randomized Controlled Dietary Modification Trial. *JAMA* 295(6):629–642.

54. Beresford, S. A. A., K. C. Johnson, C. Ritenbaugh, N. L. Lasser, L. G. Snetselaar, H. R. Black, E. Whitlock. 2006. Low-fat dietary pattern and risk of colorectal cancer. The Women's Health Initiative Randomized Controlled Dietary Modification Trial. *JAMA* 295(6):643–654.

55. Howard, B. V., J. E. Manson, M. L. Stefanick, S. A. Beresford, G. Frank, B. Jones, R. Prentice. 2006. Low-fat dietary pattern and weight change over 7 years. The Women's Health Initiative Randomized Controlled Dietary Modification Trial. *JAMA* 295(6):39–49.

56. Harvard School of Public Health. 2012. Low-fat diet not a cure-all. *The Nutrition Source.*

InDepth: Disordered Eating

1. American Psychiatric Association. 2013. *Diagnostic and Statistical Manual of Mental Disorders, 5th Edition, DSM-5.* Washington, DC: American Psychiatric Association.

2. Grave, R. D. 2011. Eating disorders: Progress and challenges. *Eur. J. Intern. Med.* 22:153–160.

3. Treasure, J., A. M. Claudino, and N. Zucker. 2010. Eating disorders. *Lancet* 375:583–593.

4. Treasure, J., A. R. Sepulved, P. MacDonald, W. Whitaker, C. Lopez, M. Zabala, O. Kyracou, and G. Todd. 2008. The assessment of the family of people with eating disorders. *Eur. Eat. Disord. Rev.* 16:247–255.

5. Strasburger, V. C., A. B. Jordan, and E. Donnerstein. 2010. Health effects of media on children and adolescents. *Pediatrics* 125(4):756–767.

6. Hogan, M. J., and V. C. Strasburger. 2008. Body image, eating disorders, and the media. *Adolesc. Med. State Art Rev.* 19(3):521–546.

7. Stice, E. 2002. Sociocultural influences on body image and eating disturbances. In: Fairburn, D. G., and K. D. Brownell, eds. *Eating Disorders and Obesity: A Comprehensive Handbook,* 2nd edn. New York: Guilford Press. pp. 103–107.

8. Costa-Font, J., and M. Jofre-Bonet. 2011, November. Anorexia, body image, and peer effects: evidence from a sample of European women. *Centre for Economic Performance*: CEP Discussion Paper No. 1098.

9. Keel, P. K., T. A. Brown, L. A. Holland, and L. D., Bodell. 2012. Empirical classification of eating disorders. *Annu. Rev. Clin. Psychol.* 8:381–404.

10. Wonderlich, S. A. 2002. Personality and eating disorders. In: Fairburn, D. G., and K. D. Brownell, eds. *Eating Disorders and Obesity: A Comprehensive Handbook,* 2nd edn. New York: Guilford Press. pp. 204–209.

11. U.S. Department of Human Services, Office of Women's Health. 2009. Anorexia nervosa.

12. National Association of Anorexia Nervosa and Associated Disorders. 2012. Eating disorder statistics.

13. *Diagnostic and Statistical Manual of Mental Disorders, Fifth Edition, DSM-5,* © 2013 American Psychiatric Association.

14. Robb, A. S., and M. J. Dadson. 2002. Eating disorders in males. *Child Adolesc. Psychiatric. Clin. N. Am.* 11:399–418.

15. Beals, K. A. 2004. *Disordered Eating in Athletes: A Comprehensive Guide for Health Professionals.* Champaign, IL: Human Kinetics.

16. Weltzin, T. E. 2013. A silent problem: males with eating disorders in the workplace. National Association of Anorexia Nervosa and Associated Disorders.

17. Murray, S. B., E. Rieger, S. W. Touyz, and Y. de la Garza Garcia. 2010. Muscle dysmorphia and the DSM-V conundrum: where does it belong? A review paper. *Int. J. Eat. Disord.* 43(6):483–491.

18. *Diagnostic and Statistical Manual of Mental Disorders, Fifth Edition, DSM-5,* © 2013 American Psychiatric Association.

19. National Institutes of Health. 2011. Eating disorders.

20. Grilo, C. M. 2002. Binge eating disorder. In: Fairburn, D. G., and K. D. Brownell, eds. *Eating Disorders and Obesity: A Comprehensive Handbook,* 2nd edn. New York: Guilford Press. pp.178–182.

21. Vander Wal, J. S. 2012. Night eating syndrome: a critical review of the literature. *Clin. Psychol. Rev.* 32:49–59.

22. Gallant, A. R., J. Lundgren, and V. Drapeau. 2012. The night-eating syndrome and obesity. *Obes. Rev.* 13:528–536.

23. Nattiv, A., A. B. Loucks, M. M. Manore, C. F. Sanborn, J. Sundgot-Borgen, and M. P. Warren. 2007. The female athlete triad. *Med. Sci. Sport Exerc.* 39(10):1867–1882.

24. Reiter, S. C., and L. Graves. 2010. Nutrition therapy for eating disorders. *Nutr. Clin. Pract.*25:122–136.

25. National Eating Disorders Association. 2013.What should I say? Tips for talking to a friend who may be struggling with an eating disorder.

Chapter 12

1. U.S. Department of Health and Human Services. 1996. *Physical Activity and Health: A Report of the Surgeon General.* Atlanta, GA: U.S. Department of Health and Human Services, Centers for Disease Control and Prevention, National Centers for Chronic Disease Prevention and Health Promotion.

2. Caspersen, C. J., K. E. Powell, and G. M. Christensen. 1985. Physical activity, exercise, and physical fitness: definitions and distinctions for health-related research. *Public Health Rep.* 100:126–131.

3. Heyward, V. H. 2010. *Advanced Fitness Assessment and Exercise Prescription*, 6th edn. Champaign, IL: Human Kinetics.

4. National Center for Health Statistics. 2012. *Health, United States, 2011: With Special Feature on Socioeconomic Status and Health.* Hyattsville, MD: National Center for Health Statistics.

5. Centers for Disease Control and Prevention. 2008. 1988–2007 No leisure-time physical activity trend chart.

6. Centers for Disease Control and Prevention. 2012. Youth risk behavior surveillance – United States, 2011. *Morb. Mortal.Wkly Rep.* 61:SS-4.

7. United States Department of Health and Human Services. 2009. 2008 physical activity guidelines for Americans.

8. Institute of Medicine, Food and Nutrition Board. 2002. *Dietary Reference Intakes for Energy, Carbohydrates, Fiber, Fat, Protein and Amino Acids (Macronutrients).* Washington, DC: The National Academy of Sciences.

9. Ryan, R. M., C. M. Frederick, D. Lepes, N. Rubio, and K. M. Sheldon. 1997. Intrinsic motivation and exercise adherence. *Int. J. Sport Psychol.* 28:335–354.

10. Buckworth, J., R. E. Lee, G. Regan, L. K. Schneider, and C. C. DeClemente. 2007. Decomposing intrinsic and extrinsic motivation for exercise: application to stages of motivational readiness. *Psychol. Sport Exerc.* 8(4):441–461.

11. Centers for Disease Control and Prevention. 2011. Physical activity for everyone. Target heart rate and estimated maximum heart rate.

12. Westerblad, H., D. G. Allen, and J. Lännergren. 2002. Muscle fatigue: lactic acid or inorganic phosphate the major cause? *News Physiol. Sci.* 17(1):17–21.

13. Brooks, G., T. Fahey, and K. Baldwin. 2005. *Exercise Physiology: Human Bioenergetics and Its Applications.* New York: McGraw-Hill.

14. Brooks, G. A. 2009. Cell-cell and intracellular lactate shuttles. *J. Physiol.* 587(23):5591–5600.

15. van Hall, G., M. Stromstad, P. Rasmussen, O. Jans, M. Zaar, C. Gam, B. Quistorff, N. H. Secher, and H. B. Nielsen. 2009. Blood lactate is an important energy source for the human brain. *J. Cerebral Blood Flow & Metab.* 29(6):1121–1129.

16. Gibala, M. J., and S. L. McGee. 2008. Metabolic adaptations to short-term high-intensity interval training: a little pain for a lot of gain? *Exerc. Sport Sci. Rev.* 36(2):58–63.

17. American College of Sports Medicine, American Dietetic Association, and Dietitians of Canada. 2009. Nutrition and athletic performance. Joint position statement. *Med. Sci. Sports Exerc.* 41:709–731.

18. Burke, L. 2010. Nutrition for recovery after training and competition. In: Burke, L., and V. Deakin, eds. *Clinical Sports Nutrition*, 4th edn. Sydney, Australia: McGraw-Hill. pp. 358–392.

19. van Hall, G., S. M. Shirreffs, and J. A. L. Calbert. 2000. Muscle glycogen resynthesis during recovery from cycle exercise: no effect of additional protein ingestion. *J. Appl. Physiol.* 88:1631–1636.

20. Jentjens, R. L., L. J. C. van Loon, C. H. Mann, A. J. M. Wagenmakers, and A. E. Jeukendrup. 2001. Addition of protein and amino acids to carbohydrates does not enhance postexercise muscle glycogen synthesis. *J. Appl. Physiol.* 91:839–846.

21. Phillips, S. M., and L. J. C. van Loon. 2011. Dietary protein for athletes: from requirements to optimum adaptation. *J. Sports Sci.* 29(S1):S29–S38.

22. Manore, M., N. L. Meyer, and J. Thompson. 2009. *Sports Nutrition for Health and Performance*, 2nd edn. Champaign, IL: Human Kinetics. p. 117.

23. Sears, B. 1995. *The Zone: A Dietary Road Map.* New York: HarperCollins.

24. Sinclair, L. M., and P. S. Hinton. 2005. Prevalence of iron deficiency with and without anemia in recreationally active men and women. *J. Am. Diet. Assoc.* 105(6):975–978.

InDepth: Do Active People Need Ergogenic Aids?

1. Heneghan, C., J. Howick, B. O'Neill, P. J. Gill, D. S. Lasserson, D. Cohen, R. Davis, A. Ward, A. Smith, G. Jones, and M. Thompson. 2012. The evidence underpinning sports performance products: a systematic assessment. *BMJ Open* 2:e001702. doi:10.1136/bmjopen-2012-001702

2. U.S. Department of Health and Human Services (HHS). 2004. News release. HHS launches crackdown on products containing andro.

3. Broeder, C. E., J. Quindry, K. Brittingham, L. Panton, J. Thomson, S. Appakondu, K. Breuel, R. Byrd, J. Douglas, C. Earnest, C. Mitchell, M. Olson, T. Roy, and C. Yarlagadda. 2000. The Andro Project: Physiological and hormonal influences of androstenedione supplementation in men 35 to 65 years old participating in a high-intensity resistance training program. *Arch. Intern. Med.* 160:3093–3104.

4. Tarnopolsky, M. A. 2010. Caffeine and creatine use in sport. *Ann. Nutr. Metab.* 57(suppl 2):1–8.

5. Reuters. 2001. Creatine use could lead to cancer, French government reports. *New York Times,* January 25.

6. Jeong, K. S., S. J. Park, C. S. Lee, T. W. Kim, S. H. Kim, S. Y. Ryu, B. H. Williams, R. L. Veech, and Y. S. Lee. 2000. Effects of cyclocreatine in rat hepatocarcinogenesis model. *Anticancer Res.* 20(3A):1627–1633.

7. Ara, G., L. M. Gravelin, R. Kaddurah-Daouk, and B. A. Teicher. 1998. Antitumor activity of creatine analogs produced by alterations in pancreatic hormones and glucose metabolism. *In Vivo* 12:223–231.

8. Manore, M. M., N. L. Meyer, and J. L. Thompson. 2009. *Sports Nutrition for Health and Performance,* 2nd edn. Champaign, IL: Human Kinetics.

9. Finn, K. J., R. Lund, and M. Rosene-Treadwell. 2003. Glutamine supplementation did not benefit athletes during short-term weight reduction. *J. Sports Sci. Med.* 2:163–168.

10. Campbell, B. I., P. M. La Bounty, and M. Roberts. 2004. The ergogenic potential of arginine. *J. Int. Soc. Sports Nutr.* 1(2):35–38.

11. Anderson, M. E., C. R. Bruce, S. F. Fraser, N. K. Stepto, R. Klein, W. G. Hopkins, and J. A. Hawley. 2000. Improved 2000-meter rowing performance in competitive oarswomen after caffeine ingestion. *Int. J. Sport Nutr. Exerc. Metab.* 10:464–475.

12. Spriet, L. L., and R. A. Howlett. 2000. Caffeine. In: Maughan, R. J., ed. *Nutrition in Sport.* Oxford: Blackwell Science. pp. 379–392.

13. Seifert, S. M., J. L. Schaechter, E. R. Hershorin, and S. E. Lipshultz. 2011. Health effects of energy drinks on children, adolescents, and young adults. *Pediatrics* 127(3):511–528.

14. Bucci, L. 2000. Selected herbals and human exercise performance. *Am. J. Clin. Nutr.* 72:624S–636S.

15. Hawley, J. A. 2002. Effect of increased fat availability on metabolism and exercise capacity. *Med. Sci. Sports Exerc.* 34(9):1485–1491.

16. Vincent, J. B. 2003. The potential value and toxicity of chromium picolinate as a nutritional supplement, weight loss agent and muscle development agent. *Sports Med.* 33(3):213–230.

17. Pliml, W., T. von Arnim, A. Stablein, H. Hofmann, H. G. Zimmer, and E. Erdmann. 1992. Effects of ribose on exercise-induced ischaemia in stable coronary artery disease. *Lancet* 340(8818):507–510.

18. Earnest, C. P., G. M. Morss, F. Wyatt, A. N. Jordan, S. Colson, T. S. Church, Y. Fitzgerald, L. Autrey, R. Jurca, and A. Lucia. 2004. Effects of a commercial herbal-based formula on exercise performance in cyclists. *Med. Sci. Sports Exerc.* 36(3):504–509.

19. Hellsten, Y., L. Skadhauge, and J. Bangsbo. 2004. Effect of ribose supplementation on resynthesis of adenine nucleotides after intense intermittent training in humans. *Am. J. Physiol. Regul. Integr. Comp. Physiol.* 286:R182–R188.

20. Kreider, R. B., C. Melton, M. Greenwood, C. Rasmussen, J. Lundberg, C. Earnest, and A. Almada. 2003. Effects of oral D-ribose supplementation on anaerobic capacity and selected metabolic markers in healthy males. *Int. J. Sport Nutr. Exerc. Metab.* 13(1):76–86.

21. Artioli, G. G., B. Gualano, A. Smith, J. Stout, and A. H. Lancha, Jr. 2010. Role of β-alanine supplementation on muscle carnosine and exercise performance. *Med. Sci. Sports Exerc.* 42(6):1162–1173.

22. Derave, W., I. Everaert, S. Beeckman, and A. Baguet. 2010. Muscle carnosine metabolism and β-alanine supplementation in relation to exercise and training. *Sports Med.* 40(3):247–263.

Chapter 13

1. U.S. Centers for Disease Control and Prevention (CDC). 2013. Notes from the field: emergence of new norovirus strain G11.4 Sydney—United States, 2012. *Morb. Mortal. Wkly. Rep.* 62(03):55.

2. U.S. Centers for Disease Control and Prevention (CDC). 2013. Surveillance for norovirus outbreaks. *CDC Features.*

3. National Food Safety Educators Network (EdNet). 2012. Advisories, alerts, and warnings. *EdNet September 2012.*

4. U.S. Centers for Disease Control and Prevention (CDC). 2012. General information: *Escherichia coli (E. coli).*

5. U.S. Centers for Disease Control and Prevention (CDC). 2012. Estimates of foodborne illness in the United States: CDC 2011 estimates: findings.

6. U.S. Government Accountability Office. 2012. Food safety: FDA's advisory and recall process needs strengthening.

7. U.S. Food and Drug Administration. 2012. Information on the recalled Jensen Farms whole cantaloupes.

8. U.S. Centers for Disease Control and Prevention (CDC). 2013. Trends in foodborne illness in the United States.

9. U.S. Food and Drug Administration. 2013. FDA proposes new food safety standards for foodborne illness prevention and food safety.

10. U.S. Centers for Disease Control and Prevention (CDC). 2013. Norovirus.

11. U.S. Centers for Disease Control and Prevention (CDC). 2011. Hepatitis A information for health professionals.

12. U.S. Centers for Disease Control and Prevention (CDC). 2013. Parasites: toxoplasmosis: toxoplasma infection.

13. U.S. Centers for Disease Control and Prevention (CDC). 2011. Parasites–Giardia.

14. U.S. Centers for Disease Control and Prevention (CDC). 2012. A-Z index for foodborne illness.

15. International Society for Infectious Diseases. 2012. Prion disease update 2012.

16. U.S. Department of Agriculture Animal and Plant Health Inspection Service. 2012. Update from APHIS regarding release of the final report on the BSE epidemiological investigation.

17. U.S. Department of Agriculture Food Safety and Inspection Service. 2011. Common questions: food safety.

18. U.S. Centers for Disease Control and Prevention (CDC). 2010. Marine toxins.

19. Habal, R. 2012. Mushroom toxicity. *Medscape Reference.*

20. Woods Hole Oceanographic Institution. 2012. Researchers report potential for a "moderate" New England "Red Tide" in 2012.

21. National Institutes of Health. 2011. Potato plant poisoning: green tubers and sprouts. *MedlinePlus.*

22. U.S. Department of Agriculture Food Safety and Inspection Service. 2011. Be food safe.

23. U.S. Department of Agriculture Food Safety and Inspection Service. 2010. Fight Bac FactSheet: Chill.

24. U.S. Department of Agriculture Food Safety and Inspection Service. 2011. Food product dating. Fact sheets: Food Labeling.

25. U.S. Food and Drug Administration. 2012. Food facts. Eating outdoors, handling food safely.

26. U.S. Centers for Disease Control and Prevention (CDC). 2012. Multistate outbreak of Salmonella Bareilly and Salmonella Nchanga infections associated with a raw scraped ground tuna product.

27. FoodSafety.gov. n.d. Checklist of foods to avoid during pregnancy.

28. U.S. Food and Drug Administration. 2012. FDA continues to study BPA.

29. U.S. Food and Drug Administration. 2012. Questions and answers about bisphenol A.

30. Center for Science in the Public Interest (CSPI). 2012. Chemical cuisine. Learn about food additives.

31. U.S. Department of Agriculture Economic Research Service. 2012. Data sets: adoption of genetically engineered crops in the U.S.

32. U.S. Environmental Protection Agency. 2012. Persistent organic pollutants: A global issue, a global response.

33. Food and Drug Administration. 2011. What you need to know about mercury in fish and shellfish.

34. U.S. Environmental Protection Agency. 2012. EPA's reanalysis of key issues related to dioxin toxicity and response to NAS comments, volume 1. EPA 600/R-10/038F.

35. U.S. Food and Drug Administration. 2012. Questions and answers about dioxins and food safety.

36. American Academy of Pediatrics. 2012. AAP makes recommendations to reduce children's exposure to pesticides.

37. Environmental Protection Agency (EPA). 2012. Pesticides and food: healthy, sensible food practices.

38. American Cancer Society. 2011. Recombinant bovine growth hormone.

39. Environmental Working Group. 2013. Superbugs invade American supermarkets.

40. Smith, T. C., M. J. Male, A. L. Harper, J. S. Kroeger, G. P. Tinkler, et al. 2009. Methicillin-resistant *Staphylococcus aureus* (MRSA) strain ST398 is present in midwestern U.S. swine and swine workers. *PLoS ONE* 4(1): e4258. doi: 10.1371/journal.pone.0004258

41. Pastagia, M., L. C. Kleinman, E. G. Lacerda de la Cruz, and S. G. Jenkins. 2012. Predicting risk for death from MRSA bacteremia. *Emerg. Infect. Dis.* 18(7).

42. Organic Trade Association. 2012. OTA's 2012 Organic Industry Survey.

43. United States Department of Agriculture Agricultural Marketing Service. 2012. National Organic Program. What is organic?

44. Reganold, J. P., P. K. Andrews, J. R. Reeve, L. Carpenter-Boggs, C. W. Schadt, J. R. Alldredge, C. F. Ross, N. M. Davies, and J. Zhou. 2010. Fruit and soil quality of organic and conventional strawberry agroecosystems. *Plos One* 5(9):e123456.

45. Asami, D. K., Y. J. Hong, D. M. Barrett, and A. E. Mitchell. 2003. Comparison of the total phenolic and ascorbic acid content of freeze-dried and air-dried marionberry, strawberry, and corn grown using conventional, organic, and sustainable agricultural practices. *J. Agric. Food Chem.* 51(5):1237–1241.

46. Dangour, A. D., S. K. Dodhia, A. Hayter, E. Allen, K. Lock, and R. Uauy. 2009. Nutritional quality of organic foods: a systematic review. *Am. J. Clin. Nutr.* doi:10.3945/ajcn.2009.28041.

47. Dangour, A. D., K. Lock, A. Hayter, et al. 2010. Nutrition-related health effects of organic foods: a systematic review. *Am. J. Clin. Nutr.* 92(1):203–210.

48. Smith-Spangler, C., M. L. Brandeau, G. E. Hunter, et al. 2012. Are organic foods safer or healthier than conventional alternatives? *Ann. Intern. Med.* 157(5):348–366.

49. International Service for the Acquisition of Agri-Biotech Applications (ISAAA). 2012. *Global Status of Commercialized Biotech/GM Crops: 2011* (ISAAA Brief No. 43-2011: Executive summary). Ithaca, NY: ISAAA.

50. World Health Organization (WHO). 2010. Twenty questions on genetically modified (GM) foods.

51. Benbrook, C. N. 2012. Impacts of genetically engineered crops on pesticide use in the U.S.—The first 16 years. *Environmental Sciences Europe.* 24:24.

52. Neuman, W. 2010. Justice Dept. tells farmers it will press agriculture industry on antitrust. *The New York Times.* March 12.

53. Shiva, V. 2011. Resisting the corporate theft of seeds. *The Nation.*

54. Center for Food Safety. 2012. Polls on GMO labeling.

InDepth: Food Ethics: Sustainability, Equity, and the New Food Movement

1. Environmental Protection Agency (EPA). n.d. What is sustainability?

2. Louis Bonduelle Foundation. 2012. Biology, varietal improvement & OMGs: summary of the green revolution.

3. Stanford University. 2010. High-yield agriculture slows pace of global warming, say researchers. *ScienceDaily.*

4. Imhoff, D., and M. Dimock. 2012. America needs a farm bill that works. *Los Angeles Times.*

5. Pollan, M. 2006. *The Omnivore's Dilemma: A Natural History of Four Meals.* New York: Penguin.

6. United States Department of Agriculture. 2008. 2007 Census of Agriculture.

7. LocalHarvest. 2011. Community supported agriculture.

8. U.S. Department of Agriculture Agricultural Marketing Service. 2011. Farmers market growth: 1994–2011.

9. Edwards-Jones, G. 2010. Does eating local food reduce the environmental impact of food production and enhance consumer health? *Proc. Nutr. Soc.* 69:582–591.

10. Bittman, M. 2011. Food: six things to feel good about. *The New York Times.*

11. Library of Congress. 2010. School gardens with Constance Carter. *Journeys and Crossings.*

12. Eschmeyer, D. 2012. FoodCorps is one of several efforts to give children healthy foods. *Washington Post.*

13. Wortham, J., and C. Cain Miller. 2013. Venture capitalists are making bigger bets on food start-ups. *The New York Times.*

14. Walmart. 2010. Walmart sustainable agriculture: fact sheet.

15. U.S. Centers for Disease Control and Prevention. 2012. A look inside food deserts.

16. Healthy Corner Stores Network. 2012. Food Deserts.

17. World Hunger Education Service. 2012. 2012 World hunger and poverty facts and statistics.

18. Fanzo, J. C., and P. M. Pronyk. 2011. A review of global progress toward the Millennium Development Goal 1 Hunger Target. *Food Nutr. Bull.* 32(2):144–158.

19. Coleman-Jensen, A., N. Mark, M. Andrews, and S. Carlson. 2012. Household food security in the United States in 2011. U.S. Dept. of Agriculture, Economic Research Service.

20. Moore Lappé, F. 2011. The food movement: its power and possibilities. *The Nation.*

21. Fair Trade USA. 2010. Impact: what is fair trade?

Chapter 14

1. Centers for Disease Control and Prevention (CDC). 2011. Pregnancy nutrition surveillance: Nation Summary of Health Indicators, Table 2D.

2. Central Intelligence Agency. 2012. *The World Factbook.* Washington, DC: Central Intelligence Agency, 2009.

3. Spitz, A. 2013. Male fertility and nutrition. The American Fertility Association.

4. Robbins, W. A., L. Zun, L. Z. FitzGerald, S. Esguerra, S. M. Henning, and C. L. Carpenter. 2012. Walnuts improve semen quality in men consuming a western-style diet: randomized control dietary intervention trial. *Biol. Reprod.* 87(101):1–8.

5. Rasmussen, K. M., and A. L. Yaktine, eds. 2009. *Weight Gain During Pregnancy: Reexamining the Guidelines.* Institute of Medicine; National Research Council. Washington, DC: National Academies Press.

6. Catalano, P. 2012. Impact of maternal GDM and obesity on mother and fetus. In: Gussler, J., and M. A. Graham, eds. *Pregnancy Nutrition and Later Health Outcomes.* Report of the 112th Abbott Nutrition Research Conference. Columbus, OH: Abbott Nutrition.

7. U.S. Department of Agriculture and U.S. Department of Health and Human Services. 2010. *Dietary Guidelines for Americans 2010,* 7th edn. Washington, DC: U.S. Government Printing Office.

8. Institute of Medicine, Food and Nutrition Board. 2002. *Dietary Reference Intakes for Energy, Carbohydrate, Fiber, Fat, Fatty Acids, Cholesterol, Protein, and Amino Acids.* Washington, DC: National Academies Press.

9. Spina Bifida Association. *Why Folic Acid.*

10. Institute of Medicine, Food and Nutrition Board. 1998. *Dietary Reference Intakes for Thiamin, Riboflavin, Niacin, Vitamin B_6, Folate, Vitamin B_{12}, Pantothenic Acid, Biotin, and Choline.* Washington, DC: National Academies Press.

11. Institute of Medicine, Food and Nutrition Board. 2000. *Dietary Reference Intakes for Vitamin C, Vitamin E, Selenium, and Carotenoids.* Washington, DC: National Academies Press.

12. Institute of Medicine, Food and Nutrition Board. 2001. *Dietary Reference Intakes for Vitamin A, Vitamin K, Arsenic, Boron, Chromium, Copper, Iodine, Iron, Manganese, Molybdenum, Nickel, Silicon, Vanadium, and Zinc.* Washington, DC: National Academies Press.

13. Institute of Medicine, Food and Nutrition Board. 2011. *Dietary Reference Intakes for Calcium and Vitamin D.* Washington, DC: National Academies Press.

14. Institute of Medicine, Food and Nutrition Board. 2004. *Dietary Reference for Water, Potassium, Sodium, Chloride, and Sulfate.* Washington, DC: National Academies Press.

15. Chan, R. L., A. F. Olshan, D. A. Savitz, A. H. Herring, J. L. Daniels, H. B. Peterson, and S. L. Martin. 2011. Maternal influences on nausea and vomiting in early pregnancy. *Matern Child Health J.* 15:122–127.

16. Uher, R., and M. Rutter. 2012. Classification of feeding and eating disorders: review of evidence and proposals for ICD-11. *World Psychiatry* 11:80–92.

17. Malcolm, J. 2012. Preventing diabetes in women with gestational diabetes. Through the looking glass: gestational diabetes as a predictor of maternal and offspring long-term health. *Diabetes Metab. Res. Rev.* 28:307–311.

18. Baptiste-Roberts, K., W. K. Nicholson, N. Wang, and F. L. Brancati. 2012. Gestational diabetes and subsequent growth patterns of offspring: the National Collaborative Perinatal Project. *Matern. Child Health J.* 16:125–132.

19. Jutcheon, J. A., S. Lisonkova, and K. S. Joseph. 2011. Epidemiology of pre-eclampsia and the other hypertensive disorders of pregnancy. *Best Pract. Res. Clin. Obstet. Gynaecol.* 25:391–403.

20. Hamilton, B. E., and S. J. Ventura. 2012. *Birth Rates for U.S. Teenagers Reach Historic Lows for All Age and Ethnic Groups.* NCHS Data BriefNo. 89. Hyattsville, MD: National Center for Health Statistics.

21. Zavorsky, G. S., and L. D. Longo. 2011. Exercise guidelines in pregnancy: new perspectives. *Sports Med.* 41:345–360.

22. The American College of Obstetricians and Gynecologists. 2011. *Frequently Asked Questions: Exercise During Pregnancy.*

23. Jarosz, M., R. Wierzejska, and M. Siuba. 2012. Maternal caffeine intake and its effect on pregnancy outcomes. *Eur. J. Obstet. Gynecol. Reprod. Biol.* 160:156–160.

24. Sengpiel, V., E. Elind, J. Bacelis, S. Nilsson, J. Grove, R. Myhre, M. Haugen, H. M. Meltzer, J. Alexander, B. Jacobsson, and A. Brantsaeter. 2013. Maternal caffeine intake during pregnancy is associated with birth weight but not with gestational length: results from a large prospective observational cohort study. *BMC Med.* 11:42. doi:10.1186/1741-7015-11-42

25. Riley, E. P., M. A. Infante, and K. R. Warren. 2011. Fetal alcohol spectrum disorders: an overview. *Neuropsychol. Rev.* 21:73–80.

26. Centers for Disease Control and Prevention. 2012. Tobacco use and pregnancy.

27. Committee on Health Care for Underserved Women and Committee on Obstetric Practice of the American College of Obstetricians and Gynecologists. 2010. Committee opinion: smoking cessation during pregnancy. *Obstet. Gynecol.* 116:1241–1244.

28. Substance Abuse and Mental Health Services Administration. 2012. *Results from the 2011 National Survey on Drug Use and Health: Summary of National Findings.* NSDUH Series H-44, HHS Publication No. (SMA) 12-4713. Rockville, MD: Substance Abuse and Mental Health Services Administration.

29. U.S. Food & Drug Administration. 2011. Food safety for moms-to-be.

30. K. Tsukimori, H. Uchi, C. Mitoma, F. Yasukawa, T. Chiba, T. Todaka, J. Kajiwara, T. Yoshimura, T. Hirata, K. Fukushima, N. Wake, and M. Furue. 2012. Maternal exposure to high levels of dioxins in relation to birth weight in women affected by Yusho disease. *Environ. Int.* 38:79–86.

31. Centers for Disease Control and Prevention. 2012. Breastfeeding report card 2012, United States, outcome indicators.

32. Holick, M. F., N. C. Binkley, H. A. Bischoff-Ferrari, C. M. Gordon, D. A. Hanley, R. P. Heaney, M. Hassan Murad, and C. M. Weaver. 2011. Evaluation, treatment, and prevention of vitamin D deficiency: an Endocrine Society clinical practice guideline. *J. Clin. Endocrinol. Metab.* 96:1911–1930.

33. American Academy of Pediatrics, Section on Breastfeeding. 2012. Breastfeeding and the use of human milk policy statement. *Pediatrics* 129:e827–841.

34. Bartick, M., and A. Reinhold. 2010. The burden of suboptimal breastfeeding in the United States: a pediatric cost analysis. *Pediatrics* 125:e1048–1056.

35. Cabrera-Rubio, R., M. C. Callado, K. Laitinen, S. Salminen, E. Isolauri, and A. Mira. 2012. The human milk microbiome changes over lactation and is shaped by maternal weight and mode of delivery. *Am. J. Clin. Nutr.* 96:544–555.

36. U.S. Department of Health & Human Services. *Bisphenol A (BPA) Information for Parents.*

37. Kotsopoulos, J., J. Lubinshi, L. Salmena, H. T. Lynch, C. Kim-Sing, W. D. Foulkes, P. Ghadirian, S. L. Neuhausen, R. Demsky, N. Tung, P. Ainsworth, L. Senter, A. Eisen, C. Eng, C. Singer, O. Ginsburg, J. Blum, T. Huzarski, A. Poll, P. Sun, and S. A. Narod for the Hereditary Breast Cancer Clinical Study Group. 2012. Breastfeeding and the risk of breast cancer in *BRAC1* and *BRAC2* mutation carriers. *Breast Cancer Res.* 14:R42.

38. Kindra, G., A. Coutsoudis, F. Exposito, and T. Esterhuizen. 2012. Breastfeeding in HIV exposed infants significantly improves child health: a prospective study. *Matern. Child Health J.* 16:632–640.

39. Adgent, M. A., J. L. Daniels, W. J. Rogan, L. Adair, L. J. Edwards, D. Westreich, M. Maisonet, and M. Marcus. 2012. Early-life soy exposure and age at menarche. *Paediatr. Perinat. Epidemiol.* 26:163–175.

40. Boletzko, B. 2012. Impact of maternal obesity on long-term health outcomes. In: Gussler, J., and M. A. Graham, eds. *Pregnancy Nutrition and Later Health Outcomes.* Report of the 112th Abbott Nutrition Research Conference. Columbus, OH: Abbott Nutrition.

41. Crume, T. L., L. G. Ogden, E. J. Mayer-Davis, R. F. Hamman, J. M. Norris, K. J. Bischoff, R. McDuffies, and D. Dabelea. 2012. The impact of neonatal breast-feeding on growth trajectories of youth exposed and unexposed to diabetes *in utero*: the EPOCH study. *Intern. J. Obesity* 36:529–534.

42. Khuc, K., E. Blanco, R. Burrows, M. Reyes, M. Castillo, B. Lozoff, and S. Gahagan. 2012. Adolescent metabolic syndrome risk is increased with higher infancy weight gain and decreased with longer breast feeding. *Intern. J. Pediatr.* doi:10.1155/2012/478610

43. Cawley, J., and C. Meyerhoefer. 2012. The medical care costs of obesity: an instrumental variables approach. *J. Health Econ.* 31:219–230.

44. Landau, E. 2012. Health care costs to bulge along with U.S. waistlines.

InDepth: The Fetal Environment: A Lasting Impression

1. Roseboom, T. J., R. C. Painter, A. F. M. van Abeelen, M. V. E. Veenedaal, and S. R. de Rooij. 2011. Hungry in the womb: what are the consequences? Lessons from the Dutch famine. *Maturitas* 70:141–145.

2. Veenendaal, M. V. E., R. C. Painter, S. R. de Rooij, P. M. M. Bossuyt, J. A. M. van der Post, P. D. Gluckman, M. A. Hanson, and T. J. Roseboom. 2013. Transgenerational effects of prenatal exposure to the 1944–45 Dutch famine. *BJOG* 120:548–554.

3. Kaijser, M., A. K. E. Bonamy, O. Akre, S. Cnattingius, F. Granath, M. Norman, and A. Ekbom. 2009. Perinatal risk factors for diabetes in later life. *Diabetes* 58:523–526.

4. Barker, D. J. P., M. Lampl, T. Roseboom, and N. Winder. 2012. Resource allocation in utero and health in later life. *Placenta* 33:e30–e34.

5. Stanner, S. A., K. Bulmer, C. Andres, O. E. Lantseva, V. Borodina, V. V. Poteen, and J. S. Yudkin. 1997. Does malnutrition in utero determine diabetes and coronary heart disease in adulthood? Results from the Leningrad siege study, a cross sectional study. *BMJ* 315:1342–1348.

6. Stanner, S. A., and J. S. Yudkin. 2001. Fetal programming and the Leningrad siege study. *Twin Research* 4:287–292.

7. Juonala, M., C. G. Magnussen, G. S. Berenson, A. Venn, T. L. Burns, M. A. Sabin, S. R. Srinivasan, S. R. Daniels, P. H. Davis, W. Chen, C. Sun, M. Cheung, J. S. Viikari, T. Dwyer, and O. T. Raitakari. 2011. Childhood adiposity, adult adiposity, and cardiovascular risk factors. *N. Engl. J. Med.* 365:1876–1885.

8. Maret, W., and H. H. Sandstead. 2008. Possible roles of zinc nutriture in the fetal origins of disease. *Exp. Gerontol.* 43:378–381.

9. Catalano, P. M., K. Farrell, A. Thomas, L. Huston-Presley, P. Mencin, S. Hauguel de Mouson, and S. B. Amini. 2009. Perinatal risk factors for childhood obesity and metabolic dysregulation. *Am. J. Clin. Nutr.* 90:1303–1313.

10. Stuebe, A. M., M. R. Forman, and K. B. Michels. 2009. Maternal-recalled gestational weight gain, pre-pregnancy body mass index, and obesity in the daughter. *Int. J. Obes. (Lond.)* 33:743–752.

11. Bouret, S. G. 2010. Role of early hormonal and nutritional experiences in shaping feeding behavior and hypothalamic development. *J. Nutr.* 140:653–657.

12. McMahon, D. M., J. Liu, H. Zhang, M. E. Torres, and R. G. Best. 2013. Maternal obesity, folate intake, and neural tube defects in offspring. *Birth Defects Res. A Clin. Mol. Teratol.* 97:115–122.

13. Garcia-Vargas, L., S. S. Addison, R. Nistala, D. Kurukulasuriya, and J. R. Sowers. 2012. Gestational diabetes and the offspring: implications in the development of the cardiorenal metabolic syndrome in offspring. *Cardiorenal. Med.* 2:134–142.

14. Nielsen, G. L., C. Dethlefsen, S. Lundbye-Christensen, J. F. Pedersen, L. Mølsted-Pedersen, and M. W. Gillman. 2012. Adiposity in 277 young adult male offspring of women with diabetes compared with controls: a Danish population-based cohort study. *Acta Obstet. Gynecol. Scand.* 91:838–843.

15. Cetin, I., C. Berti, and S. Calabrese. 2009. Role of micronutrients in the periconceptual period. *Hum. Reprod. Update* 16:80–95.

16. Dixon, M. J., M. L. Marazita, T. H. Beaty, and J. C. Murray. 2011. Cleft lip and palate: understanding genetic and environmental influences. *Nat. Rev. Genet.* 12:167–178.

17. Zucker, M. 2002. Smoking during pregnancy: even worse than you think. *Pulmonary Reviews.com* 7(3).

18. Zhang, A., H. Hu, B. N. Sánchez, A. S. Ettinger, S. K. Park, D. Cantonwine, L. Schnass, R. O. Wright, H. Lamadrid-Figueroa, and M. M. Tellez-Rojo. 2012. Association between prenatal lead exposure and blood pressure in children. *Environ. Health Perspect.* 120:445–450.

19. Sagiv, S. K., S. W. Thurston, D. C. Bellinger, C. Amarasiriwardena, and S. A. Korrick. 2012. Prenatal exposure to mercury and fish consumption during pregnancy and attention-deficit/hyperactivity disorder-related behavior in children. *Arch. Pediatr. Adolesc. Med.* 166:1123–1131.

20. Centers for Disease Control and Prevention. 2009. Chronic disease and health promotion. *Chronic Disease Overview*.

Chapter 15

1. Ogden, C. L., M. D. Carroll, B. K. Kit, and K. M. Flegal. 2012. Prevalence of obesity and trends in body mass index among US children and adolescents, 1999–2010. *JAMA* 307:483–490.

2. Institute of Medicine, Food and Nutrition Board. 2002. *Dietary Reference Intakes for Energy, Carbohydrates, Fiber, Fat, Protein and Amino Acids (Macronutrients)*. Washington, DC: National Academies Press.

3. Kleinman, R. E., ed. 2009. *Pediatric Nutrition Handbook*, 6th edn. Elk Grove Village, IL: American Academy of Pediatrics.

4. Ross, A. C., C. L. Taylor, A. L. Yaktine, and H. B. Del Valle, eds., Committee to review dietary reference intakes for vitamin D and calcium. 2011. *Dietary Reference Intakes for Calcium and Vitamin D*. Washington, DC: National Academies Press.

5. Institute of Medicine, Food and Nutrition Board. 2001. *Dietary Reference Intakes for Vitamin A, Vitamin K, Arsenic, Boron, Chromium, Copper, Iodine, Iron, Manganese, Molybdenum, Nickel, Silicon, Vanadium, and Zinc*. Washington, DC: National Academies Press.

6. Institute of Medicine, Food and Nutrition Board. 2004. *Dietary Reference Intakes for Water, Potassium, Sodium, Chloride, and Sulfate*. Washington, DC: National Academies Press.

7. Howard, A. J., K. M. Mallan, R. Byrne, A. Magarey, and L. A. Daniels. 2012. Toddlers' food preferences. The impact of novel food exposure, maternal preferences and food neophobia. *Appetite* 59:818–825.

8. U.S. Department of Agriculture, Food and Nutrition Service. 2013. National School Lunch Program: Participation and lunches served.

9. Skroza, N., E. Tolino, L. Semyonov, I. Proietti, N. Bernardini, F. Nicolucci, G. La Viola, G. Del Prete, R. Saulee, C. Potenza, and G. La Torre. 2012. Mediterranean diet and familial dysmetabolism as factors influencing the development of acne. *Scand. J. Pub. Health* 40:466–474.

10. Hong, T., J. Rice, and C. Johnson. 2011. Social environmental and individual factors associated with smoking among a panel of adolescent girls. *Women Health* 51:187–203.

11. National Archives and Records Administration. 2012. Nutrition standards in the National School Lunch and School Breakfast Programs; Final Rule. *Federal Register* 77(17, pt. II).

12. Rangan, A. M., V. M. Flood, G. Denyer, K. Webb, G. B. Marks, and T. P. Gill. 2012. Dairy consumption and dietary quality in a sample of Australian children. *J. Am. Coll. Nutr.* 31:185–193.

13. Fiese, B. H., C. Gundersen, B. Koester, and L. Washington. 2011. Household food insecurity—serious concerns for child development. *Social Policy Report* 25:3–19.

14. Sebastian, R. S., J. D. Goldman, C. Wilkinson Enns, and R. P. LaComb. 2010. Fluid milk consumption in the United States: What we eat in America, NHANES 2005–2006. Food Surveys Research Group Dietary Data Brief No. 3.

15. Burris, J., W. Rietkerk, and K. Woolf. 2013. Acne: the role of medical nutrition therapy. *J. Acad. Nutr. Diet.* 113:416–430.

16. Jamal, M., A. J. W. Van der Does, B. W. J. H. Penninx, and P. Cuijpers. 2011. Age at smoking onset and the onset of depression and anxiety disorders. *Nicotine & Tob. Res.* 13:809–819.

17. Centers for Disease Control and Prevention. 2012. Teen drivers: fact sheet.

18. Ogden, C. L., M. D. Carroll, B. K. Kit, and K. M. Flegal. 2012. Prevalence of obesity and trends in body mass index among US children and adolescents, 1999–2010. *JAMA* 307:483–490.

19. Bibbins-Domingo, K., P. Coxson, M. J. Pletcher, J. Lightwood, and L. Goldman. 2007. Adolescent overweight and future adult coronary heart disease. *N. Engl. J. Med.* 357:2371–2379.

20. U.S. Census Bureau. 2012. Statistical Abstract of the United States: 2012. Table 104. Expectation of life at birth, 1970 to 2008, and projections, 2010 to 2020.

21. Sealey, G. 2013. U.S. elderly to double in 25 years. *ABC News*, February 6.

22. Federal Interagency Forum on Aging-Related Statistics. 2012. *Older Americans 2012: Key Indicators of Well-Being*. Federal Interagency Forum on aging-related statistics. Washington, DC: U.S. Government Printing Office.

23. Fagan, K. 2013. Number of centenarians grows in U.S. *SFGate*, February 8.

24. Beavers, K. M., D. P. Beavers, D. K. Hlouston, T. B. Harris, T. F. Hue, A. Koster, A. B. Newman, E. M. Simonsick, S. A. Studenski, B. J. Nicklas, and S. B. Kritchevsky. 2013. Associations between body composition and gait-speed decline: results from the Health, Aging, and Body Composition study. *Am. J. Clin. Nutr.* 97:552–560.

25. Tieland, M., K. J. Borgonjen-Van den Berg, L. J. C. van Loon, and L. C. P. G. M. de Groot. 2012. Dietary protein intake in community-dwelling, frail, and institutionalized elderly people: scope for improvement. *Eur. J. Nutr.* 51:173–179.

26. Grossman, A. 2012. Higher but not lower doses of vitamin D are effective in fracture risk reduction in older adults. *TuftsNow*, July 12.

27. Institute of Medicine, Food and Nutrition Board. 2000. *Dietary Reference Intakes for Vitamin C, Vitamin E, Selenium, and Carotenoids*. Washington, DC: National Academies Press.

28. Saito, K., T. Yokoyama, H. Yoshida, H. Kim, H. Shimada, Y. Yoshida, H. Iwasa, Y. Shimizu, Y. Kondo, S. Handa, N. Maruyama, A. Ishigami, and T. Suzuki. 2011. A significant relationship between plasma vitamin C concentration and physical performance among Japanese elderly women. *J. Gerontol. A. Biol. Sci. Med. Sci.* doi:10.1093/Gerona/glr174

29. Juraschek, S. P., E. Guallar, L. J. Appel, and E. R. Miller, III. 2012. Effects of vitamin C supplementation on blood pressure: a meta-analysis of randomized controlled trials. *Am. J. Clin. Nutr.* 95:1079–1088.

30. Klein, R., Ch. Chou, B. E. K. Klein, X. Zhang, S. M. Meuer, and J. B. Saaddine. 2011. Prevalence of age-related macular degeneration in the US population. *Arch. Opthalmol.* 129:75–80.

31. Sun, Y., A. Ma, Y. Li, X. Han, Q. Wang, and H. Liang. 2012. Vitamin E supplementation protects erythrocyte membranes from oxidative stress in healthy Chinese middle-aged and elderly people. *Nutr. Res.* 32:328–334.

32. Evans, J. R., and J. G. Lawrenson. 2012. Antioxidant vitamin and mineral supplements for preventing age-related macular degeneration. *Cochrane Database Syst. Rev.* 6:CD000253. doi: 10.1002/14651858.CD000253.pub3

33. Institute of Medicine, Food and Nutrition Board. 1998. *Dietary Reference Intakes for Thiamin, Riboflavin, Niacin, Vitamin B_6, Vitamin B_{12}, Pantothenic Acid, Biotin, and Choline.* Washington, DC: National Academies Press.

34. Hooshmand, B., A. Soloman, I. Kåreholt, M. Rusanen, T. Hänninen, J. Leiviskä, B. Winblad, T. Laatikainen, H. Soininen, and M. Kivipelto. 2012. Associations between serum homocystein, holotranscolbalamin, folate and cognition in the elderly: a longitudinal study. *J. Int. Med.* 271:204–212.

35. Moorthyl, D., I. Peter, T. M. Scott, L. D. Parnell, C. Lai, J. W. Crott, J. M. Ordovás, J. Selhub, J. Griffith, I. H. Rosenberg, K. L. Tucker, and A. M. Troen. 2012. Status of vitamins B-12 and B-6 but not of folate, homocysteine, and the methylenetetrahydrofolate reductase C677T polymorphism are associated with impaired cognition and depression in adults. *J. Nutr.* 142:1554–1560.

36. Sunzunegui, M. V., M. T. Sanchez, A. Garcia, J. M. R. Casado, and A. Otero. 2012. Body mass index and long-term mortality in an elderly Mediterranean population. *J. Aging Health* 24:29–47.

37. Van Lancker, A., S. Verhaeghe, A. Van Hecke, K. Vanderwee, J. Goossens, and D. Beeckman. 2012. The association between malnutrition and oral health status in elderly in long-term care facilities: a systematic review. *Int. J. Nurs. Stud.* doi: 10.1016/j.ijnurstu.2012.04.001

38. Aslam, T., C. Delcourt, R. Silva, F. G. Holz, A. Leys, A. G. Layana, and E. Souied. 2013. Micronutrients in age-related macular degeneration. *Ophthalmologica* 229:75–79.

39. Qato, D. M., G. C. Alexander, R. M. Conti, M. Johnson, P. Schumm, and S. T. Lindau. 2008. Use of prescription and over-the-counter medications and dietary supplements among older adults in the United States. *JAMA* 300:2867–2878.

40. Heuberger, R. A., and K. Caudell. 2011. Polypharmacy and nutritional status in older adults. *Drugs Aging* 28:315–323.

41. Rodriguez-Fragoso, L., J. L. Martinez-Arismendi, D. Orozco-Bustos, J. Reyes-Esparza, E. Torres, and S. W. Burchiel. 2011. Potential risks resulting from fruit/vegetable-drug interactions: effects on drug-metabolizing enzymes and drug transporters. *J. Food Sci.* 76:R112–R124.

42. Agarwal, S. K. 2013. Grapefriut: a nutritional fruit fraught with danger of severe drug interactions. *Drug Discoveries* 3:43–44.

43. Ziliak, J., and C. Gundersen. 2009. Senior hunger in the United States: differences across states and rural and urban areas. *University of Kentucky Center for Poverty Research Special Reports.*

44. Hartline-Grafton, H. 2013. SNAP and public health: the role of the supplemental nutrition assistance program in improving the health and well-being of Americans. *Food Research and Action Center* 1–12.

45. Schoenborn, C. A., and P. F. Adams. 2010. Health behaviors of adults: United States, 2005–2007. National Center for Health Statistics. *Vital Health State* 10(245).

46. Barnes, P. M., and C. A. Schoenborn. 2012. *Trends in Adults Receiving a Recommendation for Exercise or Other Physical Activity from a Physician or Other Health Professional.* NCHS Data Brief, No. 86. Hyattsville, MD: National Center for Health Statistics.

47. Centers for Disease Control and Prevention. 2011. How much physical activity do older adults need?

48. Batt, M. E., J. Tanji, and M. Börjesson. 2013. Exercise at 65 and beyond. *Sports Med.* doi: 10.1007/s40279-013-0033-1

InDepth: Searching for the Fountain of Youth

1. Omodei, D., and L. Fontana. 2011. Calorie restriction and prevention of age-associated chronic disease. *FEBS Lett.* 585:1537–1542.

2. Kemnitz, J. W. 2011. Calorie restriction and aging in nonhuman primates. *ILAR J.* 8:66–77.

3. Speakman, J. 2010. Can calorie restriction increase the human lifespan? Experimental Biology Meeting, Anaheim, CA, April 24, 2010.

4. Spindler, S. R. 2010. Caloric restriction: from soup to nuts. *Ageing Res. Rev.* 9:324–353.

5. Ahmet, I., H. Tae, R. de Cabo, E. G. Lakatta, and M. I. Talan. 2011. Effects of calorie restriction on cardioprotection and cardiovascular health. *J. Mol. Cell. Cardiol.* 51:263–271.

6. Varady, K. A., S. Bhutani, E. C. Church, and M. C. Klempel. 2009. Short-term modified alternate-day fasting: a novel dietary strategy for weight loss and cardioprotection in obese adults. *Am. J. Clin. Nutr.* 90:1138–1143.

7. Varady, K. A. 2012. Alternate day fasting: effects on body weight and chronic disease risk in humans. In: McCue, M. D., ed. *Comparative Physiology of Fasting, Starvation and Food Limitation.* Berlin: Springer-Verlag.

8. Varady, K. A., S. Bhutani, M. C. Klempel, and B. Lamarche. 2010. Improvements in LDL particle size and distribution by short-term alternate day modified fasting in obese adults. *Br. J. Nutr.* 105:580–583.

9. Fontana, L., L. Partridge, and V. D. Longo. 2010. Extending healthy life span—from yeast to humans. *Science* 328:321–326.

10. Joshi, Y. G., and D. Praticò. 2012. Vitamin E in aging, dementia, and Alzheimer's diseaes. *BioFactors.* doi:10.1002/biof.195

11. Harrison, F. E. 2012. A critical review of vitamin C for the prevention of age-related cognitive decline and Alzheimer's disease. *J. Alzheimers Dis.* 29:711–726.

12. Hammar, M., and C. J. Östgren. 2013. Healthy aging and age-adjusted nutrition and physical fitness. *Best Pract. Res. Clin. Obstet. Gynaecol.* doi:10.1016/j.bpobgyn.2013.01.004

13. Bjelakovic, G., D. Nikolova, L. L. Gluud, R. G. Simonetti, and C. Gluud. 2012. Antioxidant supplements for prevention of mortalitiy in healthy participants and patients with various diseases. *Cochrane Database Syst. Rev.:* CD007176.

14. Rabin, R. C. 2013. New doubts about ginkgo biloba. *New York Times*, April 29.

15. WebMD. 2012. Human Growth Hormone (HGH).

answers

Answers to Review Questions and Math Review

Note: Review Questions and Math Review items are included in the end-of-chapter matter for main chapters only; the questions do not appear in the In Depth chapters. Math Review questions will vary in number. Answers to Review Questions and Math Review can also be found in the MasteringNutrition Study Area.

Chapter 1

1. **c.** identifying and preventing diseases caused by dietary deficiencies.
2. **a.** Pellagra is caused by a nutrient deficiency.
3. **d.** micronutrients.
4. **b.** the RDA for vitamin C.
5. **d.** "A high protein diet increases the risk for porous bones" is an example of a hypothesis.
6. **b.** National Institutes of Health
7. **True.**
8. **True.**
9. **False.** The Adequate Intake is a recommended intake level that is assumed, not known, to be adequate.
10. **True.**

Math Review

11. 24.5% of Kayla's diet comes from fat; this percentage is within the AMDR for fat.

Chapter 2

1. **b.** provides enough energy, nutrients, and fiber to maintain a person's health.
2. **d.** the % Daily Values of select nutrients in a serving of the packaged food.
3. **c.** replacing solid fats with vegetable oils.
4. **d.** fruits and vegetables.
5. **b.** a serving that is 1 ounce or equivalent to an ounce for either grains or protein foods.
6. **a.** MyPlate easily accommodates ethnic diets, vegetarian diets, and other healthful dietary variations.
7. **c.** At fast-food restaurants, a large beverage can provide a greater number of Calories than a hamburger.
8. **False.** Structure-function claims can be made without approval from the FDA; while they can be generic statements about a food's impact on the body's structure and function, they cannot refer to a specific disease or symptom.
9. **True.**
10. **True.**

Math Review

11. Total Calories = 646; Total fat content = 33 g; Percentage of Calories from fat = 46%; item contributing the highest amount of fat to the lunch = ranch salad dressing. Hannah can skip the salad dressing or ask for a low-fat dressing, if available, to make a healthier change to this lunch.

Chapter 3

1. **c.** atoms, molecules, cells, tissues, organs, systems.
2. **b.** two flexible layers of phospholipid molecules.
3. **c.** hypothalamus.
4. **c.** the middle segment of the small intestine.

5. **c.** small intestine.
6. **a.** collectively known as the enteric nervous system.
7. **a.** gastric juice in the esophagus.
8. **False.** Vitamins and minerals do not require digestion. They are absorbed directly.
9. **False.** Bile is produced by the liver and stored in the gallbladder.
10. **True.**

Math Review

11. The difference between pH 9 and pH 2 is 7. The alkalinity of baking soda as compared to gastric juice can be expressed as: $7 = \log_{10}(10,000,000)$. In other words, baking soda is 10 million times more alkaline than gastric juice.

Chapter 4

1. **a.** monosaccharides.
2. **d.** Consuming a diet high in fiber-rich carbohydrates may reduce the level of cholesterol in the blood.
3. **b.** is converted to glycogen and stored in the liver and muscles.
4. **b.** the potential of foods to raise blood glucose and insulin levels.
5. **c.** up to 65% of our daily energy intake as carbohydrate.
6. **d.** sweetened soft drinks.
7. **c.** whole-oat cereal.
8. **a.** phenylketonuria.
9. **False.** Plants store carbohydrate as glucose.
10. **True.**

Math Review

11. The AMDR for carbohydrate for adults is 45-65% of total daily energy. If Simon wants to make sure he is meeting the minimum (45%), the answers are: a) 3,500 kcal per day × 0.45 = 1,575 kcal per day of carbohydrate, preferably from fiber-rich sources; and b) 1,575 kcal per day ÷ 4 kcal per gram of carbohydrate = 393.75 grams. Thus Simon should consume at least 394 grams of carbohydrate per day.

Chapter 5

1. **a.** monounsaturated fats.
2. **b.** saturated and unsaturated fats.
3. **d.** found in leafy green vegetables, flaxseeds, soy milk, walnuts, and almonds.
4. **b.** are a major source of fuel for the body at rest.
5. **a.** lipoprotein lipase.
6. **d.** none of the above.
7. **c.** vegetables, fish, and nuts.
8. **d.** all of the above.
9. **False.** Triglycerides are composed of three fatty acid chains chemically bonded to a molecule of glycerol.
10. **True.**

Math Review

11. Answers will vary; however, notice that the table lists amounts of EPA and DHA in g/serving, not mg. Thus, eating one small (3 oz) serving of salmon would more than meet your need for EPA and DHA today.

12.

Type of Fat	Maximum Recommended Intake (% of total energy intake)	Maximum Recommended Calorie Intake
Saturated fat	7%	140 Calories/day
Linoleic acid	10%	200 Calories/day
Alpha-linolenic acid	1.2%	24 Calories/day
Trans fatty acids	0%	9 Calories/day
Unsaturated fat	None; amount equal to remainder of total fat Calories after you account for intake of saturated fat and linoleic and alpha-linolenic acids.	336 Calories/day

Calculations needed:
- Total energy needs = 2,000 Calories/day
- Maximum AMDR for fat = 35% of total energy intake = 0.35 × 2,000 = 700 Calories
- Saturated fat = 7% of total energy intake = 0.07 × 2,000 = 140 Calories
- Linoleic acid = 10% of total energy intake = 0.10 × 2,000 = 200 Calories
- Alpha-linolenic acid = 1.2% of total energy intake = 0.012 × 2,000 = 24 Calories
- *Trans* fatty acids = 0 Calories

Chapter 6

1. **c.** hydrogen, carbon, oxygen, and nitrogen.
2. **d.** None of the above.
3. **d.** mutual supplementation.
4. **a.** exert presuure that draws fluid out of tissue spaces, preventing edema.
5. **c.** protease.
6. **c.** The RDA for protein is higher for children and adolescents than for adults.
7. **a.** rice, pinto beans, acorn squash, soy butter, and almond milk.
8. **b.** Protein levels in the blood must be adequate to transport fat.
9. **False.** After leaving the small intestine, amino acids are transported via the portal vein into the liver. Once in the liver, amino acids may be converted to glucose or fat, combined to build new proteins, used for energy, or released into the bloodstream and transported to other cells as needed, but there is no storage form for amino acids in the liver.
10. **False.** Denaturation does not affect the primary structure of proteins. However, when a protein is denatured, its function is lost.

Math Review

11. **(a)** The AMDR for protein is 10% to 35% of total daily energy intake. Thus the lower level of AMDR for Barry is equal to 3,000 kcal × 0.10 = 300 kcal protein. This is equivalent to 75 g of protein (300 kcal ÷ 4 kcal/g protein). The upper level of AMDR for Barry is equal to 3,000 kcal × 0.35 = 1,050 kcal protein. This is equivalent to 262.5 g of protein (1,050 kcal ÷ 4 kcal/g protein). Barry is meeting the AMDR for protein.
(b) Assuming Barry is not an athlete, his RDA for protein is 0.8 g of protein per kg body weight per day × 75 kg = 60 g per day. Barry is exceeding the RDA for protein.

Chapter 7

1. **a.** extracellular fluid.
2. **c.** They provide protection for the brain and spinal cord.
3. **b.** It is freely permeable to water but not to electrolytes.
4. **d.** all of the above.
5. **a.** tap water.
6. **c.** Increased plasma (or serum) sodium draws water out of cells and into the extracellular fluid.
7. **b.** It can be found in fresh fruits and vegetables.
8. **b.** sweating and breathing heavily while active in a hot environment.
9. **False.** Surface water comes from lakes, rivers, and reservoirs. Groundwater comes from aquifers.
10. **False.** Chloride is also a component of hydrochloric acid and assists in immune function and nerve impulse transmission.

Math Review

11. 3 lb weight loss × 2 cups/lb = 6 cups of fluid lost. 6 cups × 1.5 = 9 cups of fluid needed to fully rehydrate.

Chapter 8

1. **b.** an atom loses an electron.
2. **a.** cardiovascular disease.
3. **d.** all of the above.
4. **b.** Both vitamins donate electrons to free radicals.
5. **c.** promotes the synthesis of collegen in connective tissues in skin, bone, and other organs.
6. **b.** Beta-carotene is a provitamin A carotenoid.
7. **c.** contains vitamin A in the form of retinal.
8. **a.** vitamin A.
9. **True.**
10. **False.** Beef liver is very high in preformed vitamin A, which can build to toxic levels very quickly and cause birth defects and spontaneous abortions. As a result, pregnant women are advised to avoid eating liver on a daily or even weekly basis.

Math Review

11. **(a)** Each tablet contains 400 IU of the synthetic form of vitamin E. In supplements containing the synthetic form of vitamin E, 1 IU is equal to 0.45 mg α-TE. To convert IU to mg α-TE = 400 IU X 0.45 = 180 mg α-TE, which is equal to 180 mg of active vitamin E.
(b) The RDA for vitamin A is 15 mg alpha-tocopherol per day. To calculate the percentage of the RDA for vitamin E coming from the supplements = (180 mg α-TE ÷ 15 mg α-TE) × 100 = 1200%
(c) The tolerable upper intake level is 1,000 mg alpha-tocopherol per day, and thus the amount coming from the supplement is relatively small at 180 mg. Although in the past up to 18 times the RDA has been shown to be safe (18 × 15 mg = 270 mg of alpha-tocopherol per day), recent evidence suggests that even 400 IU per day could increase the risk for premature mortality. Thus it would be safest for Joey's mother to obtain adequate vitamin E from her diet. If she is taking aspirin each day as prescribed, it is imperative that she stop taking vitamin E supplements, as aspirin is an anticoagulant and taking vitamin E supplements could enhance its action and result in uncontrollable bleeding and hemorrhaging.

Chapter 9

1. **d.** It provides the scaffolding for cortical bone.
2. **b.** remodeling.
3. **c.** has normal bone density as compared to an average, healthy 30-year-old.
4. **d.** structure of bone, nerve transmission, and muscle contraction.

5. **a.** broccoli.
6. **b.** increases the activity of osteoclasts.
7. **c.** a fair-skinned retired teacher living in a nursing home in Ohio
8. **a.** vitamin K.
9. **False.** Our bodies make vitamin D by converting a cholesterol compound in our skin to the active form of vitamin D.
10. **True.**

Math Review

11. As shown in the table, 96 mg of calcium are absorbed in 1 cup of skim milk. In contrast, only 37 mg of calcium are absorbed in 1 cup of broccoli. To absorb 96 mg of calcium, you would need to consume 96 mg ÷ 37 mg = 2.6 times as much broccoli; 2.6 × 1 cup = 2.6 cups of broccoli.

Chapter 10

1. **c.** a molecule that combines with and activates an enzyme.
2. **d.** thiamin, pantothenic acid, and biotin.
3. **a.** it reduces the risk for giving birth to an infant with a neural tube defect.
4. **c.** an amino acid.
5. **b.** erythrocytes, leukocytes, platelets, and plasma.
6. **b.** About two-thirds of the body's iron is found in hemoglobin, the oxygen-carrying compound in red blood cells.
7. **b.** vitamin K.
8. **a.** iron-deficiency anemia.
9. **False.** Heme iron is found only in animal-based foods; however, non-heme iron is available from a wide variety of plant foods.
10. **True.**

Math Review

11. This statement is false. Although 20 mg/day × 100 days = 2,000 mg, or 2 g, zinc absorption rates range from just 10–35% of dietary intake.

Chapter 11

1. **b.** appropriate for your gender, age, genetics, physical development, and family history.
2. **d.** body mass index.
3. **a.** basal metabolic rate, thermal effect of food, and effect of physical activity.
4. **c.** the body raises or lowers energy expenditure in response to changes in food intake and physical activity.
5. **c.** making gradual changes in energy intake, engaging in regular and appropriate physical activity, and applying behavioral modification techniques.
6. **b.** Obesity is associated with a risk of premature death that is 18% higher than that of someone of normal weight.
7. **d.** All of the above are true.
8. **False.** Apple-shaped fat patterning is associated with an increased risk for chronic disease.
9. **True.**
10. **True.**

Math Review

11. **(a)** To calculate Misty's BMI: Convert Misty's height to meters and her weight to kg. Her height is 5'8" or 68 inches, which is equal to 1.727 meters (68 inches × .0254 cm/inch). Her weight is 148 lb, which is equal to 67.27 kg (148 lb × 0.4545 kg/lb). Thus her BMI is equal to 22.6 kg/m² (67.27 kg/2.982529 meters). Misty's BMI falls into the normal weight category.
(b) There are many questions and bits of advice that you could share with Misty. You could inquire as to why she feels she is overweight, and suggest she explore the various definitions of a healthy body weight listed in this chapter. You could point out that as she exercises regularly, she is promoting overall health, and she might get her body composition measured to reassure her that her weight is in the healthful range. You could also suggest that she schedule an appointment with a registered dietitian to discuss her dietary intake and views on her personal body image.
12. **(a)** First, calculate Misty's BMR = 0.9 kcal per kg body weight per hour = 0.9 kcal/body weight/hour × 67.27 kg × 24 hours/day = 1,453 kcal/day.
(b) Second, you need to estimate the energy cost of Misty's activity level. Being moderately active, Misty's energy needed to perform activities will range from 50% to 70% of her BMR, or 726 kcal (0.50 × 1,453 kcal) and 1,017 kcal (0.70 × 1,453 kcal).
(c) Finally, add together Misty's BMR and energy needed to perform daily activities: 1,453 kcal/day + 726 kcal/day = 2,179 kcal/day to 1,453 kcal/day + 1,017 kcal/day = 2,470 kcal/day.

Chapter 12

1. **d.** all of the above.
2. **a.** cardiorespiratory fitness, musculoskeletal fitness, flexibility, and body composition.
3. **c.** reduces anxiety and mental stress.
4. **c.** 50 to 70% of your estimated maximal heart rate.
5. **a.** 1 to 3 seconds.
6. **b.** fat.
7. **d.** drink a beverage containing carbohydrate and electrolytes both before and during the event in amounts that balance hydration with energy, carbohydrate, and electrolyte needs.
8. **b.** Carbohydrate loading results in increased storage of glycogen in muscles and the liver.
9. **True.**
10. **False.** Sports anemia is not a true anemia, but rather is a transient decrease in iron stores that occurs due to an increase in plasma volume. It occurs at the start of an exercise program or in some athletes who increase their training intensity.

Math Review

11. **(a)** Liz's suggested intake for protein is identified as 1.5 grams per kg body weight. Her body weight is equal to 105 lbs ÷ 2.2 = 47.7 kg. Her protein intake (in grams) is equal to 1.5 grams protein/kg body weight × 47.7 kg = 71.6 grams.
(b) Liz's preferred fat intake is 20% of her total daily energy intake, thus 1,800 kcal × 0.20 = 360 kcal. Because the energy value of fat is 9 kcal per gram, her total intake of fat in grams = 360 kcal ÷ 9 kcal/gram = 40 grams of fat.
(c) To calculate Liz's carbohydrate intake, you must first determine the amount of kcal of her total energy intake that remains once her protein and fat intake are accounted for.
- Liz's protein intake is 71.6 grams; as the energy value of protein is 4 kcal per gram, her kcal intake from protein = 71.6 grams × 4 kcal/gram = 286.4 kcal
- Liz's fat intake has already been calculated as 360 kcal
- As Liz's total energy intake is 1,800 kcal per day, the amount of kcal she'll consume from carbohydrate = 1,800 kcal – 286.4 kcal – 360 kcal = 1,153.6 kcal of carbohydrate.
- The energy value of carbohydrates is 4 kcal per gram, and thus Liz's intake of carbohy-drate in grams is equal to 1,153.6 kcal ÷ 4 kcal/gram = 288.4 grams
(d) To determine if Liz's carbohydrate intake falls within the AMDR = (1,153.6 kcal of carbohydrate ÷ 1,800 kcal) × 100 = 64%. Thus her carbohydrate intake does fall within the AMDR.

Chapter 13

1. **a.** Federal inspections of food production facilities has decreased over the last few decades.
2. **b.** norovirus and *Toxoplasma gondii*.
3. **c.** 40°F.
4. **c.** modified atmosphere packaging.
5. **b.** sulfites and nitrites.
6. **d.** recombinant DNA technology.
7. **d.** Industrial contaminants become more concentrated in animal tissues as they move up the food chain.
8. **a.** contain only organically produced ingredients, excluding water and salt.
9. **False.** It is safe to leave the salad at room temperature for no longer than two hours total; however, it is safest to refrigerate the salad immediately after preparing and until serving.
10. **True.**

Math Review

11. On average, of the 48 million Americans who contract a foodborne illness each year, 3,000 people die. Thus: 3,000 ÷ 48,000,000 = .0000625. Multiply by 100 to derive a percentage: *.00625 percent.* Are you surprised that such a miniscule percentage of people who experience a foodborne illness die from it? This suggests that the body's mechanisms for defending against pathogens and their toxins (mainly expelling them via vomiting and diarrhea and mounting an immune response against those that remain) are generally effective.

Chapter 14

1. **b.** neural tube defects
2. **b.** women who begin their pregnancy underweight.
3. **c.** Nibble on dry cereal or crackers before bedtime to ease nighttime nausea and before rising to prevent morning nausea.
4. **c.** oxytocin
5. **d.** All of the above.
6. **a.** Certain proteins in breast milk improve the absorption of iron.
7. **c.** iron.
8. **d.** none of the above.
9. **False.** Major developmental errors and birth defects are most likely to occur in the first trimester of pregnancy.
10. **False.** If not controlled, gestational diabetes can result in a baby who is too large as a result of receiving too much glucose across the placenta during fetal life.

Math Review

11. **(a)** To calculate the % of kcal in breast milk that come from fat, first convert grams of fat to fat kcal: 35 g fat/liter × 9 kcal/g = 315 fat kcal/liter. Then calculate the % of total breast milk kcal from fat: [315 fat kcal ÷ 700 total kcal] × 100 (to convert to percentage) = 45% of kcal in breast milk are from fat.

(b) To calculate the % of kcal in breast milk that come from protein, first convert grams of protein to protein kcal: 9 g protein × 4 kcal/g = Then calculate the % of total breast milk kcal from protein: [36 kcal ÷ 700 total kcal] × 100 (to convert to percentage) = 5% of kcal from protein.

(c) 45% of kcal from fat is much higher than the range that is recommended for healthy young adults (20–35% of total kcal from fat), but a high fat diet is needed to meet the energy needs of rapidly growing infants. 5% of kcal from protein is much lower than what is recommended for most young adults (10–35% of kcal from protein), but the kidneys of young infants are immature and not able to excrete large amounts of nitrogen. The small gastric capacity of infants and their relatively immature kidneys explain why the proportions of Calories from fat and protein in breast milk are ideally suited for young infants.

Chapter 15

1. **a.** 1/2 cup of iron-fortified cooked oat cereal, 2 tbsp. of mashed pineapple, and 1 cup of whole milk
2. **c.** iron and zinc.
3. **c.** 45–65%
4. **b.** the epiphyseal plates close.
5. **c.** both boys and girls, beginning at age 9.
6. **d.** None of the above.
7. **a.** Absorption of vitamin B_{12} from the gastrointestinal tract is reduced.
8. **d.** the prevalence of obesity declines after age 75.
9. **True.**
10. **True.**

Math Review

11. To calculate the total vitamin A intake of Kristina's grandmother, add up the amount of vitamin A in one dose of each of the three supplements: 3,333 + 1,500 + 2,200 = 7,033 µg of vitamin A per day.

To calculate the % of the RDA consumed by Kristina's grandmother, take her daily total intake, divide by the RDA, and multiply by 100 to convert to a percent: [7,033 µg ÷ 700 µg] × 100 = 1,005% of the UL, or ten times more than the recommended amount.

To calculate the % of the vitamin A UL consumed by Kristina's grandmother each day, take her total daily intake, divide by the UL, and multiply by 100 to convert to a percent: [7,033 µg ÷ 3,000 µg] × 100 = 234% of the UL, or more than twice the recommended upper limit. This amount of vitamin A, taken on a regular basis, could certainly lead to vitamin A toxicity over time. The UL for adults, including the elderly, is 3,000 µg per day.

NOTE: These calculations reflect the % of the RDA, not % above the RDA.

glossary

A

absorption   The physiologic process by which molecules of food are taken from the gastrointestinal tract into the circulation.

Acceptable Daily Intake (ADI)   An FDA estimate of the amount of a non-nutritive sweetener that someone can consume each day over a lifetime without adverse effects.

Acceptable Macronutrient Distribution Range (AMDR)   The range of macronutrient intakes that provides adequate levels of essential nutrients and is associated with a reduced risk for chronic disease.

acetylcholine   A neurotransmitter that is involved in many functions, including muscle movement and memory storage.

acidosis   A disorder in which the blood becomes acidic; that is, the level of hydrogen in the blood is excessive. It can be caused by respiratory or metabolic problems.

added sugars   Sugars and syrups that are added to food during processing or preparation.

adenosine triphosphate (ATP)   The common currency of energy for virtually all cells of the body.

adequate diet   A diet that provides enough of the energy, nutrients, and fiber needed to maintain a person's health.

Adequate Intake (AI)   A recommended average daily nutrient intake level based on observed or experimentally determined estimates of nutrient intake by a group of healthy people.

aerobic exercise   Exercise that involves the repetitive movement of large muscle groups, increasing the body's use of oxygen and promoting cardiovascular health.

alcohol   Chemically, a compound characterized by the presence of a hydroxyl group; in common usage, a beverage made from fermented fruits, vegetables, or grains and containing ethanol.

alcohol abuse   A pattern of alcohol consumption, whether chronic or occasional, that results in harm to one's health, functioning, or interpersonal relationships.

alcohol dependence   A disease state characterized by chronic dependence on alcohol; commonly called *alcoholism*.

alcohol hangover   A consequence of drinking too much alcohol; symptoms include headache, fatigue, dizziness, muscle aches, nausea and vomiting, sensitivity to light and sound, extreme thirst, and mood disturbances.

alcohol poisoning   A potentially fatal metabolic state in which an overdose of alcohol results in cardiac and/or respiratory failure.

alcoholic hepatitis   Inflammation of the liver caused by alcohol; other forms of hepatitis can be caused by a virus or toxin.

alkalosis   A disorder in which the blood becomes basic; that is, the level of hydrogen in the blood is deficient. It can be caused by respiratory or metabolic problems.

alpha-linolenic acid (ALA)   An essential fatty acid found in leafy green vegetables, flaxseed oil, soy oil, and other plant foods; an omega-3 fatty acid.

amenorrhea   The absence of menstruation. In females who had previously been menstruating, it is defined as the absence of menstrual periods for 3 or more continuous months.

amino acids   Nitrogen-containing molecules that combine to form proteins.

amniotic fluid   The watery fluid contained within the innermost membrane of the sac containing the fetus. It cushions and protects the growing fetus.

anabolic   The term applied to a substance that builds muscle and increases strength.

anaerobic   Means "without oxygen;" the term used to refer to metabolic reactions that occur in the absence of oxygen.

anencephaly   A fatal neural tube defect in which there is partial absence of brain tissue, most likely caused by failure of the neural tube to close.

anorexia   An absence of appetite (Ch. 3).

anorexia nervosa   A potentially life-threatening eating disorder that is characterized by self-starvation and leads to a deficiency in energy and essential nutrients (Ch. 11.5).

antibodies   Defensive proteins of the immune system. Their production is prompted by the presence of bacteria, viruses, toxins, allergens, and other antigens.

antioxidant   A compound that has the ability to prevent or repair the damage caused by oxidation.

appetite   A psychological desire to consume specific foods.

ariboflavinosis   A condition caused by riboflavin deficiency.

atherosclerosis   A condition characterized by accumulation of cholesterol-rich plaque on artery walls; these deposits build up to such a degree that they impair blood flow.

atrophic gastritis   A condition that results in low stomach acid secretion; is estimated to occur in about 10–30% of adults older than 50 years.

atrophy   A decrease in the size and strength of muscles that occurs when they are not worked adequately.

B

bacteria   Microorganisms that lack a true nucleus and reproduce by division or by forming spores.

balanced diet   A diet that contains the combinations of foods that provide the proper proportions of nutrients.

basal metabolic rate (BMR)   The energy the body expends to maintain its fundamental physiologic functions.

beriberi   A disease of muscle wasting and nerve damage caused by thiamin deficiency.

bile   Fluid produced by the liver and stored in the gallbladder; it emulsifies fats in the small intestine.

binge drinking   The consumption of five or more alcoholic drinks on one occasion.

binge eating   Consumption of a large amount of food in a short period of time, usually accompanied by a feeling of loss of self-control.

binge-eating disorder   A disorder characterized by binge eating an average of twice a week or more, typically without compensatory purging.

bioavailability   The degree to which our body can absorb and utilize any given nutrient.

biomagnification   Process by which persistent organic pollutants become more concentrated in animal tissues as they move from one creature to another through the food chain.

biopesticides   Primarily insecticides, these chemicals use natural methods to reduce damage to crops.

blood volume The amount of fluid in blood.

body composition The ratio of a person's body fat to lean body mass.

body image A person's perception of his or her body's appearance and functioning.

body mass index (BMI) A measurement representing the ratio of a person's body weight to his or her height.

bolus A mass of food that has been chewed and moistened in the mouth.

bone density The degree of compactness of bone tissue, reflecting the strength of the bones. *Peak bone density* is the point at which a bone is strongest.

brown adipose tissue A type of adipose tissue that has more mitochondria than white adipose tissue and which can increase energy expenditure by uncoupling oxidation from ATP production. It is found in significant amounts in animals and newborn humans.

brush border The microvilli projecting from the membrane of enterocytes of the small intestine's villi. These microvilli tremendously increase the small intestine's absorptive capacity.

buffers Proteins that help maintain proper acid–base balance by attaching to, or releasing, hydrogen ions as conditions change in the body.

bulimia nervosa A serious eating disorder characterized by recurrent episodes of binge eating and recurrent inappropriate compensatory behaviors in order to prevent weight gain, such as self-induced vomiting, fasting, excessive exercise, or misuse of laxatives, diuretics, enemas, or other medications.

C

calcitonin A hormone secreted by the thyroid gland when blood calcium levels are too high. Calcitonin inhibits the actions of vitamin D, preventing reabsorption of calcium in the kidneys, limiting calcium absorption in the small intestine, and inhibiting the osteoclasts from breaking down bone.

calcitriol The primary active form of vitamin D in the body.

calcium rigor A failure of muscles to relax, which leads to a hardening or stiffening of the muscles; caused by high levels of blood calcium.

calcium tetany A condition in which muscles experience twitching and spasms as a result of inadequate blood calcium levels.

cancer A group of diseases characterized by cells that reproduce spontaneously and independently and may invade other tissues and organs.

carbohydrate One of the three macronutrients, a compound made up of carbon, hydrogen, and oxygen, that is derived from plants and provides energy (Ch. 4).

carbohydrate loading Also known as glycogen loading. A process that involves altering training and carbohydrate intake, so that muscle glycogen storage is maximized.

carbohydrates The primary fuel source for our body, particularly for our brain and for physical exercise (Ch. 1).

carcinogen Any substance capable of causing the cellular mutations that lead to cancer.

cardiovascular disease (CVD) A general term for abnormal conditions involving dysfunction of the heart and blood vessels, which can result in heart attack or stroke.

carotenoid A fat-soluble plant pigment that the body stores in the liver and adipose tissues. The body is able to convert certain carotenoids to vitamin A.

case control studies Complex observational studies with additional design features that allow us to gain a better understanding of factors that may influence disease.

celiac disease An autoimmune disorder characterized by an inability to absorb a component of gluten called gliadin. This causes an inflammatory immune response that damages the lining of the small intestine.

cell The smallest unit of matter that exhibits the properties of living things, such as growth, reproduction, and metabolism.

cell differentiation The process by which immature, undifferentiated stem cells develop into highly specialized functional cells of discrete organs and tissues.

cell membrane The boundary of an animal cell that separates its internal cytoplasm and organelles from the external environment.

Centers for Disease Control and Prevention (CDC) The leading federal agency in the United States that protects the health and safety of people. Its mission is to promote health and quality of life by preventing and controlling disease, injury, and disability.

cephalic phase The earliest phase of digestion, in which the brain thinks about and prepares the digestive organs for the consumption of food.

cholecalciferol Vitamin D_3, a form of vitamin D found in animal foods and the form we synthesize from the sun.

chronic diseases Diseases that come on slowly and can persist for years, often despite treatment.

chylomicron A lipoprotein produced in the enterocyte; transports dietary fat out of the intestinal tract.

chyme A semifluid mass consisting of partially digested food, water, and gastric juices.

cirrhosis of the liver End-stage liver disease characterized by significant abnormalities in liver structure and function; may lead to complete liver failure.

clinical trials Tightly controlled experiments in which an intervention is given to determine its effect on a certain disease or health condition.

coenzyme A molecule that combines with an enzyme to activate it and help it do its job.

cofactor A mineral or other inorganic substance that is needed to allow enzymes to function properly.

colic A condition of inconsolable infant crying that lasts for hours at a time.

collagen A protein found in all the connective tissues in our body.

colostrum The first fluid made and secreted by the breasts from late in pregnancy to about a week after birth. It is rich in immune factors and protein.

complementary proteins Two or more foods that together contain all nine essential amino acids necessary for a complete protein. It is not necessary to eat complementary proteins at the same meal.

complete proteins Foods that contain all nine essential amino acids.

complex carbohydrate A nutrient compound consisting of long chains of glucose molecules, such as starch, glycogen, and fiber.

conception The uniting of an ovum (egg) and sperm to create a fertilized egg, or zygote. Also called *fertilization*.

conditionally essential amino acids Amino acids that are normally considered nonessential but become essential under certain circumstances when the body's need for them exceeds the ability to produce them.

conditioned taste aversion   Avoidance of a food as a result of a negative experience, such as illness, even if the illness has no relationship with the food consumed.

constipation   A condition characterized by the absence of bowel movements for a period of time that is significantly longer than normal for the individual. When a bowel movement does occur, stools are usually small, hard, and difficult to pass.

cool-down   Activities done after an exercise session is completed; should be gradual and allow your body to slowly recover from exercise.

cortical bone (compact bone)   A dense bone tissue that makes up the outer surface of all bones as well as the entirety of most small bones of the body.

creatine phosphate (CP)   A high-energy compound that can be broken down for energy and used to regenerate ATP.

cretinism   A form of mental retardation that occurs in children whose mothers experienced iodine deficiency during pregnancy.

crop rotation   The practice of alternating crops in a particular field to prevent nutrient depletion and erosion of the soil and to help with control of crop-specific pests.

cross-contamination   Contamination of one food by another via the unintended transfer of microorganisms through physical contact.

cystic fibrosis   A genetic disorder that causes an alteration in chloride transport, leading to the production of thick, sticky mucus that causes life-threatening respiratory and digestive problems.

cytoplasm   The interior of an animal cell, not including its nucleus.

D

danger zone   Range of temperature (about 40°F to 140°F, or 4°C to 60°C) at which many microorganisms capable of causing human disease thrive.

DASH diet   The diet developed in response to research into hypertension funded by the National Institutes of Health; DASH stands for "Dietary Approaches to Stop Hypertension."

deamination   The process by which an amine group is removed from an amino acid. The nitrogen is then transported to the kidneys for excretion in the urine, while the carbon and other components are metabolized for energy or used to make other compounds.

dehydration   The depletion of body fluid that results when fluid excretion exceeds fluid intake.

denaturation   The process by which proteins uncoil and lose their shape and function when they are exposed to heat, acids, bases, heavy metals, alcohol, and other damaging substances.

denature   The action of the unfolding of proteins in the stomach. Proteins must be denatured before they can be digested.

dental caries   Dental erosion and decay caused by acid-secreting bacteria in the mouth and on the teeth. The acid produced is a by-product of bacterial metabolism of carbohydrates deposited on the teeth.

diabetes   A chronic disease in which the body can no longer regulate glucose normally.

diarrhea   A condition characterized by the frequent passage of loose, watery stools.

dietary fiber   The nondigestible carbohydrate parts of plants that form the support structures of leaves, stems, and seeds.

Dietary Guidelines for Americans   A set of principles developed by the U.S. Department of Agriculture and the U.S. Department of Health and Human Services to assist Americans in designing a healthful diet and lifestyle.

Dietary Reference Intakes (DRIs)   A set of nutritional reference values for the United States and Canada that applies to healthy people.

dietary supplement   A product taken by mouth that contains a "dietary ingredient" intended to supplement the diet.

digestion   The process by which foods are broken down into their component molecules, either mechanically or chemically.

disaccharide   A carbohydrate compound consisting of two sugar molecules joined together.

disordered eating   A general term used to describe a variety of abnormal or atypical eating behaviors that are used to keep or maintain a lower body weight.

diuretic   A substance that increases fluid loss via the urine. Common diuretics include alcohol, some prescription medications, and many over-the-counter weight-loss pills.

docosahexaenoic acid (DHA)   An omega-3 fatty acid available from marine foods and as a metabolic derivative of alpha-linolenic acid.

drink   The amount of an alcoholic beverage that provides approximately 0.5 fl. oz of pure ethanol.

dual energy x-ray absorptiometry (DXA or DEXA)   Currently, the most accurate tool for measuring bone density.

E

eating disorder   A clinically diagnosed psychiatric disorder characterized by severe disturbances in body image and eating behaviors.

edema   A disorder in which fluids build up in the tissue spaces of the body, causing fluid imbalances and a swollen appearance.

eicosapentaenoic acid (EPA)   An omega-3 fatty acid available from marine foods and as a metabolic derivative of alpha-linolenic acid.

electrolyte   A substance that disassociates in solution into positively and negatively charged ions and is thus capable of carrying an electrical current.

electron   A negatively charged particle orbiting the nucleus of an atom.

elimination   The process by which undigested portions of food and waste products are removed from the body.

embryo   The human growth and developmental stage lasting from the third week to the end of the eighth week after fertilization.

empty Calories   Calories from solid fats and/or added sugars that provide few or no nutrients.

energy cost of physical activity   The energy that is expended on body movement and muscular work above basal levels.

energy expenditure   The energy the body expends to maintain its basic functions and to perform all levels of movement and activity.

energy intake   The amount of food a person eats; in other words, it is the number of kilocalories consumed.

enriched foods   Foods in which nutrients that were lost during processing have been added back, so that the food meets a specified standard.

enteric nervous system (ENS) The autonomic nerves in the walls of the GI tract.

enterocytes The cells lining the wall of the intestine.

enzymes Small chemicals, usually proteins, that act on other chemicals to speed up body processes but are not apparently changed during those processes.

epiphyseal plates Plates of cartilage located toward the end of long bones that provide for growth in the length of long bones.

ergocalciferol Vitamin D_2, a form of vitamin D found exclusively in plant foods.

ergogenic aids Substances used to improve exercise and athletic performance.

erythrocytes The red blood cells, which are the cells that transport oxygen in our blood.

esophagus A muscular tube of the GI tract connecting the back of the mouth to the stomach.

essential amino acids Amino acids not produced by the body that must be obtained from food.

essential fatty acids (EFAs) Fatty acids that must be consumed in the diet because they cannot be made by our body.

Estimated Average Requirement (EAR) The average daily nutrient intake level estimated to meet the requirement of half the healthy individuals in a particular life stage or gender group.

Estimated Energy Requirement (EER) The average dietary energy intake that is predicted to maintain energy balance in a healthy adult.

ethanol A specific alcohol compound (C_2H_5OH) formed from the fermentation of dietary carbohydrates and used in a variety of alcoholic beverages.

evaporative cooling Another term for sweating, which is the primary way in which we dissipate heat.

exchange system A diet planning tool in which exchanges, or portions, are organized according to the amount of carbohydrate, protein, fat, and Calories in each food.

exercise A subcategory of leisure-time physical activity; any activity that is purposeful, planned, and structured.

extracellular fluid The fluid outside the body's cells, either in the body's tissues or as the liquid portion of blood, called *plasma.*

F

fair trade A trading partnership that promotes equity in international trading relationships, and contributes to sustainable development by securing the rights of marginalized producers and workers.

fat-soluble vitamins Vitamins that are not soluble in water but are soluble in fat, including vitamins A, D, E, and K.

fats An important energy source for our body at rest and during low-intensity exercise.

fatty acids Long chains of carbon atoms bound to each other as well as to hydrogen atoms.

fatty liver An early and reversible stage of liver disease often found in people who abuse alcohol and characterized by the abnormal accumulation of fat within liver cells.

female athlete triad A serious syndrome that consists of three clinical conditions in some physically active females: low energy availability (with or without eating disorders), menstrual dysfunction, and low bone density.

fermentation A process in which an agent causes an organic substance to break down into simpler substances and results in the production of ATP.

ferritin A storage form of iron in our body, found primarily in the intestinal mucosa, spleen, bone marrow, and liver.

fetal adaptation The process by which fetal metabolism, hormone production, and other physiologic processes shift in response to factors, such as inadequate energy intake, in the maternal environment.

fetal alcohol syndrome (FAS) A set of serious, irreversible alcohol-related birth defects characterized by certain physical and mental abnormalities, including malformations of the face, limbs, heart, and nervous system; impaired growth; and a spectrum of mild to severe cognitive, emotional, and physical problems.

fetus The human growth and developmental stage lasting from the beginning of the ninth week after conception to birth.

FITT principle The principle used to achieve an appropriate overload for physical training; FITT stands for *f*requency, *i*ntensity, *t*ime, and *t*ype of activity.

fluid A substance composed of molecules that move past one another freely. Fluids are characterized by their ability to conform to the shape of whatever container holds them.

fluorosis A condition, marked by staining and pitting of the teeth, caused by an abnormally high intake of fluoride.

food The plants and animals we consume.

food additive A substance or mixture of substances intentionally put into food to enhance its appearance, safety, palatability, and quality.

food allergy An inflammatory reaction to food caused by an immune system hypersensitivity.

food desert An area or community in which residents lack reliable access to affordable fresh produce and other healthful foods.

food insecurity A condition in which an individual is unable to regularly obtain enough food to provide sufficient energy and nutrients to meet physical needs.

food intolerance Gastrointestinal discomfort caused by certain foods that is not a result of an immune system reaction.

food movement A group of local, regional, and national initiatives aimed at promoting sustainable agriculture, food diversity, and food equity, including affordability and fair trade.

foodborne illness An illness transmitted by food or water contaminated by a pathogenic microorganism, its toxic secretions, or a toxic chemical.

fortified foods Foods in which nutrients are added that did not originally exist in the food, or which existed in insignificant amounts.

free radical A highly unstable atom with an unpaired electron in its outermost shell.

frequency Refers to the number of activity sessions per week you perform.

fructose The sweetest natural sugar; a monosaccharide that occurs in fruits and vegetables; also called levulose, or fruit sugar.

functional fiber The nondigestible forms of carbohydrates that are extracted from plants or manufactured in a laboratory and have known health benefits.

functional foods Components of a typical diet which may have biologically active ingredients that provide health benefits beyond basic nutrition.

fungi Plantlike, spore-forming organisms that can grow as either single cells or multicellular colonies.

G

galactose   A monosaccharide that joins with glucose to create lactose, one of the three most common disaccharides.

gallbladder   A sac-like accessory organ of digestion, which lies beneath the liver; it stores bile and secretes it into the small intestine.

gastric juice   Acidic liquid secreted within the stomach; it contains hydrochloric acid and other compounds.

gastroesophageal reflux disease (GERD)   A chronic disease in which episodes of gastroesophageal reflux cause heartburn or other symptoms more than twice per week.

gastrointestinal (GI) tract   A long, muscular tube consisting of several organs: the mouth, esophagus, stomach, small intestine, and large intestine.

gene expression   The process of using a gene to make a protein.

Generally Recognized as Safe (GRAS)   List established by Congress to identify substances used in foods that are generally recognized as safe based on a history of long-term use or on the consensus of qualified research experts.

genetic modification   The process of changing an organism by manipulating its genetic material.

gestation   The period of intrauterine development from conception to birth.

gestational diabetes   A condition of insufficient insulin production or insulin resistance that results in consistently high blood glucose levels, specifically during pregnancy; the condition typically resolves after birth occurs.

ghrelin   A protein, synthesized in the stomach, that acts as a hormone and plays an important role in appetite regulation by stimulating appetite.

glucagon   The hormone secreted by the alpha cells of the pancreas in response to decreased blood levels of glucose; it causes the breakdown of liver stores of glycogen into glucose.

gluconeogenesis   The generation of glucose from the breakdown of proteins into amino acids.

glucose   The most abundant sugar molecule, a monosaccharide generally found in combination with other sugars; it is the preferred source of energy for the brain and an important source of energy for all cells.

glycemic index   The system that assigns ratings (or values) for the potential of foods to raise blood glucose and insulin levels.

glycemic load   The amount of carbohydrate in a food multiplied by the glycemic index of the carbohydrate.

glycerol   An alcohol composed of three carbon atoms; it is the backbone of a triglyceride molecule.

glycogen   A polysaccharide; the storage form of glucose in animals.

glycolysis   The breakdown of glucose; yields two ATP molecules and two pyruvic acid molecules for each molecule of glucose.

goiter   Enlargement of the thyroid gland; can be caused by either iodine toxicity or deficiency.

grazing   Consistently eating small meals throughout the day; done by many athletes to meet their high energy demands.

green revolution   The period of significant increase in global productivity between 1944 and 2000 as a result of selective cross-breeding or hybridization that produced high-yield grains and industrial farming techniques.

H

healthful diet   A diet that provides the proper combination of energy and nutrients and is adequate, moderate, balanced, and varied.

heartburn   A painful sensation that occurs over the sternum when gastric juice pools in the lower esophagus.

heat cramps   Involuntary, spasmodic, and painful muscle contractions that are caused by electrolyte imbalances occurring as a result of strenuous physical activity in high environmental heat.

heat exhaustion   A serious condition, characterized by heavy sweating, pallor, nausea and vomiting, dizziness, and moderately elevated body temperature, that develops from dehydration in high heat.

heat stroke   A potentially fatal response to high temperature characterized by failure of the body's heat-regulating mechanisms; also commonly called *sunstroke*.

helminth   A multicellular microscopic worm.

heme   The iron-containing molecule found in hemoglobin.

heme iron   Iron that is a part of hemoglobin and myoglobin; found only in animal-based foods, such as meat, fish, and poultry.

hemoglobin   The oxygen-carrying protein found in our red blood cells; almost two-thirds of all the iron in our body is found in hemoglobin.

hemosiderin   A storage form of iron in our body, found primarily in the intestinal mucosa, spleen, bone marrow, and liver.

herb   A plant or plant part used for its scent, flavor, and/or therapeutic properties (also called a *botanical*).

hidden fats   Fats that are not apparent, or "hidden" in foods, such as the fats found in baked goods, regular-fat dairy products, marbling in meat, and fried foods.

high-density lipoprotein (HDL)   A lipoprotein made in the liver and released into the blood. HDLs function to transport cholesterol from the tissues back to the liver; often called "good cholesterol."

high-fructose corn syrup   A highly sweet syrup that is manufactured from corn and is used to sweeten soft drinks, desserts, candies, and jellies.

high-yield varieties   Semi-dwarf varieties of plants that are unlikely to fall over in wind and heavy rains and thus can carry larger amounts of seeds, greatly increasing the yield per acre.

homocysteine   An amino acid that requires adequate levels of folate, vitamin B_6, and vitamin B_{12} for its metabolism. High levels of homocysteine in the blood are associated with an increased risk for vascular diseases, such as cardiovascular disease.

hormone   A chemical messenger secreted into the bloodstream by one of the many glands of the body, which acts as a regulator of physiologic processes at a site remote from the gland that secreted it.

human genome   The complete set of genes making up the DNA in the nucleus of a human cell.

human microbiome   The complete set of genes belonging to the trillions of microorganisms that inhabit the human body.

hunger   A physiologic drive for food.

hydrogenation   The process of adding hydrogen to unsaturated fatty acids, making them more saturated and thereby more solid at room temperature.

hypercalcemia   A condition marked by an abnormally high concentration of calcium in the blood.

hyperglycemia   A condition in which blood glucose levels are higher than normal.

hyperkalemia   A condition in which blood potassium levels are dangerously high.

hypermagnesemia   A condition marked by an abnormally high concentration of magnesium in the blood.

hypernatremia   A condition in which blood sodium levels are dangerously high.

hypertension   A chronic condition characterized by above-average blood pressure levels—specifically, systolic blood pressure over 140 mm Hg, or diastolic blood pressure over 90 mm Hg.

hypertrophy   The increase in strength and size that results from repeated work to a specific muscle or muscle group.

hypocalcemia   A condition characterized by an abnormally low concentration of calcium in the blood.

hypoglycemia   A condition marked by blood glucose levels that are below normal fasting levels.

hypokalemia   A condition in which blood potassium levels are dangerously low.

hypomagnesemia   A condition characterized by an abnormally low concentration of magnesium in the blood.

hyponatremia   A condition in which blood sodium levels are dangerously low.

hypothalamus   A region of the forebrain above the pituitary gland, where visceral sensations, such as hunger and thirst, are regulated.

hypothesis   An educated guess as to why a phenomenon occurs.

I

impaired fasting glucose   Fasting blood glucose levels that are higher than normal but not high enough to lead to a diagnosis of type 2 diabetes.

incomplete proteins   Foods that do not contain all of the essential amino acids in sufficient amounts to support growth and health.

inorganic   A substance or nutrient that does not contain carbon and hydrogen.

insensible water loss   The loss of water not noticeable by a person, such as through evaporation from the skin and exhalation from the lungs during breathing.

insoluble fibers   Fibers that do not dissolve in water.

insulin   The hormone secreted by the beta cells of the pancreas in response to increased blood levels of glucose; it facilitates the uptake of glucose by body cells.

intensity   The amount of effort expended during an activity, or how difficult the activity is to perform.

intracellular fluid   The fluid held at any given time within the walls of the body's cells.

intrinsic factor   A protein secreted by cells of the stomach that binds to vitamin B_{12} and aids its absorption in the small intestine.

ion   Any electrically charged particle, either positively or negatively charged.

iron-deficiency anemia   A form of anemia that results from severe iron deficiency.

irradiation   A sterilization process in which food is exposed to gamma rays or high-energy electron beams to kill microorganisms. Irradiation does not impart any radiation to the food being treated.

irritable bowel syndrome (IBS)   A bowel disorder that interferes with normal functions of the colon.

K

Keshan disease   A heart disorder caused by selenium deficiency. It was first identified in children in the Keshan province of China.

ketoacidosis   A condition in which excessive ketones are present in the blood, causing the blood to become very acidic, which alters basic body functions and damages tissues. Untreated ketoacidosis can be fatal. This condition is found in individuals with untreated diabetes mellitus.

ketones   Substances produced during the breakdown of fat when carbohydrate intake is insufficient to meet energy needs. Ketones provide an alternative energy source for the brain when glucose levels are low.

ketosis   The process by which the breakdown of fat during fasting states results in the production of ketones.

kwashiorkor   A form of protein-energy malnutrition that is typically seen in malnourished infants and toddlers and is characterized by wasting, edema, and other signs of protein deficiency.

L

lactase   A digestive enzyme that breaks lactose into glucose and galactose.

lactation   The production of breast milk.

lacteal   A small lymph vessel located inside the villi of the small intestine.

lactic acid   A compound that results when pyruvic acid is metabolized in the presence of insufficient oxygen.

lactose   A disaccharide consisting of one glucose molecule and one galactose molecule. It is found in milk, including human breast milk; also called *milk sugar*.

lactose intolerance   A disorder in which the body does not produce enough lactase enzyme to break down the sugar lactose, which is found in milk and milk products.

large intestine   The final organ of the GI tract, consisting of the cecum, colon, rectum, and anal canal and in which most water is absorbed and feces are formed.

leisure-time physical activity   Any activity not related to a person's occupation; includes competitive sports, recreational activities, and planned exercise training.

leptin   A hormone, produced by body fat, that acts to reduce food intake and to decrease body weight and body fat.

leukocytes   The white blood cells, which protect us from infection and illness.

limiting amino acid   The essential amino acid that is missing or in the smallest supply in the amino acid pool and is thus responsible for slowing or halting protein synthesis.

linoleic acid   An essential fatty acid found in vegetable and nut oils; one of the omega-6 fatty acids.

lipids   A diverse group of organic substances that are insoluble in water; lipids include triglycerides, phospholipids, and sterols.

lipoprotein   A spherical compound in which fat clusters in the center and phospholipids and proteins form the outside of the sphere.

lipoprotein lipase (LPL)   An enzyme that sits on the outside of cells and breaks apart triglycerides, so that their fatty acids can be removed and taken up by the cell.

liver   The largest accessory organ of digestion and one of the most important organs of the body. Its functions include the production of bile and the processing of nutrient-rich blood from the small intestine.

low birth weight   Having a weight of less than 5.5 pounds at birth.

low-density lipoprotein (LDL)   A lipoprotein formed in the blood from VLDLs that transports cholesterol to the cells of the body; often called "bad cholesterol."

low-intensity activities   Activities that cause very mild increases in breathing, sweating, and heart rate.

M

macrocytic anemia   A form of anemia manifested as the production of larger than normal red blood cells containing insufficient hemoglobin, which inhibits adequate transport of oxygen; also called megaloblastic anemia. Macrocytic anemia can be caused by a severe folate deficiency.

macronutrients   Nutrients that our body needs in relatively large amounts to support normal function and health. Carbohydrates, fats, and proteins are macronutrients.

major minerals   Minerals we need to consume in amounts of at least 100 mg per day and of which the total amount in our body is at least 5 g.

maltase   A digestive enzyme that breaks maltose into glucose.

maltose   A disaccharide consisting of two molecules of glucose. It does not generally occur independently in foods but results as a by-product of digestion; also called *malt sugar*.

marasmus   A form of protein-energy malnutrition that results from grossly inadequate intake of energy and protein and other nutrients and is characterized by extreme tissue wasting and stunted growth and development.

maximal heart rate   The rate at which your heart beats during maximal-intensity exercise.

meat factor   A special factor found in meat, fish, and poultry that enhances the absorption of non-heme iron.

megadose   A nutrient dose that is 10 or more times greater than the recommended amount.

megadosing   Consuming nutrients in amounts that are ten or more times higher than recommended levels.

metabolic syndrome   A cluster of risk factors that increase one's risk for heart disease, type 2 diabetes, and stroke, including abdominal obesity, higher than normal triglyceride levels, lower than normal HDL-cholesterol levels, higher than normal blood pressure (greater than or equal to 130/85 mm Hg), and elevated fasting blood glucose levels.

metabolic water   The water formed as a by-product of our body's metabolic reactions.

metabolism   The process by which large chemicals, such as carbohydrates, fats, and proteins, are broken down via chemical reactions into smaller chemicals that can be used as fuel, stored, or assembled into new compounds the body needs.

micronutrients   Nutrients needed in the daily diet in relatively small amounts; vitamins and minerals are micronutrients.

mindful eating   The nonjudgmental awareness of the emotional and physical sensations one experiences while eating or in a food-related environment.

minerals   Inorganic substances that are not broken down during digestion or absorption; they assist in regulating body processes.

moderate drinking   Alcohol consumption of up to one drink per day for women and up to two drinks per day for men.

moderate-intensity activities   Activities that cause moderate increases in breathing, sweating, and heart rate.

moderation   Eating any foods in moderate amounts—not too much and not too little.

monosaccharide   The simplest of carbohydrates, consisting of one sugar molecule, the most common form of which is glucose.

monounsaturated fatty acid (MUFA)   A fatty acid that has two carbons in the chain bound to each other with one double bond; MUFAs are generally liquid at room temperature.

morbid obesity   A condition in which a person's body weight exceeds 100% of normal, putting him or her at very high risk for serious health consequences.

morning sickness   Varying degrees of nausea and vomiting associated with pregnancy, most commonly in the first trimester.

mouthfeel   The tactile sensation of food in the mouth; derived from the interaction of physical and chemical characteristics of the food.

mutual supplementation   The process of combining two or more incomplete protein sources to make a complete protein.

myoglobin   An iron-containing protein similar to hemoglobin except that it is found in muscle cells.

MyPlate   The visual representation of the USDA Food Patterns.

N

National Institutes of Health (NIH)   The world's leading medical research center and the focal point for medical research in the United States.

neural tube   Embryonic tissue that forms a tube, which eventually becomes the brain and spinal cord.

neural tube defects   The most common malformations of the central nervous system that occur during fetal development. A folate deficiency can cause neural tube defects.

neurotransmitters   Chemical compounds that transmit messages from one nerve cell to another.

night blindness   A vitamin A deficiency disorder that results in loss of the ability to see in dim light.

night-eating syndrome   Disorder characterized by intake of the majority of the day's energy between 8:00 PM and 6:00 AM. Individuals with this disorder also experience mood and sleep disorders.

non-heme iron   The form of iron that is not a part of hemoglobin or myoglobin; found in animal- and plant-based foods.

non-nutritive sweeteners   Manufactured sweeteners that provide little or no energy; also called *alternative sweeteners*.

nonessential amino acids   Amino acids that can be manufactured by the body in sufficient quantities and therefore do not need to be consumed regularly in our diet.

nucleus   The positively charged, central core of an atom. It is made up of two types of particles—protons and neutrons—bound tightly together. The nucleus of an atom contains essentially all of its atomic mass.

nutrient density   The relative amount of nutrients per amount of energy (or number of Calories).

nutrient-dense foods   Foods that provide the most nutrients for the least amount of energy (Calories).

nutrients   Chemicals found in foods that are critical to human growth and function.

nutrigenomics   A scientific discipline studying the interactions between genes, the environment, and nutrition.

nutrition   The science that studies food and how food nourishes our body and influences our health.

Nutrition Facts panel   The label on a food package that contains the nutrition information required by the FDA.

nutritive sweeteners   Sweeteners, such as sucrose, fructose, honey, and brown sugar, that contribute Calories (energy).

O

obesity   Having an excess of body fat that adversely affects health, resulting in a person weighing substantially more than an accepted standard for a given height.

observational studies   Studies that indicate relationships between nutrition habits, disease trends, and other health phenomena of large populations of humans.

olfaction   Our sense of smell, which plays a key role in the stimulation of appetite and satiety.

organ   A body structure composed of two or more tissues and performing a specific function; for example, the esophagus.

organelle   A tiny "organ" within a cell that performs a discrete function necessary to the cell.

organic   A substance or nutrient that contains the elements carbon and hydrogen (Ch.1).

organic   Produced without the use of synthetic fertilizers, toxic and persistent pesticides, genetic engineering, or irradiation (Ch.13).

osmosis   The movement of water (or any solvent) through a semipermeable membrane from an area where solutes are less concentrated to areas where solutes are highly concentrated.

osteoblasts   Cells that prompt the formation of new bone matrix by laying down the collagen-containing component of bone, which is then mineralized.

osteoclasts   Cells that erode the surface of bones by secreting enzymes and acids that dig grooves into the bone matrix.

osteomalacia   A vitamin D–deficiency disease in adults, in which bones become weak and prone to fractures.

osteoporosis   A disease characterized by low bone mass and deterioration of bone tissue, leading to increased bone fragility and fracture risk.

ounce-equivalent (oz-equivalent)   A serving size that is 1 ounce, or equivalent to an ounce, for the grains and the protein foods sections of MyPlate.

overload principle   Placing an extra physical demand on your body in order to improve your fitness level.

overweight   Having a moderate amount of excess body fat, resulting in a person weighing more than an accepted standard for a given height but not considered obese.

ovulation   The release of an ovum (egg) from a woman's ovary.

oxidation   A chemical reaction in which molecules of a substance are broken down into their component atoms. During oxidation, the atoms involved lose electrons.

P

pancreas   An accessory organ of digestion located behind the stomach; it secretes digestive enzymes as well as hormones that help regulate blood glucose.

pancreatic amylase   An enzyme secreted by the pancreas into the small intestine that digests any remaining starch into maltose.

parasite   A microorganism that simultaneously derives benefit from and harms its host.

parathyroid hormone (PTH)   A hormone secreted by the parathyroid gland when blood calcium levels fall. Also known as parathormone, it increases blood calcium levels by stimulating the activation of vitamin D, increasing reabsorption of calcium from the kidneys, and stimulating osteoclasts to break down bone, which releases more calcium into the bloodstream.

pasteurization   A form of sterilization using high temperatures for short periods.

pellagra   A disease that results from severe niacin deficiency.

pepsin   An enzyme in the stomach that begins the breakdown of proteins into shorter polypeptide chains and single amino acids.

peptic ulcer   An area of the GI tract that has been eroded away by the acidic gastric juice of the stomach.

peptide bonds   Unique types of chemical bonds in which the amine group of one amino acid binds to the acid group of another in order to manufacture dipeptides and all larger peptide molecules.

peptide YY (PYY)   A protein, produced in the gastrointestinal tract, that is released after a meal in amounts proportional to the energy content of the meal; it decreases appetite and inhibits food intake.

Percent Daily Values (%DVs)   Information on a Nutrition Facts panel that identifies how much a serving of food contributes to your overall intake of the nutrients listed on the label; based on an energy intake of 2,000 Calories per day.

peristalsis   Waves of squeezing and pushing contractions that move food in one direction through the length of the GI tract.

pernicious anemia   A form of anemia that is the primary cause of a vitamin B_{12} deficiency; occurs at the end stage of a disorder that causes the loss of certain cells in the stomach.

persistent organic pollutants (POPs)   Chemicals released into the environment as a result of industry, agriculture, or improper waste disposal; automobile emissions also are considered POPs.

pesticides   Chemicals used either in the field or in storage to decrease destruction by predators or disease.

phospholipid   A type of lipid in which a fatty acid is combined with another compound that contains phosphate; unlike other lipids, phospholipids are soluble in water.

photosynthesis   The process by which plants use sunlight to fuel a chemical reaction that combines carbon and water into glucose, which is then stored in their cells.

physical activity   Any movement produced by muscles that increases energy expenditure; includes occupational, household, leisure-time, and transportation activities.

physical fitness   The ability to carry out daily tasks with vigor and alertness, without undue fatigue, and with ample energy to enjoy leisure-time pursuits and meet unforeseen emergencies.

phytic acid   The form of phosphorus stored in plants.

phytochemicals   Compounds found in plants believed to have health-promoting effects in humans.

pica   An abnormal craving to eat nonfood substances such as clay, paint, or chalk.

placebo   An imitation treatment having no active ingredient that is sometimes used in a clinical trial.

placenta   A pregnancy-specific organ formed from both maternal and embryonic tissues. It is responsible for oxygen, nutrient, and waste exchange between mother and fetus.

plasma   The fluid portion of the blood; needed to maintain adequate blood volume so that the blood can flow easily throughout our body.

platelets   Cell fragments that assist in the formation of blood clots and help stop bleeding.

polypharmacy   The use of five or more prescription drugs at any one time.

polysaccharide   A complex carbohydrate consisting of long chains of glucose.

polyunsaturated fatty acid (PUFA)   A fatty acid that has more than one double bond in the chain; PUFAs are generally liquid at room temperature.

prebiotics   Nondigestible food ingredients that beneficially affect the consumer by selectively stimulating the growth and/or activity of one or a limited number of bacteria in the colon.

prediabetes A term used synonymously with *impaired fasting glucose*; it is a condition considered to be a major risk factor for both type 2 diabetes and heart disease.

preeclampsia High blood pressure that is pregnancy specific and accompanied by protein in the urine, edema, and unexpected weight gain.

preterm The birth of a baby prior to 38 weeks' gestation.

prion A protein that misfolds and becomes infectious; prions are not living cellular organisms or viruses.

probiotics Foods or food supplements containing microorganisms that beneficially affect consumers by improving the intestinal microbial balance.

processed foods Foods that are manipulated mechanically or chemically.

proof A measure of the alcohol content of a liquid; 100-proof liquor is 50% alcohol by volume, 80-proof liquor is 40% alcohol by volume, and so on.

prooxidant A nutrient that promotes oxidation and oxidative cell and tissue damage.

proteases Enzymes that continue the breakdown of polypeptides in the small intestine.

protein-energy malnutrition A disorder caused by inadequate consumption of protein. It is characterized by severe wasting.

proteins Large, complex molecules made up of amino acids and found as essential components of all living cells.

protozoa Single-celled, mobile microorganisms.

provitamin An inactive form of a vitamin that the body can convert to an active form. An example is beta-carotene.

puberty The period of life in which secondary sexual characteristics develop and people become biologically capable of reproducing.

purging An attempt to rid the body of unwanted food by vomiting or other compensatory means, such as excessive exercise, fasting, or laxative abuse.

pyruvic acid The primary end product of glycolysis.

Q

quackery The promotion of an unproven remedy, such as a supplement or other product or service, usually by someone unlicensed and untrained.

R

recombinant bovine growth hormone (rBGH) A genetically engineered hormone injected into dairy cows to enhance their milk output.

recombinant DNA technology A type of genetic modification in which scientists combine DNA from different sources to produce a transgenic organism that expresses a desired trait.

Recommended Dietary Allowance (RDA) The average daily nutrient intake level that meets the nutrient requirements of 97–98% of healthy individuals in a particular life stage and gender group.

remodeling The two-step process by which bone tissue is recycled; includes the breakdown of existing bone and the formation of new bone.

residues Chemicals that remain in the foods we eat despite cleaning and processing.

resistance training Exercise in which our muscles act against resistance.

resorption The process by which the surface of bone is broken down by cells called osteoclasts.

resveratrol A phytochemical known to play a role in limiting cell damage from the by-products of metabolic reactions. It is found in red wine and certain other plant-based foods.

retina The delicate, light-sensitive membrane lining the inner eyeball and connected to the optic nerve. It contains retinal.

retinal An active, aldehyde form of vitamin A that plays an important role in healthy vision and immune function.

retinoic acid An active, acid form of vitamin A that plays an important role in cell growth and immune function.

retinol An active, alcohol form of vitamin A that plays an important role in healthy vision and immune function.

rhodopsin A light-sensitive pigment found in the rod cells that is formed by retinal and opsin.

ribose A five-carbon monosaccharide that is located in the genetic material of cells.

rickets A vitamin D–deficiency disease in children. Signs include deformities of the skeleton, such as bowed legs and knocked knees. Severe rickets can be fatal.

S

saliva A mixture of water, mucus, enzymes, and other chemicals that moistens the mouth and food, binds food particles together, and begins the digestion of carbohydrates.

salivary amylase An enzyme in saliva that breaks starch into smaller particles and eventually into the disaccharide maltose.

salivary glands A group of glands found under and behind the tongue and beneath the jaw that release saliva continually as well as in response to the thought, sight, smell, or presence of food.

satiety A physiologic sensation of fullness (from the Latin *satis* meaning enough, as in *satisfied*).

saturated fatty acid (SFA) A fatty acid that has no carbons joined together with a double bond; SFAs are generally solid at room temperature.

sensible water loss Water loss that is noticed by a person, such as through urine output and visible sweating.

set-point theory The theory that the body raises or lowers energy expenditure in response to increased or decreased food intake and physical activity. This action maintains an individual's body weight within a narrow range.

sickle cell anemia A genetic disorder that causes red blood cells to be shaped like a sickle or crescent, impeding their transport to body tissues.

simple carbohydrate Commonly called *sugar;* can be either a monosaccharide (such as glucose) or a disaccharide.

small intestine The longest portion of the GI tract, where most digestion and absorption take place.

soluble fibers Fibers that dissolve in water.

solvent A substance that is capable of mixing with and breaking apart a variety of compounds. Water is an excellent solvent.

sphincter A tight ring of muscle separating some of the organs of the GI tract and opening in response to nerve signals indicating that food is ready to pass into the next section.

spina bifida The embryotic neural tube defect that occurs when the spinal vertebrae fail to completely enclose the spinal cord, allowing it to protrude.

spontaneous abortion The natural termination of a pregnancy and expulsion of pregnancy tissues because of a genetic, developmental, or physiologic abnormality that is so severe that the pregnancy cannot be maintained. Also called *miscarriage*.

starch A polysaccharide stored in plants; the storage form of glucose in plants.

sterol A type of lipid found in foods and the body that has a ring structure; cholesterol is the most common sterol in our diets.

stomach A J-shaped organ where food is partially digested, churned, and stored until it is released into the small intestine.

stretching Exercise in which muscles are gently lengthened using slow, controlled movements.

sucrase A digestive enzyme that breaks sucrose into glucose and fructose.

sucrose A disaccharide composed of one glucose molecule and one fructose molecule; sucrose is sweeter than lactose or maltose.

sudden infant death syndrome (SIDS) The sudden death of a previously healthy infant; the most common cause of death in infants over 1 month of age.

sustainability The ability to meet or satisfy basic economic, social, and security needs now and in the future without undermining the natural resource base and environmental quality on which life depends.

sustainable agriculture Techniques of food production that preserve the environment indefinitely.

system A group of organs that work together to perform a unique function; for example, the gastrointestinal system.

T

T-score A comparison of an individual's bone density to the average peak bone density of a 30-year-old healthy adult.

teratogen A compound known to cause fetal harm or danger(Ch. 7.5).

teratogen Any substance that can cause a birth defect (Ch. 14).

theory A conclusion, or scientific consensus, drawn from repeated experiments.

thermic effect of food (TEF) The energy expended as a result of processing food consumed.

thirst mechanism A cluster of nerve cells in the hypothalamus that stimulate our conscious desire to drink fluids in response to an increase in the concentration of salt in our blood or a decrease in blood pressure and blood volume.

thrifty gene theory The theory that some people possess a gene (or genes) that causes them to be energetically thrifty, resulting in their expending less energy at rest and during physical activity.

time of activity How long each exercise session lasts.

tissue A grouping of like cells that performs a function; for example, muscle tissue.

tocopherol The active form of vitamin E in our body.

Tolerable Upper Intake Level (UL) The highest average daily nutrient intake level likely to pose no risk of adverse health effects to almost all individuals in a particular life stage and gender group.

total fiber The sum of dietary fiber and functional fiber.

toxin Any harmful substance; in microbiology, a chemical produced by a microorganism that harms tissues or causes harmful immune responses.

trabecular bone (spongy bone) A porous bone tissue that makes up only 20% of our skeleton and is found within the ends of the long bones, inside the spinal vertebrae, inside the flat bones (sternum, ribs, and most bones of the skull), and inside the bones of the pelvis.

trace minerals Minerals that must be consumed in amounts of less than 100 mg/day and that are present in the body at the level of less than 5 g.

transamination The process of transferring the amine group from one amino acid to another in order to manufacture a new amino acid.

transcription The process through which messenger RNA copies genetic information from DNA in the nucleus.

transferrin The transport protein for iron.

translation The process that occurs when the genetic information carried by messenger RNA is translated into a chain of amino acids at the ribosome.

transport proteins Protein molecules that help transport substances throughout the body and across cell membranes.

triglyceride A molecule consisting of three fatty acids attached to a three-carbon glycerol backbone.

trimester Any one of three stages of pregnancy, each lasting 13 to 14 weeks.

tumor Any newly formed mass of undifferentiated cells.

type 1 diabetes A disorder in which the body cannot produce enough insulin.

type 2 diabetes A progressive disorder in which body cells become less responsive to insulin.

type of activity The range of physical activities a person can engage in to promote health and physical fitness.

U

umbilical cord The cord containing the arteries and veins that connect the baby (from the navel) to the mother via the placenta.

underweight Having too little body fat to maintain health, causing a person to weigh less than an acceptably defined standard for a given height.

urinary tract infection A bacterial infection of the urethra, the tube leading from the bladder to the body exterior.

V

variety Eating many different foods, from different food groups, regularly.

vegetarianism The practice of restricting the diet to food substances of plant origin, including vegetables, fruits, grains, and nuts.

very-low-density lipoprotein (VLDL) A lipoprotein made in the liver and intestine that functions to transport lipids, especially triglycerides, to the tissues of the body.

vigorous-intensity activities Activities that produce significant increases in breathing, sweating, and heart rate; talking is difficult when exercising at a vigorous intensity.

viruses A group of infectious agents that are usually much smaller than bacteria, lack independent metabolism, and are incapable of growth or reproduction outside of living cells.

viscous Having a gel-like consistency; viscous fibers form a gel when dissolved in water.

visible fats Fats that are clearly present and visible in our food, or visibly added to food, such as butter, margarine, cream, shortening, salad dressings, chicken skin, and untrimmed fat on meat.

vitamins Organic compounds that assist in regulating body processes.

vomiting The involuntary expulsion of the contents of the stomach and duodenum from the mouth.

W

warm-up Also called preliminary exercise; includes activities that prepare you for an exercise bout, including stretching, calisthenics, and movements specific to the exercise bout.

water-soluble vitamins Vitamins that are soluble in water, including vitamin C and the B-vitamins.

wellness A multidimensional, lifelong process that includes physical, emotional, social, occupational, and spiritual health.

whole foods Foods that have been modified as little as possible, remaining in or near their natural state.

Z

zygote A fertilized ovum (egg) consisting of a single cell.

index

credits

Walkthrough

p. 1 Foodcollection RF/Getty Images

Chapter 1

p. 2 Image Source/Getty Images; **p. 4:** Anna Hoychuk/Shutterstock; **p. 5:** Lester V. Bergman/Encyclopedia/Corbis; **p. 6: Fig. 1.1:** Yeko Photo Studio/Shutterstock; **Fig. 1.2:** mr.markin/Fotolia; **p. 10:** Tom Stewart/CORBIS; **p. 12:** Ant Strack/CORBIS; **p. 13:** Lidante/Shutterstock; **p. 14:** matin/Shutterstock; **p. 15 Fig. 1.9:** Samuel Borges Photography/Shutterstock; **p. 16:** Comstock/Thinkstock; **p. 17:** OJO Images Ltd/Alamy; **p. 20:** Sandra Baker/Alamy; **p. 21:** Miriam Doerr/Shutterstock; **p. 22:** Pearson Education/Pearson Science; **p. 24:** Liquidlibrary/Thinkstock; **p. 25:** Michael Donne/Science Source; **p. 27:** Marcin Łukaszewicz/Alamy; **p. 30:** mark phillips/Alamy; **p. 31:** Randy L. Jirtle; **p. 32:** Science Photo Library/Alamy; **p. 33:** OJO Images Ltd/Alamy; **p. 35 Fig. 1: top:** Southern Illinois University/Science Source; **top center:** DJM-photo/Shutterstock; **center:** Image Source/Getty Images; **bottom center:** Pixtal/AGE Fotostock; **bottom:** Joy Brown/Shutterstock; **p. 36 top left:** Ian O'Leary/DK Images; **bottom left:** Rob Bartee/Alamy; **right:** Kurt Wilson/FoodPix/Getty Images

Chapter 2

p.38: Image Source/InStock/Alamy; **p. 40:** Mark Follon/Adams Picture Library/Alamy; **p. 41 left:** Photosani/Shutterstock; **p. 41 right:** Forest Badger/Shutterstock; **p. 41 bottom:** iStockphoto/Thinkstock; **p. 42:** AP Images/Janet Jensen; **p. 44:** Sky Bonillo/PhotoEdit; **p. 47:** Kzenon, 2010/Shutterstock; **p. 49 top:** Alexander Walter/Getty Images; **p. 49 bottom:** DK Images; **p. 50:** Andrew Whittuck/Dorling Kindersley; **p. 53: Fig. 2.7a:** ALEAIMAGE/Getty Images; **b:** Kelly Cline/Getty Images; **c:** iStockphoto/Thinkstock; **d:** Morgan Lane Photography/Shutterstock; **e:** Natalia Mylova/Fotolia; **page 54: Fig. 2.8:** Pearson Learning Photo Studio; **p. 55: Fig. 2.9:** Pearson Education/Pearson Science; **p. 55:** iStockphoto/Thinkstock; **p. 56: Fig. 2.10 top left:** Image Source/Alamy; **top right:** Envision/Corbis; **bottom left:** F. Schussler/PhotoLink/Getty Images; **bottom right:** Ragnar Schmuck/Getty Images; **p. 58:** Joe Raedle/Staff/Getty Images; **p. 59 top:** Sigrid Estrada/Laison/Getty Images; **bottom:** Koichi Kamoshida/Newsmakers/Getty Images; **p. 65:** IMAGEMORE Co, Ltd./Getty Images; **p. 66:** Jean Luc Morales/The Image Bank/Getty Images; **Fig. 1:** Jon Riley/Stone/Getty Images; **p. 67 top:** JoeFox/Alamy; **bottom:** photomadnz/Alamy; **p. 70:** Image Source/Alamy

Chapter 3

p. 72: Eric Audras/ONOKY/Getty Images; **p. 76:** Howard Kingsnorth/The Image Bank/Getty Images; **p. 79:** Michael Flippo/Fotolia; **p. 87:** Bon Appetit/Kröger/Alamy; **p. 88: Fig. 3.12 top:** David Musher/Science Source; **center:** Steve G. Schmeissner/Science Source; **bottom:** Don W. Fawcett/Science Source; **p. 89:** shippee/Shutterstock; **p. 91:** SPL/Science Source; **p. 92:** David Sacks/Stone/Getty Images; **p. 94 top:** Digital Vision/Getty Images; **Fig. 3.16:** Dr. E. Walker/Science Photo Library/Science Source; **p. 96:** Susan Van Ette/PhotoEdit; **p. 97:** Nataliya Peregudova/Fotolia; **Fig. 3.17 top left:** BURGER/Phanie/AGE Fotostock; **p. 99:** MedicalRF.com/Alamy; **p. 102:** FotografiaBasica/E+/Getty Images; **p. 103:** Clive Streeter/DK Images; **p. 104:** David Murray and Jules Selmes/DK Images; **p. 105:** Scott Indermaur/Workbook Stock/Getty Images; **p. 106 top:** nadi555/Shutterstock; **bottom:** Cordelia Molloy/Science Source

Chapter 4

p. 108: MIXA/Getty Images; **p. 110:** Brocreative/Shutterstock; **p. 112:** Monkey Business Images/Shutterstock; **p. 113 left:** Foodcollection/Getty Images; **right:** Danny Smythe/Shutterstock.com; **p. 114:** Pearson Education/Pearson Science; **p. 115:** George Doyle/Stockbyte/Thinkstock; **p. 116: Fig. 4.5 top:** Bernd Leitner/Fotolia; **center:** Doug Menuez/Photodisc/Getty Images; **bottom:** technotr/Getty Images; **p. 117 top:** Maridav/Fotolio; **bottom:** DK Images; **p. 123 left:** DK Images; **right:** Ryan McVay/Photodisc/Getty Images; **p. 125:** Ian O'Leary/DK Images; **p. 126:** Joe Raedle/Staff/Getty Images; **p. 128:** DK Images; **p. 130: Fig. 4.14 left:** Giuseppe_R/Shutterstock; **right:** Diana Taliun/Shutterstock; **p. 131 left:** Wiktory/Shutterstock; **center left:** Dusan Zidar/Shutterstock; **center right:** DK Images; **right:** Dmytro Mykhailov/Shutterstock; **p. 132: Fig. 4.15:** Alex459/Shutterstock; **p. 134:** Pearson Education/pearson Science; **p. 136:** Brian Buckley/Alamy; **p. 139:** Cultura/Mischa Keijser/StockImage/Getty Images; **p. 140:** Scott Camazine/Alamy; **p. 142:** bikeriderlondon/Shutterstock; **p. 143:** Scott Camazine/Science Source; **p. 145:** Nancy Kaszerman/ZUMA Wire Service/Alamy

Chapter 5

p. 146: CactuSoup/E+/Getty Images; **p. 148 top:** Dan Kosmayer/Fotolia; **center:** Steve Gorton/DK Images; **p. 151 top:** oriori/Shutterstock; **center:** nikolych/Fotolia; **p. 152 top:** Stephen VanHorn/Shutterstock; **bottom:** HLPhoto/Shutterstock; **p. 153:** Comstock/Thinkstock; **p. 156:** Andersen Ross/Photodisc/Getty Images; **p. 157 top:** Doug Pensinger/Staff/Getty Images; **center:** Amy Myers/Shutterstock; **p. 158 top:** Danny E Hooks/Shutterstock; **bottom:** Kip Peticolas/Fundamental Photographs; **p. 163:** Jeff Greenberg/AGE Fotostock; **p. 164:** Wilmy van Ulft/Shutterstock; **p. 165:** Travis Amos/Pearson Education/Pearson Science; **p. 166: Fig. 5.14:** foodfolio/Alamy; **p. 168:** Michael C. Gray/Shutterstock; **p. 171 left:** holbox/Shutterstock; **center left:** iStockphoto/Thinkstock; **center right:** Jacek Chabraszewski/Shutterstock; **right:** Anna Hoychuk/Shutterstock; **p. 173:** Richard Megna/Fundamental Photographs; **p. 174:** Yory Frenklakh/Shutterstock; **p. 177:** Image Source/Getty Images; **p. 178:** Arthur Tilley/Creatas/Jupiter/Getty Images; **p. 179: Fig. 1:** Biophoto Associates/Science Source; **p. 180:** 14ktgold/Fotolia; **p. 181:** AP Images/Rich Kareckas; **p. 187:** altafulla/Shutterstock; **p. 188: Fig. 5:** Clive Streeter/DK Images

Chapter 6

p. 190: Tanya_F/E+/Getty Images; **p. 192:** © Andresr/Shutterstock; **p. 198: Fig. 6.7:** Andrew Syred/Science Source; **bottom:** AlenaKogotkova/Shutterstock; **p. 199: Fig. 6.8:** Creative Digital Visions/Pearson Education/Pearson Science; **p. 201: Fig. 6.9a:** Falater Photo/Fotlia; **b:** Mediscan/Medical-on-Line/Alamy; **p. 206:** Ian O'Leary/DK Images; **p. 207: Fig. 6.12a:** Jupiterimages/Comstock Images/Getty Images; **b:** Mike Goldwater/Alamy; **c:** Rubberball/Alan K. Bailey/Getty Images; **p. 208:** AP Images/Lionel Cironneau; **p. 209:** Ranald MacKechnie/DK Images; **p. 214a:** Liv friis-larsen/Shutterstock; **b:** stockstudios/Shutterstock; **c:** Lisovskaya Natalia/Shutterstock; **d:** Elena Elisseeva/Shutterstock; **bottom:** Pearson Education/Pearson Science; **p. 215:** BananaStock/Alamy Images; **p. 216 top:** Glowimages/Getty Images; **center:** Danita Delimont/Alamy; **bottom:** DK Images; **p. 219: Fig. 6.13a:** Lucy Deng/FlickrVision/Getty Images; **b:** Christine Osborne Pictures/

Alamy; **p. 216: Fig. 6.14:** Eye of Science/ Science Source; **p. 221 top:** Clive Streeter/ DK Images; **bottom:** DK Images; **p. 224:** FoodCollection/SuperStock; **p. 225 top:** Alexandr Makarov/Shutterstock; **bottom:** Simon Smith/DK Images; **p. 226:** Paul prescott/Shutterstock; **p. 228:** yuris/ Shutterstock; **p. 231 top:** Safia Fatimi/The Image Bank/Getty Images; **bottom:** Diana Taliun/Shutterstock; **p. 232:** Nancy R. Cohen/Photodisc/Getty Images

Chapter 7

p. 234: marcstock/Shutterstock; **p. 237:** Vinicius Tupinamba/Shutterstock; **p. 238:** Jupiterimages/Polka Dot/Thinkstock; **p. 240: Fig. 7.4 top left:** Sergey Peterman/ Shutterstock; **a:** Peter Bernik/Shutterstock; **b:** George Dolgikh/Shutterstock; **c:** Jeremy Pembrey/Alamy; **p. 242:** iStockphoto/ Thinkstock; **p. 243: Fig. 7.6:** photo25th/ Shutterstock; **p. 244:** Stockbyte/Getty Images; **p. 245 top:** Ted Levine/Fancy/ Corbis; **Fig. 7.7:** Photodisc/Getty Images; **p. 246:** Network Productions/The Image Works; **p. 247:** Kristin Piljay/Pearson Education/Pearson Science; **p. 248:** Silberkorn/Shutterstock; **p. 250 top:** David Bro/Newscom; **bottom:** Andrea Skjold/Shutterstock; **p. 251:** Rachel Weill/Photolibrary/Getty Images; **p. 254a:** picamaniac/Shutterstock; **b:** Lorraine Kourafas/Shutterstock; **c:** barbaradudzinska/Shutterstock; **d:** Antonov Roman/Shutterstock; **bottom:** Wiktory/Shutterstock; **p. 255: Fig. 7.8:** Alex Staroseltsev/Shutterstock; **p. 256:** Foodcollection/Getty Images; **p. 257: Fig. 7.9:** Peter zijlstra/Shutterstock; **bottom:** fotogiunta/Shutterstock; **p. 258 top:** Susanna Price/DK Images; **bottom:** Travis Amos/Pearson Education/Pearson Science; **p. 260:** Carolyn A. McKeone/ Science Source; **p. 261:** Tobias Titz/Getty Images; **p. 264:** webphotographeer/E+/ Getty Images; **p. 265: Fig. 1:** Kristin Piljay/ Pearson Education/Pearson Science; **p. 266:** David R. Frazier Photolibrary, Inc./Alamy; **p. 267:** Jemma Jones/Alamy; **p. 269: Fig. 4a:** Science Photo Library/ Science Source; **b:** Martin M. Rotker/ Science Source; **p. 270:** Enigma/Alamy; **p. 271: Fig. 6:** Streissguth, A.P, Clarren, S.K., & Jones, K.L. (1985, July). Natural history of the Fetal Alcohol Syndrome: A ten-year follow-up of eleven patients. Lancet, 2, 85-91.

Chapter 8

p. 274: Daniel Loiselle/E+/Getty Images; **p. 278:** Walter Bibikow/Jon Arnold Images Ltd/Alamy; **p. 280 top:** Valentyn Volkov/ Shutterstock; **bottom:** Steve Gorton/DK Images; **p. 281: Fig. 8.6:** iStockphoto/ Thinkstock; **p. 282:** David Murray/DK Images; **p. 284:** Pia Tryde/DK Images; **p. 285: Fig. 8.7:** bluestocking/iStockphoto; **bottom a:** Bon Appetit/Alamy; **bottom b:**

foodfolio/Alamy; **bottom c:** iStockphoto/ Thinkstock; **bottom d:** Stock Foundry/ Design Pics Inc/Alamy; **p. 286 top:** Philip Wilkins/DK Images; **Fig. 8.8:** Medical-on-Line/Alamy; **p. 288 top:** Stephen Hayward/ DK Images; **Fig. 8.10 bottom:** iStockphoto/ Thinkstock; **p. 289: Fig. 8.11:** Bernardo De Niz//MCT/Newscom; **p. 290 top:** United States Department of Agriculture; **Fig. 8.12:** iStockphoto/Thinkstock; **p. 292:** JLP/Sylvia Torres/Flirt/Corbis; **p. 293: Fig. 8.14:** Siri Stafford/Getty Images; **p. 294: Fig. 8.15:** Pearson Education/Pearson Science; **p. 296: Fig. 8.16 top:** iStockphoto/Thinkstock; **bottom:** DK Images; **p. 298:** Dreamstime LLC; **p. 301:** Lee Avison/GAP Photos/Getty Images; **p. 302:** Dave King/DK Images; **p. 303: Fig. 2:** St Bartholomew's Hospital/ Science Source; **p. 305: Fig. 3a:** Edward H.Gill/Custom Medical Stock; **b:** Lauren Shear/Science Source; **Fig. 4:** NIH Custom Medical Stock Photo/Newscom; **bottom:** amriphoto/Getty Images; **p. 306: Fig. 5:** Dr. P. Marazzi/Science Source; **p. 307:** Vitalii Nesterchuk/Shutterstock; **p. 308:** Suzannah Skelton/iStockphoto/Getty Images

Chapter 9

p. 310: gordana jovanovic/E+/Getty Images; **p. 315: Fig. 9.4 left:** SPL/Science Source; **right:** Pascal Alix/Science Source; **p. 316:** auremar/Shutterstock; **p. 318:** Dave King/DK Images; **p. 319: Fig. 9.6:** istockphoto/Thinkstock; **bottom:** Peter Anderson/DK Images; **p. 320: Fig. 9.7:** Brand Z Food/Alamy; Pearson Education/ Pearson Science; Comstock/Getty Images; Pearson Education/Pearson Science; Ramon Espelt Photography/Shutterstock; DK Images; BW Folsom/Shutterstock; **p. 321:** Pearson Education/Pearson Science; **p. 322 left:** Teamarbeit/Dreamstime; **center left:** Lawton/SoFood/Alamy; **center right:** Igor Dutina/Shutterstock; **right:** Alejandro Rivera/Getty Images; **p. 325:** Peter Turnley/ Corbis; **p. 326:** DK Images; **Fig. 9.10:** Jiri Hera/Shutterstock; **p. 327: Fig. 9.11:** Biophoto Associates/Science Source; **p. 328 top:** iStockphoto/Thinkstock; **center:** DK Images; **Fig. 9.12:** iStockphoto/ Thinkstock; **p. 329:** Catherine Ledner/ Getty Images; **p. 330:** Spencer Jones/Getty Images; **p. 331: Fig. 9.13:** CanuckStock/ Shutterstock; **p. 332:** Larry Williams/ Corbis; **p. 333: Fig. 9.14:** National Institute of Dental Research; **p. 335:** Johner/ Getty Images; **p. 338:** Ty Milford/Radius Images/Getty Images; **p. 339: Fig. 1:** Michael Klein/Getty Images; **Fig. 2a:** Robert Destefano/Alamy; **2b:** Living Art Enterprises/Science Source; **2c:** Custom Medical Stock/Newscom; **p. 340: Fig. 3:** ZUMA Press/Newscom; **right:** Larry Mulvehill/Science Source; **p. 341:** Spencer Platt/Getty Images; **p. 342:** Duomo/Corbis; **p. 343:** BSIP SA/Alamy; **p. 345:** Tom Wang/Shutterstock

Chapter 10

p. 346: marco mayer/Shutterstock; **p. 348:** PhotoDisc/Getty Images; **p. 350:** Nayashkova Olga/Shutterstock; **p. 351: Fig. 10.3:** Fuat Kose/Getty Images; **p. 352 top:** Burke/Triolo Productions/ Photolibrary/Getty Images; **Fig. 10.4:** Burwell and Burwell Photography/ Thinkstock; **p. 353: Fig. 10.5:** Alex Staroseltsev/Shutterstock; **bottom:** Paul Johnson/Getty Images; **p. 354:** Youlian/Shutterstock; **p. 356: Fig. 10.8:** istockphoto/Thinkstock; **p. 357:** Jupiterimages/Creatas/Thinkstock; **p. 359:** Food Features/Alamy; **p. 360: Fig. 10.10:** istockphoto/Thinkstock; **p. 361 top:** David Murray/DK Images; **Fig. 10.11:** Shutterstock; **p. 362:** Duncan Smith/Corbis Yellow/Corbis; **p. 363 top:** Alison Wright/ Encyclopedia/Corbis; **p. 363 bottom:** Monique le Luhandre/DK Images; **p. 364:** Pearson Education/Pearson Science; **p. 365: Fig. 10.12 top:** Viktar Malyshchyts/ Shutterstock; **bottom:** Kati Molin/ Shutterstock; **p. 366:** DK Images; **p. 367:** Sebastian Kaulitzki/Shutterstock; **p. 369:** Jupiterimages/Comstock/Thinkstock; **p. 371: Fig. 10.15:** zcw/Shutterstock; **p. 372 left:** Nayashkova Olga/Shutterstock; **center left:** ENVY/Shutterstock; **center right:** jabiru/Shutterstock; **right:** Andy Dean Photography/Shutterstock; **p. 374:** Isabelle Rozenbaum & Frederic Cirou/ PhotoAlto Agency/Getty Images; **p. 375 Fig. 10.17:** OlegD/Shutterstock; **bottom:** Ian O'Leary/DK Images; **p. 376: Fig. 10.18:** Ermin Gutenberger/Getty Images; **p. 377:** Kristin Piljay/Pearson Science/ Pearson Education; **p. 380:** Bochkarev Photography/Shutterstock; **p. 381: Fig. 1:** Cordelia Molloy/Science Source; **p. 382:** Pearson Education/Pearson Science; **p. 383:** Kanusommer/Shutterstock; **p. 384:** Digital Vision/Getty Images

Chapter 11

p. 388: digitalskillet/E+/Getty Images; **p. 390:** PAUL BUCK/EPA/Newscom; **p. 391:** Ryan McVay/Photodisc/Getty Images; **p. 393: Fig. 11.2a:** Peter Menzel/Science Source; **b:** Pearson Education/Pearson Science; **c:** May/Science Source; **d:** Phanie/ Science Source; **e:** Life Measurement, Inc.; **p. 394:** Robert Harding World Imagery; **p. 395: Fig. 11.4a left:** Pearson Education/ Pearson Science; **b:** Pearson Education/ Pearson Science; **p. 396: Fig. 11.5 top:** Helder Almeida/Shutterstock; **top center:** maga/Shuterstock; **top right:** Kenneth Man/Shutterstock; **center left:** Kenneth Man/Shutterstock; **center right:** lightpoet/ Shutterstock; **bottom left:** Zurijeta/ Shutterstock; **bottom right:** Brian A. Jackson/Shutterstock; **p. 397:** DK Images; **p. 399:** Stockbyte/Thinkstock; **p. 401:** Alvis Upitis/Photographer's Choice/Getty Images; **p. 403:** iStockphoto/Thinkstock; **p. 405:** Bruce Dale/GettyImages; **p. 406:**

Norma Joseph/Alamy; **p. 407:** Mark Douet/Stone/Getty Images; **p. 413 top:** Jacek Chabraszewski/Shutterstock; **bottom:** Banana Stock/Getty Images; **p. 415: Fig. 11.8:** Pearson Education/Pearson Science; **p. 419 top:** JJAVA/Fotolia; **p. 420:** doc-stock/Alamy; **bottom:** Food Alan King/Alamy; **p. 421:** Ryan McVay/Digital Vision/Thinkstock; **p. 422 top:** ObesityImages/Alamy; **Fig. 11.10** William Thomas Cain/Stringer/Getty Images; **p. 425:** Liu Jin/AFP/Getty Images; **p. 426:** Chuck Place/Alamy; **p. 429:** Jamie Grill Photography/Getty Images; **p. 430:** AP Images/Eugenio Savio; **p. 431:** Digital Vision/Getty Images; **p. 432 left:** Pearson Education/Pearson Science; **right:** Karl Prouse/Catwalking/Getty Images; **p. 433:** Oote Boe 3/Alamy; **p. 435 left:** Blake Little/The Image Bank/Getty Images; **right:** FJM/Colorise/ZUMAPRESS/Newscom; **p. 436:** blickwinkel/Alamy; **p. 437 top:** D. Hurst/Alamy; **Fig. 3 bottom:** Photodisc/Thinkstock

Chapter 12

p. 440: Monkey Business Images/the Agency Collection/Getty Images; **p. 442 top:** Robert W. Ginn/AGE Fotostock; **bottom:** My Good Images/Shutterstock; **p. 443: Fig. 12.1 left:** © Blue Jean Images/Alamy; **right:** Stockbyte/Getty Images; **p. 445:** AP Images/Mark Lennihan; **p. 446:** Will & Deni McIntyre/Science Source; **p. 447: Fig. 12.3a:** Endostock/Fotolia; **b:** Tatyana Vychegzhanina/Shutterstock; **c:** Martin Novak/Shutterstock; **p. 449:** Moodboard/Alamy; **p. 452:** Image Source/Getty Images; **p. 453: Fig 12.7 top:** Ariwasabi/Shutterstock; **a:** Peter Bernik/Shutterstock; **b:** Koji Aoki/Getty Images; **c:** Nigel Roddis/EPA/Newscom; **d:** Colin Underhill/Alamy; **e:** maho/Fotolia; **f:** Maridav/Shutterstock; **p. 455:** Randy Faris/Corbis RF/Alamy; **p. 457:** Stephen Oliver/DK Images; **p. 458:** Jens Schlueter/DDP/Getty Images; **p 459: Fig. 12.10: 1,800 kcal/day:** Morgan Lane Photography/Shutterstock; DEAN PICTURE/Newscom; **4,000 kcal/day:** iStockphoto/Thinkstock; Pearson Education/Pearson Science **p. 461:** Stockbyte/Getty Images; **p. 462:** Val Thoermer/shutterstock; **p. 464 top:** Dave King/DK Images; **p. 464 bottom:** Denkou Images/Cultura/Getty Images; **p. 465: Fig. 12.12 right:** Dburke/Alamy;

p. 468: Stockbyte/Getty Images; **p. 471:** Milan Zeremski/E+/Shutterstock; **p. 472:** Istvan Csak/Shutterstock; **p. 474:** Derek Hall/DK Images

Chapter 13

p. 476: Mikhail Malyshev/Fotolia; **p. 478:** matka_Wariatka/Shutterstock; **p. 480: Fig. 13.1a:** Exactostock/SuperStock; **b:** avatar444/Fotolia; **c:** David Wei/Alamy; **d:** A3602 Frank Rumpenhorst/Newscom; **e:** Huntstock, Inc/Alamy; **p. 481: Fig. 13.2:** Laguna Design/Science Source; **Fig. 13.3:** Dr. Tony Brain/Science Source; **p. 483: Fig. 13.4 top:** Andrew Syred/Science Source; **Fig. 13.5:** Matt Meadows/Peter Arnold/Getty Images; **p. 484:** William Shaw/DK Images; **p. 485: Fig. 13.6 top:** Neil Fletcher/DK Images; **bottom:** Jean-Louis Vosgien/Shutterstock; **p. 487 top:** Xy/Fotolia; **bottom:** planet5D LLC/Shutterstock; **p. 489:** BlueOrange Studio/Shutterstock; **p. 491 top:** Owen Franken/Corbis; **bottom:** New York Times Co/Getty Images; **p. 492:** Monty Rakusen/Getty Images; **p. 493:** Hemera Technologies/AbleStock.com/Thinkstock; **p. 494:** Pearson Education/Pearson Science; **p. 496 top:** Cardinal/Corbis; **p. 496 bottom:** Wernher Krutein/Flame/Corbis; **p. 497: Fig. 13.13a left:** incinereigh/Fotolia; **right:** Ionescu Bogdan/Fotolia; **bottom:** Franck Boston/Fototlia; **p. 499:** Paul Gunning/Science Source; **p. 502:** AP Images/Toby Talbot; **p. 505:** R Sherwood Veith/E+/Getty Images; **p. 506:** Steve Cavalie/Alamy; **p. 507: Fig. 1:** Yann Layma/The Image Bank/Getty Images; **p. 508 left:** Randy Duchaine/Alamy; **right:** David White/Alamy; **p. 509:** Richard Wayman/Alamy

Chapter 14

p. 512: mariiya/Fotolia; **p. 514:** David Phillips/The Population Council/Science Source; **p. 517: Fig. 14.4a:** Scanpix Sweden; **b:** Scanpix Sweden; **c:** Neil Bromhall/Science Source; **d:** Kletr/Shutterstock; **p. 518: Fig. 14.5:** Ron Sutherland/Science Source; **p. 519:** Ian O'Leary/The Image Bank/Getty Images; **p. 520: Fig. 14.6:** Ingret/Shutterstock; **p. 522: Fig. 14.7a:** Biophoto Associates/Science Source; **bottom:** Dave King/DK Images; **p. 523:** Juanmonino/iStockphoto/Thinkstock; **p. 524:** Allana Wesley White/Cusp/Corbis; **p. 525 top:** MSPhotographic/Fotolia; **p. 525 bottom:** DK Images; **p. 526:**

Hero/Fancy/Alamy; **p. 527:** Andrey Bandurenko/Fotolia; **p. 532: Fig. 14.9:** Brigitte Sporrer/Cultura/Getty Images; **p. 533:** endostock/Fotolia; **p. 534:** Darama/Bridge/Corbis; **p. 536:** Chris Craymer/Stone+/Getty Images; **p. 537 top:** Gayle Shomer/KRT/Newscom; **bottom:** Andy Dean Photography/Shutterstock; **p. 539:** Mel Yates/Getty Images; **p. 540:** Radius Images/Alamy; **p. 542:** Tom Grill/Spirit/Corbis; **p. 543 top:** gerain/Shutterstock; **bottom:** Richard Cooper/Alamy; **p. 544: Fig. 14.12:** Dr. Pamela R. Erickson/Pearson; **p. 545:** Photohunter/Shutterstock; **p. 548:** OJO Images/SuperStock; **p. 549 top:** Kent Page/un Agence France Presse/Newscom; **bottom:** Mopic/Shutterstock; **p. 551 top left:** John Birdsall/AGE Fotostock; **top right:** Thomas Northcut/Photodisc/Thinkstock

Chapter 15

p. 552: MIXA/Getty Images; **p. 554:** Rebecca Erol/Alamy; **p. 557: Fig. 15.1:** Jon Schulte/E+/Getty Images; **Fig. 15.2:** Pavel L Photo and Video/Shutterstock; **p. 558 top:** Roger Phillips/DK Images; **center:** foodfolio/Alamy; **bottom:** Pearson Education; **p. 559:** Jaume Gual/AGE Fotostock; **p. 560:** debr22pics/Shutterstock; **p. 561 top:** Pearson Education; **bottom:** VStock/Thinkstock; **p. 563:** Bob Daemmrich/The Image Works; **p. 564:** RoJo Images/Fotolia **p. 566:** 2xSamara.com/Fotolia; **p. 568:** Anthony Hatley/Alamy; **p. 570:** Adam Gault/Photodisc/Getty Images; **p. 571:** Sabphoto/Fotolia; **p. 572:** Blend Images/SuperStock; **p. 573 top:** Pictor International/Alamy; **bottom:** istockphoto/Thinkstock; **p. 574:** Vladimir Voronin/Fotolia; **p. 575:** Catalin Petolea/Shutterstock; **p. 576:** pressmaster/Fotolia; **p. 577:** branex/Fotolia; **p. 578:** Richard Koek/Stone/Getty Images; **p. 579:** Jed Share/Photographer's Choice/Getty Images; **p. 580 top:** Deborah Jaffe/FoodPix/Getty Images; **bottom:** Mark Richards/PhotoEdit; **p. 582: Fig. 15.8a:** National Institute of health; **Fig. 15.8b:** National Institute of health; **p. 583:** Karen Preuss/The Image Works; **p. 584:** Donna Day/The Image Bank/Getty Images; **p. 587:** Blend Images/SuperStock; **p. 589 top:** Sandra Cunningham/Fotolia; **bottom:** Andreas Pollok/Taxi/Getty Images; **p. 590 left:** Clive Streeter/DK Images